Larsen's Human Embryology

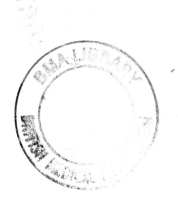

FIFTH EDITION

Larsen's Human Embryology

GARY C. SCHOENWOLF, PhD
University of Utah School of Medicine
Salt Lake City, Utah

STEVEN B. BLEYL, MD, PhD
University of Utah School of Medicine
Salt Lake City, Utah

PHILIP R. BRAUER, PhD
Creighton University School of Medicine
Omaha, Nebraska

PHILIPPA H. FRANCIS-WEST, PhD
King's College London Dental Institute
London, United Kingdom

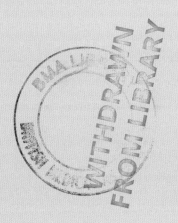

CHURCHILL
LIVINGSTONE

1600 John F. Kennedy Blvd.
Ste 1800
Philadelphia, PA 19103-2899

LARSEN'S HUMAN EMBRYOLOGY, 5TH EDITION   ISBN: 978-1-4557-0684-6

Copyright © 2015, 2009 by Churchill Livingstone, an imprint of Elsevier Inc.

Notices

Knowledge and best practice in this field are constantly changing. As new research and experience broaden our understanding, changes in research methods, professional practices, or medical treatment may become necessary.

Practitioners and researchers must always rely on their own experience and knowledge in evaluating and using any information, methods, compounds, or experiments described herein. In using such information or methods they should be mindful of their own safety and the safety of others, including parties for whom they have a professional responsibility.

With respect to any drug or pharmaceutical products identified, readers are advised to check the most current information provided (i) on procedures featured or (ii) by the manufacturer of each product to be administered, to verify the recommended dose or formula, the method and duration of administration, and contraindications. It is the responsibility of practitioners, relying on their own experience and knowledge of their patients, to make diagnoses, to determine dosages and the best treatment for each individual patient, and to take all appropriate safety precautions.

To the fullest extent of the law, neither the Publisher nor the authors, contributors, or editors, assume any liability for any injury and/or damage to persons or property as a matter of products liability, negligence or otherwise, or from any use or operation of any methods, products, instructions, or ideas contained in the material herein.

Previous editions copyrighted 2001, 1997, 1993

Library of Congress Cataloging-in-Publication Data

Schoenwolf, Gary C., author.
  Larsen's human embryology/Gary C. Schoenwolf, Steven B. Bleyl, Philip R. Brauer, Philippa H. Francis-West.—Fifth edition.
    p. ; cm.
Human embryology
Preceded by Larsen's human embryology/Gary C. Schoenwolf ... [et al.]. 4th ed. c2009.
Includes bibliographical references and index.
ISBN 978-1-4557-0684-6 (paperback : alk. paper)
  I. Bleyl, Steven B., author. II. Brauer, Philip R., author. III. Francis-West, P. H. (Philippa H.), 1964- , author. IV. Title. V. Title: Human embryology.
  [DNLM: 1. Embryonic Development—physiology. 2. Embryonic Structures—physiology. 3. Fetal Development—physiology. QS 604]

QM601
612.6'4—dc23

     2014028160

Content Strategist: Meghan Ziegler
Senior Content Development Manager: Rebecca Gruliow
Publishing Services Manager: Patricia Tannian
Senior Project Manager: Claire Kramer
Design Direction: Julia Dummitt

Printed in China

Last digit is the print number: 9   8   7   6   5   4   3   2

The fifth edition of Larsen's Human Embryology *is proudly dedicated
to the children who live with birth defects every day, hour, minute,
and second of their lives and to their families who provide loving
support and care. It is our hope that the information we have assembled here
will help the next generation of physicians and scientists make new discoveries,
resulting in better prevention, diagnosis, and treatment of birth defects.*

Content Experts

RICHARD ANDERSON
University of Melbourne, Australia

PARKER B. ANTIN
University of Arizona, USA

CAMMON ARRINGTON
University of Utah, USA

SPENCER BEASLEY
University of Otago, New Zealand

BRIAN L. BLACK
University of California at San Francisco, USA

JANICE L.B. BYRNE
University of Utah, USA

JON CLARKE
King's College London, England

MARTYN COBOURNE
King's College London, England

SIMON J. CONWAY
Indiana University School of Medicine, USA

ANDREW COPP
University College London, England

GEORGE P. DASTON
Procter & Gamble, USA

MARK DAVENPORT
King's College Hospital, England

JAMIE DAVIES
University of Edinburgh, Scotland

ELAINE DZIERZAK
Erasmus University Medical Center, The Netherlands

DARRELL J.R. EVANS
Brighton and Sussex Medical School, England

JOHN F. FALLON
University of Wisconsin Madison, USA

RICHARD H. FINNELL
The University of Texas at Austin, USA

ADRIANA GITTENBERGER-DEGROOT
Leiden University Medical Center, The Netherlands

ROBERT G. GOURDIE
Medical University of South Carolina, USA

ANNE GRAPIN-BOTTON
Swiss Institute for Experimental Cancer Research,
   Switzerland

ANNE GREENOUGH
King's College Hospital, England

BARBARA F. HALES
McGill University, Canada

HIROSHI HAMADA
Osaka University, Japan

CHRISTINE HARTMANN
Institute of Molecular Pathology, Austria

TAKAYUKI INAGAKI
University of Utah, USA

ROBYN JAMIESON
University of Sydney, Australia

CHAYA KALCHEIM
Hebrew University of Jerusalem, Israel

MATTHEW KELLEY
National Institute on Deafness and Other
   Communication Disorders/National Institutes
   of Health, USA

THOMAS KNUDSEN
U.S. Environmental Protection Agency, USA

CATHERINE E. KRULL
University of Michigan, USA

RALPH MARCUCIO
University of California at San Francisco, USA

ANTOON F. MOORMAN
Academic Medical Centre Amsterdam, The Netherlands

GUILLERMO OLIVIER
St. Jude Children's Research Hospital, USA

DAVID M. ORNITZ
Washington University, USA

MAURIZIO PACIFICI
The Children's Hospital of Philadelphia, USA

ROGER K. PATIENT
University of Oxford, England

ALAN O. PERANTONI
Frederick National Lab, USA

THEODORE PYSHER
University of Utah, USA

MARIA A. ROS
University of Cantabria, Spain

YUKIO SAIJOH
University of Utah, USA

RAMESH A. SHIVDASANI
Dana Farber Cancer Institute and Harvard Medical
  School, USA

JANE C. SOWDEN
University College of London and Institute of Child
  Health and Great Ormond Street Hospital for
  Children, National Health Service Trust, England

NANCY A. SPECK
University of Pennsylvania, USA

RAJANARAYANAN SRINIVASAN
St. Jude Children's Research Hospital, USA

MICHAEL R. STARK
Brigham Young University, USA

DAVID K. STEVENSON
University of Utah, USA

XIN SUN
University of Wisconsin Madison, USA

CHERYLL TICKLE
University of Bath, England

GIJS VAN DEN BRINK
Academic Medical Centre Amsterdam, The Netherlands

VALERIE WALLACE
University of Ottawa, Canada

JAMES M. WELLS
University of Cincinnati, USA

ARNO WESSELS
Medical University of South Carolina, USA

HEATHER M. YOUNG
University of Melbourne, Australia

Preface

The fifth edition of *Larsen's Human Embryology,* like the fourth edition, has been extensively revised.

- The number of chapters has been expanded from eighteen to twenty. This was done to organize the material better and to incorporate new information efficiently and logically.
- The text was heavily edited to increase clarity and avoid ambiguity, to improve accuracy, and to include many new scientific and medical advances since the last edition.
- Building on the success of the section called "Clinical Tasters," which was added in the fourth edition to introduce the clinical relevance of the material covered in each chapter, we added a new section—called "Embryology in Practice"—to close each chapter. The title of this section is a bit of a play on words; *practice* refers to both clinical practice and a chance for the reader to practice being a clinician and to use the material presented in the text to "walk through" a clinical scenario. As with the "Clinical Tasters," the "Embryology in Practice" section focuses on the impact of birth defects on the lives of children and their families. Although fictitious scenarios, they reflect real-life stories encountered in clinical practice with real problems that patients and their families face.
- Many new illustrations have been added; these additions reflect research advances and their clinical relevance. Many previous illustrations were thoroughly revised to facilitate student understanding. Although admittedly biased, we believe that the fifth edition of *Larsen's Human Embryology* contains the best compilation in any one textbook of illustrations on human three-dimensional descriptive embryology, animal model experimental embryology, and human birth defects.
- About fifty full-color animations have been linked directly to relevant sections of the text. These help the student understand not only the three-dimensional structure of human embryos, but also their four-dimensional structure as its complexity morphs and increases over time.
- As with the fourth edition, new Content Experts have been chosen to partner with the authors in producing the fifth edition of *Larsen's Human Embryology*. More than fifty new Content Experts are listed. With roughly the same number participating in the fourth edition, the textbook has now been critically evaluated by about 100 experts in their respective areas. Although that strengthens the book tremendously, it still does not make the book perfect, an impossible task in a complex and ever-changing field. Hence, we greatly appreciate input we receive for further improvement from students and faculty. Please continue to send your comments to schoenwolf@neuro.utah.edu.

Acknowledgments

Without students there would be no need for textbooks. Thus the authors thank the many bright young students with whom we have been fortunate enough to interact throughout our careers, as well as those students of the future, in eager anticipation of continuing fruitful and enjoyable interactions. For us as teachers, students have enriched our lives and have taught us at least as much as, if not more than, we have taught them.

For this edition, we are especially grateful to the more than fifty Content Experts who were integral partners in the preparation of the fifth edition and who, like our students, also have taught us much. Each of the Content Experts read one or more chapters, offered numerous suggestions for revision, and in some cases even provided new text and illustrations. We have pondered their many suggestions for revision, but in the end, rightly or wrongly, we chose the particular direction to go. The authors share a captivation for the embryo and have sought to understand it fully, but, of course, we have not yet accomplished this objective; thus our studies continue (we all are active researchers). Nevertheless, we took faith when writing this edition in a quote from one of the great scientific heroes, Viktor Hamburger: "Our real teacher has been and still is the embryo, who is, incidentally, the only teacher who is always right."

Finally, we must thank the many authors, colleagues, patients, and families of patients who provided figures for the textbook. Rather than acknowledging the source of each figure in its legend, we have clustered these acknowledgments into a Figure Credits section. This was done not to hide contributions but rather to focus the legends on what was most relevant.

Contents

Video Contents

Introduction

SUMMARY

As you begin your study of **human embryology**, it is a good time to consider why knowledge of the subject will be important to your career. Human embryology is a fascinating topic that reveals to each of us our own prenatal origins. It also sheds light on the **birth defects** that occur relatively frequently in humans. So the study of both normal and abnormal human embryology tells us something about every human we will encounter throughout our lives. For those seeking a career in biology, medicine, or allied health sciences, there are many other reasons to learn human embryology, which include the following:

- Knowing human embryology provides a logical framework for understanding adult **anatomy**.
- Knowing human embryology provides a bridge between basic science (e.g., anatomy and physiology) and clinical science (e.g., obstetrics, pediatrics, and surgery).
- Knowing human embryology allows the physician to accurately advise patients on many issues, such as **reproduction**, **contraception**, **birth defects**, **prenatal development**, **in vitro fertilization**, **stem cells**, and **cloning**.

In short, human embryology provides a foundation for understanding medicine and its practice by the healthcare provider: knowing embryology proffers insight into the developmental basis of pediatric and adult disease.

Human pregnancy is subdivided in many ways to facilitate understanding of the complex changes that occur in the developing organism over time. Prospective parents and physicians typically use **trimesters**: three-month periods (zero to three months, three to six months, and six to nine months) starting with the date of the onset of the last menstrual period (a memorable landmark) and ending at birth. Human embryologists sometimes use intervals called periods: **the period of the egg** (generally from fertilization to the end of the third week), **the period of the embryo** (generally from the beginning of the fourth week to the end of the eighth week), and **the period of the fetus** (from the beginning of the third month to birth).

Human embryologists also identify **phases of human embryogenesis**. Typically, six are recognized:

- **Gametogenesis**: the formation of the gametes, the egg, and sperm
- **Fertilization**: the joining of the gametes to form the zygote
- **Cleavage**: a series of rapid cell divisions that result first in the formation of the morula, a small cluster of cells resembling a mulberry, and then in the formation of the blastocyst, a hollow ball of cells containing a central cavity
- **Gastrulation**: the rearrangement of cells in the embryonic region of the implanted blastocyst into three primary germ layers—ectoderm, mesoderm, and endoderm—to form the embryonic disc
- **Formation of the tube-within-a-tube body plan**: conversion, through body folding, of the embryonic disc into a C-shaped embryonic body consisting of an outer ectodermal tube (the future skin) and an inner endodermal tube (the gut tube), with the mesoderm interposed between the two tubes
- **Organogenesis**: the formation of organ rudiments and organ systems

During gastrulation, the three cardinal **body axes** are established. In the embryo and fetus, these three axes are called the **dorsal-ventral, cranial-caudal**, and **medial-lateral** axes. They are equivalent, respectively, to the **anterior-posterior, superior-inferior**, and **medial-lateral** axes of the adult.

Clinical Taster

On a Monday morning, you get a frantic call from an uninsured 22-year-old patient who is three months pregnant. That weekend, she witnessed a car accident in which two people were badly injured, and she can't get the images of their bloodied faces out of her mind. Her neighbor told her that viewing such a shocking event could traumatize her fetus and result in the birth of a "monster." Your patient is worried that her child will now be born with a serious birth defect, and she is calling you for advice. She knows she can't afford high medical bills to care for a sick child, and she's concerned about whether her husband will love a defective child, as he is such a perfectionist. Although hesitant to ask you, she is wondering whether she should continue the pregnancy.

You tell her that her neighbor is mistaken and that there is no medical evidence to support the idea that viewing a shocking event could traumatize her fetus, resulting in a severe birth defect. She states that she is greatly relieved by talking with you and agrees to continue her pregnancy. However, she admits that she still has some misgivings. You recognize that—depending on one's culture, education, and beliefs—legend and superstition can be as powerful to some as modern medicine. You continue to try to address her concerns and reassure her over the course of her remaining prenatal visits, which include normal ultrasound examinations. The last two trimesters of her pregnancy are uneventful, and at term she delivers a vibrant, healthy, 7-pound, 6-ounce baby girl.

WHY STUDY HUMAN EMBRYOLOGY?

Quite simply put, a good reason to study human embryology is that this topic is fascinating. All of us were once human embryos, so the study of human embryology is the study of our own prenatal origins and experience. Moreover, many of us are, or someday will be, parents and perhaps grandparents. Having a child or a grandchild is an awe-inspiring experience, which once again personalizes human development for each of us and piques our curiosity about its wonders. As teachers of human embryology, one of us now well on our way toward a half-century, we still find the subject to be utterly fascinating!

Human embryology does not always occur normally. Surprisingly, 3% to 4% of all live-born children will be diagnosed eventually (usually within the first two years) with a significant **malformation** (i.e., **birth defect**). Understanding why embryology goes awry and results in birth defects requires a thorough grasp of the molecular genetic, cellular, and tissue events underlying normal human embryology. Whether someone develops normally or not has a lifelong impact on that person, as well as on the person's family.

For a student pursuing a career in biology, medicine, or allied health sciences, there are many other reasons to study human embryology based on the fact that human embryology provides a foundation for understanding medicine and its practice by the health-care provider.

- The best way to understand and remember human anatomy—microscopic anatomy, neuroanatomy, and gross anatomy—is to understand how tissues, organs, and the body as a whole are assembled from relatively simple rudiments. Knowing the embryology solidifies your knowledge of anatomy and provides an explanation for the variation that you will observe in human anatomy and surgery.
- As you continue your studies and perhaps take courses such as human genetics, pathology, organ systems, and reproductive biology, and study disease processes and aging, your knowledge of human embryology will continue to benefit you. Cancer is now widely recognized as a disease involving mutations in genes controlling development and regulating key cellular events of development, such as division and death (apoptosis).
- Many of you will become medical practitioners. Embryology will serve to bridge your basic science and clinical science courses, particularly as you start your study of obstetrics, pediatrics, and surgery. But perhaps more important, once you start your practice, your patients will have many questions about pregnancy and birth defects, and controversial and always newsworthy issues such as abortion, birth control, cryopreservation of gametes and embryos, reproductive and therapeutic cloning, in vitro fertilization, gamete and embryo donation, stem cells, storage of cord blood, and gestational surrogate mothers. Your knowledge of human embryology will allow you to provide scientifically accurate counsel, empowering your patients to make informed decisions based on current scientific understanding. Many of your patients will have reproductive concerns. As their physician, you will be their main source of reliable information.
- If you are a medical student, it is important to know that performing well on (and perhaps even passing) Step 1 National Boards involves a thorough knowledge of human embryology and the underlying developmental, molecular, and genetic principles and mechanisms. Both Dr. Larsen (the original author of this textbook) and Dr. Schoenwolf have served as Members, USMLE Step 1 Cell and Developmental Biology Test Material Development Committee, National Board of Medical Examiners (Dr. Schoenwolf joined the committee after Dr. Larsen's untimely death). Human embryology is an integral component of that examination. Moreover, because this textbook emphasizes clinical applications and developmental mechanisms (see "In the Clinic" and "In the Research Lab" sections, respectively, in each chapter), as well as descriptive aspects of development, studying human embryology and using this book can also have practical value.
- Finally, we think one of the best reasons to study human embryology is that it is a fun subject to learn. Although we now know a tremendous amount about how embryos develop, there are still many mysteries to unravel. Thus, human embryology is not a static subject; rather, our knowledge and understanding of human embryology is always evolving. As you study human embryology, be sure to pay attention to the daily news—undoubtedly, advances in human embryology will be featured several times during the course of your study.

In the Research Lab

LINKS BETWEEN DEVELOPMENT AND CANCER

The Wnt (wingless; covered in Chapter 5) family of secreted signaling molecules is one example of a signaling pathway that has multiple functions in the embryo and the adult. A major role for Wnt signaling in the embryo is to specify cell fate. In the adult, Wnt signaling maintains homeostasis in self-renewing tissues. Mutations of members of the Wnt signaling pathway result in malignant transformation (i.e., **cancer**).

These multiple roles for Wnt signaling are perhaps best understood in the gut (covered in Chapter 14). The first hint that Wnt signaling was important in gut biology came from the finding in the early 1990s that the human **tumor suppressor gene**, ADENOMATOUS POLYPOSIS COLI (APC)—a component of the Wnt signaling pathway—was mutated in **colorectal cancer**. The mutation resulted in constitutively active Wnt signaling and the subsequent development of cancer.

As covered in detail in Chapter 14, Wnt signaling also plays important roles in normal development of the gut. First, regional patterning of the gut and its folding to form the hindgut, and probably also the foregut, require Wnt signaling. Second, after the gut tube is formed, it undergoes regional histogenesis. For example, within the small intestine, villi (finger-like projections) form, which are separated by invaginations called crypts. In contrast, within the colon (large intestine), crypts also form but villi are absent. The crypts consist of highly proliferative progenitor cells, with maturating cells moving out of the crypts to the surface epithelium of the gut tube. Normal proliferation of crypt cells requires continual stimulation by the Wnt pathway.

Mutation of components of several other signaling pathways that function during development can result in cancer during postnatal life. These include the hedgehog, Tgfβ, and notch pathways, all of which are covered in detail in Chapter 5. In addition, the roles of these pathways, as well as of several other signaling pathways, in development and disease of particular organ systems are covered in the appropriate chapters.

NOTE ABOUT GENE NAMES

As you read the scientific and clinical literature to expand your knowledge of embryology, you might notice that different naming conventions and font styles are used to designate a gene, its mRNA, or its protein. Also, naming conventions are different for many animal models and in turn may differ from those used for humans. For example, the fibroblast growth factor 8 (Fgf8) gene in humans is designated as *FGF8*, its mRNA as *FGF8,* and its protein as FGF8. In mice, both the gene and its mRNA are designated as *Fgf8,* and its protein as FGF8.

For the sake of simplicity and ease of reading for the student, plain text rather than italics will be used in this textbook to designate a gene or transcript. Moreover, genes, transcripts, and proteins will be designated as lowercase text, with three exceptions. First, human genes and their transcripts will be listed in all-capital letters to make it clear that a particular gene is known to play a role in human development, or that a mutation in that gene results in a human birth defect or disease. Second, when a gene, transcript, or protein name is abbreviated, the first letter of the name will be capitalized (e.g., chicken Bmp versus chicken bone morphogenetic protein). Third, when proteins are covered in the context of their action in a process such as the menstrual cycle, rather than in a genomic/molecular genetic context, and the name is abbreviated, all-capital letters will be used. Thus, luteinizing hormone will be designated as luteinizing hormone (neither italicized nor with first letter capitalized) or by its abbreviation, LH (all capital letters). Finally, when it is important for clarity to designate whether the name indicates a gene, an mRNA, or a protein, qualifiers will be added as follows: the Fgf8 gene, the Fgf8 transcript, or the Fgf8 protein.

PERIODS OF HUMAN EMBRYOLOGY

From a medical or prospective parent's viewpoint, human prenatal development is subdivided into three main intervals called the **first**, **second**, and **third trimesters**, each consisting of three-month periods. From an embryologist's viewpoint, there are also three main subdivisions of human prenatal development, called **period of the egg, period of the embryo**, and **period of the fetus**. The first period, the period of the egg or **ovum**, is usually considered to extend from the time of **fertilization** until formation of the **blastocyst** and **implantation** of the blastocyst into the uterine wall about one week after fertilization (Fig. Intro-1). The entire **conceptus** (i.e., the product of conception or fertilization) typically is called the *egg* during this period. The conceptus at the blastocyst stage has already differentiated to give rise to tissue destined to form the embryo proper, as well as to other tissue that will form the extraembryonic layers. During the period of the egg, human embryologists identify three stages of development: **zygote** (formed at fertilization before the egg becomes multicellular), **morula** (formed after the zygote cleaves by mitosis, giving rise to a mulberry-like cluster of multiple cells or blastomeres), and **blastocyst** (a hollow ball of cells derived from the morula by the formation of a large, fluid-filled central cavity called the **blastocele**). The conceptus during this period may also be called the **preimplantation embryo**, or more accurately, the **preimplantation conceptus**. Thus, the period could also be called the period of the preimplantation embryo or preimplantation conceptus. Use of the term *egg* or *embryo* for the conceptus at these stages is particularly helpful for those conducting in vitro fertilization (eggs/embryos are collected, eggs/embryos are washed, eggs/embryos are transplanted into the uterus—try saying these phrases quickly

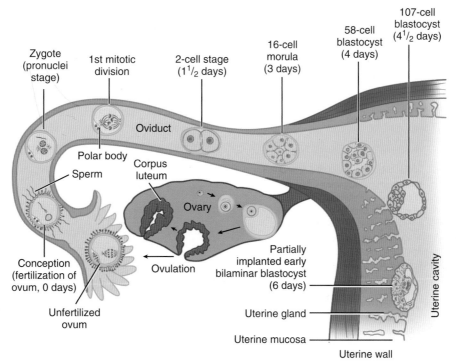

Figure Intro-1. The first week of prenatal development of the human.

using "conceptuses" or "concepti"!). But in the strictest sense, *egg* (or *oocyte*) is the name of the female gamete before fertilization, so using the term *egg* to describe later stages can lead to confusion.

The exact beginning of the period of the embryo is poorly defined, and consequently there is no universal agreement about when the period begins. Some call the cleaving morula, or even the zygote, the *embryo,* so with this classification scheme, the period of the embryo begins as early as immediately after fertilization or as late as three days after fertilization. Others use the term *embryo* only after the conceptus starts implanting into the uterine wall at the end of the first week of gestation, or becomes fully implanted into the uterine wall at the end of the second week of gestation. Still others use the term *embryo* only in the fourth week of gestation, after the embryonic disc becomes three-dimensional and a typical tube-within-a-tube body plan is established. The period of the embryo could also be called the period of the *postimplantation embryo* or *postimplantation conceptus,* if these terms are restricted to stages that follow implantation. In this textbook, the period of the embryo will be defined as beginning at the end of the first week of gestation, after implantation is initiated.

Despite lack of agreement about when the period of the embryo begins, it is universally considered to end at the end of the eighth week of gestation (i.e., at the end of the second month after fertilization), after which the period of the fetus begins. This endpoint for the period of the embryo is chosen by convention but is arbitrary, as no obvious major change occurs between the eighth and ninth weeks of gestation to mark the transition. The period of the fetus extends from the ninth week to birth and is characterized by rapid growth of the fetus and functional maturation of its organ systems (covered in Chapter 6). At birth, the baby or neonate breathes on its own, but development does not cease simply because birth has occurred. Although this textbook discusses only prenatal development, it is important to remember that development is not just a prenatal experience; rather, development is a lifelong process, with maturation during puberty and subsequent aging or senescence involving further developmental events.

In the Research Lab

WHY DO WE AGE?
Animal models have played an important role in understanding **aging**, also known as **senescence**, in humans. Using organisms as diverse as *Saccharomyces cerevisiae* (yeast), *Caenorhabditis elegans* (nematode worm), *Drosophila melanogaster* (fruit fly), and *Mus musculus* (mouse), the genetic pathways controlling aging are beginning to be elucidated. Animal models offer the key advantage that searches can be conducted for mutations in genes that affect **life span**. These studies show clearly that particular genes can be identified that extend life span in animal models—a result that is relevant for understanding human aging. For example, a locus identified on human chromosome 4 has been linked to exceptional longevity, suggesting that similar genes exist in humans. In support of this, variants of the human gene FOXO3a (a gene located on human chromosome 6 that is a homolog of a downstream transcrip-

tion factor of the first-identified longevity gene in animal models) are associated with unusual longevity in human families.

Life span and duration of good health (i.e., **healthspan**) can be extended by caloric restriction (without malnutrition) in several species of animal models, including mammals, provided that the diet includes enough nutrition for routine maintenance of the body. However, although the value of caloric restriction has been known for longer than a half century, the exact mechanism of its action remains unclear. Several factors are known to act in aging, including persistent inflammation, accumulated release of reactive oxygen species, telomere (proteins at the ends of chromosomes) shortening with each cell division, and mitochondrial dysfunction. Caloric restriction alters all of these factors. In addition, caloric restriction decreases the activity of nutrient signaling pathways such as the insulin/insulin-like growth factor pathway and the TOR pathway (both pathways are discussed below). These results collectively suggest that aging is a complex process that involves a combination of these factors, rather than just a single factor. It is interesting to note that these factors act not only in aging; increasing evidence is tying them to chronic diseases in humans such as Alzheimer's, Parkinson's, cardiac infarction, diabetes, cancer, osteoporosis, and atherosclerosis.

Puberty and menopause, two major postnatal developmental events, are controlled hormonally (covered in Chapter 1). Thus, it is not surprising that aging, a more gradual postnatal developmental event, also seems to be regulated hormonally. In particular, it has been shown that the endocrine hormone insulin/insulin-like growth factor 1 (Igf-like1) limits life span; thus, mutations in this signaling pathway extend life span. One way in which insulin/Igf-like1 hormone is regulated is through sensory neurons. Perturbations in *C. elegans* that decrease sensory perception extend life span (by up to 50%) by acting through this pathway. As surprising as it sounds, increased sensory perception leads to increased insulin/Igf-like1 hormone secretion and accelerated aging.

The germ line (covered in Chapter 1) can also regulate the rate of aging, perhaps to coordinate an animal's schedule of reproduction with its rate of aging. For example, strains of flies have been bred that produce offspring relatively late in life and have long life spans, whereas other strains have offspring at an earlier stage and are short lived. If germ cells are killed in the short-lived strain, its life span is extended. Oxidative damage also accelerates aging. *C. elegans* and fly mutants resistant to oxidative damage are long lived, whereas mutations that increase oxidative damage are short lived. This has led to the oxygen radical theory of aging, and hence, to the shelves full of antioxidants in the health food section of grocery stores. Lending credence to this theory is the demonstration that mutation of the p66[shc] gene in mice, which renders the mouse resistant to the action of oxygen radical generators, increases the life span of mice by as much as 30%.

The role of the TOR pathway in aging and chronic disease provides an interesting example of how fundamental observations in biology can lead to new understandings of human disease. In 1964, a team of scientists traveled to Easter Island to collect flora and fauna samples before the construction of an airport that would alter the island's ecosystem. A bacterium discovered in a soil sample was later shown to produce a chemical capable of prolonging life when injected into various species, including mice. The chemical was called rapamycin, after Easter Island, which is also called Rapa Nui. Subsequently, resveratrol, an ingredient in red wine, was shown to block the decreased life span of mice exposed to high-fat diets. Resveratrol seemingly works through enzymes called sirtuins, but neither resveratrol nor sirtuins seem to be very effective in extending life span in mice fed normal diets. However, rapamycin, which acts by inhibiting cell growth, is able to extend the life span of these mice significantly (approximately 10% to 15% in females and 10% in males).

Rapamycin acts on the protein TOR (target of rapamycin), inhibiting its activity. Suppressing TOR not only extends life span, it also lowers the risk of several major age-related diseases. TOR, as stated above, is a nutrient sensor providing a link to understanding the antiaging effects of caloric restriction. After feeding, insulin is released by the pancreas. One role of insulin is to increase the activity of the TOR pathway, inducing cells to grow and proliferate. Unfortunately, rapamycin cannot be used prophylactically in humans to inhibit TOR and slow aging because of its side effects. Thus, the search is on for other compounds capable of safely suppressing TOR and delaying aging and the onset of age-related disease.

In the Clinic

PROGERIA: PREMATURE AGING

A severe form of **premature aging** occurs in humans called Hutchinson-Gilford progeria syndrome (HGPS, typically called **progeria**, derived from the Greek words for early, *pro,* and old age, *geraios*). One in four to eight million children is afflicted with progeria; these children age at five to ten times the normal rate. Although they usually appear normal at birth, the growth rate of afflicted children slows, and their appearance begins to change. Children with progeria often develop baldness, aged-looking (stiff) skin, pinched noses, dwarfism, brittle bones, and small face and jaw (Fig. Intro-2). Their average life expectancy is 13 to 14 years, with death usually resulting from cardiovascular disease (heart attack or stroke).

The most common cause of progeria is a single base mutation in a gene that codes for LAMIN-A, a nuclear membrane protein. The mutation activates an aberrant cryptic splice site in LAMIN-A pre-mRNA, leading to the constitutive synthesis of a truncated protein called **progerin**. The full-length protein, together with other lamins and lamin-associated proteins of the inner nuclear membrane, has diverse functions, including promoting the physical integrity of the nucleus, regulating DNA replication and transcription, and forming complexes that function as scaffolds to form and regulate higher-order chromatin structure and the epigenetic regulation of gene expression. Cells from progeria patients have misshaped nuclear membranes, and it is speculated that tissues subjected to intense physical stress, such as those in the cardiovascular system, might undergo widespread cell death because of nuclear instability. In addition, other nuclear defects exist in progeria patients, including abnormal chromatin structure and increased DNA damage. Increasingly, lamins are being linked to a wide spectrum of diseases (e.g., Emery-Dreifuss muscular dystrophy and related myopathies; Charcot-Marie-Tooth disease type 2B1—see Chapters 4 and 10) including progeria; these diseases are collectively called **laminopathies**.

Using fibroblasts obtained from progeria patients, normal nuclear morphology (and several other critical cellular features) was restored by treating cells with a chemically stable DNA oligonucleotide (short DNA sequence, called a morpholino, that cells cannot degrade) targeted to the activated cryptic splice site (to bind to the mutated site and prevent the splicing machinery from cutting in the wrong place). This approach thus provides proof of concept for the eventual correction of premature aging with **gene therapy** in children with progeria, an exciting possibility. Other exciting avenues include treatment with rapamycin (covered in the preceding "In the Research Lab") or similar compounds, which in cultured cells promote the clearance of progerin and extend cell survival, as well as treatment with other drugs that impair progerin synthesis.

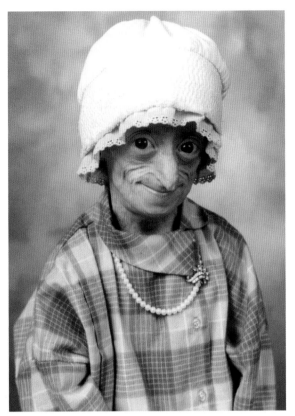

Figure Intro-2. Amy, a child with progeria, at age 16.

PERIOD OF EGG AND EMBRYO: SUMMARY OF MAIN EVENTS

The period of the egg and the embryo, collectively defined (as covered earlier) as the first eight weeks following fertilization, is characterized by a large number of rapid changes. These changes are summarized in Table Intro-1. Also listed in the table, for selected days during each of the eight weeks of gestation, are the greatest length of the embryo, the number of somites, and the Carnegie stage. The latter is the most widely used stage series for human embryos. By providing a standardized set of criteria for accurate staging, this list allows detailed comparisons to be made among different embryos in different collections around the world. Figure Intro-3 shows human embryos from the Kyoto collection at Carnegie stages 7 to 23.

PHASES OF HUMAN EMBRYOLOGY

In addition to periods of human embryology covered earlier in the chapter, embryologists subdivide human embryology into phases. These phases are introduced here to help you keep developmental events in context as you pursue your study of human embryology. Details of each of these phases are covered in subsequent chapters.

The first phase of human embryology is **gametogenesis**. This process occurs in the gonads (ovaries and testes) of females and males and involves **meiosis**. In both females and males, the main effect of meiosis is to establish a haploid cell, that is, a cell that contains half

					TABLE INTRO-1 **TIMING OF HUMAN DEVELOPMENT (WEEKS ONE THROUGH EIGHT)**
Week	Day	Length (mm)[a]	Number of Somites	Carnegie Stage	Features (Chapters in Which Features Are Discussed)[b]
1	1-7	0.1-0.2	0	1	Fertilization (1)
				2	First cleavage divisions occur (2-16 cells) (1)
				3	Blastocyst is free in uterus (1)
				4	Blastocyst hatches and begins implanting (1, 2)
2	8-14	0.1-0.2	0	5	Blastocyst fully implanted (1, 2)
				6	Primary stem villi form (2); endoderm delaminates (2); primitive streak develops (3)
3	15-21	0.4-2.5	0	7	Gastrulation commences and notochordal process forms (3)
			0	8	Primitive pit, neural plate, neural groove, neural folds, and neurenteric canal form (3, 4)
			1-3	9	Somites begin to form (4); primitive heart tube forms (12); vasculature begins to develop in embryonic disc (13)
4	22-28	1.3-5.4	4-12	10	Neural folds fuse (4); cranial end of embryo undergoes rapid flexion (4, 9); neuromeres form in presumptive brain vesicles (4, 9); optic sulci form (10, 18); otic pits form (18); heart begins to beat (12); pulmonary primordium forms (11); hepatic plate forms (14); first two pharyngeal arches form (17); tail bud forms (4)
			13-20	11	Primordial germ cells begin to migrate from wall of yolk sac (1, 16); cranial neuropore closes (4); oropharyngeal membrane ruptures (17); optic vesicles develop (18); optic pits begin to form (18)
			21-29	12	Caudal neuropore closes (4); cystic diverticulum and dorsal pancreatic bud form (14); urorectal septum begins to form (14, 15); upper limb buds form (19); pharyngeal arches 3 and 4 form (17)
5	29-35	3.9-12.0	30+	13	Dorsal and ventral columns begin to differentiate in mantle layer of spinal cord and brain stem (9); septum primum begins to form in heart (12); spleen forms (14); ureteric buds form (15); lower limb buds form (19); otic vesicles and lens placodes form (18); motor nuclei of cranial nerves form (9, 10)
				14	Spinal nerves begin to sprout (10); semilunar valves begin to form in heart (12); lymphatics and coronary vessels form (13); greater and lesser stomach curvatures and primary intestinal loop form (14); metanephric kidneys begin to develop (15); lens pits invaginate into optic cups (18); endolymphatic appendages form (18); secondary brain vesicles begin to form (9); cerebral hemispheres become visible (9)
				15	Atrioventricular valves and definitive pericardial cavity begin to form (12); cloacal folds and genital tubercle form (14, 15, 16); hand plates develop (19); lens vesicles form (18); invagination of nasal pits occur and medial and lateral nasal processes form (17); sensory and parasympathetic cranial nerve ganglia begin to form (10); primary olfactory neurons send axons into telencephalon (10)
6	36-42	10.0-21.5	30+	16	Muscular ventricular septum begins to form (12); gut tube lumen becomes occluded (14); major calyces of metanephric kidneys begin to form and kidneys begin to ascend (15); genital ridges form (16); foot plates develop (19); pigment forms in retinas (18); auricular hillocks develop (18)
				17	Bronchopulmonary segment primordia form (11); septum intermedium of heart is complete (12); subcardinal vein system forms (13); minor calyces of metanephric kidneys are forming (15); finger rays are distinct (19); nasolacrimal grooves form (17); cerebellum begins to form (9); melanocytes enter epidermis (7); dental laminae form (17)
7	43-49	18.0-26.4	30+	18	Skeletal ossification begins (8); Sertoli cells begin to differentiate in the male gonad (16); elbows and toe rays form (19); intermaxillary process and eyelids form (17); thalami of diencephalon expand (9); nipples and first hair follicles form (7)
				19	Septum primum fuses with septum intermedium in heart (12); urogenital membrane ruptures (16); trunk elongates and straightens (8)
				20	Primary intestinal loop completes initial counterclockwise rotation (14); in males, Müllerian ducts begin to regress and vasa deferentia begin to form (15); upper limbs bend at elbows (19)

Week	Day	Length (mm)[a]	Number of Somites	Carnegie Stage	Features (Chapters in Which Features Are Discussed)[b]
8	50-56	23.4-32.2	30+	21	Pericardioperitoneal canals close (11); hands and feet rotate toward midline (19)
				22	Eyelids and auricles are more developed (18)
				23	Chorionic cavity is obliterated by the growth of the amniotic sac (6); definitive superior vena cava and major branches of the aortic arch are established (12); lumen of gut tube is almost completely recanalized (14); primary teeth are at cap stage (17)

TABLE INTRO-1   TIMING OF HUMAN DEVELOPMENT (WEEKS ONE THROUGH EIGHT)—cont'd

[a]Length is the greatest length of the embryo.
[b]Timing of some events and stages can vary by up to 4-5 days during stages 10-23.

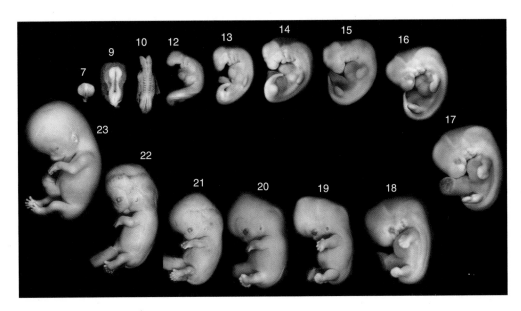

Figure Intro-3. Human embryos from the Kyoto collection at Carnegie stages 7 to 23. The embryo has been dissected from its embryonic membranes at all stages.

the number of chromosomes contained in typical body cells, such as skin cells. In addition to producing haploid cells, meiosis allows the shuffling of genetic information, thereby increasing genetic diversity. In females, gametogenesis occurs in the ovaries and is called **oogenesis**; the final cells produced by oogenesis are the eggs or oocytes. In males, gametogenesis occurs in the testes and is called **spermatogenesis**; the final cells produced by spermatogenesis are the sperm or spermatozoa. Thus, as a result of gametogenesis, gametes undergo morphologic differentiation that allows the second phase of human embryology to occur.

The second phase of human embryology is **fertilization** (see Fig. Intro-1). This process occurs in one of the oviducts of the female after the egg has been ovulated and enters an oviduct, and sperm have been deposited in the vagina at coitus. Sperm move from the vagina into the uterus and finally into the oviducts, where, if an egg is encountered, fertilization can occur. One of the main effects of fertilization is to restore the diploid number of chromosomes, that is, the normal number of chromosomes contained in typical body cells. Because egg and sperm chromosomes are united in a single cell at fertilization, establishing a new cell called the **zygote**, fertilization also results in the production of a new cell having

a unique genome, different from that of the cells of its mother or father. In addition to restoring the diploid number of chromosomes, another main effect of fertilization is to activate the egg, allowing subsequent phases of human embryology to occur.

The third phase of human embryology is **cleavage** (see Fig. Intro-1). During cleavage, the zygote divides by mitosis into two cells, each of which quickly divides into two more cells. The process continues to repeat itself, rapidly forming a solid ball of cells called a **morula**. Cleavage differs from the conventional cell division that occurs in many cell types throughout an organism's life in that during cleavage, each daughter cell formed by cleavage is roughly half the size of its parent cell. In contrast, after conventional cell division, cells grow roughly to parental cell size before undergoing the next round of division. An effect of cleavage is to increase the **nucleocytoplasmic ratio**, that is, the volume of the nucleus compared with the volume of the cytoplasm. An egg, and subsequently a zygote, has a small nucleocytoplasmic ratio because it contains a single nucleus and a large amount of cytoplasm. With each cleavage, the cytoplasm is partitioned as the nuclei are replicated so that the nucleocytoplasmic ratio approaches that of a typical body cell. Another effect of cleavage is to generate a multicellular embryo;

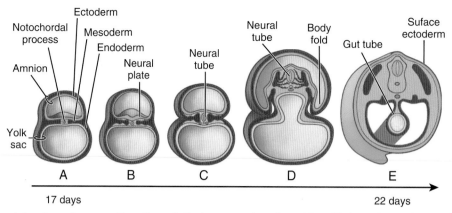

Figure Intro-4. Series of drawings of cross sections through the human embryo from 17 to 22 days of gestation. At the end of gastrulation, *A*, the conceptus consists of a trilaminar blastoderm that is composed of ectoderm, mesoderm, and endoderm, covered dorsally by amnion and ventrally by yolk sac. Body folding is well underway in *D* and is complete in *E*, establishing the tube-within-a-tube body plan (endodermal gut tube on the inside and ectodermal skin tube on the outside). For simplicity, the amnion and the yolk sac are not shown in *E*. In *B*, the midline ectoderm has thickened as the neural plate, which folds to form the neural tube in *C*. The latter is not considered to be one of the two tubes of the tube-within-a-tube body plan because it is not formed by the body folds. For further details, see Chapters 2 through 4.

the cells of the morula and the subsequent **blastocyst** (the structure formed by hollowing out the morula) are called **blastomeres**.

The fourth phase of human embryology is **gastrulation**. During gastrulation, cells undergo extensive movements relative to one another, changing their positions. This brings cells into contact with new neighbors and allows information to be passed among cells, ultimately changing their fates. An effect of gastrulation is to establish primitive tissue layers, called **germ layers** (Fig. Intro-4). Three primary germ layers are formed, called **ectoderm**, **mesoderm**, and **endoderm**. The germ layers give rise to tissues and organ rudiments during subsequent development. The three major axes of the embryo become identifiable during gastrulation (Fig. Intro-5): **dorsal-ventral axis**, **cranial-caudal axis**, and **medial-lateral axis** (including the **left-right axis**).

The fifth phase of human embryology is **formation of the body plan**. Some consider this phase to be part of gastrulation, and others call this phase **morphogenesis**. Both of these viewpoints make sense: gastrulation continues during formation of the body plan, and formation of the body plan involves morphogenesis, that is, the generation of form. However, formation of the body plan also involves extensive folding of the embryo (see Fig. Intro-4). During gastrulation, the embryo consists of a flat two- or three-layered disc of cells (depending on its exact stage of development) that is positioned at the interface between two bubble-like structures: the **amnion** (and its enclosed, fluid-filled space, the **amniotic cavity**) and the **yolk sac** (and its enclosed, fluid-filled space, the **yolk sac cavity**). Near the perimeter of the embryonic disc, where the disc joins the amnion and the yolk sac, folding begins. This is a complex process to visualize; it is covered in detail in Chapter 4. The effect of this folding, called **body folding**, is to separate the embryo from its extraembryonic membranes (i.e., amnion and yolk sac), except at the level of the future umbilical cord, and to convert the flat disc into a three-dimensional body plan,

called the **tube-within-a-tube body plan** (see Fig. Intro-4). The tube-within-a-tube body plan consists of an outer tube (formed from the ectodermal germ layer) and an inner tube (formed from the endodermal germ layer), with the two tubes separated by the mesoderm. Additional tubes (such as the neural tube, the rudiment of the central nervous system, shown in Fig. Intro-4) are formed by secondary folding of other layers of the embryo (i.e., these tubes are not formed by the action of the body folds), and they are not considered to be one of the two tubes contributing to the tube-within-a-tube body plan. In essence, with formation of the tube-within-a-tube, the embryo now has a distinctive embryo-like body shape, is protected from its outside environment by the outer tube (the primitive skin), and contains an inner tube (the primitive gut), separated by a primitive skeletal support (the mesoderm). With formation of the tube-within-a-tube body plan, the embryo now has a shape that more closely resembles that of the adult, and the three body axes are more evident (see Fig. Intro-5).

After formation of the three primary germ layers, regional changes occur in each of these layers. One such change has already been mentioned—folding of part of the ectoderm to form the neural tube. Such changes establish organ rudiments. With completion of formation of the body plan and the formation of organ rudiments, what remains to occur is the last phase of human embryology—the phase of **organogenesis**. During organogenesis, organ rudiments undergo growth and differentiation to form organs and organ systems. With continued growth and differentiation, these organs and organ systems begin to function during intrauterine life. Some organs that begin to function in the fetus need to quickly adapt to another function at the time of birth. For example, as the fetus transitions from an aqueous intrauterine life to air breathing, the functioning of the lungs (and of the cardiovascular system) needs to be rapidly altered. How this transition occurs is covered in Chapters 11 to 13.

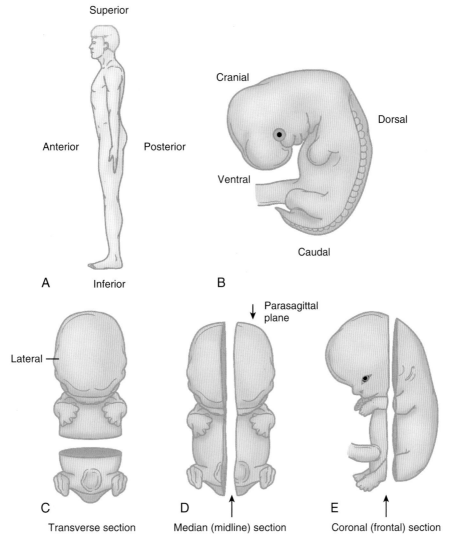

Figure Intro-5. Body axes and section planes in the human adult and embryo. *A,* Lateral view of the adult; *B,* Lateral view of the five-week human embryo; *C-D,* Ventral views of the six-week human embryo showing a transverse *(C)* and sagittal *(D)* section plane. *E,* Lateral view of the six-week human embryo showing a coronal (frontal) section plane.

BODY AXES: UNDERSTANDING EMBRYONIC COORDINATES

Understanding the structure of an embryo or fetus can be difficult and confusing, because embryos and fetuses are three-dimensional, complex objects that change their shape as they develop over time. As a metaphor, imagine examining an enlarged portion of a map without knowing the locations of north, south, east, and west. Without these coordinates, one could easily get lost trying to get from one landmark to another. Embryos and fetuses also have coordinates, and without understanding these coordinates, the study of embryos and fetuses can be perplexing. Moreover, because of our life experience, we often can use environmental clues to navigate from place to place during a journey, even if a compass or a labeled map is not available. However, for most, the embryo or the fetus is uncharted territory, and lack of life experience prevents such navigation. Because we are all familiar with the shape of the adult human body, it is useful to begin

with the coordinates of the adult human before progressing to those of the embryo and the fetus (see Fig. Intro-5).

The adult human standing erect with feet together and palms facing forward is said by anatomists to be in **anatomical position** (see Fig. Intro-5*A*). The head-feet axis represents the **superior-inferior axis**, with the head being **superior** and the feet being **inferior**. From the midline of the body (i.e., an imaginary line drawn through the center of the superior-inferior axis) toward the right and left sides runs the **medial-lateral axis**, with the midline being the most **medial** level (but note that the exact midline is called the **median plane**), and the right and left sides being the most **lateral** levels. The **left-right axis** is part of the medial-lateral axis, defining differences (i.e., asymmetries) between left and right sides of the body. From the front side of the body toward the back side of the body runs the **anterior-posterior axis**, with the front side being the **anterior** surface, and the back side being the **posterior** surface. Finally, in the adult, the terms *proximal* and *distal* are used. **Proximal** refers to close to the center of the body, whereas **distal** refers to far from the center of the body. Thus one can define, for example, the **proximal-distal axis** of the upper limb, with the shoulder being at the **proximal** end of the upper limb and the fingers being at its **distal** end.

The human embryo and fetus have a similar set of axes, again defined based on adult **anatomical position** (see Fig. Intro-5*B*). The head-tail axis of the embryo is called the **cranial-caudal axis**, with the head end being the **cranial** end, and the tail end being the **caudal** end. Sometimes this axis is referred to as the **rostral-caudal axis**, with the head end being the **rostral** end. The cranial-caudal axis can also be called the anterior-posterior axis, with the head end being the anterior end and the tail end being the posterior end. Anterior-posterior axis is often used in the developmental biology literature with animal models (especially four-legged ones), but because the anterior-posterior axis represents a totally different axis in the adult human (i.e., the front-back axis), its use with human embryos is discouraged; consequently, the anterior-posterior axis will not be used in this textbook to describe an *embryonic* axis. The axis extending from the midline to left and right sides in the embryo is called the **medial-lateral axis**, as it is in the adult. However, the axis extending from the back to the front is best called the **dorsal-ventral axis** in the embryo, with the back being **dorsal** and the front being **ventral**. It also can be called the anterior-posterior axis, as it is in the adult, although this is discouraged to prevent confusion as covered above. Finally, embryos also have a **proximal-distal axis**, which is defined in the same way as in the adult.

Because human embryos and fetuses are opaque and have complex internal structures, as well as external structures, they are often studied as sets of serial sections (see Fig. Intro-5*C-E*). Throughout this book, many sections are depicted. To understand these, it is important to know that **transverse (cross) sections** are cut perpendicularly with respect to the cranial-caudal axis of the body (i.e., within the **transverse plane**), so that a set of serial transverse sections progresses through the body in cranial-caudal (or caudal-cranial) sequence (see Fig. Intro-5*C*). **Sagittal sections** are cut in a plane that is parallel to the cranial-caudal or *long* axis of the body (i.e., the **longitudinal plane**), rather than in the transverse plane. These are oriented to cut through embryos or fetuses such that a midline (median) sagittal section (often called a **midsagittal section**) would separate the body into right and left halves (see Fig. Intro-5*D*). More lateral sagittal sections (often called **parasagittal sections**) are cut parallel to a midsagittal section but are displaced to the right or left of the midline. Serial sagittal sections can progress from the right side of the body to the midline (midsagittal) and can continue to the left side (or they can progress in the opposite direction). One further set of sections is sometimes used, but less frequently: serial **coronal (or frontal) sections**. Like sagittal sections, coronal sections are cut in a plane parallel to the cranial-caudal or long axis of the body, but in contrast to sagittal sections, coronal sections are oriented 90 degrees with respect to sagittal sections (see Fig. Intro-5*E*). In other words, serial coronal sections can progress from

the front (ventral) side of the embryo to its center (mid-coronal) and then continue to the back (dorsal) side, or they can progress in the opposite direction. Hence, a mid-coronal section would separate the body into ventral and dorsal halves.

In the Clinic

REGENERATIVE MEDICINE AND TISSUE ENGINEERING

A major goal in modern medicine is to regenerate functional cells, tissues, and organs lost through injury or disease. Approaches to achieving these goals are largely derived from embryological studies in both animal models and humans, along with advances in bioengineering and material science. Regenerative medicine and tissue engineering are largely synonymous terms, but regenerative medicine typically relies on the use of stem cells, which are covered further in Chapter 6.

Regeneration is an area of embryology concerned with the replacement of lost parts. Invertebrate animals readily regenerate lost body parts, as do some vertebrates such as fish and amphibians, but mammals are poor regenerators by comparison. Nevertheless, mammals do undergo regeneration, offering hope that the dream of regenerative medicine may be realized some day in humans. Here, we briefly cover two surprising examples of regeneration in mammals: replacement of fingertips in humans following amputation and regeneration of the heart in mouse models.

The ability of distal fingertips, that is, the terminal phalanx distal to the distal interphalangeal joint, to regenerate in children was discovered by accident. The typical treatment at the time for such amputations, when the tip was not recovered, was to close the wound with a skin flap, in which case regeneration failed to occur. A child in England in the late sixties suffered a guillotine amputation of the fingertip. The wound was covered with a simple dressing, and the child was to be referred to a plastic surgeon, but by mistake that failed to happen. When the error was discovered several days later, the wound was already healing nicely, so no further action was taken. Eventually, there was complete regrowth of the fingertip. Since then, several hundred children with fingertip amputations have been treated merely with sterile dressing and no surgery, with remarkable restoration of the fingertip.

To understand the underlying mechanism of fingertip regeneration, mouse models are used, in which a distal toe is clipped and is left surgically untreated. A typical limb regeneration blastema (a seemingly de-differentiated mass of cells that undergoes rapid proliferation) is formed in this model following amputation. Subsequently, regeneration occurs, which has been shown to require Bmp signaling (a growth factor pathway further covered in Chapter 5), apparently acting in conjunction with the transcription factors msx1/2.

It has long been believed that heart muscle in mammals is incapable of regeneration, although it has been known for several years that functional hearts can regenerate in fish and amphibians. It is now known that fetal and newborn (within the first postnatal week) heart muscle is capable of regeneration. Typically, in mammals, damaged heart muscle is replaced by scar tissue formed from cardiac fibroblasts (i.e., fibrosis occurs), but in fetal and newborn hearts, cardiomyocytes undergo proliferation to form replacement muscle. This provides hope that cardiomyocytes in adult humans might someday be reawakened to their perinatal state through appropriate treatment following cardiac infarction, thereby improving the patient's functional recovery. The search is on to identify cells capable of regenerating heart muscle; potential candidates include resident cardiac stem cells and other noncardiac cells such as bone marrow–derived cells, induced pluripotent stem cells, and embryonic stem cells (the latter two populations of stem cells are covered further in Chapter 5). Additionally, it has been suggested that fetal or placental cells might have this regenerative capability. In support of this, experimentally injured fetal mouse hearts become colonized by extracardiac fetal cells that subsequently differentiate into cardiomyocytes and two other critical populations of heart cells: endothelial cells and smooth muscle cells.

WANT TO LEARN MORE?

This textbook has been written to guide you in your study of human embryology, emphasizing important concepts, principles, and facts. Animations can be accessed on StudentConsult. Movie camera icons placed in the margin in selected regions of the text direct the reader to appropriate corresponding animations. Animations can help you understand the complex changes that occur in the morphology of the developing embryo over time. The "In the Lab" sections of each chapter emphasize the process of discovery of knowledge, and the "In the Clinic" sections emphasize the clinical application of this knowledge. The "Clinical Taster" section is designed to "whet your appetite," introducing you to material that is relevant to each chapter and emphasizing the impact of development gone awry on the persons involved. The "Embryology in Practice" section closes chapters by providing a clinical scenario that allows you to think further about some of the material presented in the chapter and situations you will encounter in the clinic in the future.

In the "Suggested Readings" at the end of each chapter, we reference mainly key review articles published during the last five years, rather than a comprehensive listing of the primary literature. This was done in part to keep the textbook from becoming too large and increasing its cost to students. But it was also done to serve as a more useful student guide to the current relevant scientific literature. Recently, there has been an explosion of journals publishing reviews in developmental biology, and most libraries throughout the world subscribe to review journals, providing easy access for students. By reading a few reviews, one can become quickly updated about a field. Also, by examining the references cited by these reviews, one can quickly find the most relevant primary literature for further detailed study.

With the advent of the worldwide web, how we find information has rapidly changed. In addition to going to the "Suggested Readings" in the text, if you wish to engage in further in-depth study, or if you want to find the very latest publications in the field (because of the delay in publication, the literature in any textbook is always at least one year out of date), online searches are the best approach. We have five suggestions for conducting these searches:

- Using key words in the textbook (i.e., those words indicated in bold type throughout the textbook and also listed in the index), go to PubMed (www.ncbi.nlm.nih.gov/pubmed) and enter one or more keywords as search terms. This will identify many articles for you to consider.
- Using PubMed, search under the names of authors of review articles listed in the "Suggested Readings." Alternatively, use Google Scholar (www.scholar.google.com); Google Scholar ranks articles based on how many times an article by a particular author is cited—one indicator of its importance in the field. Typically, the leaders in a particular area write review articles, and so this approach is likely to pull up many other articles on the same topic. Similarly, you can search under the names of other authors who are cited in the review articles.
- Again, using PubMed, scan the table of contents of recent issues of the main journals in the field by searching under journal title. In developmental biology, these include (in alphabetical order): *BioMed Central Developmental Biology; Development; Development, Genes and Evolution; Developmental Biology; Developmental Cell; Developmental Dynamics; Differentiation; Evolution and Development; Genes and Development; genesis; International Journal of Developmental Biology;* and *Mechanisms of Development* (as well as broader journals such as *Bioessays, Cell, Current Biology, Nature, Nature Genetics, Neuron, PLoS Biology, PLoS One, PNAS,* and *Science*). Many of these journals also publish review articles, which are particularly useful for beginning your study. In addition, scan the table of contents of recent issues of the review journals in the field; in developmental biology, these include *Annual Reviews of Cell and Developmental Biology, Current Opinion in Genetics and Development,* and *Current Topics in Developmental Biology.* Other useful review journals include the Trends series (e.g., *Trends in Genetics*) and the Nature Reviews series *(Nature Reviews Neuroscience).*
- "Google" (www.google.com) keywords to find other information. For example, "googling" IVF (for in vitro fertilization) results in the listing of a number of interesting sites. However, unlike information obtained in journals, which is peer-reviewed by the scientific community for validation, googled information may or may not be scientifically accurate, so it is important to verify googled information by checking it against the peer-reviewed journal literature. A monitored online encyclopedia is Wikipedia (http://www.wikipedia.org); it can be a quick and detailed source on generally any particular topic of interest.
- Seek out other useful websites and databases. For example, for genetic causes of birth defects in humans, go to the Online Mendelian Inheritance in Man (OMIM; www.ncbi.nlm.nih.gov/sites/entrez?db=OMIM); for disease-causing submicroscopic chromosome imbalances in humans, go to Database of Chromosomal Imbalance and Phenotype in Humans Using Ensembl Resources (DECIPHER; http://decipher.sanger.ac.uk/about); for an extensive database of scanning electron micrographs of mouse embryos, go to Kathy Sulik's embryo images online (www.med.unc.edu/embryo_images); and searching under topics such as "embryo" or "embryology" will locate many useful websites for further study.

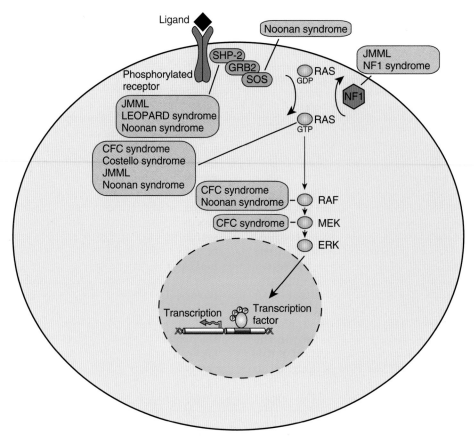

Figure Intro-6. Scheme showing the RAS-MAP kinase pathway and mutations that result in human disease. See text for abbreviations in disease names.

Embryology in Practice

ONE PATHWAY, TWO PROBLEMS

A two-year-old girl is seen by her family doctor for "fatigue and a rash." She is well known to the physician after past visits for stenosis of her pulmonary valve and issues with poor growth leading to a presumptive diagnosis of Noonan syndrome. Her exam today causes concern because it reveals lethargy, pallor, and a purple-red maculopapular (larger flat or small raised) rash on her trunk. She also has enlarged glands (lymphadenopathy) and hepatosplenomegaly (enlarged spleen and liver). The physician expresses his concern that the girl may have a serious illness, "perhaps a blood cancer," and he arranges to have the child admitted to the hospital.

On admission, a complete blood count shows anemia (a low red cell count), thrombocytopenia (low platelets), and leukocytosis (a high white cell count). The hematopathology report returns a diagnosis of juvenile myelomonocytic leukemia (JMML). The oncologist spends time with the family discussing this diagnosis and the treatments to come, which will include splenectomy, chemotherapy, radiation, and hematopoietic stem cell transplantation (bone marrow transplant). Despite intensive treatment, JMML has a high relapse rate after transplant and a poor prognosis, with a five-year survival of ≈50%.

JMML is a rare malignancy, making up only 1% to 2% of childhood leukemias. The cause of this cancer is linked to inappropriate activation of the RAS-MAP kinase pathway (Fig. Intro-6). Mutations in this pathway are also responsible for a group of genetic syndromes, including neurofibromatosis type 1 (NF1) and Noonan, cardiofaciocutaneous (CFC), LEOPARD, and Costello syndromes. Although these are distinct syndromes, the large degree of clinical overlap between them and the fact that most can be caused by mutations in an overlapping set of genes in the pathway led to a conceptual grouping of these conditions, alternatively called "RAS-opathies" or "Noonan-related disorders," among other names. Noonan syndrome is caused by mutations in at least five different genes in the RAS-MAP kinase pathway.

Mutations in this pathway also confer a high risk of JMML, and patients with NF1 and Noonan syndrome make up a significant percentage of JMML patients. RAS is a proto-oncogene—a gene that regulates cellular growth and proliferation that can become an oncogene (cancer-causing gene) if mutated or inappropriately expressed. Other examples of proto-oncogenes include MYC (linked to Burkitt's lymphoma), ERRB2 (HER2; linked to breast cancer), and CTNNB1 (β-CATENIN; linked to pancreatic cancer). The growing understanding of the genetic pathways underlying JMML gives some hope for future, more targeted therapies.

SUGGESTED READINGS

Brakenhoff R. 2011. Another NOTCH for cancer. Science 333: 1102-1103.

Burtner C, Kennedy B. 2010. Progeria syndromes and ageing: what is the connection? Nat Rev Mol Cell Biol 8:567-578.

Fontana L, Partridge L, Longo V. 2010. Extending healthy life span–from yeast to humans. Science 328:321-326.

Jopling C, Boue S, Izpisua Belmonte J. 2011. Dedifferentiation, transdifferentiation and reprogramming: three routes to regeneration. Nat Rev Mol Cell Biol 12:79-89.

Kelly D. 2011. Ageing theories unified. Nature 470:342-343.

Martin G. 2011. The biology of aging: 1985-2010 and beyond. FASEB J 25:3756-3762.

Muneoka K, Allan C, Yang X, et al. 2008. Mammalian regeneration and regenerative medicine. Birth Defects Res Pt C 84:265-280.

Polakis P. 2007. The many ways of Wnt in cancer. Curr Opin Gen Dev 17:45-51.

Rubin L, de Sauvage F. 2006. Targeting the hedgehog pathway in cancer. Nat Rev Drug Discov 5:1026-1030.

Stipp D. 2012. A new path to longevity. Sci Am 306:6-18.

Chapter 1

Gametogenesis, Fertilization, and First Week

SUMMARY

A textbook of human embryology could begin at any of several points in the human life cycle. This textbook starts with a discussion of the origin of specialized cells called **primordial germ cells (PGCs)**. PGCs can be first identified within the wall of the **yolk sac**, one of the extraembryonic membranes, during the fourth to sixth weeks of gestation. These PGCs will give rise to the **germ line**, a series of cells that form the sex cells, or **gametes** (i.e., the **egg** and **sperm**). However, these gametes will not function to form the next generation for several decades (i.e., after the onset of **puberty**). Yet, remarkably, one of the first things that happen in the developing embryo is that the germ line is set aside for the next generation. Similarly, the germ lines that gave rise to the developing embryo were established a generation earlier, when the embryo's father and mother were developing in utero (i.e., when the embryo's paternal and maternal grandmothers were pregnant with the embryo's father and mother).

From the wall of the yolk sac, PGCs actively migrate between the sixth and twelfth weeks of gestation to the dorsal body wall of the embryo, where they populate the developing gonads and differentiate into the gamete precursor cells called **spermatogonia** in the male and **oogonia** in the female. Like the normal somatic cells of the body, the spermatogonia and oogonia are **diploid**, that is, they each contain twenty-three pairs of chromosomes (for a total of forty-six chromosomes each). When these cells eventually produce **gametes** by the process of **gametogenesis** (called **spermatogenesis** in the male and **oogenesis** in the female), they undergo **meiosis**, a sequence of two specialized cell divisions by which the number of chromosomes in the gametes is halved. The gametes thus contain twenty-three chromosomes (one of each pair); therefore, they are **haploid**. The developing gametes also undergo cytoplasmic differentiation, resulting in the production of mature **spermatozoa** in the male and **definitive oocytes** in the female.

In the male, spermatogenesis takes place in the seminiferous tubules of the testes and does not occur until **puberty**. In contrast, in the female, oogenesis is initiated during fetal life. Specifically, between the third and fifth months of fetal life, oogonia initiate the first meiotic division, thereby becoming primary oocytes. However, the primary oocytes then quickly enter a state of meiotic arrest that persists until after puberty. After puberty, a few oocytes and their enclosing follicles resume development each month in response to the production of pituitary gonadotropic hormones. Usually, only one of these follicles matures fully and undergoes **ovulation** to release the enclosed oocyte, and the oocyte completes meiosis only if a spermatozoon fertilizes it. **Fertilization**, the uniting of egg and sperm, takes place in the oviduct. After the oocyte finishes meiosis, the paternal and maternal chromosomes come together, resulting in the formation of a **zygote** containing maternal and paternal chromosomes aligned on the metaphase plate. Embryonic development is considered to begin at this point.

The newly formed embryo undergoes a series of cell divisions, called **cleavage**, as it travels down the oviduct toward the uterus. Cleavage subdivides the zygote first into two cells, then into four, then into eight, and so on. These daughter cells do not grow between divisions, so the entire embryo remains the same size. Starting at the eight- to sixteen-cell stage, the cleaving embryo, or **morula**, differentiates into two groups of cells: a peripheral outer cell layer and a central **inner cell mass**. The outer cell layer, called the **trophoblast**, forms the fetal component of the placenta and associated extraembryonic membranes, whereas the inner cell mass, also called the **embryoblast**, gives rise to the embryo proper and associated extraembryonic membranes. By the thirty-cell stage, the embryo begins to form a fluid-filled central cavity, the **blastocyst cavity**. By the fifth to sixth day of development, the embryo is a hollow ball of about one-hundred cells, called a **blastocyst**. At this point, it enters the uterine cavity and begins to implant into the endometrial lining of the uterine wall.

Clinical Taster

A couple, both in their late thirties, is having difficulty conceiving a child. Early in their marriage, about ten years ago, they used birth control pills and condoms thereafter, but they stopped using all forms of birth control more than two years ago. Despite this and having intercourse three or four times a week, a pregnancy has not resulted. On routine physical examination, both the man and the woman seem to be in excellent health. The woman is an avid runner and competes in occasional marathons, and she has had regular periods since her menarche at age thirteen. The man had a varicocele, which was corrected when he was nineteen; the urologist who performed the surgery assured him that there would be no subsequent adverse effects on his fertility.

Because no obvious cause of their fertility problem is noted, the couple is referred to a local fertility clinic for specialized treatment. At the clinic, the man has a semen analysis. This reveals that his sperm count (sixty million sperm per ejaculate),

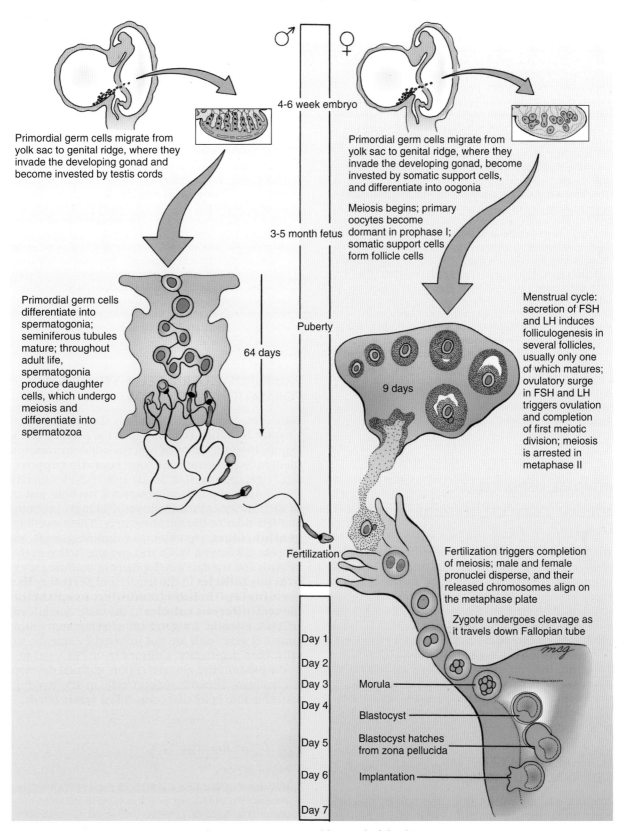

Primordial germ cells migrate from yolk sac to genital ridge, where they invade the developing gonad and become invested by testis cords

4-6 week embryo

Primordial germ cells migrate from yolk sac to genital ridge, where they invade the developing gonad, become invested by somatic support cells, and differentiate into oogonia

Meiosis begins; primary oocytes become dormant in prophase I; somatic support cells form follicle cells

3-5 month fetus

Primordial germ cells differentiate into spermatogonia; seminiferous tubules mature; throughout adult life, spermatogonia produce daughter cells, which undergo meiosis and differentiate into spermatozoa

64 days

Puberty

9 days

Menstrual cycle: secretion of FSH and LH induces folliculogenesis in several follicles, usually only one of which matures; ovulatory surge in FSH and LH triggers ovulation and completion of first meiotic division; meiosis is arrested in metaphase II

Fertilization

Fertilization triggers completion of meiosis; male and female pronuclei disperse, and their released chromosomes align on the metaphase plate

Zygote undergoes cleavage as it travels down Fallopian tube

Day 1
Day 2
Day 3   Morula
Day 4
           Blastocyst
Day 5   Blastocyst hatches
           from zona pellucida
Day 6   Implantation
Day 7

Time line. Gametogenesis and first week of development.

sperm mobility (vigorous motility and forward progression [i.e., straight swimming movement]), sperm morphology (70% with an oval head and a tail seven to fifteen times longer than the head), and semen volume (3.5 mL with a normal fructose level) are within normal ranges. Semen viscosity and sperm agglutination are also normal. As a next step, a postcoital test is planned. Using the woman's recent menstrual history to estimate the time of her midcycle, and daily basal body temperature measurements and urine LH (luteinizing hormone) tests to predict ovulation, intercourse is timed for the evening of the day on which ovulation is expected to occur. The next morning, the woman undergoes a cervical examination. It is noted that the cervical mucus contains clumped and immotile sperm, suggesting sperm-cervical mucus incompatibility.

Based on the results of the postcoital test, the couple decides to undergo **artificial insemination**. After five attempts in which the man's sperm are collected, washed, and injected into the uterus through a sterile catheter passed through the cervix, a pregnancy still has not resulted. The couple is discouraged and decides to take some time off to consider their options.

After considering adoption, gestational surrogacy, and remaining childless, the couple returns three months later and requests **IVF (in vitro fertilization)**. On the second of two very regimented attempts, the couple is delighted to learn that a pregnancy has resulted. A few weeks later, Doppler ultrasound examination detects two fetal heartbeats. This is confirmed two months later by ultrasonography. Early in the ninth month of gestation, two healthy babies are delivered—a 6-pound 2-ounce girl and a 5-pound 14-ounce boy.

PRIMORDIAL GERM CELLS

PRIMORDIAL GERM CELLS RESIDE IN YOLK SAC

Cells that give rise to **gametes** in both males and females can be identified during the fourth week of gestation within an extraembryonic membrane called the **yolk sac** (Fig. 1-1A). Based on studies in animal models, it is believed that these cells arise earlier in gestation, during the phase of gastrulation (covered in Chapter 3). These cells are called **primordial germ cells (PGCs)**, and their lineage constitutes the **germ line**. PGCs can be recognized within the yolk sac and during their subsequent migration (see next paragraph) because of their distinctive pale cytoplasm and rounded shape (Fig. 1-1B, C), and because they can be specifically labeled with a number of molecular markers.

PRIMORDIAL GERM CELLS MIGRATE INTO DORSAL BODY WALL

Between four and six weeks, PGCs migrate by ameboid movement from the yolk sac to the wall of the gut tube, and from the gut tube via the mesentery of the gut to the dorsal body wall (see Fig. 1-1A, B). In the dorsal body wall, these cells come to rest on either side of the midline in the loose mesenchymal tissue just deep to the membranous (epithelial) lining of the coelomic cavity. Most PGCs populate the region of the body wall at the level that will form the gonads (covered in Chapter 16). PGCs

continue to multiply by mitosis during their migration. Some PGCs may become stranded during their migration, coming to rest at extragonadal sites. Occasionally, stray germ cells of this type may give rise to a type of tumor called a **teratoma** (Fig. 1-1D, E).

In the Clinic

TERATOMA FORMATION

Teratomas, tumors composed of tissues derived from all three germ layers, can be extragonadal or gonadal and are derived from PGCs. Sacrococcygeal teratomas, the most common tumors in newborns, occur in 1 in 20,000 to 70,000 births (Fig. 1-1D, E). They occur four times more frequently in female newborns than in male newborns, and they represent about 3% of all childhood malignancies. Gonadal tumors are usually diagnosed after the onset of puberty. Both ovarian and testicular teratomas can form. The **pluripotency** (ability to form many cell types, not to be confused with **totipotency**, the ability to form *all* cell types) of teratomas is exhibited by the fact that they can give rise to a variety of definitive anatomic structures, including hair, teeth, pituitary gland, and even a fully formed eye.

PRIMORDIAL GERM CELLS STIMULATE FORMATION OF GONADS

Differentiation of the gonads is described in detail in Chapter 16. When PGCs arrive in the presumptive gonad region, they stimulate cells of the adjacent coelomic epithelium to proliferate and form **somatic support cells** (Fig. 1-1F; see also Figs. 16-1D and 16-5). Proliferation of the somatic support cells creates a swelling just medial to each mesonephros (embryonic kidney) on both right and left sides of the gut mesentery. These swellings, the **genital ridges**, represent the primitive gonads. Somatic support cells invest PGCs and give rise to tissues that will nourish and regulate development of maturing sex cells—**ovarian follicles** in the female and **Sertoli cells** of the **germinal epithelium (seminiferous epithelium)** of the **seminiferous tubules** in the male. Somatic support cells are essential for germ cell development within the gonad: if germ cells are not invested by somatic support cells, they degenerate. Conversely, if PGCs fail to arrive in the presumptive gonadal region, gonadal development is disrupted. Somatic support cells in the male quickly assemble into epithelial cords called **testis cords**.

In the Research Lab

ORIGIN OF PGCs

Although the exact time and place of origin of PGCs in humans are unknown, cell tracing and other experiments in the mouse demonstrate that PGCs arise from the epiblast (one of the layers of the bilaminar and trilaminar blastoderm stages; covered in Chapters 2 and 3). During gastrulation, these cells move through the caudal part of the primitive streak and into the extraembryonic area. From there, they migrate to the gut wall and through the gut mesentery to the gonadal ridges, as in humans.

Migration of PGCs to the developing gonads involves processes shared by migrating neural crest cells (see Chapter 4),

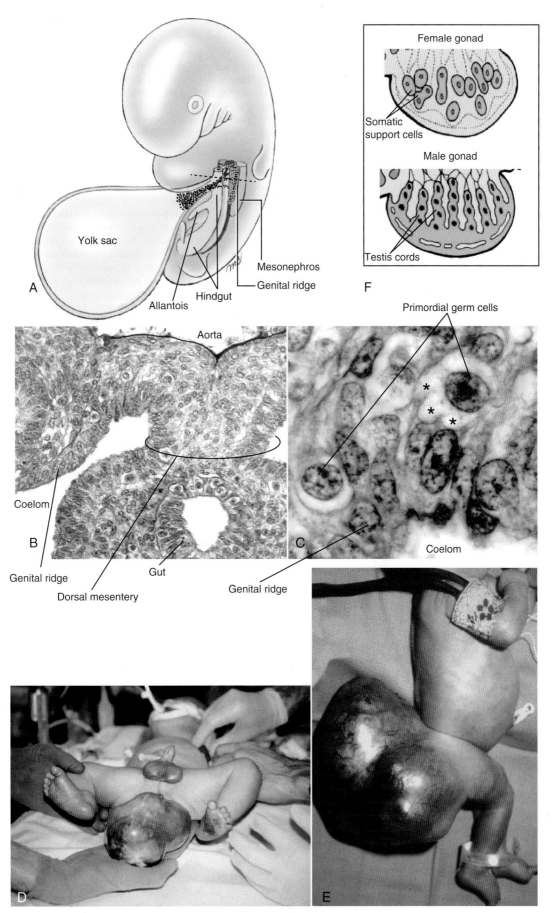

Figure 1-1. Yolk-sac origin of primordial germ cells and their migration during normal development, and formation of teratomas. *A,* Primordial germ cells (PGCs) reside in the endodermal layer of the caudal side of the yolk sac during four to six weeks of development. *B, C,* PGCs then migrate to the dorsal body wall. Asterisks indicate three pseudopodia on a migrating PGC. *D, E,* Infants with large sacrococcygeal teratomas. *F,* Between six and twelve weeks, PGCs stimulate formation of the genital ridges in the dorsal body wall. Somatic support cells differentiate and invest PGCs. In females, somatic support cells become ovarian follicle cells; in males, somatic support cells assemble in testis cords and ultimately become Sertoli cells of the seminiferous tubules.

neuronal processes (see Chapters 9 and 10), and developing blood and lymphatic vessels (see Chapter 13). These include intrinsic motility programs involving cytoskeletal dynamics (note pseudopods on one of the PGCs shown in Fig. 1-1C), adhesive substrates (such as tenascin C, β2 integrin, and laminin, all of which seem to be required for PGC migration), and extracellular attractive and repulsive cues. As covered in Chapter 10, **chemokines** (a type of **cytokine**) and their receptors direct the migration of sympathetic precursor cells. Similarly, chemokines play important roles in PGC migration by acting as **chemotropic signals** (i.e., attractive signals produced by the developing gonads) to regulate PGC honing. Such chemokines include the ligand Sdf1 (stromal cell–derived factor-1, also known as Cxcl12) and its receptor Cxcr4. PGC migration toward the gonad is disrupted in mouse or zebrafish embryos lacking the ligand or its receptor. In addition, Sdf1 acts as a PGC survival factor. Moreover, factors involved in the migration of melanocytes (covered in Chapter 4) also are involved in PGC migration. These include steel factor (also known as stem cell factor), the c-kit ligand, and its receptor c-kit.

MOLECULAR REGULATION OF PGC DEVELOPMENT

Development of the germ line involves the sequential activation of genes that direct the initial induction, proliferation, survival, migration, and differentiation of PGCs. Animal models have been very useful for understanding these events and have been used to show that the functions of many genes controlling PGC development are conserved across diverse organisms. However, mechanisms underlying the initial events of PGC formation in mammals seem to be very different from those of lower organisms.

In some model organisms, such as the fruit fly, worm, and frog, **maternal effect genes** (covered in Chapter 5) are required for initiation of germ cell formation. Activation of these maternal genes regulates the segregation of the **germ plasm** (cytoplasm containing determinants of the germ line) to a specific region of the zygote, so that it becomes incorporated during cleavage into a unique group of cells that will form the germ cell precursors.

The Drosophila gene vasa is segregated to germ cells in this fashion. Vasa transcripts are expressed ubiquitously in the oocyte cytoplasm, but vasa protein becomes specifically localized in the germ plasm. Vasa is an RNA-binding protein of the dead box family, and its possible role is to bind mRNAs involved in germ line determination, such as oskar and nanos, and to control the onset of their translation. Vertebrate orthologs of vasa exist, and in some vertebrates, vasa protein is expressed in germ cell precursors as they are forming (however, in mice, vasa is expressed in germ cells only much later, after they have differentiated and are about to colonize the gonads).

In contrast to lower organisms, in which germ cells are usually specified by the inheritance of maternal gene products, in the mouse and probably also in humans the germ line is induced. All cells of the mammalian morula are seemingly capable of forming pluripotent germ cells, but their capacity to do so becomes rapidly restricted first to the inner cell mass and then to the epiblast. Therefore, in mammals, the **initiation of germ line development** requires activation of genes that maintain pluripotency within the precursors that will form the germ line. One such gene encodes a pou domain transcription factor (Oct4, also called Pou5f1; transcription factors are covered in Chapter 5). Its activity is present initially in all cells of the morula, but then only in the inner cell mass. It is then restricted to the epiblast, and finally it is expressed only in the presumptive germ cells themselves.

Further development of the germ line requires an inductive signal from the trophoblast (induction is covered in Chapter 5). One such signal is provided by bone morphogenetic proteins (Bmps). In chimeric mouse embryos (mouse injection chimeras are covered in Chapter 5) lacking Bmp4 specifically within the trophoblast, PGCs, as well as the allantois (an extraembryonic membrane), fail to form. Bmp4 induces expression of two germ line–specific genes in mice: fragilis and stella; however, their exact roles in PGC development are unknown, as knock-outs of neither gene affect PGC cell specification.

In contrast, two other genes have been identified that are lacking in Bmp signaling mutants and when knocked out result in the loss of PGCs. One, B-lymphocyte–induced maturation protein 1, Blimp1, is a master regulator of plasma cell differentiation from B cells during development of the immune system. The other, Prdm14, has less defined roles. Both of these genes are essential for PGC differentiation.

Proliferation and survival of PGCs are ensured by the expression of **trophic factors** (factors that promote cell growth and survival) within the PGCs or within associated cells. A trophic factor expressed by PGCs and required for their early survival and proliferation is the RNA-binding protein tiar. Another is a mouse ortholog of the Drosophila gene nanos (nanos3). Many other trophic factors seem to be required for the survival and proliferation of PGCs along their migratory pathway from the yolk sac to the gut and dorsal mesentery and then to the dorsal body wall. These include several factors expressed by tissues along the pathway, including the c-kit ligand (stem cell factor or steel factor) and members of the interleukin/Lif cytokine family (a cytokine is a regulatory protein released by cells of the immune system that acts as an intercellular mediator in the generation of an immune response). Study of c-kit and steel mutants has revealed that this signaling pathway suppresses **PGC apoptosis** (cell death) during migration. This finding provides an explanation for why PGCs that stray from their normal migratory path and come to rest in extragonadal sites usually (but not always; see above discussion of extragonadal teratomas) degenerate.

Once PGCs arrive within the presumptive gonad, numerous genes must be expressed to **regulate the final differentiation of cells of the germ line**. Three new germ cell–specific genes are expressed shortly after PGCs enter the genital ridge (after which they are usually called **gonocytes**): murine vasa homolog (mVh; the vasa gene was covered above), germ cell nuclear antigen 1 (Gcna1), and germ cell–less (Gcl1). The last is expressed in the Drosophila germ line shortly after it is established and is named after the mutation in which the gene is inactivated and the germ line is lost.

GAMETOGENESIS

TIMING OF GAMETOGENESIS IS DIFFERENT IN MALES AND FEMALES

In both males and females, PGCs undergo further mitotic divisions within the gonads and then commence **gametogenesis**, the process that converts them into mature male and female gametes (**spermatozoa** and **definitive oocytes**, respectively). However, the timing of these processes differs in the two sexes (see Timeline for this chapter). In males, PGCs (usually now called **gonocytes**) remain dormant from the sixth week of embryonic development until puberty. At **puberty, seminifer-ous tubules** mature and PGCs differentiate into **spermatogonia**. Successive waves of spermatogonia undergo **meiosis** (the process by which the number of chromosomes in the sex cells is halved; see following section) and mature into spermatozoa. Spermatozoa are produced continuously from puberty until death.

In contrast, in females, PGCs (again, usually now called **gonocytes**) undergo a few more mitotic divisions after they become invested by the somatic support cells. They then differentiate into **oogonia**. By the fifth month of fetal development, all oogonia begin meiosis, after which they are called **primary oocytes**. However, during an early phase of meiosis, all sex cells enter a state of dormancy, and they remain in meiotic arrest as primary oocytes until sexual maturity. Starting at puberty, each month a few ovarian follicles resume development in response to the monthly surge of pituitary gonadotropic hormones, but usually only one primary oocyte matures into a **secondary oocyte** and is ovulated. This oocyte enters a second phase of meiotic arrest and does not actually complete meiosis unless it is fertilized. These monthly cycles continue until the onset of menopause at approximately fifty years of age. The process of gametogenesis in the male and female (called **spermatogenesis** and **oogenesis**, respectively) is covered in detail later in this chapter.

In the Research Lab

WHY IS TIMING OF GAMETOGENESIS DIFFERENT IN MALES AND FEMALES?

Experiments in mouse embryos provide insight into why the timing of gametogenesis differs in males and females. Shortly after PGCs enter the genital ridge, they stop their migration and undergo two or three further rounds of mitosis and then enter a premeiotic stage, during which they upregulate meiotic genes. In the male genital ridge, germ cells then reverse this process and arrest, but in the female genital ridge, they enter the meiotic prophase as primary oocytes and progress through meiosis until the diplotene stage, at which time they arrest. If male (XY) PGCs are transplanted into female (XX) embryos, the male PGCs follow the course just described for normal female PGCs in females. Moreover, PGCs in female or male embryos that fail to reach the gonad also progress through meiosis as oocytes, regardless of their genotype. These two results suggest that all germ cells, regardless of their chromosome constitution, are programmed to develop as oocytes and that the timing of meiotic entry seems to be a cell-autonomous property rather than being induced. In support of this, Tet1, a member of the Tet family of proteins, was recently shown to be required for the activation of meiosis in female mice. Although it is unclear how Tet1 functions, Tet proteins play a role in erasing epigenetic marks in DNA—a critical event in the development of PGCs, as covered in Chapter 2.

In males, the genital ridge prevents prenatal entry into meiosis, and experiments suggest that there is a **male meiosis inhibitor** and that this inhibitor is a diffusible signaling factor produced by Sertoli cells. Possible candidates for this factor include the protein prostaglandin D2 and the protein encoded by the Tdl gene (a gene showing sequence homology to antimicrobial proteins called beta-defensins; prostaglandins are synthesized from fatty acids and modulate several physiological functions, such as blood pressure, smooth muscle contraction, and inflammation).

MEIOSIS HALVES NUMBER OF CHROMOSOMES AND DNA STRANDS IN SEX CELLS

Although the timing of meiosis is very different between males and females, the basic chromosomal events of the process are the same in the two sexes (Fig. 1-2). Like all normal somatic (non-germ) cells, PGCs contain twenty-three pairs of chromosomes, or a total of forty-six chromosomes. One chromosome of each pair is obtained from the maternal gamete and the other from the paternal gamete. These chromosomes contain **deoxyribonucleic acid (DNA)**, which encodes information required for development and functioning of the organism. Of the total complement of forty-six chromosomes, twenty-two pairs consist of matching, homologous chromosomes called **autosomes**. The remaining two chromosomes are called **sex chromosomes** because they determine the sex of the individual. There are two kinds of sex chromosomes, X and Y. Individuals with one X chromosome and one Y chromosome (XY) are genetically male; individuals with two X chromosomes (XX) are genetically female. Nonetheless, one of the X chromosomes in the female genome is randomly inactivated, leaving only one active X chromosome in each cell (X-inactivation is covered in Chapter 2; mechanisms underlying sex determination are covered in detail in Chapter 16).

Two designations that are often confused are the **ploidy** of a cell and its **N number**. Ploidy refers to the number of copies of each *chromosome* present in a cell nucleus, whereas the N number refers to the number of copies of each unique double-stranded *DNA molecule* in the nucleus. Each chromosome contains one or two molecules of DNA at different stages of the cell cycle (whether mitotic or meiotic), so the ploidy and the N number of a cell do not always coincide. Somatic cells and PGCs have two copies of each kind of chromosome; hence, they are called **diploid**. In contrast, mature gametes have just one copy of each kind of chromosome and are called **haploid**. Haploid gametes with one DNA molecule per chromosome are said to be **1N**. In some stages of the cell cycle, diploid cells also have one DNA molecule per chromosome, and so are **2N**. However, during earlier phases of meiosis or mitosis, each chromosome of a diploid cell has two molecules of DNA, and so the cell is **4N**.

Meiosis is a specialized process of cell division that occurs only in the germ line. Figure 1-2 compares mitosis *(A)* and meiosis *(B)*. In **mitosis** (normal cell division), a diploid, 2N cell replicates its DNA (becoming diploid, 4N) and undergoes a single division to yield two diploid, 2N daughter cells. In meiosis, a diploid germ cell replicates its DNA (becoming diploid, 4N) and undergoes two successive, qualitatively different nuclear and cell divisions to yield four haploid, 1N offspring. In males, the cell divisions of meiosis are equal and yield four identical **spermatozoa**. However in females, the meiotic cell divisions are dramatically unequal and yield a single, massive, haploid definitive **oocyte** and three-minute, non-functional, haploid **polar bodies**.

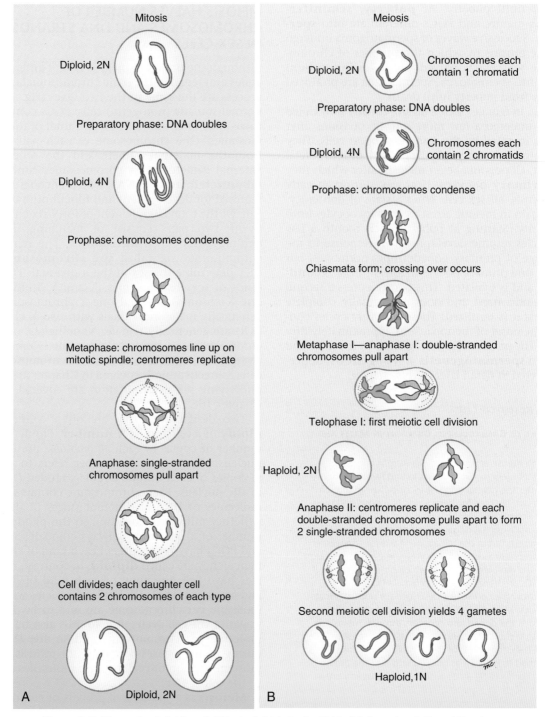

Figure 1-2. Types of cell division. *A*, Mitosis. *B*, Meiosis. See Table 1-1 for a description of the stages.

First Meiotic Division: DNA Replication and Recombination, Yielding Two Haploid, 2N Daughter Cells

The steps of meiosis are illustrated in Figure 1-2*B* and are summarized in Table 1-1. The preliminary step in meiosis, as in mitosis, is the replication of each chromosomal DNA molecule; thus, the diploid cell is converted from 2N to 4N. This event marks the beginning of gametogenesis. In the female, the oogonium is now called a **primary oocyte**, and in the male, the

spermatogonium is now called a **primary spermatocyte** (Fig. 1-3). Once the DNA replicates, each chromosome consists of two parallel strands or **chromatids** joined together at a structure called the **centromere**. Each chromatid contains a single DNA molecule (which is itself double stranded; do not confuse DNA double strands with the two chromatid strands composing each chromosome).

In the next step, called **prophase**, the chromosomes condense into compact, double-stranded structures (i.e.,

TABLE 1-1   EVENTS DURING MITOTIC AND MEIOTIC CELL DIVISIONS IN THE GERM LINE

Stage	Events	Name of Cell	Condition of Genome
Resting interval between mitotic cell divisions	Normal cellular metabolism occurs	♀ Oogonium ♂ Spermatogonium	Diploid, 2N
Mitosis			
Preparatory phase	DNA replication yields double-stranded chromosomes	♀ Oogonium ♂ Spermatogonium	Diploid, 4N
Prophase	Double-stranded chromosomes condense		
Metaphase	Chromosomes align along the equator; centromeres replicate		
Anaphase and telophase	Each double-stranded chromosome splits into two single-stranded chromosomes, one of which is distributed to each daughter nucleus		
Cytokinesis	Cell divides	♀ Oogonium ♂ Spermatogonium	Diploid, 2N
Meiosis I			
Preparatory phase	DNA replication yields double-stranded chromosomes	♀ Primary oocyte ♂ Primary spermatocyte	Diploid, 4N
Prophase	Double-stranded chromosomes condense; two chromosomes of each homologous pair align at the centromeres to form a four-limbed chiasma; recombination by crossing over occurs		
Metaphase	Chromosomes align along the equator; *centromeres do not replicate*		
Anaphase and telophase	One double-stranded chromosome of each homologous pair is distributed to each daughter cell		
Cytokinesis	Cell divides	♀ One secondary oocyte and the first polar body ♂ Two secondary spermatocytes	Haploid, 2N
Meiosis II			
Prophase	*No DNA replication takes place during the second meiotic division*; double-stranded chromosomes condense		
Metaphase	Chromosomes align along the equator; *centromeres replicate*		
Anaphase and telophase	Each chromosome splits into two single-stranded chromosomes, one of which is distributed to each daughter nucleus		
Cytokinesis	Cell divides	♀ One definitive oocyte and three polar bodies ♂ Four spermatids	Haploid, 1N

two chromatids joined by one centromere). During the late stages of prophase, the double-stranded chromosomes of each homologous pair match up, centromere to centromere, to form a joint structure called a **chiasma** (composed of four chromatids, two centromeres, and two chromosomes). Chiasma formation makes it possible for the two homologous chromosomes to exchange large segments of DNA by a process called **crossing over**. The resulting **recombination** of the genetic material

on homologous maternal and paternal chromosomes is largely random; therefore, it increases the genetic variability of future gametes. As mentioned earlier, the primary oocyte enters a phase of meiotic arrest during the first meiotic prophase.

During **metaphase**, the four-stranded chiasma structures are organized on the equator of a spindle apparatus similar to the one that forms during mitosis, and during **anaphase**, one double-stranded chromosome

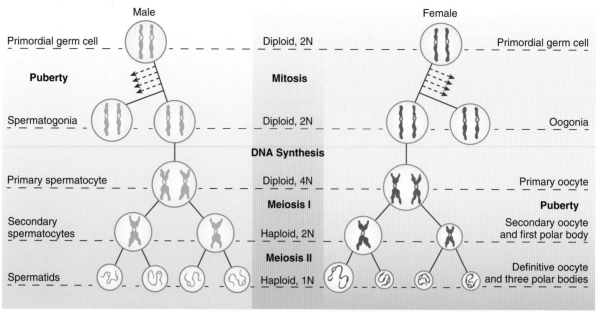

Figure 1-3. Nuclear maturation of germ cells in meiosis in the male and female. In the male, primordial germ cells (PGCs) remain dormant until puberty, when they differentiate into spermatogonia and commence mitosis. Throughout adulthood, spermatogonia produce primary spermatocytes, which undergo meiosis and spermatogenesis. Each primary spermatocyte divides to form two secondary spermatocytes, each of which forms two spermatozoa. Thus, each primary spermatocyte yields four functional gametes. In the female, PGCs differentiate into oogonia, which undergo mitosis and then commence meiosis during fetal life as primary oocytes. The primary oocytes remain arrested in prophase I until stimulated to resume meiosis during a menstrual cycle. Each primary oocyte has the potential to form a secondary oocyte and first polar body. Moreover, each secondary oocyte has the potential to form a definitive oocyte and another polar body, and the first polar body has the potential to form two polar bodies. Thus, each primary oocyte has the potential to yield a single functional gamete and three polar bodies.

of each homologous pair is distributed to each of the two daughter nuclei. During the first meiotic division, the centromeres of the chromosomes do not replicate; therefore, the two chromatids of each chromosome remain together. The resulting daughter nuclei thus are haploid but 2N: they contain the same amount of DNA as the parent germ cell but half as many chromosomes. As daughter nuclei form, the cell itself divides (undergoes **cytokinesis**). The first meiotic cell division produces two **secondary spermatocytes** in the male and a **secondary oocyte** and a **first polar body** in the female (see Fig. 1-3).

Second Meiotic Division: Double-Stranded Chromosomes Divide, Yielding Four Haploid, 1N Daughter Cells

No DNA replication occurs during the second meiotic division. The twenty-three double-stranded chromosomes condense during the second meiotic prophase and line up during the second meiotic metaphase. The chromosomal centromeres then replicate, and during anaphase, the double-stranded chromosomes pull apart into two single-stranded chromosomes, one of which is distributed to each of the daughter nuclei. In males, the second meiotic cell division produces two **definitive spermatocytes**, more commonly called **spermatids** (i.e., a total of four from each germ cell entering meiosis). In the female, the second meiotic cell division, like the first, is radically unequal, producing a large

definitive oocyte and another diminutive polar body. The first polar body may simultaneously undergo a second meiotic division to produce a third polar body (see Fig. 1-3).

In the female, the oocyte enters a second phase of meiotic arrest during the second meiotic metaphase before replication of the centromeres. Meiosis does not resume unless the cell is fertilized.

SPERMATOGENESIS

Now that meiosis has been described, it is possible to describe and compare the specific processes of spermatogenesis and oogenesis. At puberty, the testes begin to secrete greatly increased amounts of the steroid hormone **testosterone**. This hormone has a multitude of effects. In addition to stimulating development of many secondary sex characteristics, it triggers growth of the testes, maturation of seminiferous tubules, and commencement of spermatogenesis.

Under the influence of testosterone, Sertoli cells differentiate into a system of seminiferous tubules. The dormant PGCs resume development, divide several times by mitosis, and then differentiate into spermatogonia. These spermatogonia are located immediately under the basement membrane surrounding the seminiferous tubules, where they occupy pockets between Sertoli cells (Fig. 1-4A). Adjacent Sertoli cells are interconnected between the pockets by **tight junctions**, which help establish

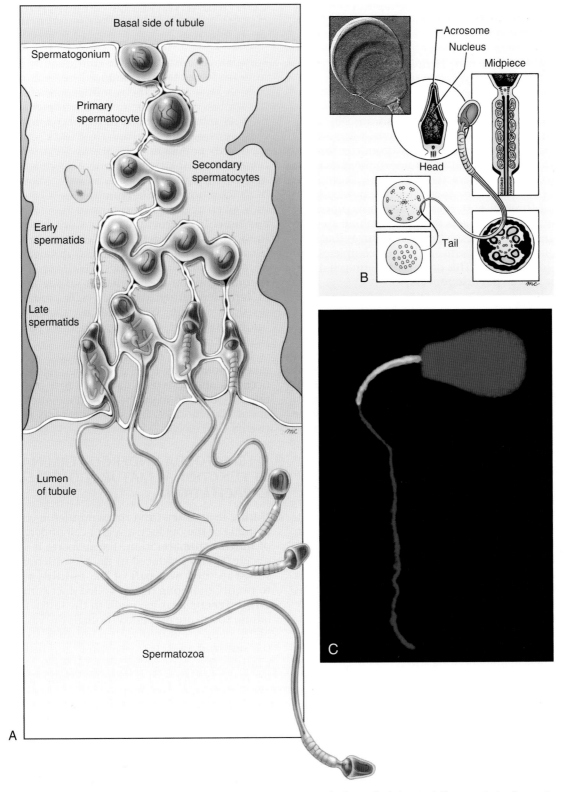

Figure 1-4. Spermatogenesis and spermiogenesis. *A,* Schematic section through the wall of the seminiferous tubule. Spermatogonium just under the outer surface of the tubule wall (basal side) undergoes mitosis to produce daughter cells, which may continue to divide by mitosis (thus renewing the spermatogonial stem cell population) or may commence meiosis as primary spermatocytes. As spermatogenesis and spermiogenesis occur, the differentiating cell is translocated between adjacent Sertoli cells to the tubule lumen. Daughter spermatocytes and spermatids remain linked by cytoplasmic bridges. The entire clone of spermatogonia derived from each primordial germ cell is linked by cytoplasmic bridges. *B,* Structure of the mature spermatozoon. The head contains the nucleus capped by the acrosome; the midpiece contains coiled mitochondria; the tail contains propulsive microtubules. The inset micrograph shows the head of a human sperm. *C,* Bull sperm labeled with fluorescent markers to reveal its nucleus (blue) in its head, mitochondria (green) in its midpiece, and microtubules (red) in its tail. The red labeling around the perimeter of the head is background labeling.

a **blood-testis barrier**. Thus, developing spermatogonia reside within an immune privileged site during their development in the testes.

MALE GERM CELLS ARE TRANSLOCATED TO SEMINIFEROUS TUBULE LUMEN DURING SPERMATOGENESIS

Cells that will undergo spermatogenesis arise by mitosis from the spermatogonia. These cells are gradually translocated between the Sertoli cells from the basal to the luminal side of the seminiferous epithelium while spermatogenesis takes place (see Fig. 1-4A). During this migratory phase, primary spermatocytes pass without interruption through both meiotic divisions, producing first two secondary spermatocytes and then four spermatids. The spermatids undergo dramatic changes that convert them into mature sperm while they complete their migration to the lumen. This process of sperm cell differentiation is called **spermiogenesis**.

SERTOLI CELLS ARE ALSO INSTRUMENTAL IN SPERMIOGENESIS

Sertoli cells participate intimately in differentiation of the gametes. Maturing spermatocytes and spermatids are connected to surrounding Sertoli cells by intercellular junctions, typical of those found on epithelial cells, and unique cytoplasmic processes called **tubulobulbar complexes** that extend into the Sertoli cells. The cytoplasm of developing gametes shrinks dramatically during spermiogenesis; the tubulobulbar complexes are thought to provide a mechanism by which excess cytoplasm is transferred to Sertoli cells. As cytoplasm is removed, spermatids undergo dramatic changes in shape and internal organization that transform them into spermatozoa. Finally, the last connections with Sertoli cells break, releasing the spermatozoa into the tubule lumen. This final step is called **spermiation**.

As shown in Figure 1-4B, C, a spermatozoon consists of a **head**, a **midpiece**, and a **tail**. The head contains the condensed nucleus and is capped by an apical vesicle filled with hydrolytic enzymes (e.g., acrosin, hyaluronidase, and neuraminidase). This vesicle, the **acrosome**, plays an essential role in fertilization. The midpiece contains large, helical mitochondria and generates energy for swimming. The long tail contains microtubules that form part of the propulsion system of the spermatozoon.

In the Clinic

SPERMATOZOA ABNORMALITIES

Errors in spermatogenesis or spermiogenesis are common. Examination of a sperm sample will reveal spermatozoa with abnormalities such as small, narrow, or piriform (pear-shaped) heads, double or triple heads, acrosomal defects, and double tails. If at least 50% of the spermatozoa in an ejaculate have a normal morphology, fertility is not expected to be impaired. Having a larger number of abnormal spermatozoa (called teratospermia if excessive) can be associated with infertility.

CONTINUAL WAVES OF SPERMATOGENESIS OCCUR THROUGHOUT SEMINIFEROUS EPITHELIUM

Spermatogenesis takes place continuously from puberty to death. Gametes are produced in synchronous waves in each local area of the germinal epithelium, although the process is not synchronized throughout the seminiferous tubules. In many different mammals, the clone of spermatogonia, derived from each spermatogonial stem cell, populates a local area of the seminiferous tubules and displays synchronous spermatogenesis. This may be the case in humans as well. About four waves of synchronously differentiating cells can be observed in a given region of the human tubule epithelium at any time. Ultrastructural studies provide evidence that these waves of differentiating cells remain synchronized because of incomplete cytokinesis throughout the series of mitotic and meiotic divisions between division of a spermatogonium and formation of spermatids. Instead of fully separating, daughter cells produced by these divisions remain connected by slender cytoplasmic bridges (see Fig. 1-4A) that could allow passage of small signaling molecules or metabolites.

In the human male, each cycle of spermatogenesis takes about sixty-four days. Spermatogonial mitosis occupies about sixteen days, the first meiotic division takes about eight days, the second meiotic division takes about sixteen days, and spermiogenesis requires about twenty-four days.

SPERMATOZOA UNDERGO TERMINAL STEP OF FUNCTIONAL MATURATION CALLED CAPACITATION

During its journey from the seminiferous tubules to the ampulla of the oviduct, a sperm cell undergoes a process of functional maturation that prepares it to fertilize an oocyte. Sperm produced in the seminiferous tubules are stored in the lower part of the **epididymis**, a fifteen- to twenty-foot long highly coiled duct connected to the **vas deferens** near its origin in the testis. During ejaculation, sperm are propelled through the vas deferens and urethra and are mixed with nourishing secretions from the **seminal vesicles, prostate**, and **bulbourethral glands** (these structures are covered further in Chapter 16). As many as three hundred million spermatozoa may be deposited in the vagina by a single ejaculation, but only a few hundred succeed in navigating through the cervix, uterus, and oviduct and into the expanded ampulla region. In the **ampulla** of the oviduct, sperm survive and retain their capacity to fertilize an oocyte for one to three days.

Capacitation, the final step of sperm maturation, consists mainly of changes in the acrosome that prepare it to release the enzymes required to penetrate the zona pellucida, a shell of glycoprotein surrounding the oocyte. Capacitation takes place within the female genital tract and is thought to require contact with secretions of the oviduct. Spermatozoa used in in vitro fertilization (IVF) procedures are artificially capacitated. Spermatozoa with defective acrosomes may be injected directly into oocytes to assist

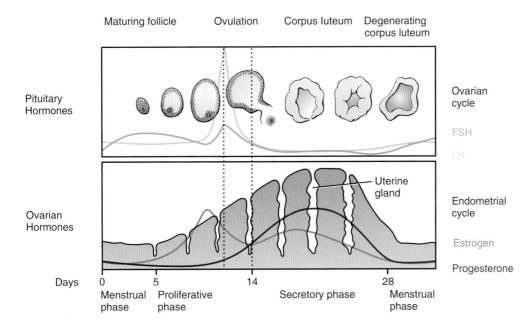

Maturing follicle   Ovulation   Corpus luteum   Degenerating corpus luteum

Pituitary Hormones

Ovarian cycle

FSH

LH

Ovarian Hormones

Uterine gland

Endometrial cycle

Estrogen

Progesterone

Days 0   5   14   28

Menstrual phase   Proliferative phase   Secretory phase   Menstrual phase

Figure 1-5. Ovarian, endometrial, and hormonal events of the menstrual cycle. Pituitary follicle-stimulating hormone (FSH) and luteinizing hormone (LH) directly control the ovarian cycle and also control production of estrogen and progesterone by responding follicles and corpus luteum of the ovary. These ovarian hormones in turn control the cycle of the uterine endometrium.

reproduction in humans (assisted reproduction technology, or ART, is covered later in the chapter in an "In the Clinic" entitled "Assisted Reproductive Technology").

OOGENESIS

PRIMARY OOCYTES FORM IN OVARIES BY FIVE MONTHS OF FETAL LIFE

As mentioned earlier, after female germ cells become invested by somatic support cells, they undergo a series of mitotic divisions and then differentiate into oogonia (see Fig. 1-3). By twelve weeks of development, oogonia in the genital ridges enter the first meiotic prophase and then almost immediately become dormant. The nucleus of each of these dormant **primary oocytes**, containing the partially condensed prophase chromosomes, becomes very large and watery and is referred to as a **germinal vesicle**. The swollen condition of the germinal vesicle is thought to protect the oocyte's DNA during the long period of meiotic arrest.

A single-layered, squamous capsule of epithelial follicle cells derived from the somatic support cells tightly encloses each primary oocyte. This capsule and its enclosed primary oocyte constitute a **primordial follicle** (covered below). By five months, when all oogonia have initiated the first meiotic division to become primary oocytes, the number of primordial follicles in the ovaries peaks at about seven million. Most of these follicles subsequently degenerate. By birth, only seven hundred thousand to two million remain, and by puberty, only about four hundred thousand.

HORMONES OF FEMALE CYCLE CONTROL FOLLICULOGENESIS, OVULATION, AND CONDITION OF UTERUS

After reaching puberty, also called **menarche** in females, and until the woman enters **menopause** several decades

later, monthly cycles in the secretion of hypothalamic, pituitary, and ovarian hormones control a **menstrual cycle**, which results each month in the production of a female gamete and a uterus primed to receive a fertilized embryo. Specifically, this twenty-eight–day cycle consists of the following:

- Monthly maturation of (usually) a single oocyte and its enclosing follicle
- Concurrent proliferation of the uterine endometrium
- Process of ovulation by which the oocyte is released from the ovary
- Continued development of the follicle into an endocrine corpus luteum
- Sloughing of the uterine endometrium and involution of the corpus luteum (unless a fertilized ovum implants in the uterus and begins to develop)

The menstrual cycle is considered to begin with menstruation (also called the menses), the shedding of the degenerated uterine endometrium from the previous cycle. On about the fifth day of the cycle (the fifth day after the beginning of menstruation), an increase in secretion by the hypothalamus of the brain of a small peptide hormone, gonadotropin-releasing hormone (GnRH), stimulates the pituitary gland to increase its secretion of two gonadotropic hormones (gonadotropins): follicle-stimulating hormone (FSH) and luteinizing hormone (LH) (Fig. 1-5). The rising levels of pituitary gonadotropins regulate later phases of folliculogenesis in the ovary and the proliferative phase in the uterine endometrium.

ABOUT FIVE TO TWELVE PRIMARY FOLLICLES RESUME DEVELOPMENT EACH MONTH

Before a particular cycle, and independent of pituitary gonadotropins, the follicular epithelium of a small group of primordial follicles thickens, converting the

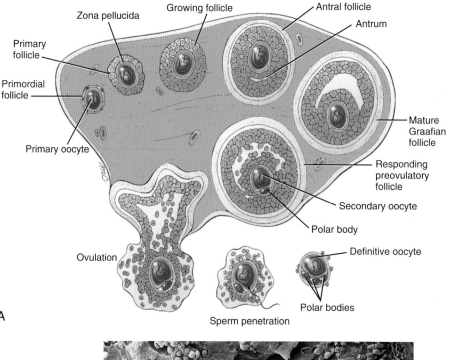

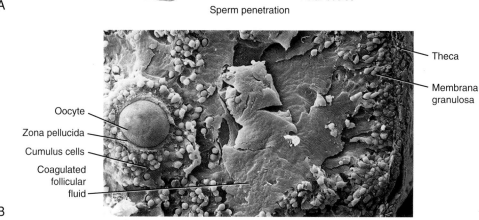

Figure 1-6. Maturation of the egg in the ovary and ovulation. *A,* Schematic depiction of the ovary showing folliculogenesis and ovulation. Five to twelve primordial follicles initially respond to the rising levels of follicle-stimulating hormone (FSH) and luteinizing hormone (LH), but only one matures. In response to the ovulatory surge in LH and FSH, the oocyte of this mature Graafian follicle resumes meiosis and ovulation occurs. Final steps of meiosis take place only if the released oocyte is penetrated by a sperm. *B,* Scanning electron micrograph of a preovulatory follicle.

single-layered follicular epithelium from a layer of squamous cells to cuboidal cells (Fig. 1-6*A*). These follicles are now called **primary follicles**. The follicle cells and the oocyte jointly secrete a thin layer of acellular material, composed of only a few types of glycoprotein, onto the surface of the oocyte. Although this layer, the **zona pellucida**, appears to form a complete physical barrier between the follicle cells and the oocyte (Figs. 1-6*B*, 1-7*A*), actually it is penetrated by thin extensions of follicle cells that are connected to the oocyte cell membrane by intercellular junctions (Fig. 1-7*B*). These extensions and their intercellular junctions remain intact until just before ovulation, and they probably convey both developmental signals and metabolic support to the oocyte. The follicular epithelium of five to twelve of these primary follicles then proliferates to form a multilayered capsule of follicle cells around the oocyte (see Fig. 1-6). The follicles are now called **growing follicles**. At this point, some of the growing follicles cease to develop and eventually degenerate, whereas a few continue to enlarge in response to rising levels of FSH, mainly by taking up fluid and developing

a central fluid-filled cavity called the **antrum**. These follicles are called **antral** or **vesicular follicles**. At the same time, the connective tissue of the ovarian stroma surrounding each of these follicles differentiates into two layers: an inner layer called the **theca interna** and an outer layer called the **theca externa**. These two layers become vascularized, in contrast to the follicle cells, which do not.

SINGLE FOLLICLE BECOMES DOMINANT AND REMAINDER DEGENERATE

Eventually, one of the growing follicles gains primacy and continues to enlarge by absorbing fluid, whereas the remainder of the follicles recruited during the cycle degenerate (undergo **atresia**). The oocyte, surrounded by a small mass of follicle cells called the **cumulus oophorus**, increasingly projects into the expanding antrum but remains connected to the layer of follicle cells that lines the antral cavity and underlies the basement membrane of the follicle. This layer is called the **membrana granulosa**. The large, swollen follicle is now called a **mature**

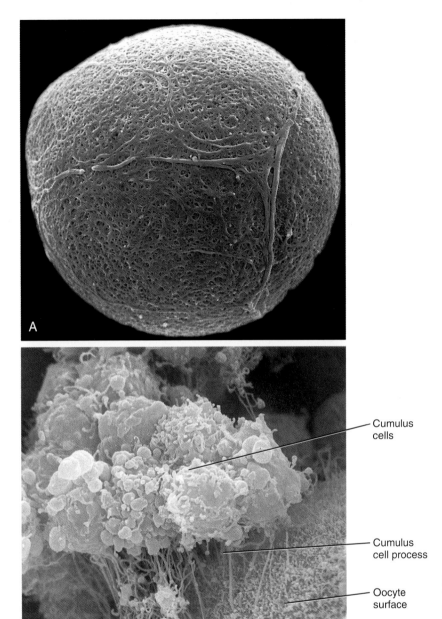

Figure 1-7. The ovulated egg and associated structures. *A*, Scanning electron micrograph of the zona pellucida after removal of the cumulus cells. The zona consists of glycoproteins and forms a barrier that the sperm penetrates by means of its acrosomal enzymes. *B*, Scanning electron micrograph of the oocyte surface and cumulus oophorus, with the zona pellucida digested away. The cumulus cells maintain contact with the oocyte via thin cell processes that penetrate the zona pellucida and form intercellular junctions with the oocyte cell membrane.

vesicular follicle or a mature Graafian follicle (see Fig. 1-6). At this point, the oocyte still has not resumed meiosis.

WHY IS FOLLICULOGENESIS SELECTIVELY STIMULATED IN ONLY A FEW FOLLICLES EACH MONTH?

The reason why only five to twelve primordial follicles commence folliculogenesis each month—and why, of this group, all but one eventually degenerate—is uncertain. One possibility is that follicles become progressively more sensitive to the stimulating effects of FSH as they advance in development. Therefore, follicles that are slightly more advanced simply on a random basis would respond more acutely to FSH and would be favored. Another possibility is that the selection process is regulated by a complex system of feedback between pituitary and ovarian hormones and growth factors.

CHROMOSOMAL ABNORMALITIES RESULT IN SPONTANEOUS ABORTION OR ABNORMAL DEVELOPMENT

It is estimated that one third of all conceptions in normal, healthy women abort spontaneously; approximately one fourth of these occur before pregnancy is detected. Chromosomal anomalies seem to cause about 40% to 50% of spontaneous abortions in those cases in which the conceptus has been recovered and examined. However, many chromosomal anomalies allow the fetus to survive to term. The resulting infants display non-random patterns of developmental abnormalities, that is, **syndromes**. One of these syndromes, Down syndrome, is covered in detail in the following section; others are covered in detail in subsequent chapters.

MANY CHROMOSOMAL ANOMALIES ARISE DURING GAMETOGENESIS AND CLEAVAGE

Abnormal chromosomes can be produced in the germ line of either parent through an error in meiosis or fertilization, or they can arise in the early embryo through an error in mitosis. Gametes or blastomeres that result from these events contain missing or extra chromosomes, or chromosomes with duplicated, deleted, or rearranged segments. Absence of a specific chromosome in a gamete that combines with a normal gamete to form a zygote results in a condition known as **monosomy** (because the zygote contains only one copy of the chromosome rather than the normal two). Conversely, the presence of two of the same kind of chromosome in one of the gametes that forms a zygote results in **trisomy**.

Down syndrome is a disorder most frequently caused by an error during meiosis. If the two copies of chromosome 21 fail to separate during the first or second meiotic anaphase of gametogenesis in either parent (a phenomenon called **non-disjunction**), half of the resulting gametes will lack chromosome 21 altogether and the other half will have two copies (Fig. 1-8A). Embryos formed by fusion of a gamete-lacking chromosome 21 with a normal gamete are called **monosomy 21 embryos**. Monosomies of autosomal chromosomes are invariably fatal during early embryonic development. If, on the other hand, a gamete with two copies of chromosome 21 fuses with a normal gamete, the resulting **trisomy 21 embryo** may survive (Fig. 1-8B). Trisomy 21 infants display the pattern of abnormalities described as **Down syndrome**. In addition to recognizable facial characteristics, mental retardation, and short stature, individuals with Down syndrome may exhibit congenital heart defects (atrioventricular septal defect is most common, that is, a failure to form both atrial and ventricular septa; covered in Chapter 12), hearing loss, duodenal obstruction, a propensity to develop leukemia, and immune system defects. Trisomy in most Down syndrome individuals is the result of non-disjunction in the mother, usually during the first meiotic division (75% to 80% of cases). Identification of the extra chromosome as maternal or paternal in origin was originally based on karyotype analysis that compared banding patterns of the extra chromosome 21 with chromosome 21 of the mother and father. These early studies concluded that about 70% to 75% of Down syndrome cases occurred as a consequence of non-disjunction in the mother. However, by the late 1980s, more sensitive karyotype analysis increased this frequency to 80%, and by the early 1990s, an even more sensitive molecular technique (Southern blot analysis of DNA polymorphisms) provided evidence that as many as 90% to 95% of Down syndrome cases arise through non-disjunction in the maternal germ line. Consequently, it is now accepted that only about 5% of cases of Down syndrome result from an error in spermatogenesis.

Occasionally, the extra chromosome 21 is lost from a subset of cells during cleavage. The resulting embryo develops as a **mosaic** of normal and trisomy 21 cells; 2% to 5% of all individuals with Down syndrome are mosaics. These individuals may show a range of Down syndrome features depending on the abundance and location of abnormal cells. If non-disjunction occurs in the germ line, a seemingly normal individual could produce several Down syndrome offspring. Meiosis of a trisomic germ cell yields gametes with a normal single copy of the chromosome, as well as abnormal gametes with two copies, so normal offspring also can be produced.

Down syndrome does not always result from simple non-disjunction. Sometimes, a copy of chromosome 21 in a developing gamete becomes attached to the end of another chromosome, such as chromosome 14, during the first or second division of meiosis. This event is called a **translocation**. The zygote produced by fusion of such a gamete with a normal partner will have two normal copies of chromosome 21 plus an abnormal chromosome 14 carrying a third copy of chromosome 21 (Fig. 1-9); 2% to 5% of all individuals with Down syndrome harbor such translocations.

Cases in which only a part of chromosome 21 is translocated have provided insight into which regions of chromosome 21 must be triplicated to produce specific aspects of Down syndrome, such as mental retardation, characteristic facial features, and cardiovascular defects. By determining which specific phenotypes occur in patients with Down syndrome having particular translocated regions of chromosome 21, **Down syndrome candidate regions** on chromosome 21 have been identified. Completion of sequencing of chromosome 21 (in May 2000) and the generation of transgenic mice (transgenic mice are covered in Chapter 5) trisomic for these candidate regions are leading to the identification of those genes responsible for specific Down syndrome phenotypes in humans.

The incidence of Down syndrome increases significantly with the age of the mother but not with the age of the father. The risk of giving birth to a live baby born with Down syndrome at maternal age thirty is 1 in 900. The risk increases to 9 in 1000 by maternal age forty. However, it is not clear whether older women actually produce more oocytes with non-disjunction of chromosome 21 or whether the efficiency of spontaneously aborting trisomy 21 embryos decreases with age.

Trisomies of other autosomes (such as chromosomes 8, 9, 13, and 18) also produce recognizable syndromes of abnormal development, but these trisomies are present much less frequently in live births than is trisomy 21. Trisomy 13 is also called **Patau syndrome**, and trisomy 18, **Edwards syndrome**. Similarly, trisomies and monosomies of sex chromosomes occur (e.g., **Klinefelter** and **Turner** syndromes, two syndromes in which there are extra or decreased numbers of sex chromosomes, respectively; covered in Chapter 16). **Triploid** or **tetraploid** embryos, in which multiple copies of the entire genome are present, can arise by errors in fertilization (covered in Chapter 2).

Several other types of chromosome anomalies are produced at meiosis. In some cases, errors in meiosis result in deletion of just part of a chromosome or duplication of a small chromosome segment. The resulting anomalies are called **partial monosomy** and **partial trisomy**, respectively. Other errors that can occur during meiosis are **inversions** of chromosome segments and the formation of **ring chromosomes**.

As covered above, maternal age is a major factor in the incidence of Down syndrome. Emerging new evidence shows that the rate of new mutations increases with paternal age, with the number of new mutations in a male's germ line doubling about every 16.5 years. Because spermatogonia

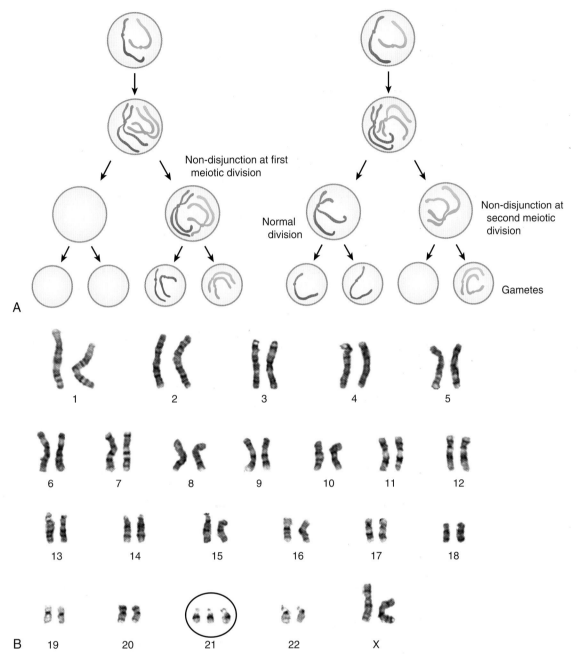

Figure 1-8. Chromosomal non-disjunction in meiosis. *A,* Failure of homologous double-stranded chromosomes to separate before cytokinesis during the first meiotic division (left-hand panel) results in their distribution to only one of the secondary gonocytes (or first polar body). Failure of the two strands of a double-stranded chromosome to separate before cytokinesis during the second meiotic division (right-hand panel) results in their distribution to only one of the definitive gonocytes (or second polar body). *B,* Karyotype of a female with trisomy 21 (circled), causing Down syndrome.

divide throughout life, replicating more than twenty times per year, they accumulate genetic copying errors such that a seventy-year-old man is about eight times more likely to pass on mutations to his offspring than is a twenty-year-old man. For example, a fifty-year-old man is about twice as likely to pass on mutations that contribute to autism than is a twenty-nine-year old man. Moreover, increased paternal age has been suggested to contribute to higher risk of other neurological disorders, such as schizophrenia, epilepsy, and bipolar disorder.

CHROMOSOME ANALYSIS CAN CHARACTERIZE DEFECTIVE GENETIC MATERIAL AND CAN GUIDE DIAGNOSIS AND TREATMENT

Genetic analysis of congenital defects is a very recent development. The normal human **karyotype** was not fully characterized until the late 1950s. Improved staining and culture conditions now allow high-resolution chromosome banding, increasing our ability to detect small deletions or duplications. Advances in molecular genetic techniques have led to a much finer analysis of DNA structure. As a result, it is possible to identify even smaller defects not evident with high-resolution

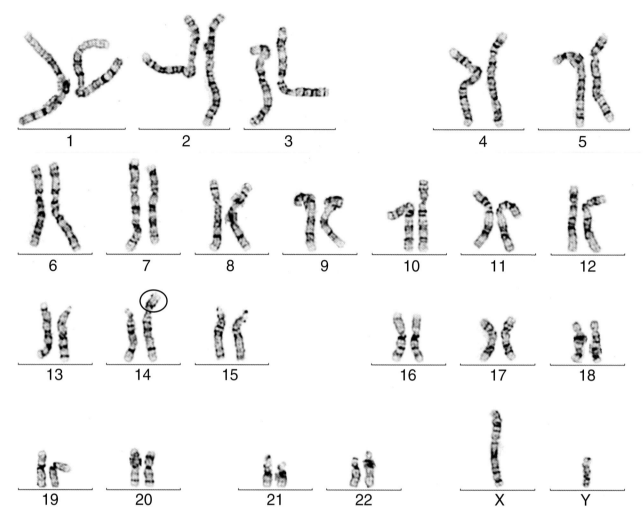

Figure 1-9. Karyotype of a male with Down syndrome caused by translocation of a third chromosome 21 onto one of the chromosomes 14 (circled).

banding. These techniques are used for both diagnosis and genetic counseling. Blood cells of a prospective parent can be checked for heritable chromosome anomalies, and embryonic cells obtained from the amniotic fluid (**amniocentesis**) or from the chorionic villi (**chorionic villous sampling**) can be used to detect many disorders early in pregnancy (covered in Chapter 6). Recent advances also allow non-invasive detection of trisomies from maternal serum through analysis of cell-free fetal DNA (see Chapter 6).

Two other molecular approaches are used routinely for chromosomal analysis (Figs. 1-10, 1-11): fluorescence in situ hybridization (FISH) and chromosome microarray (CMA). In both of these techniques, DNA probes linked to fluorescent dyes (i.e., fluorochromes, each of which emits a unique spectrum of light and is assigned a unique color by a computer) are used to probe specific loci on chromosomes. These techniques are particularly useful for detecting changes in chromosome copy number (aneuploidy) and for characterizing chromosomal material involved in translocations when paired with high-resolution chromosome banding. CMA is also useful in detecting inheritance of chromosomal material that is improperly imprinted, as in uniparental isodisomy (where entire or parts of both chromosome pairs are inherited from the same parent).

OVULATION

Animation 1-1: Ovulation.
    Animations are available online at StudentConsult.

RESUMPTION OF MEIOSIS AND OVULATION ARE STIMULATED BY OVULATORY SURGE IN FSH AND LH

On about day thirteen or fourteen of the menstrual cycle (at the end of the proliferative phase of the uterine endometrium), levels of FSH and LH suddenly rise very sharply (see Fig. 1-5). This **ovulatory surge** in pituitary gonadotropins stimulates the primary oocyte of the remaining mature Graafian follicle to resume meiosis. This response can be observed visually about fifteen hours after the beginning of the ovulatory surge, when the membrane of the swollen germinal vesicle (nucleus) of the oocyte breaks down (Fig 1-12A). By twenty hours, the chromosomes are lined up in metaphase. Cell division to form the secondary oocyte and the first polar body rapidly ensues (Fig. 1-12B). The secondary oocyte promptly begins the second

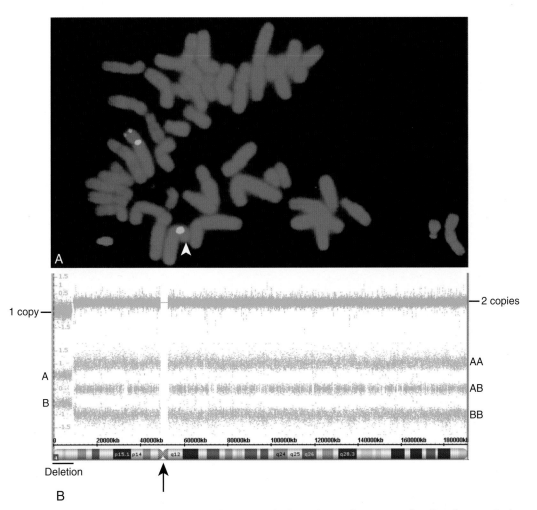

Figure 1-10. Chromosomal deletions or duplications not apparent on high-resolution chromosome banding (karyotyping) can be detected using fluorescent in situ hybridization (FISH) and/or chromosome microarray (CMA). *A,* A 4p16.2 deletion is shown using FISH on a metaphase chromosome spread. The light blue probe marks the centromeres of the homologous chromosome 4 pair. The red probe marks the two sister chromatids of one 4p16.2; this region is deleted on the other chromosome 4 (white arrowhead; tip of chromosome is folded down). *B,* Same deletion shown using CMA. This technology uses two types of probes. The first type detects DNA copy number (dosage [i.e., typically between zero and three copies], with normal being two copies, a deletion, as in this example, being one copy, or a duplication being three copies) by comparing the patient's DNA with that of a control. The signal from this type of probe is shown at the top, ranging from two copies of the chromosome (right) to one copy in the area of the deletion (left). The second type of probe analyzes single nucleotide polymorphisms (SNPs; AA, AB, and BB genotypes, resulting in three rows of signals). Each green dot represents a different DNA probe, with multiple probes placed along the entire length of chromosome 4 (chromosome bands labeled at bottom; arrow indicates the centromere). The deletion at 4p16.2 (indicated by the horizontal bar beneath the chromosome drawing) is indicated by a shift of copy number probes to a dosage of one copy and hemizygosity (A or B due to only one copy being present) for all of the SNP probes across the same region.

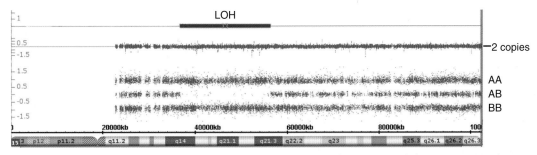

Figure 1-11. Chromosome microarray (CMA) showing loss of heterozygosity (LOH) for a portion of chromosome 11. The copy number array indicates two copies of the entire chromosome, whereas the single nucleotide polymorphism (SNP) array indicates loss of heterozygosity for bands q14-q21.3 (all genotypes are AA or BB for this approximately 20-Mb interval). This result indicates inheritance either from a common ancestor (consanguinity) or of both copies of chromosome 11 from one parent (uniparental isodisomy). In either case, genetic disease can result (recessive in the first, and errors of imprinting in the second, as in, for example, Prader-Willi or Angelman syndrome).

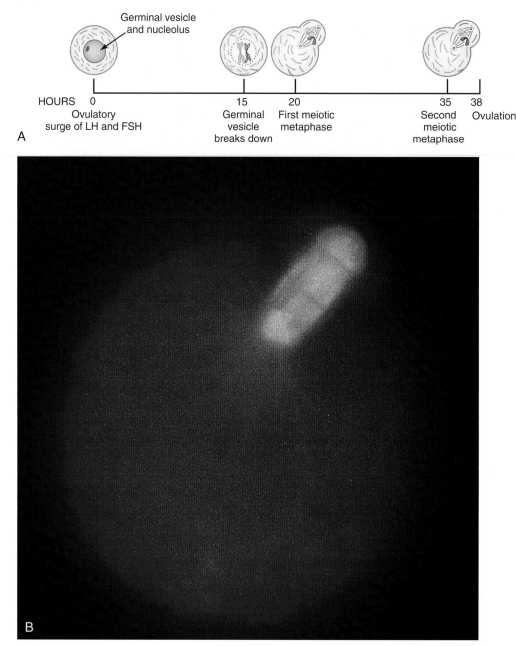

Figure 1-12. Meiotic events during the ovarian cycle. *A,* Timing. *B,* Micrograph of preovulatory oocyte at the first meiotic metaphase. The cell is stained with fluorescent antibodies specific for the spindle proteins and shows the eccentric spindle apparatus and the incipient first polar body.

meiotic division but about three hours before ovulation is arrested at the second meiotic metaphase.

CUMULUS OOPHORUS EXPANDS IN RESPONSE TO OVULATORY SURGE

As the germinal vesicle breaks down, the cumulus cells surrounding the oocyte lose their cell-to-cell connections and disaggregate. As a result, the oocyte and a mass of loose cumulus cells detach into the antral cavity. Over the next few hours, the cumulus cells secrete an abundant extracellular matrix, consisting mainly of hyaluronic acid, which causes the cumulus cell mass to expand several-fold. This process of **cumulus expansion** may play a role in several processes, including the regulation

of meiotic progress and ovulation. In addition, the mass of matrix and entrapped cumulus cells that accompanies the ovulated oocyte may play roles in the transport of the oocyte in the oviduct, in fertilization, and in early development of the zygote.

OVULATION DEPENDS ON BREAKDOWN OF FOLLICLE WALL

The process of **ovulation** (the expulsion of the secondary oocyte from the follicle) has been likened to an inflammatory response. The cascade of events that culminates in ovulation is thought to be initiated by the secretion of histamine and prostaglandins, well-known inflammatory mediators. Within a few hours after the ovulatory

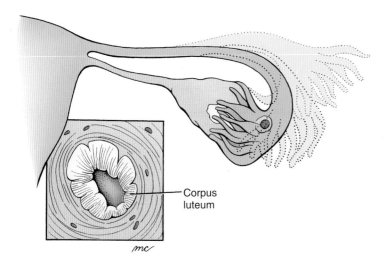

Corpus luteum

Figure 1-13. The ovulated oocyte clings to the surface of the ovary by the gelatinous cumulus oophorus and is actively scraped off by the fimbriated oviduct mouth. After ovulation, the membrana granulosa layer of the ruptured follicle proliferates to form the endocrine corpus luteum.

surge of FSH and LH, the follicle becomes more vascularized and is visibly pink and edematous in comparison with non-responding follicles. The follicle is displaced to the surface of the ovary, where it forms a bulge (see Fig. 1-6A). As ovulation approaches, the projecting wall of the follicle begins to thin, resulting in formation of a small, nipple-shaped protrusion called the **stigma**. Finally, a combination of tension produced by smooth muscle cells in the follicle wall plus the release of collagen-degrading enzymes and other factors by fibroblasts in the region causes the follicle to rupture. Rupture of the follicle is not explosive: the oocyte, accompanied by a large number of investing cumulus cells bound in hyaluronic acid matrix, is slowly extruded onto the surface of the ovary. Ovulation occurs about thirty-eight hours after the beginning of the ovulatory surge of FSH and LH.

The sticky mass formed by the oocyte and cumulus is actively scraped off the surface of the ovary by the fimbriated mouth of the oviduct (Fig. 1-13). The cumulus-oocyte complex is then moved into the ampulla of the oviduct by the synchronized beating of cilia on the oviduct wall. Within the ampulla, the oocyte may remain viable for as long as twenty-four hours before it loses its capacity to be fertilized.

RUPTURED FOLLICLE FORMS ENDOCRINE CORPUS LUTEUM

After ovulation, membrane granulosa cells of the ruptured follicular wall begin to proliferate and give rise to the **luteal cells** of the **corpus luteum** (see Figs. 1-6 and 1-13). As described later, the corpus luteum is an endocrine structure that secretes steroid hormones to maintain the uterine endometrium in a condition ready to receive an embryo. If an embryo does not implant in the uterus, the corpus luteum degenerates after about fourteen days and is converted to a scarlike structure called the **corpus albicans**.

MENSTRUAL CYCLE

Beginning on about day five of the menstrual cycle, the thecal and follicle cells of responding follicles secrete steroids called **estrogens**. These hormones in turn cause the endometrial lining of the uterus to proliferate and undergo remodeling. This **proliferative phase** begins at about day five of the cycle and is complete by day fourteen (see Fig. 1-5).

After ovulation occurs, thecal cells in the wall of the corpus luteum continue to secrete estrogens, and **luteal cells** that differentiate from remaining follicle cells also begin to secrete high levels of a related steroid hormone, **progesterone**. Luteal progesterone stimulates the uterine endometrial layer to thicken further and to form convoluted glands and increased vasculature. Unless an embryo implants in the uterine lining, this **secretory phase** of endometrial differentiation lasts about thirteen days (see Fig. 1-5). At that point (near the end of the menstrual cycle), the corpus luteum shrinks and levels of progesterone fall. The thickened endometrium, which is dependent on progesterone, degenerates and begins to slough. The four- to five-day **menstrual phase**, during which the endometrium is sloughed (along with about 35 mL of blood and the unfertilized oocyte), is by convention considered the start of the next cycle.

FERTILIZATION

Animation 1-2: Fertilization.
Animations are available online at StudentConsult.

If viable spermatozoa encounter an ovulated oocyte in the ampulla of the oviduct, they surround it and begin forcing their way through the cumulus mass (Fig. 1-14A). In vitro evidence suggests that the ovulated follicle contains a currently unknown **sperm chemotropic factor** and that only capacitated sperm are able to respond to this factor by directed swimming toward the egg. Based on this, it might be said that the human sperm finds the human egg to be "attractive" (pun intended).

When a spermatozoon reaches the tough zona pellucida surrounding the oocyte, it binds in a species- (i.e., human-) specific interaction with a glycoprotein sperm receptor molecule in the zona (ZP3, one of three glycoproteins composing the zona pellucida). Binding to ZP3 is mediated by a sperm surface protein called SED1. In addition, binding of human sperm to eggs involves a sequence of sugar

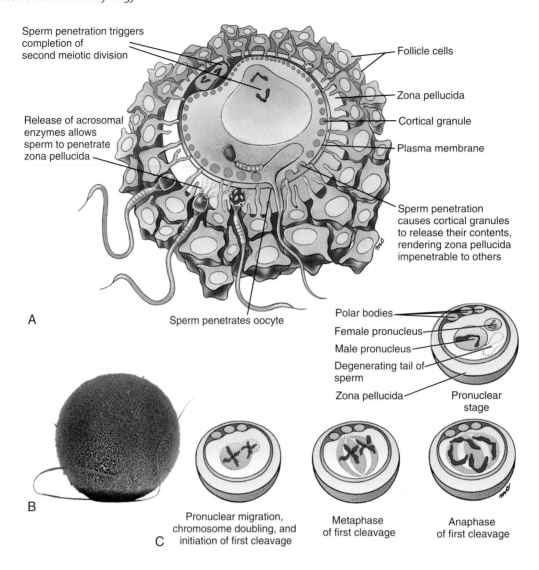

Figure 1-14. Fertilization. *A,* Spermatozoa wriggle through the cumulus mass and release their acrosomal enzymes on contact with the zona pellucida. Acrosomal enzymes dissolve the zona pellucida and allow sperm to reach the oocyte. Simultaneous with fusion of membranes of the fertilizing sperm and oocyte, cortical granules of the oocyte release their contents, which causes the zona pellucida to become impenetrable to other sperm. Entry of the sperm nucleus into the cytoplasm stimulates the oocyte to complete the second meiotic division. *B,* Scanning electron micrograph showing a human sperm fusing with a hamster oocyte that has been enzymatically denuded of the zona pellucida. The ability of a man's sperm to penetrate a denuded hamster oocyte is often used as a clinical test of sperm activity. *C,* Early events in zygote development. After the oocyte completes meiosis, the female pronucleus and the larger male pronucleus approach each other, as DNA is doubled in maternal and paternal chromosomes to initiate the first mitotic division. Pronuclear membranes then break down and maternal and paternal chromosomes assemble on the metaphase plate. Centromeres then replicate, and homologous chromosomes are distributed to the first two cells of the embryo.

molecules, called sialyl-Lewis^X at the ends of the oligosaccharides of the ZP proteins. As a result of this binding, the acrosome is induced to release degradative enzymes that allow the sperm to penetrate the zona pellucida. When a spermatozoon successfully penetrates the zona pellucida and reaches the oocyte, the cell membranes of the two cells fuse (Fig. 1-14*A, B*). The egg tetraspanin (a four-pass transmembrane protein), CD9, is required for this event, as is a sperm-specific protein named IZUMO after the Japanese shrine to marriage. (IZUMO is a member of the immunoglobulin superfamily and as such is likely to be an adhesion molecule.) Other factors implicated in fusion are members of the ADAM superfamily (all 30 or so family members contain a disintegrin and a metalloprotease

domain). FERTILINβ, also known as ADAM2, is present on the surface of mammalian sperm and interacts with an integrin (integrins are covered in Chapter 5) on the egg surface. Membrane fusion immediately causes two events to occur: formation of a calcium wave that radiates over the surface of the egg from the point of sperm contact; and release of the contents of thousands of small **cortical granules**, located just beneath the oocyte cell membrane, into the **perivitelline space** between the oocyte and the zona pellucida. These two events alter the sperm receptor molecules, causing the zona to become impenetrable by additional spermatozoa. Therefore, these changes prevent **polyspermy** or fertilization of the oocyte by more than one spermatozoon. Because a few hundred spermatozoa

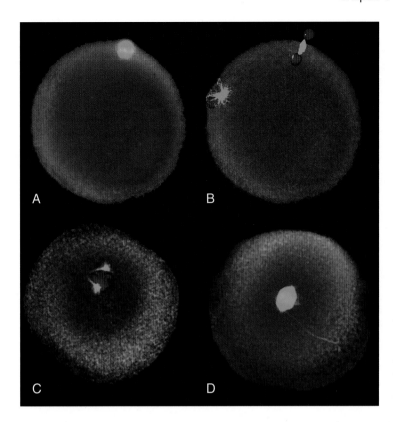

Figure 1-15. Fertilization of human eggs in vitro. *A,* The first meiotic division has occurred, forming the first polar body and secondary oocyte. *B,* The second meiotic division is completed after the sperm has entered the oocyte. This results in formation of the second polar body and female pronucleus. The male pronucleus and microtubules condensing around it are located at the nine o'clock position. *C,* The sperm centriole has split into two centrioles, which are organizing a spindle in association with merged chromosomes from the male and female pronuclei. *D,* The sperm and egg chromosomes are aligned on the metaphase plate.

reach the vicinity of the egg, the need to block polyspermy is extremely important.

Fusion of the spermatozoon cell membrane with the oocyte membrane also causes the oocyte to resume meiosis. The oocyte completes the second meiotic metaphase and rapidly proceeds through anaphase, telophase, and cytokinesis, producing another polar body. Disregarding the presence of the sperm, the oocyte is now considered to be a **definitive oocyte** (considering only the oocyte's genome, it contains a haploid complement of chromosomes and a 1N quantity of DNA after completion of the second meiotic division). However, because the sperm has now penetrated the oocyte, the fertilized oocyte can also be called a **zygote** (from Greek *zygotos,* yoked). Although a single nucleus (surrounded by a nuclear membrane) containing both the oocyte's and the sperm's chromosomes does not form in the zygote (see next paragraph and Figs. 1-14*C* and 1-15), taking into account both the oocyte's and the sperm's genomes, the zygote contains a diploid complement of chromosomes and a 2N quantity of DNA.

After penetration of the oocyte by the sperm, the nuclei of the oocyte and sperm swell within the zygote and are called the **female** and **male pronuclei,** respectively (see Figs. 1-14*C* and 1-15). Their nuclear membranes quickly disappear as both maternal and paternal chromosomes are replicated in preparation for the first cleavage (see next section).

CLEAVAGE

 Animation 1-3: Cleavage.
Animations are available online at StudentConsult.

CLEAVAGE SUBDIVIDES ZYGOTE WITHOUT INCREASING ITS SIZE

Within twenty-four hours after fertilization, the zygote initiates a rapid series of mitotic cell divisions called **cleavage** (Fig. 1-16). These divisions are not accompanied by cell growth, so they subdivide the large zygote into many smaller daughter cells called **blastomeres.** The embryo as a whole does not increase in size during cleavage and remains enclosed in the zona pellucida. The first cleavage division divides the zygote to produce two daughter cells. The second division, which is complete at about forty hours after fertilization, produces four equal blastomeres. By three days, the embryo consists of six to twelve cells, and by four days, it consists of sixteen to thirty-two cells. The embryo at this stage is called a **morula** (from Latin *morum,* mulberry).

SEGREGATION OF BLASTOMERES INTO EMBRYOBLAST AND TROPHOBLAST PRECURSORS

The cells of the morula will give rise not only to the embryo proper and its associated extraembryonic membranes but also to part of the placenta and related structures. The cells that will follow these different developmental paths become segregated during cleavage. Starting at the eight-cell stage of development, the originally round and loosely adherent blastomeres begin to flatten, developing an inside-outside polarity that maximizes cell-to-cell contact among adjacent blastomeres (Fig. 1-17). As differential adhesion develops, the outer surfaces of the cells become convex and their inner

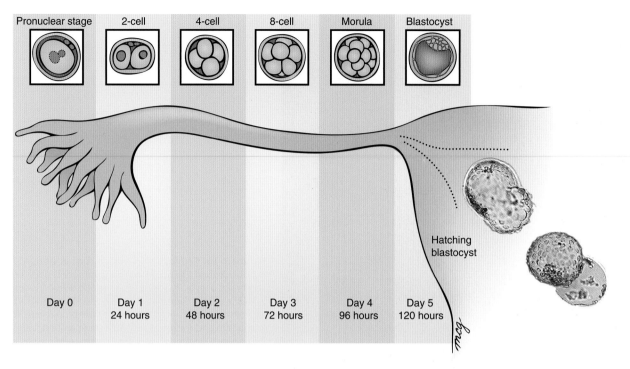

Pronuclear stage   2-cell   4-cell   8-cell   Morula   Blastocyst

Hatching blastocyst

Day 0   Day 1 24 hours   Day 2 48 hours   Day 3 72 hours   Day 4 96 hours   Day 5 120 hours

Figure 1-16. Cleavage and transport down the oviduct. Fertilization occurs in the ampulla of the oviduct. During the first five days, the zygote undergoes cleavage as it travels down the oviduct and enters the uterus. On day five, the blastocyst hatches from the zona pellucida and is then able to implant in the uterine endometrium.

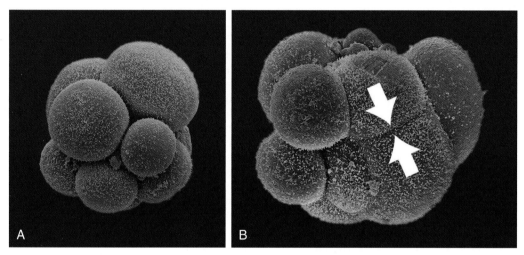

Figure 1-17. Compaction. *A*, Scanning electron micrograph of 10-cell human embryo before compaction. Note deep intercellular clefts. *B*, Scanning electron micrograph of ten-cell human embryo during process of compaction. Note absence of deep intercellular clefts between some of the blastomeres (arrows). The zona pellucida was mechanically removed from both embryos.

surfaces become concave. This reorganization, called **compaction**, also involves changes in the blastomere cytoskeleton.

With compaction, some blastomeres segregate to the center of the morula and others to the outside. The centrally placed blastomeres are now called the **inner cell mass**, whereas the blastomeres at the periphery constitute the **trophoblast**. Because the inner cell mass gives rise to the embryo proper, it is also called the **embryoblast**. The **trophoblast** is the primary source of the fetal component of the placenta (covered in Chapter 2).

In the Research Lab

WHAT DETERMINES WHETHER A BLASTOMERE WILL FORM INNER CELL MASS OR TROPHOBLAST?

The "inside-outside" hypothesis explains the differentiation of blastomeres based on their position in either inner cell mass or trophoblast—more central cells of the morula become inner cell mass, and cells on the outside of the morula become trophoblast. But how does this differentiation occur? In the morula stage, two transcription factors (transcription factors are covered in Chapter 5) are expressed uniformly throughout all blastomeres: Oct4 (covered earlier in the chapter) and nanog (a homeobox-containing transcription factor). As the inner cell mass and the trophoblast form, Oct4 and nanog expression is maintained in the inner cell mass, but expression of both is turned off in the trophoblast. Loss-of-function experiments show that commitment of cells to the lineage of the inner cell mass requires the expression of these two transcription factors. Another transcription factor, Cdx2 (like nanog, also a homeobox-containing transcription factor), is expressed in the trophoblast as it is forming as is the T box–containing transcription factor eomes (also known as eomesodermin). Loss-of-function experiments show that expression of these factors is required to downregulate expression of Oct4 and nanog. Collectively, these studies demonstrate that both expression of Oct4 and nanog in the inner cell mass and repression of expression of these two transcription factors in the trophoblast are required for the first overt differentiation event that occurs in the morula. Finally, the inner cell mass also expresses Sox2, an HMG box–containing factor highly related to SRY (covered in Chapter 16). Experiments have shown that Sox2/Oct4 regulate expression of Fgf4 protein in the inner cell mass, which is required for differentiation of the trophoblast. Thus, cell interactions occur between these two nascent populations of cells that are essential for specifying their fate.

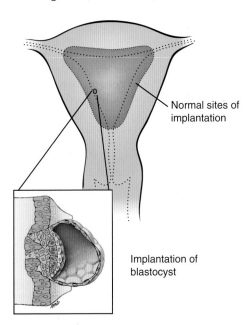

Figure 1-18. Implantation. At about six and one half days after fertilization, the trophoblast cells at the embryonic pole of the blastocyst proliferate to produce the syncytiotrophoblast, which is able to invade the uterine lining. The tan area indicates normal sites of implantation in the uterine wall, and the enlargement shows the implanting blastocyst.

MORULA DEVELOPS FLUID-FILLED CAVITY AND IS TRANSFORMED INTO BLASTOCYST

By four days of development, the morula, consisting now of about thirty cells, begins to absorb fluid. Several processes seem to be involved. First, as the trophoblast differentiates, it assembles into an epithelium in which adjacent cells are tightly adherent to one another. This adhesion results from the deposition on lateral cell surfaces of **E-CADHERIN**, a calcium-dependent cell adhesion molecule, and the formation of intercellular junctions, specifically, **tight junctions, gap junctions, adherens junctions**, and **desmosomes**. Second, forming trophoblast cells express a basally polarized membrane sodium/potassium ATPase (an energy-dependent ion-exchange pump), allowing them to transport and regulate the exchange of metabolites between the outside of the morula (i.e., the maternal environment of the oviduct) and the inside of the morula (i.e., toward the inner cell mass). The sodium/potassium ATPase pumps sodium into the interior of the morula, and water follows through osmosis to become blastocoelic fluid. As the hydrostatic pressure of the fluid increases, a large cavity called the **blastocyst cavity (blastocoel)** forms within the morula (see Fig. 1-16). The embryoblast cells (inner cell mass) then form a compact mass at one side of this cavity, and the trophoblast organizes into a thin, single-layered epithelium. The embryo is now called a **blastocyst**. The side of the blastocyst containing the inner cell mass is called the **embryonic pole** of the blastocyst, and the opposite side is called the **abembryonic pole**.

END OF FIRST WEEK: INITIATING IMPLANTATION

BLASTOCYST HATCHES FROM ZONA PELLUCIDA BEFORE IMPLANTING

The morula reaches the uterus between three and four days of development. By day five, the blastocyst hatches

from the clear zona pellucida by enzymatically boring a hole in it and squeezing out (see Fig. 1-16). The blastocyst is now naked of all its original investments and can interact directly with the endometrium.

Very soon after arriving in the uterus, the blastocyst becomes tightly adherent to the uterine lining (Fig. 1-18). Adjacent cells of the endometrial stroma respond to its presence and to the progesterone secreted by the corpus luteum by differentiating into metabolically active, secretory cells called **decidual cells**. This response is called the **decidual reaction** (covered in Chapter 6). The endometrial glands in the vicinity also enlarge, and the local uterine wall becomes more highly vascularized and edematous. It is thought that secretions of the decidual cells and endometrial glands include growth factors and metabolites that support growth of the implanting embryo.

The uterine lining is maintained in a favorable state and is kept from sloughing partly by the progesterone secreted by the corpus luteum. In the absence of an implanted embryo, the corpus luteum normally degenerates after about thirteen days. However, if an embryo implants, cells of the trophoblast produce the hormone **human chorionic gonadotropin (hCG)**, which supports the corpus luteum and thus maintains the supply of progesterone (**maternal recognition of pregnancy**). The corpus luteum continues to secrete sex steroids for eleven to twelve weeks of embryonic development, after which the placenta itself begins to secrete large amounts of progesterone and the corpus luteum slowly involutes, becoming a corpus albicans.

IMPLANTATION IN ABNORMAL SITE RESULTS IN ECTOPIC PREGNANCY

Occasionally, a blastocyst implants in the peritoneal cavity, on the surface of the ovary, within the oviduct, or at an abnormal site in the uterus. The epithelium at these abnormal sites responds to the implanting blastocyst with increased vascularity and other supportive changes, so that the blastocyst is able to survive and commence development. These **ectopic pregnancies** often threaten the life of the mother because blood vessels that form at the abnormal site are apt to rupture as a result of growth of the embryo and placenta. Typically, ectopic pregnancy is revealed by symptoms of abdominal pain and/or vaginal bleeding. Drug (methyltrexate, which blocks rapid division) or surgical intervention is usually required to interrupt the pregnancy.

In the Clinic

CONTRACEPTION

Human Reproductive Efficiency Is Very High

An average couple who does not practice contraception and has intercourse twice a week (timed randomly with respect to ovulation) has a better than 50% chance of fertilizing any given oocyte. Therefore, because (as covered earlier in this chapter) about half of all embryos undergo spontaneous abortion, the chance that one-month's intercourse will produce a term pregnancy is better than 25%. Healthy humans have astounding reproductive efficiency; it is not rare for couples who do not practice contraception to produce ten to twenty offspring in a reproductive lifetime.

Contraception has played an important role in family planning for much of human history. Some of the oldest forms are simple **barrier contraceptives**, and these methods remain among the most frequently used today. Current contraceptive research focuses on developing strategies that interfere with many of the physiological mechanisms covered earlier in this chapter that are required for successful conception.

Barrier Contraceptives Prevent Spermatozoa from Reaching Egg

One of the oldest types of contraceptive devices is the **male condom**, originally made of animal bladders or sheep cecum and now made of latex rubber and often combined with a chemical spermicide. The male condom is fitted over the erect penis just before intercourse. The **female condom** is a polyurethane sheath that is inserted to completely line the vagina as well as the perineal area. Use of the male or female condom can help prevent the spread of **sexually transmitted infections** (**STIs**; formerly called **sexually transmitted diseases**, or **STDs**). Other barrier devices, such as the **diaphragm** and the **cervical cap**, are inserted into the vagina to cover the cervix and are usually used in conjunction with a spermicide. These must be fitted by a physician to determine the proper size. The **contraceptive sponge** is a spermicide-impregnated disc of polyurethane sponge that also blocks the cervix. Its advantage over the diaphragm and the cervical cap is that the sponge does not need to be fitted by a physician because one size fits all.

Birth Control Pill Prevents Ovulation

Knowledge of the endocrine control of ovulation led to the introduction of the birth control pill ("the Pill") in the early 1960s. These early pills released a daily dose of estrogen, which inhibited ovulation by preventing secretion of the gonadotropic hormones FSH and LH from the pituitary. In modern pills, the estrogen dosage has been reduced, the progesterone analog **progestin** has been added, and the doses of estrogen and progestin are usually varied over a twenty-one-day cycle. Although the normal function of progesterone is to support pregnancy through its effect on the endometrium, it also interferes with the release of FSH and LH, thus preventing ovulation. In addition, it prevents the cervical mucus from entering its midcycle phase of becoming thin and watery (which would allow spermatozoa to pass through it more readily) and the endometrium from thickening (in preparation for implantation), and it may also interfere with oocyte transport down the oviduct or with sperm capacitation.

Injected or Implanted Sources of Progesterone Deliver a Chronic Antiovulatory Dose

A **depot preparation** of medroxyprogesterone acetate (Depo-Provera) can be injected intramuscularly and will deliver antiovulatory levels of the hormone for two to three months. Alternatively, rods or capsules have been developed (Norplant or Implanon) that are implanted subdermally and release a synthetic form of progesterone (progestin) for a period of one to five years. Another alternative is the hormone patch (Ortho Evra), which can stay in place for a week, delivering both progesterone and estrogen transdermally. Other devices act by releasing the hormone into the female reproductive tract rather than the bloodstream. Progesterone-containing **intrauterine devices (IUDs)** emit low levels of progesterone for a period of one to four years. **Vaginal rings** are inserted and removed by the user and when in place around the cervix release progestins continuously for three months.

Non-medicated IUDs May Interfere with Conception through Effects on Both Sperm and Egg

The mechanism by which non-medicated loop-shaped or T-shaped IUDs prevent conception when inserted in the uterus is unclear. Originally, they were thought to act by irritating the endometrium, resulting in an inflammatory reaction that prevented implantation of the conceptus. Because some people believe that preventing an embryo from implanting is an abortion (whereas others believe that an abortion involves removing an embryo that is already implanted), this potential mechanism of action creates ethical concerns for some. It is now thought that IUDs act mainly by inhibiting sperm migration, ovum transport, and fertilization, rather than by preventing implantation.

IUD use declined precipitously in the latter part of the 20th century because of the Dalkon Shield, an IUD blamed for a large number of pelvic infections and some deaths. Removed from the market in the mid-1970s, problems associated with the Dalkon Shield tainted all IUDs for a generation of women. However, use of IUDs is again increasing in the 21st century.

Antiprogesterone Compound RU-486 Is an Abortifacient

RU-486 (mifepristone) has potent antiprogesterone activity (its affinity for progesterone receptors is five times greater than that of endogenous progesterone) and may also stimulate prostaglandin synthesis. When taken within eight weeks of the last menses, an adequate dose of RU-486 will initiate menstruation. If a conceptus is present, it will be sloughed along with the endometrial decidua. A large-scale French study in which RU-486 was administered along with a prostaglandin analog yielded an efficacy rate of 96%.

Plan B or the Morning-After Pill Is Not an Abortifacient as Is Often Assumed

Plan B, or the so-called **morning-after pill**, contains the progestin levonorgestrel, a synthetic hormone used in birth control pills for over 40 years. Currently, in the United States, it can be obtained over-the-counter (i.e., without prescription) by women aged seventeen or older. In contrast to RU-486, Plan B will not cause a miscarriage. Instead, it seems to prevent ovulation of an egg or its fertilization, depending on where the woman is in her cycle when she has intercourse. Because Plan B will not interrupt a pregnancy after implantation has occurred, it is most effective if used as soon as possible after unprotected intercourse.

Sterilization Is Used by About One-Third of American Couples

Sterilization of the male partner (**vasectomy**) or the female partner (**ligation or "tying" of the Fallopian tubes**) is an effective method of contraception and is often chosen by people who do not want additional children. However, both methods traditionally involve surgery, and neither is reliably reversible. Recently, a non-surgical option has been developed for women. In this office procedure, called Essure, a coil-like device about 1 to 1½ inches long is inserted through the uterine cervix and is placed into each Fallopian tube using local anesthetic. The device irritates the Fallopian tube and over the next three-months or so causes it to form a scar around the device, creating a plug that blocks the passage of sperm. Like ligation, the process of blockage should be considered permanent.

How Effective is Contraception?

Sterilization and the use of hormonal contraceptives (such as the pill) have an annual pregnancy probability of from less than 1% to about 5%, whereas barrier contraception is less effective: use of the male condom has an annual pregnancy probability of about 15%—equivalent to practicing the rhythm (natural family planning) method, in which the couple practices abstinence in the days before, during, and after the expected time of ovulation; and use of the diaphragm has an annual pregnancy probability of about 25%—equivalent to practicing the withdrawal method (coitus interruptus).

By 2020, about 16% of the world's population, or about 1.2 billion people, will enter their childbearing years, raising the issue that better contraceptive methods may need to be developed. Although new approaches are being tested, tough government regulations and concerns about liability and profitability (especially when the greatest demand for products will be in poor countries) are preventing most companies from striving to develop new contraceptive products. Contraceptive research had its heyday in the 1950s and 1960s, which resulted in a major breakthrough—the development of the birth control pill. However, similar breakthroughs have not occurred since that time, and contraceptive choices remain highly limited.

Contraceptive Approaches for Males

At the time that the birth control pill was introduced, men had only two choices for birth control: condoms and vasectomy. Some fifty plus years later, these are still the only choices. Success with a male birth control pill was actually achieved in the 1950s with a drug called WIN 18,446. When tested on male prisoners, it seemed to be effective in blocking sperm development without causing significant side effects, but when moved to clinical trials, it was abandoned because men taking it became sick, exhibiting blurry vision, vomiting, headaches, and sweating. What was the cause of these side effects? Interaction with alcohol, which was used by the clinical trial population but was prohibited for use by prisoners.

Despite many obstacles, the search for new contraceptive methods slowly moves forward. For example, animal model studies have recently shown success in developing a compound, called JQI, that renders male mice infertile, without affecting their testosterone or other hormonal levels. Moreover, stopping administration of the compound allows fertility to quickly return. JQI blocks the function of BRDT, a protein essential for sperm development. JQI is one of many compounds being considered for drug repurposing. Originally developed as a cancer agent to target a protein related to BRDT (called BRD4) and shown not to have significant side effects, a potentially new use is being explored. Before clinical trials can be started on healthy men, it will be necessary to develop a more targeted version of the compound that is testis specific.

In addition to developing a male contraceptive pill to block sperm development, other strategies for developing male contraceptives are being explored based on advances in our understanding of human reproductive physiology. These include blocking the vas deferens with plugs that can be removed later if desired (surgically or by dissolving); interfering with muscular contraction in the vas deferens to pinch the tube shut, resulting in a "dry orgasm"; using special underwear to raise the temperature of the testes to inhibit sperm production; and inhibiting sperm motility to prevent them from reaching the egg after ejaculation.

ASSISTED REPRODUCTIVE TECHNOLOGY

About one in six couples have difficulty conceiving on their own. In about 30% of cases the female is infertile, in about 30% the male is infertile, and in about 30% both the male and the female are infertile. In another 10% of cases, it is unknown whether the male or the female (or both) is infertile. It is estimated that about 90% of infertile couples can conceive with medical intervention. A variety of medical options are available to help couples conceive, including artificial insemination (AI) and hormonal therapies, which are the most common procedures. In vitro techniques also can be used to assist reproduction. These techniques are referred to as **assisted reproductive technology (ART)**, and they consist of **in vitro fertilization (IVF)** and **embryo transfer, intracytoplasmic sperm injection (ICSI), gamete intraFallopian transfer (GIFT),** and **zygote intraFallopian transfer (ZIFT)**. Improved tissue culture techniques, including the use of defined culture media, have made it possible to maintain human gametes and cleavage-stage embryos outside the body. Gametes and embryos also can be successfully frozen (**cryopreserved**) and stored for later use, adding to the options for assisted reproduction.

Oocytes Can be Fertilized in Vitro and Then Implanted in Uterus

The procedure of **in vitro fertilization (IVF)** and **embryo transfer** is widely used in cases in which scarring of the oviducts (a common consequence of pelvic inflammatory disease, PID, a serious complication of sexually transmitted diseases such as gonorrhea) prevents either the sperm from reaching the ampulla of the oviduct or the fertilized oocyte from passing to the uterus. In IVF, the woman's ovaries first are induced to **superovulate** (develop multiple mature follicles) by administration of an appropriate combination of hormones, usually human menopausal gonadotropin (hMG) or FSH, sometimes combined with clomiphene citrate—a drug that blocks the ability of hypothalamic cells to detect estrogen in the blood. In the presence of clomiphene citrate, hypothalamic cells respond to the perceived deficiency of estrogen by signaling the pituitary to release high levels of FSH, which stimulates the growth of follicles and their secretion of estrogen. Once estrogen levels rise sufficiently, the pituitary gland rapidly releases LH, triggering maturation of oocytes. Sometimes to ensure that maturation of oocytes occurs, hCG is also given when follicles have attained optimal growth (determined by ultrasound examination of the ovaries and plasma estradiol concentration measurements).

Maturing oocytes are then harvested from the follicles, usually by using an ultrasonography-guided needle inserted via the vagina (transvaginal ultrasound–guided aspiration). Once retrieved, oocytes are allowed to mature in a culture medium to the second meiotic metaphase and are then fertilized with previously obtained and capacitated sperm (if obtained from the woman's partner, they are collected two hours before egg retrieval; if obtained from a sperm donor, they are obtained from a previously collected frozen aliquot). The resulting zygotes are allowed to develop in culture for about forty-eight hours and are then inserted (usually one or two) into the uterine cavity. IVF has increased our understanding of the earliest stages in human development, as embryos can be readily observed as they develop in vitro (Fig. 1-19).

Before the embryo is inserted into the uterine cavity, **assisted hatching** can be performed in cases where the zona

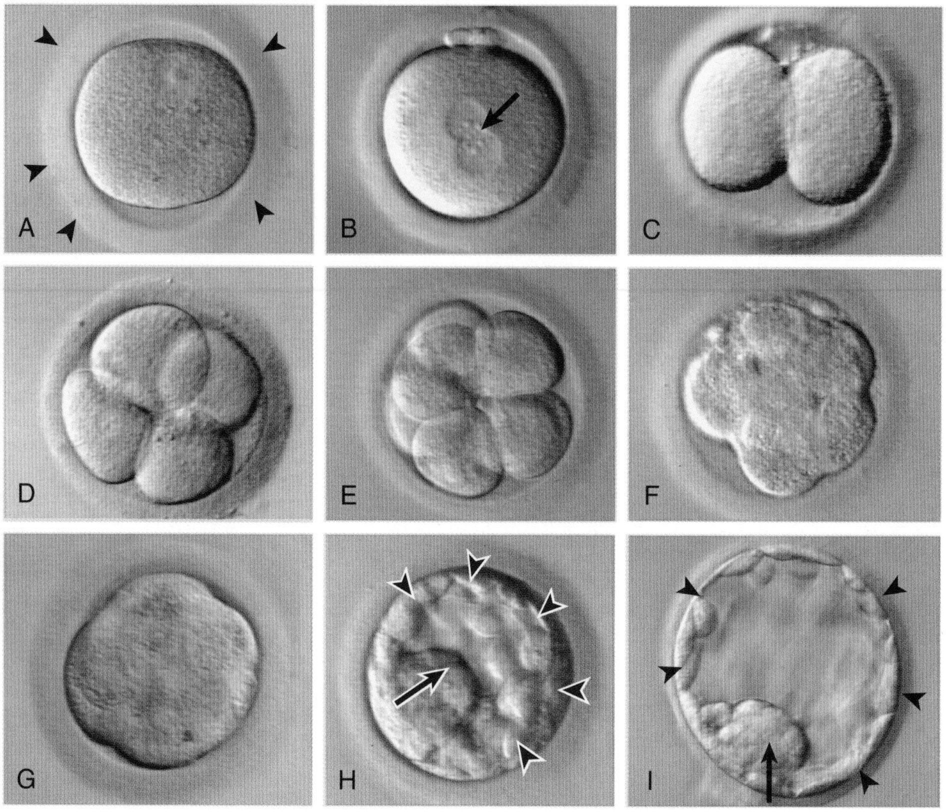

Figure 1-19. Human development in vitro. *A*, Ovulated secondary oocyte before introduction of sperm and fertilization. The oocyte containing its germinal vesicle is surrounded by the zona pellucida (arrowheads). *B*, Shortly after in vitro fertilization (IVF), the male and female pronuclei (arrow) have formed. *C*, Two-cell stage. *D*, Four-cell stage. *E*, Eight-cell stage. *F*, Morula initiating compaction. *G*, Compacted morula. *H*, Early blastocyst, with trophoblast (arrowheads) and inner cell mass (arrow). Hatching from the zona pellucida has not occurred. *I*, Hatched blastocyst, with trophoblast (arrowheads) and inner cell mass (arrow).

pellucida is tougher than normal, consequently making it more difficult for embryos to hatch. The zona pellucida ("shell") can be tougher in women older than forty and in younger woman who have a paucity of eggs. Assisted hatching involves making a small tear in the zona pellucida by using acid tyrode solution, laser ablation, or mechanical means.

The first successful case of IVF occurred in 1978 with the birth of Louise Brown, the world's first "test-tube" baby. By the time of her twentieth birthday, three hundred thousand IVF children had been born worldwide. By 2005, that number had reached more than one million. As of 2010, the number had exceeded four million. On average, IVF results in the delivery of a live baby in about 30% to 35% of attempts (i.e., live births per egg retrieval; thus, to have four million IVF children required about twelve million IVF conceptions). The success rate of IVF is remarkable considering that (as covered above) for a normal healthy couple practicing unprotected intercourse, the successful pregnancy rate is about 25% per monthly cycle.

With IVF, preimplantation diagnosis of genetic conditions (**preimplantation genetic diagnosis, PGD**) can be performed by using first or second polar bodies or blastomeres. These can be removed during IVF (Fig. 1-20), presumably without harm to further development, and then screened for aneuploidy or translocations with standard karyotypic analysis or FISH, and for mutations with techniques like the **polymerase chain reaction (PCR)**. PCR can be used to amplify DNA from a single cell, producing many copies for sequence analysis (eggs and embryos are stored until the diagnosis is made). Polar body diagnosis, unlike blastomere diagnosis, provides information about maternal contributions to the zygote but not paternal contributions, as polar bodies contain only maternal genes (i.e., they are formed by meiotic divisions of the oocyte). Hence, this method is used only when the mother is at risk for transmitting

a disease-causing mutation. If the mutation is found in a polar body, the assumption is made that the oocyte does *not* contain the mutation (if the rationale for this assumption is unclear, review meiosis). PGD offers the major advantage that it can be used to select only unaffected embryos for implanting, avoiding the later possibility of selective termination of an affected pregnancy following prenatal diagnosis.

In cases in which a partner's spermatozoa are unable to penetrate the zona pellucida, a technique called **intracytoplasmic sperm injection (ICSI)** may be used. In this procedure, a single spermatozoon is selected under a microscope, aspirated into a needle, and injected into the oocyte cytoplasm (Fig. 1-21). In one recent study, children born after ICSI were twice as likely to have major congenital anomalies as children conceived naturally. Other risks for these children include an unbalanced chromosome complement (ICSI can damage the meiotic spindle, potentially leading to aneuploidy) and male infertility. Men with cystic fibrosis (CF), an autosomal recessive disease that affects breathing and digestion, also have congenital absence of the vas deferens and are, therefore, infertile. By using microsurgical epididymal sperm aspiration (MESA), sperm can be removed from the epididymis of CF men for use in IVF. However, such sperm are unable to fertilize an egg because they have not fully matured—a process that is completed during their passage through the epididymis and vas deferens. To overcome this problem, ICSI can be used. Children born to fathers with CF using MESA and ICSI are normal CF carriers (to have CF, one must inherit a mutation in both maternal and paternal chromosomes). Because absence of the vas deferens is associated with a mild form of CF that is otherwise asymptomatic, and tests for CF mutations detect only about 87% of the mutations, it is now recommended that both parents be genetically tested for CF mutations and appropriately counseled before ICSI is used in cases in which the vas deferens is congenitally absent.

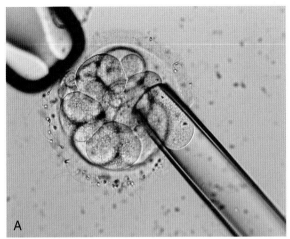

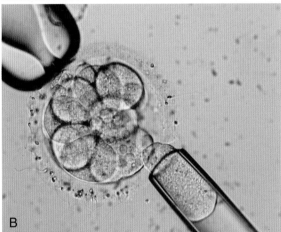

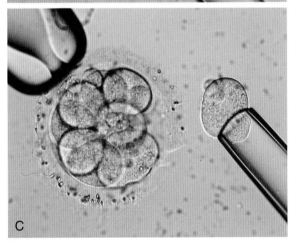

Figure 1-20. Human morula undergoing a blastomere biopsy. The temporal sequence is shown in order from top to bottom (*A-C*). The morula is held with a suction pipette, and a hole is made in the zona pellucida. A micropipette is used to remove a selected blastomere by aspiration.

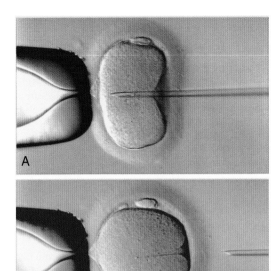

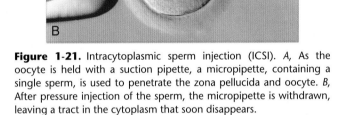

Figure 1-21. Intracytoplasmic sperm injection (ICSI). *A,* As the oocyte is held with a suction pipette, a micropipette, containing a single sperm, is used to penetrate the zona pellucida and oocyte. *B,* After pressure injection of the sperm, the micropipette is withdrawn, leaving a tract in the cytoplasm that soon disappears.

are introduced together directly into the ampulla of the oviduct, where fertilization takes place. Further development occurs by normal processes. In an alternative technique, **zygote intraFallopian transfer (ZIFT)**, the oocytes are fertilized in vitro, and only fertilized pronuclear zygotes are introduced into the ampulla.

ART in Perspective

In 1998 the following statistics were reported: in the United States, 60,000 births per year resulted from AI; 15,000 resulted from IVF; and at least 1000 resulted from surrogacy arrangements (a couple arranges for another woman to carry their child to birth following IVF and implantation of an embryo in her uterine cavity). With about four million total births in the United States per year, the use of ART (IVF and IVF plus surrogacy) thus accounts for about 0.4% of all births in the United States. An infertile couple can choose to remain childless, undergo medical therapy, including ART, or adopt a child. It was also reported in 1998 that only 30,000 healthy children were available for adoption in the United States. ART thus provides new opportunities for couples who choose not to be childless. However, ART is not without its risks: 37% of ART births are multiple as compared with 2% in the general population (risks associated with multiple births are covered in Chapter 6), and ART increases pregnancy-related risks to women, including preeclampsia, diabetes mellitus, bleeding, and anemia, as well as possible risk of ovarian cancer due to hormonal stimulation during ART. Moreover, ART-associated birth defects occur at a 1.4- to 2-fold higher rate than the overall rate of 3% to 4% of births in general.

Oocyte and Sperm Stem Cells

Recently, functional oocytes and sperm have been developed largely in vitro using stem cells derived from mouse testicles, ovaries, or skin (i.e., induced pluripotent stem cells, IPSCs; covered in Chapter 5) or from mouse embryonic stem cells (covered in Chapter 5). For example, in 2012, viable mice were produced using oocytes made from stem cells. Although this has not yet been done in humans, these results suggest the exciting possibility of new treatments for infertility in humans.

Gametes or Zygotes Can be Introduced Directly into Ampulla of Oviduct

If the woman's oviduct is normal and the couple is infertile because of an innate deficiency in spermatozoon motility or for some other reason, a technique called **gamete intraFallopian transfer (GIFT)** is often used. Oocytes are harvested as described earlier and are then placed into a laparoscope catheter along with precapacitated spermatozoa. The oocytes and spermatozoa

Embryology in Practice

EMBRYO WITH THREE PARENTS

You are a fertility specialist seeing a couple to discuss new reproductive options given the wife's medical history. She has a family history of mitochondrial disease and is herself affected with muscle weakness consistent with a slowly progressive form of MELAS (mitochondrial encephalomyopathy, lactic acidosis, and strokelike episodes).

She was diagnosed at the age of sixteen after the onset of limb weakness and exercise intolerance. She had an older sister who died at age thirteen from complications after multiple strokes, and an older brother who had seizures, weakness, and hearing loss. She was ultimately found to share a mutation in the MTTL1 gene with these two affected siblings. MTTL encodes the mitochondrial UUA/UUG tRNA for leucine required for mitochondrial protein synthesis.

This mutation was found in cultured fibroblasts from the patient's skin but was absent from her leukocytes, indicating "heteroplasmy" (a mixture of mitochondria with mutant and normal MTTL genes) and helping to explain her attenuated symptoms.

The couple had decided against children after preconception counseling, where they learned that 100% of their offspring would inherit mutant mitochondria (all of our mitochondria are maternally inherited via the cytoplasm of the oocyte) and would have some degree of mitochondrial symptoms or MELAS.

Today's visit was prompted by a story that they saw on the website of a mitochondrial disease support group about an experimental "three-parent" fertility method that would allow them to have children that were genetically "their own" but without mitochondrial disease.

You describe to them the process in which the nucleus of an embryo fertilized by the couple could be transferred to the enucleated egg of a healthy donor, taking the MTTL-mutant mitochondria out of the equation.

Proof of concept for this type of nuclear transfer has been demonstrated, but, unfortunately, you have to inform them that this treatment is still in the research phase and is currently unavailable. They are enthusiastic about research involvement, and you are able to refer them to the clinicians actively engaged in developing this technique.

SUGGESTED READINGS

Bruc, AW, Zernicka-Goetz M. 2010. Developmental control of the early mammalian embryo: competition among heterogeneous cells that biases cell fate. Curr Opin Genet Dev 20:485–491.

Gkountela S, Li Z, Vincent JJ, et al. 2012. The ontogeny of cKIT(+) human primordial germ cells proves to be a resource for human germ line reprogramming, imprint erasure and in vitro differentiation. Nat Cell Biol 15:113–122.

Handyside A. 2010. Let parents decide. Nature 464:978–979.

Laird DJ. 2012. Humans put their eggs in more than one basket. Nat Cell Biol 15:13–15.

Pearson H. 2008. Making babies: the next 30 years. Nature 454:260–262.

Richardson BE, Lehmann R. 2010. Mechanisms guiding primordial germ cell migration: strategies from different organisms. Nat Rev Mol Cell Biol 11:37–49.

Rossant J, Tam PP. 2009. Blastocyst lineage formation, early embryonic asymmetries and axis patterning in the mouse. Development 136:701–713.

Saitou M. 2009. Germ cell specification in mice. Curr Opin Genet Dev 19:386–395.

Wassarman PM. 2011. Development. The sperm's sweet tooth. Science 333:1708–1709.

Chapter 2

Second Week: Becoming Bilaminar and Fully Implanting

SUMMARY

As covered in the preceding chapter, the morula—formed by cleavage of the zygote—transforms during the first week into a blastocyst consisting of an inner cell mass, or embryoblast, and a trophoblast. At the beginning of the second week, the embryoblast splits into two layers: the **epiblast** and the **hypoblast**, or **primitive endoderm**. A cavity, called the **amniotic cavity**, develops at the embryonic pole of the blastocyst between the epiblast and the overlying trophoblast. It quickly becomes surrounded by a thin layer of cells derived from epiblast. This thin layer constitutes the lining of the **amnion**, one of the four **extraembryonic membranes**. The remainder of the epiblast and the hypoblast now constitute a **bilaminar embryonic disc**, or **bilaminar blastoderm**, lying between the amniotic cavity (dorsally) and the blastocyst cavity (ventrally). The cells of the embryonic disc develop into the **embryo proper** and also contribute to **extraembryonic membranes**. During the second week, the hypoblast apparently sends out two waves of migratory endodermal cells into the blastocyst cavity (blastocoel). The first of these waves forms the primary **yolk sac** (or the **exocoelomic membrane** or **Heuser's membrane**), and the second transforms the primary yolk sac into the secondary yolk sac.

In the middle of the second week, the inner surface of the trophoblast and the outer surface of the amnion and yolk sac become lined by a new tissue, the **extraembryonic mesoderm**. A new cavity—the **extraembryonic coelom**, or **chorionic cavity**—develops as the extraembryonic mesoderm splits into two layers. With formation and splitting of the extraembryonic mesoderm, both the amnion and yolk sac (now sometimes called the *definitive* yolk sac) become double-layered structures: amnion, consisting of ectoderm on the inside and mesoderm on the outside; and yolk sac, consisting of endoderm on the inside and mesoderm on the outside. In addition, the outer wall of the blastocyst is now called the **chorion**; like the amnion and yolk sac, it too contains a layer of mesoderm.

Meanwhile, implantation continues. The trophoblast differentiates into two layers: a cellular trophoblast, called the **cytotrophoblast**, and an expanding peripheral syncytial layer, the **syncytiotrophoblast**. These trophoblast layers contribute to the extraembryonic membranes, not to the embryo proper. The syncytiotrophoblast, cytotrophoblast, and associated extraembryonic mesoderm, together with the uterus, initiate formation of the **placenta**. During this process, the fetal tissues establish outgrowths, the **chorionic villi**, which extend into maternal **blood sinusoids**.

Many events occur in twos during the second week. Thus, a "rule of twos" constitutes a handy mnemonic for remembering events of the second week. During the second week, the embryoblast splits into two layers: the epiblast and the hypoblast. The trophoblast also gives rise to two tissues: the cytotrophoblast and the syncytiotrophoblast. Two yolk sacs form, first the primary and then the secondary. Two new cavities form: the amniotic cavity and the chorionic cavity. The extraembryonic mesoderm splits into the two layers that line the chorionic cavity, and the amnion, yolk sac, and chorion all become two-layered membranes.

Clinical Taster

A six-month-old boy is referred by his primary care physician to University Hospital for genetic evaluation because of **failure to thrive**: both his weight-for-height and height-for-age fall below the third centile for age, as assessed using standard growth charts. His mother is twenty-three and his father is twenty-nine, and the boy is their first child. The woman became pregnant two months after stopping birth control (contraceptive sponge), and her pregnancy went smoothly with only a couple of weeks of mild morning sickness. She went into labor during the thirty-ninth week of gestation, but because labor progressed poorly and abnormal fetal heart rhythms were detected, her child was delivered by cesarean section twenty-three hours later.

At the child's two-month well baby examination, his mother expressed the concern that her baby did not nurse well and seemed to have a weak cry. He also seemed not to move very much. On examination, the boy was somewhat small for his age and was hypotonic (had limp muscles). On a follow-up visit a few weeks later, the infant continued to show poor weight gain, and failure to thrive was diagnosed. To stimulate catch-up growth, the pediatrician recommended supplementing breast feeding with gavage feeding (feeding by tube) of high-calorie formula to achieve 150% of the caloric requirement for the boy's expected weight if he were at the 50th centile.

Genetic testing occurred at seven months. It revealed that the boy has a deletion of a portion of the long arm of chromosome 15, and he was diagnosed with **Prader-Willi syndrome**. The boy's parents are counseled about their son's prognosis and are given an information packet, which contains

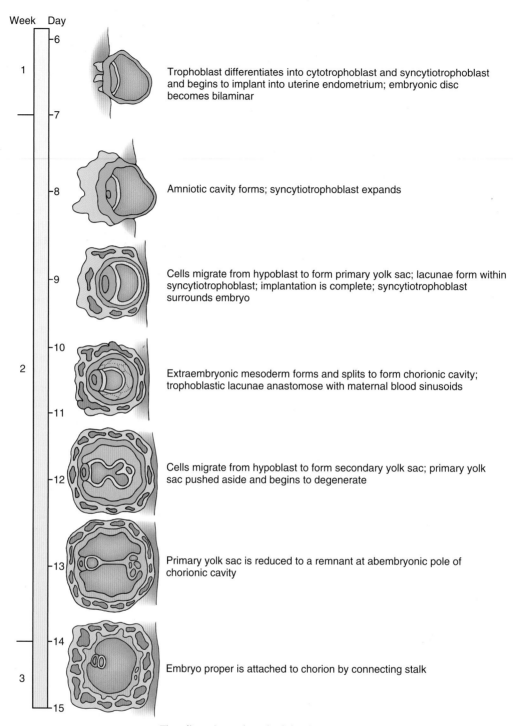

Week Day

1

6

Trophoblast differentiates into cytotrophoblast and syncytiotrophoblast and begins to implant into uterine endometrium; embryonic disc becomes bilaminar

7

8

Amniotic cavity forms; syncytiotrophoblast expands

9

Cells migrate from hypoblast to form primary yolk sac; lacunae form within syncytiotrophoblast; implantation is complete; syncytiotrophoblast surrounds embryo

2

10

Extraembryonic mesoderm forms and splits to form chorionic cavity; trophoblastic lacunae anastomose with maternal blood sinusoids

11

12

Cells migrate from hypoblast to form secondary yolk sac; primary yolk sac pushed aside and begins to degenerate

13

Primary yolk sac is reduced to a remnant at abembryonic pole of chorionic cavity

14

Embryo proper is attached to chorion by connecting stalk

3

15

Time line. Second week of development.

information about a local support group for parents of children with Prader-Willi syndrome. In meetings with the support group, they see other children of various ages with Prader-Willi, as well as their parents, and some children who are said to have the same chromosomal deletion but who act very differently than their son. They are told that these children have a different syndrome called **Angelman syndrome**. Later, by searching the web, they find that both Prader-Willi syndrome

and Angelman syndrome result from abnormalities in a process called **imprinting**, and that the difference in the two syndromes depends on whether the defect was inherited from the mother or from the father.

At nine months of age, the boy is started on growth hormone replacement therapy, which has been shown to normalize height and increase lean muscle mass in children with Prader-Willi syndrome.

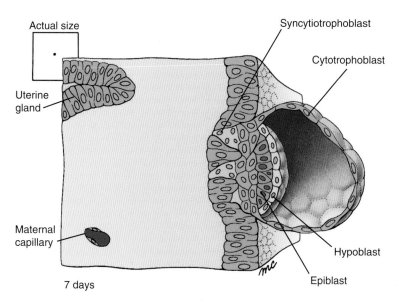

Figure 2-1. At seven days, the newly hatched blastocyst contacts the uterine endometrium and begins to implant. The trophoblast at the embryonic pole of the blastocyst proliferates to form the invasive syncytiotrophoblast, which insinuates itself among the cells of the endometrium and begins to draw the blastocyst into the uterine wall. The embryonic disc is bilaminar, consisting of epiblast and hypoblast layers.

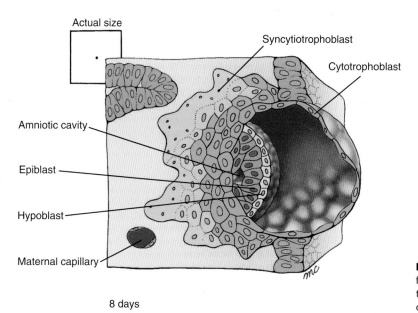

Figure 2-2. By eight days, the amniotic cavity has formed within the epiblast. Implantation continues, and the growing syncytiotrophoblast expands to cover more of the blastocyst.

BECOMING FULLY IMPLANTED

 Animation 2-1: Implantation.
Animations are available online at StudentConsult.

As described in Chapter 1, the blastocyst adheres to the uterine wall at the end of the first week. Contact with the uterine endometrium induces the trophoblast at the embryonic pole to proliferate. Some of these proliferating cells lose their cell membranes and coalesce to form a syncytium (a mass of cytoplasm containing numerous dispersed nuclei) called the **syncytiotrophoblast** (Fig. 2-1).

By contrast, the cells of the trophoblast that line the wall of the blastocyst retain their cell membranes and constitute the **cytotrophoblast**. The syncytiotrophoblast increases in volume throughout the second week as cells detach

from the proliferating cytotrophoblast at the embryonic pole and fuse with the syncytium (Figs. 2-2, 2-3).

Between days six and nine, the embryo becomes fully implanted in the endometrium. Proteolytic enzymes, including several metalloproteinases, are secreted by the cytotrophoblast to break down the extracellular matrix between the endometrial cells. Active finger-like processes extending from the syncytiotrophoblast then penetrate between the separating endometrial cells and pull the embryo into the endometrium of the uterine wall (see Figs. 2-1, 2-2). As implantation progresses, the expanding syncytiotrophoblast gradually envelops the blastocyst. By day nine, the syncytiotrophoblast blankets the entire blastocyst, except for a small region at the abembryonic pole (see Fig. 2-3). A plug of acellular material, called the **coagulation plug**, seals the small hole where the blastocyst implanted, temporarily marking this point in the endometrial epithelium.

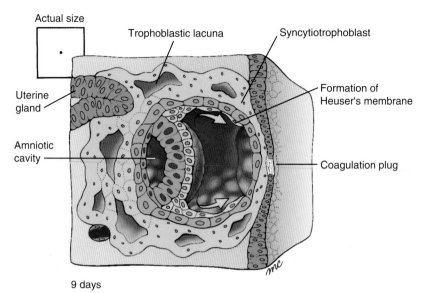

Figure 2-3. By nine days, the embryo is completely implanted in the uterine endometrium. The amniotic cavity is expanding, and cells from the hypoblast have begun to migrate to form Heuser's membrane. Trophoblastic lacunae form in the syncytiotrophoblast, which now completely surrounds the embryo. The point of implantation is marked by a transient coagulation plug in the endometrial surface.

9 days

In the Research Lab

WHAT REGULATES THE INITIAL PHASE OF IMPLANTATION: BLASTOCYST ADHERENCE TO THE UTERINE EPITHELIUM?

Before about seven days post-fertilization, both the blastocyst and the apical surface of the uterine epithelium are non-adhesive. Therefore, changes must occur in both the blastocyst and the uterine epithelium to allow blastocyst attachment and the initiation of implantation.

The uterus cycles through receptive and non-receptive stages. As covered in Chapter 1, entry into the receptive stage, during which implantation is possible, is controlled by estrogen and progesterone. For a relatively short period of time, called the **implantation window**, the uterus is receptive to implantation. **Estrogen**, acting through the **estrogen receptor**, stimulates the uterine endometrium to undergo proliferation by inducing the production of growth factors such as **insulin-like growth factor 1**. It also prevents **programmed cell death** within the uterine epithelium. **Progesterone**, in turn, acting through the **progesterone receptor**, induces the transcription factor **hand2**, which blocks continued endometrial growth and allows implantation to occur.

As the uterus enters the receptive stage, its apical **glycocalyx** (a polysaccharide matrix surface coating of epithelial cells including—in the case of the uterine epithelium—abundant high–molecular-weight mucin glycoproteins) decreases in amount and in negative charge. Moreover, apical **microvilli**, which are normally abundant, retract to establish a flattened surface in many areas of the epithelium, and large apical protrusions called **pinopodes** form.

The blastocyst undergoes maturation from an attachment-incompetent stage to an attachment-competent stage. Although the presence of the non-adhesive zona pellucida before blastocyst hatching certainly prevents blastocyst attachment, experimental removal of the zona a few days earlier demonstrates that the blastocyst itself is still at the attachment-incompetent stage. As blastocysts mature to the attachment-competent stage, they express **perlecan**, a **heparan sulfate proteoglycan**, on their surface. Heparan sulfate proteoglycans are known to have a high degree of specific binding to various extracellular matrix proteins and growth factors/cytokines and thus could serve as attachment factors. A particularly intriguing finding, with respect to the role of perlecan in attachment, is

that the uterus at the time of implantation dramatically upregulates expression of **heparin-binding epidermal growth factor–like growth factor** (**Hb-Egf**) at implantation sites, presumably in response to blastocyst signaling. Studies have shown that binding of Hb-Egf to the blastocyst requires that the blastocyst expresses both the Egf receptor and heparan sulfate proteoglycan. Perlecan-null mice do not exhibit defects in implantation, suggesting that perlecan has functional redundancy with other heparan sulfate proteoglycans that can substitute (or are compensatorily upregulated) in its absence.

In addition to heparan sulfate proteoglycans, other factors possibly involved in adhesion include selectins (a type of lectin—a sugar-binding protein), $\alpha v \beta 3$ and $\alpha v \beta 5$ integrins (transmembrane glycoproteins involved in adhesion and cell signaling; Chapter 5 provides more details), **metalloproteases** (enzymes that bind metal such as zinc and degrade proteins) and their inhibitors, **cytokines** (**Lif** and **interleukin-11**), and a cell adhesion complex called **trophinin-tastin-bystin**. Some of these latter factors (e.g., metalloproteases) play a role in trophoblast invasion of the endometrium, in addition to possibly functioning in attachment.

WHY ISN'T THE CONCEPTUS REJECTED BY ITS MOTHER?

The conceptus, which expresses both maternal and paternal genes, can be considered to be like an allograft, that is, tissue transplanted from one member of a species to another member of the same species (such as from one human to another human). Allografts typically elicit an immune response in the host, resulting in rejection of the graft. In such a host-versus-graft reaction, peptides bound to major histocompatibility complex (MHC) molecules generate tissue alloantigens that are recognized by maternal T cells. Medawar (who won the Nobel prize in 1960) proposed over fifty years ago three possibilities for why the developing conceptus is not rejected by its mother: fetal and maternal cells are physically separated from one another; the conceptus is antigenically immature; or the maternal immune system is suppressed or becomes tolerant to the conceptus during pregnancy.

It is likely that a combination of these possibilities prevents rejection of the conceptus. The trophoblast, which separates the actual tissues of the developing fetus from its mother, poorly expresses MHC molecules. Thus, the tissues are only partially separated and the conceptus is antigenically immature. However, there is evidence that maternal T cells are activated during pregnancy. Hence, because there is no completely cell-impermeable barrier between fetus and mother to prevent exposure of fetal alloantigens to maternal T cells (e.g., fetal cells can be found in maternal blood during pregnancy, and maternal cells can be found in the fetus) and because fetal tissues are antigenic, it is likely that tolerogenic mechanisms block maternal T-cell responses and prevent fetal rejection. The unique hormonal conditions of pregnancy that prepare the uterus for implantation and growth of the blastocyst apparently also induce tolerance. Such tolerance is specific for fetal antigens, for example, maternal antiviral immunity is not suppressed during pregnancy, as shown in HIV+ women who do not suffer from AIDS-like disease during pregnancy.

One way in which tolerance to paternal antigens expressed by fetal tissue might occur is through the selective loss of maternal immune cells that respond to these antigens. For example, it has been proposed that maternal-activated T cells are induced to undergo apoptosis through the Fas/Fasl system. Trophoblast cells produce Fasl, a member of the tumor necrosis factor (Tnf) and Cd40 ligand family, which signals through the Fas receptor (also called Cd95, a membrane protein of the Tnf family). In support of this possibility, mice lacking functional Fasl display extensive leukocyte infiltrates at the placental-decidual interface, and deliver small litters.

In addition to a potential host-versus-graft reaction during pregnancy, as just described, a graft-versus-host reaction could occur in which the fetus mounts an immune reaction against its mother. Why a graft-versus-host reaction does not occur is unknown, but it has been suggested that the mother's immune system interacts with the conceptus either to prevent maturation of the fetus' immune system or to evoke tolerogenic mechanisms.

Recent evidence provides insight into the suppression of both a graft-versus-host reaction and a host-versus-graft reaction during pregnancy. It is now known that immune cells, called **regulatory T cells**, are produced by both mother and fetus, and that these cells can cross the placenta, such that fetal cells reside in the mother's blood and vice versa. Maternal regulatory T cells recognize paternal antigens and suppress the mother's immune system to prevent rejection of the fetus. These cells persist in the maternal bloodstream long after birth, abrogating the immune response to other fetuses in subsequent pregnancies. Similarly, maternal regulatory T cells that cross the placental come to reside in fetal lymph nodes, where they induce the development of fetal regulatory T cells that suppress the fetus's immune response to maternal antigens. Moreover, these maternal cells persist in the child until adulthood is reached, suggesting that they continue to regulate immune responses after birth.

In the Research Lab

INITIATING ENDODERM FORMATION

The hypoblast, or primitive endoderm, is the first layer to form from the inner cell mass. Studies mainly in Xenopus and zebrafish suggest that a series of factors initiate endoderm formation. These include a T-box–containing transcription factor (VegT), which activates nodal (a member of the Tgfβ family of growth factors), which in turn induces expression of downstream transcriptional regulators (mixer, a paired-homeobox–containing transcription factor; Gata, a zinc finger GATA-binding transcription factor; and Fox, a forkhead box transcription factor). This in turn regulates expression of a relay of HMG-box–containing Sox-family transcription factors that ultimately result in the expression of Sox17, a critical factor in endoderm development.

The role of these genes in endoderm formation in mouse is less clear. Loss-of-function mutants of the mouse homolog of VegT (eomes, also known as eomesodermin) arrest very early in development, precluding analysis of their role in endoderm formation. Nodal loss-of-function mutants fail to form a primitive streak and node (covered in Chapter 3)—critical events in the genesis of not only endoderm but also mesoderm—so the exact role of nodal in mouse endoderm formation is unclear. However, the use of a hypomorphic nodal allele (i.e., a mutation in which nodal expression is severely downregulated but not completely eliminated), as well as a cripto loss-of-function mutation (cripto is an essential co-factor required for nodal signaling), provides more convincing evidence that nodal signaling is required for endoderm formation. Additional loss-of-function mutations are consistent with a role for both mixer and Sox17 in mouse endoderm formation. Hence, in conclusion, it is likely that the same general cascade of factors initiate endoderm formation in all vertebrates.

Other loss-of-function studies in mouse suggest that at least four other transcription factors are required for endoderm formation and maintenance: Gata6, (a homeobox-containing transcription factor), Hnf4 (a member of the steroid hormone vHnf1 receptor family that functions as a ligand-activated transcriptional regulator), and Foxa2 (a forkhead transcription factor previously known as Hnf3β). A regulatory hierarchy exists among some of these genes, with the first two factors (Gata6 and vHnf1) regulating expression of Hnf4. Foxa2 functions not only in formation of the endoderm but also in the formation of other lineages, such as the notochord and floor plate of the neural tube (covered in Chapter 4). Interestingly, orthologs of these genes also function in endoderm formation in other organisms (e.g., the forkhead genes in Drosophila and the Pha4 gene in *Caenorhabditis elegans* are orthologs of the Hnf3 genes; serpent in Drosophila and End1 and Elt2 in *C. elegans* are orthologs of Gata genes).

EMBRYOBLAST REORGANIZES INTO EPIBLAST AND HYPOBLAST

Even before implantation occurs, cells of the embryoblast begin to differentiate into two epithelial layers. By day eight, the embryoblast consists of a distinct external (or upper) layer of columnar cells, called the **epiblast**, and an internal (or lower) layer of cuboidal cells, called the **hypoblast**, or **primitive endoderm** (see Figs. 2-1, 2-2). An extracellular basement membrane is laid down between the two layers as they become distinct. The resulting two-layered embryoblast is called the **bilaminar embryonic disc**, or **bilaminar blastoderm**. With formation of the bilaminar embryonic disc, the primitive **dorsal-ventral axis** of the embryo is defined (i.e., epiblast is dorsal, hypoblast is ventral).

DEVELOPMENT OF AMNIOTIC CAVITY

The first new cavity to form during the second week—the **amniotic cavity**—appears on day eight as fluid begins to collect between cells of the epiblast and overlying trophoblast (see Fig. 2-2). A layer of epiblast cells expands toward the embryonic pole and differentiates into a thin membrane separating the new cavity from the cytotrophoblast. This membrane is the lining of the **amnion** (see Fig. 2-3), one of four extraembryonic membranes (i.e., amnion, chorion, yolk sac, and allantois; the first three are covered below,

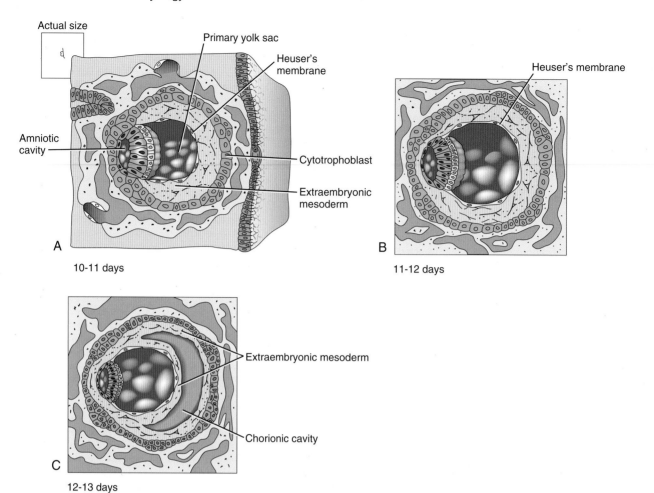

Figure 2-4. Extraembryonic mesoderm is formed in the middle of the second week. *A,* On days ten to eleven, the space between Heuser's membrane and the cytotrophoblast becomes filled with loosely associated extraembryonic mesodermal cells. At the same time, the trophoblastic lacunae begin to anastomose with maternal capillaries and become filled with blood. *B,* On days eleven and twelve, the extraembryonic mesoderm expands between the amnion and the cytotrophoblast. *C,* By days twelve and thirteen, the extraembryonic mesoderm splits into two layers: one coating the outside of Heuser's membrane, and the other lining the inside of the cytotrophoblast. The space between the two layers is the chorionic cavity.

and the allantois is covered in later chapters). Although the amniotic cavity is at first smaller than the blastocyst cavity, it expands steadily. By the eighth week, the amnion encloses the entire embryo (covered in Chapter 6).

DEVELOPMENT OF YOLK SAC AND CHORIONIC CAVITY

Proliferation of hypoblast cells, followed by two successive waves of cell migration, is believed to form the yolk sac membranes, which extend from the hypoblast into the blastocyst cavity. The first wave of migration begins on day eight and forms the primary **yolk sac** (the **exocoelomic membrane,** or **Heuser's membrane;** see Figs. 2-3, 2-4). Simultaneously, the **extraembryonic mesoderm** forms, filling the remainder of the blastocyst cavity with loosely arranged cells (see Fig. 2-4). This early extraembryonic mesoderm is believed to originate in humans from the hypoblast/primary yolk sac, in contrast to the mouse embryo, where it arises from the caudal end of the incipient primitive streak; the trophoblast may contribute

cells as well. By day twelve, the primary yolk sac is displaced (and eventually degenerates) by the second wave of migrating hypoblast cells, which forms the secondary yolk sac (Figs. 2-5, 2-6). A new space—the **extraembryonic coelom,** or **chorionic cavity**—is formed by splitting of the extraembryonic mesoderm into two layers. The extraembryonic coelom separates the embryo with its attached amnion and yolk sac from the outer wall of the blastocyst, now called the **chorion.** With splitting of the extraembryonic mesoderm into two layers, the amnion, yolk sac, and chorion all become two-layer structures: the amnion and the chorion are considered (based on comparative embryology) to consist of extraembryonic ectoderm and mesoderm, whereas the yolk sac is considered to consist of extraembryonic endoderm and mesoderm. By day thirteen, the embryonic disc with its dorsal amnion and ventral yolk sac is suspended in the chorionic cavity solely by a thick stalk of extraembryonic mesoderm called the **connecting stalk** (see Fig. 2-6).

Traditionally, the *cavity* of the yolk sac has been labeled as the yolk sac (or sometimes as the **exocoelomic cavity**) and its lining labeled as the exocoelomic

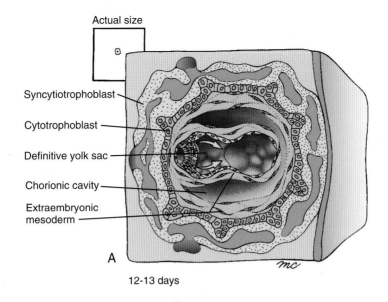

Actual size

Syncytiotrophoblast

Cytotrophoblast

Definitive yolk sac

Chorionic cavity

Extraembryonic
mesoderm

A

12-13 days

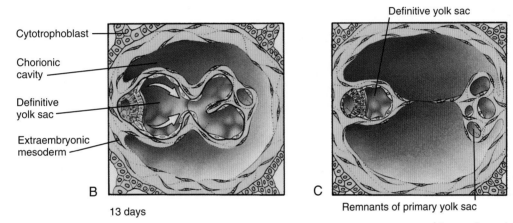

Cytotrophoblast

Chorionic
cavity

Definitive
yolk sac

Extraembryonic
mesoderm

B

13 days

Definitive yolk sac

C

Remnants of primary yolk sac

Figure 2-5. Formation of the secondary (definitive) yolk sac, and degeneration of the primary yolk sac. *A,* On days twelve and thirteen, a second wave of migration of hypoblast cells produces a new membrane that migrates out over the inside of the extraembryonic mesoderm, pushing the primary yolk sac in front of it. This new layer becomes the endodermal lining of the secondary (definitive) yolk sac. *B, C,* As the definitive yolk sac develops on day thirteen, the primary yolk sac breaks up and is reduced to a collection of vesicles at the abembryonic end of the chorionic cavity.

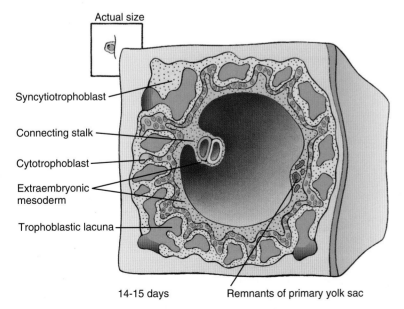

Actual size

Syncytiotrophoblast

Connecting stalk

Cytotrophoblast

Extraembryonic
mesoderm

Trophoblastic lacuna

14-15 days   Remnants of primary yolk sac

Figure 2-6. By the end of the second week, the definitive yolk sac loses contact with the remnants of the primary yolk sac, and the bilaminar embryonic disc with its dorsal amnion and ventral yolk sac is suspended in the chorionic cavity by a thick connecting stalk.

50 Larsen's Human Embryology

membrane, or Heuser's membrane; this convention has been followed in this textbook. However, it should be remembered that, like the amnion, the yolk sac is an extraembryonic membrane that contains a cavity. Thus, the **definitive yolk sac**, formed after formation and splitting of the extraembryonic mesoderm, is a two-layered structure consisting of hypoblast-derived endoderm on the inside and mesoderm on the outside (examination of sections of the very few human embryos actually available for study at this stage makes it readily understandable why the origin of the yolk sac is uncertain; Fig. 2-7).

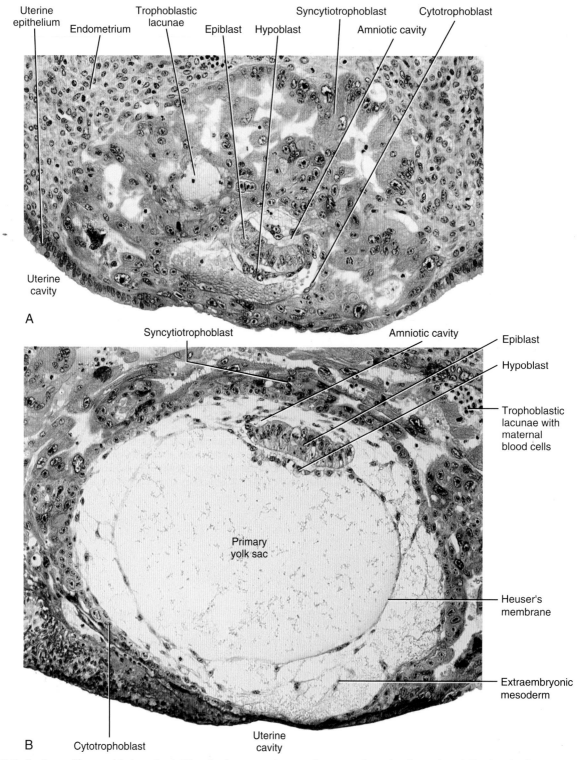

Figure 2-7. Sections of human blastocysts. *A*, Nine-day human embryo at the stage of amnion formation. *B*, Twelve-day human embryo with primary yolk sac. Both *A* and *B* are reproduced at about the same magnification, illustrating the rapid growth that occurs in the embryo in just three days.

The definitive yolk sac remains a major structure associated with the developing embryo through the fourth week and performs important early functions. Extraembryonic mesoderm forming the outer layer of the yolk sac is a major site of **hematopoiesis** (blood formation; covered in Chapter 13). Also, as described in Chapter 1, **primordial germ cells** can first be identified in humans in the wall of the yolk sac. After the fourth week, the yolk sac is rapidly overgrown by the developing embryonic disc. The yolk sac normally disappears before birth, but on rare occasions it persists in the form of a digestive tract anomaly called **Meckel's diverticulum** (covered in Chapter 14).

UTEROPLACENTAL CIRCULATORY SYSTEM BEGINS TO DEVELOP DURING SECOND WEEK

 Animation 2-2: Extraembryonic Structures.
Animations are available online at StudentConsult.

During the first week of development, the embryo obtains nutrients and eliminates wastes by simple diffusion. Rapid growth of the embryo makes a more efficient method of exchange imperative. This need is filled by the **uteroplacental circulation**—the system by which maternal and fetal blood flowing through the **placenta** come into close proximity and exchange gases and metabolites by diffusion. This system begins to form on day nine, as vacuoles called **trophoblastic lacunae** open within the syncytiotrophoblast (see Fig. 2-3). Maternal capillaries near the syncytiotrophoblast then expand to form **maternal sinusoids** that rapidly anastomose with the trophoblastic lacunae (see Figs. 2-4A, 2-8A). Between days eleven and thirteen, as these anastomoses continue to develop, the cytotrophoblast proliferates locally to form extensions that grow into the overlying syncytiotrophoblast (see Figs. 2-5A, 2-8A). The growth of these protrusions is thought to be induced by the underlying newly formed extraembryonic mesoderm. These extensions of cytotrophoblast grow out into the blood-filled lacunae, carrying with them a covering of syncytiotrophoblast. The resulting outgrowths are called **primary chorionic stem villi** (see Fig. 2-8A).

It is not until day sixteen that the extraembryonic mesoderm associated with the cytotrophoblast penetrates

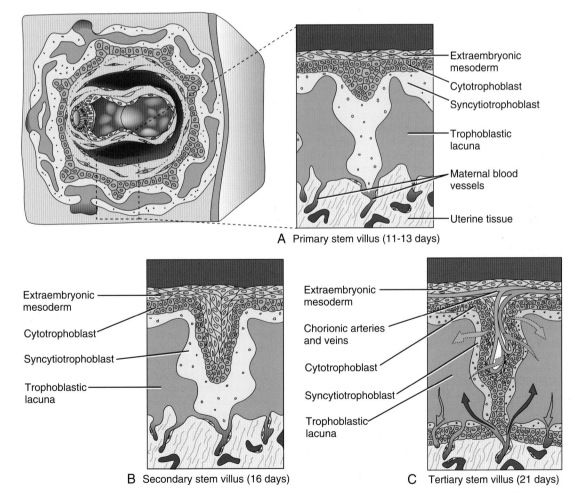

Figure 2-8. Formation of chorionic villi. *A,* Primary stem villi form on days eleven to thirteen as cytotrophoblastic proliferations that bud into the overlying syncytiotrophoblast. *B,* By day sixteen, the extraembryonic mesoderm begins to proliferate and invade the center of each primary stem villus, transforming each into a secondary stem villus. *C,* By day twenty-one, the mesodermal core differentiates into connective tissue and blood vessels, forming the tertiary stem villi.

the core of the primary stem villi, thus transforming them into **secondary chorionic stem villi** (Fig. 2-8*B*). By the end of the third week, this villous mesoderm has given rise to blood vessels that connect with the vessels forming in the embryo proper, thus establishing a working uteroplacental circulation (as covered in Chapter 12, the primitive heart starts beating on day twenty-two). Villi containing differentiated blood vessels are called **tertiary chorionic stem villi** (Fig. 2-8*C*). As can be seen from Figure 2-8*C*, the gases, nutrients, and wastes that diffuse between the maternal and fetal blood must cross four tissue layers:

- The endothelium of the villus capillaries
- The loose connective tissue in the core of the villus (extraembryonic mesoderm)
- A layer of cytotrophoblast
- A layer of syncytiotrophoblast

The endothelial lining of the maternal sinusoids does not invade the trophoblastic lacunae, so a maternal layer does not need to be crossed. Further differentiation of the placenta and stem villi during fetal development is covered in Chapter 6.

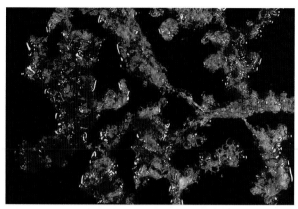

Figure 2-9. This complete hydatidiform mole has been "dissected" to show the clear, swollen villi characteristic of these structures.

In the Clinic

HYDATIDIFORM MOLES

Complete Hydatidiform Mole Is a Pregnancy without an Embryo

In a normal pregnancy, the embryoblast gives rise to the embryo, and the trophoblast gives rise to the fetal component of the placenta. However, in approximately 0.1% to 0.5% of pregnancies, the fetus is entirely missing, and the conceptus consists only of placental membranes. A conceptus of this type is called a **complete hydatidiform mole** (Fig. 2-9). Because the fetal vasculature that would normally drain the fluid taken up from the maternal circulation is absent, the placental villi of a complete mole are swollen and vesicular, resembling bunches of grapes ("hydatid" is from the Greek *hydatidos*, drop of water). Complete moles often abort early in pregnancy. If they do not abort, the physician may discover them because they result in vaginal bleeding, especially during the sixth to sixteenth weeks of pregnancy, and they often cause excessive nausea and vomiting (owing to elevated human chronic gonadotropin, hCG). Like normal trophoblastic tissue, moles secrete hCG. Moles and mole remnants are readily diagnosed on the basis of an abnormally high level of plasma hCG.

Molar pregnancies are more common in women at the extremes of reproductive age: women in their early teenage or perimenopausal years are at highest risk. Also, the risk for molar pregnancy (including choriocarcinoma; covered below) is up to fifteen-times higher for women of African or Asian ethnicity.

Definitive identification of hydatidiform moles requires cytogenetic analysis. Chromosome analysis has shown that even though the cells of a complete mole have a normal, diploid karyotype, all chromosomes are derived from the father. Further studies have demonstrated that this situation usually arises in one of two ways (Fig. 2-10). Two spermatozoa may fertilize an oocyte that lacks (or loses) its own nucleus (**dispermic fertilization**), and the two male pronuclei may then fuse to form a diploid nucleus. Alternatively, if a single spermatozoon inseminates an oocyte that lacks (or loses) its own nucleus (**monospermic fertilization**), the resulting male pronucleus may undergo an initial mitosis (doubling its DNA) without cytokinesis (division of

the single cell into two cells) to produce a diploid nucleus, which duplicates its DNA once again before the first cleavage occurs. Complete moles produced by dispermic fertilization may have either a 46,XX or 46,XY karyotype. All complete moles produced by monospermic fertilization, in contrast, are 46,XX, because 46,YY zygotes lack essential genes located on the X chromosome and cannot develop. Karyotyping surveys show that most (90%) complete hydatidiform moles are 46,XX, indicating that monospermic fertilization is the dominant mode of production.

Rarely, complete moles can have chromosomes derived from both maternal and paternal chromosomes (biparental in origin). This occurs when imprinting of maternal genes is lost from the ovum (covered in the following "In the Research Lab" entitled "Genomic Imprinting"), resulting in the functional equivalent of two paternal genomes. This type of complete mole is recurrent and is inherited as an autosomal recessive trait. A candidate region for this trait has been identified on the long arm of chromosome 19.

Partial Hydatidiform Moles Are Usually Triploid, with a Double Dose of Paternal Chromosomes, and Show Partial Development of an Embryo

In contrast to the complete hydatidiform mole, some evidence of embryonic development is usually found in **partial hydatidiform moles**. Even if no embryo remnant can be found at the time the mole aborts or is delivered, the presence of typical nucleated embryonic erythroblasts in the molar villi and the presence of fetal blood vessels indicate that an embryo was present. On rare occasions, an abnormal fetus is delivered. The swollen villi that are the hallmark of a complete mole are present only in patches, and the clinical symptoms that indicate a molar pregnancy (covered above) are usually milder and slower to develop than in the case of complete moles. Spontaneous abortion usually does not occur until the second trimester (four to six months).

Karyotype analysis indicates that conceptuses of this type are usually triploid (69,XXX; 69,XXY; or 69,XYY), with two sets of chromosomes from the father. Studies have shown that these moles result from the insemination of an oocyte containing a female pronucleus by two spermatozoa or possibly by a single abnormal diploid sperm (Fig. 2-11).

Hydatidiform Moles Can Give Rise to Persistent Trophoblastic Disease or to Choriocarcinoma

Residual trophoblastic tissue remaining in the uterus after spontaneous abortion or surgical removal of a hydatidiform mole may give rise to a condition known as **persistent trophoblastic disease**, in which the mole remnant grows to form a tumor. Tumors arising from partial moles are usually benign.

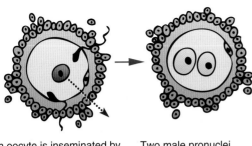

An oocyte is inseminated by two sperm and female pronucleus is lost

Two male pronuclei combine to form diploid nucleus

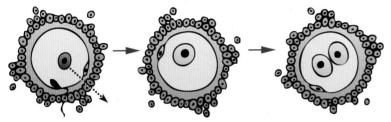

An oocyte is inseminated by a single sperm and female pronucleus is lost

Single male pronucleus divides to form two haploid nuclei, which combine to form diploid nucleus

Figure 2-10. Formation of complete hydatidiform mole. A complete mole is produced when an oocyte that has lost its female pronucleus acquires two male pronuclei. Two mechanisms are shown.

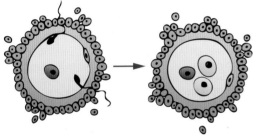

An oocyte is inseminated by two sperm (or by an abnormal diploid sperm)

Female pronucleus and two male pronuclei combine to form triploid nucleus

Figure 2-11. A partial hydatidiform mole is produced when a normal oocyte acquires two male pronuclei (or a diploid male pronucleus).

When tumors arising from complete moles become malignant, they may grow either as an **invasive mole** or as metastatic **choriocarcinoma**. Choriocarcinomas derived from moles are rare, occurring in 1 in 40,000 pregnancies. All forms of persistent mole, benign and malignant, secrete high levels of hCG.

Not long ago, the mortality rate for patients with invasive moles was about 60%, and the mortality for choriocarcinoma was approximately 100%. Today, surgery plus chemotherapy if needed has resulted in a cure rate for nonmetastatic and low-risk metastatic disease that approaches 100%, whereas the cure rate for high-risk metastatic disease is about 80% to 90%.

Cytogenetic analysis of hydatidiform moles supports the hypothesis (called the **genetic-conflict hypothesis**) that the paternal genetic complement is responsible for early development of the placenta and the maternal genetic complement is responsible for early development of the embryo. Experiments that both confirm this hypothesis and reveal molecular differences between paternal and maternal chromosomes are covered in the following section.

In the Research Lab

GENOMIC IMPRINTING

Maternal Chromosomes Regulate Embryoblast Development, and Paternal Chromosomes Regulate Trophoblast Development

As covered in the preceding section, cytogenetic analyses of human hydatidiform moles suggest that the maternal and paternal genome complements play different roles in early development. These roles have been studied with mouse oocytes experimentally manipulated to contain either two male pronuclei (androgenotes) or two female pronuclei (gynogenotes). Oocytes of this type can be produced in several ways. Fertilized mouse oocytes can be removed from the ampulla of the oviduct at the pronuclear stage of development and held by light suction at the end of a glass pipette. Either the female pronucleus or the somewhat larger male pronucleus can then be removed with a very fine pipette and replaced with a pronucleus of the opposite type. Another technique involves removing the male or female pronucleus from a fertilized oocyte and then blocking cleavage with an appropriate blocking agent while a single mitosis takes place, thus producing a diploid zygote. Removing the female pronucleus from an unfertilized oocyte and fertilizing the enucleated oocyte with an abnormal diploid sperm can also be used to produce oocytes with two male pronuclei.

When an experimental zygote containing two male pronuclei (possessing between them at least one X chromosome) is implanted into a pseudopregnant female mouse, it develops as trophoblast and gives rise to a mass of placental membranes resembling a human hydatidiform mole. Very rarely, an embryo forms and develops to a stage comparable to approximately the three-week stage of human development. In contrast, zygotes containing two female pronuclei develop as small but recognizable embryos with reduced placental membranes. These gynogenetic (or **parthenogenetic**; both terms refer to development in the absence of fertilization, or in the absence of a male pronucleus) embryos never survive to term. It is important to emphasize that these developmental patterns do not depend on the sex chromosomes present in the zygote (XX or XY), but only on the sex of the parent from whom the genome is inherited.

Early Gene Expression and Genomic Imprinting

What mechanism underlies the independent expression of maternal and paternal genomes during early development? One way that this question was approached was by studying expression of a marker viral oncogene, the Myc oncogene, which was introduced into a line of **transgenic mice** (mice whose genome contains a foreign DNA sequence; covered in Chapter 5). In theory, mice carrying this integrated transgene should express its gene product when appropriately stimulated. However, it was found that the gene product formed only when the gene had been inherited from the father, not when it had been inherited from the mother. Further investigation revealed an important difference between DNA of the male and female germ line cells: the DNA of the female germ line was more highly **methylated** (carries more methyl groups) than the DNA of the male germ line.

Further investigations were done with several different lines of transgenic mice carrying foreign transgenes at various locations in the genome. In cases where these transgenes showed a characteristic "male" or "female" degree of methylation, the pattern of methylation displayed in the somatic cells depended on the parent from which the gene had been inherited. Thus, a transgene showed the female pattern of methylation in the somatic cells of both sons and daughters if it was inherited from the mother. However, when one of these sons passed the gene to his offspring, their somatic cells showed the male pattern of methylation. The analogous reversal of methylation patterns also occurs when a grandfather's transgene is transmitted to grandchildren through a daughter.

Genomic imprinting is the process by which genes are imprinted, that is, marked so that rather than being expressed biallelically (i.e., from both maternal and paternal alleles contributed to the zygote during fertilization), they are expressed from only one allele in a parent-specific manner. One of the main ways that this marking occurs is through methylation of DNA. In addition to marking exogenously introduced transgenes as covered above, methylation marks endogenous genes, particularly several genes implicated in regulation of intrauterine growth. About eighty imprinted genes have been identified, and most are clustered. This allows groups of genes to be coordinately imprinted through specialized chromosomal regions called **imprinting centers**.

The first two imprinted endogenous genes to be discovered were Igf2 (insulin-like growth factor 2) and its receptor, Igf2r. Because of imprinting, the Igf2 allele inherited from the father is expressed in the embryo and in the adult, whereas the allele inherited from the mother is silenced. By contrast, the Igf2r allele inherited from the mother is expressed, whereas the allele inherited from the father is silenced. Imprinting occurs only in viviparous mammals, that is, mammals in which the fetus develops in utero (imprinting does not occur in egg-laying mammals). Imprinting is hypothesized to mediate a tug-of-war between maternal and paternal alleles. This hypothesis, the **genetic-conflict hypothesis** (or viviparity-driven conflict hypothesis), proposes that in polyandrous mammals (having multiple partners), there is a conflict between males and females over the allocation of maternal resources to offspring (in the hypothesis, the fetus is viewed as a parasite that competes with the mother and her future litters for resources). Fathers favor providing maximal resources for their offspring, at the expense of mothers and future offspring who

may be fathered by other males. Mothers favor providing equal resources among all their litters. The outcome for this tug-of-war is that a compromise occurs in growth rate.

In support of the genetic-conflict hypothesis, loss-of-function mutations of mouse Igf2 (a paternally expressed gene as covered above) result in a 40% reduction in growth, whereas mutations in Igf2r result in oversized offspring. Further support comes from double mutants: loss of both Igf2 and Igf2r results in normal-sized mice.

The sites of DNA methylation during imprinting are often stretches of alternating cytosine and guanosine bases (so-called **CpG islands**; p indicates that C and G are joined by a phosphodiester bond). Because CpG islands can be located around gene promoters, methylation of CpG islands often leads to gene silencing or activation. Methylation imprints go through a life cycle (Fig. 2-12). In the embryo, imprinted genes are expressed in a parent-specific manner. But in primordial germ cells, imprints are erased. During gametogenesis, imprints are once again established, so that in males undergoing spermatogenesis, the male-specific pattern is established (i.e., the pattern of the father), whereas in females, the female-specific pattern is established (i.e., the pattern of the mother). After fertilization, the parent-specific patterns are maintained in the new individual (except for in his or her primordial germ cells, where erasure once again occurs).

How does **imprinting** occur? The short answer is that it involves **epigenetic regulation** of gene expression, that is, heritable changes in gene expression that occur owing to mechanisms other than changes in the sequence of DNA. It involves changes in the genome such as **DNA methylation** (which typically blocks gene expression at an allele) and **histone modifications** (histones are basic proteins that associate with DNA), such as acetylation, phosphorylation, and methylation. Such changes in histones are mediated through the action of a number of enzymes (e.g., acetyl transferases, deacetylases, phosphorylases, methyl transferases, demethylases).

X-INACTIVATION

To compensate for the presence of only one X chromosome in the cells of males (46,XY), one of the two active X chromosomes in each cell of the female blastocyst (46,XX) is stably inactivated (the process of **dosage compensation**). The inactivation is random with respect to the parental source of the X chromosome in the embryoblast (and is, therefore, not an example of imprinting), but only paternally derived X chromosomes are inactivated in the trophoblast (an example of imprinting). Inactivation of X chromosomes in female embryos requires expression of a specific X chromosome locus, the Xist (X-inactive specific transcript gene) locus, which produces a large RNA, with no protein-coding capacity, that remains associated with ("coats") the chromosome. Moreover, the expression of Xist leads to the methylation of CpG islands at the 5′ ends of the inactivated genes on this chromosome. The inactivated X chromosome also lacks histone H4 acetylation, and, ultimately, the chromosome condenses into a recognizable structure called a **Barr body**. Although this X chromosome remains inactive in all somatic cells of the female, inactivated X chromosomes in the oogonia of the female germ line are reactivated during early fetal life. Thus, the male zygote obtains a single active X chromosome from the mother, and the female zygote obtains two active X chromosomes, one from the mother and one from the father. Both of the X chromosomes in each cell of the early female embryo then remain active until one of them is again inactivated at the blastocyst stage (as covered above).

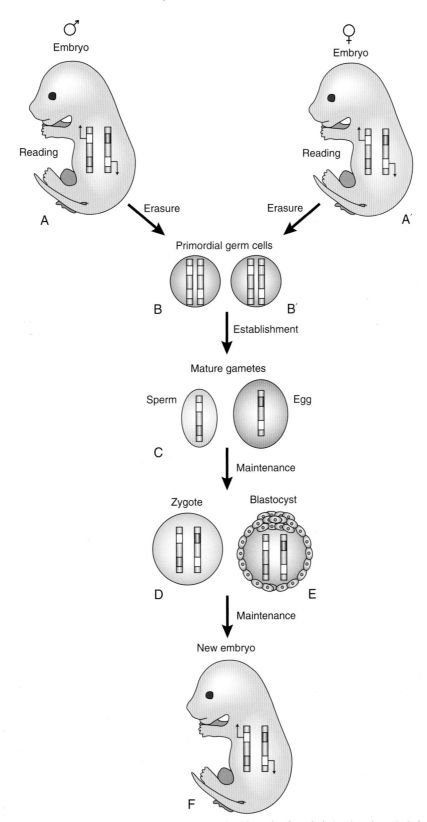

Figure 2-12. Three stages (erasure, establishment, and maintenance) in the life cycle of methylation imprints. *A, A′,* In the somatic (body) tissues of the embryo, imprinted genes are expressed from only one allele in a parent-specific manner. One chromosome pair is illustrated containing two imprinted genes (chromosome containing red mark was inherited from the mother, and blue mark from the father). In this example, methylated genes, indicated by red and blue, are silenced; therefore, the other allele of each gene is transcribed (arrows). *B, B′,* This pattern of genomic imprinting is erased in the embryo's primordial germ cells. *C,* Imprinting is established during gametogenesis (which begins in the embryo and is completed in the adult). *D-F,* From fertilization onward in development, imprinting is maintained.

In the Clinic

X-INACTIVATION AFFECTS INHERITANCE OF CONGENITAL DISEASE

One consequence of random X-inactivation in female cells is that all females are **genetic mosaics**. Some cells express only X-linked genes inherited from the mother, and some cells express only X-linked genes inherited from the father. Thus, in cases in which the female offspring inherits a *recessive* X-linked mutation from one parent and a wild-type allele from the other, she does not exhibit symptoms of the disease because of compensation by cells in her body that express the wild-type allele. This individual is called a **silent carrier**; she may transmit the disease to her sons (who inherit the X that carries the mutated gene). Examples of such X-linked recessive disease include **Duchenne muscular dystrophy** and **Simpson-Golabi-Behmel syndrome**. Duchenne muscular dystrophy results from a mutation in the gene encoding DYSTROPHIN. This mutation causes progressive dystrophy and degeneration of myofibers of skeletal or cardiac muscle, and mild mental retardation. Simpson-Golabi-Behmel syndrome results from a mutation in the GLYPICAN-3 gene. This mutation causes a protruding jaw, a broad nasal bridge, short hands and fingers, heart defects, renal defects, and hypogonadism.

Offspring who inherit a *dominant* X-linked mutation from one parent exhibit some symptoms of the disease, regardless of their gender, because the expression of the wild-type allele in other cells cannot fully compensate. These include diseases such as **Goltz syndrome** (skin atrophy and skeletal malformations) and **incontinentia pigmenti** (spotty pigmentation). The former syndrome results from a mutation in PORCN (homolog of the Drosophila porcupine gene), whereas the latter results from a mutation in IKBKG (an essential modulator of NF-KAPPAβ signaling).

GENOMIC IMPRINTING AFFECTS INHERITANCE OF CONGENITAL DISEASE

The pattern of inheritance of some human genetic disease is also dependent on **imprinting differences** in male and female autosomes. For example, deletions in a region of human chromosome 15 (15q11.2–q13) result in **Prader-Willi syndrome** when inherited from the father and **Angelman syndrome** when inherited from the mother (these syndromes are covered in the "Clinical Taster" for this chapter). These two syndromes are characterized by vastly different symptoms. Symptoms of Prader-Willi syndrome include feeding problems in infancy and rapid weight gain in childhood, hypogonadism, and mild mental retardation. Symptoms of Angelman syndrome include developmental delay, speech and balance disorders, and a unique happy demeanor. Many imprinted genes are located in the 15q11.2–q13 region of chromosome 15, including the imprinting center (IC) that controls the imprinting of imprinted genes in the 15q11.2–q13 region. Most cases of Prader-Willi syndrome and Angelman syndrome result from large deletions in the 15q11.2–q13 region of chromosome 15. However, specific mutations of the IC in the paternally inherited chromosome cause Prader-Willi syndrome, whereas mutations of the maternal IC gene cause Angelman syndrome. A small percentage of cases of Prader-Willi syndrome result from maternal uniparental disomy of chromosome 15, whereas a small percentage of cases of Angelman syndrome result from paternal uniparental disomy of chromosome 15. **Uniparental disomy** is a condition in which both chromosomes of a given pair are inherited from the same parent.

The development of several congenital **overgrowth syndromes** also results from abnormal imprinting of human autosomes. For example, translocations, duplications, or mutations of human chromosome 11p15 may lead to altered expression of INSULIN-LIKE GROWTH FACTOR 2 (ILGF2) and other genes causing **Beckwith Wiedemann syndrome**, a syndrome characterized by macrosomia (large body), renal abnormalities, and embryonal tumors. Disruption of normal imprinting may also lead to the development of cancers, including **renal (Wilms' tumor) colon**, and **cervical carcinoma**.

Embryology in Practice

HOW DO THESE CELLS ACQUIRE THEIR POSITION?

A mother brings her fourteen-year-old son to dermatology clinic because an unusual lesion has appeared on his scalp. Her comment to the nurse is, "it looks like a patch of warts on the top of his head." The mother states that the area of the lesion was a flat tan-colored patch present at birth, but it has become more textured over the last six months.

The clinician, indeed, finds a hairless lesion at the vertex of the child's scalp with a verrucous texture (i.e., scaly and wart-like) with a tan color. It does not seem to be painful to the boy. Careful examination of the rest of the child's skin reveals no similar lesions and no other skin abnormalities.

The clinician informs the mother and the boy that the lesion is benign and is called a nevus sebaceous. First described in 1895, nevus sebaceous is a hamartomatous (i.e., tumor-like) overgrowth of sebaceous glands. Like other sweat glands, sebaceous glands are hormone responsive and often become more apparent during puberty.

The main medical importance of nevus sebaceous relates to the risk of malignant transformation, which early studies reported occurs in 10% to 15% of lesions. Recent reports suggest a much lower rate, and the need for, and timing of, surgical resection remains controversial.

Most nevus sebaceous lesions are caused by postzygotic mutations in the HRAS gene, resulting in substitution of an arginine for a glycine at position 13 of the protein (p.Gly13Arg).

Although nevus sebaceous does occur elsewhere in the body, these ostensibly random mosaic mutations tend to occur most often in cells that will end up at the vertex of the scalp. The explanation for this positional predilection is unknown, but it may involve cell sorting similar to that occurring in this blastocyst to form different groups of cells, or later during gastrulation (covered in Chapter 3).

SUGGESTED READINGS

Aplin JD. 2010. Developmental cell biology of human villous trophoblast: current research problems. Int J Dev Biol 54:323–329.

Augui S, Nora EP, Heard E. 2011. Regulation of X-chromosome inactivation by the X-inactivation centre. Nat Rev Genet 12:429–442.

Betz AG. 2012. Immunology: tolerating pregnancy. Nature 490:47–48.

Daxinger L, Whitelaw E. 2012. Understanding transgenerational epigenetic inheritance via the gametes in mammals. Nat Rev Genet 13:153–162.

Hewitt SC, Korach KS. 2011. Cell biology. A hand to support the implantation window. Science 331:863–864.

Leslie M. 2008. Immunology. Fetal immune system hushes attacks on maternal cells. Science 322:1450–1451.

Li Q, Kannan A, DeMayo FJ, et al. 2011. The antiproliferative action of progesterone in uterine epithelium is mediated by Hand2. Science 331:912–916.

Mold JE, Michaelsson J, Burt TD, et al. 2008. Maternal alloantigens promote the development of tolerogenic fetal regulatory T cells in utero. Science 322:1562–1565.

Rossant J, Tam PP. 2009. Blastocyst lineage formation, early embryonic asymmetries and axis patterning in the mouse. Development 136:701–713.

Rowe JH, Ertelt JM, Xin L, Way SS. 2012. Pregnancy imprints regulatory memory that sustains anergy to fetal antigen. Nature 490:102–106.

Wang H, Dey SK. 2006. Roadmap to embryo implantation: clues from mouse models. Nat Rev Genet 7:185–199.

Zorn AM, Wells JM. 2009. Vertebrate endoderm development and organ formation. Annu Rev Cell Dev Biol 25:221–251.

Chapter 3

Third Week: Becoming Trilaminar and Establishing Body Axes

SUMMARY

The first major event of the third week, **gastrulation**, commences with the formation of a longitudinal midline structure, the **primitive streak**, in the epiblast near the caudal end of the bilaminar embryonic disc. The cranial end of the primitive streak is expanded as the **primitive node**; it contains a circular depression called the **primitive pit**, which is continuous caudally down the midline of the primitive streak with a troughlike depression called the **primitive groove**. The primitive pit and groove represent areas where cells are leaving the primitive streak and moving into the interior of the embryonic disc. Some of these cells invade the hypoblast, displacing the original hypoblast cells and replacing them with a layer of **definitive endoderm**. Others migrate bilaterally from the primitive streak and then cranially or laterally between endoderm and epiblast and coalesce to form the **intraembryonic mesoderm**. After gastrulation is complete, the epiblast is called the **ectoderm**. Thus during gastrulation, the three primary **germ layers** form: **ectoderm**, **mesoderm**, and **endoderm**. Germ layers are the primitive building blocks for formation of **organ rudiments**.

Formation of the primitive streak also defines for the first time all major **body axes**. These consist of the **cranial-caudal** (or head-tail) **axis**, the **dorsal-ventral** (or back-belly) **axis**, the **medial-lateral axis**, and the **left-right axis**. Before the flat embryonic disc folds up into a three-dimensional tube-within-a-tube body plan, these axes remain incompletely delimited; their definitive form will be better understood after Chapter 4 is studied.

As gastrulation converts the bilaminar embryonic disc into a **trilaminar embryonic disc**, it brings subpopulations of cells into proximity so that they can undergo inductive interactions to pattern layers and specify new cell types. The first cells to move through the primitive streak and contribute to the intraembryonic mesoderm migrate bilaterally and cranially to form the **cardiogenic mesoderm**. Somewhat later in development, a longitudinal thick-walled tube of mesoderm extends cranially in the midline from the primitive node; this structure, the **notochordal process**, is the rudiment of the **notochord**. Migrating bilaterally from the primitive streak and then cranially, just lateral to the notochordal process, are cells that contribute to the **paraxial mesoderm**. In the future head region, paraxial mesoderm forms the **head mesoderm**. In the future trunk region, paraxial mesoderm forms the **somites**, a series of segmental blocklike mesodermal condensations. Two other areas of intraembryonic mesoderm form from the primitive streak during gastrulation: **intermediate mesoderm** and **lateral plate mesoderm**. The intermediate mesoderm contributes to the urogenital system, and the lateral plate mesoderm contributes to the body wall and the wall of the gut (gastrointestinal system).

During gastrulation, a major inductive event occurs in the embryo: **neural induction**. In this process, the primitive node induces the overlying ectoderm to thicken as the **neural plate**, the earliest rudiment of the central nervous system.

During subsequent development, the neural plate will fold up into a **neural tube**. **Neural crest cells** arise from the lateral edges of the neural plate during formation of the neural tube. Also during subsequent development, the definitive endoderm will fold to form three subdivisions of the primitive gut: **foregut**, **midgut**, and **hindgut**. The cranial midline endoderm, just cranial to the tip of the extending notochord, forms a thickened area called the **prechordal plate**. It contributes to the **oropharyngeal membrane** during later development and is an important signaling center for patterning the overlying neural plate. With formation of endodermal, mesodermal, and ectodermal subdivisions during gastrulation, the stage is set by the end of the third week for **formation of the tube-within-a-tube body plan** and subsequent **organogenesis**—the processes by which primitive organ rudiments are established and subsequently are differentiated to form all major organ systems.

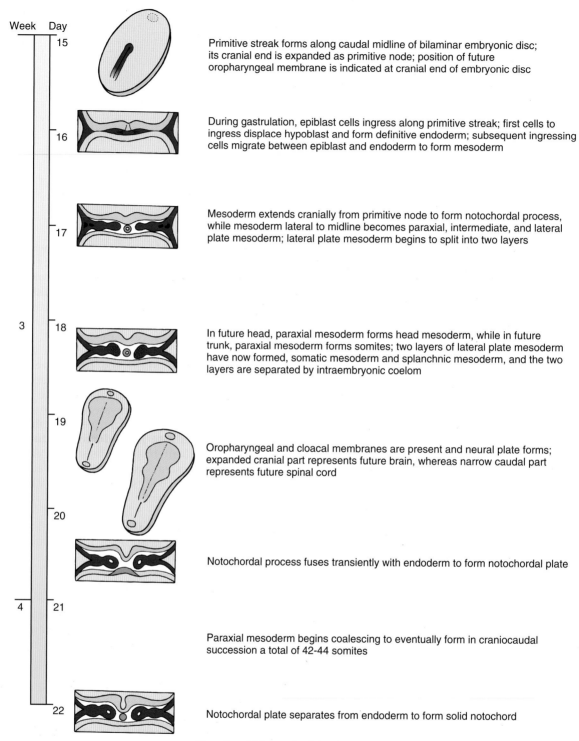

Week Day

15
Primitive streak forms along caudal midline of bilaminar embryonic disc; its cranial end is expanded as primitive node; position of future oropharyngeal membrane is indicated at cranial end of embryonic disc

16
During gastrulation, epiblast cells ingress along primitive streak; first cells to ingress displace hypoblast and form definitive endoderm; subsequent ingressing cells migrate between epiblast and endoderm to form mesoderm

17
Mesoderm extends cranially from primitive node to form notochordal process, while mesoderm lateral to midline becomes paraxial, intermediate, and lateral plate mesoderm; lateral plate mesoderm begins to split into two layers

3   18
In future head, paraxial mesoderm forms head mesoderm, while in future trunk, paraxial mesoderm forms somites; two layers of lateral plate mesoderm have now formed, somatic mesoderm and splanchnic mesoderm, and the two layers are separated by intraembryonic coelom

19
Oropharyngeal and cloacal membranes are present and neural plate forms; expanded cranial part represents future brain, whereas narrow caudal part represents future spinal cord

20
Notochordal process fuses transiently with endoderm to form notochordal plate

4   21
Paraxial mesoderm begins coalescing to eventually form in craniocaudal succession a total of 42-44 somites

22
Notochordal plate separates from endoderm to form solid notochord

Time line. Third week of development.

Clinical Taster

In 2004, a baby girl, Milagros Cerron, was born in Peru with a condition called **sirenomelia** (*siren* and *melos* are Greek, meaning "nymph limbs"). Because she is one of only three surviving children born with the "mermaid syndrome" (the oldest being sixteen years old in 2005), her birth, first birthday, and surgery at thirteen months of age received extensive press coverage.

Sirenomelia is a rare condition occurring in 1 in 70,000 births. Most babies born with sirenomelia die within a few days of birth with severe defects in vital organs. The most obvious defect in sirenomelia is a fusion of the two lower limbs at the midline (Fig. 3-1). In Milagros's case (her name is Spanish for miracles), her lower limbs were fused together from her thighs to her ankles, with her feet deviating from one another in a V-shaped pattern resembling a mermaid's tail. In the press, she is often referred to as "Peru's little mermaid." In addition to fused lower limbs, she was born with a deformed left kidney, a small right kidney that failed to ascend, and anomalies in her terminal digestive, urinary, and genital tracts. These anomalies have resulted in recurrent urinary tract infections.

For three months before her first surgery to separate her fused legs, saline-filled bags were inserted to stretch the skin to allow it to cover her legs once they were separated. She recovered quickly from surgery, and it is expected that she will need to undergo many other surgeries over the course of the next fifteen years to correct her digestive, urinary, and reproductive organs. Remarkably, a few months postsurgery, she was able to run around the school playground with her classmates and take ballet lessons.

OVERVIEW OF GASTRULATION: FORMING THREE PRIMARY GERM LAYERS AND BODY AXES

Animation 3-1: Gastrulation.
Animations are available online at StudentConsult.

PRIMITIVE STREAK FORMS AT BEGINNING OF THIRD WEEK AND MARKS THREE BODY AXES

On about day fifteen of development, a thickening containing a midline groove forms along the midsagittal plane of the embryonic disc, which has now assumed an oval shape (Fig. 3-2). Over the course of the next day, this thickening, called the **primitive streak**, elongates to occupy about half the length of the embryonic disc, and the groove, called the **primitive groove**, becomes deeper and more defined. The cranial end of the primitive streak is expanded into a structure called the **primitive node**. It contains a depression, called the **primitive pit**, which is continuous caudally with the primitive groove.

Formation of the primitive streak defines all major **body axes** (Fig. 3-3). The primitive streak forms at the caudal midline of the embryonic disc, thus defining the **cranial-caudal axis** and **medial-lateral axis** (with the primitive streak forming at the midline, that is, most medially). Because formation of the primitive streak occurs at the midline, when the epiblast is

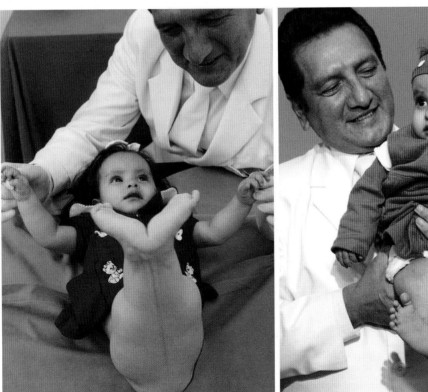
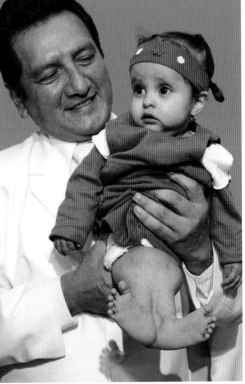

Figure 3-1. Sirenomelia. Severe reduction of caudal structures has resulted in fusion of the lower limb buds. Shown is Milagros Cerron at about one year of age with her physician.

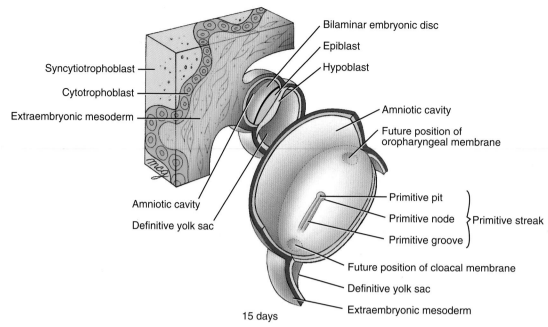

Figure 3-2. View of dorsal surface of bilaminar embryonic disc through sectioned amnion and yolk sac. Inset at upper left shows relation of the embryo to the wall of the chorionic cavity. The primitive streak, now one day old, occupies 50% of the length of the embryonic disc. The future positions of oropharyngeal and cloacal membranes are indicated.

viewed looking down at it from inside the amniotic cavity and facing its cranial end, what lies to the right of the primitive streak represents the right side of the embryo, and what lies to the left represents its left side. Thus, formation of the primitive streak also defines the **left-right axis**. At the time of primitive streak formation, the future **dorsal-ventral axis** of the embryonic disc is roughly equivalent to its ectoderm-endoderm axis. Later, with body folding and formation of the tube-within-a-tube body plan (covered in Chapter 4), the dorsal-ventral axis becomes better defined.

Formation of the primitive streak also heralds the beginning of **gastrulation**. During gastrulation, epiblast cells move toward the primitive streak, enter the primitive streak, and then migrate away from the primitive streak as individual cells (see Fig. 3-3). The movement of cells through the primitive streak and into the interior of the embryo is called **ingression**.

In the Research Lab

INDUCTION OF PRIMITIVE STREAK

Experiments in chick suggest that the primitive streak is induced by cell-cell interactions at the caudal end of the embryonic disc. Although the exact tissue interactions are disputed, it is clear that extraembryonic tissues induce the adjacent epiblast to form primitive streak (Fig. 3-3A), and that this process of induction continues as the extraembryonic endoderm (hypoblast) migrates from caudal to cranial.

Misexpression studies (gain-of-function and loss-of-function; covered in Chapter 5) in both mouse and chick suggest that Tgfβ and Wnt family members induce the primitive streak (Fig. 3-3A, B). In chick, Vg1 (a Tgfβ family member) in conjunction with Wnt8a (formerly called Wnt8c) induces the epiblast to express another

Tgfβ family member—nodal. Nodal in turn, along with Fgf8 (and likely other Fgfs), causes epiblast cells to de-epithelialize and form the primitive streak. Finally, inhibition of endogenous Bmp signaling (through its antagonist chordin; covered in Chapters 4 and 5) also seems to be required for primitive streak formation.

In mouse, Wnt3 and its downstream target brachyury (a T-box–containing transcription factor) are expressed in both future cranial and caudal prestreak epiblast (see Fig. 3-3B). During subsequent development, Wnt3 is downregulated cranially by signals from a specialized region of extraembryonic endoderm called the **anterior visceral endoderm**, and it is upregulated caudally (note: "anterior" in the mouse is equivalent to cranial in the human). Finally, expression of Wnt3, brachyury, and nodal becomes consolidated within the primitive streak. Loss-of-function mutations of genes expressed by the anterior visceral endoderm (e.g., Cer2 [Cerberus-like 2], Lefty1—both inhibitors of Tgfβ and Wnt signaling) result in formation of extra primitive streaks. Moreover, embryos with loss-of-function mutations of nodal (or its co-factor cripto) fail to form a primitive streak. Further studies in mouse (using injection chimeras; covered in Chapter 5) reveal that formation of the primitive streak involves signaling of Tgfβ family members from extraembryonic tissues (as in chick).

CELLULAR BASIS OF PRIMITIVE STREAK FORMATION

Studies in chick have revealed the cellular basis of primitive streak formation (Fig. 3-4). Four major processes are involved: **cell migration, oriented cell division**, progressive **delamination** from the epiblast, and **convergent extension**. As covered above, during formation of the primitive streak, cells are induced from the epiblast by the caudal extraembryonic region. As induction occurs, these cells delaminate (de-epithelialize or undergo an epithelial-to-mesenchymal transition) from the epiblast and migrate cranially and medially. Analyses of labeled clones of cells show that cells are displaced mainly cranially as they undergo division, suggesting that their division plane is preferentially oriented in the medial-lateral plane, so that daughters are displaced cranially. As extraembryonic endoderm

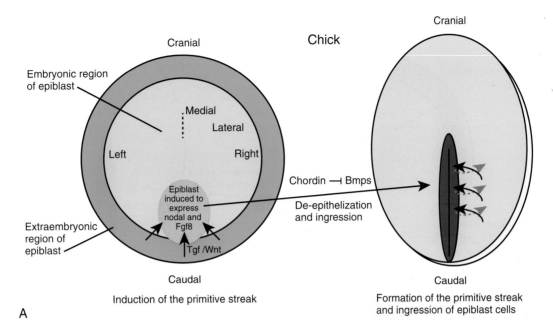

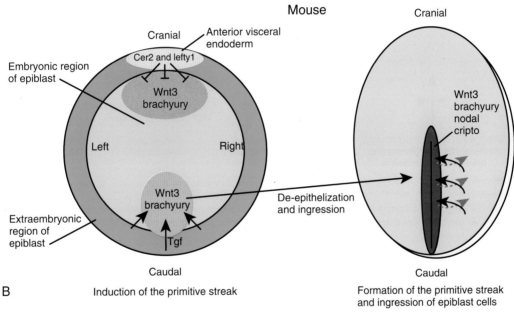

Figure 3-3. Induction and formation of the primitive streak and ingression of epiblast cells. *A,* Our current understanding based on the chick model. The left side of the figure shows the embryonic axes (cranial-caudal, medial-lateral, and left-right; dashed line marks the midline or median plane) that are visible by viewing the dorsal (upper or epiblast) surface of the blastoderm, as well as the interacting tissue regions (straight arrows) and the growth factors involved in induction of the primitive streak. The right side shows formation of the primitive streak and the directions of cell movement (curved arrows) as epiblast cells move toward, into, and away from the primitive streak to form endoderm and mesoderm. Inhibition of Bmp signaling (by antagonists such as chordin) is also required in chick for formation of the primitive streak. *B,* Our current understanding based on the mouse model. Primitive streak formation is inhibited in the cranial (anterior) blastoderm by signals emanating from the cranial extraembryonic endoderm, known as the anterior visceral endoderm. Other labeling as in *A.*

migrates cranially, progressively more cranial epiblast cells along the midline are induced to delaminate, extending the cranial end of the primitive streak more cranially. Finally, cells within the forming streak merge medially, and consequently the streak extends craniocaudally to accommodate the merging cells. Thus, convergent extension contributes to the later aspects of primitive streak formation and elongation.

ESTABLISHING LEFT-RIGHT AXIS

As covered above, with formation of the primitive streak during gastrulation, the embryonic axes—cranial-caudal, dorsal-ventral, medial-lateral, and left-right—become defined. In mouse embryos, cranial patterning actually occurs before formation of the primitive streak as a result of signaling from the anterior visceral endoderm (covered in preceding section). Whether a

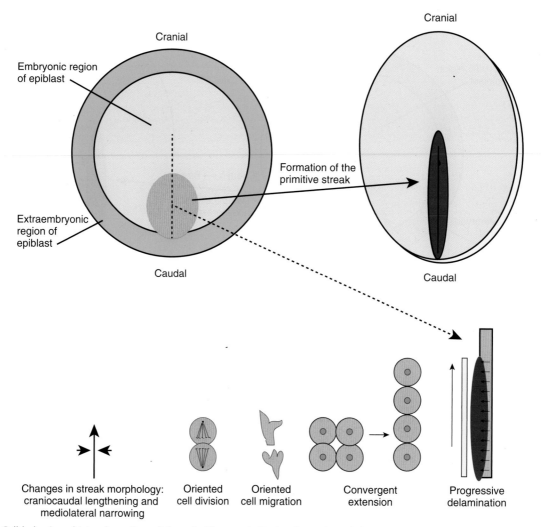

Figure 3-4. Cell behaviors driving formation of the primitive streak. During formation of the primitive streak, its overall morphology changes from wide (in the mediolateral plane) and short (in the craniocaudal plane) to narrow and long. This change in overall shape is due to oriented cell division, oriented cell migration, convergent extension, and progressive delamination. Progressive delamination is viewed in a longitudinal section (dashed arrow). As the hypoblast migrates cranially (long arrow), delamination (short, multiple arrows) progresses from caudal to cranial.

similar signaling center exists in humans to provide early cranial patterning information is unknown. With formation of the primitive streak and subsequently three primary germ layers, cell-cell interactions occur among the three layers and within different subdivisions of these layers to pattern the germ layers in both cranial-caudal and dorsal-ventral planes. This patterning is covered later in this chapter and in Chapter 4. Here, we discuss a third type of patterning—formation of the **left-right axis**, which begins at about the time that the primitive node forms at the cranial end of the primitive streak.

Handed asymmetry, as opposed to **mirror (or mirror-image) symmetry**, is the term that denotes anatomic differences on left and right sides of the body. For example, in humans, the gastrointestinal tract rotates during development so that the stomach is on the left and the liver is on the right. Also, the heart loops so that its apex points to the left, whereas its base is directed to the right. Furthermore, the right lung has three lobes and the left lung has two lobes. How is handed asymmetry initiated in the embryo?

Molecular Basis of Left-Right Asymmetry: A Simplified Scheme

Left-right asymmetry is established during gastrulation through cell-cell interactions centered at the primitive node (see Fig. 3-2)—defined as the cranial end of the primitive streak and the region of the streak that has **organizer** activity (covered later in the chapter), or the homologous structure in animal models (e.g., embryonic shield in zebrafish, dorsal lip of the blastopore in *Xenopus*, Hensen's node in chick, node in mouse). In chick, a secreted molecule, sonic hedgehog (Shh), is expressed symmetrically in Hensen's node as it forms, but shortly thereafter, expression of Shh becomes restricted to the left side. This is followed by left-sided expression of the Tgfβ family member, nodal (within both the left side of the node and the left lateral plate mesoderm; covered in mesodermal divisions, below), and subsequently, by left-sided expression of a transcription factor, Pitx2. Gain-of-function experiments in chick have revealed that Shh induces left-sided expression of nodal, which in turn induces left-sided expression of

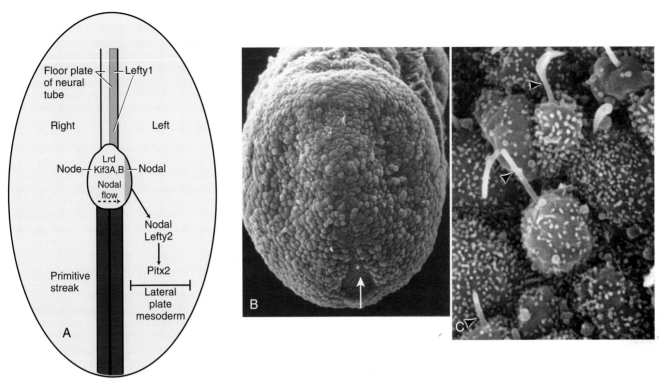

Figure 3-5. Cilia and nodal flow in the mouse node. *A*, Diagram illustrating a simplified scheme of key genes involved in establishing left-right asymmetry. The blastoderm, including the primitive streak, node, and early floor plate of the neural tube, is viewed from the ventral side. Motor proteins (Lrd, Kif3A, B) expressed by the node regulate ciliary movement and leftward (dashed arrow) nodal flow. As a result of nodal flow, the protein nodal becomes expressed by the left side of the node. This in turn results in left-sided expression of lefty2 and Pitx2 in left lateral plate. Lefty1 is expressed in the left floor plate of the neural tube, where it serves a barrier function, allowing information that specifies left and right sides to remain separate. *B*, Scanning electron micrograph of a gastrulating mouse embryo viewed from its endodermal surface. Arrow marks the node. *C*, Enlargement of nodal cilia (arrowheads).

Pitx2. Pitx2 regulates the transcription of downstream targets (mostly unknown), presumably changing cell behaviors and resulting in asymmetric morphogenesis, leading to handed asymmetry.

The scheme just outlined is a simplified version, as many other molecules are known to be asymmetrically expressed at this time, and is based mainly on experiments in the chick. Experiments in mouse have revealed that roles for some of these molecules are conserved (e.g., nodal and Pitx2), but not for others (e.g., Shh). With regard to Shh, although overexpression in chick induces ectopic nodal expression, silencing Shh in mouse shows that Shh is not required for nodal expression. However, Shh null mice do have laterality defects, presumably because Shh plays a role in development of the lateral plate mesoderm at later stages. Because of these differences between chick and mouse embryos, and because other experiments in mouse have provided considerable additional insight into how left-right asymmetry is established, further coverage of the development of left-right asymmetry will focus on the mouse model (Fig. 3-5).

Experiments in mouse have revealed that in addition to nodal, which is expressed both in the left side of the node and in the left lateral plate mesoderm, two other Tgfβ family members that are highly related to one another have left-sided expression and play essential roles in establishing left-right asymmetry (Fig. 3-5*A*). They are appropriately named lefty1 and lefty2. To set the stage for the rest of the story on how left-right asymmetry is established, we must first digress briefly to provide some additional background.

In the rare human disorder, **situs inversus viscerum totalis**, the handedness of all of the viscera is reversed. However, the

reversal is rarely complete or exact, and errors in morphogenesis often produce subsidiary malformations such as the **malrotations of the midgut** (covered below and in Chapter 14). More often, the different organ systems exhibit a discordance of sidedness, or **heterotaxy**. For example, the looping of the heart may be reversed (**dextrocardia**; covered in Chapter 12), whereas lobulation of the lungs may be normal (three lobes on the right and two lobes on the left). More than forty years ago, a mouse mutant was discovered that exhibits situs inversus, the iv/iv mouse (iv stands for inversus viscerum). The phenotype is inherited as an autosomal recessive single-gene trait, and it has been mapped to chromosome 12. But only half the mice homozygous for the mutant iv allele exhibit situs inversus; the other half show normal left-right asymmetry (**situs solitus totalis**). Thus, the gene product of the wild-type locus seems to be an essential component of the mechanism that *biases* the development of handed asymmetry in the correct direction, and thus determines the correct handedness or **situs** of the viscera. If this gene product is absent or defective (as in the iv/iv mouse), normal or inverted situs is apparently adopted at random.

Cloning of the iv mutation provided interesting clues that led to better understanding of the early stages of left-right development. The iv mutation occurs in a dynein gene designated left-right dynein, or Lrd. Dyneins are molecular motors composed of heavy and intermediate polypeptide chains. Dyneins use energy from ATP hydrolysis to move cargo toward the minus end of microtubules, or cause bending of cilia and flagella by creating a sliding force between microtubules. Thus, there are two kinds of dyneins: cytoplasmic and axonemal. The sequence of the Lrd gene suggests that it encodes an axonemal dynein, but the functions of the two kinds of dyneins probably are not completely independent of one another, as suggested from mouse loss-of-function mutations (in which mutations in single motor proteins affect both ciliary action and intracellular transport).

This connection between dynein and laterality in mice was reminiscent of a previous connection between dynein and laterality in humans. Patients with **Kartagener syndrome** have inverted laterality as well as immotile respiratory cilia and sperm flagella. They often exhibit male infertility and chronic respiratory tract infection. Kartagener syndrome patients have mutations in DYNEIN genes (both heavy and intermediate chain mutations have been identified), as well as deficiencies in their ciliary DYNEIN arms (DYNEINS form armlike projections that interconnect the outer microtubule doublets, as viewed ultrastructurally in electron micrographs). Kartagener syndrome is covered further in Chapters 11 and 12.

Nodal Flow Model

In gastrulating mouse embryos, expression of the Lrd gene is restricted to the node (Fig. 3-5A), an important organizer region (covered below). Each of the cells of the node contains a single cilium, called a **monocilium** (Fig. 3-5B, C). The monocilia of the central nodal cells are motile, in contrast to those of the peripheral nodal cells. The central cilia rotate in a vortical fashion and generate a leftward flow of fluid across the node (as demonstrated experimentally by the displacement of fluorescent beads across the node). Based on this finding and on the experimental reversal of flow in cultured embryos, the **nodal flow model** of left-right development was proposed (note: nodal in the model refers to the node and should not be confused with the gene named nodal). According to the original formulation of the model, leftward movement of fluid across the node generates an asymmetric distribution of an unknown **morphogen**, that is, a diffusible protein that affects tissue development based on its concentration. The resulting left-right morphogen concentration gradient is believed to break symmetry and initiate left-right development. Several candidate proteins have been proposed for this morphogen, including nodal, Shh, Fgf8, retinoic acid, Bmp, and Gdf1 (growth differentiation factor 1), but several have been eliminated as candidates based on genetic experiments (i.e., Shh, Fgf8, and retinoic acid). Whether the primitive node of humans contains monocilia (and if it does, whether some are motile) is unknown; however, nodal monocilia have been identified in several species.

Loss-of-function experiments in mice provide compelling support for the nodal flow model. Mice mutant for the kinesin gene Kif3A or Kif3B, both of which are expressed in the node at gastrula stages but not exclusively as is Lrd (see Fig. 3-5A), have nodal cells without cilia and altered left-right development. Kinesins are functionally similar to dyneins in that they generate motive force along microtubules (although in the opposite direction). These results indicate that the Kif3A and Kif3B genes are required for node cilia assembly and suggest that cilia, in turn, are necessary for normal left-right development. In addition, mice with a mutation in the Lrd gene have immotile nodal cilia. This shows that not just the presence but the movement of the nodal cilia is critically important for normal left-right development—again consistent with the nodal flow model.

Currently, left-right asymmetry is believed to involve several steps beginning with ciliary action in the node during gastrulation. These steps include establishing rotating cilia within the node (requiring Lrd and Kif3A, B), which in turn generates nodal flow (from the right to the left side), nodal expression in the cells on the left side of the node (these cells, as well as similarly located cells on the right side of the node, contain non-motile cilia and constitute the so-called **crown cells** of the node), nodal expression in the left lateral plate (recent studies have shown that the endoderm plays an important role in transferring left-right information, likely from the node to the left lateral plate for nodal expression), and expression of lefty2 and pitx2 in the left lateral plate (which presumably orchestrate left-right-specific morphogenesis; e.g., see Chapter 14 on mechanisms of gut rotation). In addition, lefty1, which is expressed in the left-half of the floor plate overlying the notochord, acts as a barrier, preventing diffusion of left-right information across the midline.

Additionally, it is known that as a result of nodal flow, Cer2 (a nodal antagonist) is downregulated on the left side of the node but not on the right side, resulting in a higher level of active nodal protein on the left side than on the right side. This is important, as active nodal protein is the "left-side determinant" of the lateral plate mesoderm, and its expression results in left-right morphogenesis of lateral plate–derived organs. Moreover, recent studies have shown that the endoderm plays an important role in transferring left-right information, likely a nodal-Gdf1 (growth differentiation factor 1) heterodimer, from the node to the left lateral plate, where it self-induces nodal expression by activating the nodal-responsive enhancer of the nodal gene.

Finally, for ciliary rotation to result in a directional nodal flow, individual motile cilia must have a particular orientation, and all motile cilia must have the same orientation. In the mouse node, cilia are tilted caudally. How is this orientation achieved? Recent studies show that the planar cell polarity pathway and, in particular, non-canonical Wnt signaling (both covered in Chapter 5) establish this orientation. The position of the basal body in a cell determines the position of its cilium. Within the node, the basal bodies of motile cilia are initially positioned centrally but gradually shift caudally. This shift is impaired in mutations of genes in the non-canonical Wnt pathway (e.g., Dvl or disheveled genes).

An Important Variation on the Nodal Flow Model

As originally formulated and covered above, nodal flow was proposed to transport a morphogen to the left side of the node. More recent studies have supported a variation of the nodal flow model called the **mechanosensory model**, in which it is proposed that motile cilia drive nodal fluid flow, which in turn mechanically activates a **calcium flux** on the left side of the node, with the immotile crown cell cilia acting like sensory antennae (Fig. 3-6). In support of this model, both centrally located motile cilia and peripherally located immotile cilia of the node contain a cation channel protein called polycystein2, which is the product of the polycystic kidney disease type 2 gene, Pkd2. By contrast, only motile cilia express the Lrd protein. Imaging of calcium levels (using a fluorescent reporter dye and confocal microscopy) revealed that asymmetric calcium signaling appears at the left margin of the node, coincident with the onset of nodal flow. Thus, the immotile cilia act as mechanosensors to detect fluid flow.

Ordering Genes in a Genetic Hierarchy

The order of genes in a genetic program is often determined by examination of gene expression patterns in mutants. For example, if gene A activates gene B, which activates gene C in a program, then mutation of gene B would alter the expression of gene C but not gene A. In this manner, the Lrd gene was shown to occupy a high-level position in the genetic hierarchy of left-right development. In Lrd loss-of-function mutants, the expression patterns of nodal, lefty1, lefty2, and pitx2 are all altered, indicating that they are downstream of Lrd. The expression of nodal, for example, is randomized in mice with an Lrd loss-of-function mutation. One fourth of these mutant embryos show normal nodal expression only on the left, one fourth show reversed expression only on the right, one fourth show expression on both sides, and one fourth show expression on neither side.

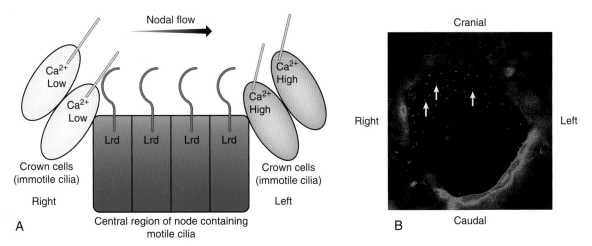

Figure 3-6. The mechanosensory model of nodal flow. *A*, Model showing that nodal flow, generated by motile monocilia in cells expressing Lrd, stimulates calcium flux in cells (i.e., crown cells) containing non-motile cilia that sense flow on the left side. *B*, Mouse node viewed from its endodermal side showing calcium signaling predominantly at the left side of the node. Arrows indicate motile cilia expressing Lrd fused with a fluorescent reporter gene.

In the Clinic

CILIOPATHIES

Not only do cilia function in the embryo in establishing left-right asymmetry, they also function in several developing organ systems such as the trachea, kidney, olfactory system, retina, testis, and oviduct. Defects in cilia structure and function that result in disease are called **ciliopathies**. Several ciliopathies occur in humans, including some forms of polycystic kidney disease, Meckel syndrome, Bardet-Biedl syndrome, and Joubert syndrome. Many ciliopathies also result in situs inversus or heterotaxy (covered earlier in the chapter).

FORMATION OF DEFINITIVE ENDODERM

On day sixteen, epiblast cells lateral to the primitive streak begin to move into the primitive streak, where they undergo an **epithelial-to-mesenchymal transformation (EMT)**. An **epithelium** consists of a sheet of regularly shaped (often cuboidal) cells tightly interconnected to one another at their lateral cell surfaces; a **mesenchyme** consists of much more irregularly shaped (often stellate) and loosely connected cells. During EMT, epiblast cells often elongate and become flask or bottle shaped (Fig. 3-7), detaching from their neighbors as they extend footlike processes called **pseudopodia** (as well as thinner processes called **filopodia** and flattened processes called **lamellipodia**), which allow them to migrate through the primitive streak into the space between the epiblast and the hypoblast (or into the hypoblast itself). This collective movement of cells through the primitive streak and into the interior of the embryo to form the three primary germ layers constitutes **gastrulation**. The first ingressing epiblast cells invade the hypoblast and displace its cells, so that the hypoblast eventually is completely replaced by a new layer of cells—the **definitive endoderm** (Fig. 3-7*A*). The definitive endoderm gives rise to the lining of the future gut and to gut derivatives.

FORMATION OF INTRAEMBRYONIC MESODERM

Starting on day sixteen, some epiblast cells migrating through the primitive streak diverge into the space between epiblast and nascent definitive endoderm to form a third germ layer—the **intraembryonic mesoderm** (Figs. 3-7*B*, *C*, 3-8). These cells migrate bilaterally from the primitive streak and initially form a loose mat of cells between epiblast and endoderm. Shortly thereafter, the mat reorganizes to form four main subdivisions of intraembryonic mesoderm: **cardiogenic mesoderm**, **paraxial mesoderm**, **intermediate mesoderm** (also called **nephrotome**), and **lateral plate mesoderm**. In addition, a fifth population of mesodermal cells migrates cranially from the primitive node at the midline to form a thick-walled midline tube called the **notochordal process**.

During the third week of development, two faint depressions form in the ectoderm: one at the cranial end of the embryo overlying the prechordal plate and the other at the caudal end behind the primitive streak. Late in the third week, the ectoderm in these areas fuses tightly with the underlying endoderm, excluding the mesoderm and forming bilaminar membranes. The cranial membrane is called the **oropharyngeal membrane**, and the caudal membrane is the **cloacal membrane**. The oropharyngeal and cloacal membranes later become the blind ends of the gut tube. The oropharyngeal membrane breaks down in the fourth week to form the opening to the oral cavity, whereas the cloacal membrane disintegrates later, in the seventh week, to form the openings of the anus and the urinary and genital tracts (covered in Chapters 14 through 16).

FORMATION OF ECTODERM

Once formation of the definitive endoderm and intraembryonic mesoderm is complete, epiblast cells no longer move toward and ingress through the primitive streak. The remaining epiblast now constitutes the **ectoderm**, which quickly differentiates into the central **neural plate** and the peripheral **surface ectoderm**. However, the embryo develops in a cranial-to-caudal sequence, so that once epiblast is no longer present cranially, for some time it still will be present caudally where cells continue to move into the primitive streak and undergo ingression (Fig. 3-9). Eventually, the process of gastrulation is complete. At that time, formation of the three definitive germ layers of the **trilaminar embryonic disc**—ectoderm, mesoderm, and definitive endoderm—will be complete throughout the disc. Thus, all three germ layers derive from epiblast during gastrulation (note: some textbooks call the epiblast the primitive ectoderm, but because epiblast gives rise to mesoderm and endoderm as well as ectoderm, the term epiblast is a more appropriate one).

Morphogenetic changes (i.e., shape-generating events) occur in each of these germ layers to form the primitive

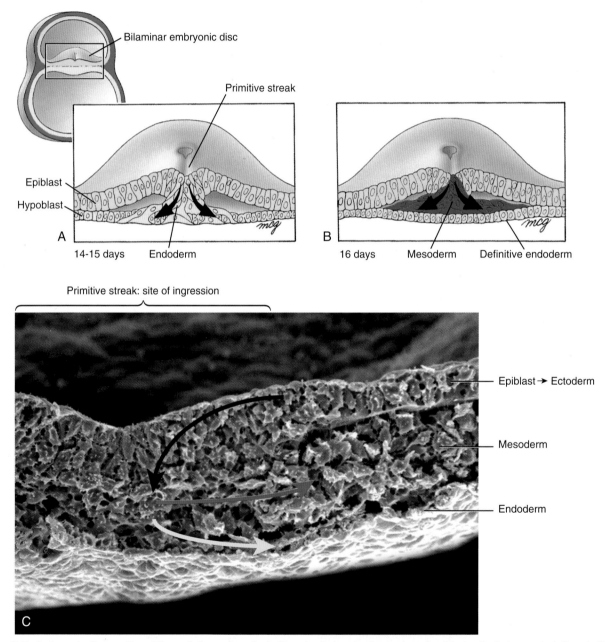

Figure 3-7. Embryonic discs sectioned through the region of primitive streak showing ingression of epiblast cells during gastrulation. *A*, On days fourteen and fifteen, ingressing epiblast cells displace hypoblast and form definitive endoderm. *B*, Epiblast that ingresses on day sixteen migrates between endoderm and epiblast layers to form intraembryonic mesoderm. *C*, Scanning electron micrograph of a cross section through the chick primitive streak. Arrows indicate the directions of cell movement during ingression from the epiblast, through the streak, and into the hypoblast to form the endoderm, and into the middle layer to form the mesoderm. After ingression at a particular craniocaudal level is completed, the epiblast forms the ectoderm.

organ rudiments. Thus, we often speak about ectodermal, mesodermal, and endoderm derivatives. In reality very few organ rudiments form from only one germ layer; rather two or more layers often collaborate (e.g., the gut tube is derived from endoderm and mesoderm). Formation of organ rudiments during the formation of the tube-within-a-tube body plan (see Chapter 4) is followed by the transformation of organ rudiments into organ systems, that is, the process of **organogenesis**; organogenesis is the major topic of most of the remaining chapters of this textbook.

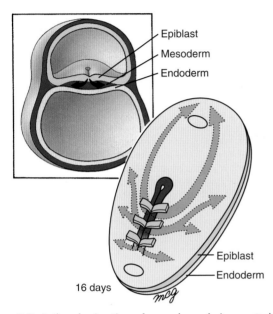

Epiblast
Mesoderm
Endoderm

Epiblast
Endoderm

16 days

Figure 3-8. Paths of migration of mesoderm during gastrulation. Cells of the primitive node migrate cranially at the midline to form the notochordal process (not shown, as it occurs later). Cells that ingress more caudally through the primitive streak migrate to form the mesoderm lying on either side of the midline. The most cranially migrating of these cells form the cardiogenic mesoderm, which moves cranial to the future position of the oropharyngeal membrane (cranial oval structure). The more laterally migrating of these cells form the paraxial, intermediate, and lateral plate mesoderm.

In the Research Lab

CELLULAR BASIS OF GASTRULATION

The cellular basis of gastrulation has been studied in a large variety of animal models. During gastrulation, cells undergo four types of coordinated group movements, called **morphogenetic movements: epiboly** (spreading of an epithelial sheet), **emboly** (internalization), **convergence** (movement toward the midline), and **extension** (lengthening in the cranial-caudal plane). The last two movements occur in conjunction with one another as a coordinated movement and are called **convergent extension**. Thus, convergent extension involves cell rearrangement to narrow the medial-lateral extent of a population of cells and concomitantly increase its cranial-caudal extent. Morphogenetic movements are generated by a combination of **changes in cell behaviors**. These behaviors include **changes in cell shape, size, position**, and **number**. These changes are often associated with **changes in cell-to-cell** or **cell-to-extracellular matrix adhesion**.

Changes in cell shape involve cell flattening (from columnar or cuboidal to squamous), cell elongation or shortening (from cuboidal to columnar or from columnar to cuboidal), and cell wedging (from columnar to wedge shaped). Changes in cell size may involve an increase in cell volume (**growth**) or a decrease. Changes in cell position involve the active (i.e., **migration**) or passive displacement of cells from one region of an embryo to another, and changes in cell number may involve an increase (**mitosis**) or a decrease (**apoptosis**, also called **programmed cell death**).

Both epiboly and emboly are involved in human gastrulation as cells move toward, into, and through the primitive streak. Epiboly involves the spreading of a sheet of cells, generally on the surface of an embryo. Epiblast cells undergo epiboly to move toward and into the primitive streak. Emboly involves the movement of cells into the interior of an embryo and is also called **internalization**. Emboly can involve the movement of individual cells or sheets of cells. Movement of cells through the primitive streak and into the interior involves a type of emboly called **ingression**—the internalization of individual cells undergoing an epithelial-to-mesenchymal transformation (EMT).

EMT involves changes in both **cell-to-cell adhesion** and **cell shape**, with the latter mediated by changes in the **cytoskeleton**. During EMT, epiblast cells within the primitive streak shift their predominant adhesive activity from cell-to-cell to cell-to-substratum (basement membranes and

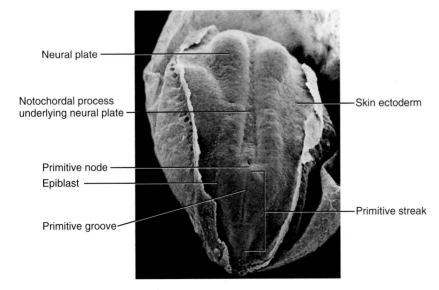

Neural plate

Notochordal process underlying neural plate

Primitive node
Epiblast

Primitive groove

Skin ectoderm

Primitive streak

Figure 3-9. Scanning electron micrograph of a Macaque embryo comparable with a nineteen-day human embryo showing the ectodermal surface of a trilaminar embryonic disc (cranial end at top). Even though the neural plate and the surface ectoderm are well formed throughout the cranial two thirds of the embryo, a regressing primitive streak and a flanking epiblast are still present caudally.

extracellular matrix). One gene responsible for repressing epithelial characteristics in the mesenchymal cells of the streak is snail, a zinc-finger transcription factor. Under its influence, expression of certain cell-to-cell adhesion molecules such as E-cadherin ceases, whereas expression of cytoskeletal proteins, such as vimentin, is induced. In addition, the cytoskeleton is altered by expression of members of the Rho family of GTPases such as RhoA and Rac1. These are required to regulate actin organization and the development of lamellipodia of gastrulating cells within the primitive streak. When GTPases are disrupted, cells accumulate and die within the space between epiblast and hypoblast. Similarly, loss-of-function mutations of a variety of adhesion and cytoskeletal molecules disrupt EMT. These include N-cadherin, a cell-cell adhesion molecule, and β-catenin, a cytoplasmic component of the cadherin/catenin adhesion complex, as well as afadin, an actin filament–binding protein. In addition to changes in adhesion and cytoskeleton, Fgf signaling plays a role in EMT. In loss-of-function mutations of fibroblast growth factor receptor 1 (Fgfr1), involuting cells lose their ability to ingress and, as a consequence, accumulate within the primitive streak.

ESTABLISHING MEDIAL-LATERAL SUBDIVISIONS OF MESODERM

Before formation of the mesoderm and its medial-lateral subdivisions is discussed, it is important to identify two areas of the early embryo that exert inductive influences across the embryo: the **Nieuwkoop center** and the **organizer** (often called the Spemann-Mangold organizer). The Nieuwkoop center is an early-forming organizing center that induces the organizer. The organizer in turn sends out signals to pattern the newly formed mesoderm into its medial-lateral subdivisions. These two signaling centers were first discovered in amphibians, but homologous centers exist in all vertebrate embryos. The Nieuwkoop center is not structurally distinct; rather it is defined by location in the early embryo and by its ability to induce the organizer. With molecular characterization of the Nieuwkoop center, gene expression patterns are used to identify it. In contrast to the Nieuwkoop center, the organizer is structurally distinct; it consists of the dorsal lip of the blastopore in amphibians, the embryonic shield in fish, Hensen's node in chick, the node in mouse, and the primitive node in humans. It also can be defined by its position in the early embryo, its ability to induce and pattern an embryonic axis (covered later in the chapter), and its gene expression patterns.

As covered earlier in the chapter, the mesoderm, after it moves between endoderm and ectoderm, quickly subdivides into several medial-lateral subdivisions. How are these subdivisions established? Experiments originally conducted in amphibian embryos suggest that gradients of secreted growth factors (i.e., **morphogens**) induce the mesodermal subdivisions. Because the early amphibian embryo is spherical rather than flat like the human embryo, formation of the medial-lateral subdivisions of the mesoderm is often referred to as dorsal-ventral patterning, with the most dorsal mesodermal subdivision being notochord, and the most ventral being lateral plate mesoderm (Fig. 3-10). Thus, to understand medial-lateral patterning of mesodermal subdivisions in the human embryo, it must be understood that dorsal mesoderm of the amphibian is equivalent to medial mesoderm of the human, and ventral mesoderm of the amphibian is equivalent to lateral mesoderm of the human. With formation of the body folds and establishment of the three-dimensional tube-within-a-tube body plan (covered in Chapter 4), the mesoderm that was originally most medial in the human (notochord) becomes the most dorsal mesoderm, and the mesoderm that was originally lateral in the human (lateral plate mesoderm) becomes the most ventral mesoderm.

Gradients involved in mesodermal patterning involve synergistic interactions between dorsalizing factors and ventralizing factors. **Dorsalizing factors** include protein products of the noggin, chordin, nodal, follistatin, and cerberus genes, whereas Bmps and Wnts act as **ventralizing factors**. These dorsalizing factors are secreted by the organizer and its derivatives (notochord and floor plate of the neural tube), and they act by antagonizing Bmp and/or Wnt signaling. Thus, each mesodermal subdivision is patterned by the specific level of Bmp and Wnt signaling that occurs in that subdivision, based on its position in relation to the organizer. In the presence of low Bmp and Wnt signaling, notochord forms; in the presence of high Bmp and Wnt signaling, lateral plate mesoderm forms. Bmp and Wnt signaling in the somites is attenuated with respect to that occurring in the lateral plate mesoderm but is enhanced relative to that occurring in the notochord. As one example, overexpression of Bmp or Wnt ventralizes the mesoderm and suppresses formation of the notochord, whereas overexpression of Bmp or Wnt antagonists (e.g., cerberus) induces ectopic notochords.

Loss-of-function experiments in mouse have identified transcription factors involved in the specification of intraembryonic mesoderm. For example, with loss of Foxa2 (a forkhead transcription factor previously known as Hnf3β) function, the node is not maintained as a distinct structure, and the notochord subsequently fails to form. Moreover, loss of Tbx6 function (a T-box–containing transcription factor gene closely related to the prototypical T-box gene brachyury) is required for the formation of paraxial mesoderm (i.e., somites). Thus, in addition to gradients of diffusible factors controlling specification of intraembryonic mesoderm, expression of transcription factors is required for differentiation and maintenance of cell fate.

SPECIFICS OF GASTRULATION: MOVING CELLS TO NEW LOCATIONS AND MAKING ORGAN RUDIMENTS THAT UNDERGO INDUCTIVE INTERACTIONS

FATE OF EPIBLAST CELLS DEPENDS ON THEIR SITE OF ORIGIN

Fate mapping and **cell lineage studies** in animal models have revealed the sites of origin of epiblast cells that give rise to various subdivisions of ectoderm, endoderm, and mesoderm. In fate mapping, groups of cells are marked in some manner (often with fluorescent dyes) and then are followed over time. In cell lineage studies, individual cells are marked (often genetically with reporter genes), rather than groups of cells, and their descendants are then followed over time. Both techniques allow construction of **prospective fate maps** (Fig. 3-11)—diagrams that show the locations of prospective groups of cells before the onset of gastrulation. Prospective fate maps show that cells of different germ layers and different subdivisions within germ layers are partially segregated from one another in the epiblast and primitive streak, although overlap between adjacent groups of cells is usually seen. Prospective fate maps reveal only which groups of cells in a particular region of the epiblast (or primitive streak) form during normal development. They reveal nothing about whether these cells are committed to a particular

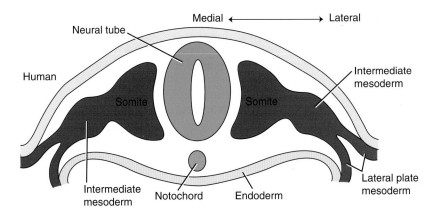

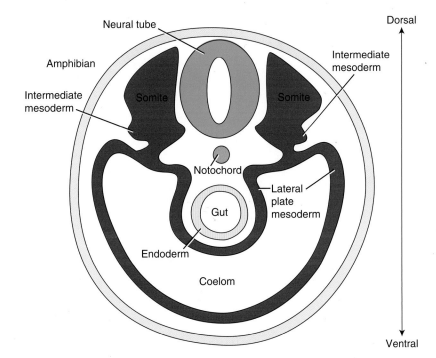

Figure 3-10. Diagrammatic cross-sectional views showing that the medial-lateral axis of the mesodermal subdivisions (notochord, somites, and intermediate mesoderm) of a flat embryo, like that of the early human (embryonic disc), is equivalent to the dorsal-ventral axis of the same mesodermal subdivisions in tubular amphibian embryos.

fate or are still **pluripotent**—that is, innately capable of developing into almost any cell type of the organism. Experiments have shown that most cells within the epiblast and primitive streak are indeed pluripotent and that their fates are specified by cell-cell interactions that occur during their migration or shortly after they arrive at their final destination. Thus, during gastrulation, the **prospective potency** of a group of epiblast cells, that is, what they are capable of forming at a particular stage of development, is typically far greater than their **prospective fate**, that is, what they are destined to form during normal development based on their place of origin.

Gastrulation involves a highly choreographed series of movements that occur over time (see Fig. 3-11). Beginning at the early primitive streak stage (Fig. 3-11*A*), **prospective gut (definitive) endoderm** moves from the epiblast surrounding the cranial half of the primitive streak into the primitive streak. It then migrates into the hypoblast to displace that layer and form a new layer of **definitive endoderm**. This process of endoderm formation occurs as late as the fully elongated primitive streak

stage. Additionally, at the early primitive streak stage, **prospective prechordal plate** within the cranial end of the primitive streak is ingressing at the cranial midline to form **prechordal plate**. The prechordal plate is one of the most misunderstood structures in human embryology. Experiments in chick and mouse provide strong evidence that the prechordal plate arises from the cranial end of the streak and intercalates into the endodermal layer, where it forms a thickening. The prechordal plate (some textbooks refer to it as *prochordal* plate) contributes to the **oropharyngeal membrane**—a two-layered membrane (ectoderm and endoderm) that ruptures to form the **mouth** opening. In addition, it forms an important signaling center involved in patterning the cranial end of the neural tube (future forebrain; covered in Chapter 4). Finally, evidence from animal models suggests that part of the prechordal plate undergoes an **epithelial-to-mesenchymal transformation** to form head mesenchyme cells that eventually reside at the cranial midline beneath the forebrain, just cranial to the notochord. Because the prechordal plate forms both mesodermal (part of head mesenchyme) and endodermal (part of oropharyngeal membrane) derivatives, it is often considered to be a **mesendodermal** structure.

Formation of the mesoderm also begins during the early primitive streak stage (Fig. 3-11*B*). **Prospective cardiogenic mesoderm** from the epiblast moves into the middle part of the primitive streak and then migrates cranially to form **cardiogenic mesoderm** flanking the oropharyngeal membrane. **Prospective extraembryonic mesoderm** moves from the epiblast into the caudal end of the primitive streak to contribute to the **extraembryonic mesoderm** of the amnion, yolk sac, and allantois (covered in Chapter 6).

At the mid-primitive streak stage (Fig. 3-11*C*), **prospective notochord** migrates cranially at the midline

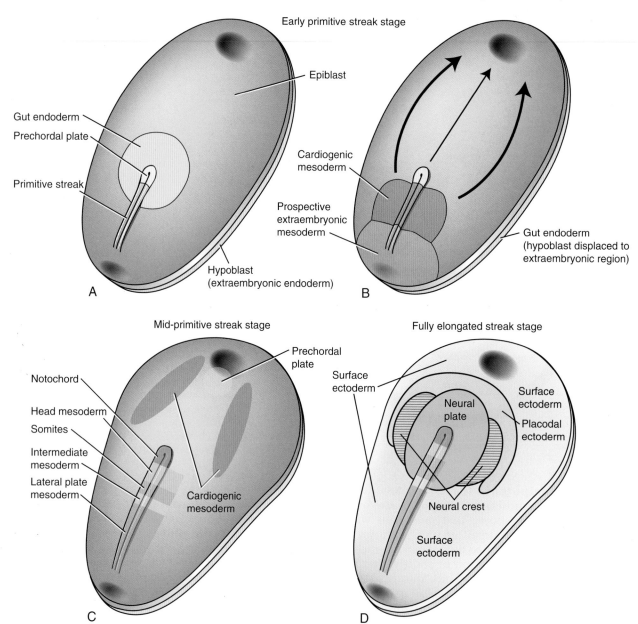

Figure 3-11. Prospective fate maps of the epiblast (based on data obtained from chick and mouse embryos), showing the regions of epiblast that ingress through the primitive streak and form the major subdivisions of the trilaminar embryonic disc. *A,* Early primitive streak stage. At this stage, the blastoderm consists of an upper epiblast and a lower hypoblast. The locations of the prospective gut endoderm in the epiblast and the prospective prechordal plate in the cranial end of the primitive streak are shown. Oval at the cranial end of the epiblast indicates the location of the future oropharyngeal membrane; caudal oval indicates future cloacal membrane. *B,* Early primitive streak stage showing the locations of the prospective cardiogenic mesoderm and the prospective extraembryonic mesoderm in the epiblast and primitive streak. Curved arrows indicate the directions of migration of the cardiogenic mesoderm. Straight arrow indicates the direction of migration of the prechordal plate. At this stage, the gut endoderm has ingressed and replaced the hypoblast as the lower layer beneath the epiblast. *C,* Mid-primitive streak stage showing the locations of the prospective mesoderm in the epiblast and primitive streak. These include prospective notochord, head mesoderm, somites, intermediate mesoderm, and lateral plate mesoderm. Note that the prechordal plate and the cardiogenic mesoderm have ingressed and lie deep to the epiblast. *D,* Fully elongated primitive streak stage showing the locations of the neural plate, surface ectoderm, neural crest cells, and placodal ectoderm after cells in the cranial half of the embryonic disc have completed their ingression into the primitive streak. Some epiblast still remains caudally at this stage, where cells are moving into and ingressing through the primitive streak.

to form the **notochordal process**. More caudally, and in cranial-to-caudal succession, **prospective head mesoderm** in the epiblast moves into and through the primitive streak to form the **head mesoderm**; **prospective somites** in the epiblast move into and through the primitive streak to form the **somites**; **prospective intermediate mesoderm** moves into and through the primitive streak to form **intermediate mesoderm**; and **prospective lateral plate mesoderm** moves into and through the primitive streak to form **lateral plate mesoderm**. Collectively, the prospective head mesoderm and prospective somites constitute the **paraxial mesoderm**.

At the fully elongated primitive streak stage, when the primitive streak has reached its maximal length and has not yet initiated its regression (Fig. 3-11*D*), movement of epiblast cells into the primitive streak is completed, except adjacent to the caudal end of the primitive streak. Thus, most of the epiblast now consists of **ectoderm**. The **prospective neural plate** is located cranial and lateral to the cranial end of the primitive streak. **Prospective neural crest cells**, a migratory population of ectodermal cells (covered in Chapter 4), flank the lateral sides of the neural plate. The **prospective placodal ectoderm**, a horseshoe-shaped area that forms sensory placodes (covered in Chapters 4 and 18), lies peripheral to the craniolateral borders of the neural plate, and the **prospective surface ectoderm** constitutes the remaining areas of the ectoderm. At this stage, only the neural plate and the surface ectoderm can be distinguished from one another when the ectoderm is viewed with scanning electron microscopy (see Fig. 3-9).

NOTOCHORD IS FORMED IN MULTIPLE STEPS

Animation 3-2: Formation of Notochord.
   Animations are available online at StudentConsult.

Formation of the notochord begins with cranial midline extension from the primitive node of a hollow tube, the **notochordal process**. This tube grows in length as primitive node cells are added to its proximal end, concomitant with regression of the primitive streak (Fig. 3-12).

When the notochordal process is completely formed, on about day twenty, several morphogenetic transformations are believed to take place to convert it from a hollow tube, to a flattened plate, to a solid rod (summarized in Fig. 3-13*C*). First, the ventral floor of the tube fuses with the underlying endoderm and the two layers break down, leaving behind the flattened **notochordal plate** (Fig. 3-13*A, B*). At the level of the primitive pit, the yolk sac cavity now transiently communicates with the amniotic cavity through an opening called the **neurenteric canal** (Fig. 3-13*B*). The **notochordal plate** then completely detaches from the endoderm, and its free ends fuse as it rolls up into the mesoderm-containing space between ectoderm and endoderm, changing as it does so into a solid rod called the **notochord** (Fig. 3-13*C*). Because the notochord derives from the primitive node and because it ends up in the mesodermal layer, it is considered to be a mesodermal derivative.

During later development, the rudiments of the vertebral bodies coalesce around the notochord, and it is commonly stated that the notochord forms the nucleus pulposus at the center of the vertebral discs. Certainly,

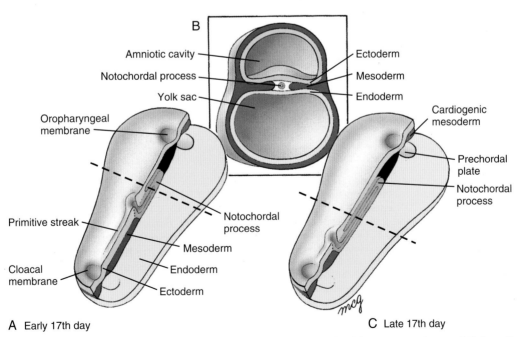

Figure 3-12. Formation of the notochordal process. *A, C,* Stages showing hollow notochordal process growing cranially from the primitive node (dissected in the midsagittal plane). Note changes in the relative length of the notochordal process and primitive streak as the embryo grows. Also note the fusion of ectoderm and endoderm in the oropharyngeal and cloacal membranes. *B,* Cross section of the embryonic disc at the level indicated by the dotted lines.

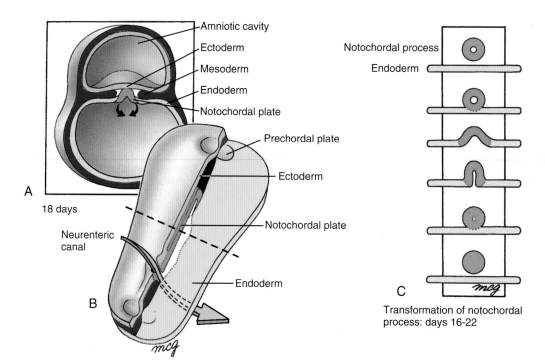

Figure 3-13. The process by which the hollow notochordal process is transformed into a solid notochord between days sixteen and twenty-two. *A, B,* First, the ventral wall of the notochordal process fuses with the endoderm, and the two layers break down, leaving behind the flattened notochordal plate. As shown in *B,* this process commences at the caudal end of the notochordal process and proceeds cranially (the dotted line marks the level of *A*). An open neurenteric canal is briefly created between the amniotic cavity and the yolk sac cavity. *C,* Series of events by which the notochordal process becomes the notochordal plate and then the notochord.

this is true in the embryo, the fetus, and young children. However, in early childhood, the nucleus pulposus cells of notochordal origin degenerate and are replaced by adjacent mesodermal cells. Thus, the notochord does not contribute to the bony elements of the spinal column. Rather, the notochord plays important inductive and patterning roles in early development (covered in Chapter 4) and is also involved in induction of the vertebral bodies (covered in Chapter 8).

In the Research Lab

CELLULAR BASIS OF CONVERGENT EXTENSION

In addition to epiboly and emboly, covered earlier in the chapter, convergent extension plays a role during gastrulation. In particular, formation of the notochordal plate involves convergent extension—the coordinated narrowing of a cluster of node-derived cells in the medial-lateral plane and concomitant lengthening in the cranial-caudal plane as the notochordal plate forms. Detailed studies of the process in amphibian embryos have revealed that convergent extension of the notochord is driven by **cell-to-cell intercalation**, that is, medial-lateral interdigitation of cells. As a metaphor, imagine four lanes of traffic merging into two lanes. If each lane contains five cars, to accommodate all twenty cars in two lanes each lane would need, on average, to double its length (and the number of cars it contains) as the number of lanes is halved. In other words, a concomitant increase in the length of the column of cars would be seen as the width of the merging traffic column was decreased.

Amphibians differ from birds and mammals in that early development of amphibians involves virtually no growth, whereas in birds and mammals, extensive growth occurs. Studies of notochord elongation in birds and mammals have revealed that, in addition to convergent extension generated by cell-to-cell intercalation, **oriented cell division** plays a role in convergent extension. Thus, mitotic division planes (i.e., metaphase plates) are positioned in dividing notochordal cells to separate daughter cells preferentially in the cranial-caudal plane, rather than in the medial-lateral plane. Modeling studies suggest that about half of the convergent extension that occurs in notochordal formation in birds and mammals is driven by cell-to-cell intercalation, whereas the other half is driven by oriented cell division.

PARAXIAL MESODERM DIFFERS IN HEAD AND TRUNK

The mesoderm that begins ingressing through the middle part of the primitive streak in mid-primitive streak stage embryos gives rise to the paraxial mesoderm that immediately flanks the notochord. In the future head region, this mesoderm forms bands of cells that remain unsegmented as the **head mesoderm** (Fig. 3-14*A*). The mesoderm becomes more dispersed with development to loosely fill the developing head as the **head mesenchyme**. Later, once neural crest cells start to migrate (covered in Chapter 4), the head mesenchyme becomes supplemented with **neural crest cells**. Thus, the head mesenchyme is derived from both head mesoderm and ectodermal neural crest cells (and at the most cranial midline, from the prechordal plate, as covered earlier in the chapter).

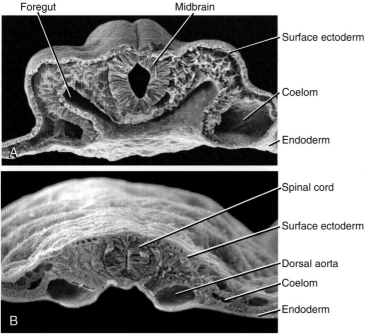

Foregut   Midbrain

Surface ectoderm

Coelom

Endoderm

A

Spinal cord

Surface ectoderm

Dorsal aorta

Coelom

Endoderm

B

Figure 3-14. Scanning electron micrographs of transversely sectioned chick embryos showing the head (*A*) and trunk (*B*) neural tube (midbrain and spinal cord) and subdivisions of the mesoderm (colored on left side, but uncolored on right side): notochord (flesh), paraxial mesoderm (orange), intermediate mesoderm (light green), and lateral plate mesoderm consisting of somatic mesoderm (purple) and splanchnic mesoderm (dark green). In the head, the lateral plate mesoderm (sometimes called the lateral mesoderm) is equivalent to the cardiogenic mesoderm. The splanchnic layer forms the heart wall, and the somatic layer forms part of the lining of the pericardial cavity.

The head mesoderm eventually gives rise to the striated muscles of the face, jaw, and throat. As described in Chapter 17, these muscles differentiate within the segmental pharyngeal arches, which develop on either side of the pharynx. The pharyngeal arches are central elements in the development of the neck and face.

In the future trunk region, the paraxial mesoderm also forms bands of cells, but these bands soon segment into **somites**, blocklike condensations of mesoderm (Figs. 3-14*B*, 3-15, 3-16). The first pair of somites forms on about day twenty at the head-trunk border. The remainder form in cranial-caudal progression at a rate of about three or four a day, finishing on about day thirty. Approximately forty-two to forty-four pairs of somites form, flanking the notochord from the occipital (skull base) region to the tip of the embryonic tail. However, the caudalmost several somites eventually disappear, giving a final count of approximately thirty-seven pairs.

Somites give rise to most of the axial skeleton, including the vertebral column and part of the occipital bone of the skull; to the voluntary musculature of the neck, body wall, and limbs; and to the dermis of the body. Thus, formation and segmentation of somites are of major importance in organization of the body structure.

The first four pairs of somites form in the occipital region. These somites contribute to the occipital part of the skull; to the extrinsic ocular muscles; and to muscles of the tongue (covered in Chapters 8 and 17). The next eight pairs of somites form in the presumptive **cervical** region. The most cranial cervical somites also contribute to the occipital bone, and others form the cervical vertebrae and associated muscles, as well as part of the dermis of the neck (covered in Chapters 8 and 17). The next twelve pairs, the **thoracic somites**, form thoracic vertebrae; the musculature and bones of the thoracic wall; the thoracic dermis; and part of the abdominal wall. Cells from cervical and thoracic somites also invade the

upper limb buds to form the limb musculature (covered in Chapters 8 and 20).

Caudal to the thoracic somites, the five **lumbar somites** form abdominal dermis, abdominal muscles, and lumbar vertebrae, and the five **sacral somites** form the sacrum with its associated dermis and musculature. Cells from lumbar somites invade the lower limb buds to form the limb musculature (covered in Chapters 8 and 20). Finally, the three or so **coccygeal somites** that remain after degeneration of the caudalmost somites form the coccyx.

In the Research Lab

MOLECULAR MECHANISM OF SOMITOGENESIS

Animation 3-3: Somitogenesis, Clock and Waveform Model.

  Animations are available online at StudentConsult.

Somites form rhythmically from the trunk and tail paraxial mesoderm—often referred to as the **presomitic mesoderm**—through the process of **segmentation**. Segmentation involves the formation of serially repeated, functionally equivalent units or **segments**, and segmentation is a common process occurring throughout much of the animal kingdom. Invertebrates and vertebrates seem to have developed somewhat different developmental strategies for segmentation. In *Drosophila*, for example, the entire blastoderm segments all at once, whereas during somitogenesis in vertebrates, segmentation occurs in a cranial-to-caudal wave. As a metaphor to visualize the difference between invertebrate and vertebrate segmentation, think of a bread-slicing machine in which the entire loaf of bread is sliced into "segments" all at the same time, as compared with using a bread knife to slice a loaf into segments beginning at one end of the loaf and progressing slice by slice to the other end.

  A breakthrough in our understanding of somitogenesis came with the discovery that certain genes, particularly those

Cranial

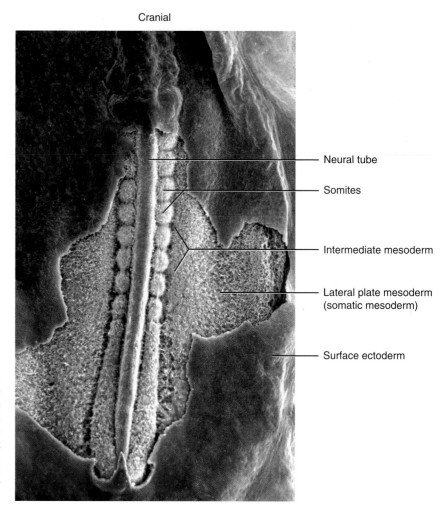

Neural tube

Somites

Intermediate mesoderm

Lateral plate mesoderm
(somatic mesoderm)

Surface ectoderm

Figure 3-15. Scanning electron micrograph of the trunk region of a chick embryo with the surface ectoderm partially removed to show the underlying neural tube and mesoderm (cranial is toward the top). Note the somites and, more caudally, the paraxial mesoderm that has not yet segmented. Lateral to the somites, the mesoderm has subdivided into the intermediate and lateral plate mesoderm (somatic mesoderm, the layer just deep to the surface ectoderm, is visible).

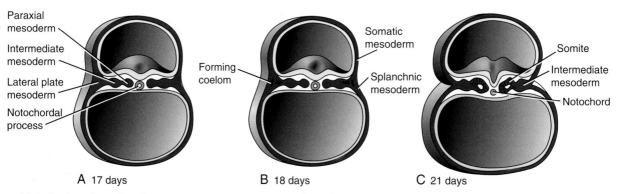

Figure 3-16. Sections through embryos at seventeen to twenty-one days of gestation showing the differentiation of mesoderm on either side of the midline. *A,* On day seventeen, the mesoderm has begun to differentiate into paraxial, intermediate, and lateral plate mesoderm. *B,* On day eighteen, the lateral plate begins to split to form intraembryonic coelom and somatic and splanchnic mesoderm. *C,* On day twenty-one, notochord, somites, and intermediate mesoderm are well formed, and splitting of the lateral plate mesoderm is complete.

in the notch signaling pathway (covered in Chapter 5), cycle in their expression in the presomitic mesoderm in concert with somitogenesis (Fig. 3-17). Specifically, expression of members of the notch family (such as lunatic fringe) spreads through the presomitic mesoderm in caudal-to-cranial sequence in a cycle that is synchronized with formation of each pair of somites. Thus, at a given axial level of presomitic mesoderm, cyclic gene expression seems to turn on and off when examined with in situ hybridization as each pair of somites form. Cycling can be very rapid, occurring every ninety minutes in chick and every twenty minutes (at 25° C) in zebrafish—the exact time it takes to from a new pair of somites in these organisms.

A number of years before cyclic genes were identified in the presomitic mesoderm, a model was proposed to explain somitogenesis. According to this model, called the **clock and wavefront model**, formation of somites involves an oscillator,

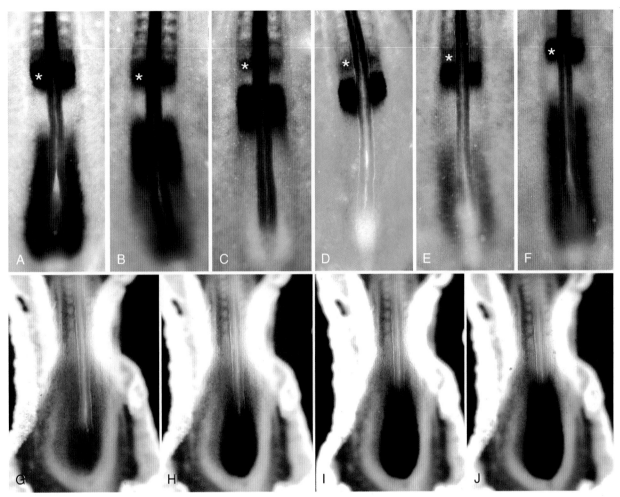

Figure 3-17. Cyclical expression of the gene lunatic fringe (*A-F*) and the Fgf8 protein gradient (*G-J*) during somitogenesis in the caudal region of the chick embryo (cranial is toward the top of each figure). *A-F*, Time course over the ninety-minute cycle of somite pair formation. Note the wave of lunatic fringe mRNA expression moving from caudal-to-cranial (*A-E*) in the unsegmented paraxial mesoderm, and into the last pair of newly formed somites (*F*). *G-J*, Increasing time of exposure of an antibody to Fgf8 protein. With a short exposure time to the antibody (*G*), only the tail bud and the most caudal segmental plate are labeled, indicating that a high concentration of protein is present in this region. With longer exposures (*H-J*), increasingly more cranial areas of segmental plate are labeled, demonstrating a caudal-to-cranial concentration gradient. Asterisk, level of last somite pair.

the so-called **segmentation clock**, whose periodic signal is used to specify somite boundaries at progressively more caudal levels, where the signal coincides in both time and space with a traveling threshold level of expression of another signaling molecule (Fig. 3-18). The segmentation clock controls expression of cyclic genes, the first of which to be identified was the hairy1 gene, an ortholog of the Drosophila segmentation gene hairy and a member of the notch family. Many other members of the notch family are now known to be part of the segmentation clock, and Wnt signaling also plays a role, such that the clockwork of the oscillator apparently involves a series of negative feedback loops between notch and Wnt signaling. Thus, this interaction establishes the rhythm of the clock and consequently the rhythm of somitogenesis.

Spacing of the somites is achieved by controlling the positioning of somite boundaries along the cranial-caudal axis using the wavefront. The wavefront is generated by a gradient of Fgf8, which is transcribed in the tail bud as the embryo undergoes cranial-caudal elongation. As cells migrate out of the tail bud into the presomitic mesoderm (covered in Chapter 4), transcription of Fgf8 stops. Moreover, Fgf8 progressively decays over time

in the cranially-caudally elongating presomitic mesoderm such that a concentration gradient of Fgf8 protein is established that is low cranially and high caudally in the presomitic mesoderm (see Fig. 3-17). This gradient is further refined by a gradient of retinoic acid that extends caudally from the previously formed somites into the presomitic mesoderm. The retinoic acid gradient antagonizes Fgf8 signaling in the cranial presomitic mesoderm and activates somitic genes such as the Mesp genes (bHLH transcription factors), the earliest-expressed somitic genes. As expression of cycling genes crosses the threshold-level point in the presomitic mesoderm, a region called the **determination** or **maturation wavefront**, the caudal boundary of a new pair of somites is specified. This is followed by new gene expression, as well as by changes in cell shape, position, and adhesion—all of which results in formation of somites.

The clock and wavefront model is supported by several experiments. For example, implantation of beads coated with Fgf8 protein into the cranial presomitic mesoderm of chick embryos prevents activation of their segmentation program. Furthermore, loss-of-function mutations in mouse cycling genes result in segmentation anomalies, including misplaced

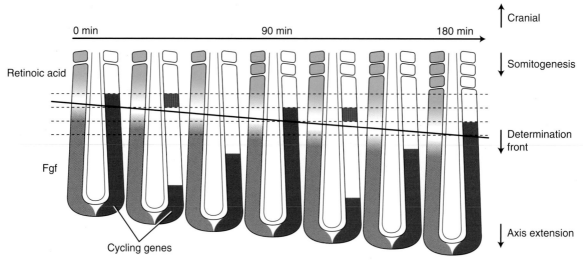

Figure 3-18. The molecular basis of the clock and wavefront model. Diagrams of the caudal end of chick embryos during two rounds of somitogenesis. Retinoic acid (blue) and Fgf8 (gray) gradients move caudally as the embryo elongates (axis extension) during somitogenesis. In chick, a somite pair forms every ninety minutes, which constitutes the length of the clock cycle. Expression of cycling genes (red) extends from caudal to cranial, and when expression of these genes spreads cranially to cross the threshold level of Fgf8 signaling (called the determination wavefront; diagonal line), somites are established (indicated by expression of Mesp genes; purple).

somitic boundaries and malformations of the vertebral column and ribs. Similarly, mutations in NOTCH signaling family in humans result in segmentation defects. Specifically, mutation of the NOTCH pathway ligand DELTA-LIKE3 gene results in an autosomal recessive condition called **spondylocostal dysostosis syndrome** (Jarcho-Levin syndrome), a condition in which abnormal segmentation of the vertebral column and ribs occurs. Moreover, **Alagille syndrome**, which includes segmentation defects, results from mutations of the NOTCH pathway ligand JAGGED1 or the NOTCH receptor NOTCH2. (Alagille syndrome is also mentioned in Chapters 5 and 12 through 14.)

As an interesting aside, the clock and wavefront model has been adjusted during evolution to give rise to differing numbers of somites (and hence vertebrae) in different organisms. For example, typical animal models used in developmental biology generate a relatively small number of somite pairs (zebrafish, 31; chicken, 55; mouse, 65), as does the human (33), but snakes can generate in excess of 300 somite pairs, and even up to 500 pairs. How is this number controlled? Experiments reveal that the snake segmental plate develops more slowly during somitogenesis than it does in embryos that develop far fewer somites, and it has a longer life span in which to contribute cells to the somites. In addition, its clock "ticks" about four times faster, generating many more somites. Adjustments in the timing of developmental events that give rise to morphological changes during evolution are referred to as **heterochrony**. The change that occurred in somite number during the evolution of snakes provides a dramatic example of this process.

INTERMEDIATE AND LATERAL PLATE MESODERM FORMS ONLY IN TRUNK

In addition to the notochord and paraxial mesoderm, both of which form in the head and trunk, two other subdivisions of mesoderm form in the trunk only: **intermediate mesoderm** and **lateral plate mesoderm** (see

Figs. 3-14*B*, 3-15, 3-16). The mesoderm lying immediately lateral to each somite also segments and forms a small cylindrical condensation—the **intermediate mesoderm**. The **intermediate mesoderm** produces the urinary system and parts of the genital system (covered in Chapters 15 and 16). Lateral to the intermediate mesoderm, the mesoderm remains unsegmented and forms a flattened sheet—the **lateral plate mesoderm**. Starting on day 17, the **lateral plate mesoderm** splits into two layers: a ventral layer associated with the endoderm and a dorsal layer associated with the ectoderm (see Figs. 3-14*B*, 3-16*B*, *C*). The layer adjacent to the endoderm gives rise to the mesothelial covering of the visceral organs (viscera), as well as to part of the wall of the viscera; hence, it is called the **splanchnic mesoderm** (from the Greek *splanchnon*, viscera). The layer adjacent to the ectoderm gives rise to the inner lining of the body wall and to parts of the limbs; hence, it is called the **somatic mesoderm** (from the Greek *soma*, body). Because the splanchnic mesoderm and adjacent endoderm act together to form structures, they are collectively called the **splanchnopleure**. Similarly, the somatic mesoderm and adjacent ectoderm act together to form structures; they are collectively called the **somatopleure**.

In the Clinic

ABNORMAL GASTRULATION LEADS TO CAUDAL DYSPLASIA

Caudal dysplasia, also called **caudal regression syndrome**, **caudal agenesis**, or **sacral agenesis**, is characterized by varying degrees of (1) flexion, inversion, and lateral rotation of the lower extremities; (2) anomalies of lumbar and sacral vertebrae; (3) imperforate anus; (4) agenesis of the kidneys and urinary tract; and (5) agenesis of the internal genital organs except for the gonads. In extreme cases, the deficiency in caudal development leads to fusion of the lower limb buds during early development, resulting in a "mermaid-like" habitus called **sirenomelia** (see Fig. 3-1; also see the "Clinical Taster" for this chapter).

In some individuals, caudal malformations are associated with more cranial abnormalities. One of these associations is called the **VATER association** because it includes some or all of the following anomalies: vertebral defects, anal atresia, tracheal-esophageal fistula (covered in Chapter 11), and renal defects and radial forearm anomalies. An extension of this association, the **VACTERL association**, also includes cardiovascular anomalies with renal and limb defects. A number of other syndromes may be related to these associations.

Although the anomalies found in these associations are diverse, it is believed that they all arise from defects resulting from abnormal growth and migration during gastrulation. Mesodermal structures formed during the third and fourth weeks participate in the development of most of the structures involved in caudal dysplasia and associated malformations. For example, the sacral and coccygeal vertebrae form from structures called **sclerotomes** that develop from the sacral and caudal somites (covered in Chapters 4 and 8). The intermediate mesoderm differentiates into kidneys in response to induction by the ingrowing mesoderm ureteric buds (covered in Chapter 15). Imperforate anus may result from the improper migration of caudal mesodermal in relation to the forming anal membrane (covered in Chapter 14), whereas tracheoesophageal fistulas may be caused by defective interaction between endodermal foregut rudiment and mesoderm (covered in Chapter 11). Radial forearm malformations apparently result from anomalous migration and differentiation of lateral plate mesoderm (covered in Chapter 20).

In animal models, caudal dysplasia can be induced by both environmental factors and mutations. For example, insulin, when injected into the chick egg during gastrulation, causes caudal dysplasia, thereby acting as a **teratogen**—a substance that causes malformation of the embryo or fetus (**teratogenesis** and teratogens are further covered in Chapters 5 and 6). Similar defects are observed in mice with mutations in the brachyury gene, a T-box–containing transcription factor expressed throughout the primitive streak during gastrulation (Fig. 3-19). Analysis of such mice indicates that the mutation interferes with gastrulation by preventing the normal ingression of epiblast cells through the primitive streak, thus providing insight into how widespread mesodermal anomalies could result in humans with caudal dysplasia. In humans, caudal dysplasia is a common manifestation of **maternal (gestational) diabetes** with elevated INSULIN levels (covered in Chapter 6).

FORMATION OF NEURAL PLATE

The first event in the development of the future central nervous system is the formation on day eighteen of a thickened **neural plate** in the ectoderm just cranial to the **primitive node** (Figs. 3-20, 3-21, 3-22). Formation of the neural plate is induced by the primitive node, the human equivalent of the **organizer** covered early in the chapter. Thus, the process of neural plate formation is called **neural induction**. As a result of neural induction, ectodermal cells differentiate into a thick plate of pseudostratified, columnar **neuroepithelial cells (neuroectoderm)**. The neural plate forms first at the cranial end of the embryo and then differentiates in a cranial-to-caudal direction. As described in Chapter 4, the neural plate folds during the fourth week to form a neural tube, the precursor of the central nervous system. The lateral lips of the neural plate also give rise to an extremely important population of cells, **neural crest cells**, which

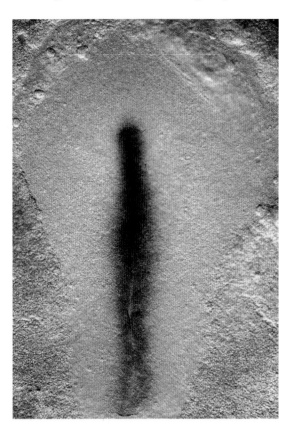

Figure 3-19. In situ hybridization showing localization of chick brachyury mRNA, a T-box–containing transcription factor that is expressed throughout the primitive streak.

detach during formation of the neural tube and migrate in the embryo to form a variety of structures.

The neural plate is broad cranially and is tapered caudally. The expanded cranial portion gives rise to **brain**. Even at this very early stage of differentiation, the presumptive brain is visibly divided into three regions: the future **forebrain**, **midbrain**, and **hindbrain** (see Figs. 3-20, 3-21). The narrower caudal portion of the neural plate (continuous cranially with the hindbrain) gives rise to the **spinal cord**. Eventually, this level of the developing nervous system will be flanked by somites. The notochord lies at the midline just deep to the neural plate. It extends cranially from the primitive node to end near the future juncture between forebrain and midbrain.

In the Research Lab

NEURAL INDUCTION

As in dorsal-ventral patterning of the mesoderm, induction of the neural plate involves the secretion of antagonists by the **organizer** to inhibit signaling. Recall that the **Nieuwkoop center** induces the organizer, which patterns the mesoderm in the dorsal-ventral plane. In addition, the organizer induces the **neural plate**. Although the location of the **Nieuwkoop center** is well established in amphibians, its location in birds and mammals remains uncertain. Nevertheless, loss-of-function experiments in mouse suggest that similar molecules induce the organizer in both lower and higher vertebrates. These include members of the Tgfβ (e.g., nodal) and Wnt families.

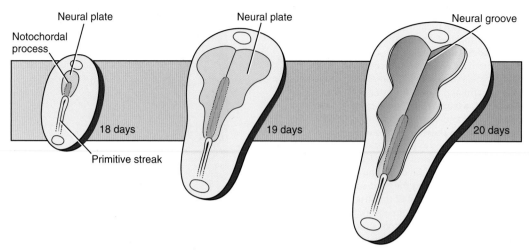

Figure 3-20. Schematic sequence showing growth of the neural plate and regression of the primitive streak between day eighteen and day twenty. The primitive streak shortens only slightly, but it occupies a progressively smaller proportion of the length of the embryonic disc as the neural plate and the embryonic disc grow.

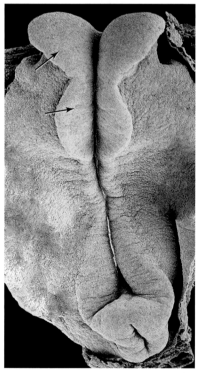

Figure 3-21. Scanning electron micrograph of a macaque embryo comparable with a twenty-day human embryo. The neural plate is clearly visible, and the expansions that will become the major subdivisions of the brain are apparent (arrows). Only a small region of the primitive streak remains. The primitive streak will disappear on day twenty-five.

The **organizer** has the amazing capacity to induce an entire secondary embryonic axis if grafted to an ectopic site of another embryo (Fig. 3-23A). This phenomenon was first discovered in the 1920s by Hilde Mangold and Hans Spemann, who were working with amphibian embryos. More than one dozen molecules are secreted by the organizer, and many of these, especially chordin (covered earlier in the chapter), have the capacity to induce secondary axes when ectopically expressed. In addition to secreted factors, the organizer expresses about ten transcription factors. Ectopic expression of some of these, such as goosecoid, also induces secondary axes (Fig. 3-23B).

The organizer induces neural plate by antagonizing the Bmp signaling pathway. In the presence of Bmp signaling, ectoderm forms **surface ectoderm**, but when Bmp signaling is inhibited, ectoderm forms **neural plate**. Bmp signaling is antagonized by the secretion of Bmp antagonists (covered earlier in the chapter) such as noggin, chordin, follistatin, and cerberus, all of which bind Bmp in the extracellular space and prevent Bmp from binding to its receptors.

In addition to antagonizing the Bmp signaling pathway, the organizer induces neural plate by secreting other growth factors, such as Fgf8 and members of the Igf (insulin-like growth factor) family. It is interesting to note that Fgf, Igf, and Bmp pathways intersect at a common point during neural induction: Smad1 phosphorylation. Both Fgf/Igf and Bmp signaling result in Smad1 phosphorylation, although at different sites. Phosphorylation as a result of Fgf/Igf signaling causes inhibition of Smad1 activity, whereas phosphorylation as a result of Bmp signaling causes stimulation of Smad1 activity. Consequently, the combined effect of Fgf/Igf signaling (inhibition of Smad1 activity) and antagonism of Bmp signaling (non-stimulation of Smad1 activity) results in a low level of Smad1 activity and neural induction.

HEAD, TRUNK, AND TAIL ORGANIZERS

Once the primitive streak has formed, it will give rise to endoderm and mesoderm of three distinct regions of the body: head, trunk, and tail. Neural induction results in formation of the neural plate, and, as covered in Chapter 4, neurulation subsequently converts the neural plate into a neural tube. The latter is quickly regionalized along the cranial-caudal axis into forebrain, midbrain, hindbrain, and spinal cord. Similarly, the mesoderm is regionalized along the cranial-caudal axis (e.g., unsegmented head paraxial mesoderm versus segmented trunk paraxial mesoderm). How does this regionalization occur?

Our understanding of cranial-caudal patterning comes from a large series of experiments in four vertebrate models: Xenopus, zebrafish, chick, and mouse. Thus cranial-caudal patterning of the embryo is typically called anterior-posterior patterning because the cranial-caudal axis of human embryos is equivalent to the anterior-posterior axis of vertebrate embryo

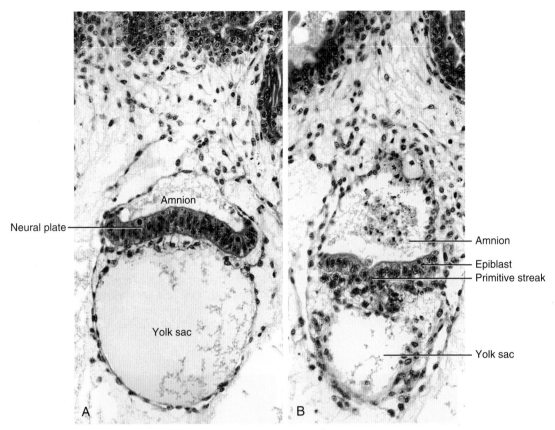

Figure 3-22. Cross sections through early human embryos. *A*, Level of neural plate. Note yolk sac cavity and amniotic cavity. *B*, Level of primitive streak. Note that the epiblast is not as thickened as the neural plate.

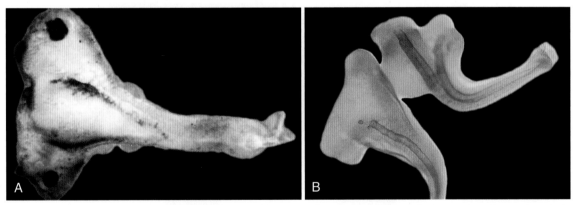

Figure 3-23. Experiments on the role of the organizer. *A*, Donor blastopore (i.e., the organizer) grafted onto a host frog embryo induces formation of a complete secondary body axis, resulting in the formation of "conjoined" twins. *B*, A frog embryo was irradiated with ultraviolet light to abolish "organizer" activity, and then two blastomeres were injected with goosecoid mRNA, resulting in induction of two embryonic axes.

models (covered in Introduction). In some of the vertebrate embryo models, separate **organizing centers** exist to pattern different levels of the cranial-caudal axis. For example, in mouse the head is patterned by the **head organizer**, also known as the **anterior visceral endoderm (AVE)**, a specialized region of extraembryonic endoderm (covered earlier in the chapter), whereas the **node** functions as a **trunk organizer**. In zebrafish, a separate **tail organizer** has been identified and is called the **ventral margin**. In other vertebrate models, these organizers seem to be combined, at least partly, in the classic organizer. For example, in chick, the

cranial end of the primitive streak first contains cells that pattern the head and later contains cells that pattern the trunk and tail. Thus, the organizer in chick is a dynamic structure in which cell populations contained within it change over time, and as a result of this change in populations, changes occur in the molecules secreted by the organizer that act to pattern the overlying neural plate along the cranial-caudal axis.

Regardless of where the signals originate during cranial-caudal patterning, comparison of results from gain-of-function and loss-of-function experiments in all four vertebrate models (covered above) has revealed that mechanisms of head, trunk, and tail patterning are highly conserved among species. Formation of all three levels of the body involves a common theme: **combinatorial signaling**, in which the amount of three signaling molecules expressed varies at different levels. The signaling molecules consist of Wnts, Bmps, and nodal.

Formation of the **head** requires inhibition of Wnt and Bmp signaling. Thus, the head organizer, be it a separate signaling center or part of the organizer itself depending on the organism, secretes Wnt and Bmp signaling antagonists. Loss-of-function of these inhibitors results in loss of head structures. For example, loss-of-function in mouse of the Wnt signaling inhibitor dickkopf1, which is expressed by the AVE, results in loss of the most cranial part of the head (Fig. 3-24A). In addition to factors secreted by the AVE, transcription factors are required for head development. One of these is the homeobox-containing gene Lim-1 (Fig 3-24B). Similar experiments suggest that nodal signaling plays little if any direct role in patterning of the head.

Formation of the trunk, in contrast to that of the head, requires Wnt and nodal signaling, as well as inhibition of Bmp signaling. Similarly, formation of the tail requires Wnt and nodal signaling, but in contrast to that of the trunk, formation of the tail also requires Bmp signaling.

PRIMARY VERSUS SECONDARY BODY DEVELOPMENT

On day sixteen, the primitive streak spans about half the length of the embryo. However, as gastrulation proceeds, the primitive streak regresses caudally, becoming gradually shorter. By day twenty-two, the primitive streak represents about 10% to 20% of the embryo's length, and by day twenty-six, it seems to disappear. However, on about day twenty, remnants of the primitive streak swell to produce a caudal midline mass of mesoderm called the **tail bud** or **caudal eminence**, which will give rise to the most caudal structures of the body. Formation of the tail bud provides a reservoir of cells that allow the embryo to extend caudally during formation of its rudimentary and transient tail. In particular, the tail bud contributes cells to the caudal end of the **neural tube** and **neural crest cells** (sacral and coccygeal), as well as the caudal **somites**. By contrast, the **notochord** of the tail extends into this region from more cranial levels, rather than forming from the tail bud, and may serve a role in organizing and patterning caudal organ rudiments.

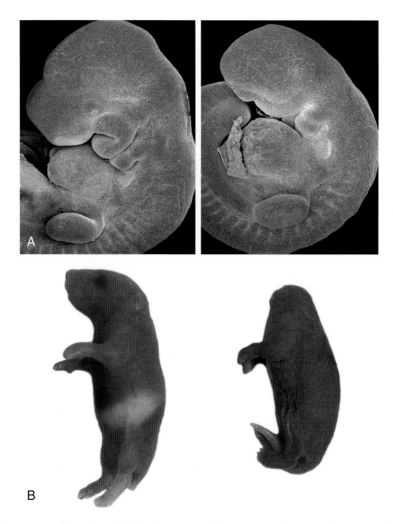

Figure 3-24. "Headless" mice. *A*, Loss-of-function of dickkopf1, a secreted antagonist of Wnt signaling, causes loss of the most cranial end of the head in mice (shown on right; left, wild-type control mouse). *B*, Similarly, loss-of-function of the homeobox-containing gene Lim-1 results in a more dramatic loss (shown on right; left, wild-type control mouse).

Gastrulation occurs during a period of development called **primary body development**. During primary body development, the primitive streak gives rise to the three primary germ layers, which subsequently assemble into organ rudiments. Formation of the rudimentary tail occurs after gastrulation is complete, during a period of development called **secondary body development**. In contrast to primary body development, secondary body development involves the direct formation of organ rudiments from the tail bud without the prior formation of distinct germ layers.

spectrum. As covered in this chapter, Shh is expressed by the notochord, the floor plate of the neural tube, and the prechordal plate—structures that interact with the overlying ectoderm to establish the midline.

Now researchers have seized on this plant poison as a treatment in a number of human cancers where overproliferation of cells mediated by the Shh pathway leads to cancer. Cyclopamine is being investigated as a chemotherapeutic drug for medulloblastoma, basal cell carcinoma, rhabdomyosarcoma, and breast and prostate cancers. Drugs like cyclopamine that specifically target signaling pathways in tumors promise better cancer treatments with fewer side effects than traditional broad-spectrum cytotoxic chemotherapy.

Embryology in Practice

LAMBS AND HEDGEHOGS

The intersection of two scientific stories that began in the1960s and the 1970s is today yielding a promising antitumor drug.

The first story began in Idaho in the late 1950s when multiple lambs were born with a single eye in the middle of their foreheads (a defect called **cyclopia** after the Cyclops of Greek mythology). By following the sheep day and night, researchers identified the culprit: the plant *Veratrum californicum*, also known as the corn lily, which when eaten by pregnant ewes caused cyclopia. After eleven years of painstaking research, the plant compound specifically responsible was purified and named "cyclopamine," but exactly how the compound caused cyclopia remained unknown for many years.

The other story had its origins in the 1970s with the description of a Drosophila mutant that was covered with pointy projections of denticle. Consequently, the mutant was named the "hedgehog" mutant, and the mutated gene, the hedgehog gene. The hedgehog gene, as covered in Chapter 5, is a secreted signaling molecule. Extensive study of the hedgehog signaling pathway led to the discovery that mutations in one of its mammalian orthologs, called **sonic hedgehog** (Shh), resulted in **holoprosencephaly** and **cyclopia** in humans (also covered in Chapters 5, 17, and 19). This important finding helped form the link between cyclopamine and the Shh pathway.

Cyclopamine inhibits the function of **smoothened**, an activator of the Shh pathway, which normally acts to switch on cell division. During embryonic development, inhibition of the Shh pathway with cyclopamine slows cell division in midline structures, resulting in smaller brains with fused anterior structures (holoprosencephaly) and reduced space between the eyes (hypotelorism) or even cyclopia at the severe end of the

SUGGESTED READINGS

Bettencourt-Dias M, Hildebrandt F, Pellman D, et al. 2011. Centrosomes and cilia in human disease. Trends Genet 27:307–315.

De Robertis EM. 2009. Spemann's organizer and the self-regulation of embryonic fields. Mech Dev 126:925–941.

Dequeant ML, Pourquie O. 2008. Segmental patterning of the vertebrate embryonic axis. Nat Rev Genet 9:370–382.

Fliegauf M, Benzing T, Omran H. 2007. When cilia go bad: cilia defects and ciliopathies. Nat Rev Mol Cell Biol 8:880–893.

Gibb S, Maroto M, Dale JK. 2010. The segmentation clock mechanism moves up a notch. Trends Cell Biol 20:593–600.

Goetz SC, Anderson KV. 2010. The primary cilium: a signalling centre during vertebrate development. Nat Rev Genet 11:331–344.

Gomez C, Ozbudak EM, Wunderlich J, et al. 2008. Control of segment number in vertebrate embryos. Nature 454:335–339.

Hildebrandt F, Benzing T, Katsanis N. 2011. Ciliopathies. N Engl J Med 364:1533–1543.

Hirokawa N, Tanaka Y, Okada Y. 2012. Cilia, KIF3 molecular motor and nodal flow. Current opinion in cell biology 24:31–39.

Revenu C, Gilmour D. 2009. EMT 2.0: shaping epithelia through collective migration. Curr Opin Genet Dev 19:338–342.

Rogers CD, Moody SA, Casey ES. 2009. Neural induction and factors that stabilize a neural fate. Birth Defects Res C Embryo Today 87:249–262.

Rossant J, Tam PP. 2009. Blastocyst lineage formation, early embryonic asymmetries and axis patterning in the mouse. Development 136:701–713.

Shiratori H, Hamada H. 2006. The left-right axis in the mouse: from origin to morphology. Development 133:2095–2104.

Skoglund P, Keller R. 2010. Integration of planar cell polarity and ECM signaling in elongation of the vertebrate body plan. Curr Opin Cell Biol 22:589–596.

Vonk FJ, Richardson MK. 2008. Developmental biology: Serpens clocks tick faster. Nature 454:282–283.

Chapter 4

Fourth Week: Forming the Embryo

SUMMARY

During the fourth week, the tissue layers laid down in the third week differentiate to form the primordia of most of the major organ systems of the body. Simultaneously, the embryonic disc undergoes a process of folding that creates the basic vertebrate body form, called the **tube-within-a-tube body plan**. The main force responsible for embryonic folding is the differential growth of different portions of the embryo. The embryonic disc grows vigorously during the fourth week, particularly in length, whereas the growth of the yolk sac stagnates. Because the outer rim of the embryonic endoderm is attached to the yolk sac, the expanding disc bulges into a convex shape. Folding commences in the cranial and lateral regions of the embryo on day twenty-two, and in the caudal region on day twenty-three. As a result of folding, the cranial, lateral, and caudal edges of the embryonic disc are brought together along the ventral midline. The endodermal, mesodermal, and ectodermal layers of the embryonic disc fuse to the corresponding layer on the opposite side, thus creating a tubular **three-dimensional body form**. The process of midline fusion transforms the flat embryonic endoderm into a **gut tube**. Initially, the gut consists of cranial and caudal blind-ending tubes—**foregut** and **hindgut**, respectively—separated by the future **midgut**, which remains open to the yolk sac. As the lateral edges of the various embryonic disc layers continue to join together along the ventral midline, the midgut is progressively converted into a tube, and, correspondingly, the yolk sac neck is reduced to a slender **vitelline duct**. When the edges of the ectoderm fuse along the ventral midline, the space formed within the lateral plate mesoderm is enclosed in the embryo and becomes the **intraembryonic coelom**. The lateral plate mesoderm gives rise to the **serous membranes** that line the coelom—the **somatic mesoderm** coating the inner surface of the body wall and the **splanchnic mesoderm** ensheathing the gut tube.

Neurulation converts the neural plate into a hollow **neural tube** covered by **surface ectoderm**. The neural tube then begins to differentiate into **brain** and **spinal cord**. Even before the end of the fourth week, the major regions of the brain—**forebrain, midbrain,** and **hindbrain**—become apparent, and neurons and glia begin to differentiate from the neuroepithelium of the neural tube. As neurulation occurs, **neural crest cells** detach from the lateral lips of the neural folds and migrate to numerous locations in the body, where they differentiate to form a wide range of structures and cell types.

Somites continue to segregate from the paraxial mesoderm in cranial-caudal progression until day thirty. Meanwhile, beginning in the cervical region, the somites subdivide into two kinds of mesodermal primordia: **dermamyotomes** and **sclerotomes**. Dermamyotomes contribute to the dermis of the neck and trunk, as well as to the **myotomes**, which form the segmental musculature of the back and the ventrolateral body wall; additionally, myotomes give rise to cells that migrate into the limb buds to form the **limb musculature**. Sclerotomes give rise to vertebral bodies and vertebral arches and contribute to the base of the skull.

Clinical Taster

A twenty-year-old university sophomore is surprised to learn that his nineteen-year-old girlfriend is pregnant. They have been having sex for only three months and have timed intercourse using the **rhythm method** of **birth control**, at least most of the time. On their first visit to student health services, they are told that the pregnancy is now in the eighth week and all seems normal. They decide to wait two months until spring break, when they will visit with their families, who live in neighboring towns, to inform them about the pregnancy.

Although both sets of parents are shocked by the news, they are supportive and arrange an immediate appointment with an obstetrician. Ultrasound examination reveals that the fetus is growing normally. However, a mass of bowel is detected protruding from the ventral (anterior) body wall into the amniotic cavity. The diagnosis of **gastroschisis** is made (Fig. 4-1*A*). On a follow-up visit, the young mother-to-be is very anxious. She's concerned that perhaps she did something to cause her baby to have gastroschisis. The doctor assures her that this is not the case and that sometimes developmental events just go awry, resulting in birth defects.

The couple decides to return to school to complete the semester and then to move back home, where they can receive more intensive prenatal care. Beginning at thirty weeks of gestation, weekly ultrasounds are scheduled to examine the thickness of the bowel wall. Based on evidence that the wall is beginning to thicken and thus is becoming damaged by exposure to the amniotic fluid, labor is induced at thirty-five weeks. At delivery, a three-centimeter opening in the abdominal wall is noted to the right of the baby's umbilicus, along with multiple loops of protruding bowel (Fig. 4-1*B*). The newborn baby is taken immediately to surgery to return the bowel to the abdominal cavity and to repair the body wall defect. Although it is a relatively common birth defect, the cause of gastroschisis remains unknown.

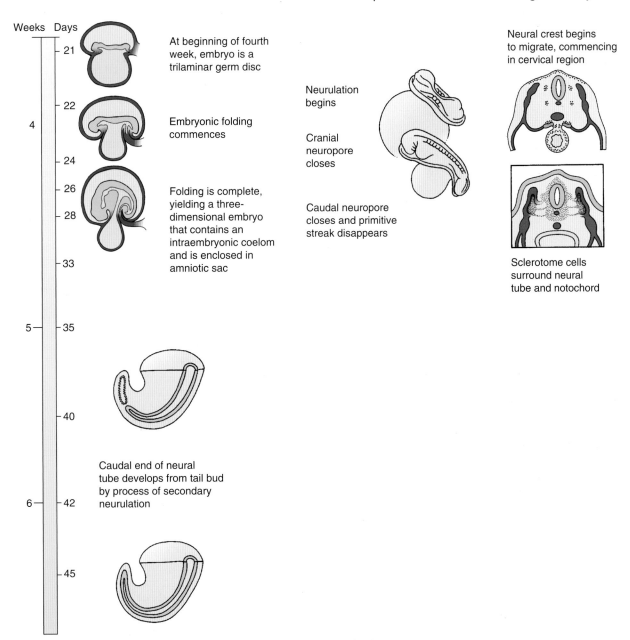

Weeks Days

21 At beginning of fourth week, embryo is a trilaminar germ disc

22

4

Embryonic folding commences

24

26

28 Folding is complete, yielding a three-dimensional embryo that contains an intraembryonic coelom and is enclosed in amniotic sac

33

Neurulation begins

Cranial neuropore closes

Caudal neuropore closes and primitive streak disappears

Neural crest begins to migrate, commencing in cervical region

Sclerotome cells surround neural tube and notochord

5 — 35

40

Caudal end of neural tube develops from tail bud by process of secondary neurulation

6 — 42

45

Time line. Fourth week of development.

TUBE-WITHIN-A-TUBE BODY PLAN ARISES THROUGH BODY FOLDING

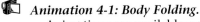 *Animation 4-1: Body Folding.*
   Animations are available online at StudentConsult.

At the end of the third week, the embryo is a flat, ovoid, trilaminar disc. During the fourth week, it grows rapidly, particularly in length, and undergoes a process of folding that generates the recognizable vertebrate body form (Figs. 4-2, 4-3). Although some active remodeling of tissue layers takes place, including localized changes in cell shape within the **body folds**, the main force responsible for embryonic folding is the differential growth of various tissues. During the fourth week, the embryonic disc and the amnion grow vigorously, but the yolk sac hardly grows at all. Because the yolk sac is attached to the ventral rim of the embryonic disc, the expanding disc balloons into a three-dimensional, somewhat cylindrical shape. The developing notochord, neural tube, and somites stiffen the dorsal axis of the embryo; therefore, most of the folding is concentrated in the thin, flexible outer rim of the disc. The cranial, caudal, and lateral margins of the disc fold completely under the dorsal axial structures and give rise to the ventral surface of the body. The areas of folding are referred to as **cranial (head)**, **caudal (tail)**, and **lateral body folds**, respectively. The cranial and caudal folds are best viewed in midsagittal sections (Fig. 4-2A-C; arrows in B), and the paired lateral body folds are best viewed in cross sections (Fig. 4-2D, E; arrows in D). Although in sections these folds have different names, it is important to realize that these folds become continuous

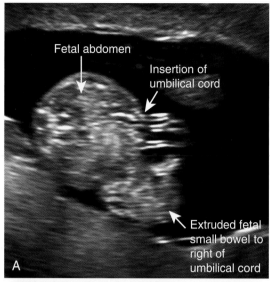

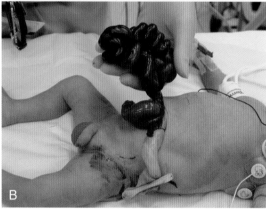

Figure 4-1. Gastroschisis. *A,* Sonogram showing the defect in a six-teen-week fetus. *B,* Newborn. The bowel herniates through an open-ing in the body wall to the right of the umbilical cord (the umbilical cord is clamped just proximal to its level of transection) and is not contained within a membranous sac.

mouth and carries the cardiogenic area and septum trans-versum toward the future chest (see Fig. 4-2*A-C*).

Starting on about day twenty-three, a similar process of folding commences in the caudal region of the embryo as the rapidly lengthening neural tube and somites over-grow the caudal rim of the yolk sac. Because of the relative stiffness of these dorsal axial structures, the thin caudal rim of the embryonic disc, which contains the cloacal membrane, folds under and becomes part of the ventral surface of the embryo (see Fig. 4-2*A-C*). When the caudal rim of the disc folds under the body, the connecting stalk (which connects the caudal end of the embryonic disc to the developing placenta) is carried cranially until it merges with the neck of the yolk sac, which has begun to lengthen and constrict (see Figs. 4-2, 4-3). The root of the **connecting stalk** contains a slender endodermal hind-gut diverticulum called the **allantois** (see Fig. 4-2*A-C*). The fate of the allantois is covered in Chapter 15.

Simultaneously with cranial-caudal body folding, the right and left sides of the embryonic disc flex sharply ven-trally, constricting and narrowing the neck of the yolk sac (see Fig. 4-2*D*). At the head and tail ends of the embryo, these lateral edges of the embryonic disc make contact with each other and then zip up toward the site of the future **umbilicus**. When the edges meet, the ectodermal, meso-dermal, and endodermal layers on each side fuse with the corresponding layers on the other side (see Fig. 4-2*D, E*). As a result, the ectoderm of the original embryonic disc covers the entire surface of the three-dimensional embryo except for the future **umbilical region**, where the yolk sac and the connecting stalk emerge. The ectoderm, along with contributions from the dermamyotomes, lateral plate mesoderm, and neural crest cells, will eventually form the skin (covered in Chapter 7).

The endoderm of the trilaminar embryonic disc is des-tined to give rise to the lining of the gastrointestinal tract. When the cranial, caudal, and lateral edges of the embryo meet and fuse, the cranial and caudal portions of the endoderm are converted into blind-ending tubes—the future **foregut** and **hindgut**. At first, the central **mid-gut** region remains broadly open to the yolk sac (see Fig. 4-2*A-D*). However, as the gut tube forms, the neck of the yolk sac is gradually constricted, reducing its communica-tion with the midgut. By the end of the sixth week, the gut tube is fully formed, and the neck of the yolk sac has been reduced to a slim stalk called the **vitelline duct** (see Fig. 4-2*C*). The cranial end of the foregut is capped by the oropharyngeal membrane, which ruptures at the end of the fourth week to form the mouth. The caudal end of the hindgut is capped by the cloacal membrane, which ruptures during the seventh week to form the orifices of the anus and the urogenital system (covered in Chapters 14 through 16).

As described in Chapter 3, the lateral plate meso-derm splits into two layers: the **somatic mesoderm**, which associates with the ectoderm, and the **splanch-nic mesoderm**, which associates with the endoderm. The space between these layers is originally open to the chorionic cavity. However, when the folds of the embryo fuse along the ventral midline, this space is enclosed within the embryo and becomes the **intraembryonic coelom** (see Fig. 4-2*E*). The **serous membranes** lining

with one another as a ring of tissue at the position of the future umbilicus.

As described in Chapter 3, the cranial rim of the embry-onic disc—the thin area located cranial to the neural plate—contains the oropharyngeal membrane, which represents the future mouth of the embryo. Cranial to the oropharyn-geal membrane, a second important structure has begun to appear: the horseshoe-shaped **cardiogenic area**, which will give rise to the heart (covered in Chapter 12). Cranial to the cardiogenic area, a third important struc-ture forms: the **septum transversum**. This structure appears on day twenty-two as a thickened bar of meso-derm; it lies just caudal to the cranial margin of the embryonic disc. The septum transversum forms the ini-tial partition separating the coelom into thoracic and abdominal cavities and gives rise to part of the diaphragm and the ventral mesentery of the stomach and duodenum (covered in Chapters 11 and 14).

Forward growth of the neural plate causes the thin cranial rim of the disc to fold under, forming the ventral surface of the future face, neck, and chest. This process translocates the oropharyngeal membrane to the region of the future this cavity form from the two layers of the lateral plate mesoderm: the inside of the body wall is lined with the somatic mesoderm, and the visceral organs derived from the gut tube are invested by splanchnic mesoderm.

As a result of body folding, the **tube-within-a-tube body plan** is established (see Fig. 4-2E). This plan consists of an embryo body design composed of two main tubes: an outer ectodermal tube forming the external layer of the skin (epidermis) and an inner endodermal tube forming the inner layer of the gut. The space between the two tubes is filled mainly with mesoderm, the lateral plate mesodermal part of which splits to form the body cavity, or **coelom**. The neural tube, derived from the outer ectodermal tube, becomes internalized during the process of neurulation (covered below).

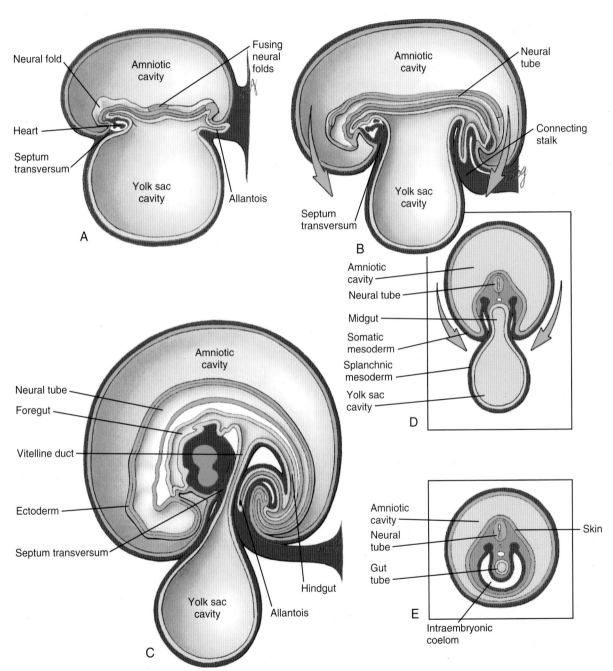

Figure 4-2. The process of craniocaudal and lateral folding that transforms the embryo from a flat embryonic disc to a three-dimensional tube-within-a-tube body plan. As folding occurs, the embryo grows more rapidly than the yolk sac, the cavity of which remains continuous with the developing gut tube through the narrowing vitelline duct. A-E, The septum transversum forms cranial to the cardiogenic area in the embryonic disc (A), and both it and the cardiogenic area are translocated to the future thoracic region through folding of the cranial end of the embryo (B, C). The allantois and the connecting stalk combine with the yolk sac and the vitelline duct through folding of the caudal end of the embryo. Fusion of ectoderm, mesoderm, future coelomic cavities, and endoderm from opposite sides is prevented in the immediate vicinity of the vitelline duct (D) but not in the more cranial and caudal regions (E). The outer ectodermal (skin) and inner endodermal (gut) tubes of the tube-within-a-tube body plan are formed by body folding (E).

In the Clinic

ANTERIOR BODY WALL DEFECTS

Failure of the anterior (ventral) body wall to form properly during body folding or subsequent development results in anterior body wall defects. Anterior body wall defects can occur in the abdominal (common) or thoracic (rare) region.

The most common anterior body wall defects include **omphalocele** and **gastroschisis**, which when grouped together occur in 1 in 2500 live births. In both of these defects, a portion of the gastrointestinal system herniates beyond the anterior body wall in the abdominal region. However, in omphalocele (Fig. 4-4B-D), the bowel is membrane covered, in contrast to gastroschisis, in which the bowel protrudes through the body wall (see Fig. 4-1B).

Two other anterior body wall defects occur in the abdominal region: **prune belly syndrome (Eagle-Barrett syndrome)** and **exstrophy of the bladder** (also known as **cloacal exstrophy**). Although the anterior body wall closes in individuals with prune belly syndrome, the abdomen becomes distended by bladder outlet obstruction, and the abdominal muscles fail to develop. Consequently, there is marked wrinkling of the anterior abdominal wall. This syndrome occurs almost exclusively in males and is associated with undescended testicles, suggesting a complex etiology. In exstrophy of the bladder, the bladder epithelium is exposed on the surface of the lower abdomen, and the bladder consists of an open vesicle (reminiscent of an open neural tube defect). Exstrophy of the bladder is covered further in Chapter 15.

Anterior body wall defects can also occur in the thoracic wall. For example, the heart can be exposed on the surface, resulting in **ectopia cordis** (about 5:1,000,000 live births). In the extremely rare **pentalogy of Cantrell**, which is considered an anterior body wall defect, five major anomalies occur together: (1) midline abdominal wall defect, (2) anterior diaphragmatic hernia, (3) cleft sternum, (4) pericardial defect, and (5) intracardiac defects such as ventricular septal defect. Thus, this defect, which occurs mainly in the thoracic region, also involves the abdominal region.

A final anterior body wall defect with a complex etiology involving multiple structures is called **limb-body wall complex (LBWC; amniotic band syndrome)**. At least in some cases, LBWC results from rupture of the amnion and constriction of the limbs by fibrous amniotic bands (hence its alternative name, although not all cases of LBWC exhibit amniotic bands). In addition to limb defects (covered in Chapter 20) and sometimes craniofacial defects (covered in Chapter 17) and exencephaly or encephalocele (covered later in this chapter), anterior body wall defects such as omphalocele or gastroschisis are present in LBWC.

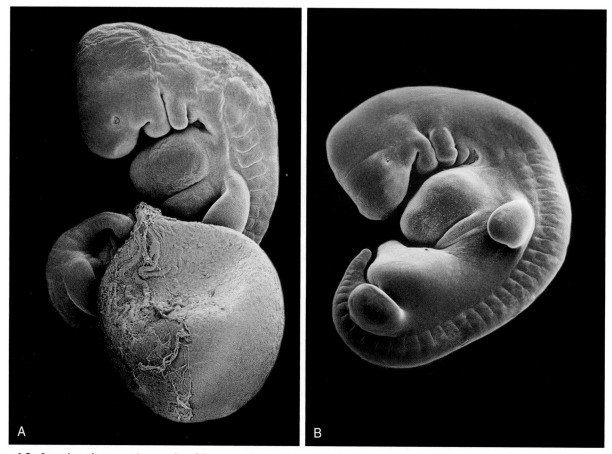

Figure 4-3. Scanning electron micrographs of human embryos. *A,* The form of this embryo is characteristic of that of a four-week human embryo, just subsequent to body folding. Note the relatively large yolk sac. *B,* The yolk sac has been removed in this five-week embryo.

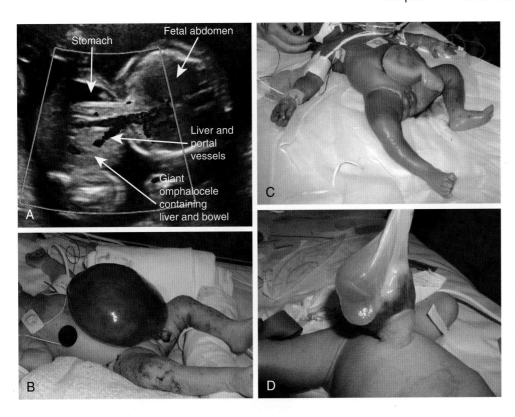

Figure 4-4. Omphalocele. *A,* Sonogram showing the defect in a twenty-two–week fetus. Blood flow in large fetal blood vessels is shown using ultrasound color Doppler. *B,* Large omphalocele containing both liver and intestines. *C, D,* Smaller omphalocele (enlarged in *D*) containing only intestines.

NEURULATION: ESTABLISHING NEURAL TUBE, RUDIMENT OF CENTRAL NERVOUS SYSTEM

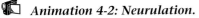 *Animation 4-2: Neurulation.*

Animations are available online at StudentConsult.

As covered in Chapter 3, by the end of the third week, the neural plate consists of a broad cranial portion that will give rise to the brain and a narrow caudal portion that will give rise to the spinal cord (see Chapter 3, Figs. 3-20, 3-21). On day twenty-two (eight pairs of somites), the narrow caudal portion of the neural plate—the future spinal cord—represents only about 25% of the length of the neural plate. However, as somites continue to be added, the spinal cord region lengthens faster than the more cranial neural plate. By day twenty-three or twenty-four (twelve and twenty pairs of somites, respectively), the future spinal cord occupies about 50% of the length of the neural plate, and by day twenty-six (twenty-five pairs of somites), it occupies about 60%. Rapid lengthening of the neural plate during this period is driven by **convergent extension** (covered in Chapter 3) of the **neuroepithelium** and underlying tissues.

Formation of the neural tube occurs during the process of **neurulation** (Fig. 4-5). Neurulation involves four main events: formation of the neural plate, shaping of the neural plate, bending of the neural plate, and closure of the neural groove (Fig. 4-6). Formation of the neural plate was covered in Chapter 3 under the topic of neural induction. The main morphogenetic change that occurs during formation of the neural plate is apicobasal elongation of ectodermal cells to form the thickened, single-layered

neural plate (Fig. 4-6*A, B*). Shaping of the neural plate involves the process of convergent extension. During shaping, the neural plate narrows in the transverse plane and lengthens in the longitudinal plane. Because the neural plate is initially broader cranially than caudally and convergent extension occurs at a greater rate at the future spinal cord level of the neural plate than at the future brain level, the future brain level of the neural plate remains much broader than the future spinal cord level.

Bending of the neural plate involves formation of **neural folds** at the lateral edges of the neural plate, consisting of both **neuroepithelium** and adjacent **surface ectoderm** (Fig. 4-6*C*). During bending, the neural folds elevate dorsally by rotating around a central pivot point overlying the notochord called the **median hinge point**. The groove delimited by the bending neural plate is called the **neural groove**. Bending around the median hinge point resembles closing of the leaves of a book. Because the neural plate/groove at the future brain level is much broader than that at the future spinal cord level, additional hinge points form in the brain neural plate to bring the neural folds together at the dorsal midline. These hinge points, called **dorsolateral hinge points**, allow neural folds at the future brain level to converge medially toward one another (Fig. 4-6*D, E*). As a result of bending, the paired neural folds are brought into apposition at the dorsal midline.

Closure of the neural groove involves the adhesion of neural folds to one another and the subsequent rearrangement of cells within the folds to form two separate epithelial layers: the **roof plate of the neural tube** and the overlying **surface ectoderm**. Forming at the interface between these epithelial layers are **neural crest cells** (Fig. 4-6*F*). These arise from the neural folds

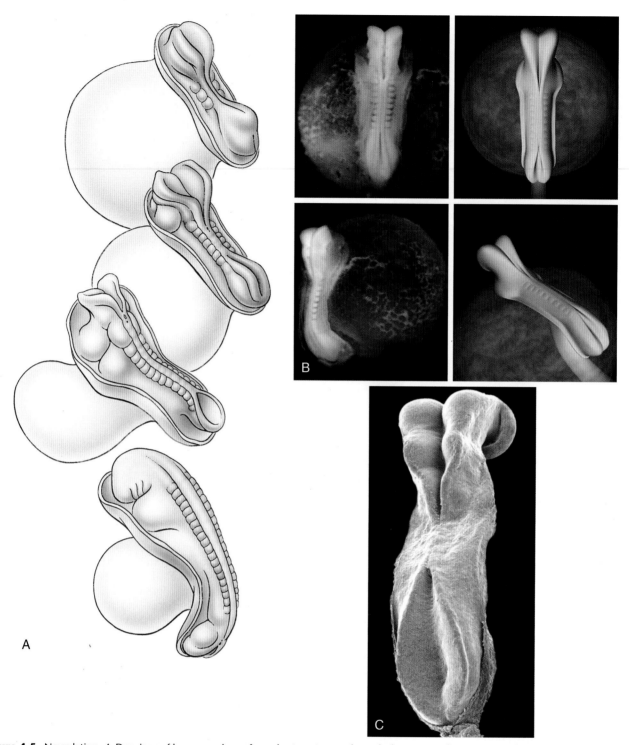

Figure 4-5. Neurulation. *A,* Drawings of human embryos from day twenty-one through days twenty-four to twenty-five (top to bottom, respectively). The lateral edges of the neural folds first begin to fuse in the occipitocervical region on day twenty-two, leaving the cranial and caudal neuropores open at each end. The neural tube lengthens as it zips up both cranially and caudally, and the neuropores become progressively smaller. The cranial neuropore closes on day twenty-four, and the caudal neuropore closes on day twenty-six. *B,* Photographs of human embryos from the dorsal (top) or lateral (bottom) side and comparable computer-generated images. *C,* Scanning electron micrograph of a mouse embryo comparable with a day twenty-one or day twenty-two human embryo. Both cranial and caudal neuropores are open.

by undergoing an **epithelial-to-mesenchymal transformation (EMT.** discussed later in the chapter); neural crest cells are also covered later in the chapter. In humans, closure of the neural groove begins on day twenty-two at the future occipital and cervical region (i.e., adjacent to the four occipital somites and first cervical somite) of the neural tube (see Fig. 4-5). From this level, closure progresses both cranially and caudally; eventually the **cranial** and **caudal neuropores**, respectively, close on day twenty-four and day twenty-six.

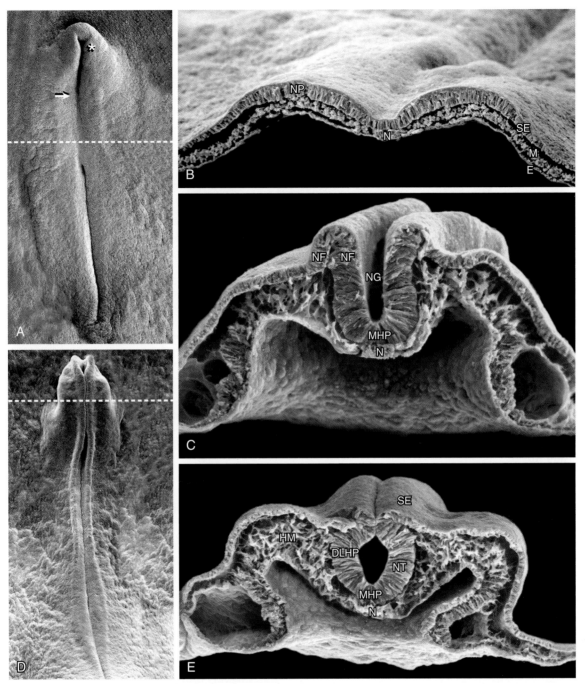

Figure 4-6. Neurulation in the chick. *A,* Dorsal view showing that neurulation occurs in cranial-to-caudal sequence such that at the level of the line in *A,* the neural plate is forming. More cranially (arrow), the neural plate is shaping, and still more cranially, the neural plate is bending (asterisk) and a neural groove and paired neural folds have formed. *B,* Level of the forming neural plate (NP) at the level of the line in *A.* E, Endoderm; M, mesoderm; N, notochord; SE, surface ectoderm. *C,* Transverse section through neural groove (future midbrain level) at a stage midway between *A* and *D.* MHP, Median hinge point; N, notochord; NF, neural fold; NG, neural groove. *D,* Dorsal view during closure of the neural groove. In contrast to humans, the neural groove in chick first closes at the future midbrain level (rather than at the occipitocervical level) and then progresses cranially and caudally to close, respectively, the small cranial neuropore and the elongated caudal neuropore/neural groove. The line indicates the level of transverse section in *E. E,* Transverse section through the incipient neural tube (NT). DLHP, Dorsolateral hinge point; HM, head mesoderm; MHP, median hinge point; N, notochord; SE, surface ectoderm.

Continued

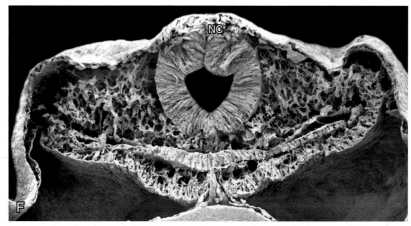

Figure 4-6 *Cont'd F,* Transverse section showing a slightly later stage in neurulation than is shown in *E.* Neural crest cells (NC) are beginning to form and emigrate from the fusing neural folds.

In the Research Lab

MECHANISMS OF NEURULATION
Tissue and Cellular Events

Neurulation, in particular shaping and bending of the neural plate, involves a number of different forces that act in concert. These forces are generated by changes in cell behavior, particularly changes in cell shape, position, and number. Some of these forces are generated within the neural plate itself, whereas other forces are generated in surrounding tissues. Forces arising within the neural plate are called **intrinsic neurulation forces**, as opposed to those arising outside the neural plate, which are called **extrinsic neurulation forces**.

The cellular basis of neurulation has been mechanistically examined most thoroughly in chick embryos (see Fig. 4-6). Although shaping and bending of the neural plate occur simultaneously, to understand their mechanisms it is best to consider them separately. As covered earlier in this chapter, shaping involves **convergent extension**, that is, transverse narrowing and longitudinal lengthening. In addition, the neural plate thickens apicobasally during shaping as its cells get taller (i.e., change shape to high columnar), continuing the process of cell elongation initiated during neural plate formation. Apicobasal elongation requires the presence of paraxial microtubules, that is, microtubules oriented along (parallel to) the apicobasal axis of the cell. **Cell elongation** contributes not only to neural plate thickening but also to its narrowing, because as cells get taller, they reduce their diameters to maintain their size (this would also reduce the length of the neural plate but is compensated for by cell rearrangement and oriented cell division; covered below). However, the major factor that narrows the neural plate is not cell elongation. Rather it is **cell rearrangement** (also called **cell intercalation**). During cell rearrangement, cells move from lateral to medial within the neural plate, thereby narrowing the neural plate and stacking up in the cranial-caudal plane, increasing the length of the neural plate. Moreover, **cell division** occurs rapidly during neurulation such that the neural plate continues to grow during shaping and bending. Many of these cell divisions are oriented to place daughter cells into the length of the neural plate rather than into its width, resulting in cranial-caudal extension of the neural plate. Thus, shaping of the neural plate involves changes in cell shape, position, and number within the neural plate. Experiments have shown that shaping is largely autonomous to the neural plate, that is, intrinsic forces drive neural plate shaping.

As covered earlier in this chapter, bending of the neural plate involves the formation of hinge points. The single **median hinge point** forms at all craniocaudal levels of the bending neural plate, whereas the paired **dorsolateral hinge points** form at future brain levels, where the neural plate is much broader than it is more caudally. Hinge points involve localized regions where neuroepithelial cells change their shape from column-like to wedgelike and where wedge-shaped cells become firmly attached to an adjacent structure through the deposition of extracellular matrix. Thus, the median hinge point cells of the neural plate are firmly attached to the underlying **notochord**, and the dorsolateral hinge point cells of the neural plate on each side are firmly attached to the adjacent surface ectoderm of the **neural folds**. Cell wedging within the hinge points is generated by both apical constriction and basal expansion. The apices of neuroepithelial cells contain a circumferential ring of microfilaments whose contraction leads to apical narrowing. In addition, bases of neuroepithelial cells simultaneously expand as the nucleus moves basally. Recall that neuroepithelial cells are dividing throughout neurulation. As these elongated cells divide, their nuclei undergo a to-and-fro movement called **interkinetic nuclear migration**. During the G1/S phase of the cell cycle, nuclei move basally. After DNA synthesis is completed during the S phase, cells round up at the apex of the neuroepithelium, where mitosis (**cytokinesis**) occurs. After division, cells elongate once again, and their nuclei move basally. During wedging, the cell cycle of neuroepithelial cells is prolonged so that cells spend more time in G and S phases and, consequently, more time with their bases expanded. This is because each neuroepithelial cell is very narrow, except at the level where the nuclei reside. Thus, basally expanded neuroepithelial cells are wedge shaped.

Historically, most studies on neurulation have focused on changes in neuroepithelial cell shapes (i.e., wedging), which generate intrinsic forces for neurulation. But more recent studies have shown that **extrinsic forces** are both sufficient and necessary for neurulation. These studies have revealed that tissues lateral to the neural plate (surface ectoderm and mesoderm) generate extrinsic forces for bending of the neural plate. Like intrinsic forces that act during shaping, these extrinsic forces are generated by changes in cell behavior and involve changes in cell shape, position, and number. Lateral tissues, like the neural plate, also undergo convergent extension driven by both oriented cell division and cell rearrangement. This results in their medial expansion, which pushes the neural folds, resulting in their elevation and convergence toward the dorsal midline. Lateral cells also exhibit changes in cell shape that contribute to medial expansion. For example, surface ectodermal cells transform from cuboidal to squamous (i.e., they flatten), increasing their surface area.

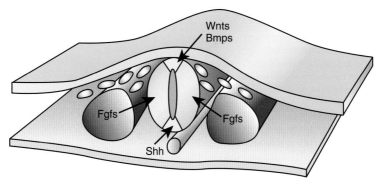

Figure 4-7. Diagram showing factors involved in dorsal-ventral patterning of the neural tube. The neural tube is dorsalized by surface ectoderm, which secretes both orthologs of the *Drosophila*, wingless family (Wnts), and bone morphogenetic proteins (Bmps), resulting in formation of the roof plate of the neural tube (lighter triangular area dorsally) and neural crest cells (migrating away from dorsal neural tube). The neural tube is ventralized by the notochord, which induces the floor plate (lighter triangular area ventrally) of the neural tube through the secretion of sonic hedgehog (Shh). Subsequently, both the notochord and the floor plate secrete Shh. Additional patterning signals are provided by the somites (fibroblast growth factors or Fgfs). Arrows indicate signaling.

The cellular basis of neural groove closure, specifically fusion of the neural folds, is poorly understood. Some studies suggest that apical extracellular adhesive coats are involved, but their molecular nature remains uncharacterized. In addition, cell rearrangements occur as epithelial sheets (i.e., neural folds) fuse and then reorganize into new epithelial (i.e., roof of neural tube and overlying surface ectoderm) and mesenchymal (i.e., neural crest cell) structures. However, precisely how cells accomplish these feats remains largely unstudied.

Molecular Mechanisms

The molecular basis of neurulation is being studied increasingly. More than two hundred mutations in mouse have been shown to result in defective neurulation and, consequently, to result in **neural tube defects (NTDs)**; thus, these mutations provide insight into which genes are involved in both normal and abnormal neurulation. Because neurulation is driven by changes in cell behavior, it is not surprising that mutation of cytoskeletal, extracellular matrix/cell adhesion, cell cycle, and cell death genes results in NTDs. Neurulation is a highly choreographed morphogenetic event that must be precisely timed and coordinated across multiple tissues. This presumably involves signaling among tissues. It is the hope of studies using mouse mutations that such signaling pathways will be identified, ultimately leading to an understanding of the molecular basis of neurulation and the formation of NTDs both in animal models and ultimately in humans.

Planar cell polarity pathway and convergent extension

As covered early in this chapter and in Chapter 3, convergent extension plays a major role in vertebrate gastrulation and neurulation. Recent studies have revealed that convergent extension is regulated by the Wnt signaling pathway. During development, epithelial sheets become polarized not only apicobasally but also within the plane of the epithelium itself. In *Drosophila*, the **planar cell polarity (PCP) pathway** functions in this latter polarization of the epithelium. Thus, for example, the orientation of wing hairs is established by the PCP pathway. In vertebrates, the PCP pathway is required for proper orientation of stereociliary bundles in the outer hair cells of the mouse inner ear (covered in Chapter 18) and for convergent extension during gastrulation and neurulation. How are the PCP and Wnt signaling pathways related?

The *Drosophila* PCP pathway consists of several core proteins that collectively act to convert an extracellular polarity cue to specific changes in the cytoskeleton. These core proteins are now known to be components of the Wnt signaling pathway, and orthologs of several of the *Drosophila* components are conserved in vertebrates. Thus, convergent extension during gastrulation and neurulation is blocked in loss-of-function mutations of the cytoplasmic protein dishevelled in *Xenopus* and its two orthologs in mouse (dishevelled 1 and 2). As covered in Chapter 5, Wnt signaling involves both a so-called canonical Wnt pathway and non-canonical Wnt pathways. The PCP pathway utilizes the non-canonical pathway in which certain Wnts, such as Wnt 11, bind to their receptors (known as frizzleds). Several other proteins, including dishevelled, must interact in this pathway for proper signaling and, consequently, for proper convergent extension to occur. In addition to double dishevelled 1 and 2 mutants, four other mouse mutants exhibit convergent extension defects: circletail, crash, spin cycle, and loop-tail. Loop-tail mice have a mutation in the ortholog of the strabismus/van Gogh gene, which encodes a transmembrane protein that interacts with dishevelled. Both crash and spin cycle mice have a mutation in the ortholog of the *Drosophila* protocadherin flamingo gene, called Celsr1. In *Drosophila*, flamingo is required for PCP signaling. Circletail mice have a mutation in the ortholog of the *Drosophila* scribble gene. Scribble interacts with strabismus. Thus, developing an understanding of the PCP pathway in *Drosophila* has had a surprising result—a better understanding of vertebrate gastrulation and neurulation and, potentially, a better understanding of how NTDs form in humans.

ACTIN-BINDING PROTEINS AND APICAL CONSTRICTION

Several actin-associated proteins when genetically ablated in mice result in NTDs. One of these, the actin-binding protein shroom, has received considerable study. Overexpression of shroom in cultured epithelial cells is sufficient to cause apical constriction. Shroom causes apical constriction by altering the distribution of F-actin to the apical side of epithelial cells and by regulating the formation of a contractile actomyosin network associated with apical intercellular junctions. When shroom is inactivated in *Xenopus* embryos, hinge point formation is drastically altered and neural tube closure fails to occur, providing further evidence for a role of cell shape changes in generating intrinsic forces important for neurulation.

DORSAL-VENTRAL PATTERNING OF NEURAL TUBE

As the neural tube is forming, it receives signals from adjacent tissues that result in its patterning in the dorsal-ventral axis. Three tissues provide patterning signals: surface ectoderm, paraxial mesoderm, and notochord. Thus, these signals originate dorsally, laterally, and ventrally, respectively (Fig. 4-7).

Ventral signals are the best understood. Several micro-surgical experiments in which notochords were removed (extirpated) from the ventral midline or were transplanted adjacent to the lateral wall of the neural tube revealed that the notochord was both sufficient and necessary for formation of the **median hinge point** and, subsequently, for formation of the **floor plate of the neural tube** (the floor plate derives from the median hinge point during subsequent development). Using loss-of-function and gain-of-function experiments mainly in chick and mouse, it was shown that sonic hedgehog (Shh), secreted initially by the notochord, was the signal that induced the median hinge point and floor plate. As the floor plate is induced, it also secretes Shh (Fig. 4-8), which in turn induces **neurons** in the ventral neural tube (e.g., motoneurons in the ventral spinal cord; covered in Chapter 9). Shh acts as a **morphogen**, such that high concentrations induce ventral neurons, lower concentrations induce more intermediate neurons, and the lowest concentrations induce more dorsal neurons.

In addition to producing a ventral-to-dorsal concentration gradient of Shh within the neural tube, the notochord produces a ventral-to-dorsal concentration gradient of chordin, a Bmp antagonist. The chordin gradient interacts with a dorsal-to-ventral concentration gradient of Bmp produced by the surface ectoderm. Because chordin blocks Bmp signaling, Bmp signaling is robust dorsally (where chordin concentration is weak or absent and Bmp concentration is high) and is weak or absent ventrally (where chordin concentration is high and Bmp concentration is weak or absent). A high level of Bmp signaling dorsally, along with Wnt signaling by the surface ectoderm, results in the induction of **neural crest cells** and the **roof plate of the neural tube**.

The paraxial mesoderm lying adjacent to the lateral walls of the neural tube also provides patterning signals, but these are the least understood. Among the secreted factors produced by the paraxial mesoderm are Fgfs, such as Fgf8. Both gain-of-function and loss-of-function experiments in *Xenopus* provide support for a role for paraxial mesoderm and Fgfs in neural crest cell induction.

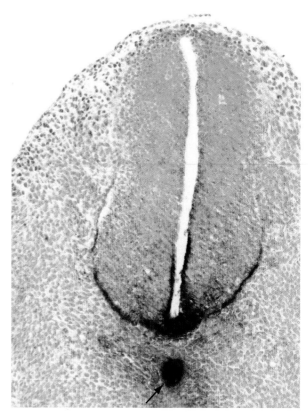

Figure 4-8. Expression of sonic hedgehog (Shh) protein (dark brown) in the eleven- to eleven-and-one-half-day postcoitum mouse notochord and overlying floor plate of the neural tube.

In the Clinic

NEURAL TUBE DEFECTS

Neural tube defects (NTDs) result when **neurulation** fails to occur normally. Thus, these defects arise during weeks three to four of gestation and can be open to the surface or covered with skin. Open NTDs are the most severe. They range from total **dysraphism**, called **craniorachischisis**, in which the entire length of the neural tube opens onto the surface of the head and back, to localized dysraphism. Total dysraphism of the brain, with normal formation of the spinal cord, is called **cranioschisis** or **anencephaly**. Infants with anencephaly lack a functional forebrain (cerebrum) and fail to gain consciousness; most do not survive longer than a few hours after birth.

Dysraphism of the spinal cord is called **myeloschisis**. Usually myeloschisis is localized rather than total, and it typically occurs at the lumbosacral level, such that only the lowermost region of the spinal cord is open (Fig. 4-9A-C). Myeloschisis is commonly referred to as **spina bifida aperta** (i.e., aperta means that the spinal cord is open to the body surface, and spina bifida means that bifid vertebral spines are present). Not all patients with spina bifida aperta have dysraphic spinal cords. Instead, membranes (**dura mater** and **arachnoid**) alone can

protrude from the vertebral canal, forming a fluid-filled sac or **cele**. When the protrusion consists solely of membranes, it is called a **meningocele** (Fig. 4-10A). When it includes an intact spinal cord, it is called a **meningomyelocele** or **myelomeningocele** (Fig. 4-10B).

Open NTDs occur in about 0.1% of all live births. Approximately four thousand pregnancies are affected by open NTDs each year in the United States, and in these cases, as many as 50% of the fetuses are electively aborted. Approximately five hundred thousand infants with spina bifida aperta are born worldwide each year. Early detection of NTDs in utero has improved greatly since the advent of **maternal serum alpha-fetoprotein** (MSAFP) screening after twelve weeks of gestation. If elevated levels of alpha-fetoprotein are detected in maternal serum, two other tests can be conducted: **ultrasound examination** of the fetal spine and head (see Fig. 4-9A) and **amniocentesis** (covered in Chapter 6); the latter procedure is used to sample and measure levels of alpha-fetoprotein contained in amniotic fluid. Alpha-fetoprotein is produced by the fetal liver and is excreted by the fetal kidneys into the amniotic fluid; eventually, it is absorbed into the maternal bloodstream. Alpha-fetoprotein levels are elevated in pregnancies affected by NTDs (and by ventral body wall defects such as **gastroschisis**) and are lower in pregnancies affected by **Down syndrome** (or other chromosomal anomalies), but why alpha-fetoprotein levels are altered in these conditions is unclear.

Skin-covered NTDs can be present at both brain and spinal cord levels. In the brain, skin-covered NTDs are called **encephaloceles**, with brain tissue protruding through the skull (Figs. 4-11, 4-12). Large encephaloceles can severely affect

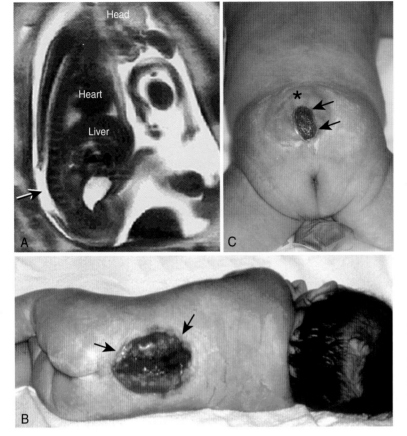

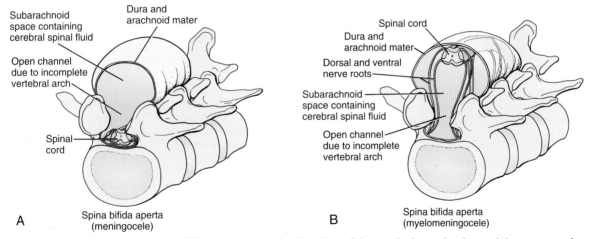

Figure 4-9. Lumbosacral myeloschisis. *A,* Magnetic resonance imaging (MRI) showing lumbosacral myeloschisis (arrow) in a fetus in utero. *B,* Newborn with a large open lesion (lumbosacral myeloschisis). Arrows mark its cranial-caudal extent. *C,* Newborn with both open (arrows mark the cranial-caudal extent of the lumbosacral myeloschisis) and closed (asterisk; meningocele or myelomeningocele) lesions.

Figure 4-10. Diagrams of two types of spina bifida aperta. Note the disruption of the vertebral neural arches and the presence of a cele. *A,* A meningocele includes dura and arachnoid but not spinal cord. *B,* A myelomeningocele or meningomyelocele contains a portion of the spinal cord and associated spinal nerves, as well as meninges.

neurological function and threaten survival. In the spinal cord, skin-covered NTDs are referred to as **spina bifida occulta** (i.e., occulta means that the defect is hidden; Fig. 4-13*A*); they occur in about 2% of the population. Typically, the location of spina bifida occulta is marked externally on the back by a tuft of hair, a pigmented nevus (mole), an angioma (port wine–colored birth mark of the skin), a lipoma (skin doming caused by an underlying mass of fatty tissue; Fig. 4-13*B*), or a dimple.

NTDs can result in serious health problems that require lifelong management. For example, the spinal cord and

spinal nerves affected by a meningomyelocele fail to develop normally, resulting in dysfunction of pelvic organs and lower limbs. In general, higher and larger defects result in greater neurological deficit than lower and smaller defects. In as many as 90% of infants with meningomyelocele, **hydrocephalus** develops (commonly referred to as water on the brain). This occurs because the meningomyelocele is associated for unknown reasons with an abnormality at the base of the brain called **Arnold-Chiari malformation** (Fig. 4-14). This malformation disrupts the normal drainage of cerebrospinal fluid (CSF) from the brain ventricles to the subarach-

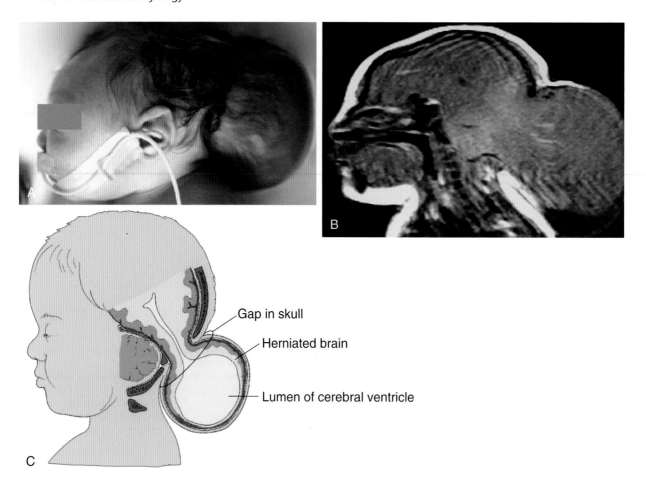

Gap in skull

Herniated brain

Lumen of cerebral ventricle

Figure 4-11. Newborns with large encephaloceles. *A,* Lateral view. *B,* Magnetic resonance imaging (MRI) showing brain tissue herniating through the back of the skull into a cele. *C,* Diagram illustrating the herniated structures.

noid space surrounding the spinal cord. This in turn increases the volume and pressure of CSF in the cerebral ventricles, causing their enlargement at the expense of more peripheral brain tissue. Hydrocephalus usually is controlled by implanting a shunt—an inert, flexible plastic tube about one-eighth of an inch thick and containing a unidirectional flow valve—into the lateral ventricles to allow fluid to drain into a body cavity (typically the abdominal cavity) where it can be resorbed. Another complication of NTDs is a **tethered spinal cord**, a condition in which the lower end of the spinal cord is attached to the skin as a result of an open or closed NTD. As the child grows and his/her vertebral column elongates, the restricted cord is stretched and damaged, resulting in neurological deficit. It is important to identify tethered cords and to surgically untether them before such neurological damage occurs, as this damage is not reversible. In infants with skin-covered NTDs, the presence of a tethered cord would not be evident. However, as covered earlier in this section, infants born with a hairy tuft, a pigmented nevus, an angioma, a lipoma, or a dimple—so-called **neurocutaneous signatures**—in the lumbosacral region might have an underlying NTD. These infants should be examined with magnetic resonance imaging (MRI) or with ultrasound to identify tethered cords associated with a closed NTD so that the cord can be untethered before neurological damage occurs.

NTDs have no single genetic or teratogenic cause and are believed to be multifactorial, that is, to arise from the interaction of both genetic and environmental factors. About 95% of babies with NTDs are born to parents with no family history of these disorders. However, if one child in the family has an NTD, the risk of a recurrence in any subsequent pregnancy rises to about 1 in 40, and if two children are affected, the incidence rises to 1 in 20, strongly suggesting a genetic predisposition. The frequency of NTDs varies by race, again suggesting a genetic predisposition. For example, in the United States as a whole, the frequency of NTDs is approximately 0.1%, but the frequency of NTDs is 0.035% among African Americans. In contrast, the frequency of NTDs in some parts of India and in Ireland is on the order of 1.1%, and in Shanxi Province in Northern China, the frequency approaches 1.6% to 1.8%.

In support of a genetic predisposition for neural tube defects in humans, mutations have been reported recently in PCP genes (covered above), such as van Gogh 1 and 2, in families having elevated risks for neural tube defects. These findings emphasize the importance of convergent extension and other tissue and cellular events in human neurulation, as well as in animal models.

Teratogens that induce NTDs in animals and humans have also been identified, opening the possibility that some human NTDs may be caused by environmental toxins or nutritional deficiencies. For example, studies on experimental animals have implicated retinoic acid, insulin, and high plasma glucose in the formation of NTDs. Factors implicated in the induction of

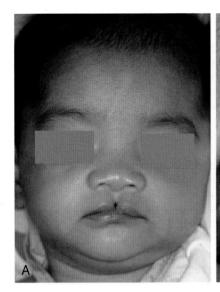 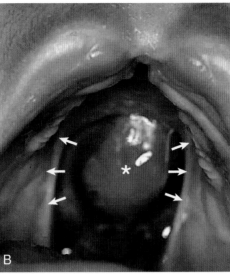

Figure 4-12. Midline defects of the orofacial region. *A,* Newborn with a midline cleft lip. *B,* Examination of the oral cavity revealed the presence of a cleft palate (arrows mark non-fused palatal shelves) and an encephalocele (asterisk) herniating into the nasal cavity.

NTDs in humans include the antiepileptic drug **valproic acid,** **maternal diabetes,** and **hyperthermia.**

    Folic acid (vitamin B9) supplementation (400 micrograms of synthetic folic acid per day in a prenatal multivitamin) can reduce the incidence of NTDs by up to 75%. However, in a 2000 Gallup poll, only 13% of women of childbearing age in the United States were aware of this fact. Moreover, to be most effective in preventing an NTD, folic acid should be taken by women of reproductive age, so that folate supplementation has already started by the time of conception. In fact, some birth control pills now contain folic acid, so that if pregnancy occurs while on birth control or shortly after stopping birth control, some level of folate supplementation already exists.

    If a mother has previously had a child with spina bifida, it is recommended that she take a prenatal multivitamin with a 10-fold higher concentration of folic acid (that is, 4 milligrams). The role of folic acid in developmental processes is complex, including the regulation of DNA synthesis, mitosis, protein synthesis, and DNA methylation, so the actual mechanism(s) by which folic acid supplementation prevents NTDs (and likely other birth defects) remains unclear.

SECONDARY NEURULATION

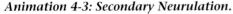 *Animation 4-3: Secondary Neurulation.*
    Animations are available online at StudentConsult.

As covered in Chapter 3, gastrulation ends with formation of the tail bud. And as covered earlier in this chapter, the neural tube develops through the process of neurulation. Neurulation is completed with closure of the caudal neuropore at about the level of somite thirty-one. Yet in the fetus, the neural tube extends caudal to this level into the sacral and coccygeal levels. This occurs because the level of the closing caudal neuropore is merged with the forming tail bud, and the latter undergoes morphogenesis to form the most caudal extent of the neural tube. Formation of the neural tube from the tail bud is called

secondary neurulation, as opposed to *neurulation* (or **primary neurulation**), which involves formation of the neural tube from the neural plate, as covered earlier in the chapter.

    Experimental studies have shown that caudal levels of neural tube, neural crest cells, and somites develop from the tail bud (Figs. 4-15, 4-16). Secondary neurulation involves the condensation of central tail bud cells into a solid mass called the **medullary cord.** Subsequently, the medullary cord undergoes cavitation to form a lumen, which quickly merges with the neural canal of the more cranial neural tube. Neural crest cells then arise from the roof of the neural tube and undergo migration to form the caudal spinal ganglia. Lateral tail bud cells undergo segmentation to form the caudal somites, and, as mentioned in Chapter 3, the caudal end of the notochord grows into the sacral, coccygeal, and tail regions. Secondary neurulation is completed by about eight weeks of development.

CRANIAL-CAUDAL REGIONALIZATION OF NEURAL TUBE

Shortly after the neural tube forms, it becomes subdivided in the cranial-caudal axis into **forebrain, midbrain, hindbrain,** and **spinal cord.** Concomitantly, the embryo becomes shaped through the process of body folding and flexure of the neural tube. Thus, by the end of the first month of development, the embryonic body is well formed, and the basic body plan is well established (Fig. 4-17). Midsagittal sections through the cranial end of the embryo at this stage reveal forebrain (also called **prosencephalon**), midbrain (also called **mesencephalon**), and hindbrain (also called **rhombencephalon**). The sharp flexure separating the prosencephalon from the mesencephalon is the **mesencephalic flexure.** Further development of the neural tube and its cranial-caudal regionalization is covered in Chapter 9.

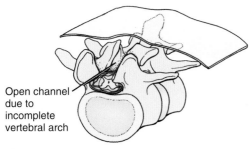

Open channel
due to
incomplete
vertebral arch

A   Spina bifida occulta

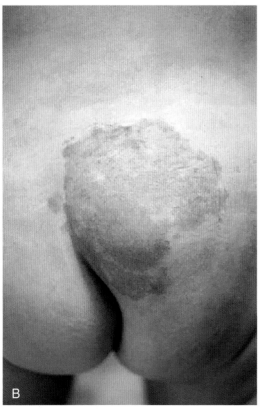

B

Figure 4-13. *A,* Spina bifida occulta may involve minor anomalies of neural arch formation and may not result in malformations of the neural tube. This condition often occurs in the midsacral region and may be indicated by a small dimple, a tuft of hair, a lipoma, or a nevus overlying the defective vertebra. *B,* Lumbosacral spina bifida occulta in a newborn with associated lipoma and angioma.

NEURAL CREST CELLS

Animation 4-4: Formation of Neural Crest.
Animations are available online at StudentConsult.

NEURAL CREST CELLS ORIGINATE DURING NEURULATION

Neural crest cells are a unique population of cells that arise from the dorsal part of the forming neural tube during neurulation. These cells undergo an **epithelial-to-mesenchymal transformation** (see following "In the Research Lab" entitled "Epithelial-to-Mesenchymal Transformation"), as they detach from the neural tube (Fig. 4-18). Subsequently, they migrate to many specific

locations in the body, where they differentiate into a remarkable variety of structures.

Neural crest cells differentiate first in the mesencephalic zone of the future brain. These cranial or cephalic neural crest cells associated with the developing brain begin to detach and migrate before closure of the cranial neuropore, even while the **neural folds** are fusing at the dorsal midline. In the spinal cord portion of the neural tube, the neural crest cells detach after the neural folds have fused.

Neural crest cells at the very caudal end of the neural tube are formed from the **medullary cord** after the caudal neuropore closes on day twenty-six. Thus, detachment and migration of the neural crest cells occur in a craniocaudal wave, from the mesencephalon to the caudal end of the spinal neural tube.

> ### In the Research Lab
>
> #### EPITHELIAL-TO-MESENCHYMAL TRANSFORMATION
> Formation of neural crest cells involves an epithelial-to-mesenchymal transformation (EMT) not unlike that occurring as cells undergo ingression through the primitive streak (covered in Chapter 3). Consequently, some of the same molecular players function in both events. Separation of the neural crest from the neural folds or neural tube is referred to as **delamination** of neural crest cells. Three key factors are known to promote neural crest cell delamination: FoxD3, a winged-helix transcription factor; snail2 (formerly called slug), a zinc-finger transcription factor; and Bmp2/4. Overexpression of FoxD3 promotes delamination of neural crest cells at all axial levels, showing that it is sufficient by itself for delamination. FoxD3 promotes delamination without upregulating the expression of snail2 (or RhoB; covered momentarily), suggesting that FoxD3 acts in parallel with (not upstream or downstream of) the other factors. Snail2 overexpression also promotes neural crest cell delamination, but only in the cranial region, not in the trunk region. Why snail2 is active only cranially in inducing neural crest cell delamination is unknown, but this experiment does show that snail2 is sufficient by itself to promote cranial neural crest cell delamination. Bmp signaling is required for delamination of neural crest cells, as overexpression of the Bmp antagonist, noggin, blocks delamination. As a result of Bmp signaling, RhoB, a small GTP-binding protein implicated in assembly of the actin cytoskeleton, is expressed by neural crest cells. Changes in the cytoskeleton are likely required for both change in cell shape, which accompanies an epithelial-to-mesenchymal transformation, and subsequent neural crest cell migration.

NEURAL CREST CELLS UNDERGO EXTENSIVE MIGRATION ALONG WELL-DEFINED PATHWAYS

Migration of neural crest cells from various craniocaudal levels of the neural folds and roof of the neural tube has been mapped by cell tracing studies in animal models. These studies reveal that neural crest cells undergo extensive migration throughout the body and subsequently differentiate into a large number of different cell types. Migration occurs along well-defined pathways or routes (Fig. 4-19). The route that particular neural crest cells take and where they stop migrating along this route determine in part what type of cell they

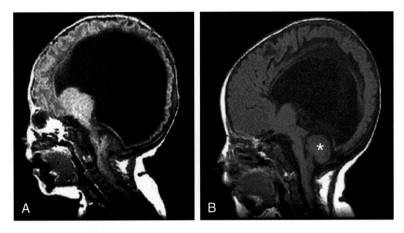

Figure 4-14. Chiari type II malformation with hydrocephalus. Magnetic resonance imaging (MRI). *A*, Infant at one month of age before shunting. Note the greatly enlarged ventricle (large black space in center), surrounded by thin, compressed cerebral tissue. In addition, the cerebellum has been pushed toward the foramen magnum. *B*, Five months after shunting. The ventricular space has reduced, the cerebral tissue has expanded, and the cerebellum (asterisk) now occupies its normal position. Currently, at eight years of age, the child uses a wheelchair and has minor finger weakness.

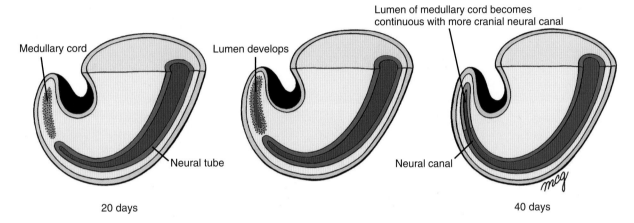

Lumen of medullary cord becomes continuous with more cranial neural canal

Medullary cord

Lumen develops

Neural tube

Neural canal

20 days

40 days

Figure 4-15. Secondary neurulation in humans. Formation of the caudal neural tube occurs by secondary neurulation. During this process, the tail bud gives rise to the medullary cord, which subsequently cavitates to form a lumen. At the end of the sixth week, this lumen merges with the neural canal of the more rostral neural tube.

will form. In addition, cranial (brain) and more caudal (spinal cord) neural crest cells give rise to some identical cell types (such as neurons) but also to some different cell types (e.g., only cranial neural crest cells form cartilage and bone). Differentiation of neural crest cells is covered in greater detail in later chapters (e.g., Chapters 10, 12, 14, and 17).

In the Research Lab

WHAT LOCAL FACTORS GUIDE MIGRATION OF NEURAL CREST CELLS?

Pathways of neural crest cell migration are established by **extracellular matrix molecules** that can be permissive for migration and hence determine the path, as well as inhibitory for migration, thereby determining the boundaries of the path. For example, neural crest cells migrate only through the cranial half of the somite and fail to enter the caudal half; in so doing, they establish the segmental patterning of the peripheral nervous system (covered in Chapter 10). Probably no one individual molecule determines the pathway. **Permissive molecules** in the cranial somite include the basement membrane proteins tenascin, fibronectin, laminin, and collagen, to name a few. **Inhibitory molecules** found in the caudal somite include proteoglycans, PNA-binding molecules (i.e., molecules that specifically bind the lectin peanut

agglutinin), F-spondin (a secreted protein produced by the floor plate of the neural tube), and ephrins (membrane-bound proteins that interact with Eph tyrosine kinases; Ephs and ephrins are covered in Chapter 5). Besides permissive molecules, there are also **chemotactic molecules** that attract neural crest cells and **negative chemotactic molecules** that repulse the crest from a distance. Gdnf (glial cell line–derived neurotropic factor) and neuregulin are examples of the former, whereas semaphorins and slits are examples of the latter (covered further in Chapter 10). Several approaches have allowed us to determine what cues guide the crest. These include the use of mouse mutants (covered in next section), in vitro studies to directly determine migratory ability on the extracellular matrix or chemotactic responses, and perturbation studies in the embryo. Determining which molecules guide the crest has been difficult because of molecular redundancy.

Recently, we have learned that not all subpopulations of neural crest cells respond the same way to these local signals. For example, neural crest cells that will become neurons or glial cells are inhibited by ephrins, whereas melanoblasts (cells derived from neural crest cells that differentiate into melanocytes, i.e., pigment cells) are stimulated to migrate on ephrins. Thus, melanoblasts are able to migrate into pathways where neurons and glial cells cannot go. Similarly, trunk neural crest cells are repulsed by slit, which is expressed in the gut mesenchyme and keeps them out of the gut, whereas vagal neural crest cells do not possess the receptor for slit and, therefore, are able to

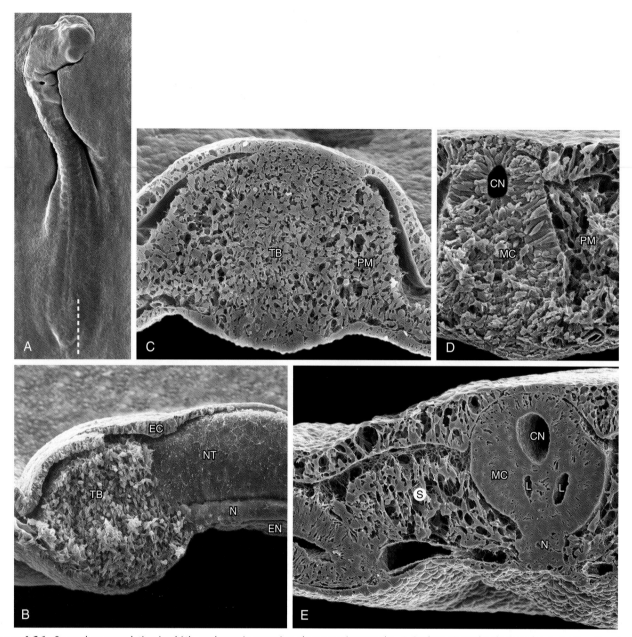

Figure 4-16. Secondary neurulation in chick, as shown in scanning electron micrographs. *A,* Surface view of a chick embryo shortly after closure of the caudal neuropore. Line indicates level of the slice shown in *B. B,* Parasagittal slice at the level shown in *A.* The lateral wall of the caudal end of the closed neural tube (NT) is shown, as is the notochord (N) and underlying endoderm (EN). Also shown are the tail bud (TB) and overlying ectoderm (EC). *C,* Transverse slice through the tail bud (TB). Also shown is the paraxial mesoderm (PM) that will form the most caudal somites. *D,* Slightly later stage than shown in *C* of a transverse slice through the medullary cord (MC), which in the chick is partially overlapped by the caudal neuropore (CN) formed during primary neurulation. Also shown is the paraxial mesoderm (PM). *E,* Slightly later stage than is shown in *D* of a transverse slice through the cavitating medullary cord (MC). CN, Caudal neuropore; L, lumina formed in the medullary cord by cavitation; N, caudal rudiment of the notochord; S, somite.

migrate into the gut to form the **enteric nervous system** (covered later in this chapter and in Chapter 10). Increasingly, we are discovering that different subpopulations of neural crest cells are specified early in their migration and respond differentially to cues in the microenvironment.

MUTANTS PROVIDE INFORMATION ABOUT MECHANISMS OF NEURAL CREST CELL MIGRATION AND DEVELOPMENTAL RESTRICTION

Several mouse mutants characterized by defects of neural crest cell development have been described. Some of these

mutations affect the proliferative activity of neural crest cell stem cell populations, whereas others are characterized by regional defects in pigmentation, innervation of the gut, or defects in the development of cranial neural crest cells.

An interesting series of mouse mutants that affect neural crest cell migration are called white-spotting and steel mutants. The white-spotting locus is a proto-oncogene that encodes a c-kit tyrosine kinase receptor (c-kit receptor), whereas the steel locus encodes the ligand for this receptor, c-kit ligand. As

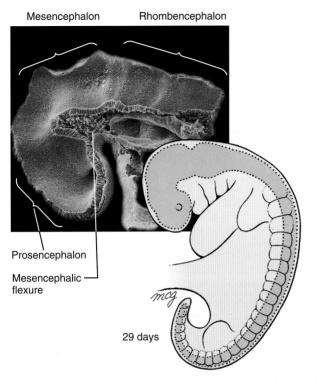

Mesencephalon   Rhombencephalon

Prosencephalon

Mesencephalic flexure

29 days

Figure 4-17. The rudiment of the central nervous system, the neural tube, is formed by the end of the fourth week. Even at this early stage, the primary vesicles of the brain can be identified. Note the sharp ventral bend in the neural tube, the mesencephalic flexure, which separates the prosencephalon from the mesencephalon.

expected, mutations of either gene produce a similar spectrum of anomalies, specifically involving migrating embryonic stem cells. For example, in severe mutations of either of these loci, **primordial germ cells** fail to populate the gonads, resulting in sterility (covered in Chapter 16), and **hematopoietic stem cells** fail to migrate from the yolk sac into the liver, resulting in severe deficiencies of blood formation (covered in Chapter 13). Less severe mutations may result in differential male or female sterility and selective loss of specific hematopoietic progenitors. In addition to disruptions of germ cell and blood cell development, these mutants display a spectrum of pigmentation defects suggesting an effect on another population of migrating embryonic cells—the neural crest cell precursors of the melanocytes.

It seems likely that c-kit ligand is a trophic factor and that it is required for survival of premelanocytes rather than for their early differentiation and migration. It has been suggested that c-kit ligand may regulate the expression of c-kit receptor by melanocyte precursors of neural crest cells and that c-kit ligand and c-kit receptor together then regulate the adhesion of these cells to the extracellular matrix. Thus, it seems that c-kit ligand must be expressed by cells along the melanocyte migration route and at its ultimate target, whereas the c-kit receptor must be expressed by the premelanocytes themselves. A **soluble form** of the c-kit ligand is apparently required for early survival of premelanocytes in a **migration staging area** between somite, surface ectoderm, and neural tube. In contrast, expression of a **membrane-associated form** of c-kit ligand seems to be required for later survival of the premelanocytes within the dermis.

A staggering array of additional genes affecting specific mechanisms of neural crest cell differentiation, migration, and survival in mice has been described within the past few years. The patch mutation affects the alpha subunit of the platelet-derived growth factor ($Pdgf_{2\alpha}$), disrupting the development of non-neuronal derivatives of neural crest cells. Null mutations of genes encoding retinoic acid receptor proteins result in defects of heart outflow tract septation (covered in Chapter 12; septation of the outflow tract requires the presence of neural crest cells, as covered below). Mice harboring the kreisler mutation exhibit wide-ranging craniofacial defects attributed to abnormal expression of several Hox genes and consequent disruption of neural crest cell development. Therefore, Hox genes apparently play pivotal roles in the signaling cascades that regulate differentiation and migration of cranial neural crest cells (covered in Chapter 17).

NEURAL CREST CELLS HAVE MANY DIVERSE DERIVATIVES

Neural crest cells are traditionally grouped into four cranial-caudal subdivisions based on their specific regional contributions to structures of the embryo (Fig. 4-20): cranial (caudal forebrain to the level of rhombomere six of the myelencephalon; rhombomeres are covered in Chapter 9); vagal (level of somites one to seven; the cranial part of the vagal level overlaps the caudal part of the cranial level, as the first few somites form adjacent to the rhombencephalon, not the spinal cord); trunk (level of somites eight to twenty-eight); and sacral/lumbosacral (level caudal to somite twenty-eight). Each of these subdivisions is covered below.

Cranial Neural Crest Cells

Neural crest cells from the caudal prosencephalon (forebrain) and mesencephalon (midbrain) regions give rise to the parasympathetic ganglion of cranial nerve III, a portion of the connective tissue around the developing eyes and optic nerves, the muscles of the iris and ciliary body, and part of the cornea of the eye; they also contribute, along with head mesoderm, to the head mesenchyme cranial to the level of the mesencephalon (covered in Chapters 10 and 17).

Neural crest cells from the mesencephalon and rhombencephalon (hindbrain) regions also give rise to structures in the developing **pharyngeal arches** of the head and neck (covered in Chapter 17). These structures include cartilaginous elements and several bones of the nose, face, middle ear, and neck. Mesencephalon and rhombencephalon neural crest cells form the dermis, smooth muscle, and fat of the face and ventral neck, and the odontoblasts of developing teeth. Neural crest cells arising from the caudalmost rhombencephalon contribute, along with vagal neural crest cells (covered later), to the **parafollicular cells of the thyroid**.

The rhombencephalic neural crest cells also contribute to some of the cranial nerve ganglia. Specifically, rhombencephalic neural crest cells give rise to some neurons and all glial cells in the sensory ganglia of cranial nerves V, VII, IX, and X (Fig. 4-21). The remaining neurons in the sensory ganglia of cranial nerves V, VII, IX, and X arise from small ectodermal placodes, called **epibranchial** or

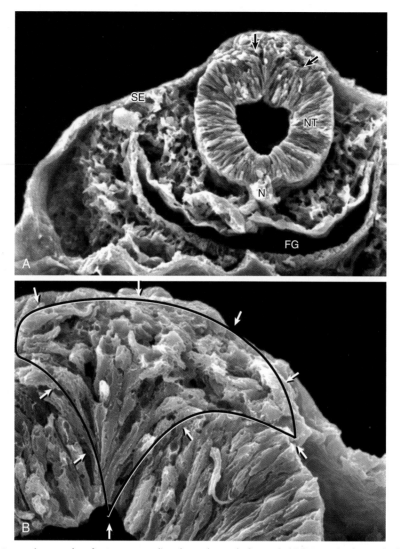

Figure 4-18. Scanning electron micrographs of a transverse slice through newly formed chick neural tube at the level of the midbrain. *B* is an enlargement of the neural crest cell–forming region of *A*. FG, Foregut; N, notochord; NT, neural tube; SE, surface ectoderm; arrows and outlined region demarcate forming and migrating neural crest cells.

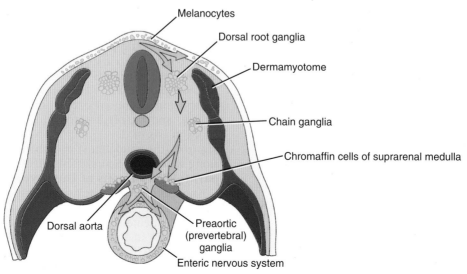

Figure 4-19. Neural crest cell migratory routes.

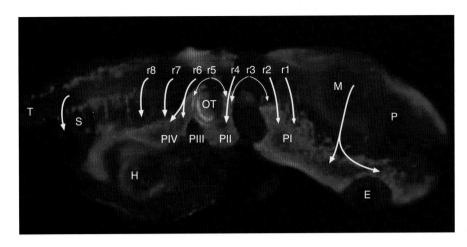

Figure 4-20. The head of a chick embryo labeled (red) with a specific neural crest cell antibody (HNK-1). Arrows show migratory routes of neural crest cells. E, Eye; H, heart; M, mesencephalon; OT, otic vesicle; P, prosencephalon; PI-PIV, pharyngeal arches I to IV; r1-r8, rhombomeres 1-8; S, somite; T, trunk (spinal cord level).

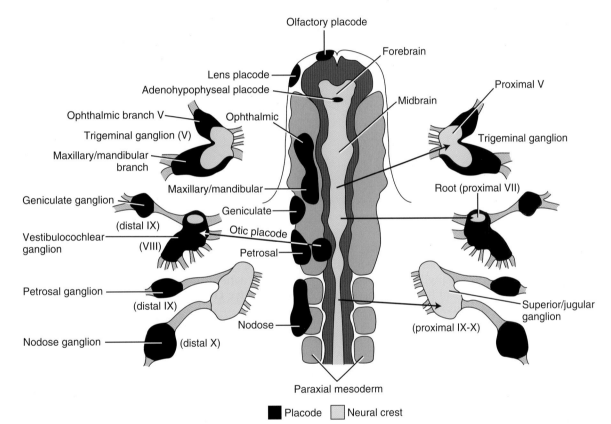

Figure 4-21. Fate map showing the contributions of placodes (left; black) and neural crest cells (center; light blue) to the cranial sensory ganglia. Note in ganglia derived from both neural crest cells and epipharyngeal placodes that the proximal (most dorsal) ganglia (and neuron cell bodies) are derived from neural crest cells. The distal (most ventral) ganglia (and neuron cell bodies) are derived from placodes. Glial cells in both proximal and distal ganglia of mixed origin are derived exclusively from neural crest cells. The special sensory nerves and associated glia (and ganglia when present) are derived from other placodes, namely, the olfactory and otic placodes, and the optic cup (derived from a portion of the forebrain adjacent to the lens placode).

epipharyngeal placodes. The special sensory nerves, associated glia, and ganglia (when present) also arise from placodes (covered in Chapters 17 through 19): cranial nerve I (olfactory) arises from the **olfactory placode**. cranial nerve II (optic) arises from the **optic cup** (the distal end of which thickens as the placode-like rudiment of the neural retina); and cranial nerve VIII (vestibulocochlear nerve) and the vestibulocochlear ganglion arise from the **otic placode**.

The rhombencephalic neural crest cells also give rise to the cranial component of the parasympathetic division of the autonomic nervous system (covered further below). Specifically, rhombencephalic neural crest cells give rise to all neurons (called postganglionic neurons; preganglionic neurons arise in the basal plate of the neural tube, as covered in Chapters 9 and 10) and glial cells in the parasympathetic ganglia of cranial nerves VII, IX, and X. Thus, in conjunction with neural crest cells derived from

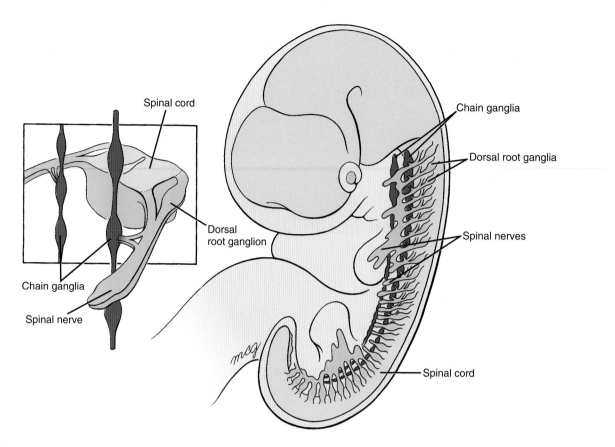

Figure 4-22. Neural crest cells form two types of segmental ganglia along almost the entire length of the spinal cord: dorsal root ganglia and chain ganglia.

the caudal prosencephalon and mesencephalon (that give rise to the parasympathetic ganglia of cranial nerve III), the entire cranial component of the parasympathetic division of the autonomic nervous system is formed from cranial neural crest cells.

Cranial neural crest cells as a group also give rise to other cell types that populate the head and neck. These include the pia mater and arachnoid—the inner and middle of the three meninges—of the occipital region; the dura mater, the outermost layer of the three meninges, arises largely or exclusively from head (paraxial) mesoderm. In addition, some cranial neural crest cells invade the surface ectoderm as they migrate away from the neural tube to form the melanocytes (pigment cells) of the skin of the head and neck.

Vagal Neural Crest Cells

Neural cells originating from the vagal region have three major contributions. Some of these neural crest cells migrate into the cranial pole of the developing heart, where they contribute to the septum (truncoconal) that forms to partition the outflow tract of the heart (covered in Chapter 12). Other vagal neural crest cells migrate more distally into the gut wall mesenchyme to form neurons, constituting the enteric nervous system, that innervate all regions of the gut tube from the esophagus to the rectum (covered later and in Chapter 14). Still other vagal neural crest cells migrate with those from the caudal

rhombencephalon (covered earlier) to the pharyngeal pouches, where they contribute to the **parafollicular cells of the thyroid** (covered in Chapter 17).

Trunk Neural Crest Cells

The peripheral nervous system of the neck, trunk, and limbs includes the following four types of peripheral neurons: peripheral sensory neurons, the cell bodies of which reside in the dorsal root ganglia; sympathetic and parasympathetic autonomic peripheral motoneurons, the cell bodies of which reside, respectively, in the sympathetic and parasympathetic ganglia; and enteric neurons, considered a third subdivision of the autonomic nervous system. All four types of peripheral neurons, plus their associated glia, are derived from neural crest cells. The following paragraphs describe the origin of these structures; their subsequent development is covered in Chapter 10.

Some of the neural crest cells arising from the trunk neural tube aggregate lateral to the neural tube, where they form small clumps in register with the somites (Fig. 4-22; see also Fig. 4-19). These clumps then differentiate into the segmental **dorsal root ganglia** of the spinal nerves, which house the sensory neurons that conduct impulses to the spinal cord from end organs in the viscera, body wall, and extremities. Fate mapping experiments demonstrate that most cells in each ganglion are derived from the neural tube at the corresponding level, although many originate from neural crest cells at adjacent cranial and caudal levels.

A pair of dorsal root ganglia develops at every segmental level except the first cervical and the second and third coccygeal levels (see Fig. 4-22). Thus, there are seven pairs of cervical, twelve pairs of thoracic, five pairs of lumbar, five pairs of sacral, and one pair of coccygeal dorsal root ganglia. The most cranial pair of cervical dorsal root ganglia (adjacent to the second cervical somite) forms on day twenty-eight, and the others form in craniocaudal succession over the next few days.

Some trunk neural crest cells migrate to a zone just ventral to the future dorsal root ganglia, where they form a series of condensations that develop into the **chain ganglia** of the **sympathetic division of the autonomic nervous system** (see Figs. 4-19, 4-22). In the thoracic, lumbar, and sacral regions, one pair of chain ganglia forms in register with each pair of somites. However, in the cervical region, only three larger chain ganglia develop, and the coccygeal region has only a single chain ganglion, which forms at the first coccygeal level. Fate mapping experiments indicate that the neural crest cells that give rise to the cervical chain ganglia originate along the cervical neural tube, whereas the thoracic, lumbar, and sacral ganglia are formed by crest cells from these corresponding levels of the neural tube.

The neurons that develop in the chain ganglia become the peripheral (postganglionic) neurons of the **sympathetic division of the autonomic nervous system**. The sympathetic division provides autonomic motor innervation to the viscera and exerts control over involuntary functions, such as heartbeat, glandular secretions, and intestinal movements. The sympathetic division is activated during conditions of "fight or flight," and this system consists of two-neuron pathways: the viscera are innervated by axons from the peripheral sympathetic neurons (whose cell bodies develop in the chain ganglia, or other ganglia described in the next paragraph), which in turn receive axons from central sympathetic motoneurons arising in the spinal cord. These central sympathetic motoneurons are located at all twelve thoracic levels and at the first three lumbar levels. For this reason, the sympathetic division (central and peripheral) is called a **thoracolumbar system**.

Not all peripheral (postganglionic) sympathetic neurons are located in the chain ganglia. The peripheral ganglia of some specialized sympathetic pathways develop from neural crest cells that congregate next to major branches of the dorsal aorta (see Fig. 4-19; covered in Chapter 10). For example, one pair of these **prevertebral** or **preaortic ganglia** forms at the base of the celiac artery. Other, more diffuse ganglia develop in association with the superior mesenteric artery, the renal arteries, and the inferior mesenteric artery. These are formed by thoracic and lumbar neural crest cells.

The **parasympathetic division of the autonomic nervous system** innervates the same structures as does the sympathetic division of the autonomic nervous system. It also consists of two-neuron (peripheral and central) pathways. Peripheral (postganglionic) parasympathetic neurons arise from neural crest cells that form ganglia. As covered above, some of these ganglia are associated with

four cranial nerves: III, VII, IX, and X. Other of these ganglia arise from neural crest cells originating from the lumbosacral neural crest cells (covered below). These neural crest cells migrate more distally to form the **parasympathetic (terminal) ganglia**, typically located near or on the wall of the viscera they innervate. Thus, the parasympathetic autonomic nervous system has a craniosacral origin. The parasympathetic division is active during periods of "peace and relaxation" and stimulates the visceral organs to carry out their routine functions of housekeeping and digestion; thus, the function of the parasympathetic division is opposite to that of the sympathetic division.

The **enteric nervous system** is derived from neural crest cells originating from both vagal and lumbosacral regions. As covered above, the vagal neural crest cells migrate into the wall of the gut tube to innervate all regions of the gut tube from the esophagus to the rectum. They invade the gut tube in a cranial-to-caudal wave. Similarly, lumbosacral neural crest cells invade the gut tube but do so in a caudal-to-cranial wave. Thus, the terminal part of the gut has a dual innervation, with its enteric nervous system originating from both vagal and lumbosacral neural crest cells (Fig. 4-23).

In addition to forming neurons and glia, trunk neural crest cells form a variety of other cell types. These include the inner and middle meningeal coverings of the spinal cord (pia mater and arachnoid mater); Schwann cells, which form the myelin sheaths (neurilemma) of peripheral nerves; and neurosecretory chromaffin cells of the suprarenal medulla. Like cranial neural crest cells, trunk neural crest cells invade the surface ectoderm as they migrate away from the neural tube to form the melanocytes of the skin of the trunk and limbs.

Sacral/Lumbosacral Neural Crest Cells

As covered above, in the most inferior regions of the gut, the enteric nervous system has a dual origin: some enteric neurons arise from the vagal neural crest cells, whereas others arise from the lumbosacral neural crest cells. These caudal neural crest cells apparently arise from both the primary and secondary portions of the neural tube. Their importance in gut innervation is exemplified by Hirschsprung disease (congenital megacolon), which results when lumbosacral neural crest cells fail to innervate the terminal portion of the colon, resulting in impaired gut motility (Hirschsprung disease is covered in Chapter 14).

As covered above, neural crest cells form a diversity of cell types. Many of the major derivatives of the cranial and trunk neural crest cells are summarized in Figure 4-24. Other contributions to derivatives of the pharyngeal pouches and associated structures are covered in Chapter 17.

In the Research Lab

SURVIVAL AND DIFFERENTIATION OF PERIPHERAL NEURONS

Experimental studies have shown that the survival and differentiation of peripheral neurons require the presence of small growth factors called **neurotrophins**. For dorsal root ganglion cells, these include nerve growth factor (Ngf), neurotrophin-3

(Nt-3), and brain-derived neurotrophic factor (Bdnf), secreted by the neural tube and the dermamyotome subdivision of the somite (covered later in the chapter). Thus, the dorsal root ganglia are virtually absent in mice lacking Ngf, Ngf receptor, or Nt-3 genes. Similarly, survival and differentiation of sympathetic chain ganglion cells depend on Ngf and Nt-3, as well as on growth factors such as insulin-like growth factor (Igf).

In the Clinic

NEURAL CREST CELL DISEASE: NEUROCRISTOPATHIES

Because neural crest cells contribute to a large diversity of structures, abnormal development of neural crest cells can affect many different organ systems. Such defects of neural crest cell development are known as **neurocristopathies**, that is, pathologies associated with neural crest cell derivatives. These occur in conditions such as **neurofibromatosis** (von Recklinghausen disease; e.g., peripheral nerve tumors), **Charcot-Marie-Tooth** (a chronic demyelinating disease of peripheral nerve, especially the peroneal nerve), **Waardenburg types I and II** and **albinism** (pigmentation defects), **pheochromocytoma** (tumors of the chromaffin cells of the suprarenal medulla), and **Hirschsprung disease** (congenital megacolon; absence of innervation of the terminal part of the colon), as well as in syndromes such as **CHARGE** (coloboma of the eye, heart defects, atresia of the choanae, retarded growth and development, genital and urinary anomalies, and ear anomalies and hearing loss) and **22q11.2 deletion syndrome** (also known as **DiGeorge** or **velocardiofacial syndrome**) that affect development of the craniofacial and cardiovascular systems. Each of these neurocristopathies is covered in the appropriate chapter covering development of the affected organ system.

In the Research Lab

INDUCTIVE INTERACTIONS UNDERLIE FORMATION OF SOMITE SUBDIVISIONS

Experiments involving tissue transplantation and ablation have shown that structures adjacent to the developing somites are responsible for patterning the somites into their subdivisions. Signals from the notochord induce the sclerotome, whereas signals from the dorsal neural tube, surface ectoderm, and adjacent lateral plate (and intermediate) mesoderm induce and pattern the dermamyotome (Fig. 4-27). More recent molecular genetic experiments have begun to elucidate the molecules mediating these signaling interactions. Notochord (and subsequently the floor plate of the neural tube) secretes sonic hedgehog (Shh), which along with noggin (a Bmp inhibitor), also secreted by the notochord, is required for induction and maintenance of the sclerotome; specifically, these factors are required for the expression of Pax1, a paired-box transcription factor. Pax1 is mutated in several of the undulated mouse mutants, characterized by vertebral body and vertebral disc defects. In the Shh null mouse, vertebrae do not form, in part because of increased cell death. Dorsal neural tube and surface ectoderm produce various Wnts (Wnt1, -3a, and Wnt4, -6, respectively), which induce dermamyotome. Formation of the dermamyotome is marked by the expression of another paired-box transcription factor, Pax3, which is required for further development of the dermamyotome, as well as for forming the myotome. Wnt6 signaling from the ectoderm also maintains the epithelial characteristics of the dermamyotome. In addition, long-range Shh signaling is needed for the initial specification of the epaxial (defined and covered below) part of the myotome.

As the dermamyotome is forming, it is further patterned by a gradient of Bmp4 signaling. This gradient is established by secretion of Bmp4 by the lateral plate mesoderm and by

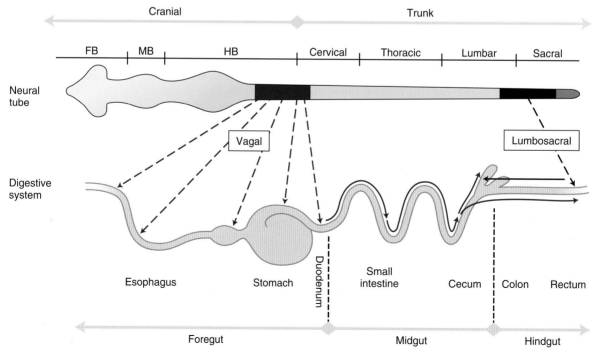

Figure 4-23. Neural crest cells invade the developing gut in two waves to form the enteric nervous system. The entire length of the gut receives contributions from vagal neural crest cells, which invade the gut in a cranial-to-caudal sequence. The terminal (caudal) part of the gut is also invaded by lumbosacral neural crest cells, which colonize the gut in a caudal-to-cranial sequence.

activation of noggin in the dorsal somite by factors secreted by the dorsal neural tube (Wnts) and notochord (Shh). Noggin, a Bmp inhibitor, attenuates Bmp signaling. Thus a gradient of Bmp signaling occurs across the dermamyotome, resulting in subsequent patterning of cells in this rudiment. Further development of the somite and its subdivisions, including myogenesis, skeletogenesis, and resegmentation, is covered in Chapter 8.

SOMITE DIFFERENTIATION: FORMING DERMAMYOTOME AND SCLEROTOME

As covered in Chapter 3, the paraxial mesoderm of the trunk undergoes segmentation to form the epithelial somites (Fig. 4-25). Shortly thereafter, each somite reorganizes into two subdivisions: the epithelial **dermamyotome** (sometimes spelled, "dermomyotome" in the

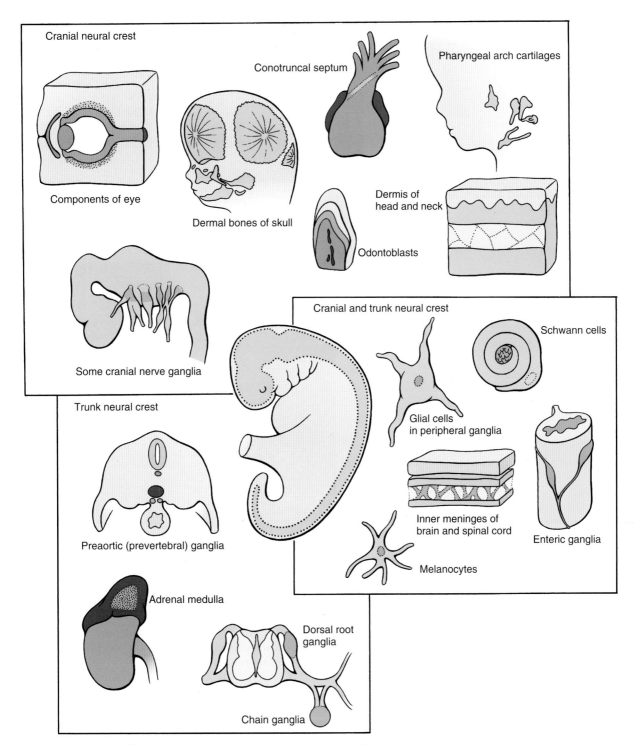

Figure 4-24. Neural crest cells migrating from both cranial and trunk regions of the neural tube give rise to a variety of tissues in the embryo.

Somite   Neural tube

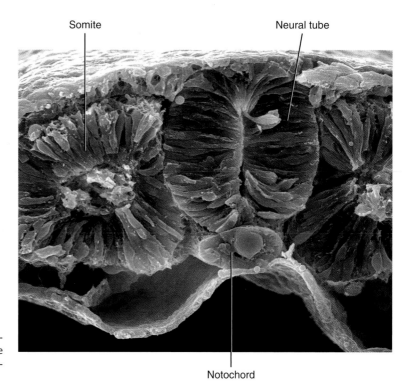

Notochord

Figure 4-25. Scanning electron micrograph of a transversely sectioned chick embryo showing the neural tube and underlying notochord and adjacent newly formed epithelial somite on one side.

Dermamyotome

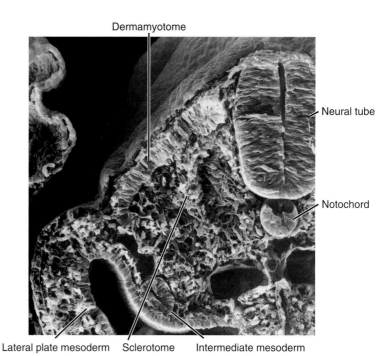

Neural tube

Notochord

Lateral plate mesoderm   Sclerotome   Intermediate mesoderm

Figure 4-26. Scanning electron micrograph of a transversely sectioned chick embryo showing the neural tube and underlying notochord and adjacent somite on one side subdivided into dermamyotome and sclerotome. Also note the intermediate mesoderm and lateral plate mesoderm.

literature) and the mesenchymal **sclerotome** (Fig. 4-26). Thus, formation of the sclerotome, like ingression of cells through the primitive streak and formation of neural crest cells, is another example of an **epithelial-to-mesenchymal transformation**.

During subsequent development, the **sclerotomes** will develop into the vertebrae. Note that the ventral portion of the sclerotome surrounds the notochord; this portion of the sclerotome will form the vertebral body. More dorsally, the sclerotome flanks the neural tube and will eventually expand dorsal to it to form the vertebral arch.

The dermamyotome contributes to the **dermis of the skin** throughout the trunk. In addition, it forms the **myotome**, which gives rise to the **epaxial** (dorsal) and **hypaxial** (ventrolateral) **muscles** of the body wall. Moreover, after formation of the limb buds, myotome cells migrate into the developing limbs to form the **limb muscles**.

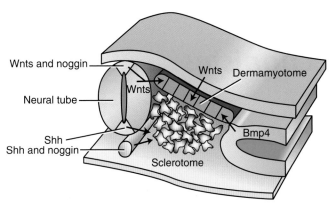

Figure 4-27. Inductive interactions involved in the formation of somite subdivisions. Arrows indicate signaling. Lighter triangular areas of the neural tube indicate the roof plate (dorsally) and the floor plate (ventrally).

In the Clinic

SPINAL ANOMALIES

A number of spinal defects are caused by abnormal formation of the sclerotomes and neural tube. Defective formation of vertebral bodies on one side of the body may result in a severe congenital **scoliosis** (lateral bending of the spinal column), which may require surgical correction. Scoliosis and other vertebral anomalies are covered further in Chapter 8. As covered earlier in the chapter, open and closed neural tube defects at the spinal cord level also result in vertebral arch and spine defects.

Embryology in Practice

LIFE WITH SPINA BIFIDA

A young man born with spina bifida is graduating from college and reflects upon his life.

His spina bifida was not a surprise to his parents, who were informed after a prenatal ultrasound. They learned all they could about the condition and met with a number of specialists in spina bifida care before his birth, which occurred before fetal surgery was used to attempt to close these defects prenatally. It was during this prenatal period that his parents learned the alternative term "neural tube defect" (NTD) used to refer to spina bifida.

He was delivered by cesarean section to minimize injury to exposed tissue, and on the first day of his life, he underwent surgical closure of a high lumbar myelomeningocele (condition in which the meningeal sac and the contained open or closed spinal cord protrude through a localized defect in vertebral elements). Profound defects in the motor and sensory function of his legs were apparent immediately to his parents and his doctors.

The boy faced multiple medical challenges in infancy and early childhood with numerous surgeries and hospitalizations. He needed surgical treatment for hydrocephalus (as is common

with NTDs) by placement of a ventriculoperitoneal or "VP" shunt (a catheter that caries CSF from the brain ventricle to the abdomen). He recalls at least one "shunt malfunction" as a child, when the passage became blocked, and surgical revision was needed. The need for shunt revision is common in these children.

Problems with bowel and bladder control also figure prominently in the boy's memory. He has ongoing constipation and needed to be hospitalized several times because of stool impaction. Besides inability to control elimination (incontinence), poor drainage of urine put excess pressure on his kidneys, requiring surgery to create a "vesicostomy" (a passage between the bladder and the body wall formed using the boy's appendix). He was left with a lifelong need for intermittent catheterization and antibiotic prophylaxis to prevent infection, but his kidneys are healthy and he is continent.

Although as a boy, he could walk short distances without the aid of braces, he now uses a wheelchair almost exclusively. He has to pay close attention to wheelchair fit and periodic repositioning to avoid skin breakdown and pressure sores where he lacks sensation. He has also dealt with other "wounds," often being the subject of teasing by other children at school and struggling with depressive symptoms.

Although many children with spina bifida have learning difficulties, this boy was always bright. And despite the many and lifelong challenges, he has succeeded in making the transition to independence in adulthood, thanks to strong support from family, community, schools, and a multidisciplinary team of health-care providers. Spina bifida is no longer exclusively a childhood disease. Advanced treatments now allow patients to achieve normal life expectancies, underscoring the need for physicians trained to care for adult patients with congenital disorders.

He wonders if one day he will marry. He is currently dating a junior at his college, and they have had long discussions about his condition and daily life. The subject of having children has come up. Although some men with spina bifida can have erections and ejaculations, allowing them to father children, others cannot. In the latter case, in vitro fertilization (IVF) is an option.

SUGGESTED READINGS

Kalcheim C. 2011. Regulation of trunk myogenesis by the neural crest: a new facet of neural crest-somite interactions. Dev Cell 21:187–188.

Kraus MR, Grapin-Botton A. 2012. Patterning and shaping the endoderm in vivo and in culture. Curr Opin Genet Dev 22:347–353.

Le Douarin NM, Dieterlen-Lievre F. 2013. How studies on the avian embryo have opened new avenues in the understanding of development: a view about the neural and hematopoietic systems. Dev Growth Differ 55:1–14.

Nitzan E, Kalcheim C. 2013. Neural crest and somitic mesoderm as paradigms to investigate cell fate decisions during development. Dev Growth Differ 55:60–78.

Suzuki M, Morita H, Ueno N. 2012. Molecular mechanisms of cell shape changes that contribute to vertebrate neural tube closure. Dev Growth Differ 54:266–276.

Vieira C, Pombero A, Garcia-Lopez R, et al. 2010. Molecular mechanisms controlling brain development: an overview of neuroepithelial secondary organizers. Int J Dev Biol 54:7–20.

Chapter 5

Principles and Mechanisms of Morphogenesis and Dysmorphogenesis

SUMMARY

Formation of the embryo and its parts involves **morphogenesis**, a form-shaping process controlled by fundamental **cell behaviors** that result in **differential growth**. Perturbation of differential growth due to a **genetic mutation**, **teratogen** exposure, or a combination of the two processes results in **dysmorphogenesis** and the formation of structural **birth defects**. Structural birth defects consist of both **malformations**—involving perturbation of developmental events directly involved in forming a particular structure—and **deformations**—involving indirect perturbation of a developing structure due to mechanical forces. Malformation can involve single organs or body parts or a constellation of organs or body parts. In the latter case, if a single cause is involved, the condition constitutes a **syndrome**. Understanding how development occurs requires the use of **animal models** in which experiments can be conducted. Because developmental mechanisms are conserved across species, the use of animal models provides insight into how normal development of the human embryo occurs and how development can be perturbed by genetic mutation or environmental insult, resulting in birth defects. The tool kit for the developmental biologist's experiments is vast, including techniques derived from the fields of **cell biology, molecular biology**, and **genetics**, combined with the classical approaches of **cut-and-paste experimental embryology**. Manipulation of the **mouse genome** has been a particularly fruitful approach for understanding how genes function during development and for developing models for human disease and birth defects. Through experimental approaches, a small number of highly conserved **signaling pathways** have been identified. These pathways are used repeatedly and in various combinations throughout embryonic development. Tools originally used to study mouse embryos have been adapted for use in human embryos. This has resulted in advances in reproductive technologies, such as in vitro fertilization (IVF), and recently in the development of **stem cells**—cells that potentially can be used to regenerate diseased or damaged organs.

Clinical Taster

A first-year medical genetics fellow is on full-time service for the month of May. Early in the month, she is asked to consult on an infant with cleft lip and palate and possible brain abnormalities that were identified on prenatal ultrasound. Review of the prenatal and postnatal history is significant only for an abnormal ultrasound during the twenty-fourth week of gestation that showed dilation and possible fusion of the lateral ventricles of the brain, and for premature birth at thirty-two weeks after the onset of preterm labor. The family history seems negative at first, but on further discussion, the fellow elicits a history of a single central incisor in the patient's father. The physical examination shows microcephaly (small head), ocular hypotelorism (closely spaced eyes), a flat nasal bridge, and bilateral **cleft lip** and **cleft palate** (Fig. 5-1*A*). Magnetic resonance imaging (MRI) of the brain shows fusion of the left and right frontal lobes and partial fusion of the parietal lobes characteristic of semilobar **holoprosencephaly**. Genetic testing discovers a deleterious mutation in the **SONIC HEDGEHOG (SHH)** gene in both the patient and her father.

Near the end of the month, the fellow is called to the nursery to examine a newborn with limb anomalies. She finds an otherwise healthy, full-term girl with **polydactyly** (extra digits) of both hands and feet occurring on the thumb and great toe side (preaxial; Fig. 5-1*B*). Chromosome analysis shows a translocation involving chromosomes 5 and 7, with the chromosome 7 breakpoint occurring distant from the SHH gene, but in a region known to affect SHH expression in the limb. Disruption of these regulatory elements is known to cause preaxial polydactyly.

The fellow is impressed by the variability of manifestations caused by different defects in the same gene (SHH), with one mutation causing brain and face abnormalities and another causing limb defects.

PRINCIPLES OF MORPHOGENESIS AND DYSMORPHOGENESIS

Having described the initial steps in embryogenesis in Chapters 1 to 4, it is appropriate to pause to lay down the basic groundwork for understanding the concepts of normal and abnormal embryology covered in later chapters. Moreover, because these concepts have been formulated using animal models for experimental studies, it is important to understand the attributes each of these models

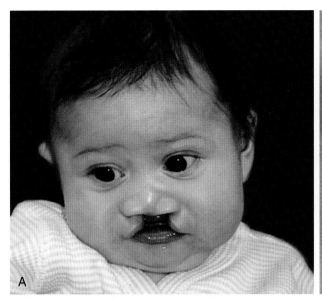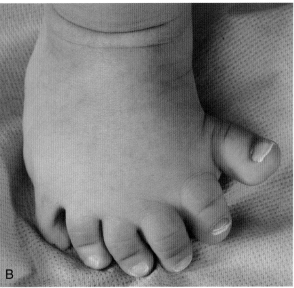

Figure 5-1. Mutations in the SONIC HEDGEHOG (SHH) gene have multiple manifestations. *A,* Infant with bilateral cleft lip and facial findings associated with holoprosencephaly. *B,* Foot of an infant with preaxial polydactyly.

provides for understanding human development. Finally, experimental techniques are described to explain how experiments are conducted in the field of developmental biology, and signaling pathways are covered to place molecules that control developmental events into context.

As covered in preceding chapters, the initially flat three-layered embryonic disc undergoes **morphogenesis** to form a three-dimensional embryo with a tube-within-a-tube body plan and the beginnings of rudiments that will form all of the adult organs and systems. In this chapter, we consider how morphogenesis occurs and how morphogenesis goes awry during the formation of **birth defects**. Morphogenesis results from **differential growth**. Differential growth is driven by a small number of fundamental **cellular behaviors**, such as changes in cell shape, size, position, number, and adhesivity. If these behaviors are perturbed during embryogenesis by a genetic mutation, environmental insult (i.e., a **teratogen**), or a combination of the two, differential growth is abnormal and **dysmorphogenesis** results with the formation of a structural birth defect.

Dysmorphogenesis can result from both **malformation** and **deformation**. Malformations consist of primary morphological defects in an organ or body part resulting from abnormal developmental events that are *directly* involved in the development of that organ or body part. For example, failure of the neural groove to close results in a malformation called a *neural tube defect*. Similarly, failure of the digits to separate fully results in *syndactyly*, that is, fusion of the digits. Deformations consist of secondary morphological defects that are imposed upon an organ or body part owing to mechanical forces, that is, deformations affect the development of an organ or body part *indirectly*. For example, if insufficient amniotic fluid forms (i.e., oligohydramnios), deformation of the feet can occur as the result of mechanical constraints, leading to club foot. Dysmorphogenesis can occur in an isolated organ or body part or as a pattern of multiple primary malformations with a single cause. In the latter case, the condition is referred to as a **syndrome**. Common examples, covered

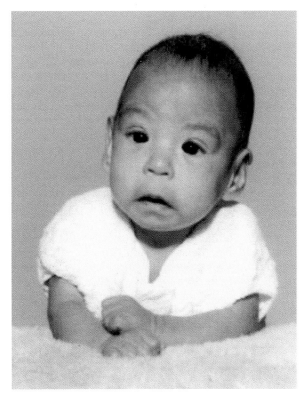

Figure 5-2. Boy with fetal alcohol syndrome. Note in particular the low nasal bridge, epicanthal folds, short palpebral fissures, indistinct philtrum, and micrognathia.

elsewhere in the text, include Down syndrome (trisomy 21) and 22q11.2 deletion syndrome—two syndromes that result from chromosomal abnormalities.

Other syndromes can result from teratogen exposure. A common example is **fetal alcohol syndrome**, also known as **fetal alcohol spectrum disorder**. This disorder affects 2 in 1000 live-born infants (Fig. 5-2). Fetal alcohol syndrome is most prevalent in alcoholic women,

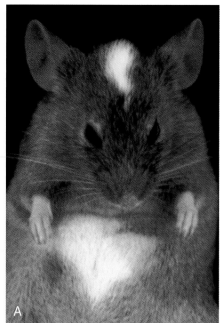 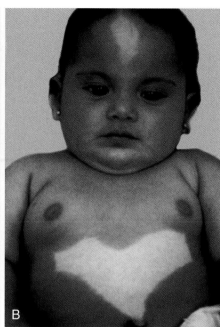

Figure 5-3. Animal models for disease can precisely phenocopy human diseases. *A,* Mouse with a mutation in the c-kit gene shows pigmentation deficits on the forehead and chest. *B,* Child with a mutation in the c-KIT gene, a condition known as piebaldism, shows pigmentation deficits that are similar to those shown by the mouse model.

especially those in their third or fourth pregnancies, suggesting that maternal health status interacts with alcohol to produce the syndrome. Nevertheless, consumption of amounts of alcohol as low as 80 g per day (i.e., between two and three shots of a grain liquor such as rum) by a non-alcoholic woman during the first month of pregnancy can cause significant defects, and it has been suggested that even a single binge may be teratogenic. In addition, chronic consumption of even small amounts of alcohol even in later pregnancy can be dangerous, as it may affect development of the fetal brain, resulting in behavioral and cognitive deficiencies that may last a lifetime. Thus, there is no known safe level of alcohol consumption during pregnancy.

Common components of the disorder include defects of brain and face development, namely, microcephaly (small head), short palpebral fissures (eye openings), epicanthal folds (folds over eye lids), a low nasal bridge with a short nose, flat midface, minor external ear anomalies, and jaw anomalies, including a thin upper lip with indistinct philtrum and micrognathia (small jaw).

ANIMAL MODELS

The aim of research in developmental biology/embryology is to understand how development occurs at tissue, cellular, and molecular levels. This aim speaks largely to our innate curiosity to understand nature and how it works. An additional aim is to understand how normal development can go awry, resulting in birth defects, particularly in humans. Understanding how both normal development and abnormal development occur could lead to ways to detect (diagnose), prevent, and cure birth defects. Thus, this aim speaks to our desire to prevent and relieve human suffering.

Although the only perfect organism for studying how the human embryo develops is the human embryo,

animal models provide useful surrogates because of the principle that **developmental mechanisms are highly conserved** from organism to organism (Fig. 5-3). Six animal models have been particularly useful for deciphering mechanisms and principles of embryogenesis: two invertebrates and four vertebrates. These models provide complementary information, which, when assembled across animal models, provides considerable insight into how the human embryo develops. All of these models are practical to obtain, use, and maintain in the laboratory, and all can be acquired and used throughout the year (i.e., they are not seasonal breeders). The unique strengths of each of these organisms for understanding mechanisms of development are covered below.

DROSOPHILA

The developing field of genetics was greatly enhanced in the early twentieth century using *Drosophila melanogaster,* the common fruit fly. Thus, the first studies to merge the burgeoning fields of genetics with developmental biology utilized Drosophila. Drosophila offers several advantages for understanding mechanisms of development. Through saturation mutagenesis using chemicals such as EMS (ethyl methane sulfonate) and subsequent screening to identify unique phenotypes, mutations have been identified in virtually every gene (Drosophila has 13,639 predicted genes). This powerful process of using random mutations in unknown genes to identify perturbed developmental events (i.e., thereby resulting in **phenotypes**), followed by identification and cloning of the mutated gene, is referred to as the **forward genetic approach**.

The life cycle of Drosophila is relatively short (about nine days; Fig. 5-4); thus, new generations can be bred very quickly (i.e., Drosophila is genetically amenable). Embryogenesis also occurs very rapidly, with embryogenesis being completed and the first larval stage forming about one day after fertilization. After formation of a

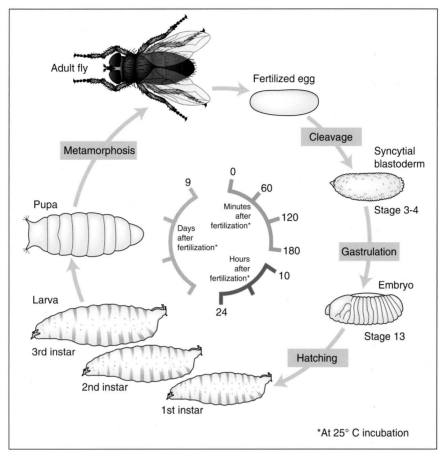

Figure 5-4. The life cycle of Drosophila.

series of larval stages, a pupa forms, which subsequently metamorphoses into the adult fruit fly.

Several techniques have been developed for gene overexpression or underexpression in Drosophila, allowing experimental analyses of gene function during development. Also, a website (FlyBase) has been developed to disseminate information on Drosophila, as a model system (flybase.org).

A surprising finding of the genomic era has been the realization that the genomes of fruit flies and humans are highly similar. Orthologs of about 60% of the genes expressed during Drosophila embryogenesis have been identified in other animal models, as well as in humans, although total gene number in humans is about double that in Drosophila (it is estimated that humans have 20,000 to 25,000 genes). Vertebrates, including humans, typically have multiple family members orthologous to each identified Drosophila gene. Thus, for example, in Drosophila, there are three Fgf ligand genes (branchless, pyramus, and thisbe) and two Fgf receptor genes (breathless and heartless), whereas in mammals, there are twenty-two Fgf genes and four Fgf receptor genes (Fgfs and Fgf receptors are covered later in this chapter; branchless and breathless are covered in Chapter 11 in the "In the Research Lab" entitled "Drosophila Tracheal System Development").

CAENORHABDITIS ELEGANS

The nematode worm, *Caenorhabditis elegans*, shares many of the features that make Drosophila an outstanding model system for understanding mechanisms of development. Like Drosophila, *C. elegans* has a short life cycle of three to four days and a short period of embryogenesis—going from fertilization to hatching (as a worm) in about one day (Fig. 5-5). Chemical mutagenesis has also been used in *C. elegans* to generate a series of mutants that have greatly advanced the field (i.e., using the forward genetic approach), particularly leading to an understanding of mechanisms underlying programmed cell death or **apoptosis**, and gene misexpression techniques are well developed (including feeding worms RNAi [interfering, double-stranded RNA]) to knock down gene expression (RNAi is covered later in the chapter). Also, a website (WormBase) has been developed to disseminate information on *C. elegans* as a model system (wormbase.org).

In addition to having many attributes shared with Drosophila, the *C. elegans* embryo is transparent. This, along with a relatively small number of cells generated during development (the adult worm is composed of only about one thousand cells, and cell number is essentially invariant between individuals), has allowed investigators to map out the complete **cell lineage** of *C. elegans* by watching cells as they divide, change position, and differentiate during embryogenesis. As a result of such study, the origin and fate of every cell in the *C. elegans* embryo are known, including one hundred thirty-one cells whose normal fate in development is to die (undergo apoptosis). The *C. elegans* genome contains 20,000 predicted genes.

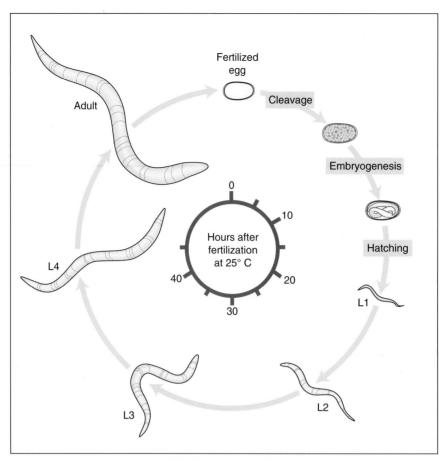

Figure 5-5. The life cycle of *C. elegans*.

ZEBRAFISH

The zebrafish model, *Danio rerio*, enables the use of muta-genesis and phenotype screening to study directly *verte-brate* development. Using ENU (N-ethyl-N-nitrosourea) mutagenesis, mutant embryos can be identified and stud-ied developmentally; more than eight thousand muta-tions have been identified using the forward genetic approach. Such study is greatly facilitated by the fact that zebrafish embryos, like *C. elegans* embryos, are transpar-ent, so internal structures can be readily visualized with-out the need in many cases for histologic study. Also, like the other model systems covered so far, zebrafish embryos develop rapidly, progressing from fertilization to free swimming fry in about two days, and fish reach sexual maturity in about three months (Fig. 5-6).

The cells (blastomeres) of cleaving zebrafish embryos are relatively large and can be injected with lineage trac-ers or RNAs for gene misexpression studies. Morpholinos (stabilized antisense RNA; covered later in the chapter) can be injected to knock down gene expression, and they can also be injected in mutant embryos to study the combined effects of loss of function of multiple genes. In addition, transgenic approaches, including generat-ing gene knockins and knockouts (covered later in the chapter), have been recently developed in zebrafish. The zebrafish genome has been sequenced and is estimated to contain 30,000 to 60,000 genes (genome duplications have occurred during zebrafish evolution). A website,

ZFIN, has been established to disseminate information on zebrafish as a model system (zfin.org).

XENOPUS LAEVIS

The field of experimental embryology began in the nine-teenth century with the use of a variety of amphibian—frog and salamander—embryos. However, during the past few decades, *Xenopus laevis*, the South African clawed toad, has become the amphibian of choice for developmental biologists. Amphibian embryos readily tolerate micro-surgical manipulation, so-called cutting-and-pasting experimental embryology (covered later in the chap-ter). In addition, because cells (blastomeres) of cleav-ing embryos are relatively large, as they are in zebrafish, they can be injected with lineage tracers. In fact, prob-ably the most precise **fate maps** produced to date using this approach are for *X. laevis*. *X. laevis*, like the models already covered, develops relatively rapidly, progressing from the fertilized egg to the tadpole in about four days (Fig. 5-7). The tadpole undergoes metamorphosis to form the adult terrestrial form, which becomes sexually mature in about two months.

Because genome duplication has occurred in *X. laevis*, this species is tetraploid. This fact makes it difficult to use *X. laevis* for gene manipulation studies. However, another species of Xenopus, *X. tropicalis*, is diploid, and it has been possible to use this species to generate **transgenic**

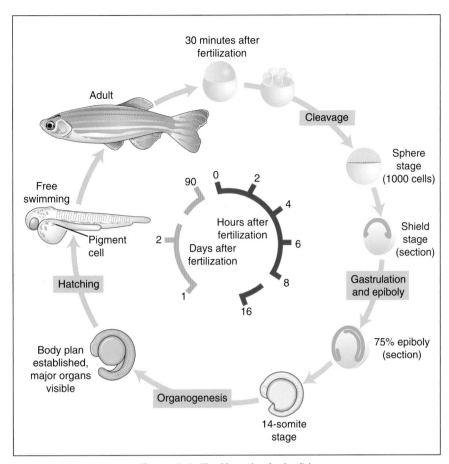

Figure 5-6. The life cycle of zebrafish.

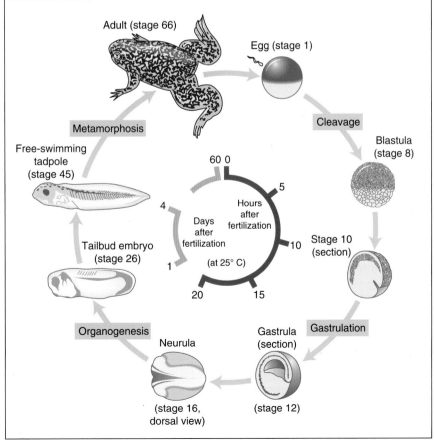

Figure 5-7. The life cycle of Xenopus.

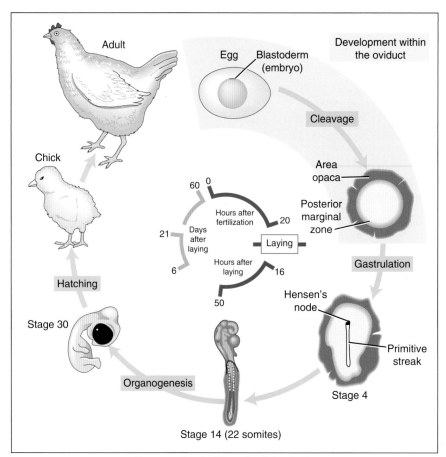

Figure 5-8. The life cycle of the chick.

animals, that is, animals in which the genome has been modified using molecular genetic techniques. Sequencing of the *X. tropicalis* genome has been completed, greatly enhancing the value of Xenopus as a model system. A website, Xenbase, has been developed to disseminate information on the Xenopus model (xenbase.org).

CHICK

Chick, or *Gallus gallus domesticus*, embryos, like Xenopus embryos, can be readily manipulated microsurgically during development. Because the chick is a warm-blooded organism (as is the human) and because it can be so readily manipulated during development, it has become over the past several decades the favored workhorse for studies utilizing cut-and-paste experimental embryology approaches (covered later in the chapter). Although currently the chicken is not used extensively for genetic studies, it was a popular model for such studies early in the twentieth century, primarily in agricultural colleges and poultry science departments. Many developmental mutants were collected, and some of these are still available today for study. As compared with the other models covered earlier in the chapter, development of the chick embryo is relatively slow, taking about twenty-one days from fertilization to hatching, and birds reach sexually maturity three to four months after hatching (Fig. 5-8).

The chicken genome has been sequenced, enhancing the use of this organism for understanding molecular

mechanisms of development. It is estimated that the chicken genome contains about 25,000 genes. Techniques have been developed for overexpressing proteins locally at specific times during chick development (e.g., using small beads coated with growth factors, injecting engineered viruses, injecting transfected cells); overexpressing genes using whole-embryo electroporation (through techniques such as sonoporation and lipofection) to target plasmids expressing the gene of interest to desired tissues in the chick embryo; and using RNAi or morpholinos (covered later in the chapter) to knockdown gene expression (typically introduced through whole-embryo electroporation). Useful websites, such as Bird Base, have been developed to disseminate information, especially genomic information and gene expression patterns, on the chick model (birdbase.arizona.edu).

MOUSE

The laboratory mouse, *Mus musculus*, was originally used for genetic studies, and hundreds of naturally occurring mutations have been identified and are available for study. Sexual maturity is reached within two to three months after birth, facilitating the breeding of mutant animals (Fig. 5-9). The time of gestation of the mouse is similar to that of the chick, ranging from nineteen to twenty-one days after fertilization.

The main strength of the mouse model is the availability of techniques to make **transgenic mice** (covered

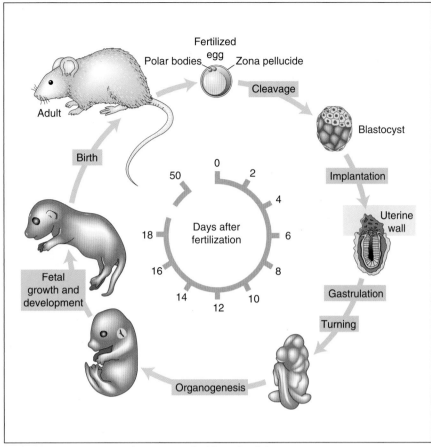

Figure 5-9. The life cycle of the mouse.

later in the chapter). Using homologous recombination, it is possible to inactivate (knock out) any gene of interest or to replace one gene with another (knock in). About 30% of mouse genes have been knocked out by this approach. In contrast to the forward genetic approach used in Drosophila, *C. elegans*, and zebrafish, the so-called **reverse genetic approach** used in mouse starts with a *known* gene and mutates it to determine its function during development. In a variation of this approach using *conditional* transgenics, it is now possible to use tissue-specific promoters to drive expression of a transgene (including reporter genes) in specific tissues (or to knock out the gene in specific tissues only), enhancing the precision of the experiment. The mouse genome has been sequenced and is predicted to contain about 30,000 genes. Useful websites include jaxmice.jax.org and ensembl.org/Mus_musculus.

USING ANIMAL MODELS TO PREDICT HUMAN RISK

Developmental toxicologists usually choose animal models different from those used by developmental biologists because the goal in their studies is different: to predict the risk to humans of exposure to drugs and potential environmental pollutants. Thus, such studies are concerned with similarities between animal models and human placentation (i.e., How similar is placental function?) or

pharmacodynamics (i.e., How similar is the metabolism of drugs?). Rodents are typically used for initial studies, but rats or rabbits may be chosen in place of mice. These model animals have a short gestation (rats, twenty-two days; rabbits, thirty-one days) and offer the advantage of a larger size, making it more likely that rare outcomes will be observed. In addition, non-human primate models are used for later studies as required based on the findings of initial studies. Non-human primate models are rarely used in developmental biology studies.

EXPERIMENTAL TECHNIQUES

Understanding how normal development and abnormal development occur requires a detailed understanding of *what* happens during development—that is, a detailed understanding of **descriptive embryology**. However, descriptive embryology alone cannot reveal *how* development occurs. Descriptive embryology provides a catalog of developmental events, which, when carefully studied and reflected upon, can lead to the formulation of **hypotheses** about how a developmental event occurs. The investigator then designs and conducts tests of the formulated hypotheses. Hypotheses are tested through a series of **experiments** (specific manipulations that usually perturb a developmental process) as compared with **controls** (non-specific manipulations used to ensure that results obtained from particular manipulations are

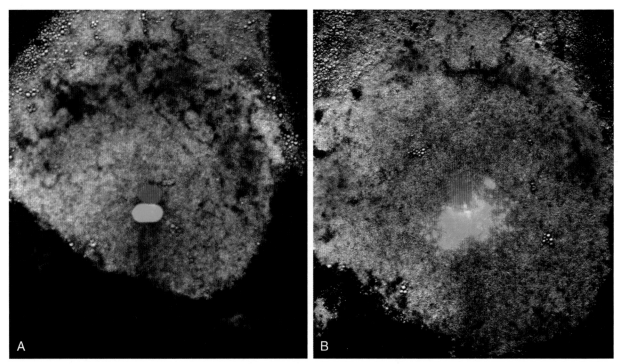

Figure 5-10. The use of fluorescent dyes to fate map cells (i.e., painting) of the primitive streak during gastrulation. Two dyes were injected into the primitive streak. *A,* Immediately after injection. *B,* Five hours after injection. Cells are now leaving the primitive streak (ingressing) to form endoderm and mesoderm.

specific and not artifactual). Through this approach, hypotheses are refuted, modified, or supported (never truly proven to be correct, but often proven to be incorrect). The cycle continues as new hypotheses are crafted, based on additional data obtained through experiments, leading to new experimental tests of their veracity.

Conducting experiments on developing model embryos constitutes the science of **experimental embryology**. Classically, experimental embryology has been used to define the tissue and cellular basis of development through a series of microsurgical manipulations. More recently, experimental embryology has merged with cell biology, molecular biology, and genetics, allowing investigators to define the molecular-genetic basis of development.

CLASSICAL EXPERIMENTAL EMBRYOLOGY

Classical experimental embryology involves three basic techniques often referred to as **cutting**, **pasting**, and **painting** (Figs. 5-10, 5-11, and 5-12). These kinds of experiments address the question of whether a tissue or a cell is **sufficient** and/or **necessary (required)** for a particular developmental event to occur. In a typical approach, a developmental biologist might ask: What is the origin of the cells that give rise to a particular region of ectoderm that forms the lens of the eye? To determine this, the ectoderm might be **fate mapped** at the gastrula stage by applying fluorescent dyes to its surface (i.e., painting) and then following the movement of patches of labeled cells over time. This not only would fate map the prospective lens ectodermal cells but would also reveal with what tissues the prospective lens cells potentially

interact (because they come in close proximity to them) during their movement to form the lens. As a second step, the prospective lens cells might be removed (extirpated or ablated; i.e., cutting) to ask whether adjacent cells could grow back, replace them, and form a lens. If so, this would suggest that the fate of lens cells is not a result of their lineage, but perhaps requires some instructive information from adjacent tissues. As another test of this, a patch of ectoderm that is not fated to form lens could be removed (cutting) from a host embryo (perhaps a chick embryo) and replaced (pasting) with a patch from a donor embryo (perhaps a quail embryo) that is fated to form lens. Also, the converse experiment could be done: a patch of ectoderm fated to form lens could be removed (cutting) from a host embryo and replaced (pasting) with a patch from a donor embryo that is not fated to form lens. If in both cases the transplanted patch of ectoderm changed its fate, this would again suggest that the fate of lens cells is not a result of their lineage, but perhaps requires some instructive information from adjacent tissues. By repeating these experiments at different times in development, it would be possible to determine approximately when signaling might occur between adjacent tissues to establish ectodermal cell fate as a lens. A third step could also be taken. Tissues adjacent to the prospective lens cells could be extirpated (cut) to determine whether the lens can form in their absence. If not, this would again suggest that lens cell fate requires some instructive information from adjacent tissues, that is, that adjacent tissues are *necessary* for acquiring lens cell fate. But the gold standard in experimental embryology is to go one step farther to take the adjacent tissue and transplant it beneath other ectoderm that never forms a lens in normal development and ask:

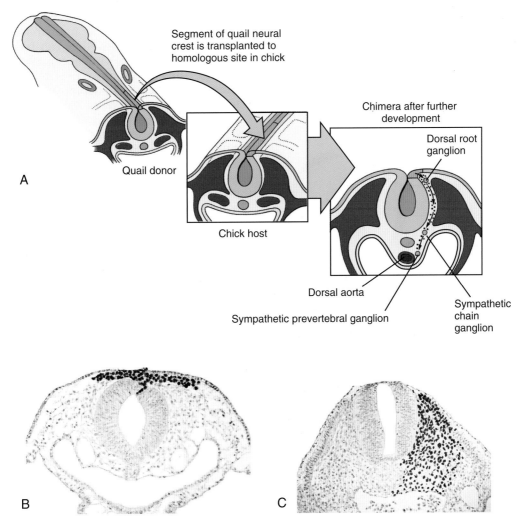

Figure 5-11. Quail-chick transplantation chimeras. *A,* Scheme illustrating the procedure. A small piece of tissue, in this case, dorsal neural tube, is removed from a chick host embryo and replaced with a comparable piece from a donor quail embryo. By using histologic staining to reveal differences in nuclear heterochromatin at the end of the experiment, or, more recently, by using chick- or quail-specific antibodies, the fate of the transplanted cells can be followed, creating prospective fate maps. This approach has been used extensively to determine the fates of neural crest cells arising from different cranial-caudal levels along the entire extent of the neural tube. *B,* Section of a chimera showing that after the graft has healed, quail neural crest cells begin to migrate. Quail cells can be easily distinguished from chick cells by using an anti-quail antibody. *C,* Another example of a quail-chick transplantation chimera in which prospective medial somitic cells of a chick embryo were replaced with those of a quail embryo. Quail cells are distinguished from chick cells by using an anti-quail antibody.

Can the transplanted tissue **induce** a lens? If so, then the experiment has revealed that the adjacent tissue is *sufficient* for conferring lens cell fate.

The situation just described is a common one in development in which one tissue acts upon another to change its fate. This process is called **induction**. It requires at least two tissues: an **inducing tissue** and a **responding tissue**. It also requires that the responding tissue be capable of responding to the inducing tissue by changing its fate. This ability is called **competence**, and it is a property that is lost over time. Thus, using the example above, transplanting tissue beneath *gastrula* ectoderm may induce a lens from cells that would never form a lens in normal development. However, repeating the experiment at the *neurula* stage may fail to induce a lens because the ectoderm may no longer be competent to be induced.

In recent years, it has become clear that **inductive interactions**, as well as so-called **suppressive interactions** that prevent a tissue from forming its "default" tissue type (e.g., Bmps prevent surface ectoderm from forming its default fate, neural ectoderm; covered in Chapter 3), depend on the secretion of small growth factors from the inducing tissue, where they bind to specific receptors present on the surface of the responding tissue. The families of growth factors involved and the cascades of signaling events evoked in the responding tissue are covered later in this chapter.

VISUALIZING GENE EXPRESSION

Techniques have been developed to reveal patterns of gene expression in developing embryos. For relatively young (and small) embryos, these techniques can be done on intact whole embryos (so-called whole mounts). If greater tissue detail is required, such embryos can be subsequently serially sectioned and studied histologically.

Although more labor intensive, for older embryos in which penetration of reagents can be a problem, tissue can first be sectioned and then labeled as sections (rather than as whole mounts) to reveal patterns of gene expression. Two techniques are used, one to visualize patterns of protein expression—immunohistochemistry—and another to visualize patterns of RNA expression—in situ hybridization.

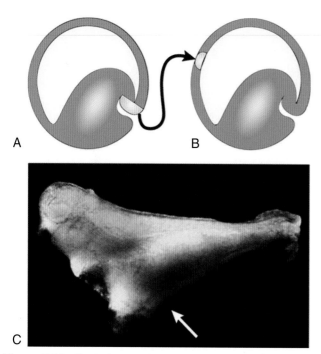

Figure 5-12. Classical cut-and-paste experimental embryology. *A*, Removal (i.e., cutting) of the dorsal lip of the blastopore of an amphibian embryo. *B*, Grafting (i.e., pasting) of the dorsal lip to the future belly ectoderm of another embryo. *C*, A secondary embryo (arrow) is induced from the belly ectoderm by the dorsal lip of the blastopore.

Both of these techniques can be used on untreated (control) embryos to reveal normal patterns of gene expression over time. Also, they can be used in experimental studies, often to visualize markers of specific tissue types. Using the example covered above, specific lens markers might be used to demonstrate that the induced ectoderm was truly forming lens and not some other ectodermal structure having a similar morphology (e.g., otic placode, the early ectodermal rudiment that forms the inner ear; covered in Chapter 18).

IMMUNOHISTOCHEMISTRY. Immunohistochemistry is used to show patterns of protein expression (Fig. 5-13). The main limitation of this technique is that it requires a specific antibody to identify the protein the investigator is interested in visualizing. Assuming that a specific antibody is available, one typical procedure (there are many variations) is to fix embryos to preserve them, treat them with detergents to make small holes in cell membranes that facilitate reagent penetration, treat with the specific antibody (e.g., an antibody to sonic hedgehog protein; often a rabbit immunoglobulin [Ig] G-type antibody), and then use a secondary antibody made against the first antibody (assuming the first or so-called *primary antibody* is a rabbit IgG, the second might be a goat anti–rabbit IgG). The secondary antibody is coupled to a marker such as peroxidase (revealed through a subsequent color reaction).

IN SITU HYBRIDIZATION. In situ hybridization is used to show patterns of RNA expression (Fig. 5-14). The approach is similar to that used in immunohistochemistry, beginning with fixation and detergent treatment. Embryos are then hybridized with a specific RNA probe (so-called riboprobe) that is complementary to the mRNA of interest (i.e., an antisense riboprobe). When the riboprobe is prepared, it is labeled with digoxigenin, a small antigenic

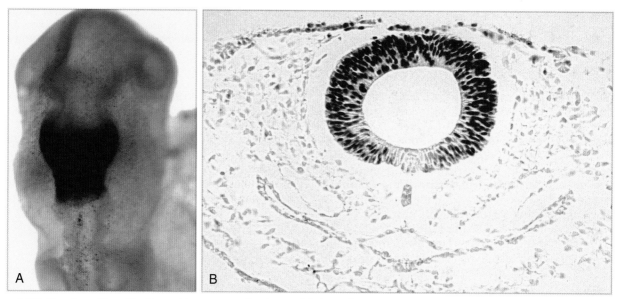

Figure 5-13. Use of specific antibodies and immunocytochemistry to label specific groups of cells. *A*, Head of a chick embryo after labeling with an antibody to engrailed-2, a transcription factor produced in cells of the future midbrain/rostral hindbrain (so-called isthmus region). *B*, A transverse section through the midbrain shows labeling in the nuclei of most of the cells of the midbrain region (except those cells in the floor plate overlying the notochord). A few cells in the surface ectoderm overlying the midbrain are also labeled.

molecule obtained from the Digitalis (foxglove) plant. After hybridization and washing to remove unbound riboprobe, digoxigenin (DIG) can be detected essentially as described above for immunohistochemistry by using an anti-DIG antibody.

When examining results from in situ hybridization, it is important to keep in mind two caveats. First, although some RNAs function in the embryo without being translated into protein (e.g., micro-RNAs), for many genes, translation of RNA into protein is required for function. For example, sonic hedgehog RNA does not function unless it is translated into sonic hedgehog protein. Typically, expression of RNA is used to infer function of the translated protein, but this may not be a valid inference because RNAs can be transcribed at a particular time in development without being translated. Second, RNAs mark cells transcribing a particular gene, but if the translated protein is secreted and diffuses, it may act at some distance from where its RNA is transcribed. Thus, the site of expression of RNA does not necessarily correspond to the site of the protein's function.

MANIPULATION OF GENE EXPRESSION

A powerful approach in developmental biology is to misexpress genes in developing embryos, that is, to ectopically (over)express genes or to block their expression (or function). Ectopically expressing genes in an embryo is the molecular equivalent of classical **pasting experimental embryology**, and often the question that is asked is, Is the gene of interest *sufficient* to cause some particular developmental event to occur (Fig. 5-15)? Knocking a gene down or out is the molecular equivalent of classical **cutting experimental embryology**, and

often the question that is asked is, Is the gene of interest *necessary* for some particular developmental event to occur? Differences and similarities between classical experimental embryology and molecular experimental embryology are illustrated in Figures 5-12 and 5-15 using a specific example: induction of a secondary embryo through transplantation of the dorsal lip of the blastopore of the frog embryo (the organizer; covered in Chapter 3), or ectopic overexpression of molecules secreted by the organizer. Many techniques have been developed for gene misexpression. These techniques take advantage of the unique experimental attributes that each of the model systems offers. Because **gene targeting** in the mouse is considered the premier approach for gene manipulation by many developmental biologists, the following section emphasizes gene manipulation in this model system.

MANIPULATION OF THE MOUSE GENOME. Over the past several years, a number of powerful molecular-genetic techniques have been developed to manipulate the mouse genome. Several lines of research have coalesced to yield techniques that make it possible to insert specific DNA sequences into their correct locations in the mouse

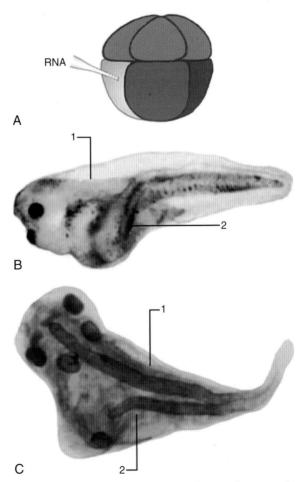

Figure 5-15. The molecular equivalent of cut-and-paste embryology. *A,* A ventral blastomere of a Xenopus early embryo is injected with an RNA encoding a protein normally expressed specifically within the dorsal lip of the blastopore. *B, C* (lateral and dorsal views, respectively), After further development, a secondary embryo (2) is induced by the ectopically (i.e., pasted) expressed gene. 1, Primary embryo.

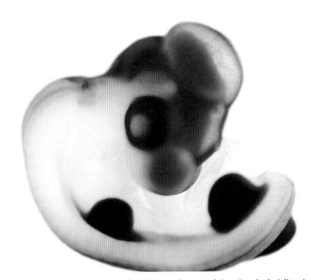

Figure 5-14. Use of specific riboprobes and in situ hybridization to label specific groups of cells. Whole chick embryo labeled with a probe for Lmx1, a transcription factor. Labeling occurs in several areas of the embryo, including much of the brain and limb buds. It is interesting to note that only the dorsal sides of the limb buds label, not their ventral sides (the ventral sides are not visible in the view shown). The eye, which also appears labeled in this photo, is not labeled by the probe (it appears dark because it contains pigmentation).

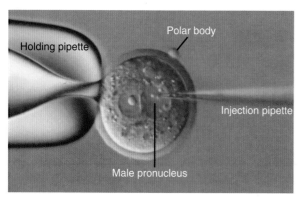

Figure 5-16. A procedure used to make a transgenic mouse. An egg is held in place using a suction (holding) pipette, and DNA is injected into the male pronucleus, the larger of the two nuclei, just after fertilization has occurred.

genome through a process called **gene targeting**. These techniques give researchers the power to alter and manipulate the genome and to investigate the function of any gene of interest. Disabling specific normal genes (by knocking *out* the desired gene) or replacing a normal gene with a mutated gene (by knocking *in* the mutated gene in place of the normal gene) can create animal models of human genetic diseases. Moreover, developing the ability to correct defective genes lays the groundwork for developing techniques to cure genetic disorders.

A **transgenic mouse** is a mouse whose genome has been altered by the integration of donor DNA sequences. The most direct way to create a transgenic mouse is to inject many copies of the donor DNA sequence into the male pronucleus of a fertilized egg; the male pronucleus is used because it is larger than the female pronucleus (Fig. 5-16). The injected DNA sometimes integrates stably into the host chromosomes, and in many cases, the donor gene is expressed. In a pioneering experiment, for example, a zinc-dependent rat growth hormone gene was introduced into the genome of a series of mice. When zinc was added to the drinking water to induce the expression of the rat growth hormone gene, these transgenic mice grew at twice the rate of control animals.

Although a simple method, the injection of DNA into the male pronucleus of the fertilized egg does not target the donor gene to a specific location in the host genome. However, targeting can be accomplished by inserting donor DNA into cells obtained from the inner cell mass of the blastocyst, and the rare cells in which the donor DNA has integrated correctly are identified and used to create a special type of transgenic animal called an **injection chimera**. With this approach, blastocysts are obtained from the oviducts of fertilized mice and are grown on a layer of fibroblasts in a culture dish. Culturing causes a cluster of cells from the inner cell mass to erupt from the blastocyst. These inner cell mass clusters are harvested and subcultured to produce stable lines of **embryonic stem (ES) cells** that are **totipotent** (able to give rise to any tissue in the body).

Donor DNA sequences can be introduced into cultured ES cells through a technique called **electroporation**, in which a suspension of ES cells is mixed with many copies of the donor DNA and subjected to an electrical current. This current facilitates movement of the donor DNA through the cell membrane, allowing the DNA to enter the nucleus. In a tiny fraction of these cells, the introduced DNA is incorporated into the desired target site on the genome by **homologous recombination**. Appropriate marker genes and screening techniques are used to isolate and subculture these rare "targeted" cells.

If introduced DNA sequences are mutated to block transcription of the targeted gene, the gene is said to be **knocked out**. Also, the allele containing the mutated sequence (or ultimately the transgenic mouse containing the mutated sequence; see next paragraph) is said to be **null** for the particular gene.

To create transgenic mice containing the new DNA, groups of eight to twelve targeted ES cells are injected into the cavity of normal mouse blastocysts, where they combine with the inner cell mass and participate in the formation of the embryo (Fig. 5-17). The resulting blastocysts (called **chimeras** because they are composed of cells from two different sources) are then implanted in the uterus of a pseudopregnant mouse, where they develop normally. Depending on their location in the embryonic disc, the ES cells may contribute to any tissue of the chimeric mouse. When they contribute to the germ line, the donor genes can be passed on to the offspring. Dominant donor genes may be expressed in the immediate offspring; if the donor genes are recessive (as they usually are), an inbreeding program is used to produce a homozygous strain that can express the phenotype.

It is not uncommon in gene knockout studies in mice to have mice born that seem to be normal despite the lack of what the scientist would have predicted (based, for example, on patterns of gene expression) to be a critical developmental gene. There are three likely reasons for such an outcome. First, many scientists believe that a mouse cannot be "normal" if it lacks any particular gene—that is, they believe that if the mouse were fully and appropriately tested, some defect (anatomic, biochemical, physiological, or behavioral) would be found. In other words, they believe that a subtle defect is present that could be easily overlooked unless appropriately tested. Second, because gene duplication has occurred during vertebrate evolution, such that critical developmental control genes in Drosophila are represented by multiple family members in mouse, **gene redundancy** exists. Thus, for example, in the absence of, say, one of the Hox genes, the animal seems normal because a second (or third) redundant Hox gene, which is still expressed, has an overlapping function with the knocked-out gene. Third, in the absence of expression of one gene, the expression of another gene can be upregulated. Thus, **compensation** can occur. Despite these possibilities, mice harboring knocked-out genes often have very obvious developmental defects that allow investigators to gain an understanding of the role(s) of the knocked-out gene in development.

Conditional transgenic mice can also be engineered such that the mutated (knocked-out) or inserted (knocked-in) gene is expressed only in particular tissues or only at desired times in development. This is important because, for example, when a gene such as an Fgf family member that is required for gastrulation and subsequently for ear development is knocked out, the embryo

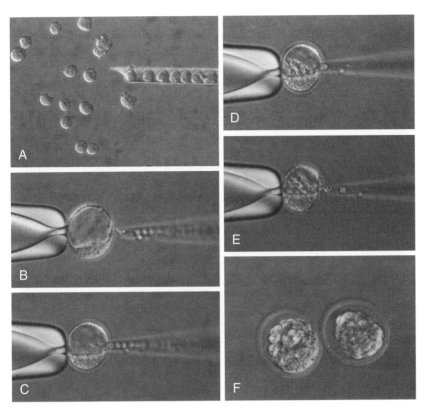

Figure 5-17. A procedure used to make chimeric mice. *A*, Blastocysts are dissociated into individual blastomeres, or, alternatively, embryonic stem (ES) cells derived from the inner cell mass are collected using a pipette. *B-E*, Using a suction pipette to hold a blastocyst, the collected cells are injected into the blastocele. *F*, Injected cells intermix randomly with both inner cell mass and trophoblast cells, and later, newly reorganized blastocysts are formed. These are injected into the uterine horns of pseudopregnant females, where they implant and undergo normal development.

might die during gastrulation. Hence, the role of this in ear development (which occurs a couple of days later) could not be studied. There are two general approaches to this problem. First, by using **tissue-specific promoters** and the **cre-lox system**, the gene of interest could be specifically knocked out only in the ear-forming region, not in the primitive streak. Second, by using **inducible promoters** and the **cre-lox system**, the time at which the gene is knocked out could be delayed until gastrulation has occurred but before ear development has been initiated. Thus, the solution to understanding the later activity of an early embryonic lethal gene is to use tissue- or time-specific knockouts.

In the first approach, the gene of interest is flanked in a targeting vector with so-called loxP sites, and transgenic mice are produced as described above. A second group of transgenic mice are engineered in which a promoter is used to drive the expression of cre recombinase to the tissue of interest. (Cre recombinase is a site-specific recombinase derived from phage; in an alternative procedure, Flp recombinase derived from yeast is used when the gene of interest is flanked with the so-called FRT sequence.) The two groups of transgenic mice are bred, and during development, the tissue-specific promoter drives expression of cre recombinase at the appropriate times and in the appropriate tissues during development. Cre recombinase acts on the loxP sites flanking the gene of interest, which is then excised, preventing its expression only in the tissue of interest (i.e., there is precise spatial control of gene inactivation).

In the second approach, an inducible promoter is used to drive cre recombinase, and the gene of interest is knocked out only in the presence of an exogenously applied reagent such as the anti–breast cancer drug

tamoxifen or the antibiotic tetracycline. Thus, at the desired time in gestation, pregnant mice are injected in their peritoneal (abdominal) cavity with tamoxifen, which quickly diffuses to the uterine horns containing the developing embryos and activates the inducible promoter. The gene of interest is excised through expression of cre recombinase, providing precise temporal control of gene inactivation.

The cre-lox system also has been used with ROSA26 transgenic mice, that is, mice that express the reporter gene lacZ in all of their tissues during development (lacZ encodes the enzyme beta-galactosidase, whose activity can be readily detected with a colorimetric reaction). However, because expression of the lacZ gene is blocked by the presence of a loxP-flanked "stop" DNA fragment that prevents transcription and translation of the lacZ gene, lacZ is expressed only in the presence of cre. By breeding mice containing a tissue-specific promoter driving cre with ROSA26 mice, cells and their descendants expressing the gene of interest will be labeled, allowing them to be followed over time to map cell **lineage**. Thus, this approach is the molecular genetic equivalent of painting used for fate mapping studies.

MANIPULATION OF GENE EXPRESSION IN OTHER MODELS. A common approach in zebrafish and Xenopus embryos is to generate **transient transgenic animals** by injecting early blastomeres with desired DNA constructs (recently, as covered above, techniques also have been developed in both *Xenopus* [*tropicalis*] and zebrafish to generate transgenic lines of animals). Using this method, genes can be ectopically expressed in embryonic tissues derived from the lineages of the injected cell. Alternatively, cells can be injected with **morpholinos** (stabilized antisense

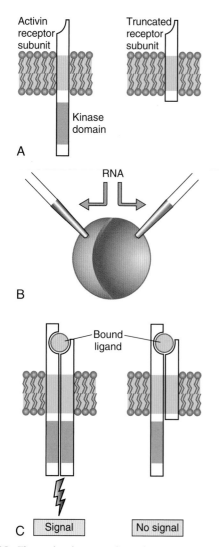

Figure 5-18. The molecular equivalent of cut-and-paste experimental embryology. *A*, In this example, truncated activin receptors lacking the intercellular signaling domain are engineered. *B*, RNA encoding the truncated (dominant negative) receptor is injected into a blastomere of an early Xenopus embryo. *C*, Because injected message for the truncated receptor is far in excess of endogenous message for the wild-type receptor, most receptors upon receptor dimerization have one or two truncated subunits and thus cannot signal.

RNA) or **RNAi** (interfering, double-stranded RNA). Both of these approaches knock *down* gene expression, rather than completely blocking it.

Recently, these approaches have been applied to chick embryos, and sometimes mouse embryos, to generate transient transgenic animals. Because chick and mouse embryos have relatively small cells, these cells cannot be injected as the cells of early zebrafish and Xenopus embryos can. Instead, genes are introduced into cells using engineered viruses or through **whole-embryo electroporation** (or other techniques such as sonoporation and lipofection). Fundamentally, whole-embryo electroporation is the same as the process used to electroporate cells in culture (covered above). Whole-embryo electroporation allows an investigator to spatially and temporally target a DNA sequence to a particular tissue at a particular time in development and to study its effects

when overexpressed (sequences consist of full-length gene) or knocked down (sequences consist of antisense, morpholino, or RNAi, specifically designed to knock down the gene of interest).

Another important approach, utilized very effectively to study growth factor signaling especially in Xenopus, is to inject **dominant negative receptors** (Fig. 5-18). These are engineered growth factor receptors that contain the ligand-binding extracellular domain, which binds the growth factor, but lack the intracellular domain necessary for signaling (i.e., the receptors are truncated). When present in excess in the extracellular space (or bound to cell surfaces in excess), dominant negative receptors bind to secreted growth factors, preventing them from binding to intact receptors, thus blocking signaling.

SIGNALING PATHWAYS

Human embryos, like those of animal models, are progressively patterned during embryogenesis, largely through **cell-cell interactions**. These interactions are a form of **intercellular communication** that is mediated by the secretion of soluble signaling molecules that diffuse within the extracellular environment to reach adjacent cells. The **cascades of signals** that cells receive during development determine their fate. Thus, early-acting regulatory genes initiate development of groups of cells by inducing expression of other "downstream" genes. The activities of these genes then induce the expression of yet additional genes, and so on, until the genes that encode the actual structural and functional characteristics of specific cells and tissues of the embryo are activated. A relatively small number of signaling pathways (fewer than twenty) act in these cascades. Many of these signaling pathways were first identified in Drosophila. Subsequently, families of orthologs of the genes encoding these signaling pathways were identified in vertebrates. Before the major signaling pathways involved in vertebrate development are addressed, the general scheme of signaling pathways acting in Drosophila development will be covered.

PATTERNING THE DROSOPHILA EMBRYO: A MAJOR ENTRY POINT INTO UNDERSTANDING HUMAN DEVELOPMENT

In Drosophila, a signaling cascade is initiated by genes expressed before fertilization, the so-called **maternal effect genes** (Fig. 5-19). These genes encode signals that establish the axes of the Drosophila embryo, namely, the anterior-posterior axis (cranial-caudal axis in humans) and the dorsal-ventral axis. In Drosophila, maternal effect genes encode proteins that impart differences to subregions of the oocyte, zygote, and early embryo along their respective axes, including **growth factors** and **transcription factors**. Although such localized **cytoplasmic determinants** are important in the development of Drosophila and some vertebrates (such as Xenopus), most evidence suggests that the mammalian oocyte cytoplasm is relatively homogeneous in composition and that

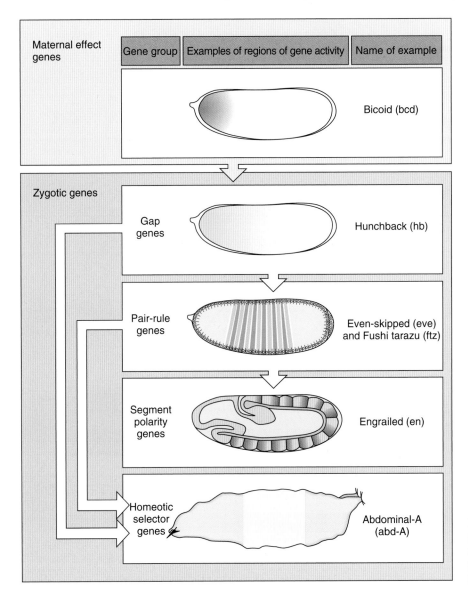

Gene group	Examples of regions of gene activity	Name of example

Figure 5-19. Genes underlying Drosophila early patterning. These consist of both maternal effect genes and four types of zygotic genes: gap genes, pair-rule genes, segment polarity genes, and homeotic selector genes.

maternal effect genes play little or no role in early patterning of the mammalian embryo.

During early embryonic development, the expression of maternal effect genes is superseded by a class of genes called **zygotic genes** (see Fig. 5-19). These genes are called *zygotic* because they are expressed after fertilization and involve both maternally and paternally inherited genes. In Drosophila, there are four classes of zygotic genes, which act in establishing the basic anterior-posterior body plan: **gap genes, pair-rule genes, segment polarity genes**, and **homeotic selector genes**. The maternal effect genes regulate the expression of the gap genes, which, in turn, regulate the expression of the pair-rule genes, which, in turn, regulate the expression of the segmental polarity genes. These genes specify the specific segments. The segment polarity genes regulate the expression of the homeotic selector genes, which provide regional identity to the different segments.

Although the cascade of expression and regulation of zygotic genes is much more varied in vertebrates, orthologs of all classes of Drosophila zygotic genes function during vertebrate patterning. Thus, our understanding of the molecular-genetic basis of patterning in Drosophila has provided a major entry point into understanding the development of vertebrates, including humans. In general, vertebrate orthologs of Drosophila patterning genes constitute two types of molecules: secreted factors that act as **signaling molecules** and **transcription factors**. Transcription factors switch other genes on or off by binding to regulatory regions of their DNA. Several transcription factors containing nucleotide sequences related to the pair-rule, segment polarity, and homeotic selector genes of Drosophila have been identified in mammals, and, as is the case in Drosophila, some of these mammalian orthologs also play a role in segmentation. For example, segmentation of the mammalian hindbrain (covered in Chapters 9, 10, and 17), the pharyngeal arches of the head and neck region (covered in Chapter 17), and the somites of the trunk (covered in Chapter 4) is regulated at least in part by these genes.

One important and well-studied group of mammalian orthologs of the homeotic selector genes of Drosophila

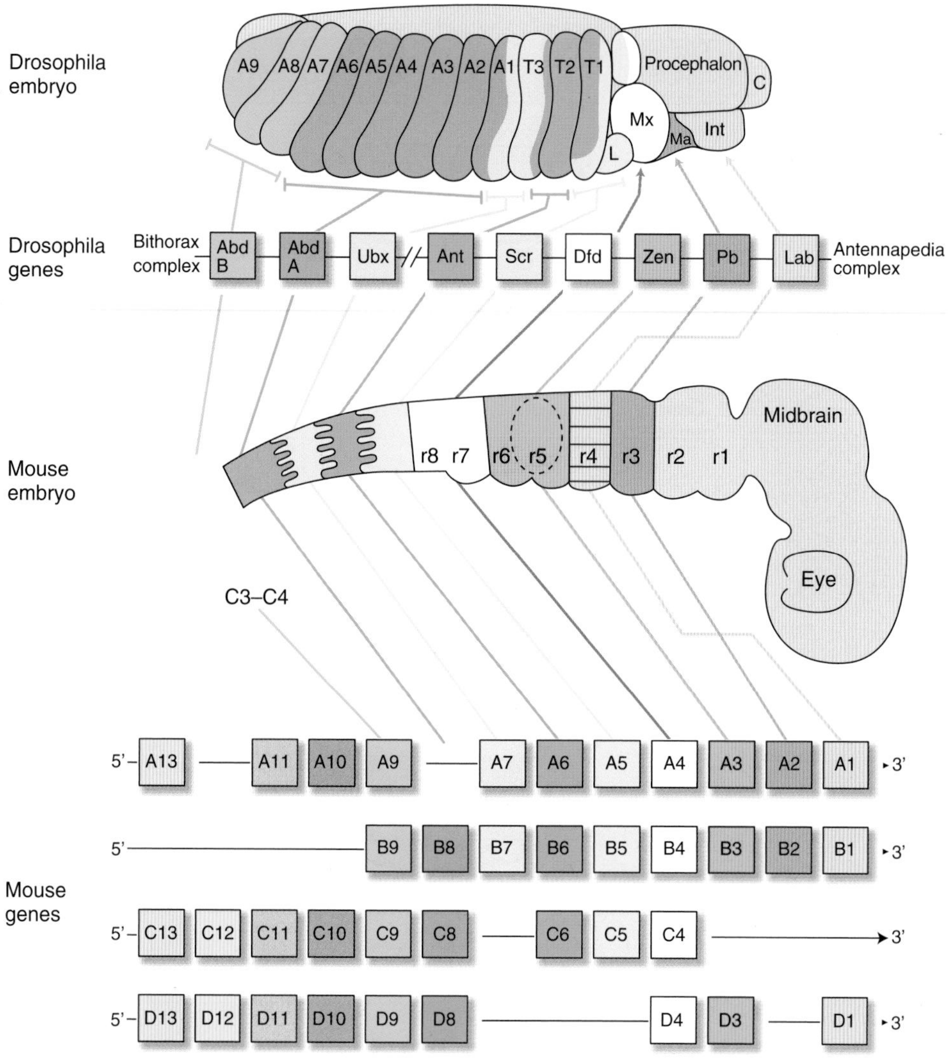

Figure 5-20. Alignment of the four vertebrate Hox complexes with the Drosophila homeotic complex. The Drosophila embryo has seven head segments (five are labeled: C, cly-polabrum; Int, intercalary; L, labial; Ma, mandibular; Mx, maxillary), three thoracic (T1-T3) segments, and nine abdominal segments (A1-A9). The genes that pattern these segments lie within two complexes on chromosome 3: the antennapedia complex, consisting of labial (Lab), proboscipedia (Pb), deformed (Dfd), sex combs reduced (Scr), and antennapedia (Ant); and the bithorax complex, consisting of ultrabithorax (Ubx), abdominal A (Abd A), and abdominal B (Abd B). Hox genes, orthologs of the Drosophila genes, are present in vertebrates, including mouse and human. There are four clusters of Hox genes (A-D), with up to 13 members per cluster. The Drosophila gene Zerknüllt (Zen) is not expressed in Drosophila head segments; it is orthologous to vertebrate Hox 3 genes.

contains a highly conserved 183–base pair region of DNA called the **homeobox**, which encodes the 61–amino acid **homeodomain**. The homeodomain recognizes and binds to specific DNA sequences of other genes. Therefore, these encoded proteins function as transcription factors that regulate the activity of many "downstream" genes and as a consequence are often referred to as **master control genes**. A special subset of Drosophila homeotic selector genes are organized into two clusters on chromosome 3 and are collectively called the **homeotic complex**, or **HOM-C** (Fig. 5-20). A common ancestor of this complex was duplicated once, and then each resulting complex was duplicated again during the evolution of mammals. The four complexes of homeobox genes in mammals are called **Hox genes**.

In Drosophila, mutations of homeotic selector genes often result in remarkable transformations of body parts. A mutation resulting in misexpression of the antenna-pedia gene during development, for example, causes cells that normally would form antennae to instead develop into legs, which now protrude from the head. Similarly, a mutation in the ultrabithorax gene results in homeotic transformation of the third thoracic segment into an additional second thoracic segment, yielding a fruit fly with four wings instead of the normal two.

The Drosophila HOM-C and mammalian Hox genes have been extremely well conserved during evolution at the levels of clustered organization, sequence, expression, and function. Although the mammalian Hox genes have been individually altered through evolution, they retain significant sequence homology to the insect HOM-C genes. The order of the Hox genes in the mammalian clusters parallels that observed in the Drosophila HOM-C. The amino acid sequences of the encoded homeodomains of the Drosophila genes and their mammalian orthologs, or corresponding genes, are often greater than 90% identical. In addition, in both mammals and fruit flies, these genes exhibit the property of colinearity, with the position of a gene within the cluster reflecting its expression domain in the developing embryo. As shown in Figure 5-20, genes located in more 5′ positions within clusters are expressed in more caudal regions of the embryo.

Transgenic fruit flies, carrying experimentally added genes, have been used to demonstrate an unexpected level of functional conservation between the Drosophila HOM-C and mammalian Hox genes. For example, misexpression of the mammalian ortholog of the antennapedia gene in the developing fruit fly also causes homeotic transformation of antennae into legs. This suggests that both Drosophila and mammalian genes are capable of recognizing the same downstream gene targets and initiating the same genetic cascade. It is interesting to note that misexpression of the Drosophila antennapedia gene or the corresponding mammalian gene results in the formation of ectopic Drosophila legs and not mammalian legs. This is because, within the genetic context of the fruit fly, the downstream target genes are capable only of programming the development of a fruit fly leg.

PATTERNING THE VERTEBRATE EMBRYO

As covered in the previous section, patterning of the vertebrate embryo occurs through signaling cascades generated by families of orthologs of genes involved in Drosophila patterning. A general scheme for how such patterning occurs is shown in Figure 5-21. An inducer cell (in vertebrates, typically a group of cells rather than a single cell) secretes a small signaling molecule, or **growth factor**. This factor diffuses through the extracellular matrix to a responding cell (in vertebrates, again, typically a group of cells rather than a single cell), where it binds to a **receptor** on the cell's surface. Binding activates (often through **phosphorylation** of intracellular proteins) an intracellular signaling cascade (a series of **signal transduction proteins**) that ultimately results in the movement of transcription factors into the nucleus, where they bind to specific regions of DNA and alter transcription. This in turn can result in cell differentiation to form a specific cell type. Often, altered transcription leads to the secretion of new growth factors that modify the fate of other cells or provide feedback to regulate the secretion of growth factors from the inducing cell.

Below, some of the major signaling pathways known to play specific roles in vertebrate development (and covered in greater detail in the appropriate chapters) will be briefly covered. A hallmark of each of these pathways is their complexity. The purpose of this section is to help you place the major players into context so that you will have a more global understanding of signaling as you encounter specific members of these pathways (e.g., sonic hedgehog) in various chapters. Each of the signaling pathways has been greatly simplified to cover only the key players covered elsewhere in the textbook. Seven major signaling pathways will be covered: Wnt signaling, hedgehog signaling, Tgfβ signaling, tyrosine kinase signaling, notch signaling, integrin signaling, and retinoic acid signaling. In addition, the relationships among cell adhesion molecules, integrins, and the cytoskeleton will be briefly covered. The wide range of developmental processes regulated by signaling pathways is reflected by the wide range of developmental disorders that result from mutations in these pathways. Examples of such disorders are listed below.

WNT SIGNALING. Vertebrate Wnts are orthologs of Drosophila wingless, a segment polarity gene. Wnts are secreted by cells into the extracellular milieu and bind to Wnt receptors (frizzleds; seven-pass transmembrane receptors) on the surfaces of other cells. In mammals, there are nineteen Wnts and ten frizzled receptors.

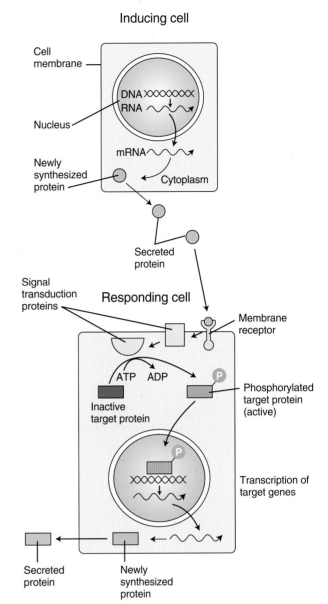

Figure 5-21. A generic cascade of signal transduction. Inducing cells influence their neighbors by secreting small proteins (growth factors) that diffuse to adjacent cells (responding cells) and bind to their membrane receptors. This initiates an intracellular signaling cascade through a series of signal transduction proteins and phosphorylation events. Phosphorylated proteins enter the nucleus, where they alter gene expression, leading to the synthesis of new proteins.

Binding of a Wnt to a frizzled receptor initiates an intracellular signaling cascade involving three pathways: the **canonical Wnt pathway**, the planar cell polarity pathway (covered in Chapter 4), and the calcium-signaling pathway. The canonical pathway is the best studied and will be the only one covered here (Fig. 5-22); it requires the co-receptor Lrp5/6 (LDL receptor–related proteins 5/6). In the canonical Wnt pathway, in the absence of Wnts, cytoplasmic β-catenin (a component of the cadherin/catenin adhesion complex) interacts with a complex of proteins, including axin (product of the mouse gene fused that regulates axis development), Apc (adenomatous polyposis coli), Gsk3 (a serine threonine

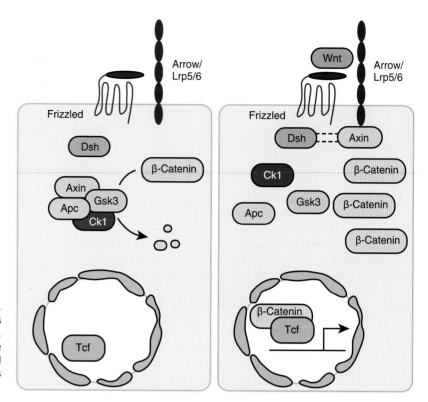

Figure 5-22. Canonical Wnt signaling pathway. In the absence of Wnt signaling (left), β-catenin is degraded, but in the presence of Wnt signaling (right), β-catenin accumulates and enters the nucleus, where in partnership with Tcf/Lef, gene expression is altered (i.e., Wnt target genes are activated). Arrow in nucleus indicates transcription.

kinase), and Ck1 (casein kinase 1). This interaction causes proteolysis of β-catenin and prevents Wnt signaling.

However, in the presence of Wnts and their binding to a frizzled/Lrp5/6 complex, a signal is transduced to dishevelled (Dsh) and axin that prevents degradation of β-catenin. β-Catenin accumulates in the cytoplasm and diffuses to the nucleus, where it acts as a transcriptional co-activator by binding to the transcriptional co-repressors Tcf/Lef. This binding de-represses the expression of Wnt-responsive genes, resulting in new transcription and Wnt signaling.

In addition to binding to frizzled receptors, Wnts can bind to soluble extracellular proteins called sFrps (secreted frizzled-like proteins). When they do so, they are no longer able to bind to frizzled receptors. Thus, sFrps act as naturally occurring inhibitors of Wnt signaling. Dickkopfs are other extracellular proteins that antagonize Wnt signaling (specifically, the canonical Wnt pathway). They do so not by binding Wnts, but by binding Lrp5/6. Cerberus is another Wnt inhibitor that acts extracellularly by binding to Wnt. In addition to inhibiting Wnt signaling, cerberus blocks nodal and Bmp signaling—both members of the Tgfβ family covered later in the chapter.

Defects in Wnt signaling that result in human disorders include cancers (APC, β-CATENIN, AXIN1, -2), osteoarthritis of the hips (FRIZZLEDB1), retinopathy (FRIZZLED4), autosomal recessive tetra-amelia (absence of all four limbs; WNT3), bone and eye disorders (LRP5), and genitourinary anomalies (WNT4).

HEDGEHOG SIGNALING. Three orthologs of the Drosophila hedgehog gene are expressed in mammals: sonic hedgehog, indian hedgehog, and desert hedgehog. In addition to these three hedgehog genes, zebrafish express two other hedgehog genes called echidna hedgehog and

tiggywinkle hedgehog. Below, only sonic hedgehog (Shh) signaling is covered because of its role in the development of a number of different systems in the vertebrate embryo, and because more is known about the role of Shh in signaling during development than is known about any other member of the hedgehog family (Fig. 5-23).

Shh is translated as a 45-kDa precursor protein, which is subsequently cleaved in the cytoplasm into a 20-kDa N-terminal signaling domain and a 25-kDa C-terminal catalytic domain. As these domains form, cholesterol binds to the 20-kDa domain in a process important for the subsequent secretion and signaling activity of Shh protein. After secretion into the extracellular milieu, the 20-kDa domain binds to a transmembrane receptor called *patched*. In the absence of Shh protein, patched interacts with another transmembrane signaling protein, smoothened, which inhibits smoothened signaling, repressing the expression of smoothened target genes.

In contrast, in the presence of Shh protein, smoothened is no longer inhibited. Instead, it is transported into a primary (non-motile) cilium projecting from the cell's surface, where it accumulates in the cilium's cell membrane. This activates an intracellular signaling cascade that results in transcriptional activation of target genes. It is interesting to note that smoothened signaling in mammals involves three proteins (called Gli proteins) that function as transcriptional activators or repressors. These proteins are orthologs of the Drosophila Ci, or cubitus interruptus protein. In vertebrates, the combination of Gli proteins expressed in a cell as a result of Shh signaling determines the fate of that cell.

Defects in SONIC signaling in humans result in several disorders, including **cancer** (PATCHED); midline defects, including **holoprosencephaly** (SHH; GLI2, -3; and PATCHED); **polydactyly** (duplicated digits; SHH;

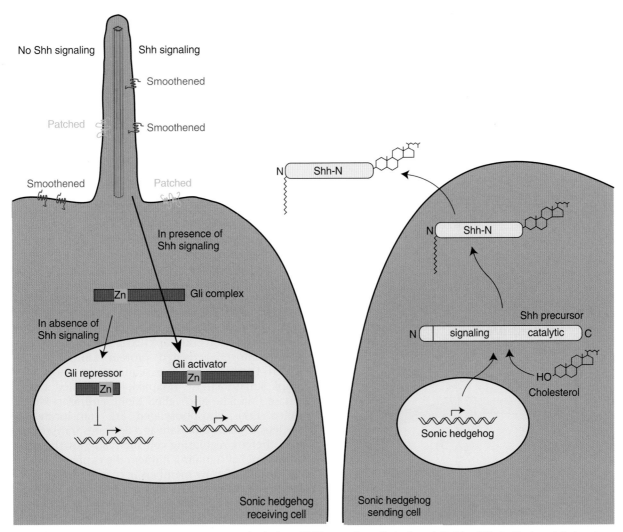

Figure 5-23. Sonic hedgehog signaling pathway. Sonic hedgehog (Shh) receptive cells (cells on left side of illustration) contain two transmembrane proteins, patched and smoothened, which occupy different locations when Shh signaling is *not* occurring (left side of left cell): patched resides within the cell's primary cilium, and smoothen resides within the non-ciliary plasma membrane. When Shh signaling is occurring, the Shh sending cell (cell on right side of illustration) synthesizes a precursor molecule that is cleaved into N- and C-terminal fragments, and cholesterol is added to the N-terminal fragment, which is then secreted. This fragment binds to patched on the Shh receiving cell and causes patched to move out of the cilium and into the plasma membrane, allowing smoothen to traffic to the primary cilium (on right side of left cell). This in turn activates a signaling cascade involving smoothened (which in the absence of the N-terminal fragment binding is blocked by patched from entering the cilium) and a zinc (Zn)-containing Gli complex. Both Gli repressors and activators exist, and their relative amounts control which target genes are expressed in the presence and absence of Shh signaling.

GLI2, -3; and PATCHED); craniofacial defects and **tracheoesophageal fistula** (GLI3); and gonadal dysgenesis (DESERT HEDGEHOG).

TGFβ SIGNALING. The Tgfβ superfamily is a large family of proteins that signals through receptors having a cytoplasmic serine/threonine kinase domain. The best-known Drosophila member is the protein decapentaplegic. Many members of this family play important roles in vertebrate development, such as the bone morphogenetic proteins (Bmps), activin, Vg1, and nodal. In addition, several inhibitors of Bmp signaling are expressed in early development and are involved in important events such as neural induction and establishment of left-right asymmetry, as covered in Chapter 3. These include chordin, noggin, follistatin, lefty, and cerberus.

Bmp signaling has been studied in detail (Fig. 5-24). A signaling cascade is initiated when a particular Bmp (several Bmps have been identified) binds within the extracellular milieu to a transmembrane Bmp receptor (Bmpr). The latter consists of heterodimers and homodimers of what are known as type I and type II Tgfβ receptors. Binding in turn results in phosphorylation of another family of nine proteins called the Smads (orthologs of the Drosophila Mad, or mothers against decapentalegic, protein). Phosphorylated Smads then enter the nucleus, where they act as transcriptional co-activators or co-repressors. Defects in Tgfβ signaling that result in human disorders include cancer and pulmonary hypertension (BMPR2) and a wide range of vascular and skeletal disorders (NOGGIN, TGFβ1, TGFβ RECEPTORS, and a TGFβ-binding protein called ENDOGLIN).

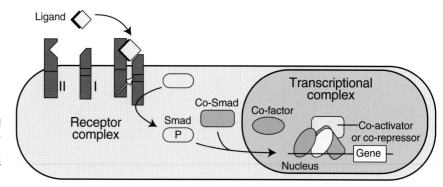

Figure 5-24. Tgfβ signaling pathway. Ligand binding activates receptor dimerization and phosphorylation of Smads. Phosphorylated Smads, along with Co-Smads, translocate to the nucleus to alter target gene expression.

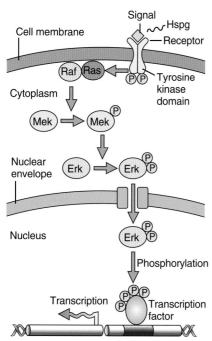

Figure 5-25. Fgf signaling pathway. Fgfs bind to Fgf receptors aided by presentation of the ligand by heparin sulfate proteoglycan (Hspg). This activates Ras as well as a phosphorylation cascade that sequentially phosphorylates Raf, Mek, and Erk. Phosphorylated Erk translocates to the nucleus, where it regulates target gene expression.

TYROSINE KINASE SIGNALING. Several families of growth factors bind to receptors that have a cytoplasmic tyrosine kinase domain. These include the fibroblast growth factors (Fgfs), epidermal growth factor (Egf), insulin-like growth factors (Igfs), platelet-derived growth factors (Pdgfs), hepatocyte growth factor/scatter factor (Hgf/Sf), vascular endothelial growth factor (Vegf), neuregulins, and ephrins. In addition, steel (stem cell factor) signals through the tyrosine kinase c-kit receptor and functions in the migration of premelanocytes (see Fig. 5-3; covered in Chapter 4). Because of the complexity of the tyrosine kinase family, only Fgfs (Fig. 5-25) and ephrins will be covered here as examples of growth factors that signal through receptors with a tyrosine kinase domain. Fgf and ephrin signaling is covered in detail in this textbook.

In mammals, the Fgfs consist of twenty-two family members (numbered 1 to 23, with species differences in the presence or absence of Fgf15 and Fgf19; i.e., mammals lack Fgf19, whereas birds lack Fgf15). Fgf ligands bind to

Fgf receptors (Fgfrs), numbered 1 to 4. Fgfr1-3 undergo alternative splicing to each form two isoforms, resulting in six Fgfrs plus Fgfr4, for a total of seven receptors. The presence of heparin sulfate proteoglycan is required for presentation of the ligand to the receptor and subsequent binding. Binding induces heterodimerization or homodimerization of the receptor and activation of the small GTPase Ras. Binding also initiates a phosphorylation cascade, known as an Erk/Mapk (extracellular signal–regulated kinase/mitogen–activated protein kinase) cascade, in which three kinases are sequentially phosphorylated: Mapk kinase kinase (Mapkkk—also called Raf); Mapk kinase (Mapkk—also called Mek); and Map kinase (also called Erk). Phosphorylated Erk translocates to the nucleus to phosphorylate and activates transcription factors, thereby regulating cell survival, growth, and differentiation. Fgf signaling induces the expression of sprouty (at least four family members in mammals), an intracellular inhibitor of Fgf signaling that establishes a regulatory feedback loop limiting the amount of Fgf signaling.

Defects in Fgf signaling result in disorders in humans that affect the skeletal system particularly and involve mutations in FGFR1-3. These mutations are covered in detail in other chapters in this textbook. Some of the more frequent mutations include **Pfeiffer syndrome** (FGFR1 or FGFR2 mutation; results in craniosynostosis with limb defects), **Apert syndrome** (FGFR2 mutation; results in **craniosynostosis** and severe fusion of digits—**syndactyly**), **Crouzon syndrome** (FGFR2 mutation; results in **craniosynostosis** without limb defects), **thanatophoric dysplasia** (FGFR3 mutation; results in severe skeletal dysplasia and is usually lethal at birth), and achondroplasia (FGFR3 mutation; results in **dwarfism**).

Ephrins are a family of proteins that bind to the so-called Eph receptors. The name "Eph" is derived from the cell line from which the first member of the family was isolated—the erythropoietin-producing human hepatocellular carcinoma line. The name "ephrin" is derived from Eph family receptor interacting proteins. Both ephrins and Eph receptors are classified into A and B subgroups consisting of ephrins A1 to A5, B1 to B3, and Ephs A1 to A8, B1 to B6. Both type A and type B Eph receptors consist of an extracellular ligand-binding domain, a transmembrane domain, and an intracellular tyrosine kinase domain. Thus, they are similar to other tyrosine kinase receptors. However, the ephrin ligands that bind to these receptors differ from other ligands that bind to tyrosine kinase receptors, such as the Fgfs, in that instead of being

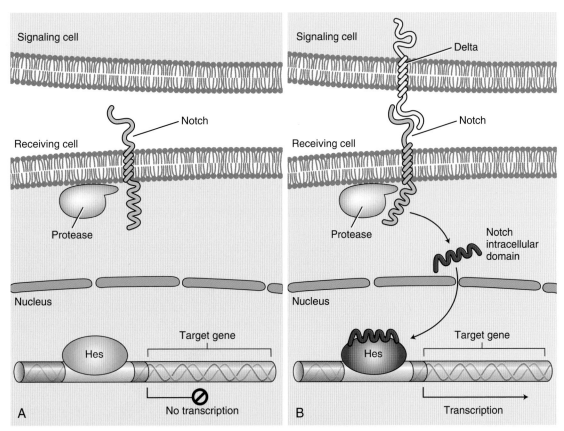

Figure 5-26. Notch signaling pathway. *A,* In the absence of a ligand, such as delta, on an adjacent cell, notch signaling does not occur and notch target genes are not regulated. *B,* In the presence of a ligand, such as delta, on an adjacent cell, notch signaling occurs when the ligand produced by the signaling cell binds to a notch receptor on the adjacent cell. Binding activates a protease that cleaves off a portion (the intracellular domain) of the notch receptor, which, in turn, translocates to the nucleus, where it regulates notch target gene expression in partnership with Hes.

secreted into the extracellular milieu, they remain bound to the cell surface that produces them.

Type A ephrins are attached to the cell surface by a GPI (glycosylphosphatidylinositol) link, whereas type B ephrins span the cell membrane. Thus, signaling occurs only between immediately adjacent cells.

Another important difference with ephrin signaling is that it occurs bidirectionally, that is, binding of the ligand to the receptor not only results in a signaling cascade within the cell containing the Eph receptor, but also signaling is activated upon binding to the Eph receptor in the cell containing the ephrin.

One human disorder that results from defects in EPHRIN signaling is **craniofrontonasal dysplasia syndrome**. This syndrome involves a mutation in EPHRIN-B1. Although this mutation affects the development of bones in the skull and face, multiple other defects occur, such as umbilical hernia; genitourinary anomalies; skin, nail, and hair anomalies; and developmental delay.

NOTCH SIGNALING. Like ephrin signaling, notch signaling can occur only between closely associated cells (Fig. 5-26). Notch proteins (numbered 1 to 4 in mammals) consist of transmembrane receptors containing an extracellular domain with Egf-like repeats for ligand binding and an intracellular domain rich with ankyrin repeats for intracellular signaling. Like the ephrins, the ligands for notch receptors are not secreted into the extracellular

milieu; rather, they consist of transmembrane proteins of the DSL family of proteins, named for the ligands delta and serrate from Drosophila (consisting of multiple delta and jagged genes in vertebrates), and Lag2 from *C. elegans*. Although these ligands are transmembrane proteins, their extracellular domain can be cleaved by proteases (such as the protease kuzbanian), allowing diffusion to adjacent cells.

Notch signaling is regulated extracellularly through actions that modify notch and its ligands. In mammals, three glycosyltransferases with whimsical names regulate notch signaling: lunatic fringe, manic fringe, and radical fringe.

Binding of delta or jagged/serrate ligands to notch receptors initiates notch signaling. Through proteolysis, the intracellular domain of notch is cleaved and migrates to the nucleus, where it interacts with Hes proteins (orthologs of Drosophila hairy and enhancer of split proteins) and/or Hes-related proteins (Hesr). This complex regulates the expression of basic helix-loop-helix (bHLH) transcriptional repressors. Thus, as mentioned in Chapters 10 and 18, selection and differentiation of neurons and glial/support cells from clusters of precursor cells involve the process of **lateral inhibition** mediated through notch signaling. As a result, the cells undergoing notch signaling repress the expression of neuronal differentiation genes (e.g., bHLH genes) and consequently differentiate as non-neuronal cell types.

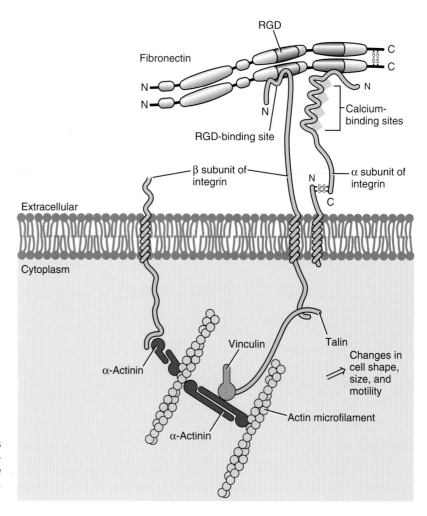

Figure 5-27. Integrin signaling pathway. Integrins form critical transmembrane links between extracellular matrix molecules such as fibronectin and the intracellular actin cytoskeleton (microfilaments). RGD, arginine-glycine-aspartate.

One human disorder that results from defects in NOTCH signaling is **Alagille syndrome** (also called **arteriohepatic dysplasia**). This syndrome, caused by mutation of the JAGGED1 or NOTCH2 genes, affects the skeletal, cardiovascular, and gastrointestinal systems (Alagille syndrome is mentioned in several chapters of this textbook). Another human skeletal disorder associated with defective NOTCH signaling is **spondylocostal dysostosis** (DELTA-3, LUNATIC FRINGE; covered in Chapter 8). Mutations in NOTCH signaling are associated with the development of cancer, namely, a NOTCH1 mutation is the cause of more than 50% of cases of T-cell acute lymphoblastic leukemia.

INTEGRIN SIGNALING. Spaces between tissue layers and between cells within tissue layers are filled with a rich extracellular matrix. This matrix consists of a number of proteins. Epithelia are lined by basement membranes. These consist largely of collagens (especially type IV), laminin, and fibronectin. A number of large complex proteoglycans are more broadly distributed within and across tissue spaces. These include syndecan, perlecan, heparan sulfate, and chondroitin sulfate.

Cells adhere to one another using intercellular junctions, such as gap and tight junctions, and calcium-dependent and calcium-independent **cell adhesion molecules**. The calcium-dependent adhesion molecules consist of the cadherins, such as N-cadherin (neural cadherin), E-cadherin (epithelial cadherin), and P-cadherin (placental cadherin). The calcium-independent adhesion molecules consist of the CAMs—e.g., N-Cam (neural cell adhesion molecule); V-Cam (vascular cell adhesion molecule); and Pe-Cam (platelet-endothelial cell adhesion molecule). Cells also adhere to their matrix. This adhesion involves integrins, which provide a link between the extracellular matrix and the cells' cytoskeletal network.

The integrins consist of non-covalently linked heterodimers of alpha and beta transmembrane subunits (Fig. 5-27). At least fifteen alpha subunits and eight beta subunits exist, but all combinations of the twenty-three subunits apparently do not exist. Collectively, the two heterodimers of each integrin form a binding domain for ligands contained in basement membrane molecules such as laminin or fibronectin. One such domain is the RGD sequence (arginine-glycine-aspartate). Upon binding of this domain to its ligand, signaling is transduced to cytoplasmic **microfilaments** via linker proteins such as alpha-actinin, vinculin, and talin. This signaling leads to cytoskeletal rearrangements that in turn lead to changes in cell shape, size, and motility.

Defects in integrin signaling result in human disorders that affect skin and connective tissues. These include **epidermolysis bullosa** (blistering skin) with **pyloric atresia** (INTEGRINβ4) and cancers of the gut, breast, and female reproductive organs.

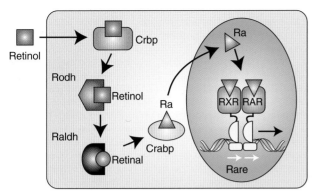

Figure 5-28. Retinoic acid (Ra) signaling pathway. Vitamin A or retinol undergoes metabolism to its biologically active form, retinoic acid (all-trans). This metabolism is mediated by a series of enzymes such as retinol dehydrogenase (Rodh) and retinaldehyde dehydrogenase (Raldh). Retinol is transported during its metabolism in the cytoplasm by a binding protein, Crbp. Retinoic acid is transported to the nucleus by another binding protein Crabp, where it binds to receptors (RXR and RAR). This results in activation of retinoic acid response elements (Rare) and regulation of target gene expression.

RETINOIC ACID SIGNALING. Retinoic acid is a powerful regulator of early development that is believed to act in a concentration-dependent manner to determine cell fate. Because it diffuses through the extracellular milieu, with its concentration decreasing with distance from its tissue of synthesis, a concentration gradient can form across an early organ rudiment such as the limb bud. This gradient is believed to provide **positional information** to cells, establishing different cell fates in different areas of an organ rudiment. Thus, retinoic acid is considered to be a **morphogen**—a diffusible substance that determines cell fate during development in a concentration-dependent manner.

Retinoic acid is derived from vitamin A (retinol). Retinol passes through the cell membrane from the extracellular milieu and binds to cytoplasmic-binding proteins called cellular retinol-binding proteins (Crbps; Fig. 5-28). Within the cytoplasm, retinol is enzymatically converted (by retinol dehydrogenases) to retinal, then to all-trans-retinoic acid (by retinaldehyde dehydrogenases), the active form of retinoic acid. Retinoic acid quickly binds to other binding proteins in the cytoplasm, the cellular retinoic acid–binding proteins (Crabps). Ultimately, retinoic acid is then released from the Crabps and enters the nucleus, where it binds to the retinoic acid receptors (RARs). These receptors are related to the steroid and thyroid hormone receptors. A second group of receptors, the retinoid X receptors (RXRs), are not as well understood. Both RARs and RXRs exist as three isoforms: alpha, beta, and gamma isoforms.

RARs, like steroid and thyroid hormone receptors, are ligand-dependent transcription factors. Upon ligand binding in the nucleus, RARs bind to a retinoic acid response element (Rare) within gene promoters, thereby regulating the expression of target genes. Several hundred genes are known to be regulated by retinoic acid signaling.

Retinoic acid signaling can be perturbed in humans by environmental and pharmacologic agents. **Accutane** and **etretinate (Tegison)**, drugs taken orally for treatment of severe acne, cause both craniofacial and limb anomalies in offspring when used by mothers during pregnancy.

EMBRYONIC STEM CELLS AND CLONING

Techniques covered earlier in this chapter to manipulate and study mouse development have been modified for use in humans, particularly for overcoming reproductive problems. As covered in Chapter 1, human eggs and sperm are now routinely manipulated during in vitro fertilization. Other techniques used in mouse can also be modified for use in humans. For example, **mouse embryonic stem cells** (called **ES cells**), derived from the inner cell mass of the mouse blastocyst, can be grown and then transplanted into tissues (such as the pancreas of diabetic mice) or manipulated genetically to form transgenic animals. Similarly, human ES cells can be derived from the inner cell mass of the human blastocyst. Such cells are potentially valuable for replacing tissues in people suffering from various diseases such as heart disease, juvenile diabetes, Alzheimer, and Parkinson disease, as well as from spinal cord injuries and resulting paralysis. Studies in animal models and a limited number of clinical trials in humans in general support this possibility. By definition, **stem cells** are cells that can self-renew under appropriate conditions and produce daughters that can differentiate into multiple cell types. Thus, stem cells are **totipotent** (i.e., capable of forming all cell types) or **pluripotent** (i.e., capable of forming many but not all cell types). One example of an adult stem cell (from the bulge of the hair follicle) is covered in the first "In the Research Lab" of Chapter 10.

In 2006, a technique was developed to produce a different kind of stem cell called **induced pluripotent stem (IPS) cells**. In this procedure, a cocktail of factors is transfected into cells obtained from an animal model or patient, for example, skin fibroblast cells. Four factors were used in the first experiments that produced pluripotent stem cells: Oct4 (also known as Pou5F1; see Chapter 1), Sox2 (see Chapter 1), Klf4, and c-Myc. In later experiments, it was shown that the last two factors could be replaced with two other factors: nanog and Lin-28. And, in human fibroblasts, the last two factors could be replaced with the drug valproic acid, a histone deacetylase inhibitor. However, both Oct4 and Sox2, which are transcription factors normally expressed by the inner cell mass of the blastocyst and the early embryo, and are known to be markers for cell pluripotency, are required to produce IPS cells (nanog is also a marker for cell pluripotency and is expressed in the early embryo, as covered in Chapter 1).

The technique to establish IPS cells has been modified in several ways and used in a variety of organisms and cell types in the past five years. It appears that IPS cells can be generated from essentially any cell type in essentially any mammal. These cells offer several advantages in that they can be readily and quickly produced in large numbers without sacrificing embryos; they can be used to generate animal- or patient-specific stem cells, avoiding immunological rejection of grafted cells; and several lines can be generated from engineered cells to establish disease-specific models, for example, for drug testing.

Many articles are published each year in the general press regarding the "cloning of humans." Two types of cloning are distinguished by scientists, and their differences are important for the public to understand: **therapeutic cloning** and **reproductive cloning**. Cloning, which has been accomplished in several plant and animal species, refers to the production of one or more individual organisms that are genetically identical to the original organism (genes can also be cloned). Both therapeutic cloning and reproductive cloning begin with an unfertilized egg of the species of choice (say a mouse) and involve the process of **somatic cell nuclear transfer (SCNT)**. In this process, the female pronucleus is removed from the egg (usually by using a suction pipette) and then is replaced with a diploid nucleus obtained from a donor cell obtained from an adult animal. In some cases, such eggs go on to develop blastocysts. In *therapeutic* cloning, ES cells are derived from the inner cell mass of such a blastocyst and then are transplanted into a tissue of the donor adult to replace a defective cell type (such as beta cells of the pancreatic islets in a diabetic mouse). Because the nucleus used for SCNT was obtained from the same animal that receives the ES cells, both the cells and the animal are genetically identical, eliminating the problem of tissue rejection. Of course, with the advent of IPS cells, these could be used instead of therapeutic cloning for tissue transplantation, also eliminating the problem of tissue rejection. However, the advantages and disadvantages of ES cells versus IPS cells for each type of tissue are currently unknown, especially in humans.

In contrast to therapeutic cloning, in *reproductive* cloning, the blastocyst that results from SCNT is transplanted into the uterus of a pseudopregnant animal (surrogate mother). If normal embryogenesis then ensues, a **clone** will be delivered, that is, an offspring genetically identical to the donor. The most famous clone to date is the sheep **Dolly**, born in 1995. No credible accounts of human reproductive cloning have been reported, although stories claiming that humans have been reproductively cloned appear from time to time in the popular press, and make entertaining novels and movies.

Embryology in Practice

VARIABILITY IS THE LAW OF LIFE

A 60-year-old Internet entrepreneur is seen by his physician and requests **whole-genome sequence** (WGS) **analysis**. He says, "I have the means and the desire to be proactive about personalizing my healthcare decisions." He also wishes to provide knowledge about "actionable genetic variants" to his adult daughters and their children.

Whole-genome sequencing is performed, whereby all nine billion base pairs of his genetic material are simultaneously sequenced and compared with the Human Genome Reference sequence to define the differences in his genome (genetic variants). These variants are analyzed and divided into bins according to clinical significance: clinically actionable variants, variants of unknown clinical significance, and benign variants (**genetic polymorphisms**).

After twelve weeks, the man returns to his physician for post-test counseling. The report contains a number of results useful for the man's health, including information about cardiovascular risk, variants that affect medication efficacy and/or toxicity (**pharmacogenomics**), and carrier status of several recessive conditions.

Among the results is a variant in the gene encoding cardiac TROPONIN T (TNNT2), a gene associated with sudden cardiac death (SCD) and adult-onset hypertrophic cardiomyopathy (HCM). This variant is reportedly novel (not seen previously in the population) and is predicted by in silico algorithms to have a deleterious effect on the TNNT2 protein function. But because the variant had not been specifically seen in other SCD/HCM patients, it was included on the report as a "variant of unknown significance," and correlation to the patient's phenotype was recommended. Adding to the patient's anxiety, further review of the patient's family history revealed two individuals in past generations who "unexpectedly died young" of unknown causes.

Concern over the significance of this TNNT2 variant prompted referral to a cardiologist and a full cardiac evaluation, including an ECG, echocardiography, cardiac MRI, and a stress test—all of which were normal. However, given the insidious onset of disease associated with TNNT2 mutations, there was discussion about the need for an implantable cardioverter-defibrillator (ICD), which the man declined.

After two years, during which interval the man was followed closely for signs of cardiac hypertrophy, the physician received a report from the lab stating that the TNNT2 variant had now been reclassified as "benign" based on its presence in a growing number of normal control individuals in the lab data base. This information was relayed to the patient, who was somewhat relieved.

Sir William Oster said, "Variability is the law of life." Nowhere has this statement proven more true than in the tremendous variation found within each of our genomes. Comparison of the genetic code from any two individuals yields between three and six million differences, many of which are unique or "private" mutations, and many more of which are present but rare in the population. These variants are found within the coding regions of known disease genes commonly enough that it not a question of *whether* a WGS test will find variants of unknown clinical significance in a patient, but *how many* will be found and *how* these variants should be followed clinically. As the case demonstrates, great care must be taken in the interpretation and application of WGS to clinical medicine.

SUGGESTED READINGS

Andersen P, Uosaki H, Shenje LT, Kwon C. 2012. Non-canonical Notch signaling: emerging role and mechanism. Trends Cell Biol 22: 257–265.

Cohen DE, Melton D. 2011. Turning straw into gold: directing cell fate for regenerative medicine. Nat Rev Genet 12:243–252.

Eichmann A, Simons M. 2012. VEGF signaling inside vascular endothelial cells and beyond. Curr Opin Cell Biol 24:188–193.

Gallet A. 2011. Hedgehog morphogen: from secretion to reception. Trends Cell Biol 21:238–246.

Goetz SC, Anderson KV. 2010. The primary cilium: a signalling centre during vertebrate development. Nat Rev Genet 11:331–344.

Guruharsha KG, Kankel MW, Artavanis-Tsakonas S. 2012. The Notch signalling system: recent insights into the complexity of a conserved pathway. Nat Rev Genet 13:654–666.

MacDonald BT, Tamai K, He X. 2009. Wnt/beta-catenin signaling: components, mechanisms, and diseases. Dev Cell 17:9–26.

Massagué J. 2012. TGFβ signalling in context. Nat Rev Mol Cell Biol 13:616–630.

Walsh DW, Godson C, Brazil DP, Martin F. 2010. Extracellular BMP-antagonist regulation in development and disease: tied up in knots. Trends Cell Biol 20:244–256.

Wickstrom SA, Fassler R. 2011. Regulation of membrane traffic by integrin signaling. Trends Cell Biol 21:266–273.

Chapter 6

Fetal Development and the Fetus as a Patient

SUMMARY

The gestation period of humans from fertilization to birth is usually 266 days, or thirty-eight weeks. As covered in the Introduction, the **embryonic period**, during which most of the major organ systems are formed, ends at the end of the eighth week of gestation. The remainder of gestation constitutes the **fetal period**, which is devoted mainly to the maturation of organ systems and to growth. For convenience, the nine-month gestation period is divided into three, three-month **trimesters**. It is not currently possible to keep alive fetuses born before about twenty-two weeks of gestation. Fetuses born between twenty-two and twenty-eight weeks have progressively increasing survival rates (from about 15% at twenty-two weeks to about 90% at twenty-eight weeks), but up to one-third of these have significant morbidity that affects their long-term survival.

Both the embryo, during weeks three to eight, and the fetus receive nutrients and eliminate their metabolic wastes via the **placenta**, an organ that has both maternal and fetal components. The mature placenta consists of a mass of feathery fetal **villi** that project into an **intervillous space** lined with fetal syncytiotrophoblast and filled with maternal blood. The fetal blood in the villous vessels exchanges materials with the maternal blood across the villus wall. However, exchange of nutrients is not the only function of the placenta; the organ also secretes a plethora of hormones, including the sex steroids that maintain pregnancy. Maternal antibodies cross the placenta to enter the fetus, where they provide protection against fetal and neonatal infections. **Cell-free fetal DNA** also crosses the placenta and can be detected in maternal blood plasma. Unfortunately, teratogenic compounds and some microorganisms also cross the placenta. The placenta grows along with the fetus; at birth it weighs about one sixth as much as the fetus.

Development of the placenta begins when the implanting blastocyst induces the **decidual reaction** in the maternal endometrium, causing the endometrium to become a nutrient-packed, highly vascular tissue called the **decidua**. By the second month, the growing embryo begins to bulge into the uterine lumen. The protruding side of the embryo is covered with a thin capsule of decidua called the **decidua capsularis**, which later disintegrates as the fetus fills the womb. The decidua underlying the embedded **embryonic** pole of the embryo—the pole at which the embryonic disc and the connecting stalk are attached—is called the **decidua basalis**, which forms the maternal face of the developing placenta. The remainder of the maternal decidua is called the **decidua parietalis**.

The **umbilical cord** forms as a result of body folding. During this process, the amnion, which initially arises from the dorsal margin of the embryonic disc ectoderm, is carried ventrally to enclose the entire embryo, taking origin from the **umbilical ring** surrounding the roots of the vitelline duct and connecting stalk. The amnion also expands until it fills the chorionic space and fuses with the chorion. As the amnion expands, it encloses the connecting stalk and yolk sac neck in a sheath of amniotic membrane. This composite structure becomes the umbilical cord.

As covered in Chapter 2, the intervillous space of the placenta originates as lacunae within the syncytiotrophoblast, which anastomose with maternal capillaries and become filled with maternal blood at about ten weeks of gestation. **Stem villi** grow from the fetal chorion into these spaces. Each villus has a core of extraembryonic mesoderm containing blood vessels and a two-layered outer "skin" of cytotrophoblast and syncytiotrophoblast. Villi originally cover the entire chorion, but by the end of the third month, they are restricted to the area of the embryonic pole that becomes the site of the mature placenta. This part of the chorion is called the **chorion frondosum**; the remaining, smooth chorion is the **chorion laeve**. The villi continue to grow and branch throughout gestation. The intervillous space is subdivided into fifteen to twenty-five partially separated compartments, called **cotyledons**, by wedgelike walls of tissue called **placental septae** that grow inward from the maternal face of the placenta.

Twins formed by the splitting of a single early embryo (monozygotic twins) may share fetal membranes to varying degrees. In contrast, twins formed by the fertilization of two oocytes (dizygotic twins) always implant separately and develop independent sets of fetal membranes. Sharing of membranes can have negative consequences when vascular connections between the two placentas exist. Although rare, this can result in vascular compromise of one fetus and subsequent loss of that fetus, or even both fetuses.

Advances in analyzing fetal products in maternal serum, the safety and sophistication of techniques for sampling fetal tissues, and the use of novel imaging techniques to examine the fetus are rapidly providing new approaches to the prenatal diagnosis and treatment of congenital disorders. Our improving ability to diagnose and treat diseases in utero and in very premature infants raises ethical and legal questions that require thoughtful debate. Questions of this nature have always arisen at the forefront of new medical techniques. What is somewhat unusual in this case is the extreme speed with which both our understanding of developmental biology and our clinical practice are advancing, along with the fact that decisions about, and solutions to, the resulting medical questions affect a new category of patient: the unborn fetus. The study and treatment of the fetus constitutes the field of **prenatal pediatrics**, or **fetology**.

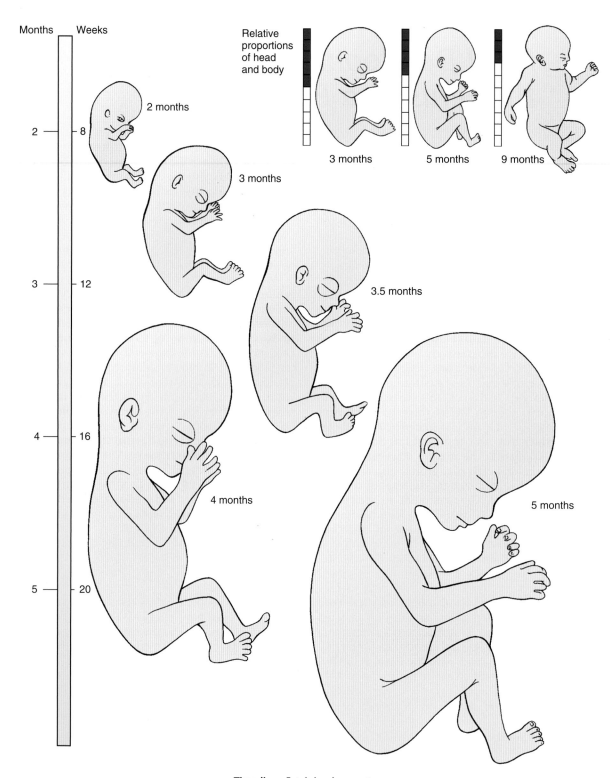

Time line. Fetal development.

Clinical Taster

A young couple is seen for a routine midgestational (week twenty) **ultrasound** during their first pregnancy. The ultrasonographer is showing the couple their child, a boy, when she pauses. After a couple of minutes, she says that there may be "abnormalities," so she will ask the doctor to take a look. After reviewing the scans, the perinatologist (an obstetric subspecialist who provides care for mother and fetus in higher-risk pregnancies) comes in and explains that the fetus has **oligohydramnios** (too little amniotic fluid), **hydronephrosis** (dilated ureters and kidneys), and **megacystis** (dilated bladder). She states her suspicion that the boy has bladder outlet obstruction due to a condition called **posterior urethral valves**. She tells them this is an abnormality of the urethra that prevents normal urine excretion and causes the urine to back up into bladder, ureters, and kidneys. She says that this backup can damage the kidneys, and the lack of amniotic fluid can prevent the lungs from developing normally. She says that if left untreated, the child will develop a condition called **Potter sequence**. The parents are warned that if nothing is done, the child will die at the time of birth as the result of **respiratory failure**.

An **amniocentesis** is performed for subsequent chromosome analysis, which shows a normal 46,XY karyotype, and in a second ultrasound, no other structural abnormalities are found. The couple is referred to a center with expertise in **fetal surgery** for correcting posterior urethral valves. After weighing the risks of surgery against the likelihood of postnatal death from **pulmonary hypoplasia**, the couple elects to undergo placement of a vesicoamniotic catheter (which shunts urine from the bladder to the amniotic cavity) at twenty-two weeks of gestation. The procedure goes well, and a follow-up ultrasound shows decompression of the bladder and urinary collecting system. The pregnancy is followed closely for signs of shunt malfunction, infection, amniotic fluid leakage, and preterm labor. The boy is delivered at thirty-six weeks of gestation, and surgery is done to create a vesicostomy (opening from the bladder to the abdominal wall), with urinary reconstructive surgery planned in the future.

Potter sequence can have multiple causes. Other clinical scenarios that result in this sequence are given in the "Embryology in Practice" and "Clinical Taster" for Chapter 15.

DURING FETAL PERIOD, EMBRYONIC ORGAN SYSTEMS MATURE AND FETUS GROWS

The preceding chapters have focused on the **embryonic period**, the period during which the organs and systems of the body are formed (Fig. 6-1A). The succeeding **fetal period**, from eight weeks to birth at about thirty-eight weeks, is devoted to the maturation of these organ systems and to growth (Fig. 6-1B; Table 6-1). The fetus grows from 14 g at the beginning of the fetal period (end of the second month) to about 3500 g at birth—a two-hundred-and-fifty-fold increase. Most of this weight is added in the third trimester (seven to nine months), although the fetus grows in length mainly in the second trimester (four to six months). The growth of the fetus is accompanied by drastic changes in proportion: at nine weeks, the head of the fetus represents about half its **crown-rump length** (the "sitting height" of the fetus), whereas at birth, it represents about one fourth of the crown-rump length.

Although all organ systems are present by eight weeks, few of them are functional. The most prominent exceptions are the heart and blood vessels, which begin to circulate blood during the fourth week. Even so, the reconfiguration of the fetal circulatory system, covered in Chapter 13, is not complete until three months. The sensory systems also lag. For example, the auditory ossicles are not free to vibrate until just before birth, and although the neural retina of the eye differentiates during the third and fourth months, the eyelids remain closed until five to seven months, and the eyes cannot focus properly until several weeks after birth.

A number of organs do not finish maturing until after birth. The most obvious example is the reproductive system and associated sexual characteristics, which, as in most animals, do not finish developing until the

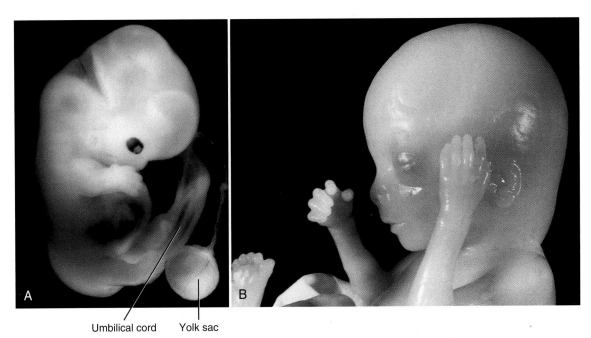

Umbilical cord   Yolk sac

Figure 6-1. Images of human embryos. *A,* Embryo at about seven weeks of gestation showing the umbilical cord and yolk sac. *B,* Head of a fetus at about sixteen weeks of gestation.

TABLE 6-1 FETAL GROWTH

Gestational Age (Completed Months of Development)	Approximate CR[1] Length (cm/in)	Approximate Weight/Mass (g/oz)
2	5.5/2	14/0.5
3	12/4.5	100/3.5
4	16.5/6.5	300/10.5

	Approximate CH[2] length (cm/in)	Approximate Weight/Mass (g/lb)
5	30/12	600/1.3
6	37.5/15	1000/2.2
7	42.5/16.5	1700/3.8
8	47/18.5	2600/5.8
9	51/20	3500/7.5

[1]Crown-rump.
[2]Crown-heel.

individual is old enough to be likely to reproduce successfully. In humans, a relatively large number of other organs are also immature at birth. This accounts for the prolonged helpless infancy of humans as compared with many mammals. The most slowly maturing organ of humans—the one that largely sets the pace of infancy and childhood—is the brain. Both the cerebrum and the cerebellum are quite immature at birth.

In the Research Lab

HOW ARE ORGAN GROWTH AND BODY GROWTH CONTROLLED DURING EMBRYOGENESIS?

What stops the continued growth of an organ, or of the fetus itself, once it reaches a particular size is a largely unanswered question. Circulating hormones and the availability of nutrients in utero clearly play an important role in growth, but how is growth regulated so that optimal size is obtained to allow the various organ systems to function in a coordinated fashion? Three factors are known to play integral roles in limiting organ growth. Two of these factors, the TOR pathway, which senses the availability of nutrients and regulates growth, and the growth factor insulin-like growth factor 1 (Igf-like1), were covered in the Introduction chapter in the context of aging. In addition to having a role in aging, it is now known that mutations in an allele of Igf-like1, which presumably regulate the functioning of the growth factor, are linked to the size of different breeds of domestic dogs. For example, little dogs, like Chihuahuas, have one gene variant that makes them small, and big dogs, like Great Danes, have another that makes them large. This correlation between type of variant and body size held when 3000 dogs from almost 150 breeds were genetically evaluated.

The third factor known to limit growth is a recently discovered pathway called the **hippo** pathway. Hippo signaling involves a kinase cascade (kinase signaling is covered in Chapter 5) with multiple other members with whimsical names such as warts, yorkie, salvador, and mats. When various members of this pathway are mutated, in organisms as diverse as Drosophila and mouse, overgrowth of organs or tissues occurs.

DEVELOPMENT OF PLACENTA

As the blastocyst implants, it stimulates a response in the uterine endometrium called the **decidual reaction**. The cells of the endometrial **stroma** (the fleshy layer of endometrial tissue that underlies the endometrial epithelium lining the uterine cavity) accumulate lipid and glycogen and are then called **decidual cells**. The stroma thickens and becomes more highly vascularized, and the endometrium as a whole is then called the **decidua**.

Late in the embryonic period, the **abembryonic** side of the growing embryo (the side opposite to the **embryonic** pole, where the embryonic disc and the connecting stalk attach) begins to bulge into the uterine cavity (Fig. 6-2). This protruding portion of the embryo is covered by a thin capsule of endometrium called the **decidua capsularis**. The embedded embryonic pole of the embryo is underlain by a zone of decidua called the **decidua basalis**, which will participate in forming the mature placenta. The remaining areas of decidua are called the **decidua parietalis**. In the third month, as the growing fetus begins to fill the womb, the decidua capsularis is pressed against the decidua parietalis, and in the fifth and sixth months, the decidua capsularis disintegrates. By this time, the placenta is fully formed and has distinct fetal and maternal surfaces (Fig. 6-3).

As covered in Chapter 2, development of the uteroplacental circulatory system begins late in the second week, as cavities called **trophoblastic lacunae** form in the syncytiotrophoblast of the chorion and anastomose with maternal capillaries. At the end of the third week, fetal blood vessels begin to form in the connecting stalk and extraembryonic mesoderm. Meanwhile, the extraembryonic mesoderm lining the chorionic cavity proliferates to form **tertiary stem villi** that project into the trophoblastic lacunae, which become blood-filled after ten weeks. By the end of the fourth week, tertiary stem villi cover the entire chorion. Hypoxia, or lower tissue oxygen content in the decidua, is critical for normal trophoblast invasion.

As the embryo begins to bulge into the uterine lumen during the second month, the villi on the protruding abembryonic side of the chorion disappear (see Fig. 6-2). This region of the chorion is now called the **smooth chorion**, or the **chorion laeve**, whereas the portion of the chorion associated with the decidua basalis retains its villi and is called the **chorion frondosum** (from Latin *frondosus*, leafy).

The placental villi continue to grow during most of the remainder of gestation. Starting in the ninth week, the tertiary stem villi lengthen by the formation of terminal **mesenchymal villi**, which originate as sprouts of syncytiotrophoblast (**trophoblastic sprouts**) similar in cross section to primary stem villi (Fig. 6-4). These terminal extensions of the tertiary stem villi, called **immature intermediate villi**, reach their maximum length in the sixteenth week. The cells of the cytotrophoblastic layer become more dispersed in these villi, leaving gaps in that layer of the villus wall.

Starting near the end of the second trimester, the tertiary stem villi also form numerous slender side branches called **mature intermediate villi**. The first-formed

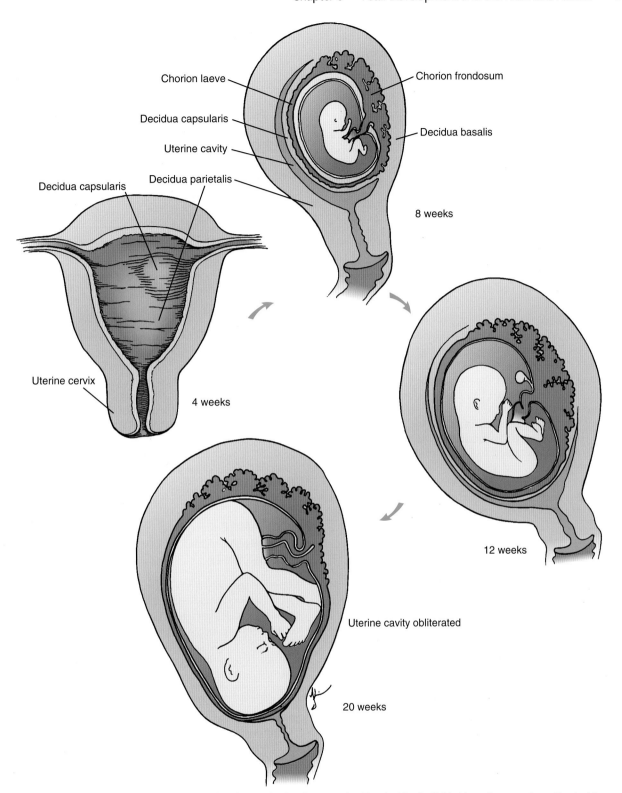

Figure 6-2. Development of the chorion and decidua during the first five months. The decidua is divided into three portions: the decidua capsularis overlying the growing conceptus, the decidua basalis underlying the placenta, and the decidua parietalis lining the remainder of the uterus. Note that the original uterine cavity is obliterated by twenty weeks owing to growth of the fetus and expansion of the amniotic cavity.

mature intermediate villi finish forming by week thirty-two and then begin to produce small, nodule-like secondary branches called **terminal villi**. These terminal villi complete the structure of the **placental villous tree**. It has been suggested that the terminal villi are formed not by active outgrowth of the syncytiotrophoblast but rather by coiled and folded villous capillaries that bulge against the villus wall.

Because the **intervillous space** into which the villi project is formed from trophoblastic lacunae that grow

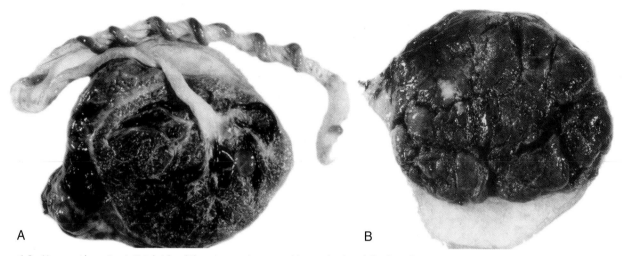

Figure 6-3. Human placenta. *A*, Fetal side of the mature placenta with attached umbilical cord. *B*, Maternal side of the mature placenta showing several cotyledons.

and coalesce, it is lined on both sides with syncytiotrophoblast (see Fig. 6-4). The maternal face of the placenta, called the **basal plate**, consists of this syncytiotrophoblast lining plus a supporting layer of decidua basalis. On the fetal side, the layers of the chorion form the **chorionic plate** of the placenta.

During the fourth and fifth months, wedgelike walls of decidual tissue called **placental (decidual) septa** grow into the intervillous space from the maternal side of the placenta, separating the villi into fifteen to twenty-five groups called **cotyledons** (see Figs. 6-3*B*, 6-4). Because the placental septa do not fuse with the chorionic plate, maternal blood can flow freely from one cotyledon to another.

DEVELOPMENT OF UMBILICAL CORD

As covered in Chapter 4, **body folding** separates the forming embryo from its **extraembryonic membranes**. As this process occurs and the embryo grows, the amnion keeps pace, expanding until it encloses the entire embryo except for the umbilical area, where the connecting stalk and the yolk sac emerge (Fig. 6-5). Between the fourth and eighth weeks, an increase in the production of amniotic fluid causes the amnion to swell until it completely takes over the chorionic space (Fig. 6-6). When the amnion contacts the soft chorion, the layers of extraembryonic mesoderm covering the two membranes fuse loosely. Thus, the chorionic cavity disappears except for a few rudimentary vesicles.

After embryonic folding is complete, the amnion takes origin from the **umbilical ring** surrounding the roots of the vitelline duct and connecting stalk. Therefore, the progressive expansion of the amnion creates a tube of amniotic membrane that encloses the connecting stalk and the vitelline duct. This composite structure is now called the **umbilical cord** (see Figs. 6-1*A*, 6-3*A*). As the umbilical cord lengthens, the vitelline duct narrows and the pear-shaped body of the yolk sac remains within the umbilical sheath. Normally, both the yolk sac and the vitelline duct disappear by birth.

The main function of the umbilical cord is to circulate blood between the embryo and the placenta. Umbilical arteries and veins develop in the connecting stalk to perform this function (covered in Chapter 13). The expanded amnion creates a roomy, weightless chamber in which the fetus can grow and develop freely. If the supply of amniotic fluid is inadequate (the condition known as **oligohydramnios**), the abnormally small amniotic cavity may restrict fetal growth, which may result in severe malformations and **pulmonary hypoplasia** (covered in the "Clinical Taster" for this chapter).

EXCHANGE OF SUBSTANCES BETWEEN MATERNAL AND FETAL BLOOD IN PLACENTA

Maternal blood enters the intervillous spaces of the placenta through about one hundred **spiral arteries**, bathes the villi, and leaves again via **endometrial veins**. The placenta contains approximately 150 mL of maternal blood, and this volume is replaced about three or four times per minute. Nutrients and oxygen pass from the maternal blood across the cell layers of the villus into the fetal blood, and waste products such as carbon dioxide, urea, uric acid, and bilirubin (a breakdown product of hemoglobin) reciprocally pass from the fetal blood to the maternal blood.

Maternal proteins are endocytosed and degraded by the trophoblast unless bound to receptors (e.g., immunoglobulin [Ig]G, transcobalamin II). Antibodies cross the placenta to enter the fetal circulation; in this way, the mother gives the fetus limited passive immunity against a variety of infections, such as diphtheria and measles. These antibodies persist in the infant's blood for several months after birth, guarding the infant against infectious diseases until its own immune system matures.

ERYTHROBLASTOSIS FETALIS

The transfer of antibodies from mother to fetus is not beneficial in one fairly common instance: when antibodies are

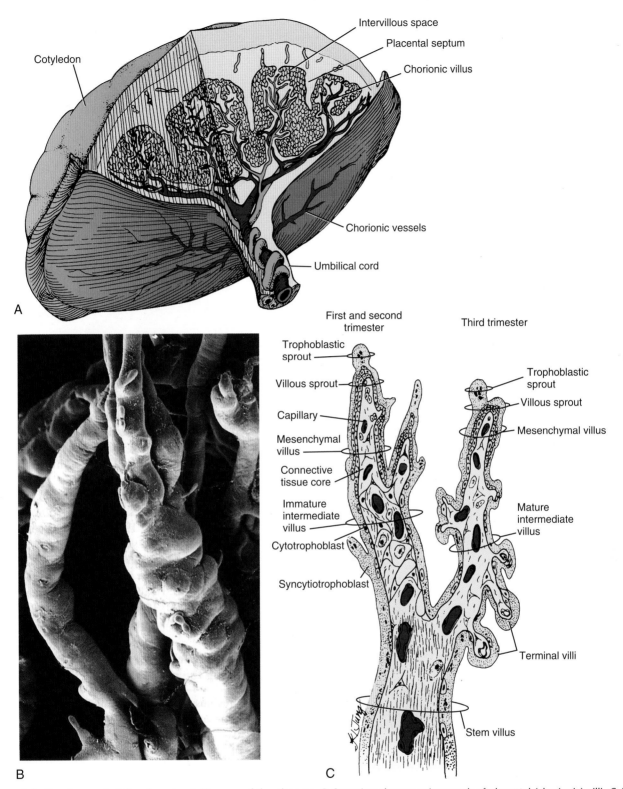

Figure 6-4. Development of the placenta. *A,* Diagram of the placenta. *B,* Scanning electron micrograph of placental (chorionic) villi. *C,* Diagram showing a stem (primary) villus, which has branched into two (secondary) villi (immature intermediate villus, left, during the first and second trimesters; mature intermediate villus, right, during the third trimester). Note that the mature intermediate villus bears several terminal (tertiary) villi.

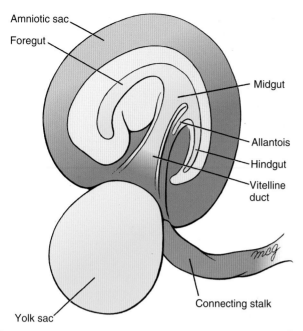

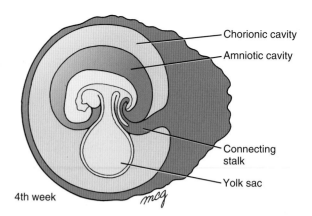

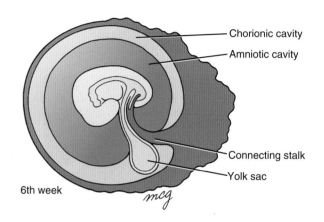

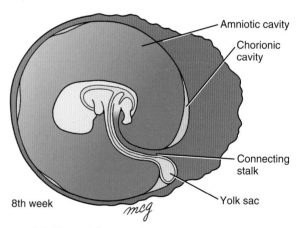

Figure 6-5. Genesis of the umbilical cord. Folding of the embryo and expansion of the amniotic cavity bring the connecting stalk and yolk sac together to form the umbilical cord. As the amnion continues to grow, a layer of amniotic membrane gradually encloses the umbilical cord.

directed against an Rh factor on the fetal red blood cells, causing hemolysis (dissolution) of the fetal red blood cells. The **Rh factors** are a group of genetically determined surface molecules that are present on the plasma membrane of red blood cells in most, but not all, individuals. Individuals whose blood cells carry an Rh factor are **Rh+**; individuals whose blood cells lack one are **Rh−**. Rh factors provoke a strong immune response in Rh− individuals. If an Rh− mother carries an Rh+ fetus, and fetal blood leaks into the maternal circulation, the mother will manufacture antibodies against the fetal red blood cells. Significant leaks of fetal blood across the placenta into the maternal circulation normally occur only at birth, so the resulting antibodies do not form in time to harm the fetus that first induces them. However, if the same mother bears a second Rh+ fetus, her anti-Rh antibodies can cross the placenta and destroy fetal red blood cells, causing anemia in the fetus and newborn. This condition is called **hemolytic disease of the newborn**, or **erythroblastosis fetalis**. The latter name comes from the fact that the destruction of red blood cells stimulates a compensatory production of large numbers of immature nucleated fetal red blood cells called **erythroblasts**. Another, sometimes fatal, consequence of the disease is **hydrops fetalis**: the accumulation of water in the fetus. Moreover, the destruction of red blood cells releases large amounts of bilirubin (a breakdown product of hemoglobin) into the fetal circulation. This substance can be deposited in the developing brain, leading to cerebral damage and, in some cases, to death.

The effects of erythroblastosis fetalis can be prevented by giving transfusions of Rh− blood to the fetus in utero and to the newborn, so that maternal antibodies find fewer cells to destroy. A more economical preventive approach is to administer anti-Rh antibodies (RhoGam) to the Rh− mother immediately after the birth of each Rh+ baby.

Figure 6-6. The rapidly expanding amniotic cavity fills with fluid and obliterates the chorionic cavity between weeks four and eight.

These antibodies destroy the fetal Rh+ red blood cells in her circulation before they stimulate her own immune system, preventing her from manufacturing anti-Rh antibodies.

TRANSFER OF CELL-FREE FETAL DNA TO MATERNAL PLASMA

Recall that the fetal side of the placenta, including the external covering of the placental villi and the entire intervillous space, is lined with a layer of syncytiotrophoblast derived from the outer layer of the blastocyst (see Fig. 6-4*C*). Apoptosis (programmed cell death) normally occurs throughout the syncytiotrophoblast during gestation, releasing fetal DNA, which enters the maternal circulation. Approximately 10% of the free-floating DNA in maternal plasma is fetal. Thus, using PCR (the polymerase chain reaction), fetal DNA can be detected in maternal plasma, beginning at about week seven of gestation and continuing to birth, after which it is rapidly cleared. PCR of fetal DNA in maternal plasma allows early and accurate prenatal genetic diagnosis of the fetus. Recently, it was shown that the entire genome sequence of a fetus could be obtained in this non-invasive manner using "a teaspoon's worth of maternal blood." Currently, fetal DNA in maternal plasma is being used to diagnose trisomies (see Chapter 1) in the fetus developing in utero.

Such analysis of fetal DNA could also be used to sex the fetus near the end of the second month of gestation by looking for the presence or absence of the SRY and other genes present on the Y chromosome (covered in Chapter 16). Using amniocentesis or chorionic villus sampling (covered later in the chapter), fetuses can be sexed near the end of the third to fourth month of gestation (i.e., one to two months later). However, both of these procedures are invasive and have a risk as high as about 1% of inducing miscarriage. Finally, fetuses can be sexed and routinely are sexed by non-invasive ultrasonography (covered later in the chapter). However, ultrasonography cannot be done until still later, that is, not until eighteen to twenty weeks of gestation.

Under what conditions would it be relevant to ascertain the sex of the fetus as early as possible? Two examples are compelling. First, if a couple already has a child with a rare genetic disorder that typically affects only boys, such as muscular dystrophy or hemophilia, they will of course be worried about having a second child with a disorder. Early sexing of the fetus would alleviate this concern early if the fetus is a girl. Second, as covered later in this chapter, women at risk of carrying a child with congenital adrenal hyperplasia (CAH) undergo preventive treatment during pregnancy with the potent corticosteroid dexamethasone to reduce masculinization of the external genitalia in affected female fetuses. If the fetus is a boy, such treatment could be stopped without ill effect on the fetus.

PLACENTA ALLOWS PASSAGE OF SOME VIRAL AND BACTERIAL PATHOGENS

Although the placenta is fairly impermeable to microorganisms, a number of viruses and bacteria can cross it and infect the fetus. Because the fetus has no functioning immune system and relies solely on maternal antibodies for protection, it is often inept at fighting infection. Therefore, a disease that is mild in the mother may damage or kill the fetus. The types of microorganisms that can cross the placenta and infect the fetus can be remembered by the acronym TORCH: ***Toxoplasma gondii*** (a protozoan that can be transmitted to humans from cat litter and soil); other agents such as **parvovirus** (a virus that causes rashes in school-aged children; the canine form

of this virus does not infect humans); ***Treponema pallidum*** (the bacterium that causes syphilis, which can result in fetal death or anomalies); **coxsackievirus** (a cause of aseptic meningitis); **varicella-zoster virus** (the agent of varicella or chickenpox); **rubella virus** (the agent of rubella or German measles); **cytomegalovirus** (infection with this virus in adults and children may be asymptomatic); and **herpes simplex virus** (the virus that causes canker sores and genital warts).

Cytomegalovirus (CMV) causes one of the most common viral infections of the fetus. In one study, 1.6% to 3.7% of women tested from high-income and low-income groups, respectively, had primary CMV infection, with risk of intrauterine transmission of 30% to 40%. If CMV infects the embryo early in development, it may induce abortion; infection that occurs later may cause a wide range of congenital abnormalities, including blindness, microcephaly (small head), hearing loss, and mental retardation.

HIV CAN BE TRANSMITTED ACROSS PLACENTA DURING PARTURITION OR IN BREAST MILK

Human immunodeficiency virus (HIV) is the agent of **acquired immune deficiency syndrome (AIDS)** and related syndromes. This virus sometimes can cross the placenta from an infected mother to infect the unborn fetus. It is important to note that 25% to 40% of babies are HIV positive if their mothers are HIV positive and remain untreated with anti-HIV therapies; with appropriate treatment (covered in the next paragraph), this number can be as low as 1%. The difference in transmission rate of 25% to 40% in untreated pregnancies is related to whether the placenta has specific co-receptors for specific strains of HIV, and whether the placenta expresses active virus. HIV is commonly transmitted during the birth process or in the mother's milk during breast feeding. Infants infected perinatally with HIV may seem healthy at birth, but they usually develop AIDS by the time they are three years old. As in adults, the disease slowly destroys a crucial component of the immune system and leaves the infant vulnerable to repeated infections. Parotid gland infection, diarrhea, bronchitis, and chronic middle ear infection are common in infants with AIDS. Pneumonia caused by the protozoan *Pneumocystis carinii*, a characteristic infection of adults with AIDS, is a particularly alarming symptom in infants: the mean survival time of infants diagnosed with AIDS and *Pneumocystis carinii* pneumonia is one to three months. HIV-1 infection is also correlated with an increased rate of low birth weight, intrauterine fetal death, and preterm birth.

In 2005 it was estimated that more than forty million people worldwide were infected with HIV. According to the Centers for Disease Control and Prevention, from approximately 1984 (roughly when the AIDS epidemic began in the United States) to 1993, a total of about fifteen thousand HIV-infected children were born to HIV-positive women in the United States (about six to seven thousand HIV-infected women give birth each year in the United States). From 1984 to 1992, the number of babies born with AIDS increased each year, but between 1992 and 1996, the number of such babies declined by 43%. This reduction occurred because of a number of factors, including enhanced prenatal care, HIV testing before or during pregnancy, and administration of antiretroviral drugs such as zidovudine (ZDV) to HIV-positive women during pregnancy and at delivery, as well as postnatal treatment with the same drugs of babies born to HIV-positive women.

TERATOGENS CROSS PLACENTA

Teratogens are environmental (i.e., non-genetic) substances that are capable of causing a **birth defect** when embryos or fetuses are exposed at critical times in development to sufficiently high doses (concentrations). The study of the role of environmental factors in disrupting development is known by the unfortunate name of **teratology**, which literally means the study of (developmental) monsters. A number of **principles of teratology** have emerged, but here only three are covered because of their direct relevance to human birth defects.

The first principle of teratology that we will discuss is that an embryonic structure is usually susceptible to teratogens only during specific **critical sensitive periods**, which usually correspond to periods of active differentiation and morphogenesis. Thus, a potent teratogen may have no effect on the development of an embryonic structure if it is administered before or after the critical period during which that structure is susceptible to its action. The time lines at the beginning of the chapters in this book generally define the sensitive periods of corresponding tissues and organ systems. During the first eight weeks of development, the major events of organogenesis occur. Thus, this is the period during which the fetus is most vulnerable to teratogens.

A second principle of teratology is that an embryonic structure is susceptible to a **critical dose** of teratogen during its specific critical sensitive period. Thus, in teratologic studies, a **dose-response curve** is constructed for a suspected teratogen in which lowest dose has no effect and the highest dose is lethal to the embryo.

A third principle of teratology is that susceptibility to a teratogen depends on the **genetic constitution** of the developing embryo or fetus. For example, if two embryos of the same age are exposed to the same dose of teratogen, one may develop severe cardiac malformations, whereas the other may remain unaffected. The molecular basis for this difference in susceptibility might, for instance, be a genetic difference in the rate at which the enzyme systems of the two embryos detoxify the teratogen. Thus, a **gene-environmental interaction** underlying susceptibility to birth defects varies from embryo to embryo.

It is not always easy to identify a compound as a teratogen. Two approaches are used: **epidemiologic studies**, which attempt to relate antenatal exposure to a suspect compound with the occurrence of various congenital anomalies in humans (so-called retrospective studies); and studies in which the compound is administered to pregnant **experimental animals** and the offspring are checked for abnormalities (so-called prospective studies). However, it is often difficult to gather enough epidemiologic data to obtain a clear result, and findings from animal studies are not necessarily applicable to humans. These difficulties are compounded by the fact that most congenital anomalies have a multifactorial etiology, that is, their pathogenesis depends on (1) the genetic makeup of the individual (third principle of teratology covered in preceding paragraph), and (2) exposure to the teratogen (i.e., dose; second principle of teratology covered in preceding paragraph). Finally, malformations of a given structure can usually be caused only during the critical sensitive period (first principle of teratology covered in preceding paragraph).

Many therapeutic drugs are known to be teratogenic; these include retinoids (vitamin A and analogs), the anticoagulant warfarin, the anticonvulsants valproic acid and phenytoin, and a number of chemotherapeutic agents used to treat cancer. Although, as stated above, most teratogenic drugs exert their main effects during the embryonic period, care must be exercised in administering certain anesthetics and other drugs, even late in pregnancy or at term, because they may endanger the health of the fetus.

Some recreational drugs are also teratogenic; these include tobacco, alcohol, and cocaine. The manifestations of fetal alcohol syndrome are covered in Chapter 5. Cocaine, used by alarming numbers of pregnant women (the drug affected three hundred thousand to four hundred thousand newborns in 1990 in the United States), readily crosses the placenta and may cause addiction in the developing fetus. In some of the major cities of the United States, as many as 20% of babies are born to mothers who abuse cocaine. Unfortunately, fetal cocaine addiction may have permanent effects on the individual, although studies suggest that early intervention with intensive emotional and educational support in the first few years of life may be helpful.

Pregnant women who use cocaine have higher frequencies of fetal morbidity (disease) and mortality (death) than pregnant women who do not. Cocaine use is associated not only with **low birth weight** but also with some specific developmental anomalies, including infarction of the cerebral cortex and a variety of cardiovascular malformations. However, it is often difficult to isolate cocaine as the teratogen responsible for a given effect because women who use cocaine often use other drugs as well, including marijuana, alcohol, tobacco, and heroin.

Children of cocaine-abusing mothers may be born prematurely as well as addicted, as cocaine-using mothers have a very high frequency of **preterm labor**. Preterm labor occurs in 25% of women who test positive for cocaine on a urine test at admission to the hospital for labor and delivery, but it occurs in only 8% of women who do not test positive for cocaine at admission. Two mechanisms have been proposed by which cocaine could cause preterm labor: cocaine, a potent constrictor of blood vessels, may cause abruption of the placental membranes (premature separation of the placenta from the uterus) by partly shutting off the flow of blood to the placenta, or, as there is evidence that cocaine directly affects the contractility of the uterine myometrium (muscle layer), it may make the myometrium hypersensitive to signals that initiate labor.

INTRAUTERINE GROWTH RESTRICTION

Intrauterine growth restriction (IUGR), often called **small for gestational age (SGA)**, is a condition in which fetal growth is markedly retarded. IUGR carries a higher risk of perinatal mortality and morbidity, so IUGR is a life-threatening birth defect. A newborn is considered to be SGA if he/she weighs less than 2500 g at term or falls below the 10th percentile for gestational age. There are many causes for IUGR, including teratogen exposure such as congenital viral or bacterial infections, fetal chromosomal anomalies (e.g., Down syndrome), maternal factors (such as **preeclampsia**, a condition affecting about 5% of pregnancies, characterized by high blood pressure and protein in the urine), and placental factors (such as **placenta previa**, or "low-lying" placenta—a condition in which the blastocyst implants near the uterine cervix and the placenta covers part of the opening of the cervix). Unlike many other birth defects covered throughout the book, IUGR is a birth defect that involves the entire fetus, rather than just one organ or organ system.

MATERNAL DIABETES AND OBESITY

Both maternal diabetes and maternal obesity during pregnancy constitute risk factors for birth defects of the fetus. Thus, the health of the mother and the resulting maternal environment impact development of the fetus (Fig. 6-7). Approximately 1 in 200 women of childbearing age have diabetes before pregnancy (preexisting diabetes), and another 2% to 5% develop diabetes during pregnancy (gestational diabetes). Women with preexisting diabetes are three to four times more likely than non-diabetic women to have a child with a major birth defect. Such defects are widespread and include neural tube defects and heart defects. Women with gestational diabetes usually do not have an increased frequency of children with birth defects. However, if diabetes in either group is poorly managed during pregnancy, the risk of delivering a very large baby (greater than 10 pounds) is increased. Such babies may have increased risk for obesity and diabetes in later life. Maternal obesity (defined in the United States as a body mass index greater than 30 kg/meter squared) is also a risk factor for birth defects. Fetuses born to obese women are 2 to 3.5 times more likely than those born to average-weight women to have neural tube defects (covered in Chapter 4), heart defects, and omphalocele (covered in Chapters 4 and 14).

PLACENTA PRODUCES SEVERAL IMPORTANT HORMONES

The placenta is an extremely prolific producer of hormones. Two of its major products are the steroid hormones **progesterone** and **estrogen**, which are responsible for maintaining the pregnant state and preventing spontaneous abortion or preterm labor. As covered in Chapter 1, the corpus luteum produces progesterone and estrogen during the first weeks of pregnancy. However, by the eleventh week, the corpus luteum degenerates and the placenta assumes its role.

During the first two months of pregnancy, the syncytiotrophoblast of the placenta produces the glycoprotein hormone **human chorionic gonadotropin (hCG)**, which supports the secretory activity of the corpus luteum. Because this hormone is produced only by fetal tissue and is excreted in the mother's urine, it is used as the basis for pregnancy tests. However, it is also produced abundantly by hydatidiform moles (see the "In the Clinic" of Chapter 2 entitled "Hydatidiform Moles"), and persistence of the hormone beyond two months of gestation may indicate a molar pregnancy.

The placenta produces an extremely wide range of other protein hormones, including, to name a few, human placental lactogen (hPL), human chorionic thyrotropin, human chorionic corticotropin, insulin-like growth factors, prolactin, relaxin, corticotropin-releasing hormone, and endothelin. It is interesting to note that hPL converts the mother from being principally a carbohydrate user to being a fatty acid user, thus sparing carbohydrates for the conceptus.

In addition to protein hormones, placental membranes synthesize **prostaglandins**, a family of compounds derived from fatty acids, which perform a range of functions in various tissues of the body. Placental prostaglandins seem to be intimately involved in maintenance of pregnancy and onset of labor. The signal that initiates

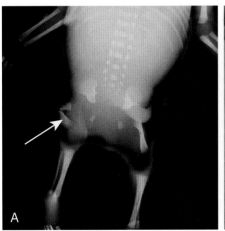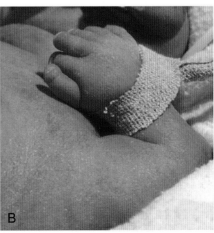

Figure 6-7. Birth defects in infants born to diabetic mothers exhibiting diabetic embryopathy. *A,* X-ray showing abnormal lower limbs in a stillborn fetus. Note the disrupted pelvis and the small and bent (arrow) femurs. *B,* Photo showing preaxial polydactyly (six digits) in the hand of an infant.

labor seems to be a reduction in the ratio of progesterone to estrogen, but the effect of this signal may be mediated by an elevation in the levels of prostaglandins produced by the placenta.

PRODUCTION AND RESORPTION OF AMNIOTIC FLUID

As described in Chapter 4 and in this chapter, embryonic folding transforms the amnion from a small bubble on the dorsal side of the embryonic disc to a sac that completely encloses the embryo. By the eighth week, the expanding amniotic sac completely fills the original chorionic cavity and fuses with the chorion. Expansion of the amnion is due mainly to an increase in the amount of **amniotic fluid**. The volume of amniotic fluid increases through the seventh month and then decreases somewhat in the last two months. At birth, the volume of amniotic fluid is typically about 1 L.

Amniotic fluid, which is very similar to blood plasma in composition, is initially produced by transport of fluid across the amniotic membrane itself. After about sixteen weeks, fetal urine also makes an important contribution to the amniotic fluid. If the fetus does not excrete urine—because of bilateral **renal agenesis** (absence of both kidneys; covered in Chapter 15) or because the lower urinary tract is obstructed (**posterior urethral valves**; covered in the "Clinical Taster" in this chapter and in Chapter 15)—the volume of amniotic fluid will be too low (a condition called **oligohydramnios**), and the amniotic cavity in consequence will be too small. A small amniotic cavity can cramp the growth of the fetus (resulting in deformations; covered in Chapter 5) and cause various congenital malformations, notably pulmonary hypoplasia (covered in the "Clinical Taster" in this chapter and in Chapter 11).

Because amniotic fluid is produced constantly, it must also be resorbed constantly. This is accomplished mainly by the fetal gut, which absorbs the fluid swallowed by the fetus. Excess fluid is then returned to the maternal circulation via the placenta. Malformations that make it impossible for the fetus to swallow fluid, for example, anencephaly or esophageal atresia (covered in Chapters 4 and 14, respectively), result in an overabundance of amniotic fluid—a condition called **hydramnios** or **polyhydramnios**.

TWINNING

Twinning occurs naturally (i.e., excluding assisted reproductive techniques [ART], in which, as described in Chapter 1, multiple blastocysts routinely are introduced into the uterus) in about 3% of births. Twins that form by the splitting of a single original embryo are called **monozygotic**, or **identical**, twins; this type of twinning occurs infrequently (i.e., about 0.4% naturally). These twins share an identical genetic makeup. Therefore, they look alike as they grow up. In contrast, **dizygotic** (i.e., **fraternal**) twins arise from separate oocytes produced during the same menstrual cycle. This type of twinning is by far more frequent (averages about 1.2% but increases with maternal age from 0.3% at age twenty to 1.4% at ages thirty-five to forty; it seems to have a genetic basis). Dizygotic twin embryos implant separately and develop separate fetal membranes (amnion, chorion, and placenta). In contrast, monozygotic twins may share none, some, or all of their fetal membranes, depending on how late in development the original embryo splits to form twins.

If the splitting occurs during cleavage—for example, if the two blastomeres produced by the first cleavage division become separated—the monozygotic twin blastomeres will implant separately, like dizygotic twin blastomeres, and will not share fetal membranes (Fig. 6-8). Alternatively, if the twins are formed by splitting of the inner cell mass within the blastocyst, they will occupy the same chorion, but they will be enclosed by separate amnions and will use separate placentas, with each placenta developing around the connecting stalk of its respective embryo. Finally, if the twins are formed by splitting of a bilaminar embryonic disc, they will occupy the same amnion. In rare cases, such twins may not fully separate, resulting in the birth of **conjoined twins** (Fig. 6-9).

Because fetal membranes fuse when they are forced together by growth of the fetus, it may not be immediately obvious whether the membranous septum separating a pair of twins represents just amniotic membranes (meaning that the twins share a single chorion; see Fig. 6-8, center image: separate amnions; common chorion and placenta) or fused amnions and chorions (meaning that the twins originally did not share fetal membranes; see Fig. 6-8, left image: separate amnions, chorions, and placentas). The clue is the thickness and opacity of the septum: amniotic membranes are thin and almost transparent, whereas chorionic membranes are thicker and somewhat opaque.

In twin pregnancies, anastomoses can form between vessels supplying the two placentas. This shared circulation usually poses no problem, but if one twin dies late in gestation or if the blood pressure of one twin drops significantly, the remaining twin is at risk. If one twin dies, the other twin may be killed by an **embolism** (blocked blood vessel) caused by bits of tissue that break off in the dead twin and enter the shared circulation. If the blood pressure of one twin falls sharply, the other twin may suffer heart failure as its heart attempts to fill both circulatory systems at once.

Two other serious complications can occur when vessels are shared between placentas: **twin-twin transfusion syndrome (TTTS)** and **twin-reversed arterial perfusion (TRAP sequence)**. In TTTS (occurs in 10% to 20% of all monochorionic, diamniotic twins and is responsible for about 15% of all perinatal deaths in twins), vascular anastomoses occur between vessels in the two placentas that result in unbalanced blood flow between the twins. One twin, the so-called donor twin, exhibits oligohydramnios and growth restriction, whereas the other, the so-called recipient twin, exhibits polyhydramnios and cardiac enlargement and eventually cardiac failure. In TRAP sequence (incidence of about 1 in 35,000 births), one twin, the so-called pump twin, provides all of the blood flow to a second acardiac/acephalic twin through placental vascular anastomoses. Because of the additional stress placed on

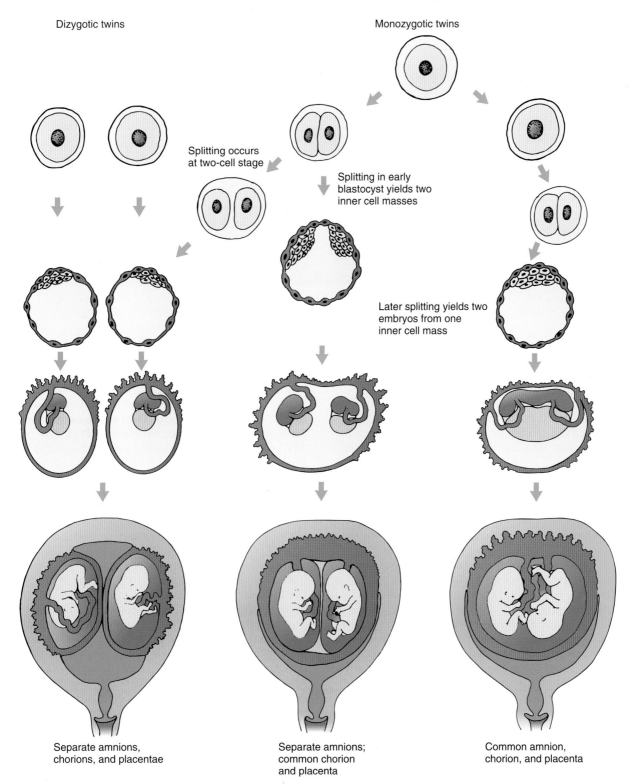

Dizygotic twins

Monozygotic twins

Splitting occurs
at two-cell stage

Splitting in early
blastocyst yields two
inner cell masses

Later splitting yields two
embryos from one
inner cell mass

Separate amnions,
chorions, and placentae

Separate amnions;
common chorion
and placenta

Common amnion,
chorion, and placenta

Figure 6-8. Development of the fetal membrane in various types of twins. The degree to which monozygotic twins share membranes depends on the stage of development at which the originally single embryo separates into two embryos: if splitting occurs at the two-cell stage of cleavage, the twins will develop as separately as dizygotic twins; if splitting yields a blastocyst with two inner cell masses, the embryos will share a single chorion and placenta but occupy separate amnions; if splitting occurs after the formation of the inner cell mass, the embryos will occupy a single amnion.

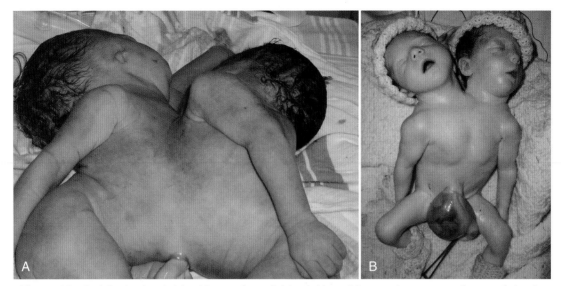

Figure 6-9. Conjoined twins. *A,* Joined front to front. *B,* Joined side to side; note the presence of an omphalocele.

the pump twin's heart, cardiac failure and the pump twin's subsequent demise occur in 50% to 75% of cases (the acardiac twin cannot survive without the pump twin, and it dies with death of the pump twin or at birth).

In the past, the only treatment for these situations was to wait until the healthy twin was old enough to have a chance of surviving outside the womb and then to perform a cesarean section. However, laser surgical techniques (see later) have been developed that may provide effective in utero treatment of these serious conditions.

PRENATAL DIAGNOSIS ASSESSES HEALTH OF UNBORN

The study and treatment of the fetus constitute the field of **prenatal pediatrics** or **fetology**. Four diagnostic techniques have revolutionized the diagnosis of fetal malformations and genetic diseases and have led to new treatments. These are **maternal serum screening, ultrasonography, amniocentesis**, and **chorionic villus sampling**. As covered earlier in the chapter, detection of **fetal DNA** in maternal plasma will further revolutionize diagnosis and treatment.

MATERNAL SERUM SCREENING

Current **maternal serum screenings** are of two types: the *triple* screen and the *quadruple* screen. These screens are sometimes referred to as the MSAFP+ screen, as they measure maternal serum **alpha-fetoprotein** plus other serum components. In the triple screen, in addition to serum levels of alpha-fetoprotein (AFP)—a protein produced by the fetal liver whose level steadily increases during pregnancy—two other serum components are measured: **human chorionic gonadotropin (hCG)**, produced by the placenta, with levels peaking at about fourteen weeks of gestation and dropping thereafter; and **estriol (uE3)**, also produced by the placenta. In the quadruple screen, **inhibin-A** is measured in addition to the other three serum components. Inhibin-A is produced by the fetus and the placenta. These screens most often are done in combination with ultrasonographic examination of the fetus (Figs. 6-10, 6-11, 6-12).

The levels of these serum components can suggest the presence of a fetus with **Down syndrome** or with a birth defect such as a **neural tube defect**. For example, AFP levels are high (when compared with normal levels at the same week of gestation) when the mother is carrying a fetus with a neural tube defect. When carrying a fetus with Down syndrome, maternal serum hCG and inhibin-A levels are elevated, and uE3 levels are low.

The maternal serum screen is not a "test" that diagnoses a birth defect; it indicates only the possibility of some types of birth defects. If abnormal results are obtained, the maternal serum screen is followed by other diagnostic procedures, including some of those described in the following paragraphs. It is important to point out to parents that the maternal serum screen has a high false-positive rate. Thus, a risk of this screen is that it can lead to unnecessary worrying by the parents. It has been estimated that the quadruple screen detects more than 80% of fetuses with Down syndrome. However, high levels of serum AFP, when assessed at sixteen to eighteen weeks of gestation—a time when the test is most accurate for predicting the presence of a fetus with a neural tube defect—are correlated with the presence of a fetus with a neural tube defect in only 1 in 16 to 1 in 33 cases. Thus, without further testing, such as ultrasonography, parents might decide unknowingly to abort a normal fetus.

ULTRASONOGRAPHY

In **ultrasonography**, the inside of the body is scanned with a beam of ultrasound (sound with a frequency of 3 to 10 MHz), and a computer is used to analyze the pattern of returning echoes. Because tissues of different density reflect sound differently, revealing tissue interfaces, the pattern of echoes can be used to decipher the inner structure of the body. The quality of the images yielded

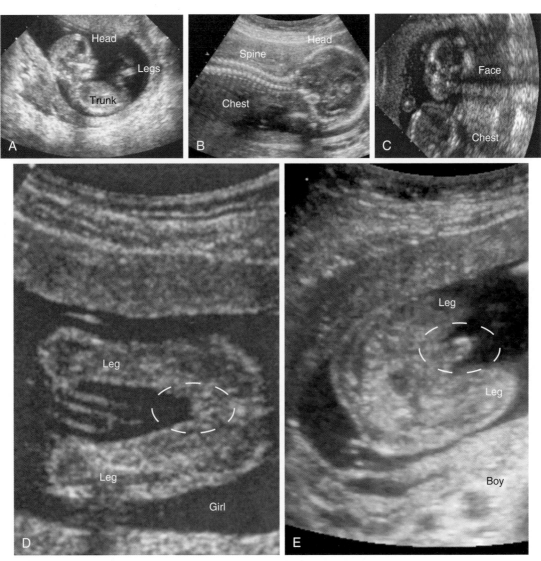

Figure 6-10. Sonograms. *A*, Lateral view of a fetus at twelve weeks of gestation. *B, C*, Views of another fetus at twenty weeks of gestation. *D, E*, Two fetuses at eighteen weeks of gestation, showing how ultrasonography reveals the sex of the fetus.

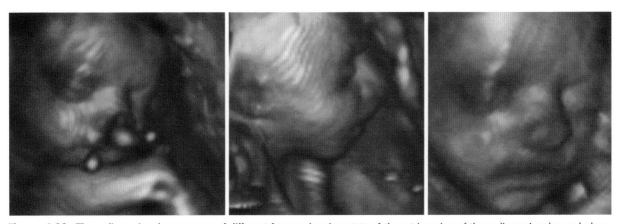

Figure 6-11. Three-dimensional sonograms of different fetuses showing state-of-the-art imaging of three-dimensional morphology.

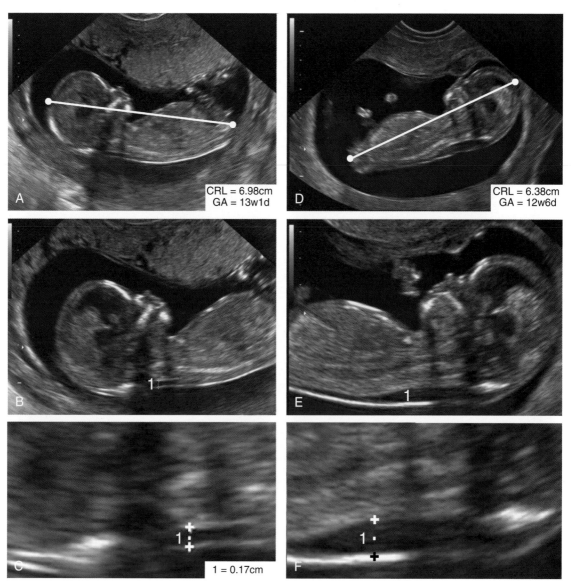

Figure 6-12. Sonograms of two fetuses showing the area measured during nuchal translucency screening. *A-C,* Overview and enlargements of a fetus with a nuchal translucency measurement (area measured indicated in *B* and *C* by the number 1) in the normal range (0.17 cm); the points of the electronic caliper are indicated by plus signs in *C. D-F,* Overview and enlargements of a fetus with a nuchal translucency measurement (more than double that shown in *C*) consistent with Down syndrome. Lines in *A* and *D* indicate the area measured to determine crown-rump length (CRL). GA, gestational age.

by ultrasonography has rapidly improved; it is now possible to visualize the structure of the developing fetus and to determine its sex (see Fig. 6-10), as well as to identify many malformations (e.g., see Fig. 6-12). Ultrasonography also is used now to guide the needles or catheters used for amniocentesis and chorionic villus sampling (amniocentesis and chorionic villus sampling are covered later in the chapter). These procedures were formerly performed unguided, with a higher consequent risk of piercing the fetus. It is important to note that ultrasound is used routinely in virtually all pregnancies in developed countries, and no evidence indicates that it is harmful to the fetus.

Various types of "display modes," or ways of analyzing and displaying ultrasound data, are used, each associated with particular advantages. **B-mode** ultrasonography

shows an image (**sonogram**) of the anatomy of a two-dimensional plane of scanning and can be performed in real time (see Fig. 6-10). Recently, it has become possible to use this type of ultrasonography with advanced equipment to obtain three-dimensional sonograms (see Fig. 6-11) and "four-dimensional" sonograms (i.e., movies of sequential images that show movement). **M-mode** ultrasonography shows changes over time in the position of a structure such as a heart valve. **Doppler ultrasonography** yields flow information and can be used to study the pattern of flow within the heart and developing blood vessels. The miniaturization of ultrasound electronics has led to the development of **endosonography**, in which a miniature ultrasound probe is inserted into a body orifice such as the vagina and is thus brought close to the structure of interest, permitting a higher-resolution image.

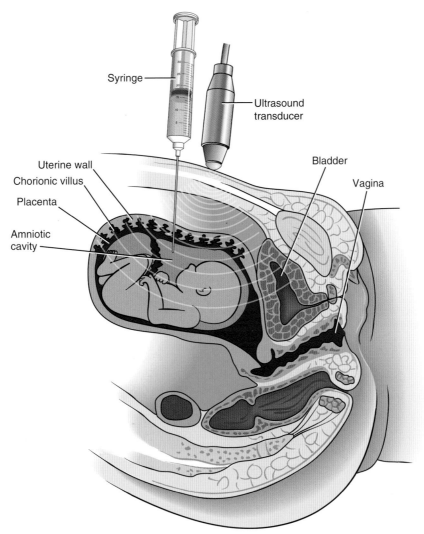

Figure 6-13. Schematic illustration of amniocentesis.

Real-time B-mode ultrasonography is the type most often used to examine the fetus (see Fig. 6-10). A wide variety of fetal anomalies can be seen and diagnosed by this technique, including craniofacial defects, limb anomalies, diaphragmatic hernias, caudal dysgenesis syndromes, teratomas, spina bifida, and renal agenesis. Abnormalities of the fetal heart and heartbeat can be analyzed using **fetal echocardiography**—more detailed ultrasonography of the heart performed by a pediatric cardiologist. Ultrasonography can also be used to measure the thickness of the clear area at the back of the neck (i.e., **nuchal region**) in a procedure known as **nuchal translucency screening** (see Fig. 6-12). Fetuses with **Down syndrome**, other chromosomal anomalies, and major heart anomalies accumulate fluid in the back of the neck during the first trimester. Thus, the thickness of the clear area provides an indication of the likelihood that such a congenital anomaly is present.

AMNIOCENTESIS

In **amniocentesis**, amniotic fluid is aspirated from the amniotic cavity (usually between fourteen and sixteen weeks of gestation) through a needle inserted via the abdominal wall (Fig. 6-13) and is examined for various clues to fetal disease. Amniotic fluid contains metabolic byproducts of the fetus, as well as cells (**amniocytes**) sloughed from the fetus (possibly the lungs) and amniotic membrane; the latter are sometimes called **amniotic stem cells** because they can give rise to multiple tissues when collected from the amniotic fluid and placed in vitro. As covered earlier, **AFP** is a useful indicator that can be assessed with amniocentesis. Elevated levels of this protein may indicate the presence of an open **neural tube defect**, such as anencephaly, or another open defect, such as **gastroschisis**. Fetal cells in the amniotic fluid can be cultured and karyotyped to determine the sex of the fetus and to detect chromosomal anomalies. Other molecular-genetic techniques can be used to screen the genome for the presence or absence of specific mutations that cause heritable disease (covered in Chapter 1). Amniocentesis has limitations early in gestation, both because it is difficult to perform when the volume of amniotic fluid is small and because a small sample may not yield enough cells for analysis. Later in pregnancy, amniocentesis

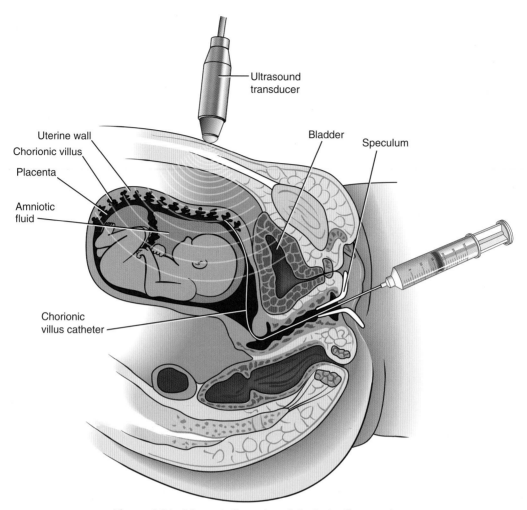

Figure 6-14. Schematic illustration of chorionic villus sampling.

is used to assess Rh sensitization and to test for fetal infection.

CHORIONIC VILLUS SAMPLING

In chorionic villus sampling (CVS), a small sample of tissue (10 to 40 mg) is removed from the chorion by a catheter inserted through the cervix or by a needle inserted through the abdominal wall (Fig. 6-14) under ultrasound guidance. This tissue may be directly karyotyped or karyotyped after culture. Chorionic villus sampling can be performed early in gestation (ten to twelve weeks) and yields enough tissue for many kinds of molecular-genetic analyses. Because placental tissue is examined directly, amniotic AFP cannot be measured by using CVS. The technique is also complicated by the fact that in 1% to 2% of cases, the results of CVS are ambiguous because of **chromosomal mosaicism** (mosaicism is covered in the "In the Clinic" of Chapter 1 entitled "Many Chromosomal Anomalies Arise During Gametogenesis and Cleavage"). This can occur with a mosaic fetus or in cases where the placental chromosome complement differs from that of the fetus—a phenomenon called **confined placental mosaicism**. Ambiguous CVS results must be further assessed by amniocentesis.

TREATING FETUS IN UTERO

If amniocentesis or chorionic villus sampling reveals that a fetus has a significant genetic anomaly, should the fetus be aborted? If ultrasonography shows a malformation serious enough to kill or deform the fetus, should corrective fetal surgery be attempted? What if fetal surgery might result in a cosmetic improvement, for example, better repair of a cleft lip with little or no scarring? The answers to these questions involve many factors, including (1) the risk to the mother of continuing the pregnancy, (2) the availability of surgeons and resources for fetal surgery, (3) the risk of the operation to the fetus and the mother, (4) the severity of the anomaly or disease, (5) the advantage of correcting the defect in utero instead of after birth, and (6) the ethical, moral, and religious beliefs of the families involved. Thus, there are no easy answers to these complex questions, and acquiring answers will require input from both the individuals involved and society as a whole.

Over the past twenty years, several approaches have been attempted to treat the fetus in utero, potentially lessening the impact of birth defects diagnosed prenatally. These treatments are of two broad types: **surgical intervention** and **drug intervention**.

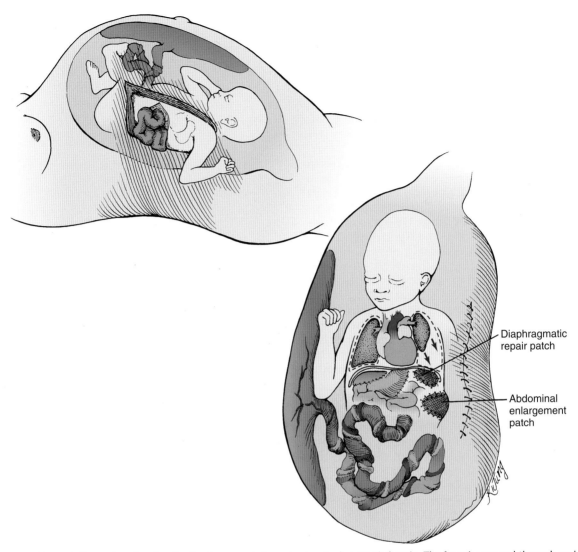

Figure 6-15. Schematic illustration showing the in utero surgical repair of a diaphragmatic hernia. The fetus is exposed through an incision in the abdominal and uterine walls (brown, v-shaped area). The fetal viscera are retracted from the left pleural cavity, and the hole in the diaphragm is repaired with a Gore-Tex patch. The left lung now has room to grow normally. Because the fetal abdominal cavity is too small for the restored viscera, a second Gore-Tex enlargement patch is placed in the fetal abdominal wall.

Surgical intervention has been used to treat **congenital diaphragmatic hernia, spina bifida (myelomeningocele), hydrocephalus** (enlargement of the brain ventricles due to blockage of the flow of cerebrospinal fluid; corrected with shunts inserted in utero or usually postnatally), **thoracic cysts** (e.g., **congenital cystic adenomatoid malformation**—a multicystic mass of pulmonary tissue that causes lung compression and resulting hypoplasia), **sacrococcygeal teratomas** (enormous tumors that require such a large blood flow that fetal heart failure can occur), vascular issues threatening fetal life in **twin** pregnancies (e.g., **TTTS, TRAP sequence**), **urinary tract obstructions** (e.g., **posterior urethral valves**), and **hypoplastic left heart syndrome** (underdeveloped left ventricle and aortic valve). These surgical procedures have had variable success, as summarized below.

Congenital diaphragmatic hernias that would result in pulmonary hypoplasia have been corrected by opening the uterus, restoring the herniated viscera to the abdominal cavity, and repairing the fetal diaphragm (Fig. 6-15). However, based on clinical trials involving multiple cases and surgical centers, no survival benefit of fetal surgery over postnatal surgery has been found, so postnatal repair remains the accepted treatment.

Prenatal surgery for the most serious form of **spina bifida, myelomeningocele** (covered in Chapter 4), has been evaluated in a clinical trial. According to this study, prenatal surgery improved leg function when assessed at 2½ years of age, as compared with children operated on postnatally. About 40% of the children having prenatal surgery could walk without crutches, but only about half that percentage having postnatal surgery could do so. Moreover, typically almost 90% of children born with this type of spina bifida develop **hydrocephalus**, which requires shunting (covered in Chapter 4). The incidence of hydrocephalus in prenatally operated children dropped to about half that in postnatally operated children. Finally, **Chiari malformations** (covered in

Chapter 4), which were present in all newborns in the study, resolved by one year in about one third of children receiving prenatal surgery but did not resolve by this age in any of the children receiving postnatal surgery. Thus, the clinical trial points to major benefits of prenatal surgery for myelomeningocele and subsequent complications. However, unfortunately, about half of fetuses receiving prenatal surgery were born quite prematurely, and other risks to both mothers and babies were increased by this approach.

Prenatal surgery to alleviate **twin-twin transfusion syndrome** (**TTTS**; covered earlier in this chapter) is now one of the most common types of prenatal surgeries, accounting for up to 50% of all fetal procedures done at some medical centers. Owing to increased use of fertility drugs for IVF and similar procedures (covered in Chapter 1), the incidence of twinning, and consequently of TTTS, is increasing. With a fetoscope equipped with a laser, endoscopic surgery is performed to map and ablate vessels on the fetal side of the placenta that connect the twins. This procedure is not without considerable risk, as one or both twins may die following surgery. However, with endoscopic surgery, the incidence of preterm birth is much lower than with the conventional abdominal surgery used for other types of prenatal surgery.

Posterior urethral valves (constriction of the lower urinary tract that prevents urine produced by the kidneys from escaping) result in oligohydramnios and consequent fetal malformations, including pulmonary hypoplasia and defects of the face and limbs (covered in "Clinical Taster" this chapter and in Chapter 15). The condition also damages the developing kidneys because of the backpressure of urine in the kidney tubules. Repair of the obstruction may prevent these problems and is now done more frequently.

Hypoplastic left heart syndrome is a serious birth defect, covered in Chapter 12, in which the left ventricle is severely underdeveloped and the aortic outflow tract is blocked. A balloon catheter is inserted into the aortic outflow tract, at twenty-two to twenty-four weeks of gestation. Inflation of the balloon opens the aortic value and tract, and allows the left ventricle to pump blood, increasing its size over time. A clinical trial has not yet been conducted to determine the efficacy of this procedure.

In addition to the prenatal surgical interventions just covered, drug intervention is used prenatally. Drug intervention has been used to prevent **neural tube defects** and to treat **congenital adrenal** (suprarenal) **hyperplasia**, **methylmalonic acidemia**, and **multiple carboxylase deficiency**. Drugs can also help prevent **congenital heart block** (a problem in the conduction system of the fetal heart that can result in a slow heart rate and, eventually, heart failure). As covered in Chapter 4, **prenatal folic acid supplementation** has been shown to prevent as many as two thirds of expected cases of neural tube defects. Like folic acid supplementation, treatment of fetal disease involves treating the mother with substances that cross the placenta. In fetal congenital adrenal (suprarenal) hyperplasia (CAH), the mother is treated during her

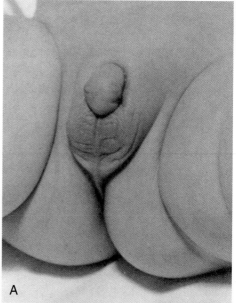

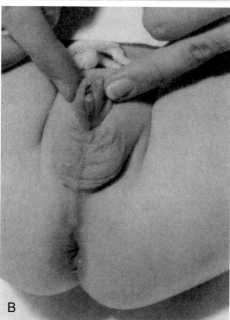

Figure 6-16. External genitalia in a newborn XX individual with congenital adrenal (suprarenal) hyperplasia. *A,* The clitoris is enlarged and the labia are partially fused as a scrotum-like structure. *B,* The urethral meatus is visible at the base of the enlarged clitoris.

pregnancy with the potent corticosteroid **dexamethasone**. CAH is caused by a deficiency in the enzyme 21-hydroxylase, which results in a reduction in cortisol production by the suprarenal cortex and accumulation of 17-hydroxyprogesterone. This in turn results in suprarenal hyperplasia and excess production of suprarenal androgens (these are negatively regulated by the presence of cortisol). In female fetuses with CAH, external genitalia are masculinized (e.g., enlargement of the clitoris and fusion of the labia; Fig. 6-16; also covered in Chapter 15). Female CAH fetuses are born with normal genitalia following appropriate maternal treatment with dexamethasone.

Dexamethasone is also being used to treat congenital heart block, especially in mothers with **lupus**. Lupus is a chronic inflammation caused by an autoimmune disease. Maternal antibodies present in lupus can affect the fetal cardiac conduction system, resulting in heart block (as covered in this chapter, maternal antibodies can cross the placental). In addition, these antibodies can cause neonatal lupus. To treat **heart arrhythmias** in fetuses, drugs such as **digoxin** and **propranolol**, both of which cross the placenta, are given to the mother.

Like CAH, methylmalonic acidemia and multiple carboxylase deficiency involve deficiencies in fetal enzymes. In some types of methylmalonic acidemia, there is a deficiency of **vitamin B$_{12}$**, a coenzyme required for the conversion of methylmalonyl coenzyme A to succinyl coenzyme A. This deficiency results in increased methylmalonic acid excretion in maternal urine. Treatment involves maternal intravenous administration of **cyanocobalamin**, which markedly raises maternal serum B$_{12}$ levels and presumably increases the amount of B$_{12}$ available to the fetus. In multiple carboxylase deficiency, there is a deficiency of the enzyme **biotinidase**. Unless treated, multiple carboxylase deficiency results in neonatal death from acidosis. Treatment involves maternal administration of the vitamin **biotin**, which readily crosses the placenta.

FETAL CORD BLOOD AND STEM CELLS

It may be feasible to apply the technique of gene therapy to correct some of the human genetic blood diseases in utero by using a procedure called **fetal liver transplant**. In preliminary trials, this procedure was used to treat fetuses diagnosed with diseases that severely cripple the white blood cells of the immune system (such as the disease suffered by the "boy in the bubble") or with **thalassemia** (a blood disease caused by a genetic error that prevents the synthesis of a protein involved in the production of hemoglobin). In these cases, cells from the fetal liver (i.e., the first major hematopoietic organ, as covered in Chapter 13) were obtained from normal aborted fetuses and were infused via an ultrasound-guided needle into the umbilical vein of the affected fetus. These cells successfully colonized the liver of the developing fetus and proceeded to manufacture the missing protein, thereby alleviating the disease. It is possible to transplant cells from one fetus to another because the immature fetal immune system does not reject foreign tissue. It is also possible to use umbilical cord blood for transplants such as these because this is an excellent source of hematopoietic stem cells.

For some disorders, it may be advantageous to use gene therapy to correct an infant's own cells. For example, the infant's own umbilical cord may provide cells that can be appropriately transfected with genes, grown up, and reintroduced without rejection. The collection and storage of fetal cells from umbilical cords is called **cord blood banking**. Advantages of the use of cord blood (compared with bone marrow or fetal liver) include (1) lack of discomfort during collection, (2) high recovery of viable **stem cells**, (3) rapid expansion of stem cells in culture, (4) high rate of recovery of viable stem cells after **cryopreservation**, (5) reduced graft versus host disease, and (6) efficiency of transfection with "corrected" genes. Umbilical cord blood has already been used in many human patients to treat diseases potentially curable with bone marrow transplants, including **severe combined immunodeficiency**.

The availability of cord blood banking has added another decision to the parenting process: Should we decide to bank cord blood in the event that my child needs it later—for example, to provide stem cells if he/she develops leukemia? And if so, should it be banked in a private or public repository? The former can be costly but guarantees that an exact genetic match will be available if the child ever needs the cells. The latter can be free and provides access to the cells to anyone who needs them if they are a genetic match. However, these cells will unlikely be available to the donor years later, so having an exact genetic match available is unlikely. Both cord blood–banking companies and the Academy of Pediatrics provide further information on the subject for parents' consideration (using a web search engine such as Google, search "cord blood banking").

PRETERM BIRTH

The greatest cause of infant mortality worldwide is preterm (also called premature) birth, with an incidence as high as 1:10. Premature babies are babies born before 37 weeks of gestation. Unfortunately, they have higher rates of perinatal death than do term babies, and they are more likely to develop lifelong disabilities, such as blindness, deafness, and cerebral palsy. Infections, such as HIV, play a role in prematurity in developing countries, yet some developed countries, such as the United States, have one of the highest rates (about 12% in the United States). Four factors seem to account for the latter: increasing numbers of mothers with obesity and diabetes, a trend toward delaying childbirth to later ages, increased use of fertility drugs, which often result in twin (or more) pregnancies, and increasing use of cesarean sections (often planned before the full-term date for convenience or for medical reasons).

Preterm births often result in babies with low birth weight. Low birth weight babies are defined as weighing less than 2500 g, and, if at term, they are considered small for gestational age (covered earlier in the chapter). Lower birth weight babies are classified as having very low birth weight (less than 1500 g) or extremely low birth weight (less than 1000 g). By two years of age, 15% to 20% of babies weighing 1000 g at birth will develop cerebral palsy, about 5% will have seizures, and 10% to 25% will have cognitive impairment. Moreover, about 3% to 5% of these babies will become blind and/or deaf. Clearly, despite major advances in neonatal intensive care over the past few decades, prematurity remains a major health issue.

Embryology in Practice

TWO PUZZLES TO SOLVE

Consider the following two scenarios.

Two brothers are separated in their teen years, when their parents become divorced. The older brother chooses to live with his father and the younger brother with his mother. The father is a U.S. army doctor and is transferred to several different bases overseas during his career. The mother is a lawyer and practices in Los Angeles, where she and her son continue to live. The two brothers never see each other again, although as adults they correspond regularly by email. The younger brother gets married to his long-term girlfriend. Five years later, the older brother dies in a car accident in Germany. Three years after that, the younger brother and his wife have a baby. The birth announcement lists both brothers as the baby's father and uncle.

Two sisters, ages four and eleven, are placed in separate foster homes after their parents are killed during a home robbery.

Eventually, both are adopted and grow up in different cities in France. At age twenty-nine, the older sister gets married. For several years, she and her husband try to conceive a baby without success, but just before her fortieth birthday, a home pregnancy test shows that she is pregnant. Nine months later, she delivers a healthy baby girl. She is overjoyed, as is her sister. Both are proud to be the baby's mother and aunt. In other words, the baby is the biologic daughter of one of the sisters and the biological niece of the other, but by relation, she is also the daughter of one sister and the niece of the other.

How are these scenarios possible? The short answer is ART, as covered in Chapter 1. The long answer is that in the first scenario, sperm were donated by the older brother before his death, and in the second, eggs were donated by the younger sister. ART certainly can challenge traditional family relationships, with the challenges beginning before conception and continuing during pregnancy and especially postnatally.

SUGGESTED READINGS

Collins SL, Impey L. 2012. Prenatal diagnosis: types and techniques. Early Hum Dev 88:3–8.

Haque FN, Gottesman II, Wong AH. 2009. Not really identical: epigenetic differences in monozygotic twins and implications for twin studies in psychiatry. Am J Med Genet C Semin Med Genet 151:136–141.

Lakhoo K. 2012. Fetal counselling for surgical conditions. Early Hum Dev 88:9–13.

Luu TM, Vohr B. 2009. Twinning on the brain: the effect on neurodevelopmental outcomes. Am J Med Genet C Semin Med Genet. 151:142–147.

Marion R. 2009. Genetic drift. Two miracles, one year later. Am J Med Genet C Semin Med Genet 151:167–172.

Rasmussen SA, Hayes EB, Jamieson DJ, O'Leary DR. 2007. Emerging infections and pregnancy: assessing the impact on the embryo or fetus. Am J Med Genet A 143:2896–2903.

Sudhakaran N, Sothinathan U, Patel S. 2012. Best practice guidelines: fetal surgery. Early Hum Dev 88:15–19.

Chapter 7

Development of the Skin and Its Derivatives

SUMMARY

The skin, or integument, consists of two layers: the **epidermis** and the **dermis**. The epidermis is formed mainly by the embryonic surface ectoderm, although it is also colonized by **melanocytes** (pigment cells), which are derived from neural crest cells, and by **Langerhans cells**, which are immune cells of bone marrow origin. The dermis of the trunk is a mesodermal tissue. The ventral dermis is derived mainly from the somatic layer of the lateral plate mesoderm, whereas the dorsal dermis is derived from the dermamyotome subdivision of the somites (covered in Chapter 8). The dermis of the face is formed from neural crest cells (covered in Chapters 4 and 17).

After neurulation, the surface ectoderm, originally consisting of a single layer of cells, forms an outer layer of simple squamous epithelium called the **periderm**. The inner layer is now called the **basal layer**. In the eleventh week, the basal layer forms a new **intermediate layer** between itself and the periderm. The basal layer is now called the **stratum germinativum**; this layer will continue to produce the epidermis throughout life. By the twenty-first week, the intermediate layer is replaced by the three definitive layers of the outer epidermis: the inner **stratum spinosum**, the middle **stratum granulosum**, and the outer **stratum corneum**, or **horny layer**. The cells of these layers are called **keratinocytes** because they contain the **keratin** proteins characteristic of the epidermis. The layers of the epidermis represent a maturation series: keratinocytes produced by the stratum germinativum differentiate as they pass outward to form the two intermediate layers and the flattened, dead, keratin-filled mature keratinocytes of the horny layer, which are finally sloughed from the surface of the skin. As the definitive epidermis develops, the overlying periderm is gradually shed into the amniotic fluid. Fetal skin cells shed into the amniotic fluid, called **amniocytes**, can be obtained from the amniotic fluid by amniocentesis and cultured to form **amniotic stem cells**, which have potential therapeutic value (covered in Chapter 6).

The dermis contains most of the tissues and structures of the skin, including its blood vessels, nerves, and muscle bundles, and most of its sensory structures. The superficial layer of the dermis develops projections called **dermal papillae**, which interdigitate with downward projections of the epidermis called **epidermal ridges**.

A number of specialized structures develop within the surface ectoderm, including hairs, a variety of epidermal glands, nails, and teeth (covered in Chapter 17). **Hair follicles** originate as rod-like downgrowths of the stratum germinativum into the dermis. The club-shaped base of each hair follicle is indented by a hillock of dermis called the **dermal papilla**, and the hair shaft is produced by the **germinal matrix** of ectoderm that overlies the dermal papilla. Various types of epidermal glands also arise as diverticula of the epidermis. Some bud from the neck of a hair follicle; others bud directly downward from the stratum germinativum. The four principal types of epidermal glands are the **sebaceous glands**, which secrete the oily sebum that lubricates the skin and hair; the **apocrine sweat glands**, found in the axillae, the pubic region, and other specific areas of skin that secrete odorous substances; the **accrine sweat glands**, which are widely distributed over the surface of the skin, where they function in body cooling; and the **mammary glands**. The primordia of the nails arise at the distal tips of the digits and then migrate around to the dorsal side. The nail plate grows from a specialized stratum germinativum located in the **nail fold** of epidermis that overlaps the proximal end of the nail primordium.

Clinical Taster

You are a pediatrician following a 3½-year-old girl with chronic constipation that started around the beginning of "potty training." You get a message from your answering service that the girl's mother called during the night from the emergency room. Apparently, they rushed the girl to the hospital in the late evening, when they found that she had rectal prolapse (protrusion of the rectum out through the anus) after straining to stool.

You see the girl with her mother later that day for follow-up. The girl was seen in the emergency room by a surgeon, who had reduced the prolapsed rectum without surgery and prescribed an enema and stool softeners. The surgeon had mentioned to the family that their pediatrician would talk to them about conditions like cystic fibrosis that can be associated with rectal prolapse and would arrange to test for such conditions.

While examining the toddler's abdomen for impacted stool, you notice that she has pale, velvety skin and an unusual number of bruises and atrophic scars (widened paper-like scars) on her shins. The mother reminds you that the girl was born one month premature after her "water broke early," and that she was a "floppy" baby who starting walking late. Her mother states that the girl inherited her father's "double-jointedness," and the girl proceeds to demonstrate just how flexible her joints are (Fig. 7-1). You also find her skin to be hyperextensible.

You tell the mother that testing for cystic fibrosis is certainly reasonable, but that you suspect the diagnosis of

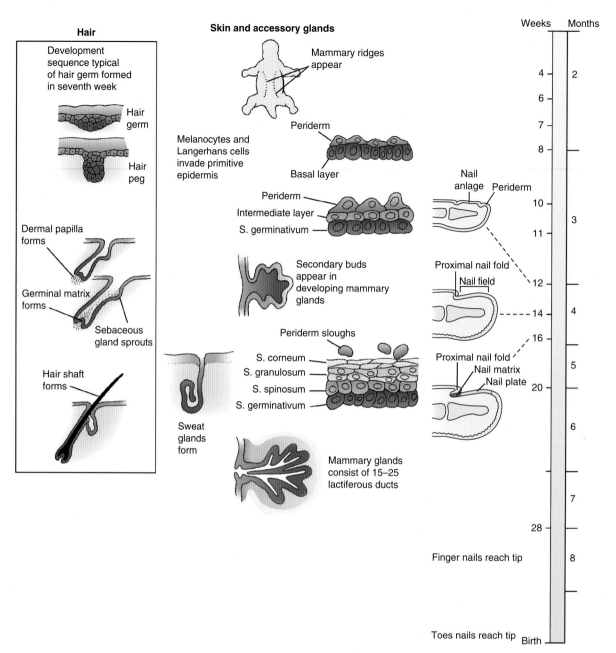

Time line. Development of the skin and its derivatives.

Ehlers-Danlos syndrome (EDS), which is a hereditary connective tissue disorder. EDS is actually a group of disorders caused by mutations in several genes involved in the formation of structural components of skin and joints. Classical EDS is caused by mutations in COLLAGEN TYPE I and V genes. You reassure the mother that her daughter's condition can be managed by restricting certain types of activities and by monitoring for more significant complications like dilation of the aortic root.

ORIGIN OF EPIDERMIS AND DERMIS OF SKIN

SURFACE ECTODERM FORMS EPIDERMIS

The surface ectoderm covering of the embryo consists initially of a single layer of cells. After neurulation in the fourth week, the surface ectoderm produces a new outer layer of simple squamous epithelium called the **periderm** (Fig. 7-2A). The underlying layer of cells is now called the **basal layer** and is separated from the dermis by the basement membrane containing proteins such as collagen, laminin, and fibronectin. The cells of the periderm are gradually sloughed into the amniotic fluid. The periderm is normally shed completely by the twenty-first week, but in some fetuses it persists until birth, forming a "shell" or "cocoon" around the newborn infant that is removed by the physician or shed spontaneously during the first weeks of life. These babies are called **collodion babies**.

In the eleventh week, proliferation of the basal layer produces a new **intermediate layer** just deep to the periderm (Fig. 7-2B). This layer is the forerunner of the outer layers of the mature epidermis. The basal layer, now called the **germinative layer** or the **stratum germinativum**, constitutes the layer of stem cells that will continue to replenish the epidermis throughout life. The cells of the intermediate layer contain the **keratin** proteins characteristic of differentiated epidermis; therefore, these cells are called **keratinocytes**.

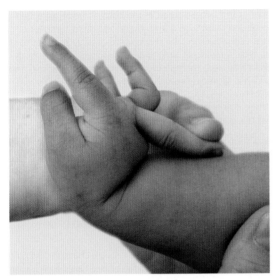

Figure 7-1. Demonstration of painless hyperflexibility of the right third metacarpal-phalangeal joint in a child.

During the early part of the fifth month, at about the time that the periderm is shed, the intermediate layer is replaced by the three definitive layers of the outer epidermis: the inner **stratum spinosum** (or **spinous layer**), the middle **stratum granulosum** (or **granular layer**), and the outer **stratum corneum** (or **horny** or **cornified layer**) (Figs. 7-3, 7-4). This transformation begins at the cranial end of the fetus and proceeds caudally. The layers of the epidermis represent a maturational series: presumptive keratinocytes are constantly produced by the stratum germinativum, they differentiate as they pass outward to the stratum corneum, and, finally, they are sloughed from the surface of the skin.

The cells of the stratum germinativum are the only dividing cells of the normal epidermis. These cells contain a dispersed network of primary keratin (krt) filaments specific to this layer, such as krt5 and krt14, and are connected by cell-to-cell membrane junctions called **desmosomes**. Together with adherens junctions, desmosomes provide a tight, impervious barrier resistant to water uptake or loss and infection. In addition, desmosomes help to distribute force evenly over the epidermis.

As the cells in the stratum germinativum move into the overlying stratum spinosum (4 to 8 cells thick; see Fig. 7-4), the krt5 and krt14 intermediate filaments are replaced by two secondary keratin proteins, krt1 and krt10. These are cross-linked by disulfide bonds to provide further strength. In addition, cells in the stratum spinosum produce the **envelope protein**, involucrin.

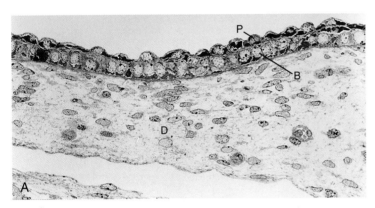

8 weeks

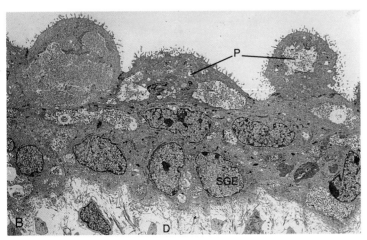

11 weeks

Figure 7-2. Differentiation of the ectoderm into the primitive epidermis. *A,* Light micrograph. Between eight and nine weeks, the surface ectoderm forms a periderm layer (P). The proliferating layer is now called the basal layer (B) and lies adjacent to the dermis (D). *B,* Transmission electron micrograph. By the eleventh week, the basal layer gives rise to an intermediate layer and is renamed as the stratum germinativum (SGE), the layer adjacent to the dermis (D). A complete but irregular outer layer of periderm (P) is still apparent.

As the cells in the stratum spinosum move into the stratum granulosum, they produce other **envelope proteins**, such as loricrin and envoplakin, which, together with the envelope protein involucrin, line the inner surface of the plasma membrane. The enzyme transglutaminase cross-links the envelope proteins. Another protein called filaggrin is produced at this time. Filaggrin aggregates with the keratin filaments to form tight bundles, helping to flatten the cell. Lipid-containing granules (**lamellar granules**) that help seal the skin are also produced. Finally, in the process called **cornification**, lytic enzymes are released within the cell, metabolic activity ceases, and enucleation occurs, resulting in loss of cell contents, including the nucleus. Consequently, the keratinocytes that enter the stratum corneum are flattened, scale-like, and terminally differentiated keratinocytes, or **squames**.

In the Research Lab

STEM CELLS IN INTEGUMENT

The skin is the largest organ of the body. It undergoes self-renewal every four weeks and, therefore, rapid turnover of cells occurs. Consequently, the skin requires a large number of **stem cells**, which, owing to their superficial location in the body, can be easily used therapeutically to regenerate the skin and its derivatives. Moreover, stem cells have the potential to regenerate other organs.

Three clearly defined populations of stem cells are found within the skin (Fig. 7-5).

- Basal stem cells, which give rise to the interfollicular skin (i.e., the skin between the hair follicles)
- The bulge, which gives rise to the hair follicle but can also give rise after severe wounding to the interfollicular epidermis and the sebaceous glands. Therefore, skin grafting is not required after tissue damage (e.g., burns) if hair follicles remain intact
- Cells at the base of the sebaceous gland, which generate the sebocytes

These three populations of stem cells are characterized by the expression of p63 (a transcription factor also called tumor protein p73-like), E-cadherin, and keratins krt5 and krt14. Although differentiation of the three stem cell populations differs in terms of their requirements for hedgehog (Hh) and Wnt signaling, in all cases stem cell differentiation requires activation of notch signaling. This is illustrated for the skin in Figure 7-4, which shows that notch signaling promotes the onset of differentiation by inducing p21 (a cell cycle inhibitor) and krt1/10 expression, while inhibiting expression of stem cell components and regulators such as krt5/14 and p63. Notch signaling also inhibits Wnt and Hh signaling, as well as expression of late differentiation markers (e.g., loricrin). In addition a new population of multipotent cells, known as skin-derived precursor (SKP) cells, has been identified. In vitro derivatives include both epidermal and mesenchymal lineages, such as neuronal cells, glia, adipocytes, smooth muscle cells, and chondrocytes. SKP cells are thought to be derived from neural crest cells (as are adult neural crest stem cells in the gut; see Chapters 4 and 14); their numbers are highest in the fetus and decline postnatally.

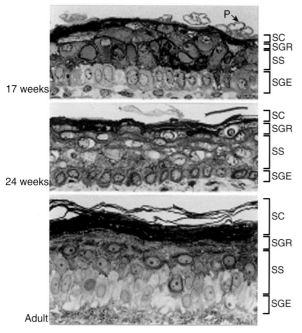

Figure 7-3. Differentiation of the mature epidermis. Light micrographs. The periderm (P) is sloughed during the fourth month and normally is absent by week twenty-one. The definitive epidermal layers, including the stratum germinativum (SGE), stratum spinosum (SS), stratum granulosum (SGR), and stratum corneum (SC), begin to develop during the fifth month and become fully differentiated postnatally.

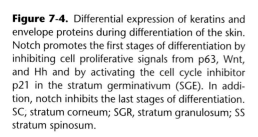

Figure 7-4. Differential expression of keratins and envelope proteins during differentiation of the skin. Notch promotes the first stages of differentiation by inhibiting cell proliferative signals from p63, Wnt, and Hh and by activating the cell cycle inhibitor p21 in the stratum germinativum (SGE). In addition, notch inhibits the last stages of differentiation. SC, stratum corneum; SGR, stratum granulosum; SS stratum spinosum.

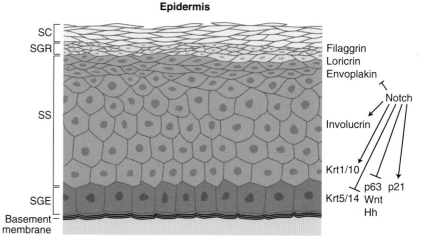

Epidermis

Recent work has focused on the induction of **pluripotent stem cells** from somatic cells. It has been shown that human dermal fibroblasts and keratinocytes can be reprogrammed to be pluripotent (i.e., capable of giving rise to many different cell types) after a combination of factors are added (e.g., Oct4, Sox2, nanog, Lin28), providing additional strategies for regenerative medicine (also see Chapter 5 on IPS cells).

In the Clinic

INHERITED SKIN DISEASES

The structural integrity of the epidermis is critical for its function and is achieved in part by the assembly of cell-type specific keratins and desmosomal proteins into a network that provides tensile strength to the epithelium. Therefore, **skin fragility syndromes** can be caused by mutations in transglutaminases, envelope proteins, desmosomes, keratins, connexins, and proteases, as well as by abnormalities in lipid metabolism. For example, mutations in various **KERATINS** can result in **epidermolysis bullosa simplex** or **epidermolytic hyperkeratosis**. These syndromes manifest as blistering or separation of the epidermis at the tissue plane in which the mutated gene plays a critical role in adhesion (Fig.7-6A, B). Both syndromes are life threatening perinatally because of the risk of infection.

Several heritable disorders result in excessive keratinization of the skin, or **ichthyosis**. For example, infants suffering from **lamellar ichthyosis** have skin that cannot be shed properly and scales off in flakes, sometimes over the whole body. These babies have defects in the mechanisms that bundle keratin fibers and regulate formation of lamellar granules in the cells of the stratum granulosum. As a consequence, keratinocytes do not mature properly and cannot be sloughed from the surface of the stratum corneum. Because of the excess skin, these infants can be born as collodion babies (i.e., encased in a shiny thin film). Infants affected by these disorders have permeability defects and require special care but are usually viable. However, **lamellar ichthyosis type 1**, or **Harlequin, fetuses** have rigid, deeply cracked skin and usually die shortly after birth.

Collagens and other matrix proteins are crucial for the elastic properties of the dermis; mutations in these proteins can result in human syndromes affecting not only the skin but additional tissues such as tendons, ligaments, joints, and connective tissues of the blood vessels and bowels. Abnormal matrix deposition may result in skin hyperextensibility, as in Ehlers-Danlos syndrome (COLLAGEN types I and IV mutations), which also results in joint hypermobility and renders the blood vessels and the bowel susceptible to rupture. Alternatively, abnormal matrix deposition may limit flexibility, as in stiff skin syndrome (FIBRILLIN 1 mutations). This syndrome is also associated with joint contractures.

In the adult, imbalances in proliferation and differentiation can result in skin disorders. For example, excessive levels of the proinflammatory cytokine tumor necrosis factor (TNF)-α can result in **psoriasis** and other hyperproliferative skin diseases. **Gorlin syndrome (nevoid basal cell carcinoma syndrome [NBCCS])** is an autosomal dominant disorder occurring in about 1:50,000 to 1:100,000 individuals. Patients are afflicted with basal cell carcinomas that begin to form early in life. NBCCS patients also have increased susceptibility to other carcinomas. Such as meningiomas, fibromas, and rhabdomyosarcomas. Non-neoplastic disorders of epidermal derivatives also characterize

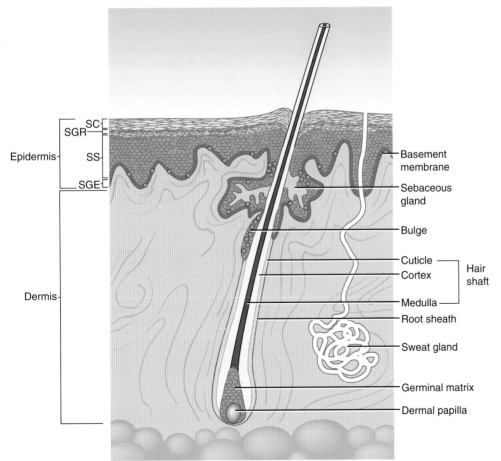

Figure 7-5. Structure of a hair follicle showing the bulge and the layers of the hair shaft. Stem cells in the bulge, stratum germinativum (SGE), and sebaceous gland are shown in green. SC, stratum corneum; SGR, stratum granulosum; SS, stratum spinosum.

Epidermis — SC, SGR, SS, SGE
Dermis

Basement membrane
Sebaceous gland
Bulge
Cuticle
Cortex — Hair shaft
Medulla
Root sheath
Sweat gland
Germinal matrix
Dermal papilla

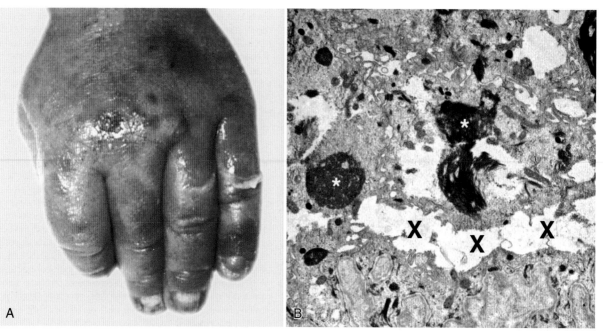

Figure 7-6. Skin fragility syndromes. *A,* Mutation in the PLAKOPHILIN gene, which encodes a desmosomal protein. *B,* Transmission electron micrograph. Mutation in KRT14, resulting in epidermolysis bullosa simplex. Xs, areas of cytolysis within the stratum germinativum; asterisks, clumped keratin fibers.

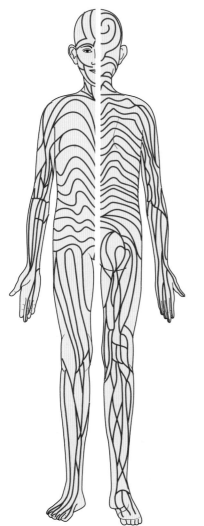

Figure 7-7. Lines of Blaschko. Mosaic skin defects typically follow these lines. Front view to left and back view to right.

NBCCS, including **odontogenic keratocysts** (arising from the dental lamina; covered in Chapter 17) and pathogno-monic **dyskeratotic pitting** of the hands and feet. NBCCS is the result of mutations in PTCH, the receptor that represses hedgehog signaling, or activating mutations in SMOOTHENED, the hedgehog receptor. Hence, the syndrome results from increased hedgehog signaling activity, which increases cell pro-liferation. These tumors have the molecular and morphologic characteristics of undifferentiated hair follicles, reflecting the major role of Shh in hair cell growth and differentiation (see Fig. 7-12). Given the key role of the hedgehog family during embry-ogenesis, developmental defects and postnatal growth defects are also present in this syndrome, including skeletal, facial, and dental anomalies, as well as neural tube closure defects.

Defects in the skin can be **mosaic** within an area. This is demonstrated by skin defects that follow the **lines of Blaschko** (originally described in 1901 by the German dermatologist Alfred Blaschko), which can occur in several human syndromes, such as **hypohidrotic ectodermal dysplasia** (see below) and basal cell carcinomas. These defects occur as "M"- or "V"-shaped patterns on the abdomen and back, as proximally and distally oriented lines along the limbs, and as anteriorly and posteriorly curved lines along the face (Fig. 7-7). These lines/patches of malformed skin reflect a common origin resulting from a defect in the development of a progenitor cell (e.g., after X-inactivation or somatic mutation).

OTHER TYPES OF EPIDERMAL CELLS

In addition to keratinocytes, the epidermis contains a few types of less abundant cells, including melanocytes, Langerhans cells, and Merkel cells. As covered in Chap-ter 4, the pigment cells, or **melanocytes**, of the skin differentiate from neural crest cells that detach from the neural tube in the sixth week and migrate to the develop-ing epidermis. Although morphologic and histochemi-cal studies do not detect melanocytes in the human

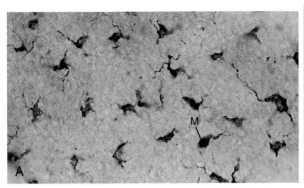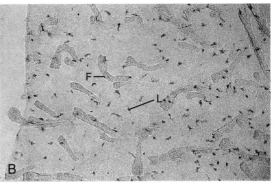

Figure 7-8. Specialized cells of the epidermis. *A,* Melanocytes (M) first appear in the embryonic epidermis during the sixth and seventh weeks. *B,* Langerhans cells (L) migrate into the epidermis from the bone marrow, starting in the seventh week. F, Hair follicle.

epidermis until the tenth to eleventh weeks, studies using monoclonal antibodies directed against antigens characteristic of melanocyte precursors have identified these cells in the epidermis as early as the sixth to seventh weeks (Fig. 7-8*A*). Thus, it may take neural crest cells only a few days to one or two weeks to migrate to the epidermis. Melanocytes are also found in the dermis during fetal life, but a vast majority of these are probably in transit to the epidermis.

Melanocytes represent between 5% and 10% of the cells of the epidermis in the adult. In the tenth week, many melanocytes become associated with developing hair follicles (covered later in the chapter), where they function to donate pigment to the hairs.

Melanocytes function as a sunscreen, protecting the deeper layers of the skin from solar radiation, which can cause not only sunburn but also, in the long run, cancer. Unfortunately, melanocytes themselves also produce tumors. Most of these remain benign, but sometimes they give rise to the highly malignant type of cancer called **melanoma**.

Langerhans cells are the macrophage immune cells of the skin, functioning both in contact sensitivity (allergic skin reactions) and in immune surveillance against invading microorganisms. They arise in the bone marrow and first appear in the epidermis by the seventh week (Fig. 7-8*B*). Langerhans cells continue to migrate into the epidermis throughout life.

Merkel cells are pressure-detecting mechanoreceptors that lie at the base of the epidermis and are associated with underlying nerve endings in the dermis. They contain keratin and form desmosomes with adjacent keratinocytes. They arise from epidermal cells and can be identified in the fourth to sixth months.

MESODERM FORMS DERMIS, EXCEPT IN FACE

The dermis, or **corium**—the layer of skin that underlies the epidermis and contains blood vessels, hair follicles, nerve endings, sensory receptors, and so forth—is a tissue with a triple embryonic origin. In the trunk, most of the dermis is derived from the somatic layer of the lateral plate mesoderm, but part of it is derived from the

dermamyotomal divisions of the somites (covered in Chapter 8). In contrast, in the face and neck, the dermis is derived from neural crest cells and thus originates from ectoderm (covered in Chapters 4 and 17).

During the third month, the outer layer of the developing dermis proliferates to form ridgelike **dermal papillae** that protrude into the overlying epidermis (Fig. 7-9). Intervening protrusions of the epidermis into the dermis are called **epidermal ridges**. This superficial region of the dermis is called the **papillary layer**, whereas the thick underlying layer of dense, irregular connective tissue is called the **reticular layer**. The dermis is underlain by subcutaneous fatty connective tissue called the **hypodermis (subcorium)**. The dermis differentiates into its definitive form in the second and third trimesters, although it is thin at birth and thickens progressively through infancy and childhood.

The pattern of external ridges and grooves produced in the skin by the dermal papillae varies from one part of the body to another. The palmar and plantar surfaces of the hands and feet carry a familiar pattern of whorls and loops, the eyelids have a diamond-shaped pattern, and the ridges on the upper surface of the trunk resemble a cobweb. The first skin ridges to appear are the whorls on the palmar and plantar surfaces of the digits, which develop in the eleventh and twelfth weeks. The entire system of surface patterns is established early in the fifth month of fetal life. Thereafter, each patch of skin retains its characteristic pattern even if it is transplanted to a different part of the body.

Blood vessels form within the subcutaneous mesenchyme, deep to the developing dermis, in the fourth week. These branch to form a single layer of vessels in the dermis by the late sixth week and two parallel planes of vessels by the eighth week. Branches of these vessels follow nerves within the dermis and enter the papillary layer to become associated with the hair follicles. These branches may disappear and reappear during different stages of hair follicle differentiation.

It is estimated that the skin of the neonate contains 20 times more blood vessels than it needs to support its own metabolism. This excess is required for thermoregulation. Much of the definitive vasculature of the skin develops in the first few weeks after birth.

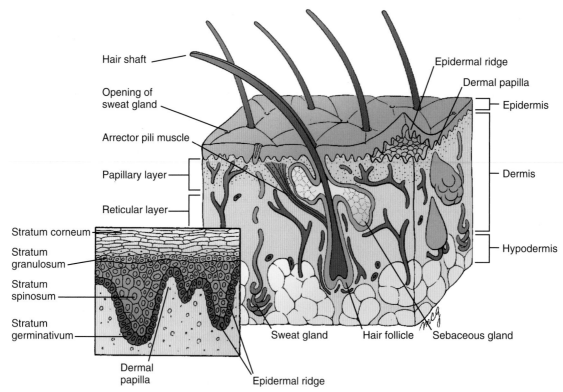

Hair shaft
Opening of sweat gland
Arrector pili muscle
Papillary layer
Reticular layer
Stratum corneum
Stratum granulosum
Stratum spinosum
Stratum germinativum
Dermal papilla
Epidermal ridge
Epidermal ridge
Dermal papilla
Epidermis
Dermis
Hypodermis
Sweat gland
Hair follicle
Sebaceous gland

Figure 7-9. Definitive organization of the dermis and epidermis. The pattern of interdigitating dermal papillae and epidermal ridges first develops during the third month. Sebaceous glands develop from the epidermal lining of the hair follicles, appearing about one month after a given hair bud is formed.

DEVELOPMENT OF SKIN DERIVATIVES

In many regions of the body, the skin gives rise to specialized structures that have a number of functions. The **sebaceous glands** produce sebum, an oily substance that protects the skin against friction and dehydration; the **hair** and **sweat glands** are involved in heat regulation; the **teeth** and **salivary glands** (covered in Chapter 17) are essential for mastication; and the **lacrimal glands** produce tears (also covered in Chapter 17). The **mammary gland** in females provides both nutrition and a source of immunity for the breast-feeding infant.

In the Research Lab

ECTODERMAL DERIVATIVES DEVELOP BY EPITHELIAL-MESENCHYMAL INTERACTIONS

Development of skin derivatives depends on reciprocal **epithelial-mesenchymal interactions**. All are characterized by the development of an ectodermal placode, followed by condensation of cells in the underlying mesenchyme, and then invagination of the epithelium into the underlying dermis to form a bud (Fig. 7-10A, B).

These morphogenetic processes in different skin derivatives are governed by many of the same signaling pathways. Overexpression of the Wnt antagonist Dkk1 arrests development at the placode stage of all ectodermal derivatives analyzed (hair, mammary gland, and tooth). Loss of function in mice of p63, or of the ectodysplasin signaling pathway (Eda), affects all ectodermal

derivatives (see the following "In the Clinic" entitled "Anomalies of Skin Derivatives"; "In the Research Lab" entitled "Regulation of Hair Patterning and Differentiation"; and "Embryology in Practice"). Ectopic expression of Eda using a keratin promoter can also induce the formation of ectopic hair, nipples, and teeth. The homeobox genes Msx1 and Msx2 are both needed for the development of placodes beyond the bud stage (Fig. 7-10B).

Recombination experiments between the dermis and the ectoderm have shown that the dermis specifies the shape and pattern of the ectodermal derivative. Therefore, mammary dermis will induce ectopic mammary glands when recombined with ventral back ectoderm. Salivary gland mesenchyme will also induce the mammary gland epithelium to form many branches characteristic of salivary glands, rather than forming a duct, although the mammary epithelium retains its original differentiation characteristics. This role of the dermis in patterning is also illustrated in Chapter 17, which covers how neural crest cells determine the pattern of feathers in birds, as well as the rate of feather growth (see Fig. 17-19C).

In the Clinic

ANOMALIES OF SKIN DERIVATIVES

Mutations in the transcription factor TUMOR PROTEIN P73-LIKE (TP73L; also known as P63) result in several syndromes that affect multiple ectodermally derived structures. Examples include **ADULT (acro-dermato-ungual-lacrimal-tooth) syndrome, ectrodactyly ectodermal dysplasia-cleft lip/palate**, or **ankyloblepharon-ectodermal dysplasia clefting**

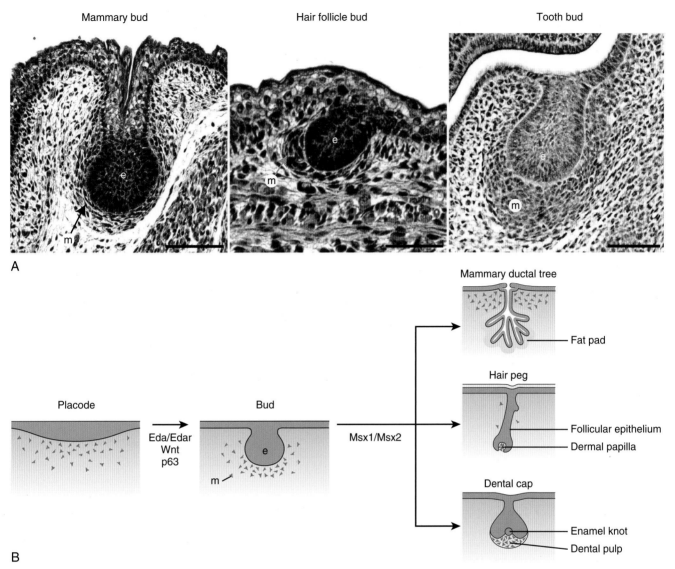

Figure 7-10. Development of the ectodermal placodes. *A,* Light micrographs. The bud stage of developing mammary glands, hair follicles, and teeth showing invaginating epithelium (e) and condensing mesenchyme (m). *B,* Differentiation of the ectodermal placodes into buds and ultimately organ rudiments requires similar molecular networks.

syndrome (AEC, also called Hay-Wells syndrome). Anky-loblepharon is fusion of the eyelids. P63, which is expressed in the stratum germinativum (see Fig. 7-4), regulates cell proliferation and differentiation. In the p63 mouse mutant, ectodermal development is normal until E13.5, at which point the developing epidermis would normally start to stratify. Stratification does not occur in the p63 null mouse, and at birth the epidermis, limbs, and all ectodermal derivatives are absent.

Different ectodermal derivatives can also be differentially affected in syndromes. Mutation in the homeobox gene DLX3 causes **tricho-dento-osseous syndrome**, affecting the hair and teeth. In addition the skull bones of those affected by this syndrome have an abnormally high density. In **nail-tooth dysplasia**, which is the result of mutations in the homeobox gene MSX1, nail and teeth are dysplastic. In contrast, in the rare syndrome **hypotrichosis-lymphedema-telangiectasia**, which results from a mutation in the transcription factor SOX18, hair is the only abnormal ectodermal derivative.

Many skin diseases occur in humans as the result of gene mutations. Several of these are summarized in Table 7-1.

DEVELOPMENT OF HAIR

Hair follicles first form at the end of the second month on the eyebrows, eyelids, upper lip, and chin. Hair follicles do not form in other regions until the fourth month. Most, if not all, hair follicles are present by the fifth month, and it is believed that novel hair follicles do not form after birth. About five million hair follicles develop in both males and females, but the distribution of the various kinds of hair differs between the sexes. These differences are caused by the different concentrations of circulating sex steroid hormones.

The hair follicle first appears as a small concentration of ectodermal cells, called a **hair germ**, in the basal layer

TABLE 7-1 SKIN DISEASES IN HUMANS

Syndrome	Phenotype	Gene	Role
Hypohidrotic ectodermal dysplasia	Sparse hair, absent or malformed teeth, hypoplasia of sweat and other glands	EDA, EDAR, EDARADD, IKK-Γ	Regulate NF-kappa-B signaling to promote the induction/stabilization of placodes during formation of ectodermal appendages
ADULT, AEC, limb-mammary syndromes	Developmental defects in ectoderm and ectodermal derivatives	P63	p63 is required for proliferation and differentiation of ectodermal cells
Focal dermal hypoplasia	Thin dermis and digit, ocular, bone, and dental defects	PORCN	Modifies Wnt proteins in endoplasmic reticulum, allowing them to be secreted
Monilethrix	Dystrophic hair, alopecia. Fragile hair with a beaded appearance	KRT81, 83, and 86 DSG4 (desmosomal component)	KRT81, 83, 86, and DSG4 are structural proteins needed for hair strength
Hypotrichosis	Premature loss of body and scalp hair	LIPASE H (generates LPA) and P2RY5 (LPA receptor) CDSN and DSG4 (desmosomal components) HAIRLESS	Expressed in inner root sheath and hair root; cell signaling to maintain hair structure. Interact with keratins to maintain hair integrity. Transcription factor required for hair cycling
Alopecia	Absence of hair in all or part of body	FOXN1	Transcription factor required for hair cell differentiation; in its absence, hairs cannot protrude above skin surface
Odonto-onycho-dermal hypoplasia	Hypotrichosis, hypodontia, keratoderma, and nail dystrophy	WNT10A	Failure of induction and differentiation of hair follicles
Tricho-dento-osseous syndrome	Hair, teeth, and bone defects	DLX3	Homeobox induced by Wnt signaling; Dlx3 is required for formation of hair shaft and inner root sheath; regulates Gata3 and Hoxc13 expression
Ulna mammary syndrome	Mammary hypoplasia, upper limb abnormalities	TBX3	Homeobox Tbx3 required for formation of the mammary placode
Blomstrand chondrodysplasia	Abnormal bone deposition in cartilage and nipple anomalies	PTHR1	Regulates Bmp signaling in mammary gland development, promoting nipple formation and duct growth
Epidermolysis bullosa simplex	Cell fragility and blistering	KRT5 and KRT14	Structural proteins required for epithelial integrity
Epidermolytic hyperkeratosis	Cell fragility and blistering, followed by hyperkeratinization	KRT1 or KRT10	Structural proteins required for epithelial integrity
Meesmann epithelial corneal dystrophy	Cell fragility and formation of cysts in cornea	KRT3 and KRT12 (cornea specific)	Structural proteins required for epithelial integrity
Epidermolytic palmoplantar keratoderma	Thickening of skin in hands and feet	KRT9 (keratin specific to palms of hands and soles of feet)	Structural proteins required for epithelial integrity
Lamellar ichthyosis (e.g., Harlequin fetus)	Thickened scale-like skin	TRANSGLUTAMINASE 1, a cross-linking enzyme (type 1); ABCA2, a keratinocyte lipid transporter (type II)	Defective keratin fibers and lamellar granule formation
Ehlers-Danlos syndrome	Fragile skin	COLLAGENS TYPE I and IV	Structural proteins required for dermis integrity
Stiff skin syndrome	Thickened skin; joint immobility/contractures	FIBRILLIN 1	Structural and signaling protein; abnormal deposition of elastin and collagens

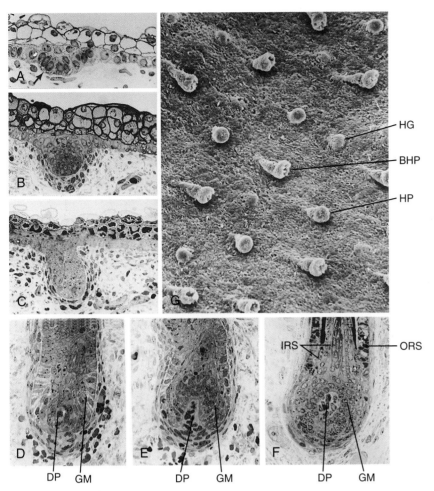

Figure 7-11. Development of the hair follicle. *A-F,* Light micrographs. *A,* Hair germ at eighty days. *B,* Elongating hair germ later in the first trimester. *C,* Hair peg in the second trimester. *D-F,* Development of the follicle base from the elongated hair peg stage to the bulbous hair peg stage. The dermal papilla (DP) at the base of the developing follicle induces the germinal matrix (GM). In *F,* the hair shaft can be seen growing up the center of the follicle, and the inner and outer epidermal root sheaths (IRS and ORS) are differentiating. *G,* Scanning electron micrograph of the undersurface of the developing epidermis, showing hair germs (HG), hair pegs (HP), and bulbous hair pegs (BHP) growing into the dermis (dermis was removed from the preparation to show the deep side of the epidermis).

of the primitive, two-layered epidermis (Fig. 7-11*A*). Hair germs are induced by the underlying dermis. The hair germ recruits dermal cells to form a dermal condensate that promotes further differentiation of the hair germ (Fig. 7-11*B, G*). The hair germ proliferates to form a rod-like **hair peg** that pushes down into the dermis (Fig. 7-11*C-G*). Within the dermis, the tip of the hair peg expands, forming a **bulbous hair peg**, and the dermis cells just beneath the tip of the bulb proliferate to form a small hillock called the **dermal papilla** (Fig. 7-11*E*), which grows into the expanded base of the hair bulb (Fig. 7-11*F*).

The layer of proliferating ectoderm that overlies the dermal papilla in the base of the hair bulb is called the **germinal matrix** (Fig. 7-11*D-F*). The germinal matrix is responsible for producing the hair shaft (Fig. 7-11*F*): proliferation of the germinal matrix produces cells that undergo a specialized process of keratinization and are added to the base of the hair shaft. The growing hair shaft is thus pushed outward through the follicular canal. If the hair is to be colored, the maturing keratinocytes incorporate pigment produced by the melanocytes of the hair bulb. The epidermal cells lining the follicular canal constitute the **inner** and **outer epidermal root sheaths** (see Fig. 7-11*F*).

Except in the case of the eyebrows and eyelashes, the dermal root sheath of the follicle becomes associated with a bundle of smooth muscle cells called the **arrector pili** muscle, which functions to erect the hair (making

so-called goose flesh or bumps) (see Fig. 7-9). The stem cells of the follicular epithelium that regenerate the follicle periodically during postnatal life are found near the site of attachment of the arrector pili muscle in the **bulge** (see Fig. 7-5; also covered in Chapter 10). There are four phases of the hair growth cycle: growth phase (**anagen**), regression phase (**catagen**), resting phase (**telogen**), and shedding phase (**exogen**).

The first generation of hairs is formed during the twelfth week; they are fine and unpigmented and are collectively called **lanugo**. They are mostly shed before birth and are replaced by coarser hairs during the perinatal period. Postnatally, there are two types of hair: the **vellus**—nonpigmented hairs that do not project deep into the dermis—and the **terminal hairs**—pigmented hairs that penetrate into the fatty dermal tissues. At puberty, rising levels of sex hormones cause fine body hair to be replaced by coarser hairs on some parts of the body: the axilla and pubis of both sexes, the face, and (in some races) the chest and back of males.

In the Research Lab

REGULATION OF HAIR PATTERNING AND DIFFERENTIATION

Establishment of the hair placode requires Eda/Edar and Wnt signaling (see Fig. 7-10), and ectopic expression of Eda or

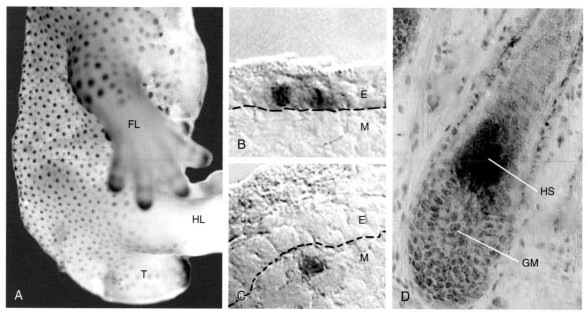

Figure 7-12. Shh and Wnt signaling pathways are active in the early development and morphogenesis of the hair follicle. *A*, Ptc1 expression, indicative of active Shh signaling, in the hair placodes (purple dots). FL, forelimb; HL, hindlimb; T, tail. *B-D*, Regions of Wnt/β-catenin signaling (purple): first in hair placodes in the ectodermal layer (E), *B*; subsequently in the underlying mesenchyme (M) in the forming germinal matrix, *C*; and then in the differentiating hair shaft (HS), just distal to the germinal matrix (GM), *D*. The dashed line in *B, C* marks the boundary between the ectoderm and the mesenchyme.

Wnt components (e.g., β-catenin, Lef-1) induces formation of ectopic placodes. Conversely, blocking Edar/Wnt signaling prevents placode formation. Consistent with this, in humans, mutations in both EDA and WNT signaling pathways are linked to hair defects (see the following "In the Clinic" entitled "Hair Anomalies"). Eda signaling is active in the ectoderm, whereas Wnt signaling is active first in the ectodermal placode and then in the underlying mesenchyme (see Fig. 7-12*B,C*). Spacing of hair follicles is controlled by the interplay of factors that promote and antagonize placode development. Eda/Wnts, with several other secreted factors, including Fgfs, follistatin, Tgfβ2, and Bmp antagonists, all promote placode development. In contrast, Bmp/Tgfβ1 signaling inhibits placode development. Localized high levels of placode inducers versus antagonists also create the correct spacing of hairs. For example, hair buds express both Bmps and Bmp antagonists. Expression of the Bmp antagonist inhibits Bmp signaling within the placode and allows placode development to proceed. Placode development is inhibited in the surrounding epithelium as Bmp molecules diffuse further than the extracellular antagonists, creating regions of high and low Bmp activity. In this way, an organized array of structures is formed. The orientation of the hair follicles is controlled by Wnt signaling via the **planar cell polarity pathway** (covered in Chapter 5). In the frizzled 6 (a Wnt receptor) knockout mouse, hairs and hair whorls are randomized and misoriented.

Once the placode has been established, the ectoderm invaginates to form the early hair follicle; this process is controlled by Shh, which is expressed in the hair placode and is mitogenic (Fig. 7-12*A*). Shh also signals to the underlying dermal papillae. In Shh mouse mutants, hair development is arrested at the early peg stage. The role of Shh during hair development is similar to that in developing teeth: in Shh mutants, tooth development is arrested at the bud stage because of decreased proliferation (covered in Chapter 17).

An individual hair consists of the hair shaft and the outer (or external) and inner (or internal) root sheaths (see Figs. 7-5, 7-11). The hair shaft consists of three concentric layers: cuticle, cortex, and medulla (from outside to inside). Each layer of the hair has a unique ultrastructure and expresses distinct keratins, which are regulated by the differential expression of growth factors and transcription factors, such as Wnts, Msx2, Foxn1, and Hoxc13, within the various layers. Fig. 7-12*D* shows the differential activation of the Wnt canonical pathway within the differentiating hair shaft. Defects in any of these layers results in monilethrix, a condition characterized by fragile and/or beaded hair (see the following "In the Clinic" entitled "Hair Anomalies"). The progenitor cells or stem cells arise in the **bulge** (see Fig. 7-5; also covered in Chapter 10 in relation to the origin of peripheral nervous system stem cells). Cells from the bulge migrate downward into the matrix of the hair follicle.

In the Clinic

HAIR ANOMALIES

Hair abnormalities range from **hypertrichosis** (excess hair) to **atrichia** (congenital absence of hair) to structural/morphologic defects. In addition, hair abnormalities can arise from (1) hair cycle defects, the most common cause of hair abnormalities in humans; (2) immunologic defects in which the skin and hair proteins become targets of the immune system; and (3) sebaceous gland abnormalities. In women, vellus hairs can be transformed at puberty into terminal hairs, for example, on the upper lip and the lower leg. This is known as **hirsutism**.

Defective hair development can encompass all stages of hair differentiation. As in the skin, mutations can occur in signaling pathways, proteases, gap junctions, and structural proteins such as desmosomes and keratins. In **hypohidrotic ectodermal dysplasia** (see "Embryology in Practice"), which affects the EDA/EDAR signaling pathway, the first stage of hair development (formation of the hair placode) does not occur (see Fig. 7-10*B*). In contrast, mutations in genes that encode structural proteins, such as PLAKOPHILIN 1 and DESMOPLAKIN 1 (both desmosomal proteins), and KERATINS affect differentiation and morphogenesis of the hair. For example, mutations in the hair KERATINS KRTB6 and KRTB1 result in **monilethrix**, in which the hair is "beaded" and fragile, and thus is easily lost.

As the hair goes through the phases of cyclic regeneration (i.e., anagen, catagen, telogen, and exogen; as discussed earlier in the chapter), a variety of stressors or illnesses (e.g., chemotherapy, pregnancy) can shift the hair cycle toward the telogen phase, resulting in excessive hair shedding—called **telogen effluvium**—several months later. Normally, during catagen, apoptosis of the matrix cells in the bulb and outer root sheath prevents further growth of the hair, but an epithelial strand between the bulge and the dermal papillae remains. This contact is necessary for the dermal papillae to induce new hair growth in the bulge, where hair progenitor cells are located. If the epithelial cord is destroyed—for example, as a consequence of mutations in the zinc-finger co-repressor HAIRLESS or the VITAMIN D RECEPTOR—the dermal papillae are stranded within the dermis and the hair cannot regrow.

Tumors may also arise within the hair. During development, Wnt signaling promotes hair placode development and differentiation of developing hair shaft cells (Fig. 17-12,*B-D*). Constitutive activation of this pathway (e.g., β-CATENIN mutations) results in **pilomatricoma**, a benign tumor of the hair follicle matrix cells.

DEVELOPMENT OF SEBACEOUS AND SWEAT GLANDS

Several types of glands are produced by downgrowth of the epidermis. Sebaceous glands and sweat glands are widespread over the body. The milk-producing mammary glands represent a specialized type of epidermal gland.

The **sebaceous glands** produce the oily **sebum** that lubricates the skin and hair. Over most of the body, these glands form as diverticula of the hair follicle shafts, budding from the side of the root sheath about 4 weeks after the hair germ begins to elongate (see Figs. 7-5, 7-9). In some areas of hairless skin—such as the glans penis of males and the labia minora of females—sebaceous glands develop as independent downgrowths of epidermis. The bud grows into the dermis tissue and branches to form a small system of ducts ending in expanded secretory acini (alveoli). The acini secrete by a **holocrine** mechanism, that is, entire secretory cells that are filled with vesicles of secretory products break down and are shed. The basal layer of the acinar epidermis consists of proliferating stem cells that constantly renew the supply of maturing secretory cells (see Fig. 7-5).

Mature sebaceous glands are present on the face by 6 months of development. Sebaceous glands are highly active in the fetus, and the sebum they produce combines with desquamating epidermal cells and remnants of the periderm to form a waterproof protective coating for the fetus called the **vernix caseosa**. After birth, the sebaceous glands become relatively inactive, but at puberty they again begin to secrete large quantities of sebum in response to the surge in circulating sex steroids.

The **apocrine sweat glands** are highly coiled, unbranched glands that develop in association with hair follicles. They initially form over most of the body, but in later months of fetal development, they are lost except in certain areas, such as the axillae, mons pubis, prepuce, scrotum, and labia minora. They begin to secrete at puberty, producing a complex mix of substances that are modified by bacterial activity into odorous compounds. These compounds may function mainly in social and sexual communication. The secretory cells lining the deep half of the gland secrete their products by an **apocrine** mechanism: small portions of cytoplasm-containing secretory vesicles pinch off and are released into the lumen of the gland.

The **eccrine sweat glands** first appear at about 20 weeks as buds of stratum germinativum that grow down into the underlying dermis to form unbranched, highly coiled glands (see Figs. 7-5 and 7-13). The central cells degenerate to form the gland lumen, and the peripheral cells differentiate into an inner layer of secretory cells and an outer layer of **myoepithelial cells**, which are innervated by sympathetic fibers and contract to expel sweat from the gland (see Fig. 7-13). The secretory cells secrete fluid directly across the plasma membrane (**eccrine** secretion). Sweat glands form over the entire body surface except in a few areas such as the nipples. Large sweat glands develop as buds of the root sheath of hair follicles, superficial to the buds of sebaceous glands, in the axilla and areola.

Sweat glands fail to develop in the X-linked genetic disorder **hypohidrotic ectodermal dysplasia** (see "Embryology in Practice"). Infants with this disorder are vulnerable to potentially lethal **hyperpyrexia** (extremely high fever) or **hyperthermia** (overheating).

DEVELOPMENT OF MAMMARY GLANDS

In the fourth week, a pair of epidermal thickenings called the **mammary ridges** develop along either side of the body from the area of the future axilla to the future inguinal region and the medial thigh (Fig. 7-14). In humans, these ridges normally disappear, except at the site of the breasts. The remnant of the mammary ridge produces a well-defined **primary bud** of the mammary gland by the seventh week (Fig. 7-14*A*, *B*). This bud grows down into the underlying dermis toward the presumptive fat pad that will induce the duct to branch. In the tenth week, the primary bud begins to branch, and by the twelfth week, several **secondary buds** have formed (Fig. 7-14*C*). These buds lengthen and branch throughout the remainder of gestation, and the resulting ducts canalize (Fig. 7-14*D*). At birth, the mammary glands consist of 15 to 25 **lactiferous ducts**, which open onto a small superficial depression called the **mammary pit** (Fig. 7-14*D*, *E*). Proliferation of the underlying mesoderm usually converts this pit to an everted nipple within a few weeks after birth, although occasionally the nipple remains depressed (**inverted nipple**). The skin surrounding the nipple also proliferates to form the areola.

On occasion, one or more supernumerary nipples (**polythelia**) or supernumerary breasts (**polymastia**)

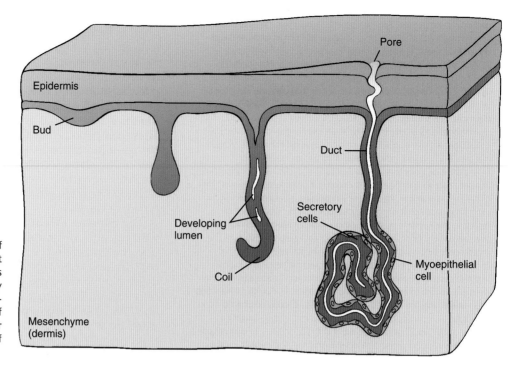

Figure 7-13. Development of sweat glands. Sweat glands first appear as elongated downgrowths of the epidermis at about twenty weeks. The outer cells of the downgrowth develop into a layer of smooth muscle, whereas the inner cells become the secretory cells of the gland.

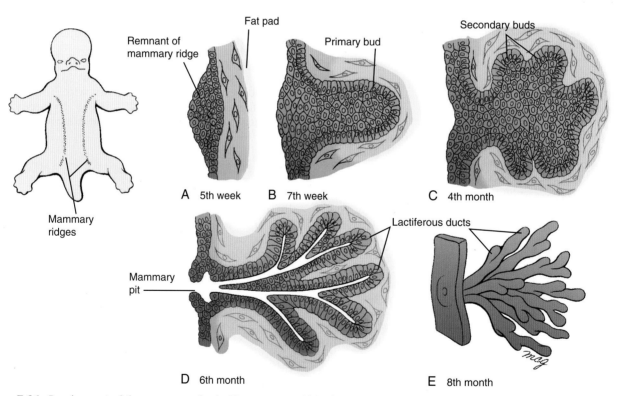

Figure 7-14. Development of the mammary glands. The mammary ridges first appear in the fourth week as thickened lines of epidermis that extend from the thorax to the medial thigh. *A, B,* In the region of the future mammary glands, the mammary ridge ectoderm then forms the primary mammary buds, which grow toward the fat pad. *C, D,* Secondary buds form during the third month and become canalized to form lactiferous ducts during the last three months of fetal life. *E,* Organization of lactiferous ducts around the developing nipple in the eighth month.

form along the line of the mammary ridges. The most common location is just below the normal breast. Supernumerary nipples are about as common in males as in females. More rarely, an ectopic nipple forms off the line of the mammary ridge as a consequence of migration of mammary tissue. Supernumerary breasts are often discovered at puberty or during pregnancy, when they enlarge or even lactate in response to stimulatory hormones.

In the Research Lab

DEVELOPMENT AND DIFFERENTIATION OF MAMMARY GLAND

As with hair follicles, development of the mammary gland is controlled by Wnt signaling. Mutation of Lef1, a transcription factor involved in Wnt/β-catenin signaling, or overexpression of the Wnt inhibitor Dkk1 results in failure of the buds to develop appropriately. The T-box transcription factor Tbx3 regulates the expression of Wnt10b and Lef1. Therefore, in Tbx3 mouse mutants, the mammary glands also do not develop. Mutations of TBX3 in humans result in **ulnar-mammary syndrome**, characterized by abnormal development of the limb, mammary gland, and other apocrine glands.

Other factors essential for mammary gland development include Bmps and Pthrp (parathyroid hormone–related peptide), which control ectoderm differentiation and duct formation. Pthrp is expressed in the ectoderm from the placode stage and signals to the underlying mesenchyme, which expresses the Pthrp receptor (r1). Pthrp signaling increases Bmp receptor expression and hence Bmp signaling, which is necessary for mammary gland specification (see later). In Pthrp and Pthrp receptor (r1) mouse mutants, the mammary bud forms, but the ductal tube and the nipples do not develop. Overexpression of Pthrp can also induce nipple formation in the ventral ectoderm. In humans, loss-of-function mutations in PTHRP RECEPTOR (R1) cause **Blomstrand chondrodysplasia**. Patients with this syndrome have endochondral bone defects and absence of the breasts and nipples. Finally, branching morphogenesis is regulated by Fgf signaling as for other branching organs, such as the lungs, kidney, and salivary glands (see Chapters 11, 15, and 17).

A crucial difference between development of the mammary gland and of the hair follicle is the requirement for higher levels of Bmp signaling and repression of Shh signaling (see Fig. 7-12A). When Shh signaling is inactivated in the ventral ectoderm, hair follicles are transformed into a mammary gland fate, whereas when Bmp signaling is reduced in the developing mammary gland, the nipple is transformed into hair follicles.

DEVELOPMENT OF NAILS

The nail rudiments (anlagen) first appear as epidermal thickenings near the distal end of the dorsal side of the digits (Fig. 7-15A, D). These thickenings form at about ten weeks on the fingers and at about fourteen weeks on the toes. Almost immediately, the nail rudiments migrate proximally on the dorsal surface of the digits. Between the twelfth and fourteen weeks, the nail rudiment forms a shallow depression called the **nail field**, which is surrounded laterally and proximally by ectodermal **nail folds** (Fig. 7-15B, E). The stratum germinativum of the proximal nail fold proliferates to become the **nail matrix**, which produces the horny **nail plate** (Fig. 7-15C, F). Like a hair, the nail plate is made of compressed keratinocytes. A thin layer of epidermis called the **eponychium** initially covers the nail plate, but this layer normally degenerates, except at the nail base.

Fate mapping studies of the ventral ectoderm have shown that the boundary between dorsal and ventral ectoderm derivatives lies at the distal tip of the **hyponychium** (the layer beneath the free edge of the nail) (Fig. 7-15G, H). The growing nails reach the tips of the fingers by the eighth month, and the tips of the toes by birth. The degree of nail growth can be used as an indicator of prematurity. WNT signaling is needed for nail development (Fig. 7-15D). In humans, mutation in a novel WNT ligand, R-SPONDIN-4, or the FRIZZLED 6 RECEPTOR, causes nail defects, including **anonychia (absence of nails)**.

Embryology in Practice

SKIN DEEP

You are a neurologist called to see a one-month-old boy who was admitted to the children's hospital for poor feeding and lethargy. The reason for the consultation is hypotonia (a neurologic reduction in muscle tone) with concern for a CNS abnormality. The child has been scheduled for an MRI of the brain under anesthesia to be done later that day. You arrive at the room and suspect the diagnosis as soon as you meet the patient and his mother.

His mother relays that after a normal pregnancy and delivery, the boy has had trouble feeding. Early on, their doctor switched him to formula because she wasn't making enough milk. Even with bottle feeds, it seems like he often chokes on his feeds and has trouble breathing through his nose. This has become worse lately, with poor weight gain and a reduced number of daily wet diapers prompting this admission. The boy often feels warm but has not had fevers, and his mother says she hasn't noted any sweating with feeds.

When asked about her health, the mother states that she is well but does have a skin condition of some sort that makes her hair thinner than normal and has given her trouble with her teeth. Her mother has the same condition, but no one else in the family has similar symptoms.

Examination of the boy is significant for very sparse hair, red circles around his eyes (periorbital hyperpigmentation), a low nasal bridge, and a raspy cry. During the visit, you note that his mother has similar facial and hair findings, although to a milder degree (see Fig. 7-16 for a patient with these features). The boy is somewhat weak and listless but is not obviously hypotonic when held prone, supported under the abdomen.

You relay to the admitting team that the boy has an ectodermal dysplasia, likely **X-linked hypohidrotic ectodermal dysplasia** (XLHED) based on your findings and on the family history. You are able to dissuade them from performing the expensive MRI. The boy's condition improves after IV hydration, and he is able to feed more effectively after nasal irrigation with saline to soften dried secretions.

Boys with XLHED have hypohidrosis (decreased sweating), hypotrichosis (reduced hair), and hypodontia (absent or small teeth). Decreased sweat production confers a risk of hyperthermia, and families must institute environmental modifications (mist sprayers, cooling vests, and avoidance of hot circumstances) to reduce this danger. Female carriers can have milder expression of any of the features of XLHED, with sparse patchy hair, small or missing teeth, and reduced production of breast milk. The combination of dry nasal mucosa in neonates with XLHED with poor milk production

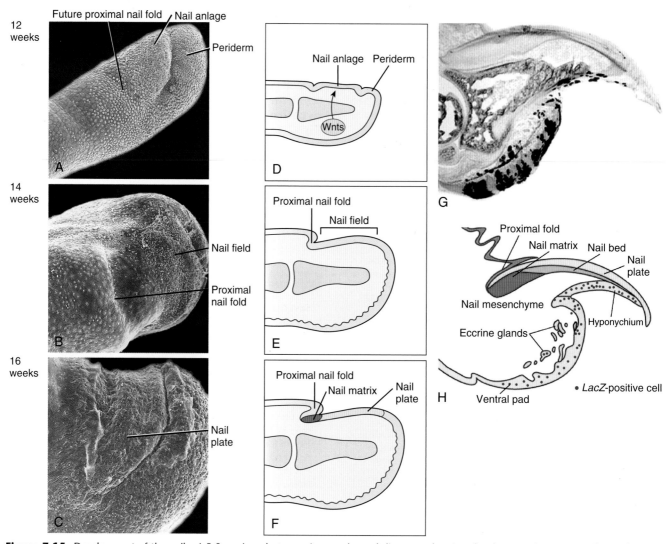

Figure 7-15. Development of the nails. *A-F,* Scanning electron micrographs and diagrams showing development between twelve and sixteen weeks. *A, D,* Formation of the nail rudiment. *B, E,* The margin of the proximal nail fold is clearly defined by fourteen weeks. *C, F,* The nail plate is apparent by sixteen weeks. *G, H,* The boundary between dorsal and ventral ectodermal derivatives in a mouse embryo is shown in the light micrograph by the presence of *LacZ*-expressing cells (dark blue) along the ventral surface. The drawing provides an explanation of the morphology seen in the light micrograph.

in carrier females can, as in this case, hinder feeding and growth. Heat intolerance is unusual in females, although a patchy distribution of sweat glands resulting from random inactivation of chromosomes carrying the normal and abnormal gene is seen.

Hypohidrotic ectodermal dysplasia is caused by mutations in the transmembrane protein, ECTODYSPLASIN (EDA), its receptor (EDAR), or components of this signaling pathway (e.g., EDAR-ADD). EDA is a member of the TNF (TUMOR NECROSIS FACTOR) family of cytokines, a pathway that is highly conserved during appendage formation, acting to control scale development in fish, feather development in birds, and hair and gland development in humans.

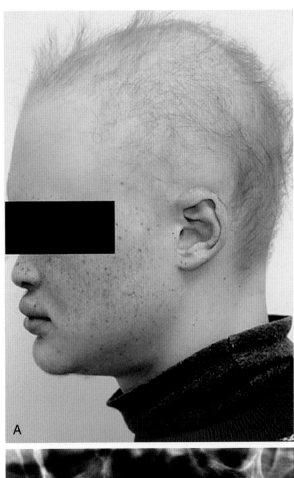

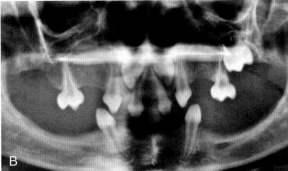

Figure 7-16. Sparse hair and dental abnormalities are characteristics of hypohidrotic ectodermal dysplasia. *A,* Patient from lateral view. *B,* X-ray of teeth.

SUGGESTED READINGS

Arin MJ. 2009. The molecular basis of human keratin disorders. Hum Genet 125:355–373.

Blanpain C, Fuchs E. 2009. Epidermal homeostasis: a balancing act of stem cells in the skin. Nat Rev Mol Cell Biol 10:207–217.

Blanpain C, Horsley V, Fuchs E. 2007. Epithelial stem cells: turning over new leaves. Cell 128:445–458.

Cowin P, Wysolmerski J. 2010. Molecular mechanisms guiding embryonic mammary gland development. Cold Spring Harb Perspect Biol 2:a003251.

Driskell RR, Clavel C, Rendl M, Watt FM. 2011. Hair follicle dermal papilla cells at a glance. J Cell Sci 124:1179–1182.

Fuchs E. 2007. Scratching the surface of skin development. Nature 445:834–842.

Fuchs E, Horsley V. 2008. More than one way to skin. Genes Dev 22:976–985.

Galach M, Utikal J. 2011. From skin to the treatment of diseases—the possibilities of iPS cell research in dermatology. Exp Dermatol 20:523–528.

Hunt DP, Jahoda C, Chandran S. 2009. Multipotent skin-derived precursors: from biology to clinical translation. Curr Opin Biotechnol 20:522–530.

Mikkola ML. 2007. Genetic basis of skin appendage development. Semin Cell Dev Biol 18:225–236.

Mikkola ML. 2008. TNF superfamily in skin appendage development. Cytokine Growth Factor Rev 19:219–230.

Mikkola ML, Millar SE. 2006. The mammary bud as a skin appendage: unique and shared aspects of development. J Mammary Gland Biol Neoplasia 11:187–203.

Robinson GW. 2007. Cooperation of signalling pathways in embryonic mammary gland development. Nat Rev Genet 8:963–972.

Schneider MR, Schmidt-Ullrich R, Paus R. 2009. The hair follicle as a dynamic miniorgan. Curr Biol 19:R132–142.

Shimomura Y, Christiano AM. 2010. Biology and genetics of hair. Annu Rev Genomics Hum Genet 11:109–132.

Uitto J, Richard G, McGrath JA. 2007. Diseases of epidermal keratins and their linker proteins. Exp Cell Res 313:1995–2009.

Chapter 8

Development of the Musculoskeletal System

SUMMARY

Development of bone and muscle occurs within mesenchymal regions of the embryo after the tube-within-a-tube body plan is established during the fourth week of gestation. Bone formation occurs in two ways. During **endochondral ossification**, a cartilage model first forms and is eventually replaced with bone. This type of ossification underlies formation of the axial skeleton (vertebral column, ribs, and sternum), cranial base, and appendicular (limb) skeleton, with the exception of part of the clavicles. During **intramembranous ossification**, bone forms directly from mesenchymal cells without the prior formation of cartilage. This type of ossification underlies formation of the cranial vault and most of the bones of the face.

Three types of cells act in endochondral bone development: **chondrocytes, osteoblasts**, and **osteoclasts**. The former two function in secreting cartilage and bone matrix, respectively, whereas the latter is involved in bone resorption. Only the latter two cell types act in intramembranous ossification.

Three types of muscles form in the embryo: skeletal, smooth, and cardiac. Skeletal, or voluntary, muscle—the focus of this chapter—develops in association with bone as part of the musculoskeletal system. Smooth muscle develops in association with formation of the walls of the viscera, blood vessels, and glands. Cardiac muscle develops only in the heart. Development of smooth and cardiac muscle is discussed in relation to development of the gut tube, urinary system, and genital system (covered in Chapters 14 through 16, respectively) and in relation to the heart (covered in Chapter 12).

Muscle development occurs in the embryo through the formation of **myoblasts**, which undergo extensive proliferation to form terminally differentiated, postmitotic **myocytes**. Myocytes express actin, myosin, and other contractile proteins and fuse to form contractile **myofibers**. Striated muscle development involves both prenatal and postnatal events: **primary myogenesis** (occurs during the stage of the embryo) and **secondary myogenesis** (occurs during the stage of the fetus) lay down the muscular system, and **satellite cells** act in muscle growth postnatally and in response to exercise or muscle damage.

The muscles and bones of the trunk derive from the **somites**. Each somite forms two distinct zones: a **sclerotome** and a **dermamyotome**. The former gives rise to the bones of the axial skeleton. The latter forms the dermis of the back skin of the trunk and neck (with the remainder of the dermis of these regions forming from **lateral plate mesoderm**), as well as the **myotome**, which forms the muscles of the trunk. The dermamyotome also gives rise to all the musculature of the limbs (covered in Chapter 20) and some of the tongue musculature (covered in Chapter 17). The **syndetome**, containing the progenitor of the tendons, develops between the myotome and the sclerotome. The **lateral plate mesoderm** forms the sternum and bones of the limbs (covered in Chapter 20) and contributes to the dermis of the trunk. As covered in Chapter 17, the bones of the face and neck arise from **neural crest cells**, as does most of the dermis of the head, whereas the facial, masticatory, and laryngeal muscles arise from unsegmented paraxial (called *head* or *cranial*) mesoderm. The bones of the cranial vault and cranial base are formed from segmented paraxial mesoderm (e.g., exoccipital bone), unsegmented paraxial mesoderm (e.g., parietal bone), or neural crest (e.g., frontal bone).

Shortly after formation of the somitic myotome, the myotome splits into a dorsal **epimere** and a ventral **hypomere**. The epimere forms the deep **epaxial muscles** of the back, which are innervated by the dorsal ramus of the spinal nerve. In contrast, the hypomere forms the **hypaxial muscles** of the lateral and ventral body wall in the thorax and abdomen, which are innervated by the ventral ramus of the spinal nerve. Therefore, like all skeletal muscles, the innervation of these muscles (covered further in Chapter 10) reflects their embryonic origin.

Formation of the vertebral column involves the process of **resegmentation** of the sclerotomes of the somites. During resegmentation, the sclerotome of each somite subdivides into cranial and caudal segments, each of which fuses, respectively, with the adjacent caudal or cranial segment. Resegmentation allows motor axons and dorsal root ganglia to lie between vertebrae, rather than running through them. In contrast, skeletal muscles keep their original segmental arrangement, connecting the two adjacent vertebrae and allowing movement.

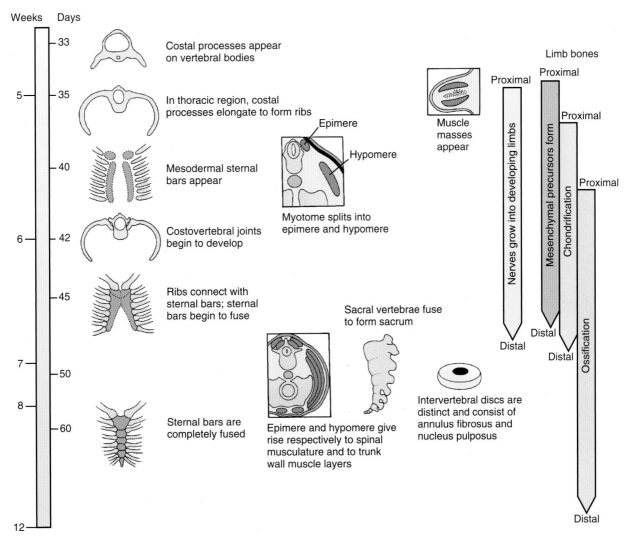

Time line. Formation of the musculoskeletal system.

A newlywed couple, both divorcees with previous children, decides to have a child together. The woman becomes pregnant within a few months of trying and, because of her "advanced maternal age" of thirty-eight, her obstetrician recommends first-trimester screening. This testing indicates an elevated chance (1 in 25) of trisomy 18. Amniocentesis shows a normal karyotype of 46,XX, and a follow-up ultrasound at twenty weeks shows that the length of the long bones is less than normal. Otherwise, the pregnancy progresses normally.

The couple delivers a healthy girl at thirty-nine weeks of gestational age without complications. Over the next few months, the family becomes increasingly concerned that their daughter seems to have short arms and legs and bears little resemblance to either parent. The girl is referred to the genetics clinic and is noted to have **rhizomelia** (shortening of the proximal limbs), short fingers, a large head, and a flat nasal bridge (Fig. 8-1). X-rays confirm the diagnosis of **achondroplasia**. The parents are told that their daughter's adult height will be around 4 feet. They are reassured somewhat when they learn that she should have normal intelligence and a normal life expectancy.

Achondroplasia, a Greek word that means "without cartilage formation," is the most common and most recognizable form of dwarfism. It is caused by mutations in the FIBROBLAST GROWTH FACTOR RECEPTOR 3 (FGFR3). In contrast to aneuploidy syndromes, like trisomy 18, in which advanced maternal age increases incidence, achondroplasia is associated with advanced *paternal* age, with 80% of cases resulting from new mutations in the FGFR3 gene.

TISSUE ORIGINS AND DIFFERENTIATION OF MUSCULOSKELETAL SYSTEM

OVERVIEW OF BONE DEVELOPMENT

There are two types of bones in the body: those that develop via **endochondral ossification** and those that develop via **intramembranous ossification**. During endochondral bone development, formation of a cartilaginous template precedes ossification. This pathway of differentiation is used by all **axial** (vertebral column, sternum, and ribs) and **appendicular** (limb) **bones** of the body, with the exception of part of the clavicle. The cranial base, sensory capsules, and pharyngeal arch cartilages also form via endochondral ossification (covered in Chapter 17).

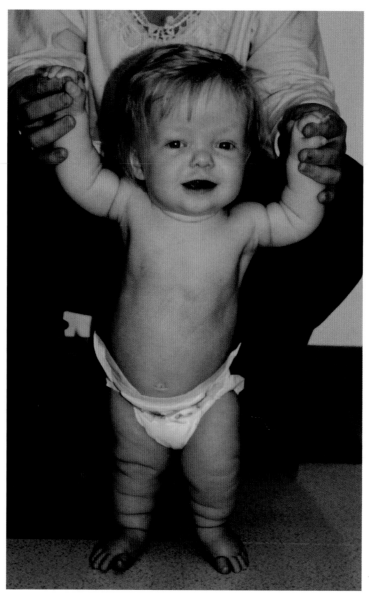

Figure 8-1. A girl with achondroplasia.

Cartilage can grow rapidly in the embryo and postnatally in the growth plates. In the adult, cartilage persists in regions of load (e.g., articular cartilage) or flexibility (e.g., laryngeal cartilages). Rather than forming from a cartilaginous template, bones may develop by intramembranous ossification, that is, directly from the mesenchyme. Intramembranous bones typify most bones of the face and cranial vault and are called **dermal** or **membrane bones**.

Endochondral bones are formed by three cell types: **chondrocytes** (cartilage cells), **osteoblasts** (bone-forming cells), and **osteoclasts** (bone-resorbing cells). Chondrocytes have three tissue origins: the **paraxial mesoderm** forms the axial skeleton, including the exoccipital portion of the cranial base; the **lateral plate mesoderm** forms the appendicular skeleton and sternum; and the **neural crest cells** (i.e., ectodermal cells) give rise to the cartilaginous elements in the face and neck. The origin of osteoblasts and osteoclasts is less diverse: osteoblasts arise from **mesenchymal stem cells**, and osteoclasts arise from the **hematopoietic** system.

Dermal bones develop from **neural crest cells** (facial bones and the frontal bone of the skull) or from unsegmented **paraxial (head/cranial) mesoderm** (e.g., parietal bone of the skull; covered in Chapter 17). In dermal bones, the osteoblasts directly differentiate within the mesenchyme.

OVERVIEW OF MUSCLE DEVELOPMENT

The striated muscles of the trunk and limb are derived from the segmented **paraxial mesoderm**, that is, the **somites**. Most of the tongue musculature also arises from the **somites** (the so-called occipital somites; covered in Chapter 17), whereas all other craniofacial muscles arise from the unsegmented cranial **paraxial mesoderm** and the **prechordal plate mesoderm** (i.e., lateral and cranial midline head mesoderm, respectively; covered in Chapter 3). The tongue and limb myoblast precursors undergo extensive migration to reach their final destination. Initially the myogenic cells, the **myoblasts**,

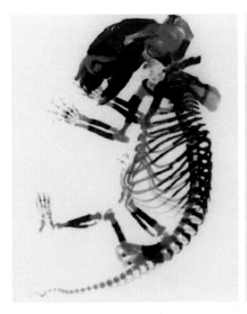
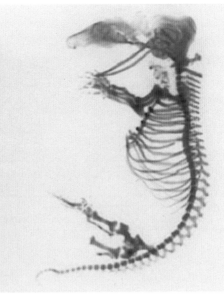

Figure 8-2. The role of Runx2 in bone development. Wild-type mouse embryo (left) and a Runx2 null embryo (right) have been stained with alcian blue and alizarin red to show cartilage (blue) and bone (red) differentiation. In the absence of Runx2, the osteoblasts (the bone-forming cells) do not develop.

proliferate. However, they soon exit the cell cycle and terminally differentiate to form **myocytes**. The myocytes express contractile proteins such as actin and myosin and fuse to form **myofibers**, each of which consists of a multinucleated **syncytium** (i.e., a cellular mass with multiple nuclei) containing the contractile **myofibrils**. The tongue and extraocular muscles express unique myosin heavy chains needed for the function of mastication and eye movement, respectively.

Striated muscle development occurs in three waves. First, there is **primary myogenesis**, which occurs in the embryo. This is followed by **secondary myogenesis**, which occurs in the fetus and gives rise to the bulk of fetal muscle. Finally, postnatal muscle growth involves **satellite cells**, small quiescent cells underlying the basal lamina of the muscle fiber. During postnatal growth and in response to exercise or muscle damage, satellite cells form myocytes, which permit further muscle growth. Satellite cells in the trunk and limb arise from the **somites**, whereas satellite cells in the head arise from the unsegmented paraxial mesoderm.

The smooth muscle of the gut and cardiac muscle form from **splanchnic mesoderm**, whereas the smooth muscle contributing to blood vessels and hair follicles arises locally within the mesoderm. Smooth muscle can also form from neural crest cells. For example, the iris and ciliary muscles (covered in Chapter 19) are derived from cranial neural crest cells, as is the smooth muscle of the dermis of the head and neck.

In the Research Lab

COMMITMENT TO MUSCULOSKELETAL LINEAGE

Commitment to the chondrogenic, osteoblastic, and myogenic lineages is determined by distinct transcription factors. Commitment to the chondrogenic lineage requires the transcription factor **Sox9**, which regulates **collagen type II** expression—a key constituent of the early cartilaginous matrix. Commitment to the osteoblastic lineage requires **Runx2** (runt-related transcription factor 2, also known as Cbfa1 or core binding factor 1),

a transcription factor. Misexpression of Runx2 in primary fibroblasts can induce the expression of bone markers, such as collagen type I, osteocalcin, bone sialoprotein, and alkaline phosphatase, required for mineralization. Gene inactivation of the transcription factor Sox9 in mice affects the early development of all cartilaginous bones. In contrast, loss of function of Runx2 in mice results in ossification defects caused by lack of osteoblasts; however, the cartilaginous templates of the endochondral bone still form (Fig. 8-2). Osterix, a zinc finger transcription factor that is downstream of Runx2, is essential for osteoblast development; in the absence of osterix, osteoblasts also do not differentiate.

Mutations in SOX9 and RUNX2 also occur in humans. Mutations in SOX9 result in **campomelic dysplasia**, typified by bowing of the long bones and defects in all endochondral bones. Campomelic dysplasia is also associated with XY sex reversal in males (covered in Chapter 16). Mutations in RUNX2 cause **cleidocranial dysplasia**, characterized by clavicular hypoplasia (which allows juxtaposition of the shoulders), large open sutures in the skull, a wide pubic symphysis, and dental abnormalities, such as delayed erupting or supernumerary teeth (covered in Chapter 17).

Striated muscle development is determined by expression of the **myogenic (or muscle) regulatory factors** (MRFs), the basic helix-loop-helix transcription factors **Myf5**, **Myf6** (previously called **Mrf4**), **MyoD**, and **myogenin (MyoG)**. A combination of Myf5, Myf6, and MyoD induces commitment of cells to the myoblast lineage, whereas myogenin, MyoD, and Myf6 are required for terminal differentiation to form **myocytes**. Myocytes are characterized by the expression of contractile proteins, such as the **myosin heavy chains** (MyHC), and they fuse to form multinucleated myofibers. The role of MRFs in muscle determination and in the molecular network regulating their expression varies in different regions of the body (see later "In the Research Lab" entitled "Regional Differences in Development of Muscles"). **Satellite cells** require the paired-box transcription factor **Pax7**; in its absence, satellite cells initiate development but fail to survive.

SOMITES DIFFERENTIATE INTO SCLEROTOME AND DERMAMYOTOME

As covered in Chapter 4, the **somites** are transient segmented structures derived from **paraxial mesoderm**.

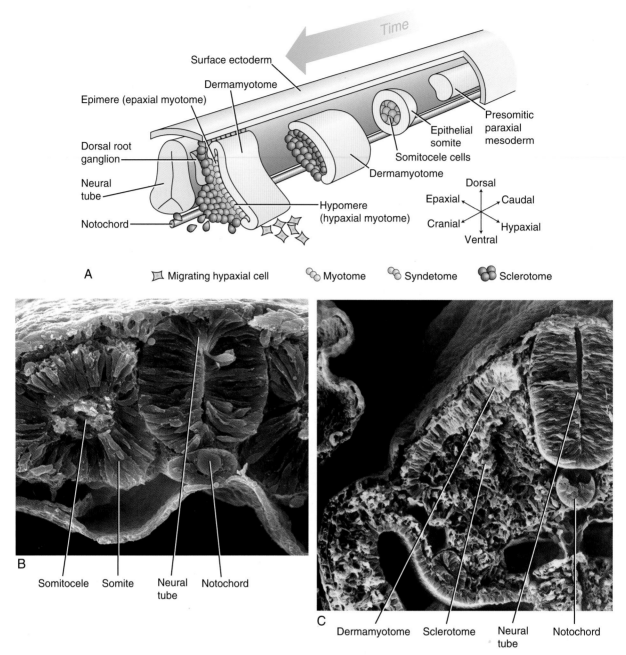

Figure 8-3. Development of the somites. *A,* With increasing time, the presomitic (unsegmented) paraxial mesoderm becomes segmented to form epithelial somites. These form two initial subdivisions: sclerotome and dermamyotome; later, the dermamyotome forms the myotome. The syndetome forms between the myotome and the sclerotome. *B, C,* Scanning electron micrographs show somites in cross-section before and after formation of the sclerotome and dermamyotome.

They contain the progenitors of the axial skeleton, trunk musculature and associated tendons, trunk dermis, endothelial cells, smooth muscle cells, brown adipose tissue, and meninges of the spinal cord. Somites are initially epithelial balls with a central cavity that contains a population of loose **core cells**—the **somitocoele** cells (Fig. 8-3*A, B*). Shortly after forming, each somite separates into subdivisions that give rise to specific mesodermal components. The ventromedial part of the somite undergoes an **epithelial-to-mesenchymal transformation**, and these cells, together with the core cells, form the **sclerotome**; after formation of the sclerotome, the remainder

of the somite consists of a dorsal epithelial layer called the **dermamyotome** (Fig. 8-3*A, C*). The sclerotome will develop into the **vertebrae** and **ribs**. As shown in Figures 8-3*A* and 8-4, cells in the ventral portion of the sclerotome migrate to surround the **notochord** and form the rudiment of the **vertebral body**; those cells in the dorsal portion of the sclerotome surround the neural tube and form the rudiment of the **vertebral arch** and **vertebral spine**; cells located more laterally in the sclerotome form the **vertebral transverse process** and **ribs**.

The dermamyotome initially retains its epithelial structure (see Fig. 8-3*C*) and contains the presumptive

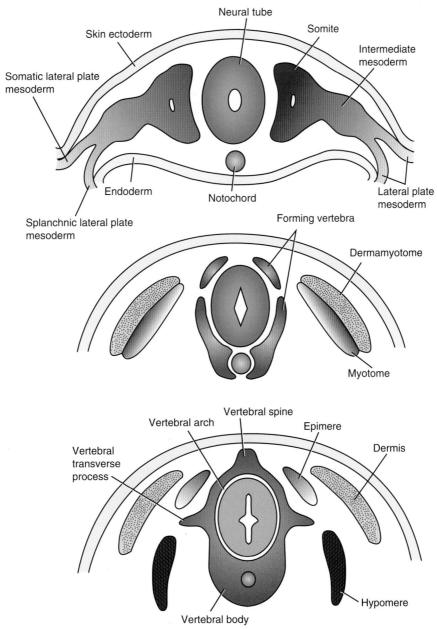

Figure 8-4. Contributions of the somites to the axial skeleton and associated structures. Subdivision of the somite involves the formation of sclerotome cells, which quickly surround the notochord, to form the rudiment of the vertebral body, and the neural tube, to form the rudiment of the vertebral arch, vertebral spine, transverse process, and ribs (not shown). With formation of the sclerotome, the dorsal part of the somite forms the dermamyotome, which quickly gives rise to the myotome. The former then forms the dermis, and the latter splits into an epimere and a hypomere, which form the epaxial and hypaxial muscles, respectively.

myogenic and dermal cells. The dermamyotome gives rise to the myotome, containing committed muscle cells (see Fig. 8-3A). The factors involved in specification and patterning of the sclerotome and myotome are covered in Chapter 4 (also see Fig. 4-27) and in the following "In the Research Lab" entitled "Subdivision of Somite."

In the Research Lab

SUBDIVISION OF SOMITE
The dermamyotome and sclerotomal compartments of the somite are specified by opposing Shh and Wnt signals from

the notochord/floor plate and the dorsal neural tube/ectoderm, respectively (see Fig. 8-15A). This is similar to the opposing roles of Shh and Wnts during specification of the dorsal-ventral axis of the neural tube (covered in Chapter 4) and otic vesicle (covered in Chapter 18). Shh, together with Bmp antagonists, is required for the early development of sclerotome, which expresses the homeobox genes, Pax1, Pax9, and Bapx1, all of which are necessary for sclerotome formation. Wnts from the roof plate and Wnts from the dorsal ectoderm specify the dermamyotome. Therefore, misexpression of Shh promotes sclerotome formation, whereas overexpression of Wnts induces a dermamyotomal fate.

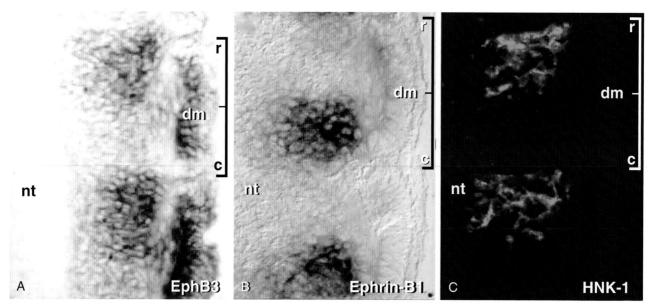

Figure 8-5. Expression patterns within the developing somites. *A, B,* EphB3 receptor and its ligand, ephrin B1, are expressed in complementary patterns in the cranial (r) and caudal (c) segments of the sclerotome. *C,* Neural crest cells (green), marked by the antibody HNK-1, migrate only through the cranial (r) half of each sclerotome and are excluded from its caudal (c) half. Brackets indicate the cranial-caudal extent of the somite. dm, dermamyotome; nt, neural tube (medial) side of each illustration.

RESEGMENTATION OF SCLEROTOMES

The sclerotome is subdivided into cranial and caudal portions based on differences in both gene expression and cell density. The caudal portion of each sclerotome is cell dense, with higher cell proliferation, whereas the cranial portion has lower cell density. These differences result in segmentation of the neural crest cells (Fig. 8-5C) and motor axons, which can migrate only toward the cranial portion of the sclerotome, as the caudal portion of the sclerotome is inhibitory for migration. This compartmentalized structure of the sclerotome is responsible for the segmentation of the peripheral nervous system (covered in Chapter 10). The division between the cranial and caudal portions of each sclerotome is characterized by a line of transversely arranged cells known as the **intrasegmental boundary**, or **von Ebner's fissure** (Fig. 8-6). In later development, the sclerotomes split along this fissure, and the caudal segment of each sclerotome fuses with the cranial segment of the sclerotome caudal to it, with each of the two segments of the sclerotome contributing to a vertebra. This process is called **resegmentation of the sclerotomes** (see Fig. 8-6). Thus, resegmentation produces vertebrae that lie **intersegmentally**.

In the Research Lab

SUBDIVISION OF SCLEROTOME
The cranial and caudal halves of each sclerotome are marked by the expression of different genes, which establish in the two halves different cell-adhesive properties. For example, the cranial half of each sclerotome expresses EphA4 and EphB3 (ephrin receptors) and Tbx18 (a T-box transcription factor), whereas the caudal half of each sclerotome expresses EphB1 and EphB4 (two other ephrin receptors), ephrin-B1 (an ephrin

ligand), delta 1 (a ligand for the notch signaling pathway), and Uncx4.1 (a homeobox-containing transcription factor); the expression patterns of EphB3 and ephrin-B1 are illustrated in Figure 8-5. It is important to note that this division of the sclerotome into cranial and caudal halves determines the migration pathway of neural crest cells and motor axons, thereby establishing the segmentation of the peripheral nervous system. Of particular relevance are the EphB3 receptor and its ligand, ephrin-B1, which together control cell mixing and segregation. As just stated, EphB3 is expressed in the cranial half of the sclerotome and in migrating neural crest cells, whereas ephrin-B1 is expressed in the caudal half of the sclerotome (see Fig. 8-5). The neural crest EphB3-expressing cells cannot mix with, and actually avoid, cells expressing the ligand ephrin-B1 (i.e., cells in the caudal half of the sclerotome). This is illustrated by plating cells on alternative strips of ephrin-B1 and non–ephrin-B1-expressing cells: neural crest cells migrate in stripes, avoiding ephrin-B1.

The fate of cells developing in different regions of the sclerotome during formation of the vertebrae is controlled by distinct genes. For example, Pax1 is required for development of the vertebral bodies and intervertebral disc, and Msx1 and Msx2 are required for the development of the vertebral spine and neural arch. Moreover, Uncx4.1 is required for the formation of the pedicles and transverse processes of the vertebrae, as well as the proximal portion of the ribs. In contrast to the regulation of Pax1 by Shh (as covered earlier in this chapter and in Chapter 4), Msx1 and Msx2 expression is regulated by Bmp4, which is expressed by the ectoderm and roof plate of the neural tube.

Development of the ribs depends on signals from the myotome, and rib anomalies are often linked to myotomal defects (e.g., in the Splotch/Pax3 mouse mutant and in Myf5/Myf6 mouse mutants). In the rib-forming regions, Myf5 and Myf6 are expressed in the hypaxial domain of the myotome, where they regulate the expression of Pdgf and Fgf4, both of which induce rib development in the underlying sclerotome. Hox genes determine the pattern of the vertebrae (see later "In the Research Lab" entitled "Specification of Vertebra Identity"), and the expression of Myf5 and Myf6 within the hypaxial domain is

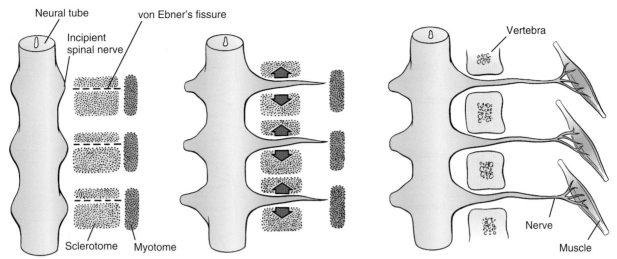

Figure 8-6. Resegmentation of the sclerotomes to form the vertebrae. Each sclerotome splits into cranial and caudal segments. As the segmental spinal nerves grow toward the cranial portion of the somite to innervate the myotomes, the cranial segment of each sclerotome recombines with the caudal segment of the next cranial sclerotome to form a vertebral rudiment.

promoted by Hox6 paralogs, which promote rib formation, and is inhibited by the Hox10 paralogs, which inhibit rib formation (see Fig. 8-11). Fgf signals from the myotome also induce scleraxis expression, which marks the **syndetome**, the tendon progenitors (see Fig. 8-3A). Therefore, the tendon progenitors are located between the developing cartilage and muscle precursors.

The sclerotomes of the most cranial four somites, the so-called occipital somites, fuse to contribute to the occipital bone of the skull base (also see Chapter 17). The more caudal somites in the series are the cervical somites. Eight cervical somites develop in the embryo, but these somites form only *seven* cervical sclerotomes. This is explained by the fact that the sclerotome of the first cervical somite is "lost" as it fuses with the caudal half of the fourth occipital sclerotome. Therefore, it contributes to the base of the skull (Fig. 8-7). The caudal half of the first cervical sclerotome then fuses with the cranial half of the second cervical sclerotome to form the first cervical vertebra (the atlas), and so on down the spine. The eighth cervical sclerotome thus contributes its cranial half to the seventh cervical vertebra and its caudal half to the first thoracic vertebra.

As a result of sclerotomal resegmentation, the intersegmental arteries, which initially passed through the sclerotomes, now pass over the vertebral body. Also, the segmental spinal nerves, which were initially growing toward the cranial portion of the sclerotome, now exit between the vertebrae. However, it is important to remember that even though there are seven cervical vertebrae, there are *eight* cervical spinal nerves. The first spinal nerve exits between the base of the skull and the first cervical vertebra (in alignment with the first cervical somite); thus, the eighth spinal nerve exits above the first thoracic vertebra (in alignment with the eighth cervical somite). From this point onward, each spinal nerve exits just below the vertebra of the same number (see Fig. 8-7). Finally, each sclerotome is associated with an overlying myotome, which contains the developing muscle plate

(see Fig. 8-6). Therefore, after resegmentation, the myotome that was initially associated with one sclerotome becomes attached to two adjacent vertebrae and crosses the intervertebral space.

The fibrous intervertebral discs develop at the intrasegmental boundary (Fig. 8-8). The original core of each disc is composed of cells of notochordal origin (see Fig. 8-4) that produce a gelatinous and proteoglycan-rich core, the **nucleus pulposus**, whereas the surrounding **annulus fibrosus** develops from sclerotomal cells that are left in the region of the resegmentating sclerotome as its cranial and caudal halves split apart.

Small lateral mesenchymal condensations called **costal processes** develop in association with the vertebral arches of all developing neck and trunk vertebrae (Fig. 8-9A). Concomitantly, transverse processes grow laterally along the dorsal side of each costal process. In the cervical vertebrae, the costal and transverse processes give rise to the lateral and medial boundaries of the **foramina transversaria** (or **transverse foramen**) that transmit the vertebral arteries. In the lumbar region, the costal processes do not project distally and contribute to the transverse processes. The costal processes of the first two or three sacral vertebrae contribute to development of the lateral sacral mass, or **ala**, of the **sacrum**.

However, in the thoracic region, the distal tips of the costal processes lengthen to form **ribs** (see Fig. 8-9A). The ribs begin to form and lengthen on day thirty-five. The first seven ribs connect ventrally to the sternum via **costal cartilages** by day forty-five and are called the **true ribs**. The five lower ribs do not articulate directly with the sternum and are called the **false ribs**. The ribs develop as cartilaginous precursors that later ossify by endochondral ossification.

The sternum develops from a pair of longitudinal mesenchymal condensations, the **sternal bars**, which form in the ventrolateral body wall (Fig. 8-9B). As the most cranial ribs make contact with them in the seventh week, the sternal bars meet along the midline and begin to fuse. Fusion commences at the cranial end of the sternal bars

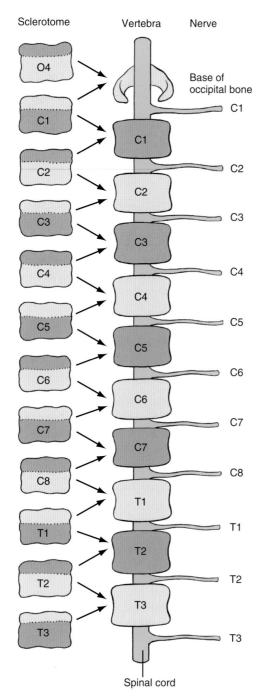

Figure 8-7. Sclerotome / Vertebra / Nerve

Figure 8-7. The mechanism by which the cervical region develops eight cervical nerves but only seven cervical vertebrae. The ventral roots of spinal nerves grow out from the spinal cord toward the sclerotome. With resegmentation of the sclerotomes, the cranial half of the first cervical sclerotome fuses with the occipital bone of the skull. As a result, the nerve projecting to the first cervical somite is now located cranial to the first cervical vertebrae. In the thoracic, lumbar, and sacral regions, the number of spinal nerves matches the number of vertebrae.

and progresses caudally, finishing with formation of the xiphoid process in the ninth week. Like the ribs, the sternal bones ossify from cartilaginous precursors. The sternal bars ossify from the fifth month until shortly after birth, producing the definitive bones of the **sternum**: **manubrium, body of the sternum**, and **xiphoid process**. The ribs inhibit ossification within the sternum.

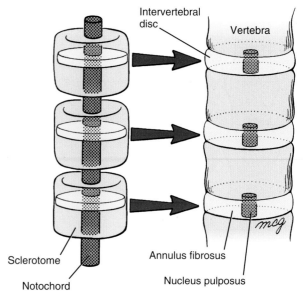

Figure 8-8. Contributions of the sclerotome and notochord to the intervertebral disc. When the sclerotome splits, cells remaining in the plane of division coalesce to form the annulus fibrosus of the disc, and the notochordal cells enclosed by this structure differentiate to form the nucleus pulposus of the disc. The regions of the notochord enclosed by the developing vertebral bodies degenerate and disappear.

In the Research Lab

SPECIFICATION OF VERTEBRA IDENTITY

Although somites throughout the trunk are morphologically indistinguishable from one another, they become specified to form structures characteristic of particular body levels. Moreover, the characteristic development of specific vertebrae seems to be related to the intrinsic properties of their particular somitic precursor. Somites transplanted to another region form structures typical of the region of their origin. For example, thoracic somites transplanted to the lumbar region form typical thoracic vertebrae and ribs at the ectopic lumbar site. Based on experiments such as these, together with more recent genetic loss and gain-of-function experiments, it is now known that somites acquire their regional specificity in the paraxial mesoderm before its segmentation into somites.

Specific numbers of presumptive cervical, thoracic, lumbar, sacral, and coccygeal somites are formed in human embryos, which results in a relatively invariant number of each type of vertebrae (seven, twelve, five, five, and four, respectively). However, significant variation in the numbers of somites and vertebrae occurs among different vertebrate organisms. For example, the number of cervical vertebrae in amphibians is only three or four, whereas the number of cervical vertebrae in geese is seventeen. Mice and even giraffes possess the same number of cervical vertebrae as humans (seven), but mice have thirteen (not twelve) thoracic vertebrae, six (not five) lumbar vertebrae, and four (not five) sacral vertebrae. Snakes have hundreds of vertebrae, whereas frogs have ten or fewer vertebrae. What factors specify regional differences in the vertebrae? And how is the number of vertebrae in any given region determined? Both of these questions can now be answered by understanding the regulation and expression of Hox genes.

It is interesting to note that a unique combination of Hox gene expression occurs at virtually every segment of the trunk, with the most cranial expression of some Hox gene paralogs, as shown by in situ hybridization or use of the LacZ reporter gene, occurring at major boundaries between trunk levels.

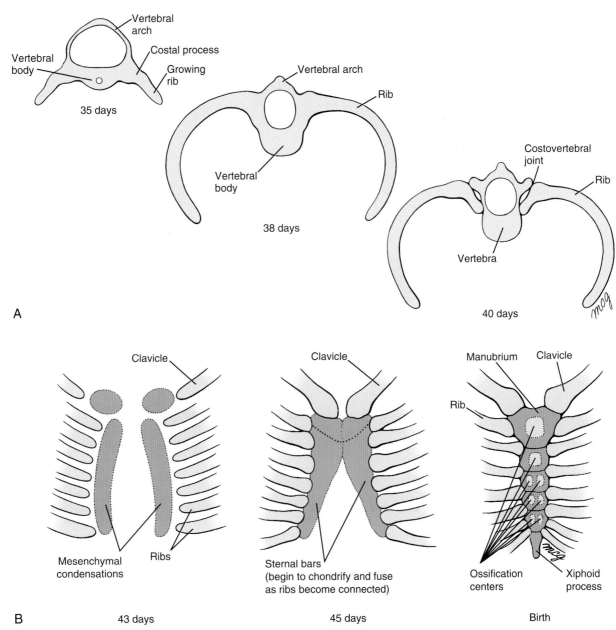

Figure 8-9. Development of the ribs and sternum. *A,* The costal processes of the vertebrae in the thoracic region begin to elongate in the fifth week to form the ribs. Late in the fifth week, the costovertebral joints form and separate the ribs from the vertebrae. *B,* Paired mesenchymal condensations called sternal bars form within the ventral body wall at the end of the sixth week. These bars quickly fuse together at their cranial ends, while their lateral edges connect with the distal ends of the growing ribs. The sternal bars then fuse across the midline in a cranial-to-caudal direction. Ossification centers appear within the sternum as early as sixty days, but the xiphoid process does not ossify until birth.

For example, during early somitogenesis, the cranial expression boundary of the Hox6 paralogs is grouped at the cervical/thoracic boundary, Hox10 paralogs tend to fall at the thoracic/lumbar transition, and Hox11 paralogs fall at the lumbar/sacral boundary (Fig. 8-10). This organization of gene expression is consistent with a leading model for the specification of Homc arthropod (i.e., insect) segments, namely, that homeotic genes specify segment diversity through a **combinatorial code**.

Consistent with this model, loss of an individual Hox gene (e.g., Hoxc9) changes the combinatorial code, resulting in the homeotic transformation of one or two vertebrae (i.e., the identity of one or two of the vertebrae transforms into that of another vertebra). Additional loss of the paralogous genes (e.g., Hoxc9 together with the loss of Hoxb9 and Hoxd9) significantly affects vertebrae

development by resulting in anterior homeotic transformations (i.e., **"cranialization"**) of several somitic segments of the trunk. The regions affected by loss of the Hox paralogous genes are summarized in Figure 8-11*A*. Following loss of Hox4 paralogs, C2-C5 vertebrae are transformed into vertebrae with C1 characteristics, and loss of Hox5 paralogs transforms the vertebrae between C3 and T2 to a C2-like morphology. The Hox9 paralogs are required for the development of floating ribs versus those attached to the sternum. Loss of all Hox10 paralogs results in loss of vertebrae with lumbar characteristics—these develop as thoracic vertebrae, complete with ribs (Fig. 8-11*B*), whereas following loss of the Hox11 paralogs, the sacral region acquires lumbar characteristics.

Conversely, gain of Hox gene expression **"caudalizes"** the vertebrae. Gain of function of Hox6 induces rib development in

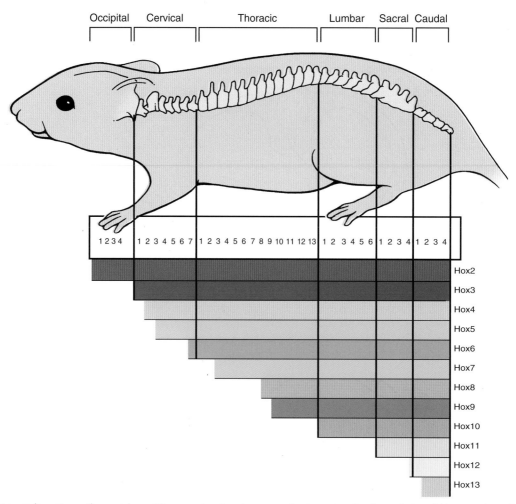

Figure 8-10. Hox code patterns the vertebrae. Diagram showing the approximate expression boundaries of Hox paralogs along the cranial-caudal axis of the body. Hox genes are expressed in nested patterns along the cranial-caudal axis, with each vertebra, or small groups of vertebrae, having a distinct combinatorial Hox code. The boundaries of some Hox genes correlate with changes in vertebrae identity and the formation of appendages (i.e., the forelimbs always form at the cervical to thoracic boundary, whereas the hindlimbs always form at the lumbar to sacral boundary). This correlation between Hox gene expression and identity of vertebrae is conserved across species.

every vertebra. Hox10 misexpression respecifies thoracic vertebrae to form vertebrae with lumbar characteristics, that is, they lack ribs (Fig. 8-11C). This effect is opposite to the effect that occurs with loss of the Hox10 paralog group described above. Misexpression of Hox6 or Hox10 in the presomitic mesoderm or later in the somites has different effects. Only when Hox6 or Hox10 is misexpressed in the presomitic mesoderm are the vertebrae transformed. In contrast, misexpression later, after somitogenesis has occurs, results in relatively minor abnormalities.

The nested anterior-posterior pattern of Hox gene expression is established during gastrulation and tail bud stages and is refined during early somitogenesis. Hox genes are expressed as the paraxial mesodermal cells ingress through the primitive streak (covered in Chapter 3). Cells that express the more 3′ Hox (i.e., anterior) genes ingress ahead of cells that express the more 5′ Hox (i.e., posterior) genes. The timing of ingression can be altered experimentally by changing Hox gene expression. Ectopic expression of the 5′ Hox genes delays ingression, whereas ectopic expression of the 3′ Hox genes promotes ingression. In this way, a nested pattern of Hox gene expression is established along the anterior-posterior axis.

In addition to controlling the specification of vertebra type, Hox genes control axis elongation. The last cells to form express the most 5′ Hox genes (e.g., Hoxb13), and this decreases the

Wnt3a expression required for cell proliferation and maintenance of the presomitic mesoderm. The decrease in Wnt3a also uncouples the balance between antagonistic Wnt/Fgf and retinoic acid signals required for somite formation (see Chapter 4), and retinoic acid now promotes apoptosis within the presomitic mesoderm, also preventing further somite formation. Premature initiation of Hoxb13 expression results in truncation of the axial skeleton. Conversely, more vertebrae are formed in the absence of Hoxb13.

During gastrulation and in the presomitic mesoderm after gastrulation, the expression of Hox genes is regulated by Wnt, Bmp11 (also known as Gdf11), and retinoid signaling. Therefore, changes in these signals can result in homeotic transformations. **Retinoic acid** regulates Hox gene expression, in part by the induction of another homeobox gene called **caudal**. Genetic loss of function of two or more members of the family of **retinoic acid receptors** results in the **cranialization** of vertebral segments (Fig. 8-12). This cranialization is similar to that observed in the homeotic null mutations of Hox genes described above. Conversely, the ectopic application of excess retinoic acid results in the **caudalization** of vertebral segments, similar to that occurring in the Hox "homeotic" gain-of-function mutant (see Fig. 8-12). This is similar to retinoic acid regulation of Hox gene expression in the hindbrain, which determines rhombomere identity (covered in Chapters 9

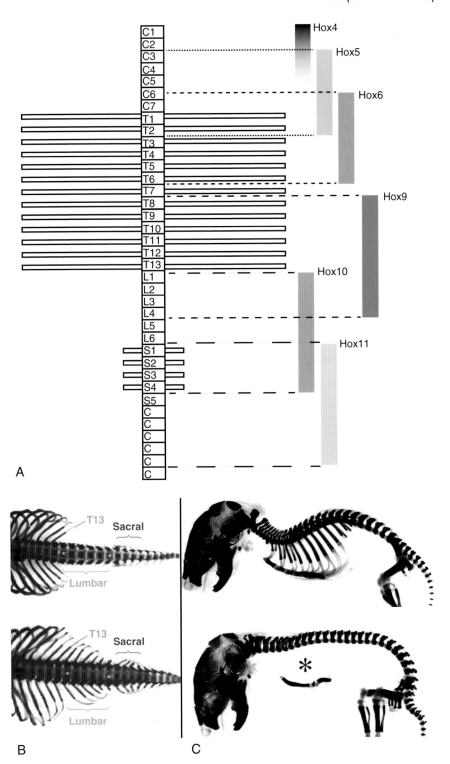

A

B

C

Figure 8-11. Homeotic transformations. *A,* Diagram showing which Hox genes specify the different types of vertebrae. *B,* Loss of the Hox10 paralogs converts lumbar and sacral vertebrae into thoracic vertebrae complete with ribs. *C,* Gain of Hoxa10 function in the presomitic mesoderm converts thoracic vertebrae into lumbar vertebrae lacking ribs. The sternum forms in the area superficial to (below) the asterisk.

and 17). Loss of Bmp11 results in the cranialization of vertebrae, whereas loss of Wnt3a differentially affects the expression of members of the Hox gene family: there is caudalization of the mid-thoracic vertebrae, together with cranialization of the sacral vertebrae.

The mechanism by which segmental identity is achieved in vertebrates is undoubtedly far more complex than is implied by this brief consideration, and neither a combinatorial Hox code nor posterior prevalence models (i.e., in which the identity of the vertebra is determined by expression of the most posterior, that is, most 5′ Hox gene) can totally explain the observations. For example, in

contrast to the loss-of-function Hox mutations covered above, a loss-of-function mutation of Hoxa6 has been shown to caudalize the seventh cervical vertebra, as indicated by its development of a rib. Some other Hox gene knockouts simultaneously cranialize one region of the spine and caudalize another region. Thus, although retinoic acid and Hox genes seem to play a role in cranial-caudal specification of the vertebrae, they may only establish the general pattern of regional specification. Other factors, including the ability of some members of the Hox family to antagonize the function of other Hox genes, may fine-tune the regulation of specific segmental differentiation.

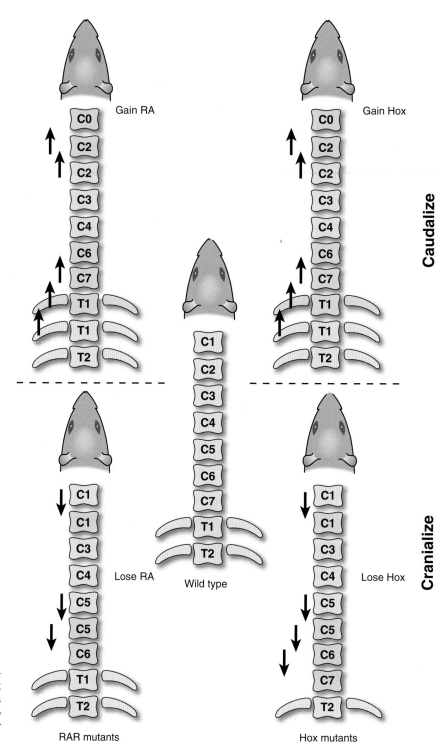

Figure 8-12. Homeotic transformations following gain (drawings at top) and loss (drawings at bottom) of either Hox gene function (drawings to right) or retinoid acid signaling (drawings to left). Wild-type condition is shown in the center drawing.

In the Clinic

VERTEBRAL DEFECTS

A number of spinal defects are caused by abnormal induction of the sclerotomes. **Spina bifida occulta** or **cleft vertebrae**, wherein the neural tube itself is morphologically unaffected (i.e., it is closed), is caused by abnormal induction of the vertebral arch rudiments by the neural tube/ectoderm. Defective induction and morphogenesis of vertebral bodies on one side of the body may result in a severe congenital **scoliosis** (lateral bending of the spinal column), which may require surgical correction. Cleft vertebrae may be a secondary consequence of failure of neural tube closure, as in **spina bifida aperta**. Spina bifida is further covered in Chapter 4.

Vertebrae, together with rib anomalies, may show isolated defects, such as in a heterogeneous group of conditions including **spondylothoracic** and **spondylocostal dysostosis**. Typically, spondylocostal dysostosis is characterized by vertebral defects throughout the spine, such as hemivertebrae, rib fusions, and kyphoscoliosis (spine curvature in both lateral and anterior-posterior planes) (Fig. 8-13A). Mutations in DELTA-3, a ligand for the NOTCH signaling pathway; LUNATIC FRINGE, an intracellular factor that modulates NOTCH receptors, thereby altering their affinity for their ligands; and two downstream transcriptional targets of NOTCH signaling, HES7 and MESP2, can cause spondylocostal dysostosis (see Fig. 8-13A). All of the above-mentioned genes are linked to the notch signaling pathway and are necessary for functioning of the segmentation clock and, consequently, somitogenesis (covered in Chapter 4).

Vertebral defects may also be restricted to specific regions of the spine, such as **cervicothoracic dysostosis** (previously known as **Klippel-Feil anomaly**) (Fig. 8-13B), which affects the cervical and thoracic vertebrae such that the neck is shorter with restricted movement (cervical vertebrae are sometimes fused). Vertebral defects, which are easily identifiable in prenatal screens, may also indicate an organized condition such as **VATER/VACTERL** (vertebral-anal-cardiac-tracheo-esophageal-renal-limb), **Alagille**, and **CHARGE** syndromes (these conditions are also covered in Chapters 3, 5, and 12 through 14). In **Alagille syndrome** (resulting from mutations in JAGGED1, a NOTCH ligand, or NOTCH2), butterfly vertebrae are a feature in approximately 60% of cases (Fig. 8-13C).

MYOTOMES DEVELOP AT SEGMENTAL LEVELS

As mentioned above, as the sclerotome forms, the dorsal part of the somite remains epithelial and is called the **dermamyotome**. This structure then gives rise to the **myotome** (Fig. 8-14; also see Figs. 8-3A and 8-4) and the dermis (including fat and connective tissue) of the neck and the back. However, as covered in Chapter 7, most of the dermis is derived from somatopleuric lateral plate mesoderm (also, as covered in Chapter 17, the dermis of the face is derived from neural crest cells).

The myotomes consist of myogenic (muscle-producing) cells (see Fig. 8-14). Each myotome splits into two structures: a dorsal **epimere** and a ventral **hypomere** (see Figs. 8-3A and 8-4). The epimeres give rise to the deep **epaxial muscles** of the back, including the **erector spinae** and **transversospinalis** groups. These are innervated by the **dorsal ramus of the spinal nerve**. The hypomeres form the **hypaxial muscles** of the lateral and ventral body wall in the thorax and abdomen. These are innervated by the **ventral ramus of the spinal nerve**. The hypaxial muscles include three layers of **intercostal muscles** in the thorax (**external** and **inner intercostals**, and **innermost intercostals**), the homologous three layers of the abdominal musculature (**external oblique, internal oblique**, and **transversus abdominis**), and the **rectus abdominis** muscles that flank the ventral midline. The rectus column is usually limited to the abdominal region, but occasionally it develops on either side of the sternum as a **sternalis muscle**. In the cervical region, hypaxial myoblasts, together with the occipital lateral plate mesoderm, form the strap muscles of the neck, including the **scalene** and **infrahyoid** muscles. In the lumbar region, the hypomeres form the **quadratus lumborum** muscles. The limb and tongue muscles arise from the hypaxial dermamyotome. At limb-forming levels, premyogenic cells

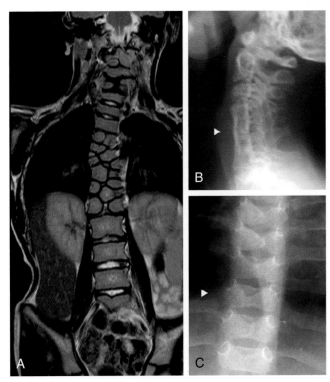

Figure 8-13. Different types of vertebral defects. *A*, Patient with an MESP2 mutation showing severe vertebral segmentation defects. *B*, Cervical dysostosis showing fused cervical vertebral bodies (arrowhead). *C*, Alagille syndrome showing "butterfly" vertebrae (arrowhead marks one vertebra; note the deep midline cleft in each vertebra).

arise from the hypaxial dermamyotome and invade the developing limb buds to give rise to the **limb** musculature (see Figs. 8-21 and 8-23). In the occipital region, somitic (i.e., occipital; covered in Chapter 17) myoblasts arise from the hypaxial dermamyotome and migrate along the hypoglossal cord to form the **intrinsic** and **extrinsic tongue musculature**. The tendons connecting the muscle and vertebrae arise from the **syndetome** region of the somite between the developing sclerotome and the myotome (see Fig. 8-3A).

In the Research Lab

DEVELOPMENT OF DERMAMYOTOME AND MYOTOME

The dermamyotome is a transient multipotent structure that gives rise, under the control of different signaling factors, to endothelial cells, vascular smooth muscle cells, skeletal muscle including satellite cells, dorsal dermis, and brown adipose tissue. Initial myogenic commitment occurs with the dorsomedial lip (DML) in response to Wnt signals from the dorsal neural tube, notch signals from the migrating neural crest, Shh from the notochord and floor plate, and activation of noggin expression within the DML (Fig. 8-15A). Noggin blocks the repressive action of Bmps (produced by both the dorsal neural tube and the ectoderm), resulting in the onset of Myf5 expression. During primary myogenesis, myogenic cells from the DML (the "pioneer cells") delaminate and enter the myotome to form postmitotic myocytes. This is followed by the entry of myogenic cells from all edges of the dermamyotome (Fig. 8-15A). These myogenic cells fuse with the pioneer cells to form multinucleated

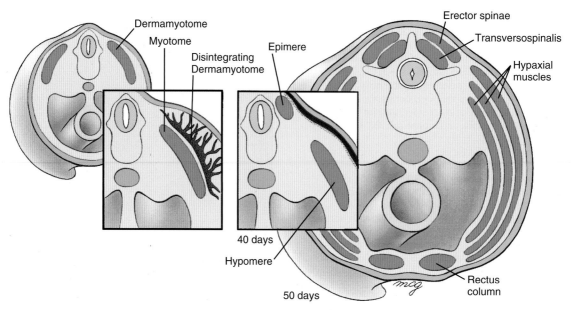

Figure 8-14. Fate of the dermamyotome and myotome. The dermamyotome gives rise to the subjacent myotome and dermis. Dermal precursor cells migrate to the surface ectoderm of the corresponding segmental region. There, with cells from the lateral plate mesoderm, they form the dermis. Each myotome splits first into a dorsal epimere and ventral hypomere. The epimere forms the deep muscles of the back. In the thoracic region, the hypomere splits into three layers of the anterolateral muscles (external oblique, internal oblique, and transversus abdominis); in the abdominal region, a fourth ventral segment also differentiates and forms the rectus abdominis muscle.

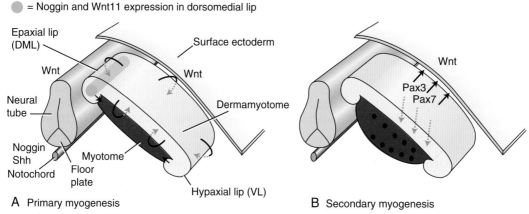

Figure 8-15. Development of the myotome. *A,* Myogenic cells in the myotome first form from the edges of the dermamyotome (i.e., the epaxial or dorsomedial lip, DML, and the hypaxial or ventrolateral lip, VL, and cranial and caudal borders) in response to Wnt signals from the dorsal neural tube and ectoderm, Shh from the notochord and floor plate, and notch from migrating neural crest (not shown), together with noggin antagonism of Bmp signaling. Arrows indicate the directions of cell movements from the dermamyotome into the myotome during primary myogenesis. Wnt11 (within the DML) controls the polarized migration and elongation of the myocytes during the establishment of the myotome. *B,* Myogenic precursors populate the myotome from the central region of the dermamyotome, which expresses Pax3 and Pax7. These contribute to later phases of growth. The dermamyotome also gives rise to cells in the dermis. Arrows indicate cell movements from the dermamyotome into the myotome (curved and straight arrows) during primary myogenesis (*A*), and from the dermamyotome into the myotome (dashed arrows giving rise to cells colored black) and from the dermamyotome into the dermis (solid arrows) during later development (*B*).

myofibers. The myocytes are aligned and elongate along the anterior-posterior axis of the myotome. This polarized behavior is controlled by Wnt11 expression in the DML, which acts through the PCP signaling pathway. During secondary myogenesis, uncommitted proliferative cells enter the myotome from the central region of the dermamyotome, which expresses Pax3 and Pax7. The cells in the central dermamyotome are bipotential and divide perpendicularly to the dermamyotome: those that enter the myotome give rise to muscle cells during secondary myogenesis in the fetus, as well as to satellite cells, which will give rise to myocytes postnatally. These cells maintain Pax3 and

Pax7 expression. The other cells arising from these divisions do not express these genes and form the dermis under the control of canonical Wnt signaling.

Proliferation and differentiation of Pax3/Pax7 expressing cells is controlled by notch, Fgfs, and myostatin. Notch is required for the self-renewal of cells, whereas Fgfs and myostatin (also known as Gdf8, growth differentiation factor 8, a member of the Tgfβ family) promote terminal differentiation. Naturally occurring mutations in **myostatin** happened in large doubled-muscled cattle, such as Belgian Blue and Piedmontese, and in the Texel breed of sheep. The large muscles in these breeds

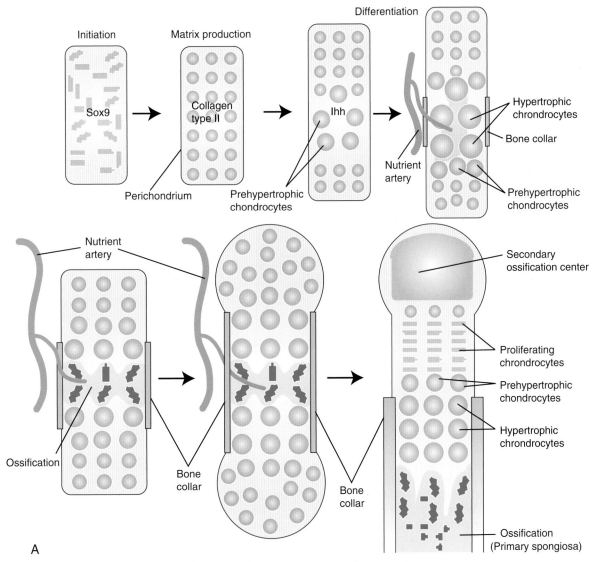

Figure 8-16. Long bone development. *A,* Summary of events.

Continued

are a result of muscle hyperplasia and hypertrophy. Myostatin mutations also occur in the Whippet breed of dogs; Whippets heterozygous for myostatin mutations are able to run faster. MYOSTATIN mutations have also been reported in humans and are linked to increased muscle strength.

LONG BONE AND JOINT DEVELOPMENT

With the exception of part of the clavicle, the bones of the limbs and girdles (constituting the **appendicular skeleton**) form by **endochondral ossification**. Part of the clavicle, in contrast, is a **membrane bone**.

Most of the endochondral bones of the limb are long bones. Their development begins as mesenchymal cells condense, which is characterized by the expression of Sox9 (long bone development is summarized in Fig. 8-16A). In response to growth factors, **chondrocytes** differentiate within this mesenchyme and begin to secrete molecules characteristic of the extracellular matrix of cartilage, such as collagen type II and proteoglycans.

Distinct layers of chondrocytes appear with formation of the prehypertrophic and then hypertrophic chondrocytes (see Fig. 8-16A). Progenitor cells for cartilage growth, the resting chondrocytes, are located at the ends, or **epiphyses**, of the long bone (Fig. 8-16B). Toward the center, or **diaphysis**, of the long bone is a proliferating layer of chondrocytes, then a **prehypertrophic** zone in which the chondrocytes have enlarged. Finally, at the center are enlarged, terminally differentiated, or **hypertrophic** chondrocytes that are surrounded by calcified matrix (see Fig. 8-16A, B). Hypertrophic chondrocytes express collagen type X.

Following terminal differentiation (i.e., hypertrophy), the process of **ossification** commences in the **primary ossification center** at the center of the long bone (see Fig. 8-16A). Ossification begins when the developing bone is invaded by multiple blood vessels that branch from the limb vasculature (covered in Chapter 13). One of these vessels eventually becomes dominant and gives rise to the **nutrient artery** that nourishes the bone. Establishment of the vasculature brings in the preosteoblastic cells that differentiate into osteoblasts and replace

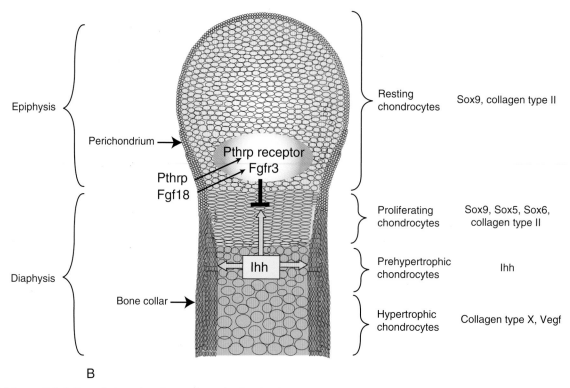

B

Figure 8-16, cont'd *B,* Four distinct chondrocyte layers in the developing cartilage element. Indian hedgehog (Ihh), parathyroid hormone–related protein (Pthrp), and Fgf18 are three of the crucial genes that regulate the differentiation of the chondrocytes.

the hypertrophic chondrocytes forming the **primary spongiosa.** The osteoblasts lay down collagen type I and mineralized matrix. Ossification spreads from the primary ossification center toward the epiphyses of the rudiment to form a loose **trabecular network** of bone.

In addition to osteoblasts, the blood vessels bring in cells called **osteoclasts,** which break down previously formed bone. These are important for remodeling of the growing bone. Bone is continually remodeled throughout development and adult life.

The region surrounding the diaphysis ossifies to form a **primary bone collar** around the circumference of the bone. This primary bone collar thickens as osteoblasts differentiate in progressively more peripheral layers of the perichondrium to form **cortical bone.**

At birth, the **diaphyses**—or shafts of the limb bones (consisting of a bone collar and trabecular core)—are completely ossified, whereas the ends of the bones, called the **epiphyses,** are still cartilaginous. After birth, **secondary ossification centers** develop in the epiphyses, which gradually ossify (see Fig. 8-16A). However, a layer of cartilage called the **epiphyseal cartilage plate (growth plate** or **physis)** persists between the epiphysis and the growing end of the diaphysis (**metaphysis).** In the epiphyseal cartilage plate, distinct zones of chondrocytes are present (proliferating and flattened, prehypertophic and hypertrophic), which are arranged in columns directing growth along the long axis (see Fig. 8-16A). Continued proliferation of the chondrocytes, followed by differentiation and replacement by bone in this growth plate, allows the diaphysis to lengthen. Finally,

when growth of the body is complete at about twenty years of age, the epiphyseal growth plate completely ossifies.

The process of ossification is similar in other endochondral bones, although some cartilage elements such as cartilages of the larynx, intervertebral discs, and pinna do not ossify. The chondrocostal cartilages also remain unossified until about fifty years of age.

Figure 8-17 illustrates the process of development of the **diarthrodial (synovial) joints,** which connect the limb bones. First, the mesenchyme of the interzones between the chondrifying bone primordia differentiates into **fibroblastic tissue** (undifferentiated connective tissue). Then, at the proximal and distal ends, this tissue differentiates into **articular cartilage** covering the two facing bone primordia, which are separated by a region of dense connective tissue. The connective tissue of this central region gives rise to the internal elements of the joint. Proximally and distally, it condenses to form the **synovial tissue** that will line the future joint cavity. Its central zone gives rise to the **menisci** and **enclosed joint ligaments,** such as the cruciate ligaments of the knee. Vacuoles form within connective tissue and coalesce (i.e., the central region of the dense connective tissue cavitates) to form the **synovial cavity** filled with a lubricating and anti-adhesive liquid that permits joint movement. The **joint capsule** also arises from the interzone.

Synchondroidal or **fibrous joints,** such as those connecting the bones of the pelvis, also develop from interzones. However, the interzone mesenchyme simply differentiates into a single layer of fibrocartilage.

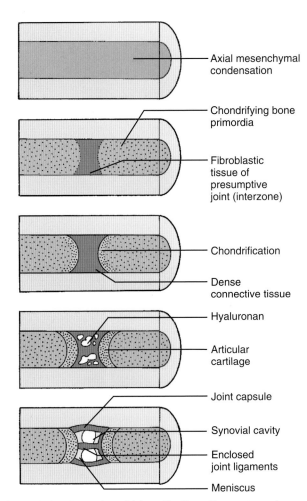

Axial mesenchymal condensation

Chondrifying bone primordia

Fibroblastic tissue of presumptive joint (interzone)

Chondrification

Dense connective tissue

Hyaluronan

Articular cartilage

Joint capsule

Synovial cavity

Enclosed joint ligaments

Meniscus

Figure 8-17. Formation of joints. Cartilage, ligaments, and capsular elements of the joints develop from the interzone regions of the axial mesenchymal condensations that form the long bones of the limbs.

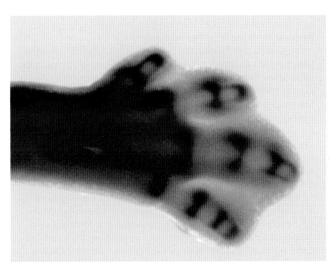

Figure 8-18. Expression of Gdf5 in the developing joint interzones of the autopod.

In the Research Lab

MOLECULAR REGULATION OF BONE AND JOINT DEVELOPMENT

Not only is an understanding of skeletal development essential for the understanding of human syndromes, it can also be used to devise strategies to repair postnatal pathologies, such as loss of bone mass following menopause and degeneration of articular cartilage that has limited capacity to repair. In addition, it is now known that hardening of the arteries occurs as the result of activation of Bmp signaling and expression of Runx2 in vascular smooth muscle cells. In this instance, embryonic processes are recapitulated erroneously in the adult, causing pathology and disease.

Chondrogenesis requires Bmp and Fgf signaling, which results in cell condensation owing to the increased expression of cell adhesion molecules such as N-cadherin. The condensing cells start to express Sox9, which in turn regulates the expression of collagen type II (Fig. 8-16A). In the absence of Sox9, cartilaginous condensations do not form. Sox5 and Sox6, which are coexpressed with Sox9 slightly later during differentiation, are also required for chondrogenesis (see Fig. 8-16B). In Sox5, 6 double mouse mutants, the early cartilage condensation forms, but the cells do not differentiate.

Once the chondrocyte layers and the perichondrium—the fibroblastic layer surrounding the cartilaginous element—have formed, development of the skeleton involves an interplay between the perichondrium and the chondrocytes (see Fig. 8-16B).

The expression of Sox9, which inhibits prehypertrophy, now becomes restricted to the epiphyseal chondrocytes. As cells divide, the orientation and stacking of chondrocytes are controlled by Wnt-PCP signaling. There are three key regulators of the rate of chondrocyte proliferation and maturation: Indian hedgehog (Ihh), parathyroid hormone–related protein (PthrP), and Fgf18. Fgf18 is expressed in the perichondrium and reduces the rate of proliferation and differentiation in the flattened/proliferating chondrocytes, which express Fgfr3. Signaling via Fgfr3 induces the expression of the cell cycle inhibitor, p21. In the absence of Fgf18 or Fgfr3, there is an expanded zone of proliferation and an increase in the length of bones, whereas gain of function of Fgf signaling results in truncation of limb bones (see the following "In the Clinic" entitled "Defects in Skeletal Development").

Ihh is expressed by the prehypertrophic chondrocytes and signals to the periarticular perichondrium to induce the expression of Pthrp. Pthrp expression in turn signals to the proliferating and prehypertrophic chondrocytes, which express the Pthrp receptor. This signaling loop prevents hypertrophy. Ihh also promotes chondrocyte proliferation independently of PthrP. In both mice and humans, mutations in Ihh or Pthrp result in short limbs due to premature hypertrophy and a depletion of the progenitor pool.

Hypertrophy requires the Runx2 and Runx3 transcription factors. Hypertrophy is induced by canonical Wnt and Ihh signaling and is inhibited by Bmps. Runx2 induces the expression of collagen type X and vascular endothelial growth factor (Vegf), which, as in other regions of the body, promotes vascularization (covered in Chapter 13).

The joints arise from the developing interzone, which is characterized by the expression of growth differentiation factors (Gdf) 5/6 (members of the Bmp family), noggin (a Bmp antagonist), and Wnts (specifically, Wnt9a—previously called Wnt14—and Wnt4), which act via the β-catenin pathway (Fig. 8-18). Fate mapping studies have shown that the interzone gives rise to the articular cartilage, synovial lining, ligaments, and capsule tissue. In the joint interzone, Bmp antagonists and Wnts regulate joint development by preventing chondrogenic differentiation, whereas Gdf5/6 promotes chondrogenesis. Thus, the joint interzone is characterized by chondrogenic and anti-chondrogenic activities that may be necessary for the development of distinct cell types (e.g., articular cartilage versus synovial lining) within the developing joint. The transcription factor Erg, which is also expressed in the interzone, is thought to maintain the articular chondrocyte phenotype, preventing terminal chondrocyte differentiation.

Following specification of the joint, its cavitation to form the joint (synovial) cavity is achieved by the secretion of hyaluronan (also called hyaluronic acid or hyaluronate, a glycosaminoglycan that readily absorbs water, thereby creating tissue spaces). Movement promotes hyaluronan synthesis; if movement is prevented during development (e.g., by neuromuscular paralysis), the joints either do not cavitate, or, if they have started to cavitate, they fuse and the joint becomes fixed. Therefore, lack of movement due to a constricted space (e.g., too little amniotic fluid) may contribute to **arthrogryposis**—fusion, stiffening, or deformation of joints.

Endochondral bone development and joint development are interconnected. For example, loss of Ihh signaling affects joint morphogenesis, as the interzone does not form appropriately. Conversely, factors from the developing joint such as Gdf5 signal to adjacent skeletal elements to control chondrocyte proliferation. This explains the shortening of the appendicular cartilage elements in Brachypod (Gdf5) mutant mice and in humans with GDF5 mutations (see the following "In the Clinic" entitled "Defects in Skeletal Development").

Osteoblast development is controlled by the transcription factors, Runx2 and osterix, and requires canonical Wnt signaling, Ihh, and Tgfβ/Bmp (see the following "In the Clinic" entitled "Defects in Skeletal Development"). Runx2 induces differentiation of the early pre-osteoblast, thereby preventing its mesenchymal cell precursor from forming other cell types, whereas β-catenin signaling and osterix are required for further differentiation into osteoblasts. Terminal differentiation of osteoblasts (i.e., the formation of osteocytes) requires the transcription factor Atf4.

Osteoclast development depends on osteoblasts. First, osteoblasts express macrophage colony-stimulating factor, which promotes the proliferation and survival of osteoclast precursors and upregulates the expression of a receptor called Rank (receptor activator of nuclear factor kappa B). Osteoblasts also express the ligand Rankl, which binds to the Rank receptor on osteoclasts and osteoclast precursors. This interaction promotes differentiation of the osteoclasts and activates mature osteoclasts. Emphasizing this importance, gene inactivation of Rank or Rankl results in a complete absence of osteoclasts.

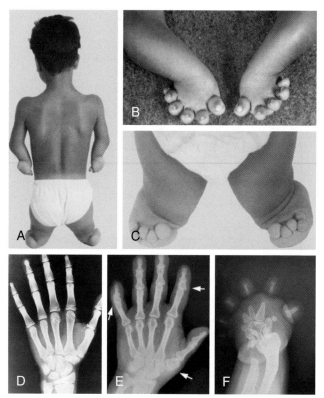

Figure 8-19. Mutations in GDF5 cause Grebe-type chondrodysplasia. All skeletal abnormalities are restricted to the limb. *A*, Ten-year-old boy with a GDF5 mutation showing severe lower limb and upper limb anomalies. *B, C*, Enlarged views of the upper and lower limbs, respectively. *D*, X-ray of a normal hand of a 10-year-old child. *E*, X-ray of a hand of a child with a heterozygous mutation; note shortened phalangeal elements (marked with arrows). *F*, X-ray of a hand of a child with a homozygous mutation; note the severe carpal and phalangeal anomalies, as well as distal anomalies of the radius and ulna.

In the Clinic

DEFECTS IN SKELETAL DEVELOPMENT

Defects in skeletal development may be the result of defects in growth factor signaling (e.g., FGF and GDF5), transcription factors (e.g., SOX9 and RUNX2), and matrix components (COLLAGENS TYPES I, II, and X). These can include syndromes where all endochondral bones are affected, such as **achondroplasia**. Alternatively, these can include conditions in which a subset of skeletal structures is affected, as in **Grebe-type chondrodysplasia** (Fig. 8-19), which specifically affects the appendicular skeleton, or as in spondylocostal dysplasia syndromes, covered earlier in this chapter. Similarly, membranous bones can be specifically affected, as in **craniosynostosis** (covered in the first "In the Clinic" of Chapter 17 entitled "Craniosynostosis"). Defects in skeletal development may be linked to changes in patterning, as in some spondylocostal abnormalities (other examples are covered in Chapter 20), or they may reflect intrinsic changes in skeletal tissues. The different skeletal syndromes are summarized in Figure 8-20.

Achondroplasia, an autosomal dominant syndrome, is the most common form of dwarfism (see Fig. 8-1). It is characterized by shortening of the long bones, a small midface resulting

from defects in the cranial base (the latter is derived from endochondral bones as covered in Chapter 17), and curvature of the spine. Achondroplasia is the result of an activating mutation of the FIBROBLAST GROWTH FACTOR RECEPTOR 3 (FGFR3). Mutations in FGFR3 can also cause the more severe, neonatally lethal syndromes such as **thanatophoric dysplasia type I** and **II**, and other skeletal syndromes. Animal models with activating Fgfr3 mutations have been used to show that abnormal skeletal growth is due to decreased chondrocyte proliferation (see previous "In the Research Lab" entitled "Molecular Regulation of Bone and Joint Development").

In contrast, some syndromes affect discrete groups of bones. This is typified by **Grebe-** and **Hunter-Thompson–type chondrodysplasias** and **brachydactyly types C** and **A2** (see Figs. 8-19, 8-20). These are all characterized by shortening of the appendicular skeleton (brachydactyly means short fingers) and loss of some joints. All can result from mutations in GDF5. Like other Bmps, GDF5 promotes chondrogenesis by increasing the size of initial chondrocyte condensations and by increasing chondrocyte proliferation. Grebe and Hunter-Thompson syndromes can affect all limb skeletal elements, with increasing severity in a proximal-to-distal direction; in the brachydactyly syndromes, only the phalanges are affected (shortened). Both Grebe and Hunter-Thompson syndromes are autosomal recessive, but Grebe-type chondrodysplasia is more severe than the Hunter-Thompson type. This is attributed to the different mutations in the GDF5 gene (so-called **genotype-phenotype correlations**). Hunter-Thompson–type

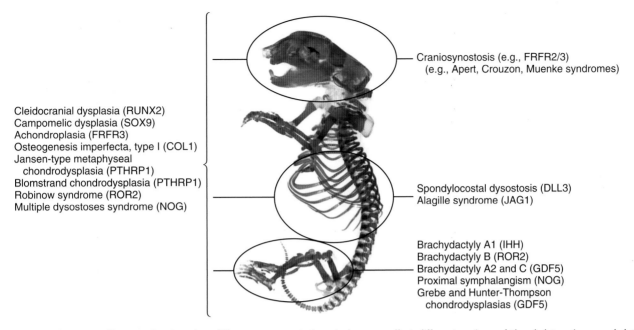

Cleidocranial dysplasia (RUNX2)
Campomelic dysplasia (SOX9)
Achondroplasia (FRFR3)
Osteogenesis imperfecta, type I (COL1)
Jansen-type metaphyseal
   chondrodysplasia (PTHRP1)
Blomstrand chondrodysplasia (PTHRP1)
Robinow syndrome (ROR2)
Multiple dysostoses syndrome (NOG)

Craniosynostosis (e.g., FRFR2/3)
   (e.g., Apert, Crouzon, Muenke syndromes)

Spondylocostal dysostosis (DLL3)
Alagille syndrome (JAG1)

Brachydactyly A1 (IHH)
Brachydactyly B (ROR2)
Brachydactyly A2 and C (GDF5)
Proximal symphalangism (NOG)
Grebe and Hunter-Thompson
   chondrodysplasias (GDF5)

Figure 8-20. Summary diagram showing that different gene mutations in humans affect different regions of the skeleton (mouse skeleton shown).

chondrodysplasia is predicted to be loss of function, whereas in Grebe-type chondrodysplasia, the mutated GDF5 protein is able to form dimers with other Bmp members, which cannot be secreted. Therefore, Grebe syndrome is the result of loss of GDF5 function, as in Hunter-Thompson syndrome, together with a dominant negative effect on other members of the Bmp family. The brachydactyly phenotypes are milder: in these syndromes, only one copy of GDF5 is mutated/nonfunctional.

GDF5 mutations are also found in autosomal dominant **proximal symphalangism**—the fusion of the interphalangeal, wrist, and ankle joints. Analysis of one of these GDF5 mutations has shown that it is a gain-of-function mutation, with the mutant protein showing increased binding to the BMPR1A receptor. Loss of the joint seems to be due to excessive chondrogenesis. Mutations in NOGGIN, a Bmp antagonist, also result in proximal symphalangism and **multiple synostoses syndrome type 1**, which is characterized by fusion of the limb joints and craniofacial anomalies that are typified by conductive hearing loss and a broad nose. This syndrome can also involve synostoses of the vertebrae. Likewise, the noggin mutant mouse has multiple fusions of the bones in both appendicular and axial skeletons. The study of these human skeletal mutations has taught us that increased Bmp/GDF5 activity causes joint fusions, and blocking Bmp activity is necessary both for normal joint development in the embryo and for maintenance of the joint cavity postnatally. Why loss of function GDF5 mutations result in the loss of some joints is currently unclear.

Another striking illustration of the role of Bmp signaling during endochondral ossification is shown in the syndrome **fibrodysplasia ossificans progressiva** (FOP), which is due to an activating mutation in the Bmp receptor, ACVR1. In FOP, following damage and inflammation, ectopic bone differentiates within muscles and connective tissues, typically resulting in death by the age of 40.

A decrease in the number of functional osteoblasts and/or an increase in the number of osteoclasts results in **osteoporosis**, the loss of bone mass associated with increased skeletal fragility and bone fracture. The converse situation results in excess bone mass, or **osteopetrosis**. Mutations in the LIPOPROTEIN RECEPTOR PROTEIN, LRP5, a Wnt co-receptor, result in

either an increase in bone mass or a decrease (**osteoporosis pseudoglioma syndrome**) in bone mass, both of which are attributed to changes in osteoblast development. Wnts and Lrp5 control osteoblast proliferation, differentiation, and survival, and LRP5 mutations that result in a decrease in bone mass are due to loss of LRP5 function. Recent research has shown that Lrp5 is also required in the enterochromaffin cells of the gastrointestinal tract to increase the levels of circulating serotonin, which directly controls osteoblast development through the Htr1B receptor.

Mutations in LRP5 that result in a gain of bone mass affect the ability of the Wnt antagonist DICKKOPF 1 to bind to the LRP5 receptor and block Wnt signaling. Hence, these mutations result in increased Wnt signaling via the β-CATENIN pathway. Other mutations that result in osteopetrosis include those that affect different aspects of osteoclast function. Mutations in the vacuolar proton pump, as in **infantile malignant osteopetrosis**, prevent the establishment of the acidic environment necessary to dissolve the mineral matrix. CATHEPSIN K is a secreted osteoclast enzyme that works at low pH to degrade exposed organic residues. Mutations in CATHEPSIN K result in **pycnodysostosis**, another condition with enhanced bone mass.

In addition to mutations in genes expressed in skeletal tissues, defects in tissues outside the skeleton may affect its development. Postnatal growth is regulated hormonally, and defects in the pituitary gland, as in **acromegaly**—a condition in which growth hormone production is increased—increase the size of the hands, feet, and face.

DEVELOPMENT OF LIMB MUSCLES

Axial muscles of the trunk and muscles of the limb develop similarly. Both groups of muscles arise from the somites and move ventrally—along the dorsolateral body wall into the ventral body wall in the case of axial muscles, and ventrally into the limb buds in the case of limb muscles. Both groups of muscles are innervated by spinal

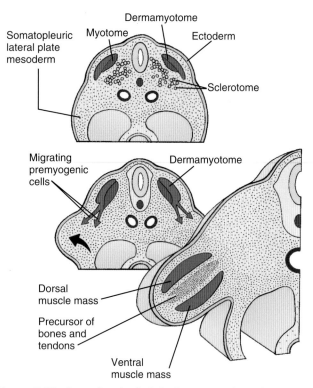

Figure 8-21. Soon after the limb bud grows out from the somatopleuric lateral plate mesoderm (dark blue arrow), the muscle progenitors (i.e., the premyogenic cells) migrate from the dermamyotome and enter the limb bud, initially forming two major muscle masses. The ventral muscle mass gives rise mainly to flexors, pronators, and adductors, whereas the dorsal muscle mass gives rise mainly to extensors, supinators, and abductors.

TABLE 8-1	MUSCLES DERIVED FROM THE VENTRAL AND DORSAL MUSCLE MASSES OF THE LIMB BUDS	
Ventral Muscle Mass	**Dorsal Muscle Mass**
Upper Limb	**Upper Limb**
Anterior compartment of arm and forearm	Posterior compartment muscles of arm and forearm
All muscles on palmar surface of hand	Deltoid
	Lateral compartment muscles of forearm and hand
	Latissimus dorsi
	Rhomboids
	Levator scapulae
	Serratus anterior
	Teres major and minor
	Subscapularis
	Supraspinatus
	Infraspinatus
Lower Limb	**Lower Limb**
Medial compartment muscles of thigh	Anterior compartment muscles of thigh and leg
Posterior compartment muscles of thigh except for short head of biceps femoris	Tensor fascia latae
	Short head of biceps femoris
Posterior compartment muscles of leg	Lateral compartment muscles of leg
All muscles on plantar surface of foot	Muscles of the dorsum of foot
Obturator internus	Gluteus maximus, medius, and minimus
Gemellus superior and inferior	Piriformis
	Iliacus
Quadratus femoris	Psoas

nerves bordering their level of origin (by dorsal and ventral rami in the case of axial muscles, and by ventral rami only in the case of limb muscles). As covered in Chapters 10 and 11, the muscle of the diaphragm also arises from somitic myotomes (specifically, cervical myotomes 3, 4, and 5). Thus, as the diaphragm descends to form a partition separating the pleural and abdominal cavities, it carries its innervation—the **phrenic nerves**—with it, explaining why a thoracic/abdominal structure is innervated by nerves originating from the cervical region.

In human embryos, migration of the myogenic precursors into the limb buds starts during the fifth week of development. The invading myoblasts form two large condensations in the dorsal and ventral limb bud (Fig. 8-21). The dorsal muscle mass gives rise in general to the **extensors** and **supinators** of the upper limb and to the **extensors** and **abductors** of the lower limb, whereas the ventral muscle mass gives rise to the **flexors** and **pronators** of the upper limb and to the **flexors** and **adductors** of the lower limb (Table 8-1). Experimental studies in animal models have shown that as these progenitor cells migrate toward the limb bud, they are bipotential and can form myocytes and/or endothelial cells (see the following "In the Research Lab" entitled "Migration of Muscle Progenitors"). In contrast to limb muscles, which arise from the somitic myotomes, the limb tendons arise from the lateral plate mesoderm.

In the Research Lab

MIGRATION OF MUSCLE PROGENITORS

Classical quail-chick recombination experiments (covered in Chapter 5) showed that limb myogenic cells arise from the somites. Therefore, if a quail somite is transplanted into a chick host, the limb muscles will be of quail origin (Fig. 8-22). Experiments such as these have shown that the limb muscles are patterned by surrounding connective tissues, as in other regions of the body.

As covered earlier in this chapter, the myogenic cells that give rise to the limb, tongue, and diaphragm muscles delaminate from the dermamyotome to migrate into their respective final environments. Delamination and migration of muscle progenitors require several factors. In the limb bud (Fig. 8-23), these include Pax3 (a paired-box transcription factor), c-Met (a proto-oncogene, that is, a normal gene that when mutated can become an oncogene, resulting in the development of cancer), Hgf (hepatocyte growth factor)/scatter factor, and Lbx1 (homolog of the Drosophila lady bird late gene, a homeobox transcription factor). In response to Hgf signaling in the early limb bud, c-Met–expressing cells in the somitic dermamyotome delaminate and start to migrate. Pax3 regulates the expression of c-Met—the Hgf receptor that is necessary for migration. Therefore, in the **Splotch** mouse (Pax3 mutant), the limb (and also the diaphragm) muscles are absent. The transcription factor Lbx1 is also required. In Lbx1 mutants, myogenic precursors delaminate but do not migrate

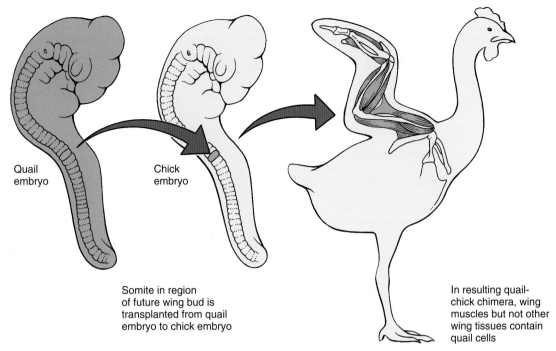

Quail
embryo

Chick
embryo

Somite in region
of future wing bud is
transplanted from quail
embryo to chick embryo

In resulting quail-
chick chimera, wing
muscles but not other
wing tissues contain
quail cells

Figure 8-22. Summary diagram showing a cell-tracing experiment using quail-chick transplantation chimeras. This experiment demonstrated that the musculature of the limbs forms from somitic mesoderm, whereas the limb bones form from lateral plate mesoderm. Quail somites, transplanted to the axial level at which development of the limb bud occurs, give rise to limb myocytes.

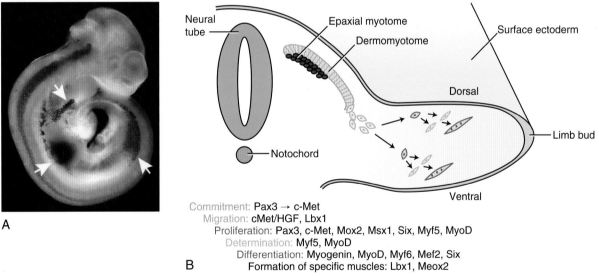

Neural
tube

Epaxial myotome

Dermomyotome

Surface ectoderm

Dorsal

Limb bud

Notochord

Ventral

A

Commitment: Pax3 → c-Met
Migration: cMet/HGF, Lbx1
Proliferation: Pax3, c-Met, Mox2, Msx1, Six, Myf5, MyoD
Determination: Myf5, MyoD
Differentiation: Myogenin, MyoD, Myf6, Mef2, Six
Formation of specific muscles: Lbx1, Meox2

B

Figure 8-23. Regulation of limb myogenesis. *A*, Expression of Lbx1, a gene necessary for migration in the migratory limb and tongue muscle precursors (arrows). *B*, Summary diagram showing the molecular regulators of limb myogenesis.

appropriately; consequently, hindlimb muscles are totally absent, but flexor muscles (ventral muscle mass) form in the forelimb. Once within the limb bud, the premyogenic cells proliferate (requires several genes, as listed in Fig. 8-23) and become committed to the myogenic pathway. This commitment requires Pax3, which regulates the expression of Myf5 (covered earlier in this chapter). Meox2 (a homeobox gene; also called Mox2) is needed for development of the appropri-

ate number of myogenic cells in the limb; this in turn leads to formation of the full range of normal limb muscles; in the absence of Meox2 function, some of the limb muscles do not form or are abnormally patterned.

Fate mapping studies have shown the surprising result that the ventral muscle mass of the hindlimb also gives rise to the perineal muscles (i.e., the muscles located in the perineal region). These muscles include external anal sphincter, superficial transverse perineal muscle, ischiocavernosus muscle, bulbospongiosus muscle, deep transverse perineal muscle, and sphincter urethrae muscle. During their formation, the prospective perineal muscles move caudally from the hindlimbs to the forming perineal region.

MUSCLE CELL AND FIBER TYPE COMMITMENT

Cell lineage studies in which an individual premigratory hypaxial cell is labeled with a unique molecular tag have shown that as the cells leave the somite, they are not yet committed to an endothelial or myogenic cell fate (as covered in Chapter 13, paraxial mesoderm also contributes to the endothelium of intraembryonic blood vessels). Thus, endothelial and myogenic differentiation occurs as a result of local environmental cues within the limb bud. Similarly, early myogenic cells are not yet committed to becoming **slow** or **fast** myocytes. The distribution of slow and fast myotubes determines how a muscle functions. Simplistically, slow myocytes are characterized by the expression of slow myosin heavy chain (MyHC); slow myocytes contract slowly and have oxidative metabolism (i.e., aerobic metabolism). Consequently, these fibers do not fatigue quickly and are involved in the maintenance of posture. In contrast, "fast" fibers tend to express fast MyHCs, contract rapidly with high force, and have glycolytic metabolism (i.e., anaerobic metabolism). "Fast" fibers are needed for movement. As in cell fate determination, local environmental cues also control slow and fast fiber differentiation within the limb bud during primary myogenesis. However, during secondary myogenesis and postnatally, fiber type is also influenced by innervation.

REGIONAL DIFFERENCES IN MUSCLE DEVELOPMENT

The development of axial and limb muscles has been emphasized in this chapter on musculoskeletal development. However, it is important to point out that differences exist between what has been described here for the development of axial and limb muscles and for the development of craniofacial muscles (covered in Chapter 17). For example, as covered earlier in

this "In the Research Lab: Migration of Muscle Progenitors," Pax3 mutations affect the development of the trunk and limb muscles. However, the craniofacial musculature is unaffected. Conversely, inactivation of capsulin (also known as Tcf21) and MyoR, two transcription factors related to the myogenic regulatory factors (covered earlier in the chapter), results in loss of the muscles of mastication, leaving most axial muscles unaffected. The homeobox gene, Pitx2, is required for the development of the extraocular muscles (Fig. 8-24). Thus, the axial, branchiomeric, and extraocular muscles are distinct and seem to be controlled by different networks of signaling molecules. Moreover, whereas Wnt signaling is necessary for myogenic commitment in the trunk and limb, Wnt signaling is inhibitory for myogenesis in the pharyngeal arches. The regulatory network that controls the expression of the Mrfs also varies regionally, as illustrated by the regulation of MyoD. MyoD is activated by a combination of Myf5 and Myf6 in extraocular muscles, Tbx1 and Myf5 in the pharyngeal arches, and Myf4, Myf5, and Pax3 in the trunk. Therefore, in the Myf5/Myf6 double knockout mouse, the extraocular muscles are absent, whereas other muscles can develop as a result of the ability of Tbx1 and Pax3 to activate MyoD expression independently of Myf5/Myf6. These molecular differences are also found in the satellite cells, which share the same tissue origin, and may explain, in part, the various susceptibilities of different muscles in myopathies.

A subset of the pharyngeal arch muscles (e.g., mylohyoid, stylohyoid, and digastric) arise within the secondary heart field and share molecular characteristics with the developing cardiac cells (Tbx1, Pitx2) (see Fig. 8-24). During development, skeletal muscle development is initially suppressed by Bmps in the secondary heart field to allow for expansion of the cardiac progenitors (also covered in Chapter 12). Satellite cells from these muscles retain some plasticity and, unlike satellite cells from the axial muscles, can be induced to express cardiac markers. It has been proposed that cranial satellite cells may be used to repair cardiac muscle damage following cardiac infraction.

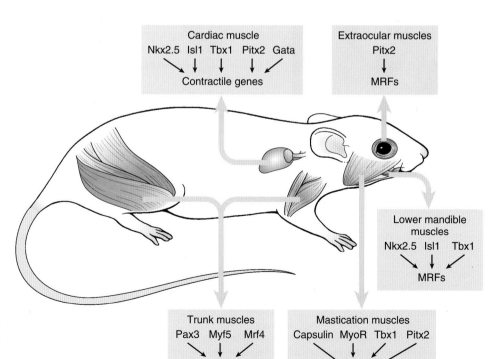

Figure 8-24. Comparison of craniofacial and trunk/limb myogenesis. Some craniofacial muscles share tissue origins with the second heart field. MRFs, muscle regulatory factors.

In the Clinic

MUSCULAR DYSTROPHY

Muscular abnormalities include the devastating muscular dystrophies in which functional muscle mass is not maintained, or the satellite cells—the progenitors for postnatal growth and muscle repair—are defective. Both X-linked **Duchenne muscular dystrophy** and the milder condition, **Becker-type muscular dystrophy**, are due to mutations in DYSTROPHIN, a large protein (encoded by the largest gene in the human genome) that links intracellular cytoskeletal proteins with the sarcolemma, the plasma membrane of the muscle fiber. Duchenne muscular dystrophy occurs in 1 in 3500 male infants and affects most of the muscles of the body, including the cardiac and respiratory muscles, thereby typically resulting in death by the age of thirty. The truncated form of dystrophin has some function, as shown by the much less severe phenotype observed in Becker-type muscular dystrophy, and this has provided clues to therapies to treat the much more severe Duchenne myopathy. Other dystrophies may affect a subset of muscles, such as **oculopharyngeal muscular dystrophy** (due to mutations in PABPN1, POLYADENYLATE-BINDING PROTEIN, NUCLEAR 1), which affects the neck, face, and proximal limb muscles. Many strategies are being taken to try to repair these myopathies, several of which have entered clinical trials. In Duchenne muscular dystrophy, one approach has been to generate a truncated form of dystrophin through gene therapy, where a truncated dystrophin is misexpressed using adeno-associated vectors, or a truncated form of dystrophin from the mutated gene, achieved by exon splicing. In exon splicing, the mutated exons are removed during RNA splicing to restore the open reading frame. Other strategies include drug treatments that allow read-through of a premature stop codon, blocking of antibodies against myostatin to induce muscular hypertrophy, and cell therapies such as treatment with wild-type mesoangioblasts expressing dystrophin, which fuses with the muscle cells.

Muscular defects can also include the absence of specific muscles, for example, in the sporadic **Poland anomaly**, in which the pectoralis major muscle is absent on one side of the body, or in **prune-belly syndrome**, in which the abdominal wall muscles fail to develop. Finally, muscle weakness may have an extrinsic component resulting from defects in motor nerve innervation. This is typified by **Duane anomaly**, characterized by lateral gaze palsy (abnormal eye movements). In Duane anomaly, there are abnormalities in cranial nerve VI (abducens nerve), which innervates the lateral rectus, the extraocular eye muscle that moves the globe laterally.

Embryology in Practice

BRITTLE BONES

A primigravida twenty-nine-year-old woman is seen for a mid-gestation ultrasound. The pregnancy had been progressing without incident. Unfortunately, the images suggest that her fetus has a severe **skeletal dysplasia**. Specifically, the ultrasound reveals very short, bowed upper and lower limbs and a markedly reduced chest circumference. The long bones are suspicious for fractures. In addition, there is a reduction of the amniotic fluid (**oligohydramnios**), with evidence of premature rupture of the membranes. An amniotic fluid sample is taken and sent for a chromosome study.

One week later, the chromosomes are reported as normal. However, the ultrasound examination continues to be extremely worrisome, revealing a very small fetus for date of gestation, little or no fetal movement, and worsening of the oligohydramnios. The decision is made to induce delivery of the twenty-week-gestational-age, non-viable fetus. The parents request an autopsy to determine, if possible, the etiology of their pregnancy loss, and to inform them of their recurrence risk in the future.

The autopsy shows a very small fetus with short bowed limbs. The hips are held in the "frog-leg" position (flexed and abducted). The thorax diameter measures much smaller than the second centile, with very hypoplastic lungs. X-rays (Fig. 8-25A, B) show multiple fractures, with a crumpled appearance of the long bones and small "beaded" ribs. The skull is not ossified. The scapulae are irregularly shaped and under-ossified. Histologic examination of the ribs (Fig. 8-25C) shows orderly endochondral ossification, with columns of proliferating chondrocytes (to the left of the image and toward the costochondral joint) becoming progressively larger toward the conversion line. This rules out a **chondrodysplasia**. Moving toward the shaft of the bone (to the right of the conversion line in the image), the chondrocytes are replaced by invading osteoblasts laying down osteoid on the edges of chondroid matrix. Within the shaft of the bone (further to the right in the image), the bony trabeculae and the rim of cortical bone at the lateral edges of the ribs are thin and fragmented, indicative of multiple small fractures. These distort the longitudinal contour of the bone, resulting in the "crumpled" appearance on the radiographs.

The pathologist makes the diagnosis of **osteogenesis imperfecta** (OI) **type II** based on gross, X-ray, and histologic examinations. OI type II is considered a "lethal skeletal dysplasia," as it is almost always fatal in the neonatal period, often from resulting **lung hypoplasia**. The family sees a genetic counselor and is told that OI type II is an autosomal dominant condition caused by mutations in the gene encoding type I collagen, either COL1A1 or COL1A2. However, they are reassured that in almost all cases, the causative mutation occurs de novo in the affected individual. The recurrence risk for future pregnancies is usually quoted at 2% to 4% because of the chance that a mutation would be inherited from a parent who carries the mutation only in the sperm or egg (**germline mosaicism**).

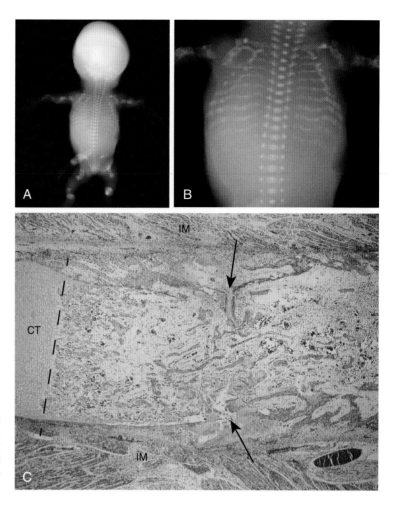

Figure 8-25. Stillborn twenty-week fetus with osteogenesis imperfecta type II. *A, B,* X-rays. *C,* Histologic section of rib and surrounding tissues. CT, cartilage of costochondral junction; IM, intercostal muscles. Dashed line indicates the approximate location of the rib conversion line (interface between cartilage and forming bone). Arrows indicate large fractures of the rib.

SUGGESTED READINGS

Alexander T, Nolte C, Krumlauf R. 2009. Hox genes and segmentation of the hindbrain and axial skeleton. Annu Rev Cell Dev Biol 25:431–456.

Baldridge D, Shchelochkov O, Kelley B, Lee B. 2010. Signaling pathways in human skeletal dysplasias. Annu Rev Genomics Hum Genet 11:189–217.

Bryson-Richardson RJ, Currie PD. 2008. The genetics of vertebrate myogenesis. Nat Rev Genet 9:632–646.

Buckingham M, Vincent SD. 2009. Distinct and dynamic myogenic populations in the vertebrate embryo. Curr Opin Genet Dev 19:444–453.

Cossu G, Sampaolesi M. 2007. New therapies for Duchenne muscular dystrophy: challenges, prospects and clinical trials. Trends Mol Med 13:520–526.

Edwards JR, Mundy GR. 2011. Advances in osteoclast biology: old findings and new insights from mouse models. Nat Rev Rheumatol 7:235–243.

Giampietro PF, Dunwoodie SL, Kusumi K, et al. 2009. Progress in the understanding of the genetic etiology of vertebral segmentation disorders in humans. Ann N Y Acad Sci 1151:38–67.

Lefebvre V, Bhattaram P. 2010. Vertebrate skeletogenesis. Curr Top Dev Biol 90:291–317.

Mallo M, Wellik DM, Deschamps J. 2010. Hox genes and regional patterning of the vertebrate body plan. Dev Biol 344:7–15.

Murphy M, Kardon G. 2011. Origin of vertebrate limb muscle: the role of progenitor and myoblast populations. Curr Top Dev Biol 96:1–32.

Pourquie O. 2011. Vertebrate segmentation: from cyclic gene networks to scoliosis. Cell 145:650–663.

Sambasivan R, Kuratani S, Tajbakhsh S. 2011. An eye on the head: the development and evolution of craniofacial muscles. Development 138:2401–2415.

Chapter 9

Development of the Central Nervous System

SUMMARY

Even before neurulation begins, the primordia of the three **primary brain vesicles—prosencephalon**, **mesencephalon**, and **rhombencephalon**—are visible as broadenings of the neural plate. During the fifth week, the prosencephalon subdivides into the **telencephalon** and **diencephalon**, and the rhombencephalon subdivides into the **metencephalon** and **myelencephalon**. Thus, along with the mesencephalon, there are five **secondary brain vesicles**. During this period, the hindbrain is divided into small repetitive segments called **rhombomeres**. The extension of the neural tube caudal to the rhombomeres constitutes the **spinal cord**.

The primordial brain portion of the neural tube undergoes flexion at three points. At two of these—**mesencephalic (cranial) flexure** and **cervical flexure**—the bends are ventrally directed. At the **pontine flexure**, the bend is dorsally directed.

Cytodifferentiation of the neural tube begins in the rhombencephalon at the end of the fourth week. During this process, the neural tube neuroepithelium proliferates to produce the neurons, glia, and ependymal cells of the central nervous system. The young neurons, born in the **ventricular zone** that surrounds the central lumen, migrate peripherally to establish the **mantle zone**, the precursor of the gray matter, wherein lie the majority of mature neurons. Axons extending from mantle layer neurons establish the **marginal zone** (the future white matter) peripheral to the mantle zone. In areas of the brain that develop a cortex, including the cerebellum and cerebral hemispheres, the pattern of generation and migration of neurons is more complex.

The mantle zone of the spinal cord and brain stem is organized into a pair of **ventral (basal) plates** and a pair of **dorsal (alar) plates**. Laterally, the two plates abut at a groove called the **sulcus limitans**; dorsally and ventrally, they are connected by non-neurogenic structures called, respectively, the **roof plate** and the **floor plate**. **Association neurons** form in the dorsal plates, and one or two cell columns (depending on the level) form in the ventral plates: the **somatic motor column** and the **visceral motor column**.

The nuclei of the third to twelfth cranial nerves are located in the brain stem (mesencephalon, metencephalon, and myelencephalon). Some of these cranial nerves are motor, some are sensory, and some are mixed, arising from more than one nucleus. The cranial nerve motor nuclei develop from the brain stem basal plates, and the associational sensory nuclei develop from the brain stem alar plates. The brain stem cranial nerve nuclei are organized into seven longitudinal columns, which correspond closely to the types of functions they subserve. From ventromedial to dorsolateral, the three basal columns contain **somatic efferent**, **branchial (or special visceral) efferent**, and **(general) visceral efferent motoneurons**, and the four alar columns contain **general visceral afferent**, **special visceral afferent** (subserving the special sense of taste), **general somatic afferent**, and **special somatic afferent** (subserving the special senses of hearing and balance) **associational neurons**.

The myelencephalon gives rise to the **medulla oblongata**, the portion of the brain most similar in organization to the spinal cord. The metencephalon gives rise to the **pons**, a bulbous expansion that consists mainly of the massive white matter tracts serving the cerebellum, and to the **cerebellum**. A specialized process of neurogenesis in the cerebellum gives rise to the gray matter of the **cerebellar cortex**, as well as to the **deep cerebellar nuclei**. The cerebellum controls posture, balance, and the smooth execution of movements by coordinating sensory input with motor functions.

The mesencephalon contains nuclei of two cranial nerves as well as various other structures. In particular, the alar plates give rise to the **superior** and **inferior colliculi**, which are visible as round protuberances on the dorsal surface of the midbrain. The superior colliculi control ocular reflexes; the inferior colliculi serve as relays in the auditory pathway.

The forebrain has no basal plate. The alar plate of the diencephalon is divided into a dorsal portion and a ventral portion by a deep groove called the **hypothalamic sulcus**. The **hypothalamic swelling** ventral to this groove differentiates into the nuclei collectively known as the **hypothalamus**, the most prominent function of which is to control visceral activities such as heart rate and pituitary secretion. Dorsal to the hypothalamic sulcus, the large **thalamic swelling** gives rise to the **thalamus**, by far the largest diencephalic structure, which serves as a relay center, processing information from subcortical structures before passing it to the cerebral cortex. Finally, a dorsal swelling, the **epithalamus**, gives rise to a few smaller structures, including the **pineal gland**.

A ventral outpouching of the diencephalic midline, called the **infundibulum**, differentiates to form the **posterior pituitary**. A matching diverticulum of the stomodeal roof, called **Rathke's pouch**, grows to meet

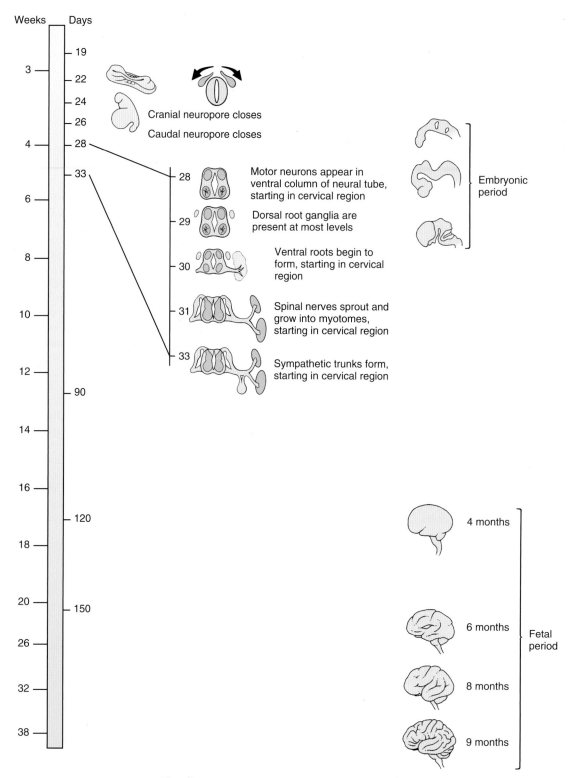

Time line. Development of the brain and spinal cord.

the infundibulum and becomes the **anterior pituitary**. Cranial diencephalic outpouchings also form the eyes, as covered in Chapter 19.

The telencephalon is subdivided into a dorsal **pallium** and a ventral **subpallium**. The latter forms the large neuronal nuclei of the **basal ganglia (corpus striatum, globus pallidus)**—structures crucial for

executing commands from the **cerebral hemispheres**. These cortical structures arise as lateral outpouchings of the pallium and grow rapidly to cover the diencephalon and mesencephalon. The hemispheres are joined by the cranial **lamina terminalis** (representing the zone of closure of the cranial neuropore) and by axon tracts called **commissures**, particularly the massive **corpus**

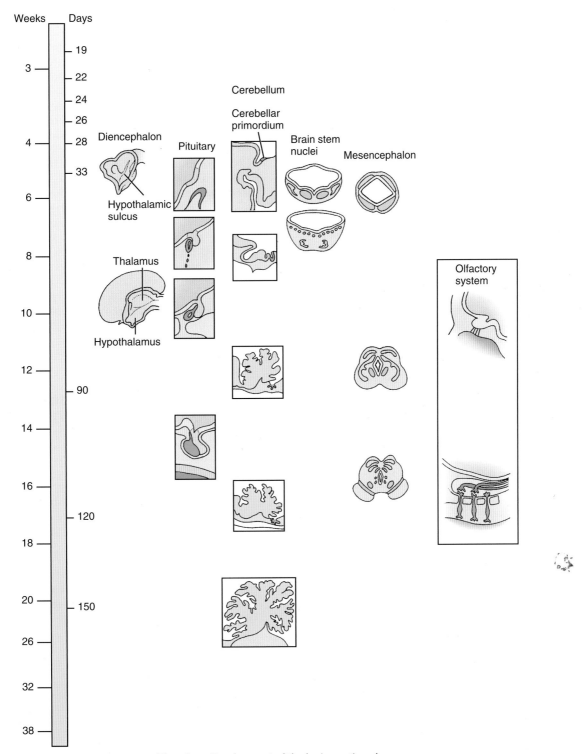

Time line. Development of the brain continued.

callosum. The **olfactory bulbs** and the **olfactory tracts** arise from the cranial telencephalon and receive input from the primary olfactory neurosensory cells, which differentiate from the nasal placodes and line the roof of the nasal cavity.

The expanded **primitive ventricles** formed by the neural canal in the secondary brain vesicles give rise to the ventricular system of the brain. The cerebrospinal fluid that fills the ventricle system is produced mainly by secretory **choroid plexuses** in the lateral, third, and fourth ventricles, which are formed by the ependyma and overlying vascular pia. The third ventricle also contains specialized ependymal secretory structures called **circumventricular organs**.

STRUCTURAL DIVISIONS OF NERVOUS SYSTEM

The nervous system of vertebrates consists of two major *structural* divisions: a **central nervous system (CNS)** and a **peripheral nervous system (PNS)**. The CNS consists of the brain and spinal cord. The development of the CNS is covered in this chapter. The PNS consists of all components of the nervous system outside of the CNS. Thus, the PNS consists of cranial nerves and ganglia, spinal nerves and ganglia, autonomic nerves and ganglia, and the enteric nervous system. The development of the PNS is covered in Chapter 10.

FUNCTIONAL DIVISIONS OF NERVOUS SYSTEM

The nervous system of vertebrates consists of two major *functional* divisions: a **somatic nervous system** and a **visceral nervous system**. The somatic nervous system innervates the skin and most skeletal muscles (i.e., it provides both sensory and motor components). Similarly, the visceral nervous system innervates the viscera (organs of the body) and the smooth muscle and glands in the more peripheral part of the body. The visceral nervous system is also called the **autonomic nervous system**. It consists of two components: the **sympathetic division** and the **parasympathetic division**. The somatic and visceral nervous systems are covered both in this chapter (CNS components) and in Chapter 10 (PNS components).

Both divisions of the autonomic nervous system consist of two-neuron pathways. Because the peripheral autonomic neurons reside in ganglia, the axons of the central sympathetic neurons are called **preganglionic fibers**, and the axons of the peripheral sympathetic neurons are called **postganglionic fibers**. This terminology is used for both sympathetic pathways and parasympathetic pathways (discussed later in the chapter). Sometimes preganglionic fibers are also called *presynaptic fibers*, and postganglionic fibers, *postsynaptic fibers*. They are so called because the axons of the preganglionic fibers *synapse* on the cell bodies of postganglionic neurons in the autonomic ganglia.

PRIMARY BRAIN VESICLES SUBDIVIDE TO FORM SECONDARY BRAIN VESICLES

Animation 9-1: Neurulation.
    Animations are available online at StudentConsult.

Chapters 3 and 4 describe how during neurulation, the rudiment of the central nervous system arises as the neural plate from the ectoderm of the embryonic disc and folds to form the neural tube. The presumptive brain is visible as the broad cranial portion of the neural plate (see Fig. 3-20). Even on day nineteen, before bending of the neural plate begins, the three major divisions of the brain—**prosencephalon (forebrain)**, **mesencephalon (midbrain)**, and **rhombencephalon (hindbrain)**—are demarcated by indentations in the neural plate. The future eyes appear as outpouchings from the forebrain neural folds by day twenty-two (covered in Chapter 19). Bending of the neural plate begins on day twenty-two, and the cranial neuropore closes on day twenty-four. The three brain divisions are then marked by expansions of the neural tube called **primary brain vesicles** (Fig. 9-1A, B).

An additional series of narrow swellings called **neuromeres** becomes apparent in the future brain (see Fig. 9-1A, B). These are prominent in the hindbrain, where seven or eight **rhombomeres** (depending on the species) partition the neural tube into segments of approximately equal size. The rhombomeres are transient structures that become indistinguishable by early in the sixth week.

During the fifth week, the mesencephalon enlarges and the prosencephalon and the rhombencephalon each subdivide into two portions, thus converting the three primary brain vesicles into five **secondary brain vesicles** (Fig. 9-1C, D). The prosencephalon divides into a cranial

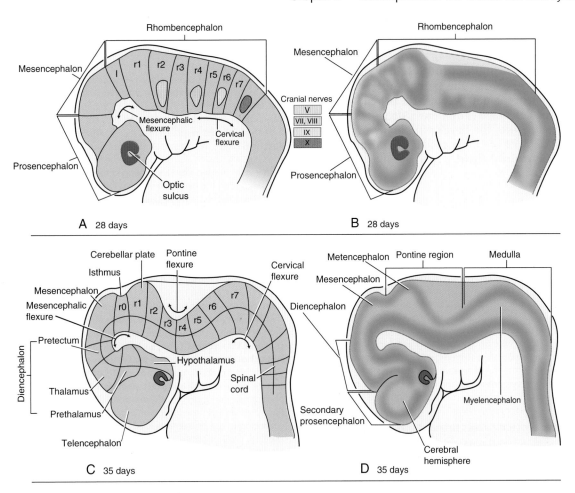

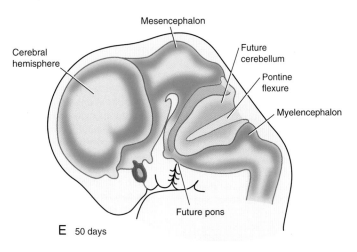

Figure 9-1. Early development of the brain. *A, B,* By day twenty-eight, the future brain consists of three primary brain vesicles (prosencephalon, mesencephalon, and rhombencephalon). The locations of the mesencephalic and cervical flexures are indicated, as are the positions of the isthmus (I), rhombomeres (r1-r7), and some cranial nerve ganglia (roman numerals). *C-E,* Further subdivision of the brain vesicles creates five secondary vesicles: the enlarged mesencephalon, the metencephalon and myelencephalon (that arise from the rhombencephalon), and the diencephalon and telencephalon (that arise from the prosencephalon). The cerebral hemispheres appear and expand rapidly. The pontine flexure folds the metencephalon back against the myelencephalon.

telencephalon ("end-brain") and a caudal **diencephalon** ("between-brain"). The diencephalon, like the rhombencephalon, becomes subdivided into a series of three or four units called **prosomeres**. The rhombencephalon divides into a cranial **metencephalon** ("behind-brain,"

consisting of rhombomeres one and two) and a caudal **myelencephalon** ("medulla-brain," consisting of the remaining rhombomeres). Within each of the brain vesicles, the neural canal is expanded into a cavity called a **primitive ventricle**. These primitive ventricles will become the definitive ventricles of the mature brain (see Fig. 9-23). The cavity of the rhombencephalon becomes the **fourth ventricle**, the cavity of the mesencephalon becomes the **cerebral aqueduct (of Sylvius)**, the cavity of the diencephalon becomes the **third ventricle**, and the cavity of the telencephalon becomes the paired **lateral ventricles** of the cerebral hemispheres. After the closure of the caudal neuropore, the developing brain ventricles and the central canal of the more caudal **spinal cord** are filled with **cerebrospinal fluid**, a specialized dialysate of blood plasma.

In the Research Lab

One of the major challenges facing the embryo is how to generate a very large number of different neuronal cell types while at the same time ensuring that each of them forms at its correct position in the neural tube. Distinguished and defined by the specificity of their connections with other neurons, the neuronal cell types of the CNS number in the many hundreds, or even thousands, and the embryo has to get the right cells in the right places for the system to wire up appropriately and function correctly. The highly elaborate patterning of cell specification and the subsequent formation of precise connections between remote cells during development set the CNS far apart from other organ systems; how these processes are controlled is thus an important question for researchers.

POSITIONAL INFORMATION PATTERNS NEURAL PLATE AND TUBE

In addressing the issue of **cell patterning**, it is helpful to think in terms of a Cartesian system of **positional information**, in which undifferentiated precursor cells may sense their position on orthogonal gradients of **morphogens** acting along the cranial-caudal (CrCd) and medial-lateral (ML) axes of the neural plate. Cells would acquire a unique "grid reference" by measuring the ambient concentration of morphogen on each of the intersecting axes and would then interpret this, their **positional value**, by selecting an appropriate fate from the range made available in the genome. This concept is undoubtedly simplistic but not wholly unrealistic.

The events of pattern formation can be summarized as follows: first, polarization of the entire CrCd axis of the CNS primordium; and next, the setting up of discrete morphogen sources at particular positions along the axis that act as local **signaling centers**, informing neighboring cells about their position and fate (Fig. 9-2A, B). Similar events occur on the ML axis of the neural plate (later the dorsal-ventral [DV] axis of the neural tube) except that, because it is considerably shorter than the CrCd axis, morphogen sources established at the dorsal and ventral poles are sufficient to pattern the entire axis (Fig. 9-2C).

At gastrulation, when a region of the dorsal ectoderm is set aside to be the **neural plate** (see Chapter 3), the CrCd axis is polarized by a gradient of **Wnt** molecules diffusing from the caudal pole of the neural plate, and by counteracting Wnt inhibitors at the cranial pole. In the absence of Wnt signaling, the default neural fate of cranial is realized. Higher Wnt levels effectively confer successively more caudal neural fates. Gradients of **retinoid** signaling, also high at the caudal end of the embryo, operate in addition to Wnts to polarize the CrCd axis. The initially coarse regional subdivision of the CrCd axis is manifest by the expression of **transcriptional control genes** in distinct domains that dictate the direction of their subsequent development. For example, Otx2 is expressed only in the cranial neural plate (forebrain or prosencephalon and midbrain or mesencephalon), whereas Hox genes are expressed in nested

subdomains of the caudal neural plate (hindbrain and spinal cord). Another transcriptional control gene, Gbx2, is expressed between the Otx2 and Hox expression domains.

Gbx2 and Otx2 proteins mutually repress each other's expression, so their domains abut at a sharp line—this will become the midbrain/hindbrain boundary (see Fig. 9-2A). At this interface between gene expression domains (an area known as the **isthmus**), a band of cells differentiates that secrete **fibroblast growth factor 8** (Fgf8), which signals the formation of optic tectum in the Otx2 expression domain and cerebellum in the Gbx2 domain. Fgf8 is also released from a signaling center at the cranial pole of the axis (called the **anterior neural ridge** [ANR]), inducing the local expression of transcription factors such as Bf1 (also known as FoxG1) that establish the telencephalon as a distinct region of the forebrain (see Fig. 9-2A). Similarly, a further signaling center that develops in the middle of the diencephalon (at the **zona limitans intrathalamica** [ZLI]) releases another morphogen, **sonic hedgehog** (Shh), which signals the formation of prethalamus cranially and thalamus caudally (see Fig. 9-2A).

As the initially flat neural plate neurulates to form the neural tube, distinct signaling centers form at both ventral and dorsal midlines, along almost the entire length of the CrCd axis (also covered in Chapter 4). The ventral pole cells, constituting the **floor plate of the neural tube**, secrete Shh (as does the underlying **notochord** and **prechordal plate**, more rostrally), whereas the dorsal cells, constituting the **roof plate of the neural tube**, secrete **bone morphogenetic proteins** (Bmps). In the context of midbrain, hindbrain, and spinal cord, Shh signaling from the floor plate induces the formation of a variety of neuronal cell types according to the concentration of Shh—at high levels, close to the floor plate, motoneurons are induced, whereas a diversity of interneurons is induced at successively lower Shh levels, impinging on precursor cells at successively more dorsal positions in the basal plate (see Fig. 9-2C). The Bmp gradient from the roof plate counteracts the Shh gradient and is responsible for the elaboration of a range of alar plate cell types (see Fig. 9-2C).

How CrCd and DV signals interact to confer position in two dimensions is not fully understood. However, it is clear that signals from the dorsal and ventral poles are essentially uniform along the length of the CrCd axis, yet they induce different cell types at different CrCd positions. For example, Shh from the midbrain floor plate induces the formation of oculomotor neurons at one CrCd position and dopaminergic neurons of the substantia nigra at another CrCd position. One explanation is that the uniform ventral signal in this case acts on a preexisting bias, or **competence**, of the receiving cells that is conferred during patterning of the CrCd axis.

Having achieved a correct spatial pattern of differentiation, with individual neuronal subtypes either in their correct positions or specified to migrate into new settling positions, the next major event in brain development is the outgrowth of axons to form connections with other neurons—the substrate of forming neural networks. A well-studied example is the visual system, where all sequential processes of cell patterning, axon outgrowth, and formation of appropriate connections are accessible. The development of the visual system will be considered later in this chapter.

FORMATION OF BRAIN FLEXURES

Between the fourth and eighth weeks, the brain tube folds sharply at three locations (see Fig. 9-1). The first of these folds to develop is the **mesencephalic flexure (cranial or cephalic flexure)**, centered at the midbrain region. The second fold is the **cervical flexure**, located

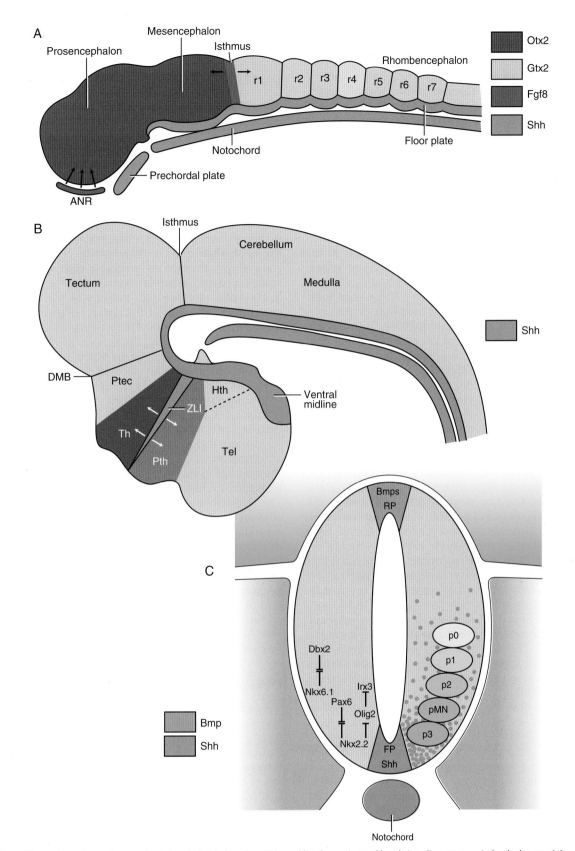

Figure 9-2. The early embryonic neural axis is subdivided and partitioned by the actions of local signaling centers in both the cranial-caudal (*A, B*) and dorsal-ventral (*C*) axes. In the earlier embryo (*A*), signaling boundaries develop between rhombomeres (r1-r7) and at the midbrain-hindbrain boundary (isthmus). The latter expresses the signaling molecule Fgf8, which triggers development of the optic tectum in the caudal midbrain and cerebellum in r1. At the cranial tip of the neural plate, a row of cells that earlier expressed Wnt inhibitors develops into the anterior neural ridge (ANR); the Fgfs released by ANR cells are involved in specifying development of the telencephalon (Tel). Later in development (*B*), another major signaling center (the zona limitans intrathalamica, ZLI) develops in the mid-diencephalon and regulates the development of thalamus (Th) and prethalamus (Pth). DMB, diencephalic/mesencephalic boundary; Hth, hypothalamus; Ptec, pretectum. *C*, Cross section through the dorsal-ventral (DV) axis of the neural tube. Ventral midline cells (floor plate [FP]) express the morphogen sonic hedgehog (Shh), which diffuses through the ventral regions forming a concentration gradient. Different transcription factors are induced at different Shh concentrations, such that their expression domains subdivide the DV axis. Some of these factors (*shown on left of figure*) mutually repress each other's expression, effectively sharpening the interfaces between their domains. The transcription factors expressed in each domain direct the expression of downstream genes that regulate progenitor cell identity. Shown on the right side are the progenitors for motoneurons (pMN) and for four different types of interneuron (p0-p3). Bmps are expressed in the roof plate (RP) and induce dorsal interneurons.

near the juncture between the myelencephalon and the spinal cord. Both of these flexures involve a ventral folding of the brain tube. The third fold, a reverse, dorsally directed flexion called the **pontine flexure**, begins at the location of the developing pons. By the eighth week, deepening of the pontine flexure has folded the metencephalon (including the developing cerebellum) back onto the myelencephalon.

CYTODIFFERENTIATION OF NEURAL TUBE

Cytodifferentiation of the neural tube commences in the rhombencephalic region, just after the occipitocervical neural folds fuse, and proceeds cranially and caudally as the groove closes at these levels to form the neural tube. The precursors of most cell types of the future central nervous system—neurons, some types of glial cells, and ependymal cells that line the central canal of the spinal cord and the ventricles of the brain—are produced by proliferation in the layer of neuroepithelial cells that immediately surrounds the neural canal (Fig. 9-3). Early neuroepithelial cells share some glial characteristics and are often called **radial cells** when they span most of the wall of the early neural tube (e.g., the left-most cell in Fig. 9-3*A*). These cells undergo proliferation to give rise to both neuronal and glial cell progenitors. Proliferating neuroepithelial cells are contained within the **ventricular layer** of the differentiating neural tube, with mitosis occurring at the luminal surface. The first wave of cells produced in the ventricular layer consists of postmitotic **young neurons**, which migrate peripherally to establish a second layer containing cell bodies, the **mantle layer**, external to the ventricular layer. This **neuron**-containing layer develops into the **gray matter** of the central nervous system. The neuronal processes (axons) that sprout from the mantle layer neurons grow peripherally to establish a third layer, the **marginal layer**, which contains no neuronal cell bodies and becomes the **white matter** of the central nervous system. The white matter is so called because of the whitish color imparted by the fatty myelin sheaths that wrap around many of the axons. In the CNS, these sheaths are formed by oligodendrocytes (discussed in the next section; in the PNS, myelin sheaths are formed by neural crest cell–derived Schwann cells; Schwann cells are covered in Chapter 10). The marginal layer contains axons entering and leaving the CNS, as well as axon tracts coursing to higher or lower levels in the CNS.

After production of neurons is waning in the ventricular layer, this layer begins to produce a new cell type, the **glioblast** (see Fig. 9-3*A*). These cells differentiate into the **glia** of the CNS—**astrocytes** and **oligodendrocytes**. Glia provide metabolic and structural support to the neurons of the central nervous system. The last cells produced by the ventricular layer are the **ependymal cells**; these line the brain ventricles and the central canal of the spinal cord (see Fig. 9-3*A, C*). Elaborations of the ependyma are responsible for producing **cerebrospinal fluid (CSF)**, which fills the brain ventricles, the central canal of the spinal cord, and the subarachnoid space that surrounds the CNS. The CSF is under pressure and thus provides a fluid jacket that protects and supports the brain.

DIFFERENTIATION OF SPINAL CORD

The differentiation of the spinal cord is relatively simple compared with that of the brain, so we will begin our discussion with the spinal cord. Starting at the end of the fourth week, the neurons in the mantle layer of the spinal cord become organized into four plates that run the length of the cord: a pair of **dorsal** or **alar plates (columns)** and a pair of **ventral** or **basal plates (columns)** (Fig. 9-4). Laterally, the two plates abut at a groove called the **sulcus limitans**; dorsally and ventrally, they are connected by non-neurogenic structures called, respectively, the **roof plate** and the **floor plate**. The cells of the ventral columns become the **somatic motoneurons** of the spinal cord and innervate somatic motor structures such as the voluntary (striated) muscles of the body wall and extremities. The cells of the dorsal columns develop into **association neurons**. These neurons receive synapses from *afferent* (incoming) fibers from the sensory neurons of the dorsal root ganglia (covered in Chapter 10). In addition, the axon of an association neuron may synapse with motoneurons on the same (ipsilateral) or opposite (contralateral) side of the cord, forming a reflex arc—or it may ascend to the brain. The outgoing (*efferent*) motor neuron fibers exit via the ventral roots.

In most regions of the cord—at all 12 thoracic levels, at lumbar levels L1 and L2, and at sacral levels S2 to S4—the neurons in more dorsal regions of the ventral columns segregate to form **intermediolateral cell columns**. The thoracic and lumbar intermediolateral cell columns contain the **visceral motoneurons** that constitute the central **autonomic motoneurons of the sympathetic division**, whereas the intermediolateral cell columns in the sacral region contain the **visceral motoneurons** that constitute the central **autonomic motoneurons of the parasympathetic division**. The structure and function of these systems are covered in Chapter 10 (where the peripheral components are described). In general, at any given level of the brain or spinal cord, the motoneurons form before the sensory elements.

OVERVIEW OF SPINAL NERVES

Spinal nerves (see Fig. 9-4) consist of (1) a dorsal root, containing axons whose cell bodies reside in the dorsal root ganglion; (2) a ventral root, containing axons whose cell bodies reside in the ventral spinal cord gray matter (ventral columns); and (3) at levels in which intermediolateral cell columns are present, a visceral root, containing axons that connect preganglionic autonomic neuronal cells bodies within the spinal cord (intermediolateral cell columns) with postganglionic autonomic cell bodies in the periphery (autonomic ganglia). The region where these roots join and extend peripherally constitutes the spinal nerve. Spinal nerves are covered in greater detail in Chapter 10.

DIFFERENTIATION OF BRAIN

For purposes of description, the brain can be divided into two parts: the **brain stem**, which represents the cranial continuation of the spinal cord and is similar to

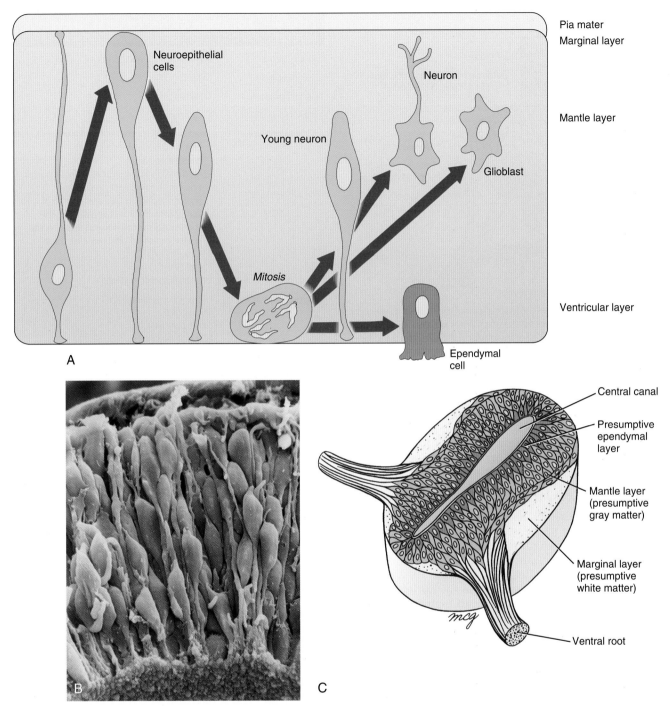

Figure 9-3. Cytodifferentiation of the neural tube. *A, B,* Neuroepithelial cells are elongated and span the entire thickness of the wall of the early neural tube before rounding up at the luminal side for mitosis. Waves of mitosis and differentiation form postmitotic young neurons, which migrate away from the luminal side to form definitive neurons and glioblasts, some of which form radial glia (or Bergmann glia in the cerebellum). Such a wave is illustrated in *A,* which shows progression in time from left to right. *A, C,* As neurons form, the neural tube becomes stratified into a ventricular layer (adjacent to the neural canal), a mantle layer (containing neuronal cell bodies), and a marginal layer (containing nerve fibers).

it in organization, and the **higher centers**, which are extremely specialized and retain little trace of a spinal cord–like organization. The brain stem consists of the **myelencephalon**, the **metencephalon** derivative called the **pons**, and the **mesencephalon**. The higher centers consist of the **cerebellum** (derived from the metencephalon) and the **forebrain**.

BRAIN STEM

The fundamental pattern of alar columns, basal columns, dorsal sensory roots, and ventral motor roots described earlier in the chapter for the spinal cord also occurs, albeit more elaborately, in the brain stem. This pattern is altered during development as some groups of neurons migrate

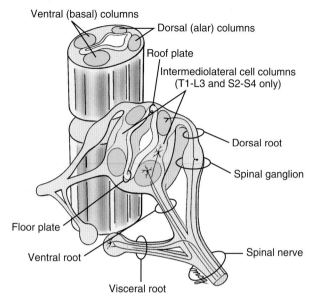

Ventral (basal) columns
Dorsal (alar) columns
Roof plate
Intermediolateral cell columns (T1-L3 and S2-S4 only)
Dorsal root
Spinal ganglion
Floor plate
Ventral root
Spinal nerve
Visceral root

Figure 9-4. Neurons within the mantle layer of the neural tube become organized into two ventral motor (basal) columns and two dorsal sensory (alar) columns throughout most of the length of the spinal cord and hindbrain. Intermediolateral cell columns also form at spinal levels T1-L3 and S2-S4 (the slice showing the intermediolateral cell columns is taken from the midsection of the spinal cord shown in the background of the figure).

Brain Region	Associated Cranial Nerves
	TABLE 9-1 LOCATION OF THE CRANIAL NERVE NUCLEI
Telencephalon	Olfactory (I)
Diencephalon	Optic (II)
Mesencephalon	Oculomotor (III)
Metencephalon	Trochlear (IV) (arises in the metencephalon but is later displaced into the mesencephalon)
	Trigeminal (V) (trigeminal sensory nuclei arise in the metencephalon and myelencephalon but are later displaced partly into the mesencephalon; the trigeminal motor nucleus arises in the metencephalon and remains there)
	Abducens (VI)*
	Facial (VII)*
	Vestibulocochlear (VIII)*
Myelencephalon	Glossopharyngeal (IX)
	Vagus (X)
	Accessory (XI)
	Hypoglossal (XII)

*The origin of these three nerves is uncertain, and it may differ among species. Thus, it is unclear in human embryos whether these nerves originate from the caudal metencephalon or the cranial myelencephalon.

away from their site of origin to establish a nucleus elsewhere. Also, as in the spinal cord, the brain stem is organized into a ventricular zone (containing proliferating neuroepithelial cells that generate young neurons and glioblasts), a mantle zone, and a marginal zone.

Overview of Cranial Nerves

All of the twelve cranial nerves except the first (olfactory) and second (optic) have nuclei located in the brain stem. These nuclei are among the earliest structures to develop in the brain and hence are discussed here; cranial nerves are covered in greater detail in Chapter 10. The basal plates of the rhombencephalon form the earliest neurons in the CNS. By day twenty-eight, all brain stem cranial nerve motor nuclei are distinguishable. As in the spinal cord, the alar plates of the brain stem form somewhat later than the basal plates, appearing in the middle of the fifth week. The cranial nerve associational nuclei are all distinguishable by the end of the fifth week.

Although cranial nerves show homologies to spinal nerves, they are much less uniform in composition. Three cranial nerves are exclusively sensory (I, II, and VIII); four are exclusively motor (IV, VI, XI, and XII); one is mixed sensory and motor (i.e., mixed; V); one is motor and parasympathetic (III); and three include sensory, motor, and parasympathetic fibers (VII, IX, and X). Nevertheless, the motor and sensory axons of the cranial nerves bear the same basic relation to the cell columns of the brain that the ventral and dorsal roots bear to the cell columns of the spinal cord. Table 9-1 summarizes the relations of the cranial nerves to the subdivisions of the brain.

Organization of Columns

In the same way that the basal plates of the spinal cord are organized into somatic motor and autonomic (visceral)

motor columns (covered earlier in the chapter), the basal and alar cranial nerve nuclei of the brain stem are organized into seven columns that subserve particular functions. Although seven columns form, some textbooks described only *six* functions, three motor and three sensory. The columns are as follows (Fig. 9-5; numbers listed below correspond to the numbers shown in Figs. 9-5 and 9-6).

MOTOR FUNCTIONS (BASAL COLUMNS)

1. *Somatic efferent* neurons in the brain innervate the extrinsic ocular muscles and the muscles of the tongue (III, IV, VI, and XII).
2. *Branchial efferent* (alternatively called *special visceral efferent*) neurons serve the striated muscles derived from the pharyngeal arches and ensheathed by connective tissue derived from cranial neural crest cells (V, VII, IX, X). The motor nucleus of the accessory nerve (XI) is branchial efferent because it forms part of this column; even though the trapezius and sternocleidomastoid muscles that it innervates are not obviously derived from pharyngeal arch mesoderm, their connective tissue derives from cranial neural crest cells.
3. *Visceral efferent* (alternatively called *general visceral efferent*) neurons serve the parasympathetic pathways innervating the sphincter pupillae and ciliary muscles of the eyes (III) and (via the glossopharyngeal nerve, IX, and the vagus nerve, X) the smooth muscle and glands of the thoracic, abdominal, and pelvic viscera, including heart, airways, and salivary glands.

SENSORY FUNCTIONS (ALAR COLUMNS)

4. *Visceral afferent* (alternatively called *general visceral afferent*) association neurons receive impulses via the

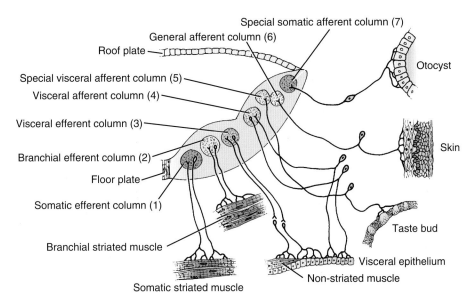

Figure 9-5. Organization of the brain stem cranial nerve nuclei. The basal columns give rise to motor (efferent) cranial nerve nuclei, and the alar columns to associational (afferent) cranial nerve nuclei. These nuclei can be grouped into seven discontinuous columns (numbers in parentheses correspond to the numbering describing these columns in the text), each subserving a specific type of function.

vagus nerve from sensory receptors in the walls of the thoracic, abdominal, and pelvic viscera (referred to as *interoceptive sensory receptors*).

5. *Special afferent* association neurons subserve the special senses. This function is sometimes subdivided into two functions—*special visceral afferent* (taste; VII, IX) and *special somatic afferent* (hearing and balance; VIII)—to match the two columns of special afferent nuclei that develop in the brain stem.

6. *General afferent* (alternatively called *general somatic afferent*) association neurons in the brain subserve "general sensation" (e.g., touch, temperature, pain) over the head and neck, as well as for the mucosa of the oral and nasal cavities and the pharynx (V, VII, IX).

The number of columns present at different levels of the brain stem varies, with all columns present in the rhombencephalon and only two columns present in the mesencephalon (see Fig. 9-6). The distribution of columns in the brain stem is as follows (columns are numbered as described immediately above and as labeled in Figs. 9-5 and 9-6):

1. The *somatic efferent* column consists of the nucleus of the hypoglossal nerve (XII) in the caudalmost rhombencephalon, that of nerve VI more cranially in the rhombencephalon, that of nerve IV in the most cranial rhombencephalon (later displaced into the caudal midbrain), and that of nerve III in the mesencephalon.

2. The *branchial efferent* column contains three nuclei serving nerves V, VII, and IX through XI and is confined to the rhombencephalon. The branchial efferent nuclei serving nerves V and VII are located cranially in the rhombencephalon; caudally, the elongated nucleus ambiguus supplies branchial efferent fibers for nerves IX, X, and XI.

3. The *visceral efferent* column includes two nuclei located in the rhombencephalon. The salivatory nuclei provide preganglionic parasympathetic innervation to the salivary and lacrimal glands via nerves VII and IX. Just caudal to this nucleus is the dorsal nucleus of the

vagus, which contains preganglionic parasympathetic neurons innervating the viscera. The Edinger-Westphal nucleus (III) is located in the mesencephalon.

4. The general *visceral afferent* column consists of the nucleus that receives interoceptive information via the glossopharyngeal nerve (IX) and the vagus nerve (X).

5. The first *special afferent* column (sometimes called the *special visceral afferent* column) consists of the nucleus of the tractus solitarius, which receives taste impulses via the facial (VII), glossopharyngeal (IX), and vagus (X) nerves.

6. The *general afferent* column consists of the neurons that receive impulses of general sensation from areas of the face served by the trigeminal (V) and facial (VII) nerves and from the oral, nasal, external auditory, and pharyngeal and laryngeal cavities (V, VII, IX, and X).

7. The second *special afferent* column (sometimes called the *special somatic afferent column*) consists of the cochlear and vestibular nuclei, which subserve the special senses of balance and hearing (VIII).

Not all nuclei that develop within the basal and alar columns remain where they form. For example, the branchial efferent nucleus of the facial nerve travels first caudally and then laterally, circumnavigating the abducens nucleus, to form the internal genu of the facial nerve. The nucleus ambiguus also migrates, as do some of the noncranial nerve nuclei of the rhombencephalon, such as the olivary and pontine nuclei, which arise from the rhombic lip but migrate to a ventral position (Fig. 9-7). Many CNS neurons "reel out" their axons behind them as they migrate; thus, the migratory path of a nucleus often can be reconstructed by tracing its axons.

Rhombencephalon

In contrast to the spinal cord, where the roof and floor plates are narrow and lie at the bottom of deep grooves (see Fig. 9-4), in the rhombencephalon, the walls of the neural tube splay open dorsally so that the roof plate is stretched and widened and the two sides of the hindbrain

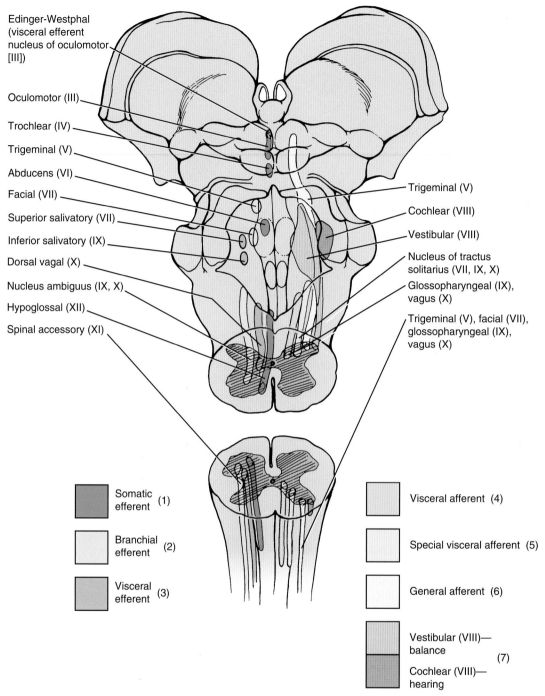

Figure 9-6. View of the brain stem showing the locations of the cranial nerve nuclei making up the seven columns (numbers in parentheses correspond to the numbers describing these columns in the text). The efferent nuclei are shown on the left and the afferent nuclei on the right.

become disposed at an obtuse angle to one another (see Fig. 9-7). The rhombencephalic neural canal (future fourth ventricle) is rhombus (diamond)-shaped in dorsal view, with the widest point located at the pontine flexure. The dorsal margin of the alar plate, adjoining the massively expanded roof plate, is called the **rhombic lip**. Its metencephalic portion contributes to the granule cells of the cerebellum (covered later).

The thin rhombencephalic roof plate consists mainly of a layer of ependyma and is covered by a well-vascularized layer of pia mater called the **tela choroidea**. On either side of the midline, the pia and ependyma form a zone of minute, finger-like structures projecting into the fourth ventricle. This zone, called a **choroid plexus**, is specialized to secrete cerebrospinal fluid. Similar choroid plexuses develop in the ventricles of the forebrain (covered later in the chapter). Cerebrospinal fluid circulates constantly through the central canal of the spinal cord and the ventricles of the brain and also through the subarachnoid space surrounding the CNS, from which it is

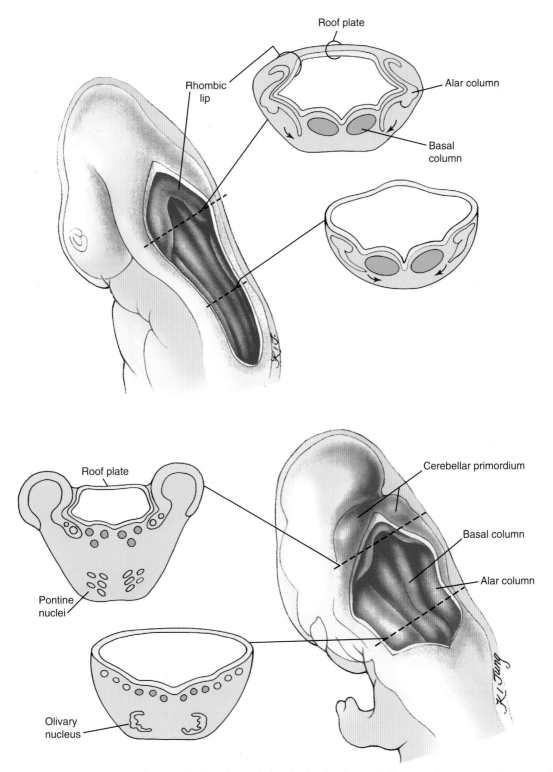

Figure 9-7. Early differentiation of the rhombencephalon. The roof plate in the rhombencephalic region forms a wide, transparent membrane over the fourth ventricle. The basal and alar columns give rise to the motor and associational nuclei, respectively, of most of the cranial nerves, as well as to other structures. Extensions of the alar columns also migrate ventrally to form pontine and olivary nuclei.

reabsorbed into the blood. The fluid gains access to the subarachnoid space via three holes that open in the roof plate of the fourth ventricle: a single **median aperture (foramen of Magendie)** and two **lateral apertures (foramina of Luschka)**.

Formation of Medulla Oblongata, Pons, and Cerebellum

The myelencephalon (consisting of rhombomeres three to eight) differentiates to form the **medulla oblongata**, which is the portion of the brain most similar to the

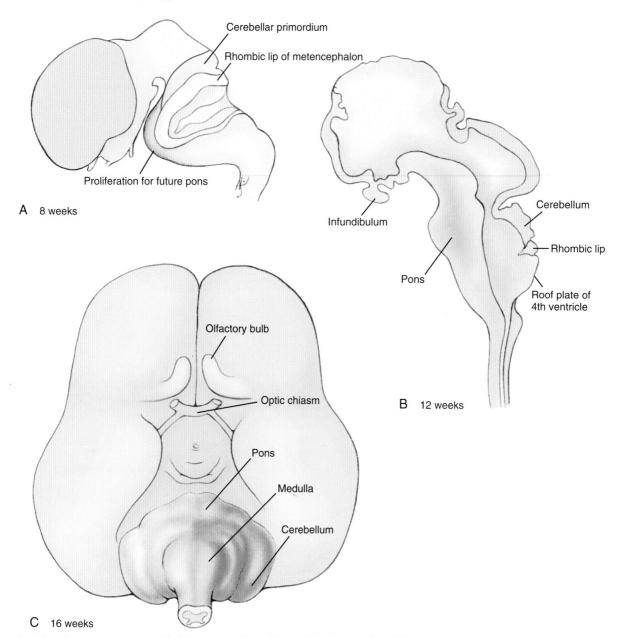

Figure 9-8. Development of the pons (*A-C*). The pons is formed by proliferation of cell and fiber tracts on the ventral side of the metencephalon.

spinal cord. In addition to housing many cranial nerve nuclei, the medulla serves as a relay center between the spinal cord and the higher brain centers and contains centers and nerve networks that regulate respiration, heartbeat, reflex movements, and a number of other functions.

The metencephalon (rhombomeres one and two) gives rise to two structures: the **pons**, which functions mainly to relay signals that link both the spinal cord and the cerebral cortex with the cerebellum; and the **cerebellum**, which is a center for balance and postural control. (Although the cerebellum is part of the higher centers, rather than part of the brain stem, it is covered here because it is derived from the rhombencephalon.) The pons (Latin, for "bridge") contains massive axon tracts (Fig. 9-8) that arise mainly from the marginal layer of the basal columns of the metencephalon. In addition,

ventrally located **pontine nuclei** relay input from the cerebrum to the cerebellum (see Fig. 9-7).

The cerebellum is derived from both the alar plates of the metencephalon and the adjacent rhombic lips; the latter give rise to **cerebellar granule cells** and the deep cerebellar nuclei (covered later). The rudiment of the cerebellum is first recognizable as a pair of thickened **cerebellar plates** or **cerebellar primordia** (Fig. 9-9; see also Fig. 9-7). By the second month, the cranial portions of the growing cerebellar plates meet across the midline, forming a single primordium that covers the fourth ventricle. This primordium initially bulges only into the fourth ventricle and does not protrude dorsally. However, by the middle of the third month, the growing cerebellum begins to bulge dorsally, forming a dumbbell-shaped swelling at the cranial end of the rhombencephalon.

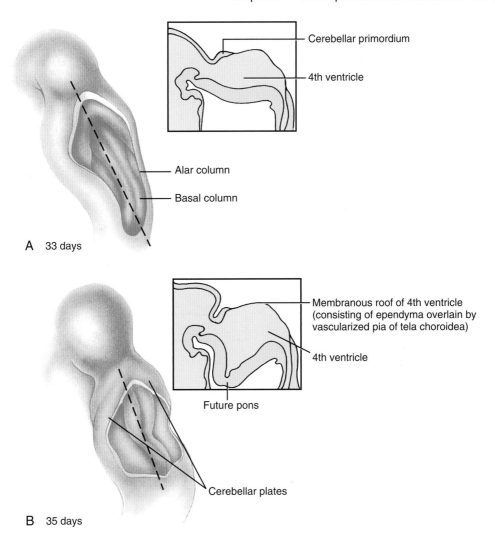

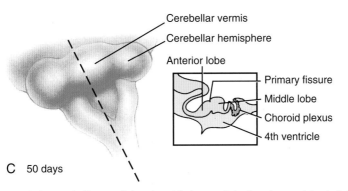

Figure 9-9. Development of the cerebellum and the choroid plexus of the fourth ventricle. *A, B,* Proliferation of cells in the metencephalic alar plates and adjacent rhombic lips forms the cerebellar plates. *C,* Further growth creates two lateral cerebellar hemispheres and a central vermis. The primary fissure forms and divides the cerebellum into anterior and middle lobes. A choroid plexus develops in the roof plate of the fourth ventricle.

Continued

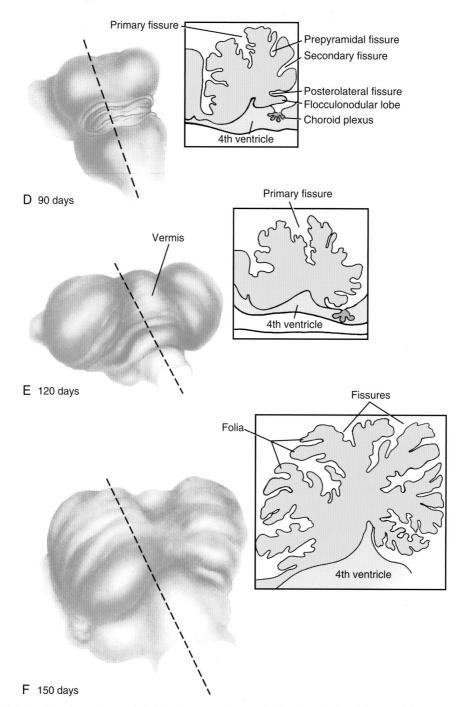

Figure 9-9, cont'd *D-F,* Continued fissuration subdivides the expanding cerebellum into further lobes, and then, starting in the third month, into lobules and folia. This process greatly increases the area of the cerebellar cortex.

At this stage, the developing cerebellum is separated into cranial and caudal portions by a transverse groove called the **posterolateral fissure** (Fig. 9-9D). The caudal portion, consisting of a pair of **flocculonodular lobes**, represents the most primitive part of the cerebellum. The larger cranial portion consists of a narrow median swelling called the **vermis**, connecting a pair of broad **cerebellar hemispheres**. This cranial portion grows much faster than the flocculonodular lobes and becomes the dominant component of the mature cerebellum.

The cerebellar vermis and hemispheres undergo an intricate process of transverse folding as they develop. The major **primary fissure** deepens by the end of the third month and divides the vermis and hemispheres into a cranial **anterior lobe** and a caudal **middle lobe** (see Fig. 9-9C, D). These lobes are further divided into a number of **lobules** by the development of additional transverse fissures (starting with the **secondary** and **prepyramidal fissures**), and the surface of the lobules is thrown into closely packed, leaflike transverse gyri called

Parasagittal sections through the roof of the 4th ventricle

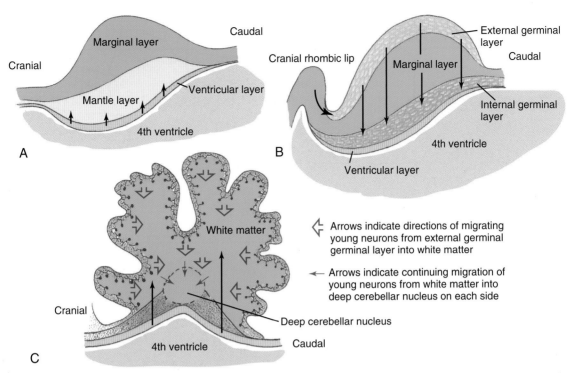

Figure 9-10. Cytodifferentiation of the cerebellum. *A*, During the second month, typical ventricular, mantle, and marginal zones have formed throughout the metencephalon region, the dorsal part of which (alar plates and associated rhombic lips) forms the cerebellum. Arrows indicate movement of cells from the ventricular to the mantle layer. *B*, During the third month, two additional layers have formed: an external germinal layer (derived from the metencephalic, cranial, rhombic lips; *curved arrow*) and an internal germinal layer (composed of granule cells born in the external germinal layer that subsequently migrate toward the ventricle to form this layer; *straight arrows*). Neurons residing earlier in the mantle zone (and born in the ventricular zone, namely, stellate, basket, Golgi, and Purkinje cells) have dispersed into the marginal zone, where they will subsequently arrange into a distinct pattern. *C*, Neurons (granule cells) produced by the external germinal layer continue to migrate inward (*red open arrows*), while neurons produced by the ventricular zone continue to migrate outward (*black closed arrows*). Some of the inwardly migrating neurons continue their migration ventrally to form the deep cerebellar nuclei (*red closed arrows*).

Continued

folia. These processes of fissure formation and foliation continue throughout embryonic, fetal, and postnatal life, and they vastly increase the surface area of the cerebellar cortex (Fig. 9-9*E, F*).

The cerebellum has two types of gray matter: a group of internal **deep cerebellar nuclei** and an external **cerebellar cortex**. Four deep nuclei form on each side: **dentate**, **globose**, **emboliform**, and **fastigial nuclei**. All output from the cerebellar cortex is relayed through these nuclei. The cerebellar cortex has an extremely regular cytoarchitecture that is similar over the entire cerebellum. The cell types of the cortex are arranged in layers.

The deep nuclei and cortex of the cerebellum are produced by a complex process of neurogenesis and neuronal migration (Fig. 9-10). As elsewhere in the neural tube, the neuroepithelium of the metencephalon undergoes an initial proliferation to produce ventricular, mantle, and marginal layers (Fig. 9-10*A*). However, in the third month, a second layer of proliferating cells forms over the marginal zone. It is derived from the most cranial rhombic lips. This new outer layer of proliferation and neurogenesis is called the **external germinal layer** (or, sometimes, the **external granular layer**; Fig. 9-10*B*).

Starting in the fourth month, the germinal layers undergo highly regulated cell divisions that produce the various populations of cerebellar neurons (Fig. 9-10*C*). The *ventricular* layer produces four types of neurons that migrate to the cortex: **Purkinje cells, Golgi cells, basket cells**, and **stellate cells**, as well as their associated glia (astrocytes—including Bergmann glia, which are discussed below—and oligodendrocytes). The remaining cells of the cerebellar cortex, the **granule cells**, arise from the *external germinal* layer. The external germinal layer also gives rise to the **primitive nuclear neurons**, which migrate to form the **deep cerebellar nuclei** (Fig. 9-10*D*).

As each newly born Purkinje cell migrates from the ventricular layer toward the cortex, it reels out an axon that maintains synaptic contact with neurons in the developing cerebellar nuclei. These axons will constitute the only efferents of the mature cerebellar cortex. The Purkinje cells form a distinct **Purkinje cell layer** just underlying the external germinal layer, which is initially multilayered but becomes a single layer when foliation is complete. Basket and stellate cells also migrate radially from the ventricular layer, closely associated with the Purkinje cells, and form the **molecular layer** of the

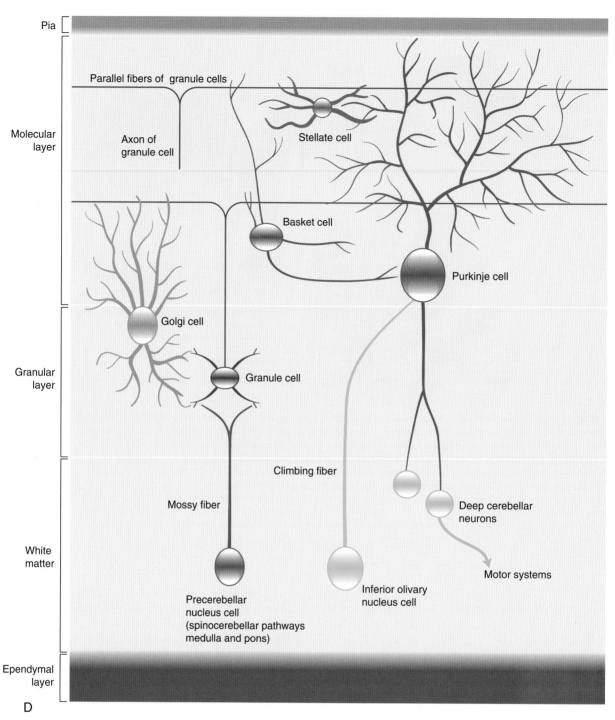

Pia

Molecular layer

Parallel fibers of granule cells

Axon of granule cell

Stellate cell

Basket cell

Purkinje cell

Granular layer

Golgi cell

Granule cell

White matter

Climbing fiber

Mossy fiber

Deep cerebellar neurons

Motor systems

Precerebellar nucleus cell (spinocerebellar pathways medulla and pons)

Inferior olivary nucleus cell

Ependymal layer

D

Figure 9-10, cont'd *D,* Histologic structure of the mature cerebellar cortex showing the four types of neurons that originate from the ventricular zone (Purkinje cells, Golgi cells, basket cells, and stellate cells) and a granule cell neuron, which originates from the external germinal (granular) layer. Each granule cell extends an axon vertically, which splits into two branches known as parallel fibers. Also shown are the connections of the neurons with one another and with mossy fibers (from precerebellar nucleus cells), climbing fibers (from inferior olivary nucleus cells), and deep cerebellar neurons. Bergmann glia and oligodendrocytes are not shown.

definitive cortex. Once the granule cells begin to differentiate, they migrate (in a direction that is opposite of that of the Purkinje, basket, and stellate cells) from the external germinal layer through the developing molecular layer toward the ventricular layer. Here, they form the **internal germinal layer** or **internal granular layer** of the developing cortex (see Fig. 9-10*B*), simply

called the **granular layer** of the definitive cortex (see Fig. 9-10*D*). Granule cells migrate along the elongated fibers of glial cells called **Bergmann (radial) glia.** The bifurcated axons of granule cells course transversely in the outermost, molecular layer of the cortex, passing through and synapsing with the fanlike array of Purkinje cell dendrites (see Fig. 9-10*D*).

In the Clinic

CELLULAR AND MOLECULAR BASIS OF CEREBELLAR MALFORMATIONS AND DYSFUNCTION

A variety of malformations occur during the development of the human cerebellum, including **hypoplasias** (under development), **dysplasias** (abnormal tissue development), and **heterotopias** (misplaced cells). More subtle developmental defects in the organization of the cerebellar cortical circuits might underlie a plethora of other disorders. **Schizophrenia**, for instance, which affects up to 1% of adult humans, might be related to early defects in neuronal migration, the expression of neurotransmitter receptors, or myelination, not only in the forebrain (the area usually thought to be affected in most mental illnesses) but, surprisingly, also in the cerebellar cortex. Another subset of cerebellar abnormalities result from **degeneration**. Cerebellar disorders often result in **ataxias** (disruptions of coordination).

Cerebellar ataxias can be caused by either environmental toxins or genetic anomalies. Mercury, an environmental toxin, may cause focal damage to the granular layer of the cerebellum and ataxia in humans following exposure. Genetic causes of ataxia include both chromosomal anomalies and single-gene mutations. Trisomy 13 results in gross brain abnormalities affecting the cerebellum and cerebrum. In the cerebellum, the vermis is hypoplastic and neurons are heterotopically located in the white matter. Cerebellar dysplasia, usually of the vermis, is also characteristic of trisomy 18, and Down syndrome (trisomy 21) may involve abnormalities of the Purkinje and granule cell layers. A variety of chromosome deletion syndromes, including 5p– (**cri du chat**), 13q–, and 4p–, also may cause cerebellar anomalies.

A large number of cerebellar ataxias are inherited, with autosomal recessive, autosomal dominant, X-linked, and mitochondrial inheritance all observed. Several autosomal recessive cerebellar ataxias are known; one of the most common is **Friedreich ataxia**, which affects the dorsal root ganglia, spinal cord, and cerebellum. It is a progressive disorder with onset in childhood characterized by clumsy gait, ataxia of the upper limbs, and dysarthria (disturbed speech articulation). Other autosomal recessive cerebellar ataxia syndromes include **ataxia-telangiectasia**, **Marinesco-Sjögren syndrome**, **Gillespie syndrome**, **Joubert syndrome**, and the growing class of disorders termed **congenital disorders of glycosylation**. The latter three disorders often present with gross cerebellar malformations that can be diagnosed after birth with CT (computed tomography) or MRI (magnetic resonance imaging).

More than thirty autosomal dominant **spinocerebellar ataxia syndromes** have been mapped, and the gene has been identified in about half of these. Many of these conditions are caused by unstable CAG **trinucleotide repeat** tracts within the coding region of the genes. CAG codes for the amino acid glutamine, and these **polyglutamine disorders** occur when the tract of glutamine residues reaches a disease-causing threshold. Expanded CAG trinucleotide repeats are unstable and can increase in size as they are passed from one generation to the next, with earlier onset and more severe disease. This worsening of the disease in successive generations is called **genetic anticipation**.

The mutations that cause some of the recessive heritable cerebellar ataxias are known to affect the metabolism of mucopolysaccharides, lipids, and amino acids. In the cerebellum, these mutations cause effects such as a deficiency of Purkinje cells (mucopolysaccharidosis III), abnormal accumulation of lipid (juvenile gangliosidosis), and reduced myelin formation (phenylketonuria). The disorder called **olivopontocerebellar atrophy** seems in some cases to be caused by a deficiency in the excitatory neurotransmitter glutamate, resulting in turn from a deficiency in the enzyme glutamate dehydrogenase.

In the Research Lab

MOUSE MUTANTS WITH CEREBELLAR ATAXIAS

A more detailed understanding of the cellular and molecular mechanisms that cause various cerebellar anomalies has been gained by research on a series of mouse mutants that display a broad array of cerebellar ataxias. The strange gaits of many of these mouse mutants can be correlated with defects in cerebellar cytoarchitecture. For example, the high-stepping, broad-based gait of the stumbler mutant is apparently caused by defects in Purkinje cells. The meander tail mutant also has Purkinje cell deficits, but only in the anterior lobe of the cerebellum. The vibrator mouse displays a rapid postural tremor caused by progressive degeneration of cerebellar neurons. This phenotype has been linked to mutations in the gene encoding phosphatidylinositol transfer protein alpha. Tottering and leaner mice exhibit symptoms of ataxia and epilepsy, which are likely due to mutations in the calcium channel alpha (1A) subunit gene. In humans, mutations in this gene have been linked to familial hemiplegic migraine, episodic ataxia type 2, and chronic spinocerebellar ataxia type 6.

Normally, the granule cells that arise in the external germinal layer of the developing cerebellum produce bipolar processes and then migrate inward along Bergmann glia (astrocyte) fibers to populate the internal granule cell layer, reeling out an axon behind them as they travel. In the homozygous recessive weaver mutant, the granule cells fail to produce processes, fail to migrate, and then die prematurely.

Weaver mice harbor a missense mutation in the gene coding for the G protein–coupled inward-rectifying potassium channel (Girk2). How this defect leads to granule cell death remains unclear. However, a series of experiments, using wild-type and weaver astrocytes and granule cells mixed in vitro, showed that wild-type granule cells interact normally with weaver astrocytes, but weaver granule cells do not interact with wild-type astrocytes and do not migrate along astrocyte processes. Thus, the weaver mutation has a direct effect on granule cells but not on astrocytes.

Granule cells also interact with Purkinje cells as well as astrocytes, and this interaction is required for granule cell survival. In the normal cerebellum, the relative number of granule cells is matched to the number of Purkinje cells. This matching is accomplished by a process of **histogenetic cell death**, by which the great overabundance of granule cells initially produced by the external germinal layer is reduced to the correct number. Various experiments have indicated that this process is automatically controlled by the number of Purkinje cells: apparently, granule cells die unless they make contact with the dendritic arbor of a Purkinje cell. Sonic hedgehog is expressed by Purkinje cells and is required for granule cell proliferation and, likely, survival.

The role of Purkinje cells in granule cell survival was examined in two ways. In one experiment, staggerer–wild-type chimeras were made by aggregating eight-cell staggerer mutant mouse embryos with wild-type embryos and then reinserting them into the uterus of a pseudo-pregnant mother (**aggregation chimeras** are an alternative to injection chimeras, covered in Chapter 5, for making mouse chimeras). The death of Purkinje cells in the staggerer mouse embryos beginning in late gestation (staggerer mice harbor a mutation in RAR-related orphan receptor alpha, but the cause of Purkinje cell death is unknown) resulted in the birth of animals with widely different numbers of normal and wild-type Purkinje cells. Examination revealed a linear relationship between the number of granule cells and the number of wild-type Purkinje cells, confirming the hypothesis that granule cell survival depends on the presence of appropriate Purkinje cell targets. In another experiment, transgenic technology was used to kill Purkinje cells. It was found that overlying granule cells stopped their proliferation, and the internal granule layer of the cerebellar cortex (normally formed by migrating granule cells; discussed above) failed to form.

Mesencephalon

Much of the mesencephalon is composed of white matter, principally the massive tracts that connect the forebrain with the hindbrain and spinal cord. The midbrain also contains a number of important neuronal centers, including four cranial nerve nuclei.

As mentioned earlier in the chapter, the motor nuclei of the oculomotor (III) and trochlear (IV) nerves are located in the mesencephalon, as is a portion of the sensory nucleus of the trigeminal nerve (V) called the **mesencephalic trigeminal nucleus** (Fig. 9-11). However, of these nuclei, only those serving the oculomotor nerve and the trigeminal nerve arise from mesencephalic

neuroepithelial cells; the trochlear nuclei originate in the metencephalon and are secondarily displaced into the mesencephalon. The two nuclei of the oculomotor nerve are the somatic motor **oculomotor nucleus**, which controls the movements of all but the superior oblique and lateral rectus extrinsic ocular muscles, and the general visceral efferent **Edinger-Westphal nucleus**, which supplies parasympathetic pathways to the pupillary constrictor and the ciliary muscles of the globe.

The **superior** and **inferior colliculi** are visible as four prominent swellings on the dorsal surface of the midbrain (Fig. 9-11C). The superior colliculi receive axons from the retinae and mediate ocular reflexes. In

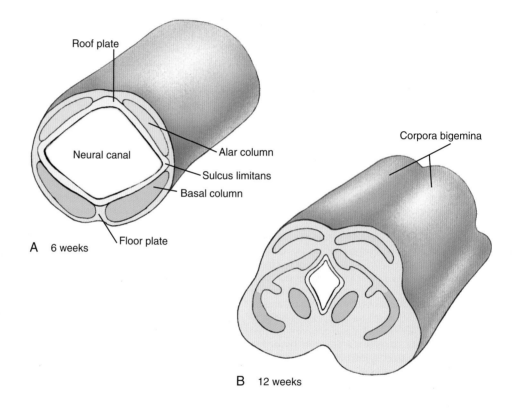

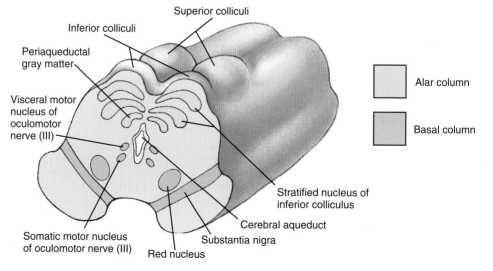

Figure 9-11. Development of the mesencephalon. *A, B,* A shallow longitudinal groove develops on the dorsal surface of the mesencephalon between weeks six and twelve, creating the corpora bigemina. *C,* Over the next month, a transverse groove subdivides these swellings to produce the superior and inferior colliculi. The mesencephalic alar columns form the stratified nuclear layers of the colliculi, the periaqueductal gray matter, and the substantia nigra. The mesencephalic basal columns form the red nuclei and nuclei of the oculomotor nerve.

contrast, the inferior colliculi form part of the perceptual pathway by which information from the cochlea is relayed to the auditory areas of the cerebral hemispheres. The colliculi are formed by mesencephalic alar plate cells that proliferate and migrate medially. The dorsal thickening produced by these cells is subsequently divided by a midline groove into a pair of lateral **corpora bigemina** (Fig. 9-11*B*), which are later subdivided into inferior and superior colliculi by a transverse groove. The synapses of axons from retinal ganglion cells form precise spatial maps in the superior colliculi of the corresponding sensory fields of the retina.

During development, the primitive ventricle of the mesencephalon becomes the narrow **cerebral aqueduct** (see Fig. 9-11*C*). The cerebrospinal fluid produced by the choroid plexuses of the forebrain normally flows through the cerebral aqueduct to reach the fourth ventricle. However, various conditions can cause the aqueduct to become blocked during fetal life. Obstruction of the flow of cerebrospinal fluid through the aqueduct results in the congenital condition called **hydrocephalus**, in which the third and lateral ventricles are swollen with fluid, the cerebral cortex is abnormally thin, and the sutures of the skull are forced apart, allowing the calvarial bones to increase in size (Fig. 9-12).

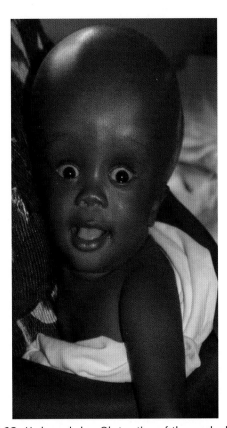

Figure 9-12. Hydrocephalus. Obstruction of the cerebral aqueduct causes the developing forebrain ventricles to become swollen with cerebrospinal fluid. If not corrected, either prenatally or typically soon after birth, by insertion of a shunt to drain cerebral spinal fluid from the ventricles and relieve excess pressure, the skull can undergo extreme enlargement as illustrated.

HIGHER CENTERS: FOREBRAIN

As covered earlier, the higher centers consist of the cerebellum (derived from the metencephalon) and the forebrain. The development of the cerebellum was discussed in the preceding section as part of the discussion of development of the rhombencephalon; hence, this section discusses only the development of the forebrain and its derivatives.

The forebrain or prosencephalon consists of two secondary brain vesicles: the diencephalon and the telencephalon. The walls of the diencephalon differentiate to form a number of neuronal centers and tracts that are described later. In addition, the roof plate, floor plate, and ependyma of the diencephalon give rise to several specialized structures through mechanisms that are relatively unique. These structures include the **choroid plexus** and **circumventricular organs**, **posterior lobe of the pituitary gland (neurohypophysis)**, and **optic vesicles**. The origin of the optic cups from the diencephalic neural folds is covered in Chapter 19.

The thin dorsal telencephalon **(pallium)** gives rise to the **cerebral hemispheres** and to the commissures and other structures that join them. It also forms the **olfactory bulbs** and **olfactory tracts**, which, along with the olfactory centers and tracts of the cerebral hemispheres, constitute the **rhinencephalon** ("nose-brain"). The thicker ventral part of the telencephalon, the **subpallium**, budges into the neural canal to form the ganglion eminences that later make up the **basal ganglia**.

Diencephalon

As mentioned earlier in the chapter, the walls of the diencephalon are formed by alar plates; basal plates are lacking. The alar plates form three subdivisions that have been described as neuromeres (called **prosomeres**), similar to the rhombomeres of the hindbrain: a rostral neuromere that forms the **prethalamus** and **hypothalamus**, a middle neuromere that forms the **thalamus** and **epithalamus**, and a caudal neuromere that forms the **pretectum** (Fig. 9-13; also see Fig. 9-2*B*). The thalamus and the hypothalamus differentiate to form complexes of nuclei that serve a diverse range of functions. The thalamus acts mainly as the relay center for the cerebral cortex: it receives all information projecting to the cortex from subcortical structures, processes it as necessary, and relays it to the appropriate cortical area(s). Within the thalamus, the sense of sight is handled by the **lateral geniculate nucleus** and the sense of hearing by the **medial geniculate nucleus**. The hypothalamus regulates the endocrine activity of the pituitary as well as many autonomic responses. It participates in the limbic system, which controls emotion and coordinates emotional state with appropriate visceral responses. The hypothalamus also controls the level of arousal of the brain (sleep and waking). The small epithalamus gives rise to a few more minor structures covered later in the chapter.

At the end of the fifth week, the thalamus and the hypothalamus are visible as swellings on the inner surface of the diencephalic neural canal, separated by a deep groove called the **hypothalamic sulcus** (Fig. 9-13*A*). The thalamus grows disproportionately after the seventh week and becomes the largest element of the diencephalon.

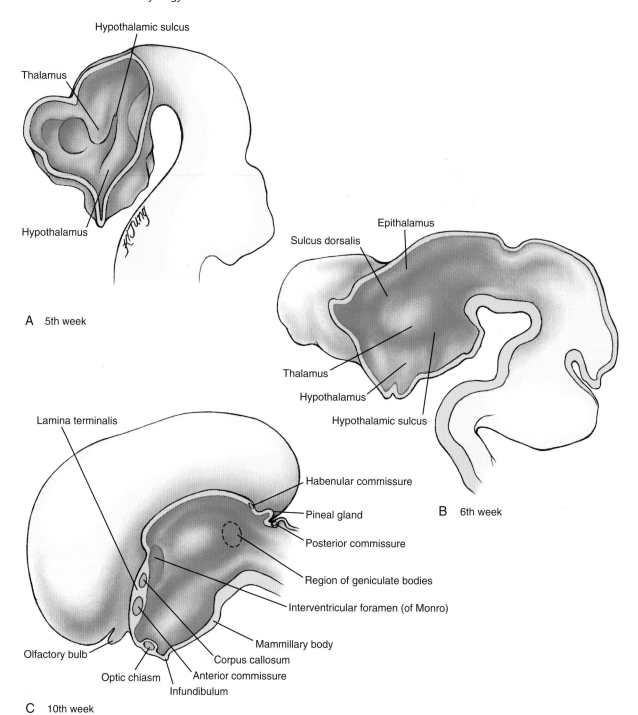

Figure 9-13. Development of the diencephalon. *A,* The thalamus and the hypothalamus become demarcated by a hypothalamic sulcus during the fifth week. *B,* By the end of the sixth week, the thalamus is clearly differentiated from the more dorsal epithalamus by a shallow groove called the sulcus dorsalis. *C,* By ten weeks, additional specializations of the diencephalon are apparent, including the mammillary body, the pineal gland, and the posterior lobe of the pituitary. The optic sulci, the posterior and habenular commissures, and the geniculate bodies are also specializations of the diencephalon.

The two thalami usually meet and fuse across the third ventricle at one or more points called **interthalamic adhesions** (Fig. 9-14*C*).

By the end of the sixth week, a shallow groove called the **sulcus dorsalis** separates the thalamus from the epithalamic swelling, which forms in the dorsal rim of the diencephalic wall and the adjoining roof plate (see Fig. 9-13*B*, *C*). The epithalamic roof plate evaginates to form a midline diverticulum that differentiates into the endocrine **pineal gland**. The epithalamus also forms a neural structure called the **trigonum habenulae** (including the **nucleus habenulae**) and two small commissures, the **posterior** and **habenular commissures**. Growth of the thalamus eventually obliterates the sulcus dorsalis and displaces the epithalamic structures dorsally.

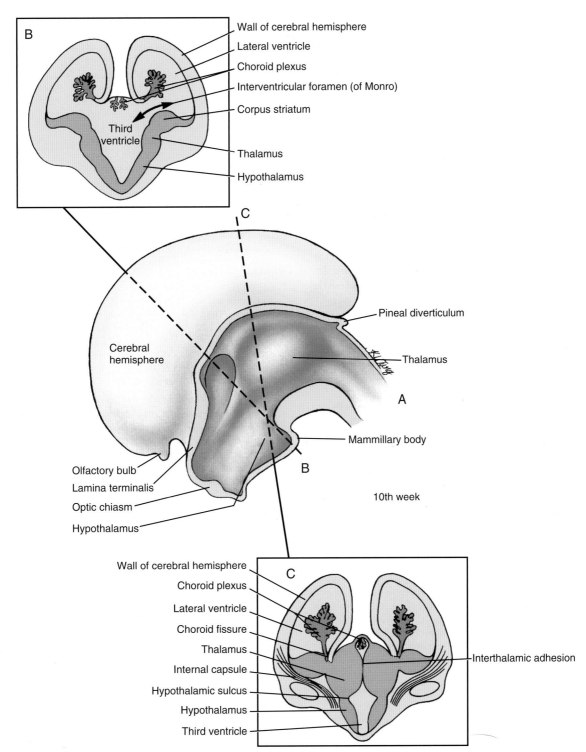

Figure 9-14. Development of the cerebral hemispheres and lateral ventricles (*A-C*), as seen in sagittal view (*A*) and in sections (*B, C*) at the levels indicated in *A*. The lateral ventricle in each hemisphere communicates with the third ventricle through an interventricular foramen (of Monro). The choroid fissure running the length of each lateral ventricle contains a choroid plexus, which produces cerebrospinal fluid. The fibers growing to and from the cerebral cortex form the massive fiber bundle called the internal capsule. The thalami function mainly as relay centers that process information destined for the cerebral hemispheres. The growing thalami meet across the third ventricle, forming the interthalamic adhesion.

Retinal fibers from the optic cups project to the lateral geniculate nuclei. As covered in Chapter 19, the axons from the retinal ganglion cells grow back through the optic nerves to the diencephalon. Just before they enter the brain, axons growing from both eyes meet to form the **optic chiasm** (Fig. 9-14*A*; also see Fig. 9-13*C*), a joint midline structure in which the axons from the inner (nasal) side of each eye cross over to the other side of the brain (decussate), whereas those of the outer (temporal) side of each eye remain on the same side; axons relaying information from the left half of the visual field of both eyes project to the right side of the brain and vice versa. The resulting bundles of ipsilateral and contralateral fibers then project back to the lateral geniculate nucleus, where they synapse to form a map of the visual field. Not all retinal fibers project to the lateral geniculate nuclei; as mentioned earlier in the chapter, some of them terminate in the superior colliculus, where they mediate ocular reflex control.

Cranial to the epithalamus, the diencephalic roof plate remains epithelial. This portion of the roof plate differentiates along with the overlying pia to form the paired **choroid plexuses** of the third ventricle (see Fig. 9-14C). Elsewhere in the third ventricle, the ependyma forms a number of unique secretory structures that add specific metabolites and neuropeptides to the cerebrospinal fluid. These structures, collectively known as the **circumventricular organs**, include the **subfornical organ**, the **organum vasculosum of the lamina terminalis**, and the **subcommissural organ**.

In the Research Lab

DEVELOPMENT OF VISUAL SYSTEM: EXAMPLE OF HOW NERVOUS SYSTEM WIRES ITSELF

The projection neurons of the retinae (**retinal ganglion cells**) produce axons that grow across the retinae and thence through the optic nerves and tracts to synapse in the **lateral geniculate nucleus** (or **body** [LGN]) of the thalamus and the superior colliculi (SC) of the dorsal midbrain (tectum). Lateral geniculate axons then relay visual information to the visual cortex (Fig. 9-15). Development of this system, which is characterized by highly precise, point-to-point mapping of retinal cells to higher brain centers, raises a number of key questions about **axonal guidance** and the formation of **topographic neural connections**.

It will become apparent below that among the molecules used to guide axons to their targets are some of the same molecules that the embryo uses earlier as morphogens to pattern cell differentiation—an example of how a relatively small set of signaling molecules is used repeatedly for different tasks at different times and in different developmental contexts. However, before considering neuronal connectivity in the visual system, we must first examine how the cell pattern is formed in the retinae and how this translates into the transcriptional control of molecules involved in the navigation of retinal axons.

Cell Pattern in Neural Retinae

As covered in Chapter 19, each retina consists of two components: the **neural retina**, which receives visual information and transmits it to the brain via the retinal ganglion cells, and the pigment epithelium, which lies behind the neural retina. The neural retina itself consists of several cell layers in all, but here we will consider only that which lines its inner surface: the layer of retinal ganglion cells (RGCs) that project in point-to-point fashion to the visual centers, creating a map of visual space in the brain. To ensure this precisely patterned connectivity, individual neurons in the RGC layer must be endowed with positional identity. Just as for the CNS axis as a whole, this is achieved by patterning along each of its planar axes: CrCd (cranial-caudal; alternatively referred to as nasal-temporal, to denote its orientation in the skull) and DV (dorsal-ventral). Both axes of the neural retina are specified before neurogenesis, even before the retina emerges as a distinct layer of the optic vesicle.

An early step in the subdivision of the optic vesicles involves the expression of two forkhead genes, Bf1 and Bf2, in complementary fashion along the CrCd axis; Bf1 is highly expressed at the cranial (nasal) pole of the retina and Bf2 at the caudal (temporal) pole. The cranial domain is then further subdivided by the expression of two homeobox genes, Soho (for sense organ homeobox) and Gh6 (Gallus homeobox 6). Each of these transcriptional control genes plays a part in patterning the CrCd axis, as both knockout and overexpression studies result in altered positional identity of RGCs, revealed by their aberrant projections. However, it remains unclear how the patterned expression of these genes is directed by upstream signals.

The DV axis is patterned slightly later than the CrCd axis, at the optic cup stage. Here, it seems that the governing mechanism involves a gradient of Bmp4 (bone morphogenetic protein 4) diffusing from the dorsal pole and a complementary gradient of a Bmp antagonist (ventroptin) diffusing from the ventral pole. High levels of Bmp signaling induce the expression of a transcriptional control gene, Tbx5, in the dorsal retina, whereas high levels of ventroptin associate with expression of the homeobox gene Vax2 and the paired box gene Pax2 in the ventral retina. Ectopic misexpression of Tbx5 dorsalizes the retina. Conversely, misexpression of Vax2 results in ventralization, including downregulation of the dorsal factors Bmp4 and Tbx5, and misprojection of dorsal RGC axons. How the retinal polarity conferred by these transcription factors translates into the graded expression of axon guidance receptor molecules is considered next.

Spatial Targeting of Retinal Axons

As covered further in Chapter 10, a specialized structure at the tip of the axon called the **growth cone** is responsible for neuronal pathfinding (Fig. 9-16; also see Fig. 10-12). The first task for the retinal ganglion cell growth cones, after they enter the axon layer that lines the inner surface of the retina, is to grow to the **optic disc** and then turn sharply to funnel into the **optic nerve** (Fig. 9-17). Outgrowth of retinal ganglion cell axons and guidance of their growth cones to the optic disc seem to require interaction with radial glia endfeet (specializations of the luminal side of radial glia) within the inner layer of the neural retina and associated cell adhesion and extracellular matrix molecules. Indeed, many such substratum-associated or diffusible factors seem to play a role in the guidance of RGC growth cones, either within the retina or in the optic nerve. These include laminin, L1, axonin-1, Ncam, netrins, slits, semaphorins, ephrins, hedgehogs, and sFrps. Some of these molecules act as attractants, whereas others act as repellents, serving to restrict axons to a localized pathway by surround repulsion. In addition, the survival of RGCs within the retina may be supported by **trophic factors**, including a factor produced by pigment epithelial cells. Other trophic factors that support survival of RGCs include Bdnf and neurotrophin 4/5.

Directional growth by RGC growth cones toward the centrally located optic disc is particularly influenced by attractive interactions involving the **laminin** and **netrin** signaling pathways but is also regulated by their repulsion from the periphery of the neural retina. A zinc-finger gene, **Zic3**, which is expressed strongly in the peripheral retina with a decreasing gradient toward the optic disc, seems to regulate the expression of (so far unidentified) axon repellent factors. When the growth cone reaches the optic disc, its morphology changes from a simple tapered cone to a complex, actively pleomorphic structure that puts out numerous cell processes called **filopodia** (see Fig. 9-16). The filopodia, especially, have been implicated in the sensing and transducing of environmental signals that guide the growth cone to its target. The increased morphologic complexity of the growth cone at such **choice points** reflects its response to the environmental signals that determine its behavior. The retinal axon growth

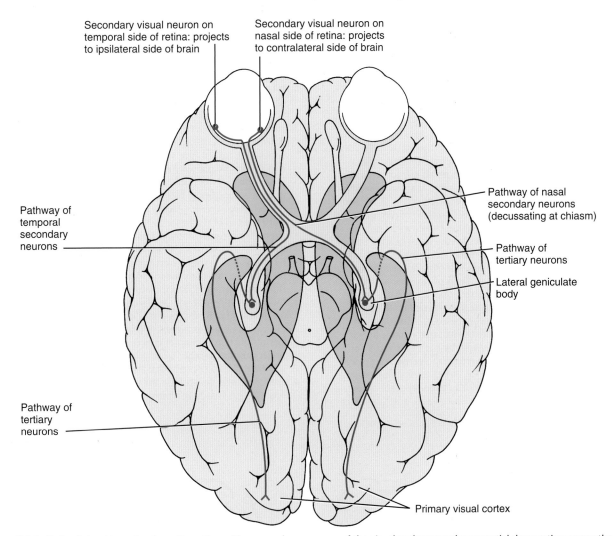

Figure 9-15. Path of visual impulses from the retinae. The secondary neurons of the visual pathway undergo partial decussation across the optic chiasm so that each visual cortex receives information from the contralateral visual field. As shown, axons from the nasal half of each retina cross over in the chiasm to enter the contralateral visual tract, whereas axons from the temporal half of each retina enter the ipsilateral visual tract. These secondary axons synapse in the lateral geniculate bodies with the tertiary neurons of the visual pathway, which project to the primary visual cortex in the occipital lobe. The synapses in the lateral geniculate bodies and the visual cortex are arranged so as to form a spatial map of the visual field. Dark blue marks the position of the lateral ventricles.

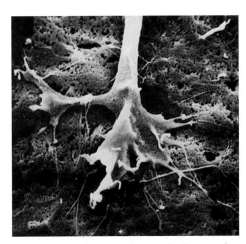

Figure 9-16. Scanning electron micrograph of a growth cone. Note numerous filopodia and lamellipodia.

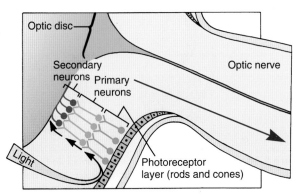

Figure 9-17. Organization of neurons in the retina and optic nerve. Photoreceptor cells—rods and cones—form the deepest layer of the neural retina (the layer farthest from the vitreous humor). Information from the rods and cones is gathered by a layer of short primary visual neurons, which synapse in the retina with the secondary visual neurons. The axons of these secondary neurons traverse the surface of the retina and then travel via the optic nerve to the brain.

cones change back to a simple, tapered shape once they have plunged into the optic nerve, but they become complex again when they reach the **optic chiasm**, where they must decide whether to cross into the other side of the brain.

Half of the Retinal Ganglion Axons Cross Midline

In most submammalian vertebrates, whose left and right visual fields are separate, all retinal axons cross at the optic chiasm and innervate the contralateral side of the brain. In humans, half the axons from each retina (those of the medial or nasal half) cross over to the other side and form the contralateral optic tract, whereas axons from the lateral (or temporal) half turn into the ipsilateral optic tract, where they join axons that have already crossed over from the contralateral nasal retina (Fig. 9-18; also see Fig. 9-15). The decision for an RGC axon to remain ipsilateral rather than to cross (**decussate**) at the chiasm exists only for animals with **binocular** vision, where the visual fields of left and right eyes overlap, and information from the visual field is relayed from both eyes to one side of the brain. How in the case of binocularity do some retinal axons know to cross at the optic chiasm whereas others know not to cross?

The mouse optic chiasm has featured prominently as a model for addressing this question, being particularly amenable to genetic manipulation, despite the fact that in mice only a small part of the visual field is shared by both eyes and a correspondingly small region of the retina (the **ventrotemporal crescent**) projects ipsilaterally (Fig. 9-19). Recent studies have revealed the matched expression of an axon-repellent molecule (ephrin-B2) by midline glial cells at the chiasm, and a receptor

(EphB1) for this ligand exclusively on RGC of the ventrotemporal retina. **Ephrins** are a large family of ligands that may cause collapse of the growth cone with loss or slowing of its locomotor activity when sensed by a neuron that expresses a receptor tyrosine kinase of the **Eph** family (ephrins are covered in greater detail in Chapter 5). Significantly, when the function of ephrin-B2 is blocked, all axons project contralaterally, recapitulating the primitive "default" condition for the monocular visual pathway. Normally, ephrin-B2 function causes those growth cones that are sensitive to it to be repelled from the midline and to join the pathway provided by axons crossing from the other side. It is interesting to note that the metamorphosis of frogs is accompanied by the acquisition of an ipsilateral visual projection: as the side-facing eyes of a tadpole rotate up toward the top of the head, so the originally separate visual fields overlap to some extent and retinal axons begin to project to the ipsilateral tectum. This correlates with the onset of ephrin-B2 expression in the chiasm and of EphB1 in the ventrotemporal retina—again consistent with a pivotal role for Eph/ephrin signaling in effecting the ipsilateral routing of axons. Regulating the noncrossing phenotype of ventrotemporal RGC, and likely upstream of EphB1 expression, is a zinc-finger transcription factor, Zic2, which is expressed exclusively in these cells. In genetic loss-of-function experiments in mice, the ventrotemporal RGC project contralaterally.

The deflection of temporal axons back into the ipsilateral optic tract also depends on the presence of the axons from the opposite eye that have already crossed over in the chiasm and

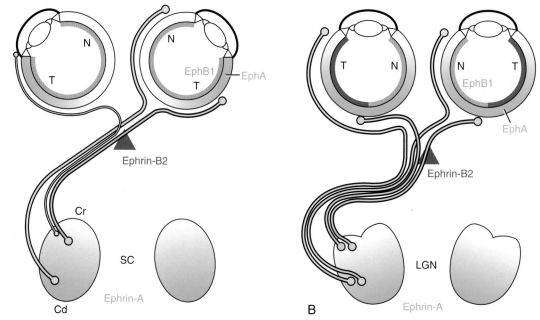

Figure 9-18. Visual mapping in mouse and human. In the mouse (*A*), a large majority of retinal ganglion cells (RGC) project to the mesencephalic superior colliculus (SC), and a minority project to the diencephalic lateral geniculate nucleus (LGN; *not shown*). The visual field is only partly binocular, so that only a small contingent of axons from the temporal hemiretina (T) project to the ipsilateral SC, whereas all the others project contralaterally. The ipsilateral RGC express EphB1 receptors, which regulate their exclusion from the midline chiasm cells that express ephrin-B2. EphA receptors are expressed in a decreasing temporal-to-nasal gradient, complementary to the gradient of ephrin-A ligands in the SC. Axons from the temporal hemiretina (T) are excluded from caudal (Cd) SC by repulsive interactions between EphAs and ephrin-As and thus project to the cranial SC (Cr). Nasal RGC (N) project to the caudal SC (Cd). In humans *(B),* a large majority of RGC project to the LGN, and only a minority project to the SC *(not shown)*. The visual field is binocular, so that the entire temporal hemiretina projects ipsilaterally, and the entire nasal hemiretina projects contralaterally. Ipsilateral and contralaterally projecting RGC from both eyes that see the same point in space terminate at the same craniocaudal position in the LGN but in adjacent eye-specific layers.

constructed a **preformed pathway** to which ipsilateral axons can adhere. If the opposite eye is removed in a mouse embryo, so that the crossing axons never develop, the ipsilaterally targeting axons of the remaining eye pause for a long period at the chiasm and may never project further. Normal formation of the ipsilateral tract seems to depend on adhesive interactions with the already crossed axons, for which a candidate is the immunoglobulin family cell adhesion molecule L1. In mice lacking this protein, the ipsilateral projection is severely diminished. Another factor influencing the choice of axonal pathway at the chiasm is the presence of melanin, which is normally expressed by chiasm cells. In ocular albinos of numerous species, many axons go to the wrong side of the brain, resulting in targeting anomalies that degrade visual acuity, and may alter the visible morphology of the lateral geniculate nuclei.

Retinal Ganglion Cell (RGC) Axons Form Precise Map of Visual Space When They Synapse in Tectum and Lateral Geniculate Nucleus

Each retinal axon courses to the correct region in the **lateral geniculate nucleus** (LGN) and synapses with the correct target neurons, thus reproducing in the LGN the spatial information from the retina, point-to-point. A similar feat is accomplished by the axons of the LGN, which grow back to the occipital lobe of the cerebrum, where they map onto the **primary visual (striate) cortex**. Axons from right and left eyes synapse in distinct, eye-specific layers of the LGN. By means of these neural maps, passed on between successive stages in the neural pathway, a representation of the visual world is transmitted to the cortex, which integrates the right and left visual fields and forms an image that is congruent between the two eyes (see Fig. 9-18).

Precise visual maps are also reproduced by the targeting of specific populations of RGC axons to the **superior colliculi** (SC)—the homolog of the submammalian tectum. In humans and other primates, for which vision is a dominant sense, only a small minority of RGC axons project to the SC, whereas a large majority of RGC axons project to the LGN. In rodents, which lack high visual acuity, the situation is reversed—with a large majority of RGC axons projecting to the SC. The SC, along with other regions of the tectum, including the inferior colliculi, integrates visual, auditory, and somatosensory information and coordinates reflex responses to movement, sound, and somatic sensation.

The question of how visual mapping is achieved is of interest not only in itself but also because spatial maps are a common and characteristic feature of the CNS, especially the sensory systems. A number of studies have begun to shed light on the intricate puzzle of how maps are formed, most of which have involved experimenting with the retinotectal/retinocollicular projection of zebrafish, Xenopus, chick, and mouse embryos. The visual map is created in two steps. First, a number of **activity-independent cues** guide the growing retinal axons to the approximately correct point (**termination zone**) in the tectum/SC where they arborize extensively and synapse to form a rough map. Second, these initial, somewhat unfocused synapses are then sharpened by **activity-dependent** pruning of axonal arbors, by secondary axonal reconnection, and by cell death of inappropriately targeted cells to form a highly tuned point-to-point map.

The synapses of RGC axons in the optic tectum reproduce the spatial order of the retina on two orthogonal axes, such that the temporonasal (TN) axis of the retina maps to the cranial-caudal (CrCd) axis of the tectum, and the dorsoventral (DV) axis

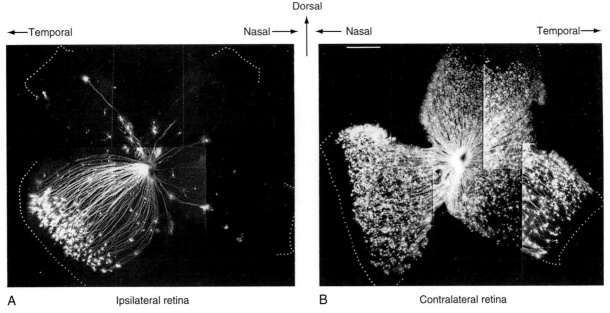

A   Ipsilateral retina   B   Contralateral retina

Figure 9-19. A "tract-tracing" technique used to show the projection of secondary retinal neurons to a particular locus in the optic tract. The use of dyes to analyze the arrangement of the axons projected by distant neurons is a time-honored neurobiologic technique. In this example, a crystal of the carbocyanine dye DiI was inserted into the optic tract of a sixteen-and-one-half-day mouse embryo at a site caudal to the optic chiasm. After the dye had time to diffuse along the axons, the ipsilateral (A) and contralateral (B) retinae were mounted flat on a microscope slide and were examined with a fluorescence microscope to determine which of the axons were back-filled with dye. The back-filled axons can be assumed to represent the axon population that projects to the site of the crystal in the optic tract. In the ipsilateral retina (A), secondary neurons located mainly in the ventrotemporal crescent project to the site of the crystal, whereas in the contralateral retina (B) neurons from all areas project to this site. This pattern is characteristic of the adult retina. Fibers from the ipsilateral and contralateral retinae are intermingled in the optic tract at the site of the crystal.

of the retina maps to the medial lateral (LM) axis of the tectum (see Fig. 9-18). The relationship is such that the axes of retina and tectum are in inverse orientation, that is, nasal retina (originally cranial on the neuraxis) maps to caudal tectum and ventral retina maps to medial (originally dorsal) tectum. This inversion effectively corrects the inversion of the visual field produced by the lens.

Having traversed the surface of the diencephalon to reach the dorsal midbrain, retinal axon growth cones enter the tectum at its cranial border and grow toward its caudal border, that is, they grow near parallel to the midline (Fig. 9-20). In chick and mouse embryos, axons may overshoot their termination zone by a considerable distance, and appropriate retinotopic connectivity occurs through the interstitial branching of collaterals from the main axon shaft. Interstitials bud off at roughly the correct position on the CrCd axis, which may be some distance back from the growth cone, and then grow at right angles to the axon shaft to reach their correct termination zone on the ML axis. In fish and frog, by contrast, the correct termination zone is reached directly by the primary growth cone. In these species, which grow continuously throughout life, the retinotectal projection changes constantly to incorporate the radial increments of retinal growth into a tectal map with two orthogonal dimensions.

However, in all species, once an axon or collateral reaches the CrCd and ML position that maps to the position of the parent neuron in the retina, it invades the tectum and arborizes extensively in the retinorecipient layers. This point-to-zone mapping is thought to be controlled, at least in part, by complementary gradients of ephrins expressed in the tectum and of Eph receptors expressed in the retina. For example, ephrin-A2 and ephrin-A5 are expressed in increasing cranial-to-caudal gradients, whereas their EphA receptor is expressed in an increasing nasal-to-temporal gradient. The ephrin-As are powerful repellents of growth cones and inhibitors of interstitial branching. Because the level of EphA receptor on a cell determines the degree to which its axon (or branching capacity) is inhibited by ephrin-As, temporal axons are subject to more intense repulsion than nasal axons and are thereby confined to the anterior tectum. Countergradients of receptor and ligand may sharpen the ability of axons across the

nasal-temporal axis to find their correct termination zone in the tectum according to particular thresholds of inhibition.

A similar mechanism involving complementary gradients of ephrin-B ligands and EphB receptors operates in mapping the DV axis of the retina onto the LM axis of the tectum. Here, however, evidence from both frogs and mice points to an attractant interaction rather than a repellent one, with high EphB expressing ventral RGC projecting to high ephrin-B expressing medial tectum.

Almost 50 years ago, work on the visual system of frogs led Sperry to propose a **chemoaffinity hypothesis** for topographic mapping, which held that each position in the optic tectum has a unique address dictated by the gradient distribution of molecular labels along orthogonal axes, matched by an equivalent distribution of labels in the retina. This hypothesis, long neglected in favor of more mechanical mechanisms for axon guidance, has been substantially vindicated by the discovery of Eph/ephrin gradients and their central role in retinotectal mapping.

We saw above how certain transcription factors may confer polarity on the neural retina and positional identity on the RGC. However, in only a few examples is it yet seen that these factors regulate the Eph/ephrin system, which is the essential readout of retinal position information. For example, overexpression of Soho and Gh6 on the CrCd axis can repress expression of EphAs, leading to pathway errors and mapping defects. On the DV axis, ectopic expression of Vax induces EphB in the dorsal retina, whereas knocking out Vax2 leads to loss of EphB expression, dorsalization of the ventral retina, and the shift of ventrotemporal axon terminations from medial to lateral regions of the superior colliculus. The search for genes involved in upstream regulatory control of the tectal gradients has revealed few candidates: the most prominent of these is the homeobox gene **engrailed**, which regulates the expression of ephrin-A ligands in the caudal midbrain and has a similarly graded expression pattern.

Binocular Visual System of Humans Also Involves Ephs and Ephrins in Guidance and Mapping

Retinal mapping in humans and other primates with fully binocular vision is characterized by congruent mapping of

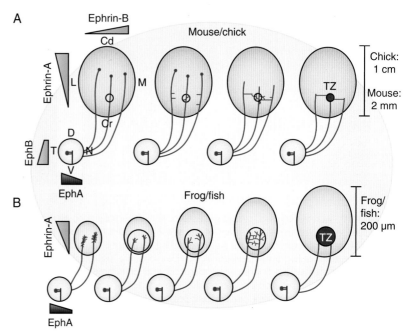

Figure 9-20. Development of visual projections in amniotes (chick, mouse) (A) and in anamniotes (frog, fish) (B). In all species, the temporonasal axis of the retina (TN) maps to the cranial-caudal axis of the tectum/superior colliculus (CrCd), and the dorsal-ventral axis of the retina (DV) maps to the medial-lateral axis (ML) of the tectum/superior colliculus. The termination zones (TZ) of retinal ganglion cells (RGC) are established according to position on orthogonal gradients of ephrin-As (CrCd axis) and ephrin-Bs (LM axis). In amniotes, the termination zones are set up by collaterals that bud interstitially from the main axon shaft, which itself may extend well beyond the TZ. In anamniotes, the TZs are set up directly by the growth cones of RGC. In both cases, extensive arborization in the TZ before final point-to-point mapping is achieved by secondary refinement of activity-dependent pruning.

hemiretinas from both eyes onto the same target—the LGN on one side of the thalamus. Just as in rodents, where EphB1 expression in the ventrotemporal retina regulates ipsilateral passage at the chiasm, so in humans this receptor is expressed in the entire temporal hemiretina, and its repellent ligand, ephrin-B2, is expressed at the optic chiasm (see Fig. 9-18). Similarly, the ephrin-A gradients that segregate temporal and nasal axons in the tectum of birds and the mouse SC are also formed in the human LGN, in complementary fashion to EphA gradients in the retina.

Fine-Tuning the Visual Map Depends on Neuronal Activity

Several studies indicate that feedback in the form of neural impulses from the retina is important in refining the coarse-grained visual map formed by **activity-independent** axon guidance mechanisms. Fine-tuning the visual map depends as much on retraction from inappropriate targets as it does on growth to appropriate targets. Indeed, when correlated electrical activity is inhibited within the visual system by sodium channel blockers such as tetrodotoxin (TTX), axons are not retracted from inappropriate targets, and large, more diffuse termination zones persist. Moreover, it has been demonstrated in cultured neurons that neurite retraction depends on the density of voltage-activated calcium channels following stimulation. It has been demonstrated in several vertebrate systems that the final pattern of point-to-point synaptic connections depends on matching the frequency and duration of impulse activity—cells that fire together wire together. Matching coactive retinal inputs to the tectum/SC requires the activity of the N-methyl-D-aspartate (NMDA) receptor: blocking excitatory transmission with NMDA receptor inhibitors such as 2-amino-5-phosphonovalerate (APV) disorganizes the retinotopic map.

It is also becoming clear that the visual system is extensively modified by the **death of neurons** even as it is being formed. As in other areas of the nervous system, far more neurons are initially produced than survive in the mature system. For example, it is estimated that three- to four-million ganglion cells arise in the human retina, but only just over one-million survive in the adult. Many of the original synaptic connections made by these cells are eliminated by a pruning process that participates in tuning the visual maps in the LGN and superior colliculus.

Pituitary Gland

During the third week, a diverticulum called the **infundibulum** develops in the floor of the third ventricle and grows ventrally toward the stomodeum (Fig. 9-21; see also Fig. 9-13C). Simultaneously, an ectodermal placode appears in the roof of the stomodeum (an ectodermal lined space near the future mouth opening, between the maxillary and mandibular processes; covered in Chapter 17) and invaginates to form a diverticulum called **Rathke's pouch**, which grows dorsally toward the infundibulum. Rathke's pouch eventually loses its connection with the stomodeum and forms a discrete sac that is apposed to the cranial surface of the infundibulum. This sac differentiates to form the **adenohypophysis** of the pituitary. The cells of its anterior surface give rise to the **anterior lobe** proper of the pituitary, and a small group of cells on the posterior surface of the pouch form the functionally distinct **pars intermedia**. Meanwhile, the distal portion of the infundibulum differentiates to form the **posterior pituitary (neurohypophysis)**. The lumen of the infundibulum is obliterated by this process, but a

small proximal pit, the **infundibular recess**, persists in the floor of the third ventricle.

Telencephalon

The cerebral hemispheres first appear on day thirty-two as a pair of bubble-like outgrowths of the telencephalon. By sixteen weeks, the rapidly growing hemispheres are oval and have expanded back to cover the diencephalon. The thin roof and lateral walls of each hemisphere represent the future **cerebral cortex** (Fig. 9-22A). The floor is thicker and contains neuronal aggregations called **ganglionic eminences**, which give rise to the **basal ganglia (corpus striatum** and **globus pallidus)** (see Fig. 9-14B). As the growing hemispheres press against the walls of the diencephalon, the meningeal layers that originally separate the two structures disappear, so that the neural tissue of the thalami becomes continuous with that of the floor of the cerebral hemispheres. This former border is eventually crossed by a massive axon bundle called the **internal capsule**, which passes through the corpus striatum (giving it its striated appearance) and carries axons from the thalamus to the cerebral cortex (and vice versa), as well as from the cerebral cortex to lower regions of the brain and spinal cord (see Fig. 9-14C).

The cerebral hemispheres are initially smooth surfaced. However, like the cerebellar cortex, the cerebral cortex folds into an increasingly complex pattern of gyri (ridges) and sulci (grooves) as the hemispheres grow. This process begins in the fourth month with the formation of a small indentation called the **lateral cerebral fossa** in the lateral wall of each hemisphere (Fig. 9-22B; also see Fig. 9-22A). The caudal end of each lengthening hemisphere curves ventrally and then grows forward across this fossa, creating the **temporal lobe** of the cerebral hemisphere and converting the fossa into a deep cleft called the **lateral cerebral sulcus**. The portion of the cerebral cortex that originally forms the medial floor of the fossa is covered by the temporal lobe and is called the **insula**.

By the sixth month, several other cerebral sulci have formed. These include the **central sulcus**, which separates the frontal and parietal lobes, and the **occipital sulcus**, which demarcates the occipital lobe. The detailed pattern of gyri that ultimately forms on the cerebral hemispheres varies somewhat from individual to individual. The gyri and sulci effectively increase the surface area of the brain such that when fully grown, it is the size of a pillowcase.

Each cerebral hemisphere contains a diverticulum of the telencephalic primitive ventricle called the **lateral ventricle**. The lateral ventricle initially occupies most of the volume of the hemisphere but is progressively constricted by thickening of the cortex. However, along the line between the floor and the medial wall of the hemisphere, the cerebral wall does not thicken but instead remains thin and epithelial. This zone forms a longitudinal groove in the ventricle; the groove is called the **choroid fissure** (see Fig. 9-14C). A choroid plexus develops along the choroid fissure. As shown in Figure 9-23, the lateral ventricle extends the whole length of each hemisphere, reaching anteriorly into the frontal lobe and, at its posterior end, curving around to occupy the temporal lobe. The opening between each lateral ventricle and the third ventricle persists as the **interventricular foramen (foramen of Monro)**.

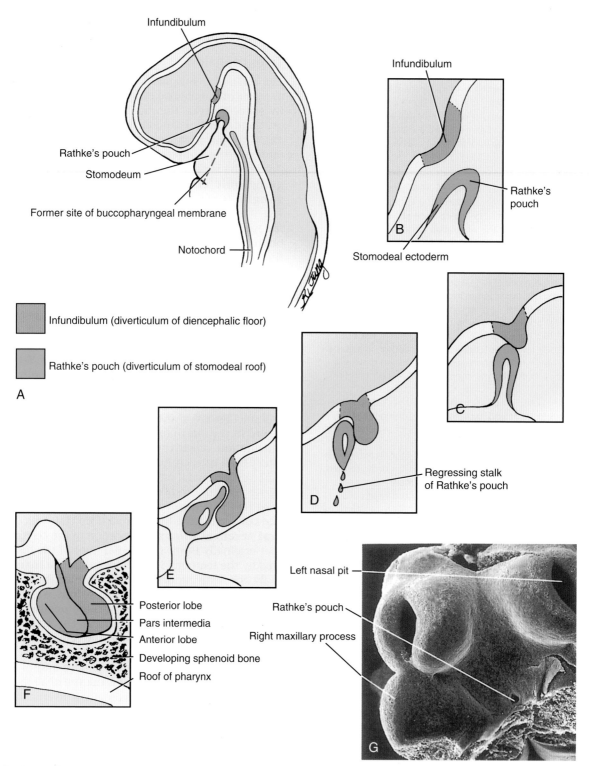

Figure 9-21. Development of the pituitary (*A-F*). The pituitary gland is a compound structure. The posterior lobe forms from a diverticulum of the diencephalic floor called the infundibulum, whereas the anterior lobe and the pars intermedia form from an evagination of the ectodermal roof of the stomodeum called Rathke's pouch. Rathke's pouch detaches from the stomodeum and becomes associated with the developing posterior pituitary. *G*, Scanning electron micrograph of the roof of the embryonic oral cavity, showing the opening to Rathke's pouch.

The neuroepithelium of the cerebral hemispheres is initially much like that of other parts of the neural tube. However, studies on cerebral histogenesis have shown that the process of proliferation, migration, and differentiation by which the mature cortex is produced is unique.

The cerebral cortex is made up of several cell layers (or laminae) that vary in number from three in the phylogenetically oldest parts to six in the dominant **neocortex**. In other regions of the CNS, the white matter (axons) forms outside the gray matter (neuronal cell bodies); this

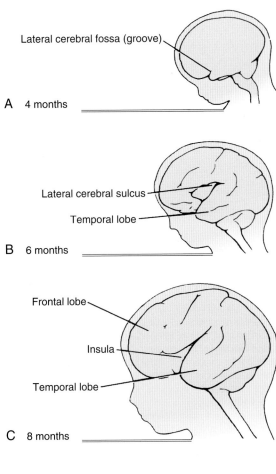

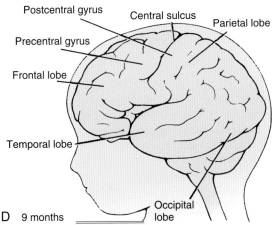

Figure 9-22. Growth and folding of the cerebral hemispheres during fetal life. Growth of the cerebral hemispheres is continuous throughout embryonic and fetal development and continues after birth. *A, B,* In the fourth month, formation of the narrow lateral cerebral fossa delineates the temporal lobe of the cerebral hemisphere. By the sixth month, additional clefts delineate the frontal, parietal, and occipital lobes. *C, D,* Additional sulci and gyri form throughout the remainder of fetal life.

cells of the ventricular layer undergo a series of regulated divisions to produce waves of neurons that migrate peripherally and establish the neuronal layers of the cortex. Axons extend from these cells on the inner or deep surface of the neuronal layers, between them and the ventricular zone. Furthermore, the cortical layers are laid down in a sequence from *deep* to *superficial*, that is, the neurons of each wave migrate through the preceding layers to establish a more superficial layer. As the production of neurons tapers off, the ventricular layer gives rise to various kinds of glia and then to the ependyma.

Let us now examine the process in greater detail (Fig. 9-24*A*). The first neurons produced from the ventricular zone form a superficial layer, the **preplate**, which immediately underlies the developing pia. Axons extend from these neurons on the *inner* side of the preplate, establishing an **intermediate zone**. The next neurons to be born migrate into the middle of the preplate and split it into a superficial **marginal zone** (future lamina I) and deep **subplate**, forming a middle layer called the **cortical plate**. Young neurons migrate on the surfaces of a preformed array of **radial glial cells**, whose processes span the full thickness of the cortex. Axons from neurons in the cortical plate and subplate join those already in the intermediate zone, which will later become the **white matter** of the cortex. The early neurons of the cortical plate form the deep layers (laminae VI and V) of the finished cortex, whereas later-born cells migrate radially from the ventricular zone across the intermediate zone and subplate, through the earlier layers VI and V of the cortical plate. In the process they establish, in sequence, the more superficial laminae IV, III, and (finally) II. As neurogenesis proceeds, new neurons are increasingly formed in an accessory germinative zone lying deep to the ventricular zone, called the **subventricular zone**.

The above describes the generation of the principal excitatory neurons of the neocortex—the **pyramidal cells**—the large neurons that project to subcortical targets and to the contralateral hemisphere. More numerous but smaller than the pyramidal neurons are the inhibitory interneurons—the **granule cells**. Most of the latter do not arise from either the ventricular zone or the subventricular zone of the cortical area in which settle; rather, they originate in the ganglionic eminences of the ventral telencephalon and migrate dorsally into the cortex via a tangential route (Fig. 9-24*B*).

Whereas laminae II to VI are the principal constituents of the gray matter in the adult neocortex, the first-born neurons that contribute to lamina I and the subplate disappear later in development; however, their transient existence is crucial to normal cortical histogenesis. Lamina I, the marginal zone, contains transient neurons called **Cajal-Retzius cells**, most of which originate in a dorsal midline structure of the telencephalon (the cortical hem) and migrate tangentially into lamina I. Through their secretion of the large glycoprotein **reelin**, Cajal-Retzius cells are believed to orchestrate the inside-to-outside migration of neurons into the cortical plate. In the absence of reelin, or of other proteins in the reelin signaling pathway, successive waves of young neurons pile up on the inside of their predecessors rather than passing through to form a more superficial layer. The neurons of

situation is reversed in the cerebral cortex. Here, axons enter and leave through an intermediate zone that lies deep to the gray matter and thus forms the outer surface of the brain. The details of how this inside-out arrangement of gray and white matter develops are complex and are still poorly understood. To summarize, proliferating

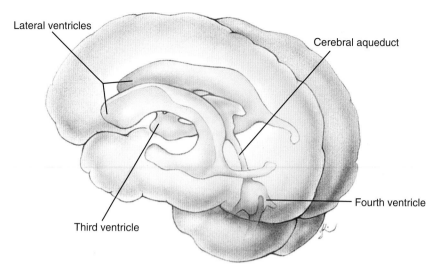

Figure 9-23. The cerebral ventricles. Expansions of the neural canal in the primary and secondary brain vesicles and cerebral hemispheres give rise to the cerebral ventricles. The ventricle system consists of the lateral ventricles in the cerebral hemispheres, the third ventricle in the diencephalon, the narrow cerebral aqueduct (of Sylvius) in the mesencephalon, and the fourth ventricle in the rhombencephalon.

the subplate, which are the first of the cerebral cortex to extend axons, are thought to be crucial in guiding the ordered ingrowth of thalamic axons toward their appropriate presumptive cortical area.

In the Clinic

CONGENITAL MALFORMATIONS OF CEREBRAL CORTEX

Like the human cerebellum, the human cerebrum is subject to a variety of developmental disorders that result from abnormal cell migration, differentiation, survival, or proliferation. The most severe of these abnormalities are obvious in early development, but some do not manifest until later in life. Diagnosis can be made from gross specimens or by MRI, CT, or ultrasonography.

Classical lissencephaly (incidence of at least 1 in 100,000 live births) is a condition that results from incomplete neuronal migration to the cerebral cortex during the third and fourth months of gestation. Brains from patients with lissencephaly have a smoothened cerebral surface as the result of a combination of **pachygyria** (broad, thick gyri), **agyria** (lack of gyri), and widespread neuronal **heterotopia** (cells in aberrant positions compared with those of normal brain). Enlarged ventricles and malformation of the corpus callosum are common. As newborns, these patients often appear normal but sometimes have apnea, poor feeding, or abnormal muscle tone. Patients typically later develop seizures, profound mental retardation, and mild spastic quadriplegia.

Subcortical band heterotopia (SBH) is also believed to result from aberrant migration of differentiating neuroepithelial cells. These patients have bilateral circumferential and symmetric ribbons of gray matter located just beneath the cortex and separated from it by a thin band of white matter, which led to the term *double cortex syndrome*. Seizures, mild mental retardation, and some behavioral abnormalities are often present in infancy. However, intelligence can be normal and seizures may begin later in life. A related syndrome, **X-linked lissencephaly** and **SBH**, also occurs in which homozygous males have lissencephaly and heterozygous females have SBH.

Recent studies have identified two genes that are linked to lissencephaly and SBH. One, LIS1, maps to chromosome 17p13 and encodes a protein that functions as a regulatory subunit of PLATELET-ACTIVATING FACTOR ACETYLHYDROLASE, which degrades PLATELET ACTIVATING FACTOR and is involved in

microtubule dynamics. With regard to its latter role, PLATELET-ACTIVATING FACTOR ACETYLHYDROLASE controls the distribution and function of the microtubule motor DYNEIN, thereby controlling the movement of the nucleus during neuronal migration. Studies of mice with targeted Lis-1 mutations suggest that this protein is necessary for normal pyramidal cell migration and neurite outgrowth. Another gene, called DOUBLECORTIN, is located on the X chromosome and is mutated in patients with X-linked lissencephaly and SBH. The protein product of DOUBLECORTIN is highly expressed in fetal neurons and their precursors during cortical development. Like PLATELET-ACTIVATING FACTOR ACETYLHYDROLASE, the DOUBLECORTIN protein is associated with microtubules, suggesting that it is also involved in cell migration through interactions with the cytoskeleton.

As covered in Chapter 17, the nasal placodes form at the end of the fourth week. Very early, some cells in the nasal placode differentiate to form the **primary neurosensory cells** of the future olfactory epithelium. At the end of the fifth week, these cells sprout axons that cross the short distance to penetrate the most cranial end of the telencephalon (Fig. 9-25A). Subsequent ossification of the ethmoid bone around these axons creates the perforated cribriform plates.

In the sixth week, as the nasal pits differentiate to form the epithelium of the nasal passages, the area at the tip of each cerebral hemisphere (where the axons of the primary neurosensory cells synapse) begins to form an outgrowth called the **olfactory bulb** (Fig. 9-25B-D). The cells in the olfactory bulb that synapse with the axons of the primary sensory neurons differentiate to become the secondary sensory neurons (mitral cells) of the olfactory pathways. The axons of these cells synapse in the olfactory centers of the cerebral hemispheres. As the changing proportions of the face and brain lengthen the distance between the olfactory bulbs and their point of origin on the hemispheres, the axons of the secondary olfactory neurons lengthen to form stalk-like CNS **olfactory tracts**. Traditionally, the olfactory tract and bulb together are referred to as the **olfactory nerve**.

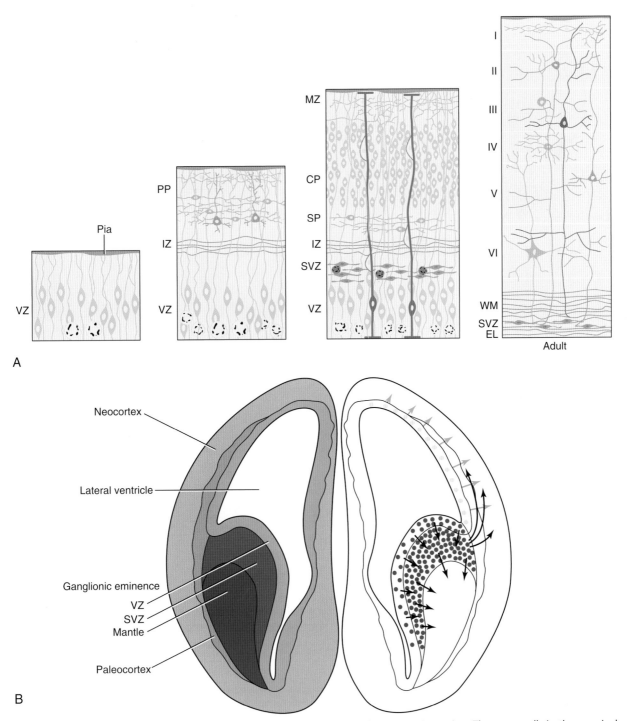

Figure 9-24. Cytodifferentiation and lamination of the neocortex. *A,* A series of four stages in section. The green cells in the marginal zone (MZ) are the Cajal-Retzius cells. CP, cortical plate; EL, ependymal layer; IZ, intermediate zone; PP, preplate; SP, subplate; WM, white matter; I-VI, numbered layers of neocortex. *B,* Migration of interneurons (nonpyramidal cells) from their origin in the ventricular and subventricular zones (VZ, SVZ) of the ganglionic eminences via tangential pathways (*arrows on right side*) to the neocortex. A small minority of cortical interneurons arise from the cortical germinative zones (*yellow*). The germinative zones of the ganglionic eminences also produce the neurons of the corpus striatum and the globus pallidus (basal ganglia).

In the Clinic

KALLMANN SYNDROME

Kallmann syndrome is characterized by **anosmia** (loss of sense of smell) or **hyposmia** (diminished sense of spell) and **hypogonadism** (small gonads). It affects between 1 in 10,000 and 1 in 60,000 people and occurs five times more frequently in males than in females. Anosmia or hyposmia results because the olfactory bulbs and the olfactory nerves fail to develop properly. Hypogonadism results because the hypothalamus fails to produce sufficient GnRH (gonadotropin-releasing hormone), a hormone required for normal development of the gonads (covered in Chapter 16).

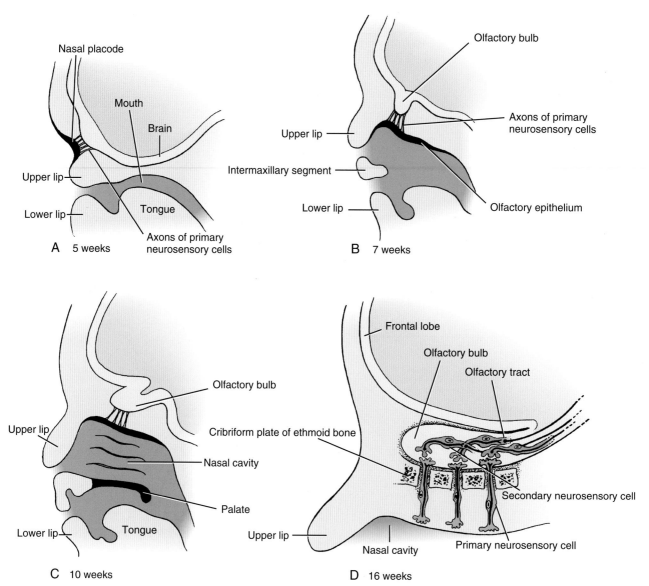

Figure 9-25. Formation of the olfactory tract as seen in sagittal views. *A*, During the fifth week, cells of the nasal placode differentiate into the primary neurosensory cells of the olfactory tract and produce axons that grow into the presumptive olfactory bulb of the adjacent telencephalon. There they synapse with secondary neurons. *B-D*, As development continues, the elongating axons of the secondary olfactory neurons in the olfactory bulb produce the olfactory tract.

Failure of the hypothalamus to produce sufficient GnRH is secondary to a neuronal migration defect. GnRH neurons originate in the olfactory placodes and migrate to the developing hypothalamus via the olfactory bulbs. The gene responsible for the X-linked form of Kallmann syndrome, KAL1, has been identified. It encodes an extracellular matrix glycoprotein protein called ANOSMIN-1. Kallmann also results from mutations in other genes including FGFR1, PROKINETICIN2, and its receptor (a cysteine-rich protein secreted by the suprachiasmatic nucleus and involved in the circadian clock). The syndrome can be inherited as an autosomal dominant or autosomal recessive trait, or as a digenic trait. With identification of the genes involved, Kallmann syndrome can be diagnosed during in vitro fertilization and preimplantation genetic diagnosis (covered in Chapter 1).

The commissures that connect the right and left cerebral hemispheres form from a thickening at the cranial end of the telencephalon, which represents the zone of final neuropore closure. This area can be divided into a dorsal **commissural plate** and a ventral **lamina terminalis**.

The first axon tract to develop in the commissural plate is the **anterior commissure**, which forms during the seventh week and interconnects the olfactory bulbs and olfactory centers of the two hemispheres (Fig. 9-26). During the ninth week, the **hippocampal**, or **fornix commissure**, forms between the right and left hippocampi (a phylogenetically old portion of the cerebral hemisphere that is located adjacent to the choroid fissure). A few days later, the massive, arched **corpus callosum** begins to

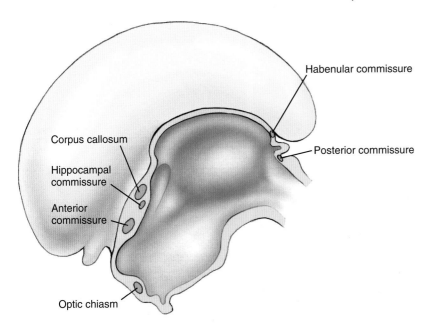

A   10 weeks

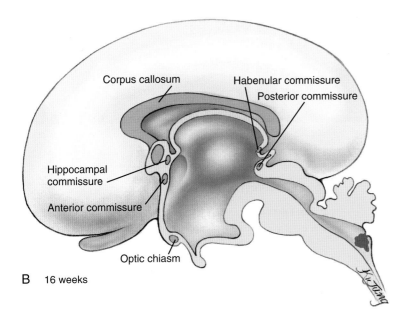

B   16 weeks

Figure 9-26. Formation of the commissures at ten (*A*) and sixteen (*B*) weeks. The telencephalon gives rise to commissural tracts that integrate the activities of the left and right cerebral hemispheres. These include the anterior and hippocampal commissures and the corpus callosum. The small posterior and habenular commissures arise from the epithalamus.

form, linking together the right and left neocortices along their entire length. The most anterior part of the corpus callosum appears first, and its posterior extension (the **splenium**) forms later in fetal life.

GROWTH OF BRAIN

Although growth of the brain is rapid during fetal life (see Fig. 9-22), the brain at birth is only about 25% of its adult volume. Some of the postnatal growth of the brain is the result of increases in the size of neuronal cell bodies and the proliferation of neuronal processes. However, most of this growth results from the myelination of nerve fibers. The brain reaches its final size at around seven years of age.

The manner in which the ten billion to one trillion neurons of the human brain become organized and interconnected is a problem of daunting complexity. As covered in this chapter, not only do the neurons themselves proliferate, migrate, and differentiate according to a precise pattern, but their cell processes display phenomenal pathfinding abilities.

In the Clinic

BRAIN SIZE

Microcephaly, typically defined as small head, results from the formation of a small brain (Fig. 9-27). Recently, genes have been identified that play roles in dramatically regulating brain

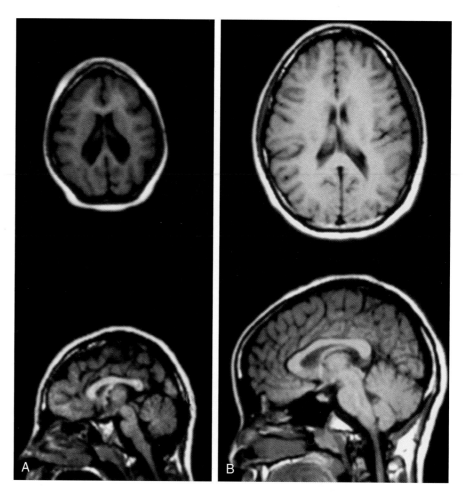

Figure 9-27. MRIs showing the head of an adolescent with microcephaly (*A*) compared with that of an adolescent with a head of normal size (*B*). The top row shows images taken in the coronal plane; the bottom row shows images taken in the sagittal plane.

growth. One gene, ASPM (ABNORMAL SPINDLE-LIKE MICRO-CEPHALY ASSOCIATED), a homolog of the Drosophila abnormal spindle gene, is mutated in the most common form of autosomal recessive primary microcephaly in humans. ASPM plays an essential role in embryonic neuroblasts in normal mitotic spindle function, and it is expressed in proliferating regions of the cerebral cortex during neurogenesis.

Brains that are lissencephalic are also microcephalic. One link between these two brain defects involves two genes: LIS1 (as discussed earlier in the chapter, results in lissencephaly when mutated) and a second gene called NDE1. NDE1, formerly known as mNUDE and homologous to the nude gene of the filamentous fungi *Aspergillus nidulans*, has been shown to directly interact with LIS1. In *A. nidulans*, nude localizes to the microtubule organizing center and regulates microtubule organization. Genetic ablation of Nde1 function in mice results in microcephaly, with the most striking reduction in brain size occurring in the cerebral cortex. It is unknown whether NDE1 is mutated in patients with microcephaly.

Another gene that regulates brain size is β-catenin. When this gene is overexpressed in mice, the brain grows to almost twice its normal size. In addition, foliation of the brain is increased, such that the cerebral cortex of the mouse more closely resembles that of the human.

Embryology in Practice

UNDER PRESSURE

The parents of a three-month-old infant boy notice that he has no head control and does not fix visually on his parents' faces. They also recognize that his head circumference is increasing and that his "soft spot" is firm to the touch. His parents are well aware of these things because, unfortunately, they saw the same symptoms in their previous child, who eventually died.

This family lives in sub-Saharan Africa, and their son is developing **hydrocephalus** ("water on the brain"). In their small village, limited newborn care exposes infants to a high rate of infection, including meningitis. Both of their children survived this brain infection only to develop a life-threatening buildup of **cerebrospinal fluid** (CSF) in the ventricular system of their brains as the result of blockage of the cerebral aqueducts with tissue debris resulting from the infection. As did his sibling, this boy will likely die after progressive loss of brain tissue due to enlarging fluid-filled ventricles, accompanied by dramatic head enlargement (see Fig. 9-12).

Hydrocephalus is a major problem in underdeveloped countries, due both to an increased rate of acquiring the disease and to limited availability of treatment. Worldwide, more than three-hundred-thousand infants are affected—more than those affected by deafness or Down syndrome. Efforts are under way to address this problem, including outreach programs, in which surgeons from developed countries travel to treat patients and to train local surgeons. Treatment consists of providing an alternative route for CSF drainage by placing a catheter, or a shunt, into the ventricle so that it can drain into the abdomen. With early surgical drainage, a better chance of recovery is possible.

In this couple's rural village, the disorder is thought of as a curse caused by "evil spirits," and it brings shame to the family. Fortunately, this family is able to travel to an urban care facility, where their son undergoes a ventricular shunt placement. He is one of the lucky few, and within a few weeks, they notice improvement in his ability to focus and to control his head.

SUGGESTED READINGS

Borello U, Pierani A. 2010. Patterning the cerebral cortex: traveling with morphogens. Curr Opin Genet Dev 20:408–415.

Caviness Jr VS, Nowakowski RS, Bhide PG. 2009. Neocortical neurogenesis: morphogenetic gradients and beyond. Trends Neurosci 32:443–450.

Evans TA, Bashaw GJ. 2010. Axon guidance at the midline: of mice and flies. Curr Opin Neurobiol 20:79–85.

Hebert JM, Fishell G. 2008. The genetics of early telencephalon patterning: some assembly required. Nat Rev Neurosci 9:678–685.

Ming GL, Song H. 2011. Adult neurogenesis in the mammalian brain: significant answers and significant questions. Neuron 70:687–702.

Suh H, Deng W, Gage FH. 2009. Signaling in adult neurogenesis. Annu Rev Cell Dev Biol 25:253–275.

Chapter 10

Development of the Peripheral Nervous System

SUMMARY

The nervous system consists of complex networks of neurons that carry information from the sensory receptors in the body to the central nervous system (CNS); integrate, process, and store it; and return motor impulses to various effector organs in the body. The development of the CNS is covered in Chapter 9; this chapter covers the development of the peripheral nervous system (PNS).

The PNS and its central pathways are traditionally divided into two systems. The **somatic nervous system** is responsible for carrying conscious sensations and for innervating the voluntary (striated) muscles of the body. The **autonomic nervous system** is strictly motor and controls most of the involuntary, visceral activities of the body. The autonomic system itself consists of two divisions: the **parasympathetic division**, which, in general, promotes the anabolic visceral activities characteristic of periods of peace and relaxation, and the **sympathetic division**, which controls the involuntary activities that occur under stressful "fight or flight" conditions. Each of these systems is composed of two-neuron pathways consisting of **preganglionic** and **postganglionic neurons**. As covered in Chapters 4 and 14, the gut contains its own nervous system called the **enteric nervous system**.

Neurons originate from three embryonic tissues: the **neuroepithelium** lining the neural canal, **neural crest cells**, and specialized regions of ectoderm in the head and neck called **ectodermal placodes**. Neurons of the CNS arise from the neuroepithelium (covered in Chapter 9), whereas those of the PNS arise from neural crest cells and ectodermal placodes.

Trunk ganglia are formed by migrating neural crest cells. These ganglia include (1) sensory **dorsal root ganglia** that condense next to the spinal cord in register with each pair of somites and consist of sensory neurons that relay information from receptors in the body to the CNS and their supporting **satellite cells**; (2) **sympathetic chain ganglia** that also flank the spinal cord (but more ventrally) and the **prevertebral** (or **preaortic**) **ganglia** that form next to branches of the abdominal aorta and contain the peripheral (postganglionic) neurons of the two-neuron sympathetic pathways; and (3) the **parasympathetic ganglia** embedded in the walls of the visceral organs and containing the peripheral (postganglionic) neurons of the two-neuron parasympathetic division. The parasympathetic ganglia that reside within the gut are termed **enteric ganglia**.

As neural crest cells of the trunk coalesce to form spinal ganglia, somatic motor axons begin to grow out from the basal columns of the spinal cord, forming a pair of **ventral roots** at the level of each somite. These somatic motor fibers are later joined by autonomic motor fibers arising in the intermediolateral cell columns. The somatic motor fibers grow into the myotomes and, consequently, come to innervate the voluntary muscles. The autonomic (preganglionic) fibers, in contrast, terminate in the autonomic ganglia (sympathetic and parasympathetic), where they synapse with cell bodies of the peripheral (postganglionic) autonomic neurons that innervate the appropriate target organs.

The central (preganglionic) neurons of the sympathetic division develop in the intermediolateral cell columns of the **thoracolumbar** spinal cord (T1 through L2 or L3). The thinly myelinated axons of these cells leave the spinal cord in the ventral root but immediately branch off to form a **white ramus**, which enters the corresponding chain ganglion. Some of these fibers synapse with peripheral (postganglionic) sympathetic neurons in the chain ganglion; others pass onward to synapse in another chain ganglion or in one of the prevertebral ganglia. The unmyelinated axons of the peripheral (postganglionic) sympathetic chain ganglion neurons reenter the spinal nerve via a branch called the **gray ramus**.

The ganglia of the head consist of two types: **cranial nerve ganglia**, the neurons of which arise from either neural crest cells or ectodermal placodes, depending on the particular ganglion (glial cells arise exclusively from neural crest cells in all ganglia); and **cranial parasympathetic ganglia**, which arise from neural crest cells.

The central (preganglionic) neurons of the parasympathetic pathways are located in the brain stem and in the spinal cord at levels S2 through S4. The parasympathetic division is, therefore, called a **craniosacral system**. Parasympathetic fibers from the hindbrain reach the parasympathetic ganglia of the neck and trunk viscera via the **vagus nerve**, whereas sacral parasympathetic fibers innervate hindgut and pelvic visceral ganglia via the **pelvic splanchnic nerves**.

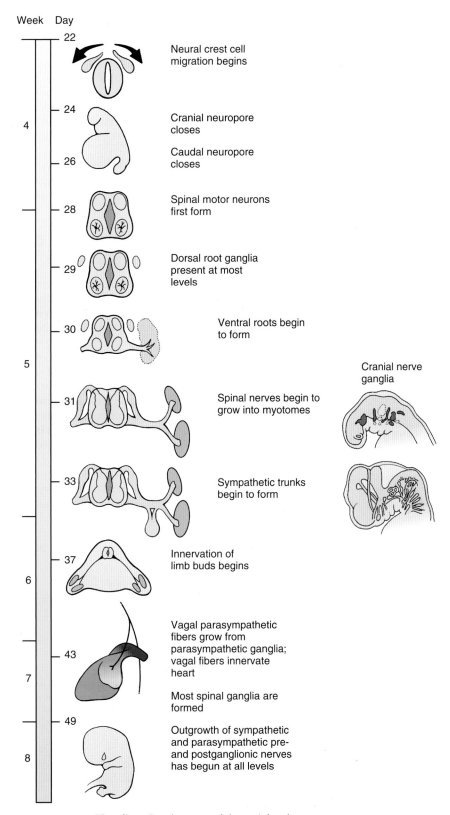

Week   Day

22   Neural crest cell migration begins

4   24   Cranial neuropore closes

26   Caudal neuropore closes

28   Spinal motor neurons first form

29   Dorsal root ganglia present at most levels

30   Ventral roots begin to form

5   Cranial nerve ganglia

31   Spinal nerves begin to grow into myotomes

33   Sympathetic trunks begin to form

37   Innervation of limb buds begins

6

43   Vagal parasympathetic fibers grow from parasympathetic ganglia; vagal fibers innervate heart

7   Most spinal ganglia are formed

49   Outgrowth of sympathetic and parasympathetic pre- and postganglionic nerves has begun at all levels

8

Time line. Development of the peripheral nervous system.

a

Clinical Taster

A toddler is brought to the emergency department after biting off the right anterolateral part of his tongue. While an oral surgeon is suturing the tongue, the staff notices other suspicious injuries. These include lacerations of the gums with missing teeth (Fig. 10-1A), a burn on the left index finger (Fig. 10-1B), and multiple other small cuts and bruises. An X-ray of the face, done to investigate the broken teeth, reveals an occult fracture of the parietal bone. An inquiry is begun by child protective services (CPS).

The parents claim that the injuries are all "self-inflicted," and describe the boy as having "no pain." They explain that the broken teeth are a result of biting on toys, and that the burned finger occurred when the child touched a hot grill. He does not cry with any of these significant injuries, including the bitten tongue, and they express their surprise when the skull fracture is discovered. His medical records show that he has been admitted to the hospital several times with high fever and presumed sepsis (severe infection) that was treated with antibiotics. The family has noticed that he becomes flushed and lethargic in the heat, and they have never seen him sweat. The boy cries little during the procedure to repair his tongue and is indifferent to the needle sticks needed to obtain lab tests. The CPS investigation uncovers no evidence of abuse. The family has two older children who are healthy and well cared for.

Neurology is consulted, and they obtain a skin biopsy that shows a paucity of small nerve fibers in the skin and absence of innervation of the sweat glands. Based on the clinical history and on these histologic findings, the diagnosis of **congenital insensitivity to pain with anhidrosis** (CIPA; anhidrosis means lack of sweating) is made. Confirmatory sequencing of the NTKR1 gene uncovers two deleterious mutations, each carried by one parent. NTKR1 is a receptor for NERVE GROWTH FACTOR and is required for the development of nociceptive (pain) sensory innervation of the skin, and for autonomic innervation of the eccrine sweat glands.

STRUCTURAL DIVISIONS OF NERVOUS SYSTEM

As covered in Chapter 9, the nervous system of vertebrates consists of two major *structural* divisions: a **central nervous system (CNS)** and a **peripheral nervous system (PNS)**. The CNS consists of the brain and spinal cord. The development of the CNS is covered in Chapter 9. The PNS consists of all components of the nervous system outside of the CNS. Thus, the PNS consists of cranial nerves and ganglia, spinal nerves and ganglia, autonomic nerves and ganglia, and the enteric nervous system. The development of the PNS is covered in this chapter.

FUNCTIONAL DIVISIONS OF NERVOUS SYSTEM

As covered in Chapter 9, the nervous system of vertebrates consists of two major *functional* divisions: a **somatic nervous system** and a **visceral nervous system**. The somatic nervous system innervates the skin and most skeletal muscles (i.e., it provides both sensory and motor components). Similarly, the visceral nervous system innervates the viscera (organs of the body) and smooth muscle and glands in the more peripheral part of the body. The visceral nervous system is also called the **autonomic nervous system**. It consists of two components: the **sympathetic division** and the **parasympathetic division**. The somatic and visceral nervous systems are covered both in Chapter 9 (CNS components) and in this chapter (PNS components).

Both divisions of the autonomic nervous system consist of two-neuron pathways. Because the peripheral autonomic neurons reside in ganglia, the axons of the central sympathetic neurons are called **preganglionic fibers** and the axons of the peripheral sympathetic neurons are called **postganglionic fibers**. This terminology

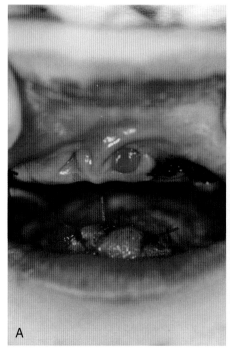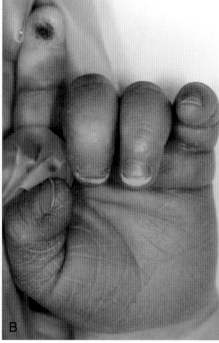

Figure 10-1. Child with congenital insensitivity to pain with anhidrosis. *A,* Mouth of a toddler showing sutured lacerations of the tongue and gums and missing teeth. *B,* Hand of a toddler showing burn on the left index finger.

is used for both sympathetic pathways and parasympathetic pathways (covered later in the chapter). Sometimes preganglionic fibers are also called *presynaptic fibers*, and postganglionic fibers, *postsynaptic fibers*, because the axons of the preganglionic fibers *synapse* on the cell bodies of postganglionic neurons in the autonomic ganglia.

ORIGIN OF PNS

 *Animation 10-1: Formation of Neural Crest.*
      Animations are available online at StudentConsult.

Chapters 3 and 4 describe how, during neurulation, the rudiment of the central nervous system arises as a neural plate from the ectoderm of the embryonic disc and folds to form the neural tube (the rudiment of the brain and spinal cord). The PNS arises from the neural tube and two groups of cells outside of the neural tube: neural crest cells and ectodermal placodes (the ectodermal placodes are covered further in Chapter 18). The PNS develops as an integrated system, essentially in cranial-to-caudal sequence. However, for the sake of simplicity, the development of the trunk (associated with the spinal cord) and of cranial (associated with the brain) portions of the PNS will be covered separately. The sympathetic division of the autonomic nervous system arises in association with the trunk (thoracolumbar levels of the spinal cord), whereas the parasympathetic division of the autonomic nervous system arises in association with the brain and caudal spinal cord (craniosacral levels of the CNS).

◼ In the Research Lab

PLASTICITY OF PRECURSOR CELLS OF PNS

As just mentioned, the PNS arises from both neural crest cells and ectodermal placodes. How are these structures determined in the early embryo and to what extent are they able to change their fate? Induction of neural crest cells is covered in Chapter 4, and induction of ectodermal placodes is covered in Chapter 18. Hence, here we will consider the plasticity of neural crest cells and ectodermal placodes.

Plasticity of Neural Crest Cells and Ectodermal Placodes

Heterotopic transplantation studies have revealed that both neural crest cells and ectodermal placodes are highly plastic at the time of their formation. In these studies, small groups of prospective neural crest cells or small patches of preplacodal ectoderm are transplanted from their normal site of origin to an ectopic site. Typically, quail tissues are transplanted heterotopically to chick embryos, so that donor and host tissues can be specifically traced during subsequent development (covered in Chapter 5; see Fig. 5-11). Preplacodal cells generally are transplanted from one prospective placode to another (e.g., lens to otic or vice versa), where they readily adapt to their new environment and change their fate, that is, they exhibit plasticity. Neural crest cells are generally transplanted from one craniocaudal level to another, including the placement of trunk neural crest cells in the head and vice versa. As covered in Chapter 4, neural crest cells give rise to a large number of cell types, including cartilage, bone, melanocytes, endocrine tissues, PNS neurons, and glial cells. Only head (cranial) neural crest cells are capable of forming bone and

cartilage in transplantation studies, although isolated trunk neural crest cells subjected to various signaling molecules in vitro are capable of forming cartilage in some cases. Thus, neural crest cells at the time of their migration also display considerable plasticity.

Despite having early plasticity at the time of their formation, generally by about late neurulation stages, the fates of both neural crest cells and placodal cells as *populations* become fixed. Hence, heterotopic transplantation typically results at these stages in the formation of ectopic structures commensurate with the *origin*—not the new position—of the transplanted tissue.

NEURAL CREST CELLS AND THEIR DERIVATIVES AS STEM-LIKE CELLS

As just covered, neural crest cells give rise to a large number of different cell types, and, consequently, they have properties similar to stem cells (embryonic stem cells are covered in Chapter 5). This stem-like cell nature not only occurs within migrating neural crest cells but also continues in their progeny (i.e., in tissues and organs formed by neural crest cells) as *individual* cells. For example, pluripotent neural crest cells (i.e., stem-like cells) have been identified in the embryonic chick dorsal root ganglion, sympathetic ganglion, and cardiac outflow tract. Neural crest cell stem-like cells are present also in the mammalian embryonic sciatic nerve, and in the embryonic and adult gut. However, the developmental potentials of these cells are more restricted than for migrating neural crest cells, and they vary according to the location of the cells.

It is surprising to note that pluripotent neural crest cells that can give rise to all cranial neural crest cell derivatives have been isolated from the bulge of adult mammalian hair follicles. The follicular bulge is an epidermal structure of the hair follicle that serves as a niche for keratinocyte stem cells, which form new epidermis, sebaceous gland, and hair (covered in Chapter 7). Thus, the bulge contains a mixed population of stem-like cells consisting of both keratinocyte stem cells and neural crest cell stem-like cells. Highly motile neural crest cell–derived stem-like cells (**epidermal neural crest cell stem-like cells**) emigrate from bulge explants dissected from adult hair follicles (Fig. 10-2). Remarkably, more than 88% of these migrating cells are pluripotent stem cells that can generate all cranial neural crest derivatives.

Because of their existence in humans, their accessibility, and their high degree of physiologic plasticity, neural crest cell stem-like cells in the periphery of the adult organism are promising candidates for cell replacement therapy.

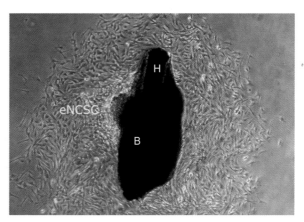

Figure 10-2. Bulge explant four days after onset of epidermal neural crest cell stem-like cell (eNCSC) emigration. The bulge (B), which was dissected from an adult mouse whisker follicle, releases numerous highly motile eNCSC, which divide rapidly in culture. The hair (H) is visible within the bulge.

NEUROFIBROMATOSIS TYPE 1 (NF-1)

Neurofibromatosis type 1 (also known as von Recklinghausen disease) is a prevalent familial tumor disposition that affects 1 in 3500 individuals worldwide. It is a progressive disease with multiple deficits, including benign and malignant tumors of the peripheral and central nervous systems. A gene mutated in neurofibromatosis type 1, NEUROFIBROMIN (NF-1), is a **tumor suppressor gene** that inactivates the **proto-oncogene** RAS. Patients with NF-1 are heterozygous for the inactivating mutations of the NF-1 gene. Thus, RAS function is upregulated in NF-1 patients. In addition, inhibitors of fibroblast growth factor (Fgf) signaling (which occurs through the Ras-Mapk pathway; see Chapter 5) such as SPRED1, a member of the sprouty/spred family of proteins, when mutated result in an NF-1–like condition.

One hallmark of NF-1 is the presence of six or more large (greater than 0.5 cm in children; greater than 1.5 cm in adults) café au lait spots—pigmented birth marks (frequently, one or two café au lait spots are present in unaffected individuals). These are non-symptomatic. A second, problematic hallmark is the presence of numerous benign cutaneous tumors, called **neurofibromas**. These tumors contain multiple cell types, including Schwann cells, neurons, fibroblasts, and mast cells. As covered in Chapter 4, the first two of these cell types are derived from neural crest cells. Evidence suggests that the second wild-type allele is lost in NF-1 patients through subsequent somatic deletion (the so-called **two-hit hypothesis**), which leads to certain types of tumors (e.g., malignant peripheral nerve sheath tumor). However, because of the infrequency of somatic deletion and the frequency of neurofibromas developing in NF patients, second mutations are likely not required for neurofibroma formation.

Both paracrine and/or cell-autonomous events are known to trigger neurofibroma formation. For example, the onset of puberty and of pregnancy is often associated with a major increase in the number and size of neurofibromas. Both circumstances involve hormonal changes and an increase in subcutaneous adipose tissue deposits. Therefore, potentially hormonal and/or paracrine mechanisms may be responsible for tumorigenesis in some NF-1 patients. In this regard, there is an interesting convergence of two observations: first, hair follicles from normal-looking skin of NF-1 patients are often surrounded by numerous S100-positive neural crest cell–derived Schwann cells, or Schwann cell progenitors; and second, as covered in the preceding "In the Research Lab" entitled "Plasticity of Precursor Cells of PNS," hair follicles contain neural crest cell stem-like cells. Therefore, it is conceivable that mitogens produced by adipocytes and/or female hormones promote proliferation of neural crest stem-like cells in hair follicles of NF-1 patients, leading to neurofibroma formation.

In NF-1, nerve fibers can grow uncontrollably, putting pressure on affected nerves and resulting in nerve damage, pain, and loss of nerve function. As no specific treatment for the disease is known, it is managed surgically by removing neuromas that are painful or rapidly growing, as the latter may become cancerous. Tumors can also occur in structures such as the optic nerves, subsequently resulting in blindness.

NEUROGENESIS IN PNS

The process of neurogenesis occurs similarly in the CNS and the PNS and involves a series of steps in which multipotential precursor cells (i.e., stem cells or stem-like cells) become progressively restricted in their fate over time. During this process, cells generally transform from multipotent precursors (e.g., capable of forming all types of neurons and glia) to restricted neuronal (or glial) precursors (e.g., capable of forming only neurons or only glia, but not both) to differentiated cell types (i.e., a specific type of neuron). Within the CNS, these precursors arise from the neural plate; within the PNS, they arise from neural crest cells and ectodermal placodes. Initially, cells in these rudiments rapidly divide to expand the number of cells in the population. However, over time the division of these cells becomes asymmetric such that one daughter cell derived from a particular mitotic division remains mitotically active and undifferentiated, whereas the other daughter cell becomes postmitotic, migrates away from its site of generation, and begins to differentiate.

Several genes play essential roles in regulating neurogenesis. These include both positive regulators and negative regulators. Examples of the former include the basic helix-loop-helix (bHLH) transcription factors known as the **proneural genes**. In vertebrates, these include genes such as Mash (the mammalian ortholog of Drosophila achaete-scute genes). Other vertebrate proneural genes include Math, NeuroD, and the neurogenins (the latter three are vertebrate—mammalian in the case of Math—orthologs of Drosophila atonal genes). Expression of these proneural genes is both sufficient and necessary for the formation of neurons. Examples of the negative regulators of neurogenesis include members of the notch signaling pathway (covered in Chapter 5). Through a process called **lateral inhibition** (covered in Chapters 10 and 18), which involves notch signaling, a neuronal precursor cell inhibits its neighbors from differentiating as neurons (e.g., by secreting a notch ligand such as delta, which binds to the neighbor's notch receptors). Lateral inhibition thus regulates the number of neurons born in any one region of the developing nervous system and allows for the generation of supporting glial cells. Nevertheless, many more neurons are actually born than required. Hence, through a subsequent process of **programmed cell death**, the number of definitive neurons is reduced to the characteristic number for each area of the CNS and PNS.

DEVELOPMENT OF TRUNK PNS

The trunk PNS consists of spinal nerves and ganglia, autonomic nerves and ganglia, and the enteric nervous system. Sympathetic nerves course through spinal nerves at the thoracolumbar level to reach their ganglia. In addition, parasympathetic nerves course through sacral spinal nerves to reach their ganglia. Thus, the development of spinal nerves (and ganglia) and associated autonomic nerves (sympathetic at thoracolumbar levels and parasympathetic at sacral levels) is considered together. The development of the enteric nervous system is covered in Chapter 4, as well as in Chapter 14 in the context of development of the gut wall.

DEVELOPMENT OF SPINAL NERVES AND GANGLIA

Ventral Column Motor Axons Are First to Sprout from Spinal Cord

The first axons to emerge from the spinal cord are produced by somatic motoneurons in the ventral gray columns. These fibers appear in the cervical region on about day thirty (Fig. 10-3) and (like so many other embryonic processes) proceed in a craniocaudal wave down the spinal cord.

The ventral motor axons initially leave the spinal cord as a continuous broad band. However, as they grow toward the sclerotomes, they rapidly condense to form discrete segmental nerves. Although these axons will eventually synapse with muscles derived from the developing myotomes, their initial guidance depends only on the sclerotomes and not on myotomal or dermatomal elements of the somite. As covered in Chapter 8, neural crest cells migrate within the cranial half of each sclerotome; ventral column axons migrate within the cranial half of each sclerotome as well (see Fig. 10-3). As a result, these growing axons pass close to the developing dorsal root ganglion at each level.

The pioneer axons that initially sprout from the spinal cord are soon joined by additional ventral column motor axons, and the growing bundle is now called a **ventral root** (Fig. 10-4). At spinal levels T1 through L2 or L3, the ventral root is later joined by axons from the sympathetic motoneurons developing in the intermediolateral cell columns at these levels (see Fig. 10-4; also see and later coverage in this chapter).

Somatic and Autonomic Motor Fibers Combine with Sensory Fibers to Form Spinal Nerves

As axons of the ventral motoneurons approach the corresponding dorsal root ganglion, the neurons in the dorsal root ganglion begin to extend axons bidirectionally. Each of these bipolar neurons, whose cell bodies reside within the dorsal root ganglion, has a branch that grows medially toward the dorsal column of the spinal cord and a branch that joins the ventral root and grows toward the periphery to innervate the target organ (Fig. 10-5). The bundle of axons that connect the dorsal root ganglion to the spinal cord is called the **dorsal root**. The central processes of dorsal root ganglion cells penetrate the dorsal columns of the spinal cord (Fig. 10-6), where they synapse with developing **association neurons**. These association neurons in turn sprout axons that synapse

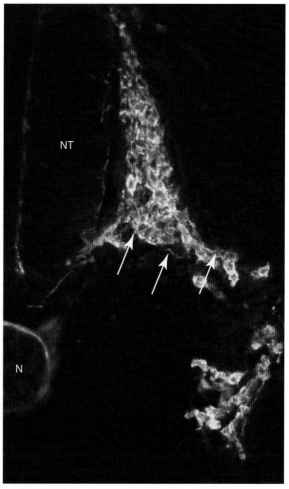

Figure 10-3. Double-stained immunochemical preparation showing neural crest cells (in a chick embryo stained with HNK-1 antibody; yellow) and ventral motoneuron fibers (labeled with E/C8, an antibody against neurofilament-binding protein; red and arrows). Neural crest cells are migrating through the cranial half of the sclerotome. N, notochord; NT, neural tube.

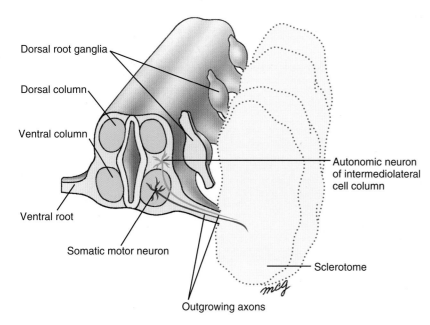

Figure 10-4. Outgrowth of the ventral roots and formation of the dorsal root ganglia. Axons growing from ventral column motoneurons at each segmental level of the spinal cord are guided by the sclerotome to form a ventral root. Dorsal root ganglia form in the same plane.

either with autonomic motoneurons in the intermedio-lateral cell columns or with somatic motoneurons in the ventral columns, or they ascend to higher levels in the spinal cord in the form of **tracts**. The axons of some association neurons synapse with motoneurons on the same, or **ipsilateral**, side of the spinal cord, whereas others cross over to synapse with motoneurons on the opposite, or **contralateral**, side of the cord.

The mixed motor and sensory trunk formed at each level by the confluence of the peripheral processes of the dorsal root ganglion cells and the ventral roots is called a **spinal nerve** (see Fig. 10-5). The sympathetic fibers (preganglionic) that exit via the ventral roots at levels

T1 through L2 or L3 soon branch from the spinal nerve and grow ventrally to enter the corresponding **sympathetic chain ganglion** (Fig. 10-7; also see Figs. 4-19, 4-22). This branch is called a **white ramus**. Some of the sympathetic fibers carried in the white ramus synapse directly with a neuron in the chain ganglion. This neuron becomes the second (peripheral or postganglionic or postsynaptic) neuron in a two-neuron sympathetic pathway and sprouts an axon that grows to innervate the appropriate peripheral target organ.

Not all preganglionic sympathetic fibers that enter a chain ganglion via the white ramus synapse there. The remainder project cranially or caudally and synapse in

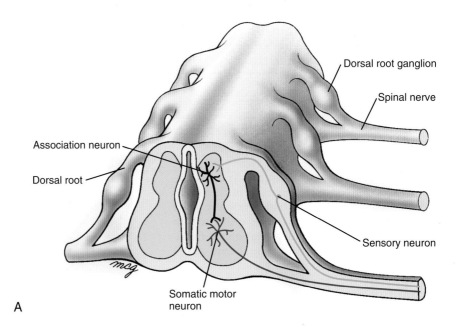

A

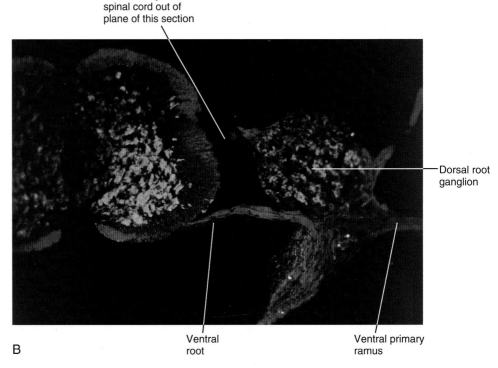

B

Figure 10-5. Spinal nerves. *A,* Once the ventral roots are formed, sensory neurons within each dorsal root ganglion sprout processes that grow into the neural tube to synapse with association neurons in the dorsal column. Other processes grow outward from the dorsal root ganglion to join the ventral root, forming a typical spinal nerve. The dorsal root connects the dorsal root ganglion to the spinal cord. The axon of the association neuron in this illustration synapses with a motor neuron on the same side of the spinal cord at the same segmental level (axons may also display other patterns of connection; discussed in text). *B,* Double-stained immunochemical preparation showing neuronal cell bodies (green) and neurofilaments within nerve cell processes (red).

a more cranial or caudal chain ganglion or in one of the prevertebral (or preaortic) ganglia (see Fig. 4-19). These fibers, plus the chain ganglia themselves, constitute the **sympathetic trunk**. They are covered later in the chapter.

The postganglionic fibers that originate in each chain ganglion form a small branch—the **gray ramus**—that grows dorsally to rejoin the spinal nerve, and then grows toward the periphery (see Fig. 10-7). Distal to the gray ramus, the spinal nerve thus carries sensory fibers, somatic motor fibers, and postganglionic sympathetic fibers.

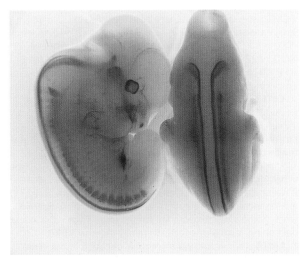

Figure 10-6. Dorsal and lateral views of transgenic mice that express the bacterial lacZ gene in tissues that also produce peripherin (a neurofilament protein characteristic of PNS, but not CNS, neurons). The enzyme encoded by the lacZ gene causes the cells producing peripherin to turn blue when appropriately processed. The blue stain is localized in small neurons of the neural crest cell–derived dorsal root ganglia and in the axons of these cells that penetrate the spinal cord in a region overlying the dorsal gray columns of the spinal cord (parasagittal stripes).

Axons in Spinal Nerves Grow to Specific Sites

Motor and sensory axons in spinal nerves grow to specific targets in the body wall and extremities. Shortly after leaving the spinal column, each axon first chooses one of two routes, growing either dorsally toward the **epimere** or ventrally toward the **hypomere**. Thus, the spinal nerve splits into two **rami**. The axons that direct their path toward the epimere form the **dorsal ramus**, and the fibers that grow toward the hypomere form the **ventral ramus** (see Fig. 10-7). The presence of the epimere is required for formation of the dorsal ramus. If a single epimere is removed from an experimental animal, the dorsal ramus of the corresponding spinal nerve will grow to innervate an adjacent epimere. However, if several successive epimeres are ablated, the corresponding dorsal rami do not form.

Axons of somatic motor fibers in the dorsal and ventral rami seek out specific muscles or bundles of muscle fibers and form synapses with the muscle fibers, whereas postganglionic sympathetic motor fibers innervate the smooth muscle of blood vessels and sweat glands and erector pili muscles in the skin. The specific signals that guide motor fibers to their targets are not known. Inhibitory signaling from ephrins in ventral muscles is thought to direct motor axons into dorsal nerve branches (also see the coverage of axonal guidance in the following two sections of "In the Research Lab" entitled "Patterning Migration of Sympathetic Precursor Cells and Sympathetic Ganglia" and "Regulating Axonal Guidance in PNS"). Moreover, it has been suggested that sympathetic fibers use the developing vascular system as a guide. Conversely, it has been suggested that peripheral nerves provide a template that determines the organotypic pattern of blood vessel branching and arterial differentiation in the skin via local secretion of vascular endothelial growth factor (Vegf).

Sensory axons grow somewhat later than motor axons. For most of their length, they follow the pathways

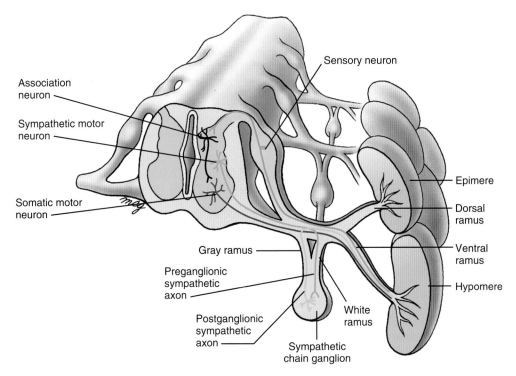

Figure 10-7. Organization of spinal nerves and associated chain ganglia at levels T1-L2 and S2-S4. In this example, the preganglionic fiber growing from the intermediolateral cell column exits the spinal nerve through a white ramus and synapses with a neuron in the chain ganglion at the same level. The postganglionic fiber then exits through the gray ramus and rejoins the same spinal nerve. Each spinal nerve splits into a dorsal primary ramus and a ventral primary ramus, which innervate the segmental epimere and hypomere, respectively. Both rami contain motor, sensory, and autonomic fibers.

Association neuron

Sensory neuron

Sympathetic motor neuron

Somatic motor neuron

Epimere

Dorsal ramus

Ventral ramus

Hypomere

Gray ramus

Preganglionic sympathetic axon

Postganglionic sympathetic axon

White ramus

Sympathetic chain ganglion

established by the somatic and sympathetic motor fibers, but eventually they branch from the combined nerves and ultimately become associated with sensory end organs, such as muscle spindles, temperature and touch receptors in the dermis of the skin, and pressure sensors and chemoreceptors in the developing vasculature. In many cases, the sensory neurons are responsible for inducing and maintaining the specialized sensory receptors.

In the Clinic

HEREDITARY PERIPHERAL NEUROPATHIES

Motoneurons, whose cell bodies lie in the anterior horns of the spinal cord, may extend their axons for up to a meter in the PNS. Sensory neurons, whose cell bodies lie in the dorsal root ganglia, extend their central processes segmentally into the spinal cord, and their peripheral processes fasciculate with the axons of motoneurons to form mixed nerves. Axons in the PNS are myelinated by **Schwann cells**. Thus, the Schwann cell performs the role in the PNS subserved by astrocytes and oligodendrocytes in the CNS (covered in Chapter 9). The signal for myelination comes from the axon, and myelination occurs in axons larger than 1 to 2 μm in diameter. Each segment of a myelinated axon is the territory of a single Schwann cell, with the length of the segments correlating with the diameter of the axon. For unmyelinated fibers, single Schwann cells usually surround multiple axons. The myelin sheath is composed of compacted layers of the Schwann cell membrane. It is predominantly lipid but contains several proteins that have key roles in maintaining the structure and compaction of the myelin and adhesion of the sheath to the axon. Several of these proteins and lipids may be important immunogens in disease.

Peripheral nerves are generally mixed nerves composed of sensory, motor, sympathetic, and parasympathetic fibers. The nerves are divided into fascicles surrounded by the **perineurium**, a connective tissue sheath, and are bound together by the **epineurium**, a similar connective tissue sheath. Individual nerve fibers are surrounded by a third sheath, the **endoneurium**. This sheath contains collagen, fibroblasts, mast cells, and resident macrophages. Endoneurial arterioles are supplied by a plexus of epineurial blood vessels with multiple systemic feeders. Circulating macromolecules are excluded from the endoneurium by the **blood-nerve barrier**, which is analogous to the blood-brain barrier and is formed by the endothelial cells and their tight junctions.

The long length of PNS axons, their dependence on axonal transport for renewal of structural membrane and cytoskeletal components, and other factors make them especially vulnerable to damage. Major pathologies of the nerve involve axonal degeneration and demyelination. Damage to Schwann cells or myelin can result in segmental demyelination. In this process, the myelin sheath is stripped from a complete segment up to 1 mm in length. Macrophages remove myelin debris, and Schwann cells divide after segmental demyelination. Remyelination can begin quickly, within a few days, producing shorter segments of myelin, usually about 300 μm long.

Certain demyelinating diseases are hereditary. Specific diagnosis is now possible by genetic analysis of appropriate phenotypes, obviating the need for nerve biopsy in many cases. Diagnosis guides neurologic assessment and counseling of at-risk family members.

Charcot-Marie-Tooth Hereditary Neuropathy

Charcot-Marie-Tooth (CMT) hereditary neuropathy, also called hereditary motor-sensory neuropathy (HMSN), is a group of chronic demyelinating polyneuropathies (i.e., motor and sensory) that present in the first and second decades with slowly progressive distal weakness, wasting, and sensory loss, which is worse in the legs. High arches (pes cavus), hammer toes, ankle instability, and eventual deformity are common. Nerve hypertrophy may be seen. Slowed nerve conduction velocities, usually to 20 to 30 m/sec (normal ≥40 m/sec), without conduction block are typical. Biopsies show loss of myelinated fibers, signs of demyelination and remyelination, and onion bulbs (concentric laminar structures formed by Schwann cells). Ankle braces, special shoes, and corrective foot and ankle surgery are often helpful. Most patients remain ambulatory. Four separate types are currently recognized: types **CMT1, -2, -4**, and **-X**. Mutations that result in CMT have been identified in more than thirty genes.

CMT1 is an autosomal dominant disease occurring in 50% of CMT patients. Mutations have been identified in five different genes encoding **myelin** or myelin-related proteins, with most (70% to 80%) occurring in the PMP22 (PERIPHERAL MYELIN PROTEIN 22) gene and 5% to 10% occurring in the MPZ (MYELIN PROTEIN ZERO) gene. Demyelination affects both motor and sensory nerves and results in muscle atrophy and sensory deficits.

CMT2 is predominantly an autosomal dominant disease causing chronic motor-sensory polyneuropathy of **axons**, without demyelination. It occurs in 20% to 40% of CMT patients. Electrophysiologic studies show signs of chronic distal muscle denervation and minor slowing of nerve conduction velocities. CMT1 and CMT2 patients present similarly with high arches and hammer toes, along with a distal predominance of wasting, weakness, and sensory loss. CMT2 is genetically heterogeneous, with mutations identified in thirteen different genes. Some of these genes are known to be involved in axonal functioning, such as the KINESIN family member KIF1B.

CMT4 is a rare autosomal recessive disease that can cause abnormalities of **myelin** and/or **axons**. Patients present with typical CMT symptoms, including muscle weakness and sensory loss. Mutations have been identified in nine different genes.

CMTX is an X-linked condition affecting 10% to 20% of CMT patients. Axonopathy and demyelination occur more severely in male subjects, who clinically resemble patients with CMT1 and CMT2. About half of female carriers are mildly affected. Slowing of nerve conduction velocities to 30 to 40 m/sec is seen. Pathologic changes suggest an **axon** defect, but the abnormal protein CONNEXIN-32 is a gap junction protein found in compacted **myelin**.

In addition to the four types of CMT, other CMT-like hereditary peripheral neuropathies exist, such as **Refsum disease**. This disease is distinguished from CMT by the presence of additional symptoms including anosmia, deafness, retinitis, ichthyosis, and ataxia. It is caused by the accumulation of **phytanic acid** (a substance commonly present in foods) resulting from mutations in the gene encoding the enzyme PHYTANOYL-CoA HYDROXYLASE. Mutations have been identified in two different genes.

PATTERN OF SOMATIC MOTOR AND SENSORY INNERVATION IS SEGMENTAL

Motor and sensory nerves innervate the body wall and limbs in a pattern that is based on the segmental organization established by the somites. For example, the intercostal muscles between a given pair of ribs are innervated by the spinal nerve that grows out at that level. The sensory innervation of the skin is also basically segmental: each dermatome is innervated by the spinal nerve growing out at the same level (also covered in Chapter 7). However, the sensory component of each spinal nerve spreads to some extent into the adjacent dermatomes, so some overlap in dermatomal innervation is evident (Fig. 10-8).

PATTERN OF SYMPATHETIC INNERVATION IS NOT ENTIRELY SEGMENTAL

Sympathetic fibers traveling in the spinal nerves share the segmental distribution of the somatic motor and sensory fibers. Therefore, segments of the body wall and extremities developing at levels T1 through L2 or L3 are innervated by postganglionic fibers originating from chain ganglia at corresponding levels of the spinal cord. However, another pattern is required to provide sympathetic innervation to remaining levels of the body wall and extremities, which correspond to cord levels lacking central sympathetic neurons. Chain

ganglia develop in the cervical, lower lumbar, sacral, and coccygeal regions in addition to the thoracic and upper lumbar regions. How do these ganglia receive central sympathetic innervation? The answer (as hinted earlier) is that some of the preganglionic sympathetic fibers that enter chain ganglia at levels T1 through L2 or L3 travel cranially or caudally to another chain ganglion before synapsing. Some of these ascending or descending fibers supply the chain ganglia outside of T1 through L2 or L3 (Fig. 10-9).

Postganglionic fibers from each chain ganglion enter the corresponding spinal nerve via a gray ramus. As a result, the spinal nerves at levels T1 through L2 or L3

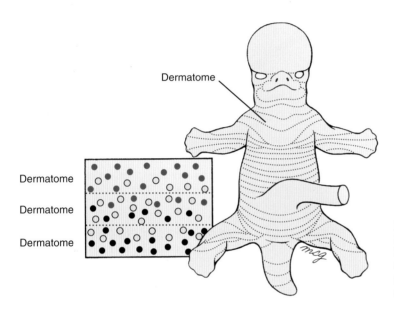

Figure 10-8. Dermatomal distribution of sensory innervation. Sensory fibers of each spinal nerve innervate receptors mainly in the corresponding body segment or dermatome. However, the innervation of adjacent dermatomes shows some overlap, so that ablation of a dorsal root does not entirely obliterate sensation in the corresponding dermatome.

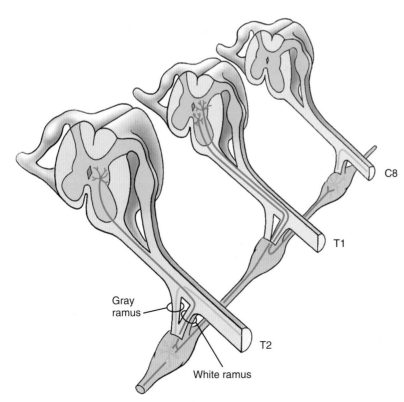

Figure 10-9. Preganglionic fibers growing from the intermediolateral cell column may synapse with a neuron in a chain ganglion at their own level, a lower level, or a higher level. This mechanism provides sympathetic innervation to spinal levels other than T1-L2, which lack a white ramus (i.e., C1-C8, L3 and L5, S1-S5, and the first coccygeal nerve).

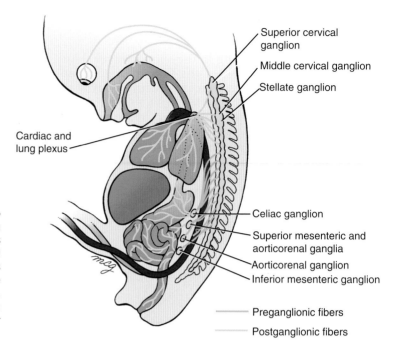

Figure 10-10. Some postganglionic sympathetic fibers do not join with spinal nerves. Postganglionic fibers emanating from cervical and thoracic chain ganglia follow blood vessels to structures in the head and pharynx and to the heart and lungs. The splanchnic nerves are preganglionic fibers that pass directly out of the chain ganglia at levels T5 to L2 to innervate neurons within the celiac, superior mesenteric, aorticorenal, and inferior mesenteric ganglia. Postganglionic fibers from these ganglia grow out along blood vessels to innervate their visceral end organs.

have both white and gray rami, whereas all other spinal nerves have just a gray ramus. Thus, the motor fibers linking chain ganglia to one another are exclusively preganglionic sympathetic fibers.

Sympathetic Innervation of Organs of Thorax and Head

The sympathetic supply to the heart originates at cord levels T1 through T4 (Fig. 10-10). Some of the fibers from T1 travel up the sympathetic trunk to synapse in the three cervical chain ganglia—the **inferior cervical ganglion** (which is sometimes fused with the chain ganglion at T1 to form the **stellate ganglion**), the **middle cervical ganglion**, and the **superior cervical ganglion**. Postganglionic fibers from these ganglia join postganglionic fibers emanating directly from nerves T1 through T4 to form the cardiac nerves, which innervate the heart muscle.

Postganglionic sympathetic fibers exiting directly from chain ganglia associated with levels T1 through T4, or from cervical ganglia innervated by preganglionic fibers originating at cord levels T1 to T4, also innervate the trachea and lungs.

Some postganglionic fibers arising from the superior cervical ganglion project to various structures in the head that receive sympathetic innervation. These structures include the lacrimal glands, the dilator pupillae muscles of the iris, and the nasal and oral mucosa.

Sympathetic Innervation of Abdomen

The preganglionic sympathetic fibers destined to supply the gut arise from cord levels T5 through L2 or L3 and enter the corresponding chain ganglia. However, instead of synapsing there, they immediately leave the sympathetic trunk via the **splanchnic nerves**, which emerge directly from the chain ganglia (see Fig. 10-10). The splanchnic nerves innervate the various prevertebral (or

preaortic) ganglia, which, in turn, send postganglionic fibers to the visceral end organs. The pattern of distribution is as follows:

Fibers from levels T5 through T9 or T10 come together to form the **greater splanchnic nerves** serving the **celiac ganglion**.

Fibers from T10 and T11 form the **lesser splanchnic nerves** serving the **superior mesenteric** and **aorticorenal ganglia**.

Fibers from T12 alone form the **least splanchnic nerves** serving the **renal plexus**.

Fibers from L1 and L2 form the **lumbar splanchnic nerves** serving the **inferior mesenteric ganglion plexus**.

The prevertebral (or preaortic) ganglia develop next to major branches of the descending aorta (i.e., the celiac, superior mesenteric, and inferior mesenteric arteries; covered in Chapter 13, and in relation to regions of the gut in Chapter 14). The postganglionic sympathetic axons from the prevertebral ganglia grow out along these arteries and thus come to innervate the same tissues that the arteries supply with blood (see Fig. 10-10). Thus, postganglionic fibers from the celiac ganglia innervate the distal foregut region vascularized by the celiac artery—that is, the portion of the foregut from the abdominal esophagus through the duodenum to the entrance of the bile duct. Similarly, fibers from the superior mesenteric ganglia innervate the **midgut** (the remainder of the duodenum, the jejunum, and the ileum) plus the ascending colon and about two-thirds of the transverse colon. The aorticorenal ganglia innervate the kidney and suprarenal gland, and the inferior mesenteric ganglia innervate the **hindgut**, including the distal one third of the transverse colon, the descending and sigmoid colons, and the upper two thirds of the anorectal canal.

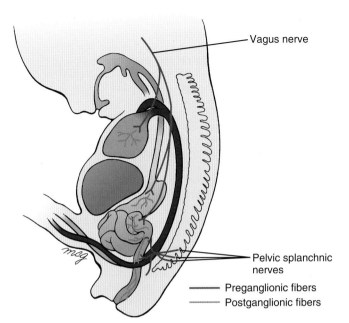

Vagus nerve

Pelvic splanchnic
nerves

——— Preganglionic fibers
········· Postganglionic fibers

Figure 10-11. The vagus nerve and pelvic splanchnic nerves provide preganglionic parasympathetic innervation to ganglia embedded in the walls of visceral organs. The preganglionic fibers originating at cord levels S2 through S4 issue from the cord at those levels and then branch off to form pelvic splanchnic nerves. The latter innervate the parasympathetic ganglia of the target viscera. The postganglionic parasympathetic fibers are relatively short.

Parasympathetic Innervation of Lower Abdomen, Pelvis, and Perineum

Parasympathetic preganglionic fibers arising in the sacral spinal cord emerge from the ventral rami of the cord and join together to form the **pelvic splanchnic nerves**. These nerves ramify throughout the pelvis and lower abdomen, innervating ganglia embedded in the walls of the descending and sigmoid colons, rectum, ureter, prostate, bladder, urethra, and phallus. Postganglionic fibers from these ganglia innervate smooth muscle or glands in the target organs (Fig. 10-11).

■ *In the Research Lab*

PATTERNING MIGRATION OF SYMPATHETIC PRECURSOR CELLS AND SYMPATHETIC GANGLIA

Ventrally migrating neural crest cells in the trunk region sort into two functionally different populations: dorsal root ganglia and sympathetic ganglia. How is this choice made? Sophisticated cell lineage and live-imaging experiments in chick, combined with gene mis-expression studies, have revealed that a subset of such migrating neural crest cells express the chemokine receptor Cxcr4. Chemokines are a family of small proteins that were named for their ability to induce chemotaxis in neighboring cells containing chemokine receptors. Many chemokines are pro-inflammatory and act to recruit cells to sites of infection postnatally. However, chemokines and their receptors also play a role in development. In the case of neural crest cells, the subset expressing Cxcr4 forms the core of the sympathetic ganglia, and these cells are directed to this site, adjacent to the developing dorsal aorta, during their migration by the Cxcr4 ligand, stromal-derived factor-1 (Sdf-1), which is a cytokine that

acts as a chemoattractant. Thus, two populations are selected from the trunk neural crest migrating stream: those expressing Cxcr4, which are attracted to the site of the forming sympathetic ganglia, and those not expressing Cxcr4, which stop their migration more dorsally and coalesce as the dorsal root ganglia.

Once neural crest cells populate the level of the developing sympathetic ganglia, they form a continuous band of cells, yet in the adult, the sympathetic ganglia are segregated into distinct clusters of cells. How is this pattern generated? Similar experiments to those just described provide the answer: cells are dispersed into islands distributed along the craniocaudal axis by inhibitory interactions between cells expressing Ephs and other expressing ephrins, and those within the islands establish adhesive intercellular contacts with one another, mediated by the cell adhesion molecule N-cadherin. Such interactions establish the characteristic morphology of the sympathetic chain ganglia.

Once the sympathetic precursor cells reach their destination lateral to the developing dorsal aorta, they still must undergo differentiation into the correct neuronal type to function properly. As just mentioned, these cells contribute to the sympathetic chain ganglia. In addition, some of these cells contribute to the medulla of the adrenal gland, another component of the sympathetic nervous system. How are these separate neuronal lineages generated? Experiments, again using chick embryos, have revealed the answer. Bone morphogenetic proteins (Bmps) produced by the dorsal aorta, are required for production of the chemoattractant cytokine Sdf-1 (covered earlier) and neuregulin1 (a member of the epidermal growth factor family; covered in Chapter 5), which also acts as a chemoattractant; these two chemoattractants direct neural crest cells to their final locations adjacent to the dorsal aorta (see previous section), confirming and expanding our understanding of this process.

At later stages in development, Bmps produced by the dorsal aorta play another role in cell specification: they act to segregate sympathetic ganglion cells from adrenal medullary cells. Once the sympathetic chain precursor cells reach the level of the dorsal aorta, they become refractory to Bmp signaling, but adrenal medullary precursor cells still respond. In a clever set of experiments using tetracycline (tet)-controlled gene expression to precisely regulate temporally the ability of precursor cells to respond to Bmp signaling, it was shown that Bmp signaling was essential for the formation of adrenal medullary cells, but that extinguishing Bmp signaling was essential for the formation of sympathetic chain ganglia cells.

Finally, how do sympathetic neurons navigate their axons across large distances to reach their correct target sites? Students of anatomy know that nerves, arteries, veins, and lymphatics often travel together as a neurovascular bundle. Hence, it is not surprising that factors produced by blood vessels have a role in axonal guidance. Endothelins are one such factor. Endothelins are proteins produced by blood vessels that have a role in controlling blood pressure by causing the constriction of blood vessels. They signal through endothelin receptors. Experiments using mouse mutants have shown that endothelin 3 acts through endothelin receptor A to guide a subset of sympathetic neurons to their preferred intermediate target, the external carotid artery.

Regulating Axonal Guidance in PNS

As was just introduced for the sympathetic chain ganglia neurons, sensory neurons and motoneurons of the brain and spinal cord become interconnected in functional patterns, and axons grow out of the CNS and peripheral ganglia to innervate appropriate **target (end) organs** in the body. Peripheral axons travel to their target structures, as they do within the CNS (covered in Chapter 9) —that is, through active locomotion of an apical structure called the **growth cone** (Fig. 10-12; see also

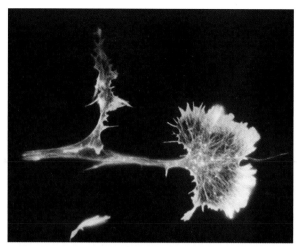

Figure 10-12. Axonal growth cone. The nerve cell body has been removed but would have been toward the left. The actin filaments in the fan-shaped growth cone (toward the right of the illustration) are stained with rhodamine-labeled phalloidin. Rhodamine is a fluorescent molecule, and phalloidin (the toxin in the poisonous green fungus *Amanita phalloides*) binds strongly to actin filaments.

Fig. 9-16). The growth cone guides the axon along the correct trajectory to its target by detecting and integrating various molecular guidance cues in and around the axon pathways. This activity of the growth cone is called **pathfinding**. Once the growth cone reaches its target, it halts and forms a synapse. Somatic motor and sensory fibers synapse directly with their target organs. In contrast, the axons of central autonomic neurons terminate in peripheral autonomic ganglia, where they synapse with the peripheral neuron of the two-neuron autonomic pathway.

The process of axon pathfinding is orchestrated by a complex interplay between highly conserved families of attractive and repulsive guidance molecules, among which the **netrins, Slits, semaphorins**, and **ephrins** are best understood. Netrins can guide axons from distances of up to a few millimeters, but in other cases they act only short-range. Netrins signal through the transmembrane proteins Unc5 and Unc40. The latter belongs to the Dcc (deleted in colorectal carcinoma) family of genes. Slits are large secreted proteins that can act as repellents and that signal through the roundabout (Robo) family of receptors. In mammals, three Slit and four Robo genes are present. Because Slit1 and Slit2 are expressed in cells that border the optic chiasm, the idea emerged that Slits may form a repulsive border and thus a corridor to guide retinal axons through the chiasm (covered in Chapter 9). Semaphorins are a large family of cell surface and secreted guidance molecules (more than thirty have been identified to date), defined by the presence of a conserved "sema" domain. They signal through the **neuropilin** family of receptors, which, in turn, bind to a second family of receptors called the **plexins**. Semaphorin is thought to act as a short-range inhibitory cue that deflects growth cones away from inappropriate regions or guides them through repulsive corridors. Conversely, for certain axons, semaphorins may act as attractants. Ephrins form a family of membrane-bound ligands for the Eph family of receptors that mainly act as repellents. Ephrin-A ligands in the superior colliculi and EphA receptors in the retinae, respectively, form complementary gradients, thus directing topographically correct connections (covered in Chapter 9). Both "forward" signaling from ligand to receptor and "reverse" signaling from Eph receptors to their membrane-bound ligands occur. The

ability to mediate either attraction or repulsion is a common theme among guidance molecules.

A few years ago, the prevailing view was that neuronal activity plays a role only during the terminal stages of target selection. This notion has now been challenged by evidence of **early episodes of spontaneous rhythmic electrical activity** in the embryonic spinal cord that depend on GABA-mediated excitatory currents (i.e., currents resulting from the release of the neurotransmitter gamma-aminobutyric acid) and appear to be required for motor axons to navigate correctly to their peripheral targets. Inhibiting this early bursting activity with picrotoxin perturbs axonal guidance and causes a marked reduction in the expression of polysialylated neural cell adhesion molecule (Psa-Ncam) and EphA4. These intriguing results suggest that early neuronal activity contributes to axonal pathfinding by regulating Psa-Ncam and guidance molecule expression on motor axons.

A newer hypothesis on axonal pathfinding suggests a role for morphogens, including the **hedgehog, Wnt**, and **Bmp** families of proteins. Evidence comes from netrin-deficient ventral spinal cord explants that were challenged with a local source of sonic hedgehog (Shh). Shh attracted the growth cone. This event could be prevented by blocking the hedgehog transducer smoothened. Conversely, Bmp repulses commissural fibers in the dorsal spinal cord. Mice that lack the Wnt receptor frizzled3 show aberrant commissural neuron trajectories. These morphogens have an attractive feature that is desirable for guidance cues: they form gradients within the spinal cord. Bmp, which initially has a dorsalizing role, forms a dorsoventral gradient; Shh, having a ventralizing activity, forms a ventrodorsal gradient; and Wnt4 forms a rostrocaudal gradient in the floor plate. Although these are exciting data, many questions remain. It is not known, for instance, how these molecules signal to the cytoskeleton to direct axon growth, rather than to the nucleus to determine cell fate.

It is thought that guidance molecules and electrical neuronal activity converge in changing **calcium homeostasis** within the growth cone to regulate growth cone turning. Hotspots of intracellular free calcium are found closest to the source of the guidance factor. The amplitude of the calcium signal seems to decide the role of the guidance factor. For example, treatments that reduce calcium signals convert netrin-1–induced growth cone steering from attraction to repulsion. Thus it is thought that a gradient of intracellular free calcium across the growth cone can mediate steering responses, with higher-amplitude calcium signals mediating attraction and lower-amplitude calcium signals mediating repulsion. Calcium signaling in turn is thought to affect the cytoskeleton in the growth cone by stabilizing the dynamically extending and retracting microtubules, which grow preferentially along the filopodial actin filaments. Subsequently, asymmetric extension of stabilized microtubule bundles within filopodia initiates growth cone turning toward the new direction.

Although many of the mechanisms discussed in this section have been elucidated in the CNS, many are likely to be conserved in the PNS. Overall, currently available information points to a complex system of diverse long-range and short-range cues, in which relative rather than absolute concentrations convey positional information.

Not all axons need to navigate pathways independently. It is likely that the first (the **"pioneer"**) growth cones to traverse a route establish a pathway that is used by later growing axons. This mechanism would account for the formation of nerves, in which many axons travel together. The phenomenon of axonal pathfinding is a very active area of research, with obvious implications for the process of nerve regeneration after injury in children and adults.

DEVELOPMENT OF CRANIAL PNS

The cranial PNS consists of cranial nerves and ganglia, as well as autonomic (parasympathetic) nerves and ganglia. Parasympathetic nerves course through cranial nerves in the head and sacral spinal nerves in the caudal trunk to reach their ganglia. Those arising with sacral spinal nerves are discussed earlier in the chapter. The development of cranial nerves (and ganglia) and the development of cranial parasympathetic nerves are considered together.

DEVELOPMENT OF CRANIAL NERVES AND SENSORY AND PARASYMPATHETIC GANGLIA

The peripheral neurons of the cranial nerve sensory and parasympathetic pathways are housed in ganglia that lie outside the CNS. The cranial parasympathetic division consists of two-neuron pathways: the central neuron of each pathway resides in a peripheral nucleus, whereas the peripheral neuron resides in a ganglion located in the head or neck. The cranial sensory (afferent) and parasympathetic (visceral efferent) ganglia (Table 10-1, Fig. 10-13) appear during the end of the fourth week and the beginning of the fifth week. The cranial nerve sensory ganglia contain the cell bodies of sensory neurons for the corresponding cranial nerves. The cranial nerve parasympathetic ganglia can be divided into two groups: the ganglia associated with the vagus nerve, which are located in the walls of the visceral organs (e.g., gut, heart, lungs, pelvic organs), and the parasympathetic ganglia of cranial nerves III, VII, and IX, which innervate structures in the head. The head receives sympathetic innervation via nerves from the cervical chain ganglia.

Origin of Cranial Nerve Sensory Ganglia

Experiments involving quail-chick transplantation chimeras (covered in Chapter 5) have shown that neurons in the cranial nerve sensory ganglia have a dual origin (see Fig. 10-13; also see Fig. 4-21). Some are formed from neural crest cells in the same way as neurons in the dorsal root ganglia of the spinal nerves, and other neurons are derived from **ectodermal placodes**. Three of these placodes—nasal placodes, retinal placodes (the thickened inner layer of the optic vesicles, also called neural retinae), and otic placodes—are covered in Chapters 17 through 19. In addition, a series of four **epipharyngeal** (also called **epibranchial**) **placodes** develop as ectodermal thickenings just dorsal to the four pharyngeal clefts, and a more diffuse **trigeminal placode** develops in the area between the epipharyngeal placodes and the lens placode. Epipharyngeal placodes give rise to neuronal precursors beginning roughly at the end of the fourth week of gestation. In contrast to neurons in the cranial nerve sensory ganglia, which can arise from neural crest cells or ectodermal placodes, all glia in these ganglia are derived from neural crest cells.

The nasal placodes give rise to the primary neurosensory cells of the olfactory epithelium, and the axons of these cells form the olfactory nerve (I), which penetrates the olfactory bulb of the telencephalon. With some exceptions, the remaining cranial nerve sensory ganglia show a regular stratification with respect to their origin: the ganglia (or portions of ganglia) that lie closer to the brain (i.e., the so-called proximal ganglia) are derived from neural crest cells, whereas the neurons of ganglia (or portions thereof) lying farther from the brain (i.e., the so-called distal ganglia) are formed by placode-derived cells. However, the supporting cells of all cranial nerve sensory ganglia are derived from neural crest cells.

TABLE 10-1	ORIGINS OF THE NEURONS IN THE CRANIAL NERVE GANGLIA	
Cranial Nerve	**Ganglion and Type**	**Origin of Neurons**
Olfactory (I)	Olfactory epithelium (primary neurons of the olfactory pathway) (special afferent)	Nasal placode
Oculomotor (III)	Ciliary ganglion (visceral efferent)	Neural crest cells of the caudal diencephalon and the cranial mesencephalon
Trigeminal (V)	Trigeminal ganglion (general afferent)	Neural crest cells of the caudal diencephalon and the cranial mesencephalon; trigeminal placode
Facial (VII)	Superior ganglion of nerve VII (general and special afferent)	Rhombencephalic neural crest cells; first epipharyngeal placode
	Inferior (geniculate) ganglion of nerve VII (general and special afferent)	First epipharyngeal placode
	Sphenopalatine ganglion (visceral efferent)	Rhombencephalic neural crest cells
	Submandibular ganglion (visceral efferent)	Rhombencephalic neural crest cells
Vestibulocochlear (VIII)	Acoustic (cochlear) ganglion (special afferent)	Otic placode
	Vestibular ganglion (special afferent)	Otic placode plus contribution from neural crest cells
Glossopharyngeal (IX)	Superior ganglion (general and special afferent)	Rhombencephalic neural crest cells
	Inferior (petrosal) ganglion (general and special afferent)	Second epipharyngeal placodes
	Otic ganglion (visceral efferent)	Rhombencephalic neural crest cells
Vagus (X)	Superior ganglion (general afferent)	Rhombencephalic neural crest cells
	Inferior (nodose) ganglion (general and special afferent)	Third and fourth epipharyngeal placodes
	Vagal parasympathetic (enteric) ganglia (visceral efferent)	Rhombencephalic neural crest cells

The **trigeminal (semilunar) ganglion** of cranial nerve V has a mixed origin: the proximal portion arises mainly from diencephalic and mesencephalic neural crest cells, whereas most neurons in the distal portion arise from the diffuse trigeminal placode. The sensory ganglia associated with the second, third, fourth, and sixth pharyngeal arches are derived from the corresponding epipharyngeal placodes and from neural crest cells. Each of these nerves has both a proximal and a distal sensory ganglion. In general, the proximal-distal rule discussed in the preceding paragraph holds for these ganglia. The combined **superior ganglion** of nerves IX and X is formed by rhombencephalic neural crest cells, whereas the neurons of the **inferior (petrosal) ganglion** of nerve IX are derived from the second epipharyngeal placode, and those of the **inferior (nodose) ganglion** of nerve X are derived from the third and fourth epipharyngeal placodes. The **superior combined ganglion** of nerves VII and VIII is derived from both the first epipharyngeal placode and the rhombencephalic neural crest cells, but the neurons of the **inferior (geniculate) ganglion** of nerve VII are derived exclusively from the

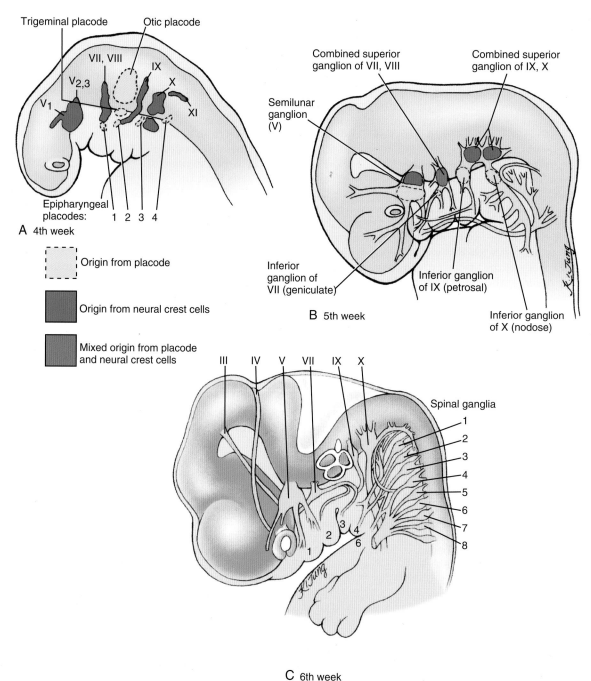

Figure 10-13. Development of the cranial nerves and their ganglia. *A, B,* Origin of cranial nerve ganglia from neural crest cells and ectodermal placodes. Cranial nerve parasympathetic ganglia arise solely from neural crest cells, whereas neurons in the cranial nerve sensory ganglia arise from either neural crest cells or placode cells. Glia in all cranial nerve ganglia are derived from neural crest cells. *C,* The definitive arrangement of cranial nerves is apparent by the sixth week.

first epipharyngeal placode. As mentioned in Chapter 18, the distal ganglia of cranial nerve VIII—the **vestibular ganglion** and the **cochlear ganglion**—differentiate from the otic placode.

Origin of Cranial Nerve Parasympathetic Ganglia

The origin of the neural crest cells giving rise to the various cranial nerve parasympathetic ganglia has been determined in experiments using quail-chick transplantation chimeras (covered in Chapter 5). The neurons and glia in each ganglion (and thus the entire ganglion) arise from neural crest cells located at roughly the same level as the corresponding brain stem nucleus (compare Figs. 10-13 and 9-6; also see Fig. 4-21). Specifically, the **ciliary ganglion** of the oculomotor nerve (III) is formed by neural crest cells arising in the caudal part of the diencephalon and the cranial part of the mesencephalon; the **sphenopalatine** and **submandibular ganglia** of the facial nerve (VII) are formed by neural crest cells that migrate from the cranial rhombencephalon; and the **otic ganglion** of the glossopharyngeal nerve (IX) and the enteric ganglia served by the vagus nerve are derived from neural crest cells originating in the caudal portion of the rhombencephalon.

DIFFERENCES IN PREGANGLIONIC AND POSTGANGLIONIC FIBER LENGTH BETWEEN PARASYMPATHETIC AND SYMPATHETIC DIVISIONS OF AUTONOMIC NERVOUS SYSTEM

Parasympathetic ganglia form close to the organs they are destined to innervate. This is in contrast to sympathetic ganglia, which form relatively far from the organs they are destined to innervate. Thus, in general, preganglionic fibers of the parasympathetic division are relatively long and their postganglionic fibers are relatively short, whereas in the sympathetic division the situation is reversed.

The central (preganglionic or presynaptic) neurons of the two-cell parasympathetic pathways reside in one of four motor nuclei in the brain (associated with cranial nerves III, VII, IX, and X) or in intermediolateral cell columns of the sacral cord at levels S2 through S4. The cranial nuclei supply the head and the viscera superior to the hindgut, whereas the sacral neurons supply the viscera inferior to this point (see Fig. 10-11).

The preganglionic parasympathetic fibers associated with cranial nerves III, VII, and IX travel to parasympathetic ganglia located near the structures to be innervated, where they synapse with the second (postganglionic or postsynaptic) neuron of the pathway. Organs receiving parasympathetic innervation in this way include the dilator pupillae muscles of the eye, the lacrimal and salivary glands, and glands of the oral and nasal mucosa (covered in Chapter 17). In contrast, the preganglionic parasympathetic fibers associated with cranial nerve X join with somatic motor and sensory fibers to form the **vagus nerve**. Some branches of the vagus nerve serve structures in the head and neck, but other parasympathetic and sensory fibers within the nerve

continue into the thorax and abdomen, where the parasympathetic fibers synapse with postganglionic neurons in numerous small parasympathetic ganglia embedded in the walls of target organs such as heart, liver, suprarenal cortex, kidney, gonads, and gut. Preganglionic vagal fibers, therefore, are very long, whereas postganglionic fibers that penetrate the target organs are very short (see Fig. 10-11).

Embryology in Practice

UNEVEN CRY

At the birth of a full-term boy, born to new parents, the delivery team notices that the infant has an asymmetric crying face. He is otherwise healthy. Very healthy indeed, tipping the scales at almost 4000 g (8 pounds 12 ounces)! His difficult arrival into this world required the assistance of instruments called "forceps," or what his father loudly called at the time "the salad tongs."

First by the nurse, and then by the doctor, the infant is scrutinized for problems. They pay particular attention to the neurologic examination of his head and neck and conclude that he has no movement of the right side of his face but has normal suck and gag reflexes. He also has normal rooting reflexes bilaterally (in which the infant turns and makes sucking motions toward the side of a rubbed cheek). Based on impaired motor function but normal sensory function, they conclude that he has facial nerve (cranial nerve VII) palsy and explain that this was likely "acquired during the difficult delivery."

Staff members observe the boy over the course of his first day of life and are encouraged by his progress. After a rocky start with breast feeding, he is able to feed normally after working with a lactation specialist. He also passes his newborn hearing screen (ruling out involvement of cranial nerve VIII), and the family is told that no further workup is indicated.

Facial nerve palsy discovered at birth has an incidence of 1.8 per 1000 births. About 90% of the time, the problem is acquired and is strongly associated with forceps-assisted delivery, primiparity, and birth weight over 3500 grams. Forceps-induced facial nerve palsy is thought to result from compression of the nerve at the stylomastoid foramen or from pressure on the bone overlying the facial canal. Outcomes for acquired facial nerve palsy are predicted to be favorable. The patient described above would be expected to recover fully in one to two months with no treatment.

In the differential for traumatic facial nerve palsy are developmental anomalies. Patients with multiple, usually bilateral, cranial nerves palsies with an expressionless face fall into a spectrum called **Mobius syndrome**. Patients with **CHARGE syndrome** can also have multiple cranial nerve anomalies including palsy of nerve VII. A non-neurologic cause of facial asymmetry is **Cayler anomaly**, which is caused by hypoplasia of the depressor anguli oris muscle and results in facial asymmetry only with crying. This condition can be associated with the more far-reaching 22q11 deletion syndrome and should prompt the clinician to evaluate the infant carefully.

SUGGESTED READINGS

Bovolenta P, Rodriguez J, Esteve P. 2006. Frizzled/RYK mediated signalling in axon guidance. Development 133:4399–4408.
Gelfand MV, Hong S, Gu C. 2009. Guidance from above: common cues direct distinct signaling outcomes in vascular and neural patterning. Trends Cell Biol 19:99–110.

Kasemeier-Kulesa JC, McLennan R, Romine MH, et al. 2010. CXCR4 controls ventral migration of sympathetic precursor cells. J Neurosci 30:13078–13088.

Lowery LA, Van Vactor D. 2009. The trip of the tip: understanding the growth cone machinery. Nat Rev Mol Cell Biol 10:332–343.

Round J, Stein E. 2007. Netrin signaling leading to directed growth cone steering. Curr Opin Neurobiol 17:15–21.

Saito D, Takase Y, Murai H, Takahashi Y. 2012. The dorsal aorta initiates a molecular cascade that instructs sympatho-adrenal specification. Science 336:1578–1581.

Takeichi M. 2007. The cadherin superfamily in neuronal connections and interactions. Nat Rev Neurosci 8:11–20.

Zou Y, Lyuksyutova AI. 2007. Morphogens as conserved axon guidance cues. Curr Opin Neurobiol 17:22–28.

Chapter 11

Development of the Respiratory System and Body Cavities

SUMMARY

As covered in Chapter 4, shortly after the three germ layers form during gastrulation, **body folding** forms the endodermal foregut at the cranial end of the embryo, thereby delineating the inner tube of the **tube-within-a-tube body plan**. On day twenty-two, the foregut produces a ventral evagination called the **respiratory diverticulum** or **lung bud**, which is the primordium of the lungs. As the lung bud grows, it remains ensheathed in a covering of splanchnopleuric mesoderm, which will give rise to the lung vasculature and to the connective tissue, cartilage, and muscle within the bronchi. On days twenty-six to twenty-eight, the lengthening lung bud bifurcates into left and right **primary bronchial buds**, which will give rise to the two lungs. In the fifth week, a second generation of branching produces three **secondary bronchial buds** on the right side and two on the left. These are the primordia of the future lung lobes. The bronchial buds and their splanchnopleuric sheath continue to grow and bifurcate, gradually filling the pleural cavities. By week twenty-eight, the sixteenth round of branching generates **terminal bronchioles**, which subsequently divide into two or more **respiratory bronchioles**. By week thirty-six, these respiratory bronchioles have become invested with capillaries and are called **terminal sacs** or **primitive alveoli**. Between thirty-six weeks and birth, the alveoli mature. Additional alveoli continue to be produced throughout early childhood.

During the fourth week, partitions form to subdivide the intraembryonic coelom into pericardial, pleural, and peritoneal cavities. The first partition to develop is the **septum transversum**, a block-like wedge of mesoderm that forms a ventral structure partially dividing the coelom into a thoracic **primitive pericardial cavity** and an abdominal **peritoneal cavity**. Cranial body folding and differential growth of the developing head and neck regions translocate this block of mesoderm from the cranial edge of the embryonic disc caudally to the position of the future diaphragm. Coronal **pleuropericardial folds** meanwhile form on the lateral body wall of the primitive pericardial cavity and grow medially to fuse with each other and with the ventral surface of the foregut mesoderm, thus subdividing the primitive pericardial cavity into a definitive **pericardial cavity** and two **pleural cavities**. The pleural cavities initially communicate with the peritoneal cavity through a pair of **pericardioperitoneal canals** passing dorsal to the septum transversum. However, a pair of transverse **pleuroperitoneal membranes** grow ventrally from the dorsal body wall to fuse with the transverse septum, thus closing off the pericardioperitoneal canals. Therefore, the septum transversum and the pleuroperitoneal membranes form major parts of the future diaphragm.

As covered in Chapter 6, as a result of folding, the amnion, which initially arises from the dorsal margin of the embryonic disc ectoderm, is carried ventrally to enclose the entire embryo, taking origin from the **umbilical ring** surrounding the roots of the vitelline duct and connecting stalk. The amnion also expands until it fills the chorionic space and fuses with the chorion. As the amnion expands, it encloses the connecting stalk and yolk sac neck in a sheath of amniotic membrane. This composite structure becomes the **umbilical cord**.

Clinical Taster

An 18-year-old construction worker undergoes surgical repair of a broken femur after falling off a roof. The surgery and initial postoperative course are uncomplicated. However, the bedridden patient experiences a prolonged postoperative oxygen requirement despite receiving appropriate respiratory care, including frequent use of incentive spirometry (the patient exhales into this device to maintain lung volume). He develops increasing cough and shortness of breath, and five nights after surgery, he spikes a high fever. The on-call resident orders a chest X-ray that shows a focal consolidation (area of dense lung tissue) in the left lower lobe consistent with a bacterial pneumonia. The patient is started on intravenous antibiotics and receives more intensive respiratory therapy.

The family tells the team that the man has had pneumonia once before, and he has also had several cases of sinusitis. He has a chronic cough that was diagnosed as "asthma," but the cough is not severe enough to prevent him from being physically active. One of the patient's older brothers has a similar respiratory issue and was found to be sterile after failing to conceive children.

The patient improves upon receiving antibiotics and respiratory therapy. After a repeat chest X-ray is done to monitor the pneumonia, the radiologist calls to inform the team that an error was made during performance of the previous chest X-ray. Apparently the patient has **situs inversus**, and the night radiology technician who performed the previous X-ray mislabeled that film. The radiologist also notes subtle changes at the bases of the patient's lung fields consistent with bronchiectasis (abnormal dilation and inflammation of airways associated with mucous blockage), similar to that seen in **primary ciliary dyskinesia** (PCD) or cystic fibrosis. The combination of recurrent sinus infections, bronchiectasis, and

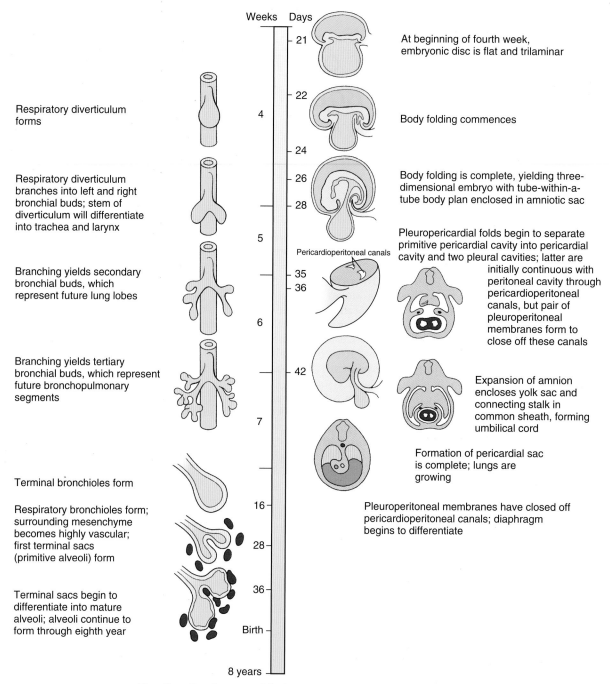

Weeks Days

21 — At beginning of fourth week, embryonic disc is flat and trilaminar

Respiratory diverticulum forms

4

22 — Body folding commences

24

Respiratory diverticulum branches into left and right bronchial buds; stem of diverticulum will differentiate into trachea and larynx

26 — Body folding is complete, yielding three-dimensional embryo with tube-within-a-tube body plan enclosed in amniotic sac

28

5

Pericardioperitoneal canals

Pleuropericardial folds begin to separate primitive pericardial cavity into pericardial cavity and two pleural cavities; latter are initially continuous with peritoneal cavity through pericardioperitoneal canals, but pair of pleuroperitoneal membranes form to close off these canals

Branching yields secondary bronchial buds, which represent future lung lobes

35
36

6

Branching yields tertiary bronchial buds, which represent future bronchopulmonary segments

42 — Expansion of amnion encloses yolk sac and connecting stalk in common sheath, forming umbilical cord

7

Formation of pericardial sac is complete; lungs are growing

Terminal bronchioles form

Respiratory bronchioles form; surrounding mesenchyme becomes highly vascular; first terminal sacs (primitive alveoli) form

16

Pleuroperitoneal membranes have closed off pericardioperitoneal canals; diaphragm begins to differentiate

28

Terminal sacs begin to differentiate into mature alveoli; alveoli continue to form through eighth year

36

Birth

8 years

Time line. Development of the lungs, respiratory tree, and body cavities.

---

situs inversus is consistent with the diagnosis of **Kartagener syndrome** (pronounced "KART-agayner"; see Chapters 3 and 12 for additional discussion of Kartagener syndrome), a variant of PCD. Kartagener syndrome is caused by autosomal recessive mutations in the DYNEIN AXONEMAL HEAVY CHAIN 5 (DNAH5) gene. Mutations in this gene result in **immotile cilia** in the respiratory tract, leading to poor mucus transport and frequent infections. Because cilia are also involved in sperm transport, affected males are sterile. During embryonic development, cilia in the node are involved in determination of the left-right axis (covered in Chapter 3). Loss of node ciliary function in PCD leads to randomization of laterality, with 50% of affected individuals having situs inversus.

DEVELOPMENT OF LUNGS AND RESPIRATORY TREE

Animation 11-1: Development of Lungs.
Animations are available online at StudentConsult.

Development of the esophagus, stomach, trachea, and lungs from the foregut region is tightly linked (Fig. 11-1A). Hence, defects in the development of the foregut region often involve both the cranial level of the gastrointestinal system and the respiratory system (see Chapters 14 and 17 for further coverage of the development of the foregut region). Development of the lungs begins on day

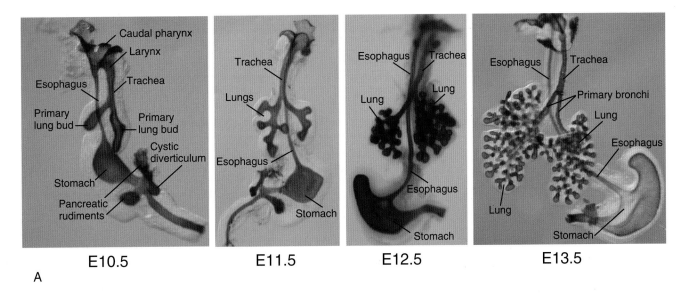

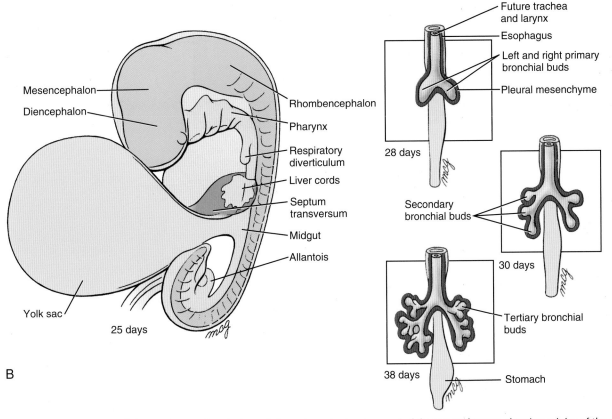

Figure 11-1. Development of the respiratory diverticulum. *A,* Four stages in development of the mouse foregut, showing origins of the esophagus, trachea, lungs, and stomach. The foregut epithelium has been stained with an antibody to E-cadherin. The branching pattern of the mouse respiratory tree differs from that of the human, which is described in the text. *B,* The respiratory diverticulum first forms as an evagination of the foregut on day twenty-two and immediately bifurcates into two primary bronchial buds between day twenty-six and day twenty-eight. Early in the fifth week, the right bronchial bud branches into three secondary bronchial buds, whereas the left bronchial bud branches into two. By the sixth week, secondary bronchial buds branch into tertiary bronchial buds (usually about ten on each side) to form the bronchopulmonary segments.

twenty-two with formation of a ventral outpouching of the endodermal foregut called the **respiratory diverticulum** (Fig. 11-1*B*). This bud grows ventrocaudally through the mesenchyme surrounding the foregut, and on days twenty-six to twenty-eight, it undergoes a first bifurcation, splitting into right and left **primary bronchial** (or **lung**) **buds**. These buds are the rudiments of the two lungs and the right and left **primary bronchi**, and the proximal end (stem) of the diverticulum forms the **trachea** and **larynx**. The latter opens into the pharynx via the **glottis**, a passageway formed at the original point of evagination of the diverticulum. As the primary bronchial

TABLE 11-1	**STAGES OF HUMAN LUNG DEVELOPMENT**	
Stage of Development	**Period**	**Events**
Embryonic	Twenty-six days to six weeks	Respiratory diverticulum arises as a ventral outpouching of foregut endoderm and undergoes three initial rounds of branching, producing the primordia successively of the two lungs, the lung lobes, and the bronchopulmonary segments; the stem of the diverticulum forms the trachea and larynx
Pseudoglandular	Six to sixteen weeks	Respiratory tree undergoes fourteen more generations of branching, resulting in the formation of terminal bronchioles
Canalicular	Sixteen to twenty-eight weeks	Each terminal bronchiole divides into two or more respiratory bronchioles. Respiratory vasculature begins to develop. During this process, blood vessels come into close apposition with the lung epithelium. The lung epithelium also begins to differentiate into specialized cell types (ciliated, secretory, and neuroendocrine cells proximally and precursors of the alveolar type II and I cells distally)
Saccular	Twenty-eight to thirty-six weeks	Respiratory bronchioles subdivide to produce terminal sacs (primitive alveoli). Terminal sacs continue to be produced until well into childhood
Alveolar	Thirty-six weeks to term	Alveoli mature

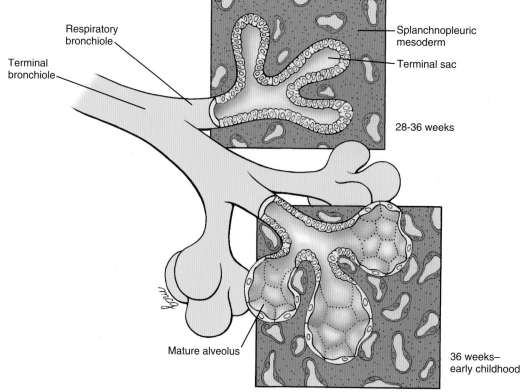

Figure 11-2. Maturation of lung tissue. Terminal sacs (primitive alveoli) begin to form between weeks twenty-eight and thirty-six and begin to mature between thirty-six weeks and birth. However, only 5% to 20% of all terminal sacs eventually produced are formed before birth. Subsequent septation of the alveoli is not shown.

buds form, the stem of the diverticulum begins to separate from the overlying portion of the pharynx, which becomes the **esophagus**. During weeks five and twenty-eight, the primary bronchial buds undergo about sixteen rounds of branching to generate the respiratory tree of the lungs. The pattern of branching of the lung endoderm is regulated by the surrounding mesenchyme, which invests the buds from the time that they first form. The stages of development of the lungs are summarized in Table 11-1.

The first round of branching of the primary bronchial buds occurs early in the fifth week (see Fig. 11-1B). This

round of branching is highly stereotypical and yields three **secondary bronchial buds** on the right side and two on the left. The secondary bronchial buds give rise to the **lung lobes**: three in the right lung and two in the left lung. During the sixth week, a more variable round of branching typically yields ten **tertiary bronchial buds** on both sides; these become the **bronchopulmonary segments** of the mature lung.

By week sixteen, after about fourteen more branchings, the respiratory tree produces small branches called **terminal bronchioles** (Fig. 11-2). Between sixteen and twenty-eight weeks, each terminal bronchiole divides into two or more **respiratory bronchioles**, and the mesodermal tissue surrounding these structures becomes highly vascularized. By week twenty-eight, the respiratory bronchioles begin to sprout a final generation of stubby branches. These branches develop in craniocaudal progression, forming first at more cranial terminal bronchioles. By week thirty-six, the first-formed wave of terminal branches are invested in a dense network of capillaries and are called **terminal sacs (primitive alveoli)**. Limited gas exchange is possible at this point, but the alveoli are still so few and immature that infants born at this age may die of respiratory insufficiency without adequate therapy (covered in a following "In the Clinic" entitled "Lung Maturation and Survival of Premature Infants").

Additional terminal sacs continue to form and differentiate in craniocaudal progression both before and after birth. The process is largely completed by two years. About twenty-million to seventy-million terminal sacs are formed in each lung before birth; the total number of alveoli in the mature lung is three-hundred million to four-hundred million. Continued thinning of the squamous epithelial lining of the terminal sacs begins just before birth, resulting in the differentiation of these primitive alveoli into mature alveoli.

The development of the lung during fetal and postnatal life is often subdivided into four phases. The **pseudoglandular phase** begins around the beginning of the fifth month of gestation. It is characterized by the presence of terminal bronchi consisting of thick-walled tubes surrounded by dense mesenchyme. The **canalicular phase** begins around the beginning of the sixth month of gestation (Fig. 11-3A). It is characterized by thinning of the walls of the tubes as the lumens of the bronchi enlarge. During the canalicular phase, the lung becomes highly vascularized. The **saccular phase** begins around the beginning of the seventh month of gestation (Fig. 11-3B). It is characterized by further thinning of the tubes to form numerous sacculi lined with type I and II alveolar cells (the former form the surface for gas exchange, and the latter respond to damage to type I cells by dividing and replacing them; as covered in the "In the Clinic" entitled "Lung Maturation and Survival of Premature Infants," type II cells are the source of pulmonary surfactant). The **alveolar phase** begins shortly before birth, typically around the beginning of the ninth month of gestation, and continues into postnatal life (Fig. 11-3C). It is characterized by the formation of mature alveoli.

An important process of **septation**, which further subdivides the alveoli, occurs after birth. Each septum formed during this process contains smooth muscle and capillaries.

The lung is a composite of endodermal and mesodermal tissues. The endoderm of the respiratory diverticulum gives rise to the mucosal lining of the bronchi and to the epithelial cells of the alveoli. The remaining components of the lung, including muscle and cartilage supporting the bronchi and the visceral pleura covering the lung, are derived from the splanchnopleuric mesoderm, which covers the bronchi as they grow out from the mediastinum into the pleural space. The lung vasculature is thought to develop via angiogenesis (i.e., sprouting from neighboring vessels; angiogenesis is covered in Chapter 13).

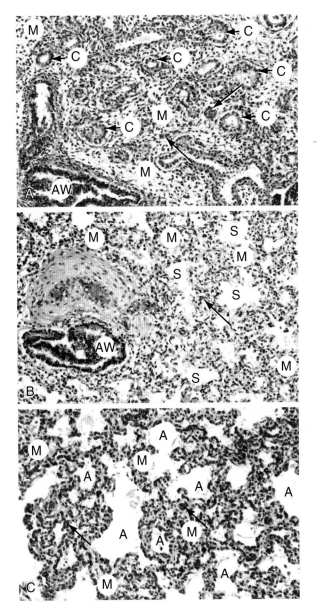

Figure 11-3. Histologic stages of normal human lung development. *A,* Canalicular stage. *B,* Saccular stage. *C,* Alveolar stage. A, alveolus; AW, airway; C, canaliculus; M, mesenchyme; S, saccule; Arrows, capillaries.

In the Research Lab

INDUCTION OF LUNGS AND RESPIRATORY TREE

Experiments in mouse embryos have revealed that induction of the respiratory tree requires Wnt signaling. After inactivation of β-catenin in the foregut endoderm, or in mice null for Wnt2/2b, the foregut fails to express the transcription factor Nkx2.1 (formerly called thyroid transcription factor-1; Titf1) —the earliest marker of the respiratory tree—and the lungs fail to form. Conversely, increasing Wnt/β-catenin signaling leads to the conversion of esophagus and stomach endoderm into lung endoderm that expresses Nkx2.1. Collectively, these experiments demonstration that Wnt signaling is both sufficient and necessary for formation of the respiratory tree, and that a choice is made during development through inductive interactions to convert the foregut endoderm into either trachea and lungs or esophagus and stomach.

In the Clinic

ESOPHAGEAL ATRESIA AND TRACHEOESOPHAGEAL FISTULA

Esophageal atresia (EA; a blind esophagus) and **tracheoesophageal fistula** (TEF; an abnormal connection between tracheal and esophageal lumens resulting from failure of the foregut to separate completely into trachea and esophagus; also called **esophagotracheal fistula**) are usually found together and occur in 1 of 3000 to 5000 births (Fig. 11-4). However, many variations in these defects are known, including an EA that connects to the trachea, forming a proximal TEF (with or without a distal TEF; the latter is illustrated in Fig. 11-4), an isolated TEF (i.e., without an EA), and an isolated EA (i.e., without a TEF). In addition, both of these defects can be associated with other defects (e.g., esophageal atresia with cardiovascular defects such as tetralogy of Fallot—covered in Chapter 12; tracheoesophageal fistula with **VATER or VACTERL association**—covered in Chapter 3). Both esophageal atresia and tracheoesophageal fistula are dangerous to the newborn because they allow milk or other fluids to be aspirated into the lungs. Hence, they are surgically corrected in the newborn. In addition to threatening survival after birth, esophageal atresia has an adverse effect on the intrauterine environment before birth: the blind-ending esophagus prevents the fetus from swallowing amniotic fluid and returning it to the mother via the placental circulation. This leads to an excess of amniotic fluid (**polyhydramnios**) and consequent distention of the uterus.

In the Research Lab

ESOPHAGEAL ATRESIA AND TRACHEOESOPHAGEAL FISTULA

The cause of **esophageal atresia** is thought to be failure of the esophageal endoderm to proliferate rapidly enough during the fifth week to keep up with the elongation of the embryo. However, the cause of **tracheoesophageal fistula** and the reason why the two defects are usually found together remain a puzzle. During development of the mouse embryo, the anterior foregut expresses the transcription factor Sox2, with highest levels of expression occurring in the future esophagus and stomach. In contrast, the future tracheal region of the foregut expresses the transcription factor Nkx2.1. Moreover, sonic hedgehog (Shh) is expressed in the ventral endoderm of the foregut, where it controls cell proliferation, and fibroblast growth factors (Fgfs) are expressed in the adjacent ventral mesenchyme. Disruption of the Shh pathway or the transcription factor Nkx2.1 causes tracheoesophageal fistula. It is believed that Sox2 expression in the foregut sets up a boundary separating the trachea and the esophagus in normal development, and organ culture experiments suggest that Fgfs expressed by the ventral mesenchyme regulate Sox2 expression. Moreover, bone morphogenetic protein (Bmp) signaling is also required to repress Sox2 expression in the future trachea. Finally, Sox2 and Nkx2.1 reciprocally inhibit each other's expression, supporting an important role for the establishment of a tissue boundary in normal tracheal and esophagus development.

In the Clinic

DEVELOPMENTAL ABNORMALITIES OF LUNGS AND RESPIRATORY TREE

Many lung anomalies result from failure of the respiratory diverticulum or its branches to branch or differentiate correctly. The most severe of these anomalies, **pulmonary agenesis**, results when the respiratory diverticulum fails to split into right and left bronchial buds and to continue growing. Errors in the pattern of pulmonary branching (**branching morphogenesis**) during the embryonic and early fetal periods result in defects ranging from an abnormal number of pulmonary lobes or bronchial segments to the complete absence of a lung. The complexity of branching morphogenesis can be appreciated by examining developing lungs in mouse

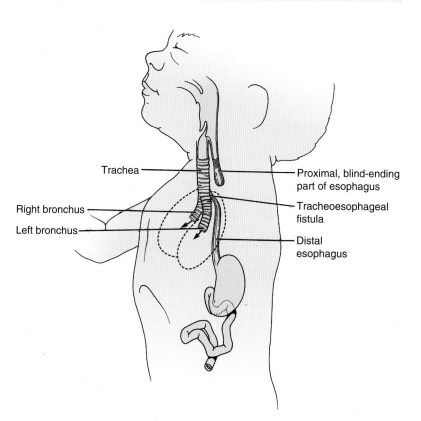

Figure 11-4. Diagram of an infant with esophageal atresia and tracheoesophageal fistula shows how the first drink of fluid after birth could be diverted into the newly expanded lungs (arrows).

embryos in which the respiratory tree has been specifically stained (Fig. 11-5); such images make clear how defects in branching morphogenesis can lead to lobe or bronchial segment anomalies.

Defects in the subdivision of the terminal respiratory bronchi or in the formation of septae after birth can result in an abnormal paucity of alveoli, even if the respiratory tree is otherwise normal. Some of these types of pulmonary anomalies are caused by intrinsic molecular and cellular defects of branching morphogenesis (see the following "In the Research Lab" entitled "Molecular and Cellular Basis of Branching Morphogenesis"). However, the primary cause of **pulmonary hypoplasia**—a reduced number of pulmonary segments or terminal air sacs—often represents a response to some condition that reduces the volume of the pleural cavity, thus restricting growth of the lungs (e.g., protrusion of the abdominal viscera into the thoracic cavity, a condition known as congenital diaphragmatic hernia; covered in a later "In the Clinic" entitled "Diaphragmatic Defects and Pulmonary Hypoplasia").

LUNG MATURATION AND SURVIVAL OF PREMATURE INFANTS

As the end of gestation approaches, the lungs undergo a rapid and dramatic series of transformations that prepare them for air breathing. The fluid that fills the alveoli prenatally is absorbed at birth, the defenses that will protect the lungs against invading pathogens and against the oxidative effects of the atmosphere are activated, and the surface area for alveolar gas exchange increases greatly. Changes in the structure of the lung take place during the last three months, accelerating in the days just preceding a normal term delivery. If a child is born prematurely, the state of development of the lungs is usually the prime factor determining whether he or she will live. Infants born between twenty-four weeks and term—during the phase of accelerated terminal lung maturation—have a good chance of survival with appropriate (including intensive medical assistance at the younger ages) neonatal support. Infants born earlier than twenty-four weeks (during the canalicular phase of lung development) currently have a poor chance of survival (in neonatal intensive care units, or NICUs, 10% to 15% of infants born at 22 to 23 weeks survive, but about 50% of these have profound impairment; recently, an infant born at twenty-one weeks was reported to survive). Unfortunately, surviving infants receiving

intensive respiratory assistance may develop lung fibrosis that results in long-term respiratory problems.

Although the total surface area for gas exchange in the lung depends on the number of alveoli and on the density of alveolar capillaries, efficient gas exchange will occur only if the barrier separating air from blood is thin—that is, if the alveoli are thin-walled, properly inflated, and not filled with fluid. The walls of the maturing alveolar sacs thin out during the weeks before birth. In addition, specific alveolar cells (alveolar type II cells) begin to secrete **pulmonary surfactant**, a mixture of phospholipids and surfactant proteins that reduces the surface tension of the liquid film lining the alveoli and thus facilitates inflation. In the absence of surfactant, the surface tension at the air-liquid interface of the alveolar sacs tends to collapse the alveoli during exhalation. These collapsed alveoli can be inflated only with great effort.

The primary cause of the **respiratory distress syndrome** of premature infants (pulmonary insufficiency accompanied by gasping and cyanosis) is inadequate production of surfactant. Respiratory distress syndrome not only threatens the infant with immediate asphyxiation, but the increased rate of breathing and mechanical ventilation required to support the infant's respiration can damage the delicate alveolar lining, allowing fluid and cellular and serum proteins to exude into the alveolus. Continued injury may lead to detachment of the layer of cells lining the alveoli—a condition called **hyaline membrane disease**. Chronic lung injury associated with preterm infants causes a condition termed **bronchopulmonary dysplasia**, in which the lungs become inflamed and ultimately scarred, compromising their ability to oxygenate the blood. In mothers at high risk for premature delivery, the fetus can be treated antenatally with steroids to accelerate lung maturation and the synthesis of surfactant.

Critically ill *newborns* were first successfully treated with **surfactant replacement therapy**—administration of exogenous surfactant—in the late 1970s. Although originally extracted from animal lungs or human amniotic fluid, synthetic surfactant preparations are now used. In addition to containing phospholipids, current preparations include some of the supplementary proteins found in natural surfactant. Four native surfactant proteins are known: hydrophobic surfactant proteins B and C (Sp-B and Sp-C, respectively) and hydrophilic surfactant proteins A and D (Sp-A and Sp-D, respectively). Sp-B seems to act by organizing the surfactant phospholipids into tubular structures, termed tubular myelin, which is particularly effective at reducing surface tension. Although Sp-C is not required for tubular myelin formation, it does enhance the function of surfactant phospholipids. Sp-A and -D apparently play important roles in innate host defense of the lung against viral, bacterial, and fungal pathogens.

A fatal disease called **hereditary surfactant protein B deficiency (hereditary SP-B deficiency)** is a rare cause of **respiratory failure** in both premature and full-term newborn infants. Alveolar air spaces are filled with granular eosinophilic proteinaceous material, and tubular myelin is absent. Even though aggressive medical interventions have been applied in these cases, including surfactant replacement therapy, infants afflicted with this disease will die, typically within the first year, if they do not receive a lung transplant.

Hereditary SP-B deficiency is an autosomal recessive condition. The genetic basis for this condition has been examined. In most cases, a **frameshift mutation** in exon 4 of the human SP-B gene has been identified. This mutation results in premature termination of translation of the SP-B protein. Other mutations of the SP-B gene have also been identified that result in synthesis of defective forms of the SP-B protein. It has been demonstrated that effects of SP-B deficiency extend beyond the disruption of translation of the SP-B gene. Results of studies of null mutations of the sp-b gene in transgenic mice, for example, show that although the amount of sp-c or sp-a mRNA is not affected, precursors of

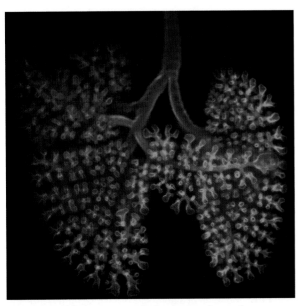

Figure 11-5. Whole mount of developing lungs from a mouse embryo at E14.5. Lung and tracheal epithelium has been labeled with an antibody to E-cadherin to show the pattern of branching (the pattern differs from the human pattern, which is described in the text).

the mature sp-c protein are not completely processed. In addition, the processing of pulmonary phospholipids is disrupted. Similar disruptions of SP-C peptide and phospholipid processing have been described in a human infant with SP-B deficiency. More than fifteen different mutations in the SP-B gene have been associated with hereditary SP-B deficiency. Mild mutations can cause chronic pulmonary disease in infants. Although these studies have been useful in diagnosis, it is hoped that they will lead to effective therapies for this usually fatal disease.

In the Research Lab

APPROACHES FOR STUDYING LUNG DEVELOPMENT AND BRANCHING MORPHOGENESIS

Organ Culture

Just after formation of the primary bronchial buds, the lung primordia can be removed from embryonic birds or mice and cultured in media free of serum and other exogenous growth factors. Under these conditions, the lung primordia will grow and branch for a few days. However, in the absence of an intact vascular system, complete development is not possible. With this limitation, it is possible to use these cultured lungs to analyze the roles of growth factors and other agents in the branching process. In one such study, a small peptide that served as a competitive inhibitor of ligand binding to integrins resulted in abnormal morphology of the developing lung primordium. In another study, incubation with monoclonal antibodies to specific sequences of the extracellular matrix protein laminin resulted in reduction of terminal buds and segmental dilation of the explanted lung primordia. In another strategy, lung explants were treated with antisense oligonucleotides, which bind with and inactivate the mRNA of the specific factor of interest. Experiments with antisense oligonucleotides against transcription factors such as Nkx2.1 resulted in a reduction in the number of terminal branches of the lung primordium. It is possible to cleanly separate the endoderm of the lung buds from the mesoderm and to culture each alone or together and in the presence of purified factors. This can reveal the mechanisms by which these layers and factors interact in vivo.

Transgenic and Gene-Targeting Technologies

Genetic strategies, including the generation of engineered loss-of-function mutations (gene knockouts) and gain-of-function transgenes, have provided important insights into lung development. Recent advances have enabled genes to be deleted only in lung epithelial cells, either in the embryo or in the adult, thus bypassing the early lethality of some null mutations. In addition, transgenes can be selected that drive expression of proteins in specific respiratory cell types. Among examples, a surfactant B gene null mutation was described in the preceding "In the Clinic" entitled "Lung Maturation and Survival of Premature Infants." Similar approaches have implicated many transcription factors in the control of lung growth, differentiation, and branching. These include the proto-oncogene N-myc, the homeodomain protein Gata6, and the Lim homeodomain factor Lhx4 (previously known as Gsh4). Similarly, the homeodomain-containing transcription factor Nkx2.1 and the winged helix transcription factors Foxa1 and Foxa2 (previously known, respectively, as hepatic nuclear factor 3α and β) have been shown to be required for the regulation of lung cell genes, including surfactant synthesis. A dramatic result was obtained by targeted disruption of the function of an Fgf receptor protein in the lung. A transgene consisting of the surfactant C promoter element and a mutant form of the Fgf receptor that lacked a kinase sequence was constructed and injected into fertilized eggs to generate transgenic mice. Inclusion of the surfactant C promoter element in the transgene resulted in its expression only in the airway epithelium. The rationale behind the experiment is that formation of a functional

Fgf receptor requires dimerization of two normal Fgf protein monomers. Therefore, dimerization of the mutant protein produced by the transgene with the endogenous wild-type (normal) Fgf protein resulted in formation of inactive receptors only in the lungs. As a consequence, other tissue of the embryos developed normally, but branching of the respiratory tree in the transgenic pups was completely inhibited. This resulted in formation of elongated epithelial tubes that were incapable of supporting normal respiratory function at birth (Fig. 11-6). Subsequent gene-targeting experiments in mice demonstrated that fibroblast growth factor 10 (Fgf10) and an isoform of its receptor in the respiratory epithelium, the Fgf-receptor2, were critical for formation of both lungs and limbs. Similarly, ablation of Nkx2.1 blocked formation of both thyroid and lung.

Genetic strategies have also been used to create models of human pulmonary disease such as **cystic fibrosis**. Mouse mutants in which the c-AMP–stimulated chloride secretory activity of the cystic fibrosis gene is absent or reduced have been created by homologous recombination. These mice express some, but not all, of the abnormal phenotypes characteristic of the human disease. In other experiments, transgenic mice have been created that carry the normal human cystic fibrosis gene to demonstrate that it is non-toxic and, therefore, probably safe to use in human therapy. Currently, various approaches to human gene therapy for cystic fibrosis are being developed with viral- and DNA-based delivery systems. The long-term goal is to insert the cystic fibrosis gene directly into the somatic airway epithelial cells of afflicted infants and children.

MOLECULAR AND CELLULAR BASIS OF BRANCHING MORPHOGENESIS

As covered earlier in the chapter, endodermal bronchial buds and subsequent airway branches grow into the mesenchyme surrounding the thoracic gut tube. Deficiencies or abnormalities in branching of the respiratory tree serve as the basis of many

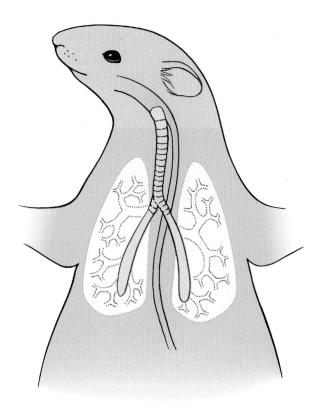

Figure 11-6. Mutation of a fibroblast growth factor receptor specifically expressed in the lungs results in inhibition of branching of the respiratory tree and formation of elongated epithelial tubes that end bluntly. Stippling indicates the outline of where the lungs would form and their branching pattern in a wild-type embryo.

forms of **pulmonary hypoplasia** (covered in the preceding "In the Clinic" entitled "Developmental Abnormalities of Lungs and Respiratory Tree"). Studies over the past several decades have demonstrated that **branching morphogenesis** of the respiratory tree is regulated by reciprocal interaction between endoderm and surrounding mesoderm. For example, when mesenchyme in the region of the bifurcating bronchial buds is replaced with mesenchyme from around the developing trachea, further branching is inhibited. Conversely, replacement of tracheal mesenchyme with that from the region of the bifurcating bronchial buds stimulates ectopic tracheal budding and branching. Based on experiments such as these, components of the **extracellular matrix** and **growth factors** have been implicated in the stimulation and inhibition of branching. For example, collagen types IV and V, laminin, fibronectin, and tenascin—all components of the extracellular matrix—are thought to play a permissive or a stimulatory role in branching of the bronchial buds. Likewise, regulation of expression of receptors for these matrix components has been implicated in control of branching morphogenesis.

Many **growth factors** have been implicated in the growth, differentiation, and branching morphogenesis of the lung. Among them are retinoic acid (RA), transforming growth factorβ (Tgfβ), Bmps, Shh, Wnts, Fgfs, epithelial growth factor (Egf), platelet-derived growth factor (Pdgf), insulin-like growth factor (Igf), and transforming growth factorα (Tgfα). These growth factors and their receptors are expressed in specific cell populations during different phases of lung growth and branching, consistent with their postulated roles in this complex process. For example, branching during the **pseudoglandular stage** is apparently influenced in part by the dynamic activity of RA, Shh, Fgf (especially Fgf10), Bmp, and Tgfβ signaling pathways. Thus, experiments have shown that Fgf10, produced by the mesenchyme overlying the tips of the outgrowing bronchial buds, promotes both proliferation of the endoderm and its outward **chemotaxis** (i.e., directed movement according to the presence of so-called chemotactic factors in the cellular environment). On the other hand, Shh, produced by the endoderm, promotes proliferation and differentiation of the overlying mesoderm. In addition, Shh negative regulates Fgf10 expression, thereby suppressing inappropriate branching.

The complex branching pattern of the mouse lung has been examined three-dimensionally (see Fig. 11-5), and it was noted that branching occurs in three geometric modes: domain branching—formation of branches arranged much like the bristles on a brush; planar bifurcation—splitting of the tip of a branch into two branchlets; and orthogonal bifurcation—involving two rounds of planar bifurcation with 90-degree rotation between rounds to form a rosette-like structure of four branches. Through iteration of these three simple branching patterns, the more than a million branches present in the mouse lung are generated. In addition, experiments support a model in which airway branching, following the establishment of left-right asymmetry in the lung (e.g., three lobes in the right lung and two in the left of humans), is controlled by a **master branch generator** served by three slaves (i.e., subroutines that control discrete patterning events). The three subroutines consist of a **periodicity clock**, which times the formation of branches, and two other routines—one that controls bifurcation, and another that controls branch-point rotation. Sprouty2, an Fgf signaling inhibitor, is a candidate gene for the periodicity clock. Interactions between sprouty2, Fgf10, and Fgf receptor2 control the master branch generator. The other two subroutines involve interactions among the myriad signaling systems covered earlier in this section. Finally, it is important to point out that the lungs in mammals and the tracheal system in flies (see next section entitled "Drosophila Tracheal System Development") undergo extensive branching to increase the surface area for gas exchange, and that Fgf signaling (and presumably branching) is regulated by oxygen levels in flies. In mammals, at least two families of factors likely act as oxygen sensors in lung branching morphogenesis: hypoxia-inducible factor (Hif) and vascular endothelial growth factor (Vegf).

DROSOPHILA TRACHEAL SYSTEM DEVELOPMENT

The respiratory organ in Drosophila, the tracheal system, consists of a branched network of tubes (Fig. 11-7). It is interesting to note that given the central role for Fgf signaling in vertebrate lung development just covered, formation of the tracheal system also involves Drosophila orthologs of the Fgf signaling system. Three components of this system have been identified during development of the tracheal system: branchless, an Fgf-like ligand; breathless, an Fgf receptor; and sprouty, an endogenous Fgf inhibitor. Although at least thirty other genes are involved in tracheal development, branchless and breathless are used repeatedly to control branch budding and outgrowth. Sprouty provides negative feedback regulation by antagonizing Fgf signaling, thereby limiting the amount of branching that occurs.

MOLECULAR AND CELLULAR BASIS OF ALVEOLAR DIFFERENTIATION

Growth factors such as Fgfs and Egf regulate not only early growth and branching of the lung, but also later formation and maturation of terminal sacs during the saccular stage. Later still, PdgfA is required for the postnatal formation of alveolar septae–containing myofibroblasts. Like Nkx2.1 and Foxa1/a2 (covered in a preceding section of this "In the Research Lab" entitled "Transgenic and Gene-Targeting Technologies"), cytokines, glucocorticoids, and thyroxine stimulate surfactant synthesis before birth. It is hoped that these findings will lead to therapeutic stimulation of adequate alveolar formation and differentiation and surfactant synthesis within the lungs of premature infants.

Considerable effort has been spent in identifying genes that regulate the differentiation of lung progenitor cells into specialized types such as ciliated, secretory (Clara), and neuroendocrine cells. For example, analysis of lungs from mice lacking the gene Mash1 (a member of the notch pathway; covered in Chapter 5) has shown that they lack neuroendocrine cells, whereas in Hes1 (another member of the notch pathway) null mutants, neuroendocrine cells form prematurely and in larger numbers than normal. The gene Foxj1 (one of the many Fox transcription factors) is required for the development of differentiated ciliated cells. The formation of submucosal glands, which are the major source of mucus production in the normal lung, is also regulated genetically. Mice lacking genes controlling the ectodysplasin (Eda/Edar) signaling pathway (a gene involved in epithelial morphogenesis; covered in Chapter 7) do not develop submuscosal glands. These glands are also absent in humans lacking the EDA gene.

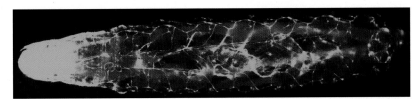

Figure 11-7. The Drosophila tracheal (respiratory) system consists of a network of interconnected epithelial tubes, visualized in a third-instar larva by expression of green fluorescent protein driven by the breathless promoter. Breathless is an Fgf receptor ortholog that is required for tracheal tube branching and outgrowth. Image shows a ventral view of the larva, with the head (anterior) to the left.

PARTITIONING OF COELOM AND FORMATION OF DIAPHRAGM

 Animation 11-2: Development of Body Cavities and Diaphragm.
  Animations are available online at StudentConsult.

At the beginning of the fourth week of development, before body folding, the **intraembryonic coelom** forms a horseshoe-shaped space that partially encircles the future head end of the embryo (Fig. 11-8).

Cranially, the intraembryonic coelom lies just caudal to the **septum transversum** and represents the future **pericardial cavity**. The two caudally directed limbs of the horseshoe-shaped intraembryonic coelom represent the continuous future **pleural** and **peritoneal cavities**. At about the mid-trunk and more caudal levels, the intraembryonic coelom on each side is continuous with the **extraembryonic coelom** or **chorionic cavity**.

With body folding, changes occur in the position of the intraembryonic coelom. The **head fold** moves the

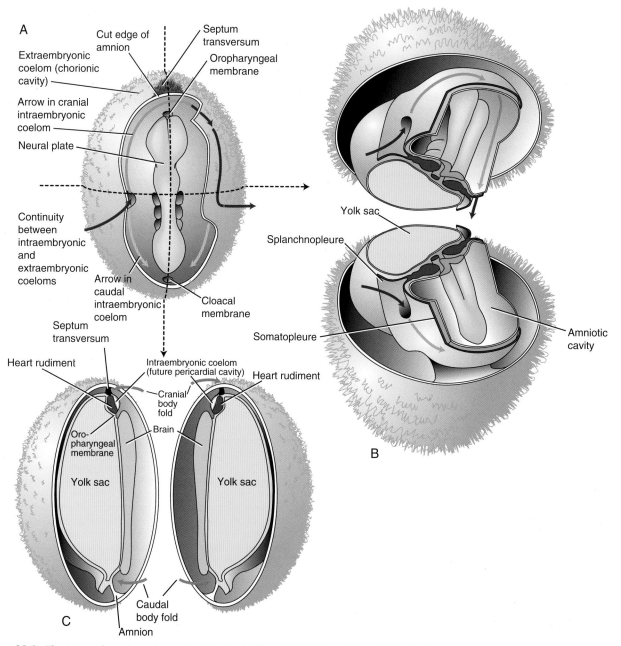

Figure 11-8. The intraembryonic coelom prior to body folding. *A*, At the beginning of the fourth week, the intraembryonic coelom forms a horseshoe-shaped space partially encircling the head end of the embryo. Diagram of the epiblast after removal of the amnion shows the position of the neural plate, oropharyngeal and cloacal membranes, and intraembryonic coelom; the latter is continuous with the extraembryonic coelom at about the mid-trunk and at more caudal levels. *B*, Cranial (top) and caudal (bottom) halves of embryos transected at the level indicated in *A*. Arrows show continuity between the intraembryonic and extraembryonic coeloms. *C*, Midsagittal view through the right side of an embryo at the level indicated in *A*. Arrows show the directions of the head and tail body folds.

future pericardial cavity caudally and repositions it on the anterior (ventral) side of the developing head (Fig. 11-9*A*). The septum transversum, which initially constitutes a partition that lies cranial to the future pericardial cavity, is repositioned by the head fold to lie caudal to the future pericardial cavity. The developing heart (covered further in Chapter 12), which initially lies ventral to the future pericardial cavity, is repositioned dorsally and quickly begins to bulge into the pericardial cavity. Thus, after formation of the head fold, the intraembryonic coelom is reshaped into a ventral cranial expansion (**primitive pericardial cavity**); two narrow canals called **pericardioperitoneal canals** (future **pleural cavities**) that lie dorsal to the septum transversum; and two more caudal areas (which merge to form the future **peritoneal cavity**), where the intraembryonic and extraembryonic coeloms are broadly continuous (Fig. 11-9*B*).

During the fourth and fifth weeks, continued folding and differential growth of the embryonic axis cause a gradual caudal displacement of the septum transversum. The ventral edge of the septum finally becomes fixed to the anterior body wall at the seventh thoracic level, and the dorsal connection to the esophageal mesenchyme becomes fixed at the twelfth thoracic level. Meanwhile, myoblasts (muscle cell precursors) differentiate within the septum transversum. These cells, which will form part of the future diaphragm muscle, are innervated by spinal nerves at a transient, cervical level of the septum transversum—that is, by fibers from the spinal nerves of cervical levels three, four, and five (C3, C4, C5). These fibers join to form the paired **phrenic nerves**, which elongate as they follow the migrating septum caudally.

PERICARDIAL SAC IS FORMED BY PLEUROPERICARDIAL FOLDS THAT GROW FROM LATERAL BODY WALL IN A CORONAL PLANE

During the fifth week, the pleural and pericardial cavities are divided from each other by **pleuropericardial folds** that originate along the lateral body walls in a coronal plane (Fig. 11-10; see Fig. 11-9*B* for orientation). These septae appear as broad folds of mesenchyme and pleura that grow medially toward each other between the heart and the developing lungs. At the end of the fifth week, the folds meet and fuse with the foregut mesenchyme,

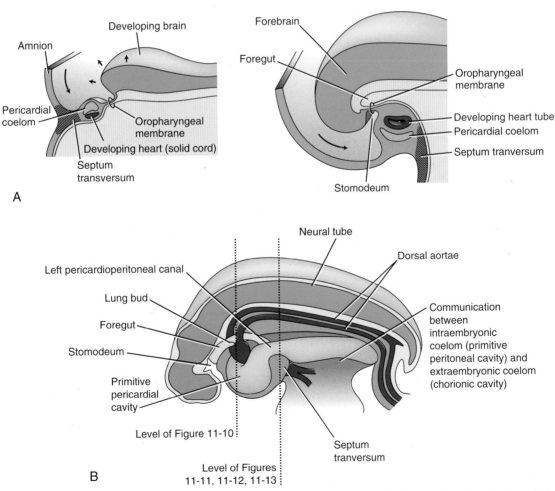

Figure 11-9. Body folding changes the shape of the intraembryonic coelom. *A*, The head end of the embryo before (left) and after (right) formation of the head fold. *B*, Initial subdivision of the intraembryonic coelom into a primitive pericardial cavity, paired pericardioperitoneal canals, and paired primitive peritoneal cavities. The latter are continuous on each side with the extraembryonic coelom. Subsequent lateral body folding progressively separates the intraembryonic and extraembryonic coeloms as the yolk stalk narrows.

thus subdividing the primitive pericardial cavity into three compartments: a fully enclosed, ventral **definitive pericardial cavity** and two dorsolateral **pleural cavities**. The latter are still continuous with the more caudal peritoneal cavities through the pericardioperitoneal canals. The name *pericardioperitoneal* is retained for these canals, even though they now provide communication between pleural and peritoneal cavities.

As the tips of the pleuropericardial folds grow medially toward each other, their roots migrate toward the ventral midline (Fig. 11-10*B, C*). By the time the tips of the folds meet to seal off the pericardial cavity, their roots take origin from the ventral midline. Thus, the space that originally constituted the lateral portion of the primitive pericardial cavity is converted into the ventrolateral part of the right and left pleural cavities.

The pleuropericardial folds are three-layered, consisting of mesenchyme sandwiched between two epithelial layers; all three layers are derived from the body wall. The thin definitive pericardial sac retains this threefold composition, consisting of inner and outer serous membranes (the inner **serous pericardium** and the outer **mediastinal pleura**) separated by a delicate filling of mesenchyme-derived connective tissue, the **fibrous pericardium**. The phrenic nerves, which originally run through the portion of the body wall mesenchyme incorporated into the pleuropericardial folds, course through the fibrous pericardium of the adult.

PLEUROPERITONEAL MEMBRANES GROWING FROM POSTERIOR AND LATERAL BODY WALL SEAL OFF PERICARDIOPERITONEAL CANALS

Recall that the **septum transversum** is repositioned by the head fold to lie ventral to the paired **pericardioperitoneal canals** (Fig. 11-11; see Fig. 11-9*B* for orientation). At the beginning of the fifth week, a pair of membranes, the **pleuroperitoneal membranes**, arise along an oblique line connecting the root of the twelfth rib with the tips of ribs twelve through seven (Fig. 11-12; see Fig. 11-9*B* for orientation). These membranes grow ventrally to fuse with the septum transversum, thus sealing off the pericardioperitoneal canals. The left pericardioperitoneal canal is larger than the right and closes later. Closure of both canals is complete by the seventh week. The membranes that close these canals are called *pleuroperitoneal membranes* because they do not contact the septum transversum until after the pericardial sac is formed; thus, after they fuse with the septum transversum, they separate the definitive pleural cavities from the peritoneal cavity.

DIAPHRAGM IS A COMPOSITE DERIVED FROM FOUR EMBRYONIC STRUCTURES

The definitive musculotendinous **diaphragm** incorporates derivatives of four embryonic structures: (1) septum

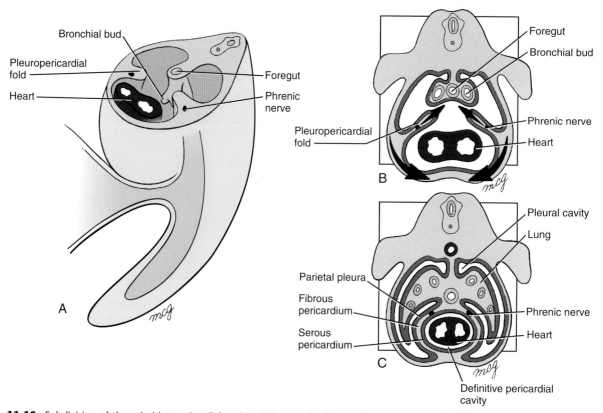

Figure 11-10. Subdivision of the primitive pericardial cavity. *A,* During the fifth week, pleuropericardial folds grow out from the lateral body wall toward the midline, where they fuse with each other and with mesoderm associated with the esophagus. Simultaneously, the roots of these folds migrate ventrally so that they ultimately connect to the ventral (anterior) body wall. *B,* The phrenic nerves initially embedded in the body wall are swept into these developing partitions. *C,* The pleuropericardial folds with their associated serous membrane form the pericardial sac and transform the primitive pericardial cavity into a definitive pericardial cavity and right and left pleural cavities.

transversum, (2) pleuroperitoneal membranes, (3) mesoderm of the body wall, and (4) esophageal mesoderm (Fig. 11-13*A*; see Fig. 11-9*B* for orientation). Some of the myoblasts that arise in the septum transversum emigrate into the pleuroperitoneal membranes, pulling their phrenic nerve branches along with them. Most of the septum transversum then gives rise to the non-muscular **central tendon** of the diaphragm (Fig. 11-13*B*).

The bulk of the **diaphragm muscle** within the pleuroperitoneal membranes is innervated by the phrenic nerve. However, the outer rim of diaphragmatic muscle arises from a ring of body wall mesoderm (see Figs. 11-12*B*, 11-13*A*); this mesoderm is derived from somatic mesoderm and is invaded by myoblasts arising from the myotomes of neighboring somites. Therefore, the peripheral musculature of the diaphragm is innervated by spinal nerves from thoracic spinal levels T7 through T12. Finally, mesoderm arising from vertebral levels L1 through L3 condenses to form two muscular bands—the **right** and **left crura** of the diaphragm, which originate on the vertebral column and insert into the dorsomedial diaphragm (see Fig. 11-13*B*). The right crus originates on vertebral bodies L1 through L3, and the left crus originates on vertebral bodies L1 and L2.

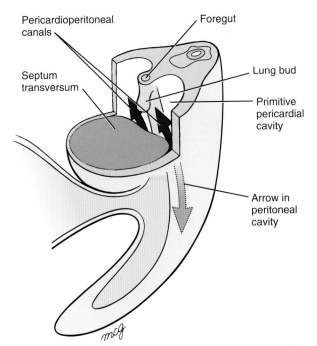

Figure 11-11. In the future thoracic region, the septum transversum forms a ventral partition beneath the paired pericardioperitoneal canals (*arrows*), which interconnect the primitive pericardial cavity cranially and peritoneal cavities caudally.

In the Clinic

DIAPHRAGMATIC DEFECTS AND PULMONARY HYPOPLASIA

As covered earlier in the chapter, **pulmonary hypoplasia** often occurs in response to some conditions that reduce the volume of the pleural cavity, thereby restricting growth of the lungs. In **congenital diaphragmatic hernia**, the developing abdominal viscera may bulge into the pleural cavity (Fig. 11-14). If the mass of displaced viscera is large enough, it will stunt growth of the lungs, typically on both sides. Congenital diaphragmatic hernia occurs in about 1 of 2500 live births. The left side of the diaphragm is involved four to eight times more often than is the right (i.e., about 80% of diaphragmatic hernias occur on the left side), probably because the left pericardioperitoneal canal is larger and closes later than the right. Most diaphragmatic hernias (i.e., 95%) occur posterolaterally within the diaphragm and are referred to clinically as Bochdalek hernias. However, diaphragmatic hernias can rarely occur through the esophageal hiatus or more anteriorly

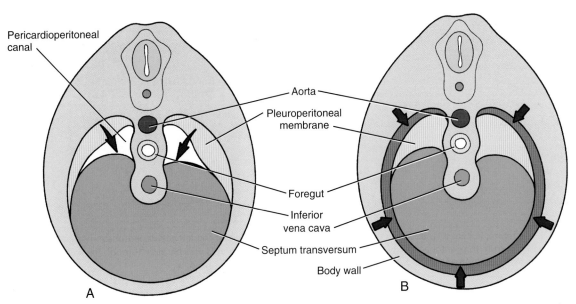

Figure 11-12. Closure of the pericardioperitoneal canals (*A, B*). Between weeks five and seven, a pair of horizontal pleuroperitoneal membranes grow from the posterior body wall to meet the septum transversum (arrows, *A*), thus closing the pericardioperitoneal canals. These membranes form the posterior portions of the diaphragm and completely seal off the pleural cavities from the peritoneal cavity. Arrows in *B* indicate invasion of the developing diaphragm by muscle fibers from the adjacent body wall.

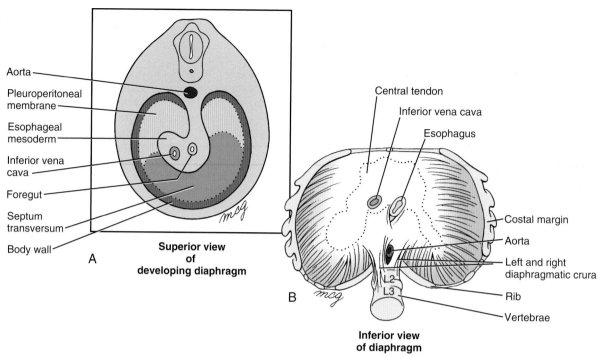

Figure 11-13. Formation of the diaphragm. The definitive diaphragm is a composite structure, including elements of the septum transversum, pleuroperitoneal membranes, and esophageal mesenchyme, as well as a rim of body wall mesoderm. A, Superior view. B, Inferior view.

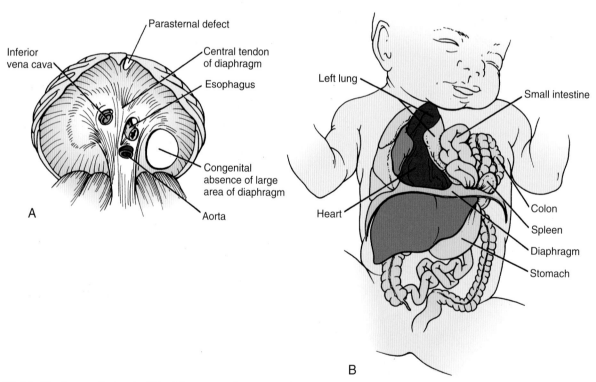

Figure 11-14. Diaphragmatic hernia. This defect most often occurs through failure of the left pleuroperitoneal membrane to seal off the left pleural cavity completely from the peritoneal cavity. A, Inferior view. B, Abdominal contents may herniate through the patent pericardioperitoneal canal, preventing normal development of the lungs on both sides, which become compressed.

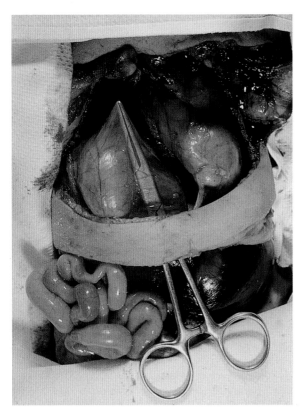

Figure 11-15. Eventration of the diaphragm. Failure of the pleuroperitoneal membranes to differentiate normally during fetal life may allow abdominal organs to dilate the abnormally thin regions of the diaphragm and eventrate into the pleural cavity.

(i.e., retrosternally or parasternally), where they are referred to clinically as Morgagni hernias. The mortality rate from diaphragmatic hernias is high, averaging about 50%, but the prognosis depends on the type of hernia. For example, right-sided Bochdalek hernias have a worse prognosis than do left-sided hernias, and Morgagni hernias usually have only minor clinical consequences. Diaphragmatic hernias can be surgically corrected at birth and have also rarely been corrected by surgery during fetal life (covered in Chapter 6). However, if the hernia has resulted in severe pulmonary hypoplasia, the newborn may die of pulmonary insufficiency or pulmonary hypertension even if the hernia is repaired.

If the development of muscle tissue in the diaphragm is deficient, the excessively compliant diaphragm may allow the underlying abdominal contents to balloon or **eventrate** into the pulmonary cavity (Fig. 11-15). This condition can also result in pulmonary hypoplasia and hypertension, which may be fatal.

OLIGOHYDRAMNIOS AND PULMONARY HYPOPLASIA

As covered earlier in the chapter, pulmonary hypoplasia can result from failure of proper branching morphogenesis during development of the lungs and respiratory tree, as well as from diaphragmatic defects as just described. Another classic cause of pulmonary hypoplasia is **oligohydramnios**, the condition in which there is an insufficient amount of amniotic fluid. The causes of oligohydramnios and how they result in pulmonary hypoplasia are complex. During in utero life, the lung acts like an exocrine gland, producing fluid that provides a substantial contribution to the amniotic fluid. In addition, once the kidneys begin to function, after about sixteen weeks, fetal urine provides a substantial

contribution to the amniotic fluid. Therefore, **bilateral renal agenesis**—failure of both kidneys to form (covered in Chapter 15)—results in oligohydramnios. Also, in a condition called **premature rupture of the membranes** (PROM), the amnion ruptures early and amniotic fluid is lost, resulting in oligohydramnios. Presumably, oligohydramnios, regardless of its cause, results in pulmonary hypoplasia due to excessive loss of fluid from the fetal lungs and resulting decreased fluid pressure within the maturing respiratory tree. Compression of the fetal chest by the uterine wall has been postulated to play a role.

In the Research Lab

CONGENITAL DIAPHRAGMATIC HERNIA

Little is known about the molecular mechanisms of diaphragm formation and how this process fails to occur, resulting in congenital diaphragmatic hernia (CDH). However, it was shown in a screen of fetal mice harboring ENU-induced genetic mutations that CDH resulted from a mutation in the Fog2 (friend of Gata2; Gata2 is a transcription factor) gene. In addition, pulmonary hypoplasia occurred early in gestation, and Fog2 was expressed throughout the pulmonary mesenchyme during stages of branching morphogenesis, suggesting a direct role of Fog2 in pulmonary development. Screening of DNA from patients with congenital diaphragramatic defects revealed mutations in FOG2, demonstrating a role for this gene in development of the diaphragm in both mouse and human.

Additional evidence that FOG2 is critical for normal diaphragm formation comes from studies that have shown that Fog2 is an important regulator of Gata4 in the developing heart, and that both genes are co-expressed during cardiac embryogenesis. Homozygous mice null for Gata4 also have CDH, suggesting that abnormal regulation of Gata4 by Fog2 might be important for diaphragm development. Furthermore, Fog2 binds to the ligand-binding domain of chicken ovalbumin upstream promoter transcription factor II (Coup-tfII). Coup-tfII has been shown to be necessary for Fog2 to repress the transcription of a Gata4. It is important to note that mice with tissue-specific mutations of Coup-TFII have CDH, and Coup-TFII is located on human chromosome 15q26.2—a genomic region that is deleted in some CDH patients.

Embryology in Practice

LUNG MASS

A mid-gestation ultrasound reveals a mass that fills much of the left hemi-thorax of a fetus at twenty weeks of gestation. The remainder of the examination and the pregnancy history are unremarkable. Chromosome studies from an earlier amniocentesis, which was done because of advanced maternal age, were normal.

Careful review of the ultrasound shows normal diaphragm and abdominal contents, which argues against the presence of a congenital diaphragmatic hernia. The two remaining considerations for an interthoracic mass include bronchopulmonary sequestration (BPS) and congenital cystic adenomatoid malformation (CCAM).

Examination of the mass by color Doppler ultrasound demonstrates lack of a systemic arterial blood supply, which is always seen in cases of BPS. The presumptive diagnosis of a CCAM is made.

The parents are counseled that the effects on the fetus depend on the size of the lesion. Smaller lesions may have no

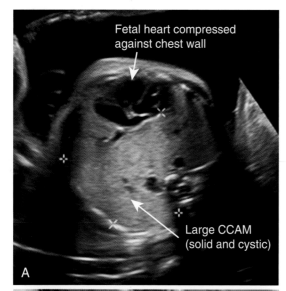

Fetal heart compressed against chest wall

Large CCAM (solid and cystic)

A

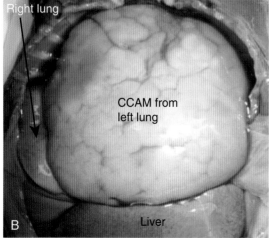

Right lung

CCAM from left lung

Liver

B

Figure 11-16. Congenital cystic adenomatoid malformation (CCAM). *A,* Sonogram at twenty-nine weeks. *B,* Autopsy photo of the stillborn fetus showing the enlarged left lung mass after removal of the chest wall.

effect on the pregnancy, but larger masses can impact the fetus by compression of the thoracic contents. Close follow-up with serial ultrasounds is planned.

Unfortunately, these ultrasounds show progressive growth of the mass, causing a mediastinal shift and resultant lung hypoplasia (Fig. 11-16*A*). The mass also impinges on the heart, leading to cardiovascular compromise and fetal hydrops. Compression of the esophagus and reduced swallowing of amniotic fluid lead to polyhydramnios. At thirty weeks of gestation, the pregnancy is spontaneously lost as the result of fetal cardiac failure. An autopsy reveals that the chest is almost completely filled with a solid mass, with compression of the lungs and heart (Fig. 11-16*B*).

As the name suggests, congenital cystic adenomatoid malformation (CCAM) consists of proliferative overgrowths of abnormal lung tissue that occur without a known cause (*adenomatoid malformation* means "a benign tumor"). CCAM is differentiated from BPS by the lack of a systemic arterial supply. BPS is typically a wedge-shaped, left-sided anomaly surrounded by its own visceral pleura. Several subtypes of CCAM (also called congenital pulmonary airway malformation, or CPAM) have been designated on the basis of cyst size. The risk of malignant transformation prompts surgical resection in surviving infants at many centers, irrespective of type.

SUGGESTED READINGS

Ahlfeld SK, Conway SJ. 2012. Aberrant signaling pathways of the lung mesenchyme and their contributions to the pathogenesis of bronchopulmonary dysplasia. Birth Defects Res A Clin Mol Teratol 94:3–15.

De Langhe SP, Reynolds SD. 2008. Wnt signaling in lung organogenesis. Organogenesis 4:100–108.

Domyan ET, Sun X. 2011. Patterning and plasticity in development of the respiratory lineage. Dev Dyn 240:477–485.

Holder AM, Klaassens M, Tibboel D, et al. 2007 Genetic factors in congenital diaphragmatic hernia. Am J Hum Genet 80:825–845.

Maeda Y, Dave V, Whitsett JA. 2007. Transcriptional control of lung morphogenesis. Physiol Rev 87:219–244.

Metzger RJ, Klein OD, Martin GR, Krasnow MA. 2008. The branching programme of mouse lung development. Nature 453:745–750.

Morrisey EE, Hogan BL. 2010. Preparing for the first breath: genetic and cellular mechanisms in lung development. Dev Cell 18:8–23.

Ornitz DM, Yin Y. 2012. Signaling networks regulating development of the lower respiratory tract. Cold Spring Harb Perspect Biol 4:1–19.

Warburton D. 2008. Developmental biology: order in the lung. Nature 453:733–735.

Chapter 12
Development of the Heart

SUMMARY

In response to inductive and permissive signals emanating from the endoderm, ectoderm, and midline mesoderm, cardiogenic precursors form a cardiac primordium within the splanchnic mesoderm at the cranial end of the embryonic disc called the **cardiac crescent**, or **first heart field**. In response to signals from the underlying endoderm, a subpopulation of cells within the first heart field form a pair of **lateral endocardial tubes** through the process of **vasculogenesis**. The cranial and lateral folding of the embryo during the fourth week results in the fusion of these tubes along the midline in the future thoracic region, where they form a single **primary heart tube**. This tube consists of a single endocardial tube with adjacent mesoderm differentiating into cardiomyocytes.

The **heartbeat** is initiated around the twenty-first day, and its continual beating is required for normal heart development. Between weeks four and eight, the primary heart tube undergoes a series of events, including **looping**, **remodeling**, **realignment**, and **septation**, eventually leading to the transformation of a single heart tube into a four-chambered heart, thus laying down the basis for the separation of pulmonary and systemic circulations at birth.

Starting at the inflow end, the primary heart tube initially consists of the **left** and **right horns of the sinus venosus**, the **primitive atrium**, the **atrioventricular canal**, the **primitive left ventricle**, and a short outflow region. Lengthening of the primary heart tube and proper cardiac bending and looping are driven through the addition of cardiac precursor cells by the **second heart field**. At the outflow end, the main additions are the **primitive right ventricle** and the **outflow tract** that connects with the **aortic sac** at the arterial orifice. As the outflow tract lengthens, proximal (conus) and distal (truncus) components can be distinguished. Septation of the outflow tract leads to separate left and right ventricular outlets and to formation of the ascending aorta and pulmonary trunk. At the inflow end, the second heart field also contributes myocardium to the sinus venosus wall, the body of the **right** and **left atrium**, and the **atrial septa**.

Venous blood initially enters the sinus horns through paired, symmetrical **common cardinal veins**. However, as covered in Chapter 13, changes in the venous system rapidly shift the entire systemic venous return to the right, so that all blood from the body and umbilicus enters the future right atrium through the developing **superior** and **inferior caval veins**. The left sinus horn becomes the **coronary sinus**, which collects blood from the coronary circulation. A process of intussusception incorporates the right sinus horn and the ostia of the **caval veins** into the posterior wall of the future right atrium. In this process, the **pulmonary vein** developing within the dorsal mesocardium shifts to the future left atrium as a result of the development of a **dorsal mesenchymal protrusion**. Subsequently, the walls of the pulmonary vein are partially incorporated into the atrial wall, forming the larger part of the dorsal left atrial wall. In the fifth and sixth weeks, the atrial septum starts to develop. This is a two-step process. It begins with the formation of the **septum primum (primary atrial septum)**, which is followed by formation of the **septum secundum (secondary atrial septum)**. The formation of this atrial septal complex results in separation of the right and left atria. However, the two septa do not fuse until after birth, allowing for right-to-left shunting of blood throughout gestation. The **mitral (bicuspid)** and **tricuspid atrioventricular valves** develop from atrioventricular cushion tissue during the fifth and sixth weeks. Meanwhile, the heart undergoes remodeling, bringing the future atria and ventricles into correct alignment with each other and aligning both ventricles with their respective future outflow vessels. During expansion of the primitive right and left ventricles, a **muscular ventricular septum** forms that partially separates the ventricles. During the seventh and eighth weeks, the outflow tract of the heart completes the process of septation and division. During this process, remodeling of the distal outflow tract cushion tissue (truncal cushions) results in the formation of the **semilunar valves** of the aorta and pulmonary artery. Fusion of the proximal outflow tract cushions (conal cushions) creates the outlet septum, resulting in the separation of left and right ventricular outlets. Complete ventricular septation depends on fusion of the outflow tract (conotruncal) septum, the muscular ventricular septum, and the atrioventricular cushion tissues.

The myocardium of the heart differentiates into working myocardium and myocardium of the **conduction system**. The **epicardium** grows out from the **proepicardial organ** covering the myocardium. It contributes to the formation of the coronary vasculature, which is necessary for oxygenation of the thickening myocardial wall and myocardial cell population.

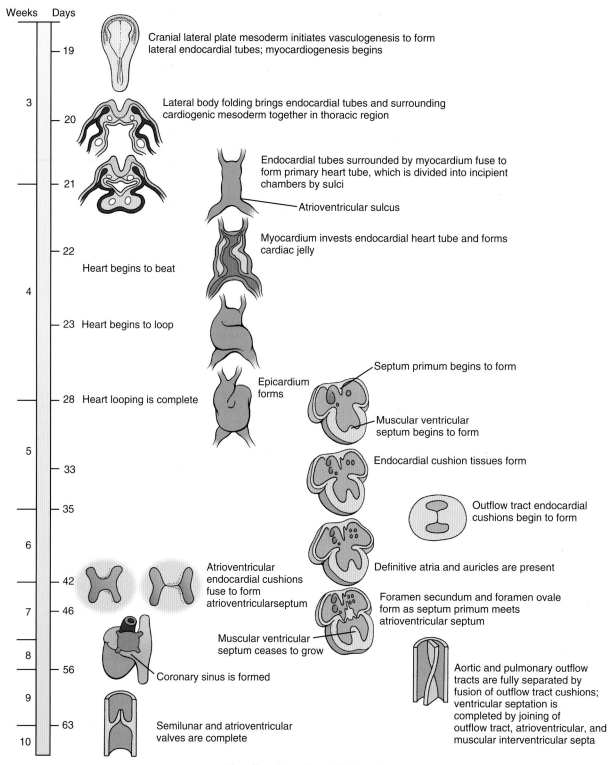

Weeks   Days

3

19   Cranial lateral plate mesoderm initiates vasculogenesis to form lateral endocardial tubes; myocardiogenesis begins

20   Lateral body folding brings endocardial tubes and surrounding cardiogenic mesoderm together in thoracic region

21   Endocardial tubes surrounded by myocardium fuse to form primary heart tube, which is divided into incipient chambers by sulci

Atrioventricular sulcus

22   Myocardium invests endocardial heart tube and forms cardiac jelly

Heart begins to beat

4

23   Heart begins to loop

28   Heart looping is complete

Epicardium forms

Septum primum begins to form

Muscular ventricular septum begins to form

5

33   Endocardial cushion tissues form

35   Outflow tract endocardial cushions begin to form

6

Definitive atria and auricles are present

42   Atrioventricular endocardial cushions fuse to form atrioventricularseptum

7   46   Foramen secundum and foramen ovale form as septum primum meets atrioventricular septum

Muscular ventricular septum ceases to grow

8   56   Coronary sinus is formed

Aortic and pulmonary outflow tracts are fully separated by fusion of outflow tract cushions; ventricular septation is completed by joining of outflow tract, atrioventricular, and muscular interventricular septa

9

63   Semilunar and atrioventricular valves are complete

10

Time line. Formation of the heart.

Clinical Taster

A full-term boy is born to a primigravid (first gestation) mother after an uncomplicated pregnancy. The delivery goes smoothly, with healthy Apgar scores of 8/10 at one minute and 9/10 at five minutes. All growth parameters (length, weight, and head circumference) are normal, ranging between the 10th and 25th centiles. The newborn examination is also normal, and the infant is returned to his mother to begin breast feeding.

The boy initially feeds well, but he becomes sleepy and disinterested in feeding as the day progresses. At twenty hours after birth, he exhibits decreased peripheral perfusion, cyanosis, and lethargy. A pulse oximeter shows oxygen saturation in the low 80% range (normal equals >90%) with increasing **respiratory distress**. Paradoxically, blood oxygen saturation worsens after administration of oxygen. The boy is emergently transferred to the neonatal intensive care unit in worsening shock. There, he is intubated, central intravascular catheters are placed, and he is started on **prostaglandins**.

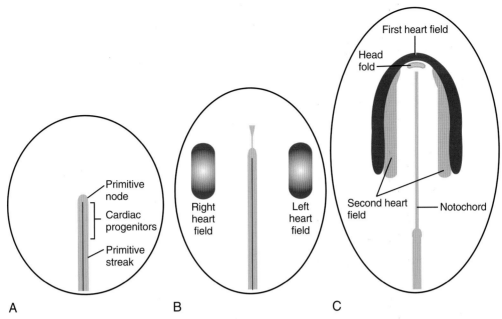

Figure 12-1. Formation of the first heart field seen in ventral views. *A*, Location of cardiogenic progenitors in the early primitive streak. *B*, Location of cardiogenic precursors (red gradated regions) within the mesoderm shortly after gastrulation and during initial specification. *C*, Location of the first heart field (red) containing specified cardiogenic cells. The crescent-like arrangement of the progenitors is due to their migration pattern, local cardiogenic induction signals, and development of the body folds. Medial and slightly caudal to the first heart field lies the second heart field (orange).

A chest x-ray shows **cardiomegaly** (enlarged heart) and increased pulmonary vascularity (indicative of increased blood flow). An **echocardiogram** shows a very small left ventricle with a small aortic outflow tract, leading to the diagnosis of **hypoplastic left heart syndrome** (HLHS).

HLHS is a shunt-dependent lesion: survival of these patients depends on maintaining a **patent ductus arteriosus** (PDA) to carry blood from the pulmonary artery to the aorta and out to perfuse the systemic circulation. Supplemental oxygen lowers resistance to pulmonary blood flow, causing blood to circulate to the lungs instead of crossing the PDA. Thus, administering supplemental oxygen actually decreases blood oxygen saturation. Administration of prostaglandins prevents the physiological closure of the ductus arteriosus, maintaining systemic perfusion until surgery can be performed. The first-stage surgery, called the Norwood procedure, connects the right ventricular outflow tract to the aorta, and a separate shunt is used to provide blood flow to the lungs. More surgeries follow at about six months and two to three years of age. Occasionally, heart transplantation is performed. The five-year survival rate for HLHS is around 70%.

ESTABLISHING CARDIAC LINEAGE

The heart is the first organ to function in human embryos. It begins beating as early as the twenty-first day, and starts pumping blood by the twenty-fourth to twenty-fifth day. Much of cardiac development, including remodeling and septation, occurs while the heart is pumping blood. This is necessary to provide nutrients and oxygen and to dispose of wastes during embryonic and fetal development, but this mechanical and electrical activity also plays an important role in the morphogenesis of the heart. The embryonic heart is first morphologically identifiable as a single tube composed of contractile myocardium surrounding an inner endocardial (endothelial) tube, with an intervening extracellular matrix. The heart is also an asymmetrical organ whose left-right patterning is established during gastrulation (left-right patterning is covered in Chapter 3 and later in this chapter).

Cardiac progenitor cells are derived from intraembryonic mesoderm emerging from the cranial third of the primitive streak during early gastrulation. These progenitors leave the primitive streak and migrate in a cranial-lateral direction to become localized on either side of the primitive streak (Fig. 12-1*A*, *B*). The cardiac progenitor cells eventually become localized within the cranial lateral plate mesoderm on both sides of the embryo, extending and arcing cranial to the developing head fold, forming a **cardiac crescent** (Fig. 12-1*C*). Cells in the cardiac crescent constitute the so-called **first heart field**. It is thought that the cardiac cell lineage is specified from mesodermal cells within the first heart field. As discussed later, the first heart field is not the sole source of cardiogenic cells for the developing heart, as medial to the first heart field, there is already a population of **second heart field** cells (Fig 12-1*C*).

In the Research Lab

SPECIFICATION OF CARDIAC PROGENITOR CELLS

To what degree cardiac progenitor cells within the epiblast and the primitive streak are specified remains unknown. Activin and Tgfβ produced by the hypoblast of the chick induce cardiogenic properties in some of the overlying epiblast cells (Fig. 12-2*A*, *B*). Other members of the Tgfβ superfamily, including nodal and Vg1, also play a role in inducing cardiogenic properties in the epiblast. During gastrulation, cardiac precursors residing in the primitive streak are uncommitted, but these progenitors become specified to become cardiogenic mesoderm soon after migrating into the lateral plate. Mesp1 (mesoderm posterior 1) and Mesp2 (mesoderm posterior 2), members of the basic HLH family of transcription factors, are expressed transiently during the primitive streak stage. Both are required for migration of the cardiac progenitor cells into the cranial region of the embryo, and both have been implicated in the specification of the early cardiovascular lineage. Interaction of cranial lateral mesoderm with the endoderm is required for this cardiac specification. The endoderm secretes several signaling molecules—including Bmp, Fgf, activin, insulin-like growth factor 2, and Shh—that promote cell survival and proliferation of cardiogenic cells. One particularly important growth factor is Bmp2, which is essential for stimulating the expression of early cardiogenic transcription factors, such as Nkx2.5 (Nkx2 transcription factor related, locus 5) and Gata (proteins that bind to a DNA GATA sequence) within the lateral mesoderm. In the chick embryo, Bmp2 can induce expression of myocardial cell markers in ectopic regions (i.e., outside their proper position), whereas mouse embryos lacking Bmp2 fail to develop hearts. However, cardiac specification of the mesoderm still occurs in these embryos, likely as the result of overlapping functions of other Bmp family members with Bmp2.

Bmp signaling specifies the cardiogenic lineage, but its effect on the mesoderm is limited to the lateral mesoderm. Why? The reason is that Bmp antagonists and inhibitors are released from midline tissues. The notochord synthesizes and releases chordin

and noggin, two proteins that sequester Bmps and prevent binding to their receptors (Fig. 12-2C). If chordin activity is inhibited in cranial paraxial mesoderm, the medial mesoderm has the capacity to form cardiac cells. In addition, the developing neural plate ectoderm releases Wnt1 and Wnt3a, which also antagonize Bmp signaling. If Wnt signaling is abrogated in mouse embryos, multiple hearts are generated. Therefore, because of the antagonizing effects of chordin/noggin and Wnt signaling on Bmp signaling, the influence of Bmp on mesoderm is limited to lateral regions.

But why is the cardiogenic region limited to the cranial portion of the lateral mesoderm? We know that the caudal lateral plate mesoderm is capable of responding to cardiac specification signals: if it is grafted into the cranial region, it transforms into cardiogenic cells. As covered above, Wnt1/Wnt3a and chordin/noggin inhibit the effects of Bmps on mesoderm. However, other Wnts (e.g., Wnt8) expressed in the cranial and caudal mesoderm also inhibit Bmp effects on the mesoderm. Knowing that Bmp signaling is required for cardiac mesoderm formation, how can Bmp still exert its influence on the cranial lateral mesoderm in the presence of these Wnts but not on the caudal lateral plate? The answer is that other molecules secreted by the cranial *endoderm* antagonize the negative effects of Wnts on Bmp-driven heart formation. These include *secreted* frizzled-like proteins (sFrps) that sequester Wnts and Dickkopfs that bind to and inhibit the Wnt co-receptors of the Lrp (low-density lipoprotein receptor–related protein) class (Fig. 12-3). Hence, in the absence of Wnt signaling, the effect of Bmp is to promote the cardiac lineage in the cranial portion of the lateral mesoderm, whereas in the presence of Wnt signaling, Bmp initiates a blood vessel–forming capacity in the caudal portion of the lateral plate mesoderm. However, recent studies suggest that canonical Wnt signaling has biphasic effects on cardiogenesis depending on the time of action, promoting cardiac specification during gastrulation but later obstructing it. Non-canonical Wnt signaling (Wnt5a and Wnt11) also promotes cardiogenesis.

Several cardiac transcription factors are activated within the first heart field. The earliest transcription factors with limited expression within the cardiac lineage include Nkx2.5, Tbx5, and members of the Gata family. Nkx2.5 is expressed in cardiac progenitor cells soon after the onset of gastrulation under the influence of endodermally derived Bmp. Downstream targets of Nkx2.5 include several other cardiac genes, such as Mef2c, ventricular myosin, and Hand1. A human ortholog of NKX2.5 has been mapped to chromosome 5q35.2, and mutations in this gene are associated with human congenital heart disease, including atrial septal defects, ventricular septal defects, and defects in the conduction system. Nkx2.5 knockout mice die in utero but still form a heart, albeit one without left ventricular markers, with incorrect looping, and with a deranged cranial-caudal identity. So Nkx2.5 expression is not solely responsible for dictating the cardiac cell lineage. Mice null for Gata4 have fewer cardiomyocytes. Mice lacking Gata5 are normal but exhibit elevated Gata4 levels, suggesting a compensatory effect for the loss of Gata5. Gata5 null mice also lacking one of the Gata4 genes exhibit profound cardiac defects, whereas mice with normal Gata5 genes lacking one of the Gata4 genes are normal. This suggests that Gata4 and Gata5 act cooperatively in directing early cardiac lineage. Nkx2.5 and Gatas may mutually reinforce cardiac expression of each other's cardiac expression, as each contains promoter regions for the other.

In summary, the program of early cardiac specification is quite flexible, but it requires the presence of particular morphogens providing a permissive environment for lineage specification. Moreover, no single transcription factor or signaling molecule has been identified that is solely responsible for encoding myocardial specification and differentiation. Rather, it seems that a combination of factors working together is needed to stably specify the cardiac cell lineage.

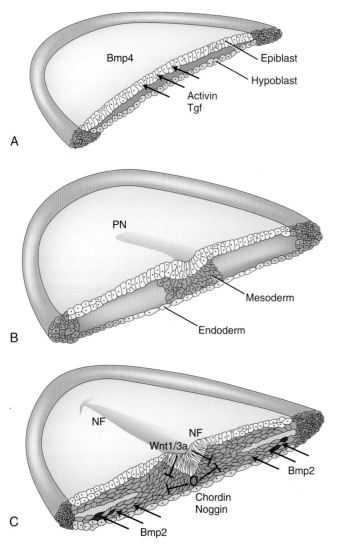

Figure 12-2. Induction of the first heart field. *A, B,* Before and during gastrulation, Tgfβ and activin released by the hypoblast induce cardiogenic potential in a subset of epiblast cells and newly forming mesodermal cells. *C,* Bmps, released from the newly formed endoderm, signal the formation of a cardiogenic lineage from the mesoderm (red cells), but their influence is limited to the lateral mesoderm because of the release of chordin and noggin from the notochord and Wnt1/3a from the forming neuroectoderm. NF, Neural fold; PN, primitive node.

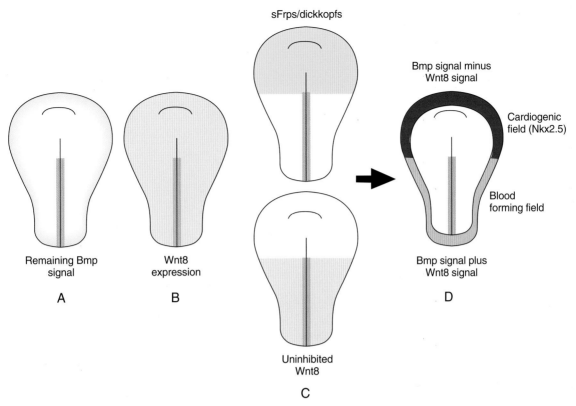

Figure 12-3. Regional specification of cardiogenic mesoderm. *A,* Pattern of Bmp signaling on the mesoderm remaining after accounting for chordin/noggin and Wnt1/3a inhibition. *B,* Pattern of Wnt8 expression in the mesoderm. *C,* Spatial distribution of secreted frizzled-related proteins (sFrps) and dickkopf expression (both Wnt antagonists) in the underlying endoderm, and remaining pattern of uninhibited Wnt8 activity in the mesoderm. *D,* Pattern of expression of the cardiogenic marker Nkx2.5 as a result of Bmp signaling in the absence of Wnt inhibition. In the presence of Bmp and Wnt8 signaling, blood-forming fields are primed.

FORMATION OF PRIMARY HEART TUBE

Animation 12-1: Formation of Primitive Heart Tube. Animations are available online at StudentConsult.

With formation of the intraembryonic coelom, the lateral plate mesoderm is subdivided into somatic and splanchnic layers; the first heart field forms within the splanchnic mesodermal subdivision. During the process of body folding (covered in Chapter 4), the cranialmost portion of the first heart field is pulled ventrally and caudally to lie ventral to the newly forming foregut endoderm (Fig. 12-4). As the lateral body folds move medially, they bring the right and left sides of the first heart field together, and the two limbs of the first heart field fuse at the midline, caudal to the head fold and ventral to the foregut (Fig. 12-5*A-D*). This fusion occurs at the site of the anterior intestinal portal and progresses in a cranial-to-caudal direction as the foregut tube lengthens. As the two limbs of the first heart field fuse, a recognizable pair of vascular elements called the **endocardial tubes** develops within each limb of the first heart field (Fig. 12-5*B, C*). These vessels form within the first heart field from a seemingly distinct progenitor population from other endothelial subtypes through mechanisms that still are not well understood. The cells of the endocardial tubes coalesce into a single tube as the limbs of the first heart field join to make the primary heart tube (Fig. 12-5*C, D*). If fusion of the first heart field limbs fails, two tube-like structures form rather than a single primary heart tube,

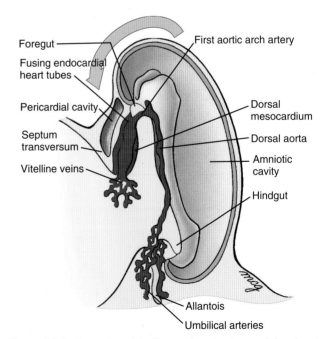

Figure 12-4. Formation of the first aortic arch artery and dorsal aorta during the third week. The paired dorsal aortae develop in the dorsal mesoderm on either side of the notochord and connect to the fusing endocardial heart tubes while body folding ensues. As flexion and growth of the head fold (large curved arrow) carry the forming primary heart tube into the cervical and then into the thoracic region, the cranial ends of the dorsal aortae are pulled ventrally until they form a dorsoventral loop—the first aortic arch artery. A series of four more aortic arch arteries will develop during the fourth and fifth weeks.

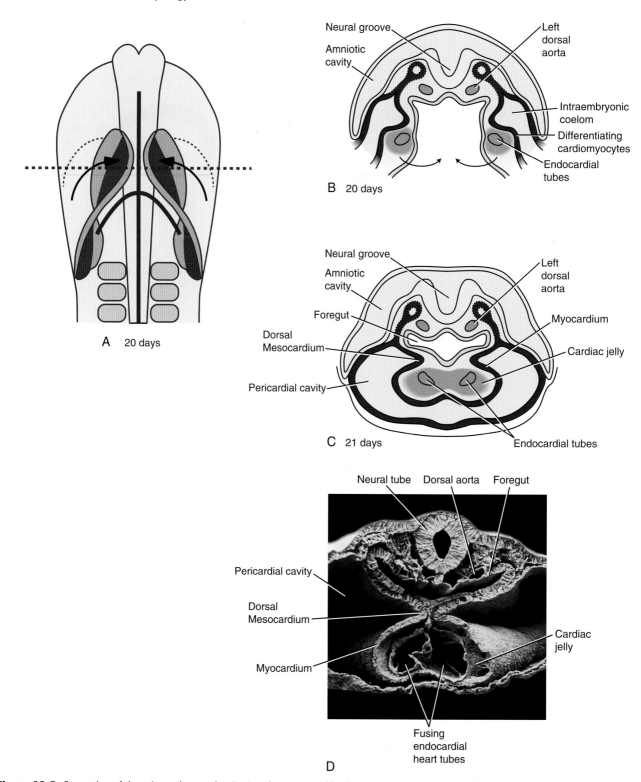

Figure 12-5. Formation of the primary heart tube. During the process of body folding in the third week, the cranialmost portion of the first heart field is pulled ventrally and caudally to lie beneath the newly forming foregut. *A*, Ventral view; dashed horizontal line indicates the level of sections illustrated in *B* and *C*; curved solid line indicates the anterior (cranial) intestinal portal of the developing foregut; vertical solid line indicates the notochord; red, first heart field; orange, second heart field. As the lateral body folds (arrows) fuse in the midline in a cranial-to-caudal progression, they also bring the right and left sides of the first heart field together (red). *B, C,* Drawings of cross sections at the level indicated by the dashed line in *A,* with *C* at a later stage than *B. D,* Scanning electron micrograph of a cross section. As the two limbs of the first heart field fuse, a recognizable pair of vascular elements called the endocardial tubes develops within each limb of the first heart field. These endocardial tubes then fuse to form the primary heart tube.

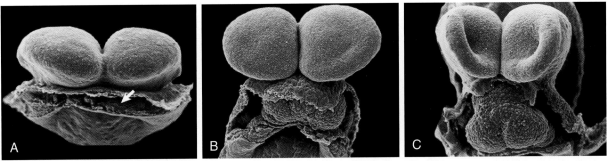

Figure 12-6. Scanning electron micrographs of developing mouse embryos. *A-C,* Head folding progressively translocates the developing endo-cardial tubes from a region initially just cranial to the neural plate to the thoracic region (arrow in *A,* cardiogenic region).

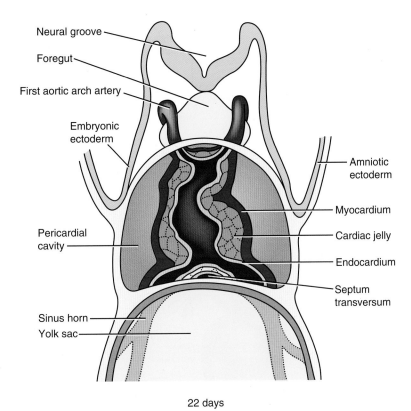

22 days

Figure 12-7. Composition of the primary heart tube walls. By twenty-two days, the endocardium of the primary heart tube is invested by an acellular layer of cardiac jelly and a layer of myocardial cells. The myocardium is derived from a mass of splanchnic mesoderm that encloses the endocardial heart tube. The myocardium then secretes the extracellular cardiac jelly between itself and the endocardium.

leading to **cardia bifida** (however, both tubes persist, contract, and continue to undergo cardiogenesis, including looping; looping is covered below). The primary heart tube harbors progenitors for the atria and left ventricle, as well as endocardium. As the fusion process continues, cell proliferation in the first heart field continues to add the more caudal segments of the heart, including the atrio-ventricular canal, the primitive atria, and a portion of the sinus venosus (covered later in the chapter). Late in the third week, cranial body folding brings the developing heart tube into the thoracic region (Figs. 12-4, 12-6; also covered in Chapters 4 and 11).

By the twenty-first to twenty-second day, the primitive endocardial tube is surrounded by a mass of splanchnic mesoderm containing myocardial progenitors that aggregate around fused endocardial tubes to form the

myocardium. A thick layer of acellular extracellular matrix, the **cardiac jelly**, is deposited mainly by the developing myocardium, separating it from the endocardial tube (Fig. 12-7). The **epicardium** (visceral lining of the pericardial cavity covering the heart) is formed later by a population of mesodermal cells that are independently derived from splanchnic mesoderm that migrates onto the outer surface of the myocardium (covered later in the chapter).

A series of constrictions and expansions develop in the primary heart tube (Fig. 12-8). Over the next five weeks, as the tubular heart lengthens, these expansions contribute to the various heart chambers. Starting at the caudal (inflow) end, the **sinus venosus** consists of the partially confluent left and right **sinus horns**, into which the common cardinal veins (covered later in the chapter)

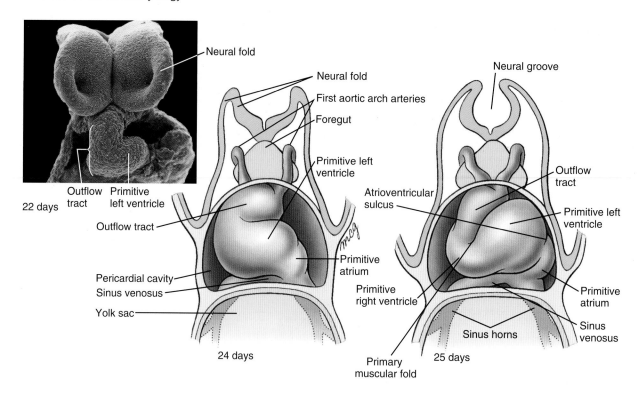

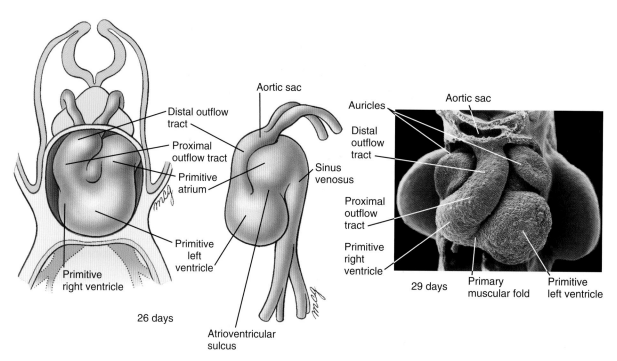

Figure 12-8. Regionalization of the heart tube during its lengthening. As the heart tube lengthens and adds to the outflow segment, looping of the heart tube repositions the outflow tract ventrally and to the right, shifts the primitive left ventricle to the left, and shifts the primitive atrium dorsally and cranially. Addition of myocardium at the arterial end forms the right ventricle and the future proximal and distal segments of the outflow tract. The primitive left ventricle will form the definitive left ventricle, and the primitive atrium will give rise to a portion of the atrial wall and auricles of the heart. During this process, deepening external folds and grooves increasingly distinguish each segment of the heart tube.

drain. Cranial to the sinus venosus, the next chamber is the **primitive** (or **common**) **atrium**, which, as a result of the subsequent formation of the atrial septal complex, eventually becomes divided into the right and left atria. Connected in series with the atrium are the **atrioventricular canal**, the **primitive left ventricle**, and the developing **primitive right ventricle** and **outflow tract**. The primitive left ventricle is separated from the primitive right ventricle by a **primary muscular fold** (formerly referred to as the **bulboventricular fold**), the latter contributing to the **muscular ventricular septum**. Whereas the atria, atrioventricular canal, and left ventricle are largely derived from the first heart field, the right ventricle and outflow tract are not. Rather, they are derived from an additional source of cardiac precursor cells, referred to as the **second heart field**. The outflow tract forms the outflow region for both the left and right ventricles. The outflow tract can be subdivided into a **proximal outflow tract** (conus arteriosus), which eventually becomes incorporated into the left and right ventricles, and the **distal outflow tract** (truncus arteriosus), which eventually splits to form the ascending aorta and pulmonary trunk. The distal outflow tract is connected at its cranial end to a dilated expansion called the **aortic sac**. The aortic sac is continuous with the first aortic arch artery and, eventually, is continuous with the other four aortic arch arteries as they develop. The aortic arch arteries form major arteries transporting blood to the head and trunk (covered in Chapter 13).

The primary heart tube is initially suspended in the developing pericardial cavity by a **dorsal mesocardium (dorsal mesentery of the heart)** formed by splanchnic mesoderm located beneath the foregut. Subsequently, this dorsal mesocardium ruptures over almost the entire length of the heart tube, with the exception of the caudalmost aspect, where a small but very important component of the dorsal mesocardium persists. As a result, the heart is left suspended in the pericardial cavity by its developing arterial and venous poles, with the region of the ruptured dorsal mesocardium becoming the **transverse pericardial sinus** within the pericardial sac of the definitive heart (Fig. 12-9). Ligatures sometimes are passed through this space and around the vessels at either pole to control blood flow in children or adults undergoing surgery.

As noted earlier, not all of the cardiac cells found in the mature heart are derived from the first heart field. Rather, additional sources of cardiogenic precursors are recruited from the mesoderm immediately adjacent and medial to the initial cardiac crescent (Fig. 12-10). While the developing primary heart tube continues to expand, there is continued recruitment of cardiac progenitor cells from outside the original first heart field at both the arterial (cranial) and venous (caudal) poles. The source of

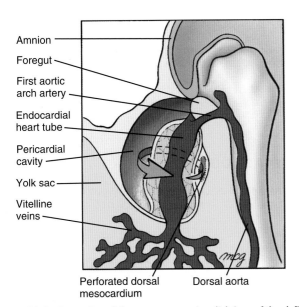

Figure 12-9. Formation of the transverse pericardial sinus of the definitive pericardial cavity by rupture of the dorsal mesocardium early in the fourth week. Arrow passes through the transverse pericardial sinus.

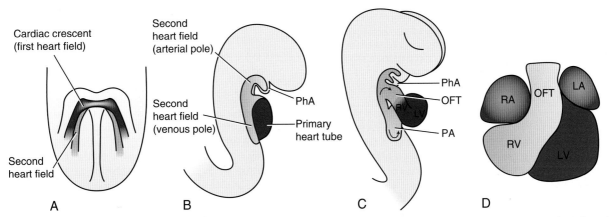

Figure 12-10. The second source of cardiogenic progenitors for the heart, the second heart field (shown in orange in *A-D*). *A,* Location of the second heart field relative to the first heart field before body folding. The second heart field is located within the splanchnic mesoderm just medial and slightly caudal to the first heart field (first heart field shown in red). *B,* After formation of the primary heart tube, the second heart field becomes located dorsal to the dorsal mesocardium and runs along the craniocaudal axis. *C,* With rupture of the dorsal mesocardium, the second heart field is divided into a caudal segment, responsible for adding to the venous pole of the heart, and a cranial segment, responsible for lengthening the heart tube at the arterial pole. *D,* Ventral view of the looped heart shows the contributions of the first and second heart fields (contributions of the second heart field to the atria are not visible in this view). *LA,* Left atrium; *LV,* left ventricle; *OFT,* outflow tract; *PA,* primitive atrium; *PhA,* pharyngeal arch; *RA,* right atrium; *RV,* right ventricle.

these cells is referred to as the **second heart field**. The primitive heart tube lengthens at both ends, particularly the outflow (arterial) end, through the addition of cardiac progenitors from the second heart field mesoderm. Lineage-tracing studies suggest that in mammals the proximal and distal outflow tract, the right ventricle, and a portion of the venous pole and atria are derived from the second heart field mesoderm (Fig. 12-10D).

In the Research Lab

ROLE OF SECOND HEART FIELD IN FORMATION OF OUTFLOW SEGMENT OF HEART

Animation 12-2: Contributions of First and Second Heart Fields.
   Animations are available online at StudentConsult.

Cells of the first and second heart fields may arise from a common precursor established before the cardiac crescent stage (likely during early gastrulation). Recent studies suggest that progenitors for the second heart field lie just medial and slightly caudal to the first heart field within the lateral plate mesoderm (see Figs. 12-1, 12-10). Like the first heart field, the second heart field is subjected to the influences of Bmps and Fgfs released by the foregut (pharyngeal) endoderm that activate cardiogenic transcription factors. However, the more medial location of the second heart field at the cardiac crescent stage also positions these cells closer to the negative influence of Wnts and chordin/noggin emanating from the developing notochord and neural plate (see Figs. 12-2, 12-10). Manifestation of the cardiac cell lineage within the second heart field is likely suspended until the primary heart tube is formed and the intervening distance between the second heart field and the midline neural tube/notochord is increased. Therefore, cells of the second heart field may not represent a distinct cardiogenic lineage from the first heart field.

   As the two limbs of the cardiac crescent move toward the midline during fusion, the second heart field cells come into contact with the dorsal surface of the primary heart tube (future inner curvature of the heart) and end up at both the cranial and caudal ends of the developing dorsal mesocardium (see Fig. 12-10B, C). It is after the second heart field cells come to lie ventral to the foregut that expression of Nkx2.5 and Gata4 increases in the second heart field (Fig. 12-11). Second heart field cells lying just cranial to the arterial outflow of the heart tube and ventral to the developing pharyngeal endoderm assume a *right* ventricular identity, whereas cells more caudal to the arterial outflow contribute to the wall of the proximal and distal outflow tracts. Those at the inflow end of the heart tube contribute myocardial cells to the wall of the atria, atrial septum, and sinus venosus. The bulk of heart tube lengthening comes from proliferation within the second heart field at the arterial pole.

GENE MUTATIONS TARGET FIRST AND SECOND HEART FIELDS
Mutations in particular genes reveal regional sensitivities of the myocardium that reflect the origin of their cardiomyocyte progenitors. For instance, in Tbx5-deficient mice (Tbx5 is a T-box transcription family member that is expressed in the primary heart tube), the atrium is abnormal and the left ventricle is hypoplastic. Yet, the right ventricle and outflow tract seem normal, suggesting that this mutation mainly targets proliferation and development of cells of the first heart field. Isl1 is expressed in the second heart field. Mice null for Isl1 typically develop only two heart chambers: the atria and the left ventricle. The outflow tract is missing, right ventricular markers are not expressed, and the posterior atrial myocardium is hypoplastic. Fgf8 is expressed in

the ectoderm and pharyngeal endoderm near the arterial pole of the heart tube. Proper Fgf8 signaling within the second heart field is necessary for continued proliferation of cranial second heart field cells at the arterial pole. Fgf8 hypomorphs (an embryo with a partial loss-of-function mutation; i.e., Fgf8 expression in the hypomorph is knocked down but is not eliminated completely) die as a result of abnormal outflow tract development. Tbx1 (lost in 22q11.2 deletion syndrome), a transcription factor expressed in the second heart field, interacts genetically with Fgf8. Again, loss of Tbx1 expression in the second heart field reduces myocardial cell number in the outflow tract and right ventricle, whereas forced Tbx1 overexpression in the second heart field causes an expansion of the outflow tract. From these studies, it is clear that in addition to a first heart field, a large portion of the definitive heart tube arises from the second heart field. Several other signaling molecules and transcription factors play important roles in mediating continued proliferation or survival of second heart field cells, including Shh, canonical Wnts, Pdgf, retinoic acid and retinoic acid receptors, Mef2c, Msx1, Msx2, Hand2, Tbx18, Shox2, Foxa2, Foxc1, and Foxc2. Once heart tube elongation is completed, studies suggest that cranial second heart field mesodermal cells in the pharyngeal arches may activate a branchiomeric skeletal muscle program (covered in Chapter 17). Lengthening of the heart tube by the second heart field plays an important role in proper cardiac looping and septation of the heart.

CARDIAC LOOPING

Animation 12-3: Looping of Primitive Heart Tube.
   Animations are available online at StudentConsult.

On day 23, the primary heart tube begins to elongate and simultaneously bend into a C-shaped structure, with the bend extending toward the right side. Formation of this bend is not simply a matter of forming a kink in the tube, with the right side of the tubular heart becoming the outer curvature and the left side forming the inner curvature. Rather, it seems that the ventral surface of the primary heart tube forms the right outer curvature of the C-shaped heart, because the ventral surface is displaced toward the right by torsional forces working along the craniocaudal axis (Fig. 12-12). With the rupture of the dorsal mesocardium, much of the dorsal side of the straight primary heart tube becomes situated on the inner curvature of the C-shaped heart. As the heart tube continues to elongate at both arterial and venous poles, it takes on an S-shaped configuration. In the process, the primitive right ventricle is displaced caudally, ventrally, and to the right; the developing primitive left ventricle is displaced to the left. The primitive atrium acquires a more dorsal and cranial position (Fig. 12-13; see also Fig. 12-8). By day twenty-eight, the elongation of the heart tube is complete, but there continues to be additional remodeling such that the outflow tract comes to lie between the presumptive future atria, and the atrioventricular canal aligns with both ventricles (see Fig. 12-8). The end result of cardiac looping is to bring the four presumptive chambers of the future heart into their correct spatial relationship to each other. The remainder of heart development consists mostly of remodeling these chambers, developing the appropriate septa and valves between them, and forming the epicardium, coronary vasculature, and cardiac innervation and conducting system.

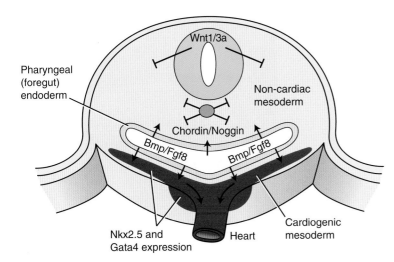

Figure 12-11. Role of growth factors in lengthening of the heart tube by the second heart field. Specification of cardiogenic precursors in the second heart field is similar to that in the first heart field. The cardiogenic promoting effect of Bmp and Fgf8 released by the endoderm on the splanchnic mesoderm is no longer antagonized after formation of the foregut by Wnts and chordin/noggin released by midline tissues. As a result, the cardiogenic mesoderm of the second heart field begins to express cardiac markers (e.g., Nkx2.5 and Gata4), proliferates, and drives the lengthening of the heart tube.

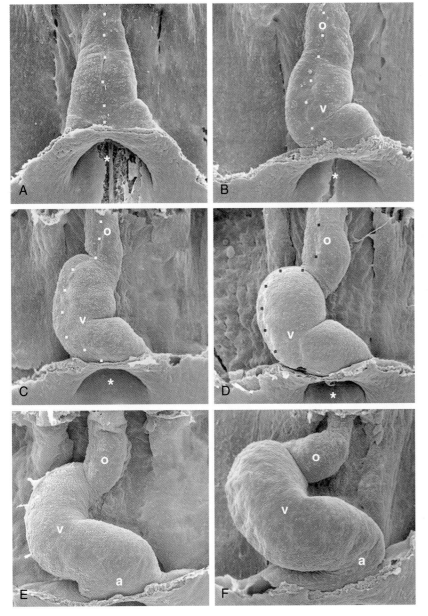

Figure 12-12. Scanning electron micrographs showing looping of the chick heart tube in ventral views (endoderm has been removed). *A, B,* Shows the primary heart tube just before overt looping. The ventral midline of the primary heart tube is marked by the dotted line. *C-F,* Cardiac looping is driven in part by cardiac lengthening from the second heart field. Note that looping to the right is accompanied by twisting, such that the original ventral surface of the primary heart tube becomes the outer curvature of the looped heart. These forces help drive the formation primary muscular fold. Several of the cardiac regions are easily identifiable during this process, including atrium (a), outflow tract (o), and primitive left ventricle (v). The asterisks demarcate the anterior intestinal portal.

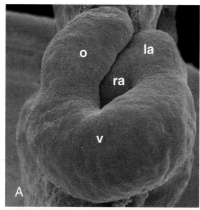

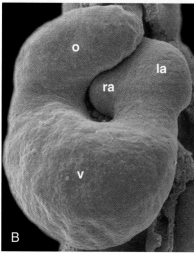

Figure 12-13. Scanning electron micrographs showing late views of looping of the chick heart tube. *A, B,* Position and morphology of the heart regions at progressively later end stages of cardiac looping. Ventral view of the outflow tract (o), non-septated ventricle (v), and non-septated right atrium (ra) and left atrium (la) showing their relative anatomical positions near the end of cardiac looping. Note that both atrial and venous poles are now adjacent to each other and that the outflow tract is moving leftward and ventral to the atria.

In the Clinic

SIDEDNESS IN HEART LOOPING

As covered in Chapter 3, abnormal left-right axis determination can lead to development of **heterotaxy** (with an estimated incidence of 3 out of 20,000 live births). This term is sometimes used to describe any defect ascribed to abnormal left-right axis formation, be it a reversal of some organs **(partial situs ambiguus)** or a reversal of all viscera **(situs inversus totalis)**. With regard to the heart, this may include abnormal looping, resulting in **ventricular inversion** (Fig. 12-14). Proper looping toward the right is a prerequisite for proper cardiac septation, as it is required to bring the primitive left ventricle toward the left, the primitive right ventricle toward the right, and the outflow tract region to the middle. Because individuals with situs inversus totalis exhibit a reversal in handedness of all organs, they exhibit few problems. In contrast, **visceroatrial heterotaxy syndrome** in humans (where the abdominal viscera and the atrial pole are oriented on opposing sides) is associated with structural defects, including a common atrium, malalignment of atrioventricular canal and outflow tract, and abnormal venous and arterial vascular connections.

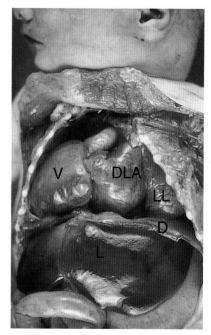

Figure 12-14. Infant with ventricular inversion, a condition in which the looping of the heart tube is reversed from its normal sinistral pattern, producing a heart that has its apex inferior and to the right (rather than left) side. D, Diaphragm; DLA, dilated left atrium; L, liver; LL, left lung; V, ventricle.

Besides inverted situs, indeterminate left-right axis formation can lead to bilateral left-sidedness or right-sidedness, so-called isomerism. For example, in the condition called right atrial isomerism, both atria have right atrial morphology. Similarly, in left pulmonary isomerism, both lungs have the lobar and hilar anatomy of the left lung.

In the Research Lab

MECHANISMS DRIVING CARDIAC BENDING AND LOOPING

Cardiac looping involves two major processes: establishing the directionality of looping, and performing the biomechanical steps that drive the looping itself. Directionality of looping reflects the left-right asymmetry established early during gastrulation (covered in Chapter 3), which is superimposed on the morphogenetic mechanisms of cardiac looping. In fact, the initial bending of the heart tube into the C shape is the first morphological evidence of embryonic left-right asymmetry.

The precise mechanisms driving the initial bending and the heart tube's continued looping into an S-shaped tube are still unclear, even though considerable effort has gone into identifying the forces responsible for the process. At one time, it was suggested that these processes occur simply because the heart tube, being anchored on both ends, outgrows the length of the primitive pericardial cavity and is forced to bend and loop. However, hearts excised from experimental animals and grown in culture demonstrate an intrinsic ability to bend, likely due to active changes in cell shape caused by forces of actin polymerization. Still, excised hearts do not exhibit rightward torsion, suggesting that forces external to the primary heart tube drive the latter. Experimental manipulations in chick embryos suggest that asymmetrical growth within

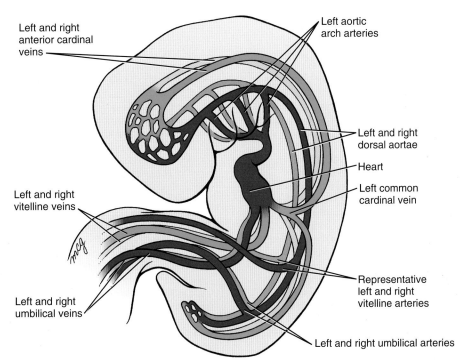

Figure 12-15. Schematic depiction of the embryonic vascular system in the middle of the fourth week. The heart has begun to beat and to circulate blood. The outflow tract is now connected to three pairs of aortic arch arteries and the paired dorsal aortae that circulate blood to the head and trunk. Three pairs of veins—umbilical, vitelline, and cardinal—deliver blood to the inflow end of the heart.

the primitive atria and the attached ventral splanchnopleure provide the torsional forces driving displacement of the heart to the right, while the dorsal mesocardium constrains this motion on the dorsal side, thereby resulting in the C-shaped bend. Other models suggest that remnants of the dorsal mesocardium shorten and force the heart tube to bend. However, the primary heart tube exhibits signs of bending before rupture of the dorsal mesocardium. Alternatively, before rupture, the dorsal mesocardium may exert tension on the future inner curvature, providing the biomechanical driving force necessary for bending. Finally, asymmetrical cell proliferation and growth within the cranial second heart field may also generate torsional forces necessary for generating the C-shaped bend.

FORMATION OF PRIMITIVE BLOOD VESSELS ASSOCIATED WITH THE ENDOCARDIAL TUBE

Many of the major vessels of the embryo, including the paired dorsal aortae, develop at the same time as the endocardial tube. The inflow and outflow vessels of the future heart make connections with the endocardium of the primary heart tube even before this tube is translocated into the thorax. The paired **dorsal aortae**, which form the primary outflow vessels of the heart, develop in the dorsal mesenchyme of the embryonic disc on either side of the notochord. As the flexion and growth of the head fold carry the heart tube into the cervical and then thoracic region, the cranial ends of the dorsal aortae are pulled ventrally until they

form a dorsoventral loop—the **first pair of aortic arch arteries**. (Fig. 12-15; see also Figs. 12-4, 12-7, 12-8, 12-9). A series of four more aortic arch arteries develop during the fourth and fifth weeks in connection with the mesenchymal pharyngeal arches (covered in Chapters 13 and 17). In addition, the craniocaudal flexure facilitates cardiac looping by bringing the venous (sinus venosus) and arterial (distal outflow tract and aortic sac) poles closer to one another in a process called **convergence**.

Six vessels, three on each side (Fig. 12-15), initially provide the inflow to the heart. Venous blood from the body of the embryo enters the heart through a pair of short trunks, the **common cardinal veins**, which are formed by the confluence of the paired **posterior cardinal veins** draining the trunk and the paired **anterior cardinal veins** draining the head region (see Fig. 12-15). A pair of **vitelline veins** drains the yolk sac, and a pair of **umbilical veins** delivers oxygenated blood to the heart from the placenta. The embryonic venous system is discussed in Chapter 13.

In the Research Lab

SUBREGIONS OF HEART ARE SPECIFIED EARLY IN DEVELOPMENT

The chambers of the heart are developmentally, electrophysiologically, and pharmacologically distinct. How does this regionalization develop within a single heart tube? Fate mapping studies show that cardiac progenitor cells within the epiblast are topologically organized such that the cardiac inflow progenitors are located more lateral, and the outflow progenitors more medial. Subsequently, during the process of gastrulation, this orientation is converted to a craniocaudal (arterial/venous) topography by the time of the cardiac crescent stage. Cells within the first heart field are still plastic with regard to chamber specification: if caudal cardiac progenitor tissue is substituted for cranial cardiogenic tissue, proper hearts are generated. However, soon afterward, commitment to particular chambers is evident by the expression of chamber-specific regulators.

Regionalization of the heart is likely an outcome of having at least two separate heart areas within the first heart field. In mice, clonal analysis suggests that the atrial region becomes clonally distinct (i.e., clones of progenitor cells become restricted to a single compartment) before the rest of the heart. Tbx5 has been linked to atrial lineage determination. Initially expressed in the entire first heart field, Tbx5 expression becomes limited to the sinus venosus and atria, with some expression in the left ventricle (i.e., first heart field derivatives; Fig. 12-16). Tbx5 knockout mice exhibit severe hypoplasia of these chambers, whereas forced expression of Tbx5 throughout the heart leads to loss of ventricular-specific gene expression, essentially "atrializing" the heart. Mutations in human TBX5 have been identified in families with **Holt-Oram syndrome**, which includes heart chamber malformations, atrial septal defects, and cardiac conduction system anomalies. Irx4, an Iroquois homeoprotein, is expressed only in the cranial portion of the first heart field (Fig. 12-16); later, it is restricted to ventricular cells, where it stimulates the expression of ventricular myosin heavy chain-1 (Mhc1v) and suppresses atrial myosin heavy chain-1 (Mhc1a). Irx4 is thought to maintain the cranial-caudal phenotype of the heart by suppressing atrial commitment, because loss of Irx4 expression in mice leads to ectopic expression of atrial markers in the ventricles. Once the initial heart tube begins to lengthen and cardiac bending and looping begin, major changes occur in the expression of several chamber/region-restricted transcription factors, with the expression of a number of genes becoming increasingly restricted to atrial, atrioventricular, ventricular, and outflow tract regions. For example, Tbx20 encodes a transcription factor with heart chamber–promoting characteristics.

Tbx20 negatively regulates Tbx2, a transcription factor normally expressed in non-chamber myocardium, such as the wall of the atrioventricular canal and outflow tract, by sequestering receptor-mediated Smad signaling. Hence, Tbx20 and Tbx2 work in concert to delineate chamber from non-chamber myocardium along the cardiac tube.

Expression of several of the chamber-specific properties depends on many of the same cranial/caudal-patterning influences driving regionalization of the neural ectoderm and paraxial mesoderm. Application of excess retinoic acid during early chick embryo cardiogenesis causes "atrialization" or "caudalization" of the primitive heart tube, as indicated by ubiquitous expression of Tbx5 throughout the heart tube, whereas treatment with retinoic acid antagonists leads to "ventricularization." Atrial gene expression in mice is similarly expanded with retinoic acid treatments in utero. A potential mechanism for localized retinoid signaling in embryos is the restricted expression of retinaldehyde dehydrogenenase-2 (Raldh-2), a limiting enzyme in retinoic acid biosynthesis. Restricted expression of Raldh-2 to the caudal border of the cardiogenic field is correlated with the caudal limit of atrial gene expression in both chick and mouse embryos. Mouse embryos deficient in Raldh-2 have reduced Tbx5 expression in the caudal heart field, lack atria and limbs, and die in utero. Recent studies support the hypothesis that retinoic acid plays an essential role in establishing the caudal boundary of the cardiogenic field.

COORDINATED REMODELING OF HEART TUBE AND PRIMITIVE VASCULATURE PRODUCES SYSTEMIC AND PULMONARY CIRCULATIONS

At day twenty-two, the primitive circulatory system is bilaterally symmetrical: right and left cardinal veins (common, anterior, and posterior) drain the two sides of the body, and blood from the heart is pumped into right and left aortic arches and dorsal aortae. The

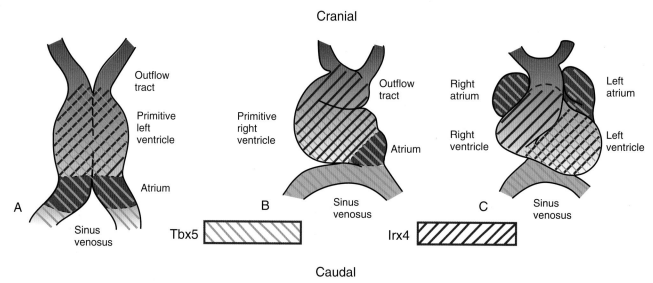

Figure 12-16. Schematic depiction of expression patterns of the transcription factors Tbx5 and Irx4 during early specification of the cardiac chambers. *A-C,* Ventral views at three stages of heart development. Tbx5, linked to the atrial phenotype, becomes increasingly restricted to the atria and the sinus venosus, whereas Irx4, a transcription factor that drives Mhc1v expression and suppresses Mhc1a expression, becomes increasingly restricted to ventricular cells. The thickness of the lines indicates the levels of gene expression, with thicker lines representing higher levels of expression than thinner lines.

paired dorsal aortae fuse at axial levels T4 to L4 during the fourth week to form a single midline dorsal aorta. The venous system undergoes a complicated remodeling (detailed in Chapter 13), with the result that all systemic venous blood drains into the right atrium through the newly formed superior and inferior caval veins.

The heart starts to beat on day twenty-one, and by day twenty-four to twenty-five, blood begins to circulate throughout the embryo. Venous return initially enters the right and left sinus horns via the common cardinal, umbilical, and vitelline veins (Fig. 12-17). Within the next few weeks, the venous system is remodeled so that all systemic venous blood enters the right sinus horn via the **superior** and **inferior caval veins** (Fig. 12-17). As venous inflow shifts to the right, the left sinus horn ceases to grow and is transformed into a small venous sac on the posterior wall of the heart (see Fig. 12-17). This structure gives rise to the **coronary sinus** and the small **oblique vein of the left atrium**. The coronary sinus will receive most of the blood draining from the coronary circulation of the heart.

As the right sinus horn and the caval veins enlarge to keep pace with the rapid growth of the rest of the heart, the right side of the sinus venosus is gradually incorporated into the right caudal/dorsal wall of the developing atrium, displacing the original right half of the primitive atrial wall farther to the right (Figs. 12-17, 12-18). The differential growth of the right sinus venosus also repositions the vestigial left sinus horn (the future coronary sinus) to the right. The portion of the atrium consisting of the incorporated sinus venosus is now called the **sinus venarum**. The original right

side of the primitive atrium can be distinguished in the adult heart by the pectinate (comb-like) trabeculation of its wall, which contrasts with the smooth wall of the sinus venarum.

Through a process of **intussusception** (folding in of an outer layer) of the right sinus venosus, the openings, or **ostia**, of the superior and inferior caval veins and future coronary sinus are incorporated into the dorsal wall of the definitive right atrium, where they form the **orifices of the superior and inferior caval veins** and the **orifice of the coronary sinus** (Fig. 12-18B). As this occurs, a pair of tissue flaps, the **left** and **right venous valves**, develops on either side of the three ostia (see Fig. 12-18B). Cranial to the sinuatrial orifices, the left and right valves join to form a transient septum called the **septum spurium**, which, along with the left venous valve, becomes part of the septum secundum, one of the septa contributing to the separation of the definitive right and left atria (covered later in the chapter). The right venous valve persists and contributes to the formation of the **terminal crest (crista terminalis)**, the **valve of the inferior caval vein**, and **valves of the coronary sinus**. Incorporation of the sinus venosus tissue into the dorsal wall of the right atrium results in remodeling of the right atrial chamber and the formation of the **right atrial appendage** (the **right auricle**).

The terminal crest now delimits the trabeculated right atrium from the smooth-walled sinus venarum (see Fig. 12-18B). The **sinoatrial node**, the cardiac pacemaker, is an important element of the cardiac conducting system and is located at the junction of the superior caval vein and the terminal crest. The cardiac impulse generated in the sinoatrial node reaches

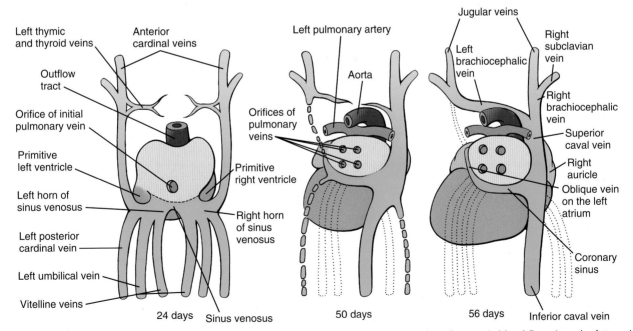

Figure 12-17. Remodeling of the inflow end of the heart between weeks four and eight so that all systemic blood flows into the future right atrium. The left sinus horn is reduced and pulled to the right side. It loses its connection with the left anterior cardinal vein and becomes the coronary sinus, draining blood only from the heart wall. The left anterior cardinal vein becomes connected to the right anterior cardinal vein through an anastomosis of thymic and thyroid veins, which form the left brachiocephalic vein. A remnant of the right vitelline vein becomes the terminal segment of the inferior caval vein (covered in Chapter 13).

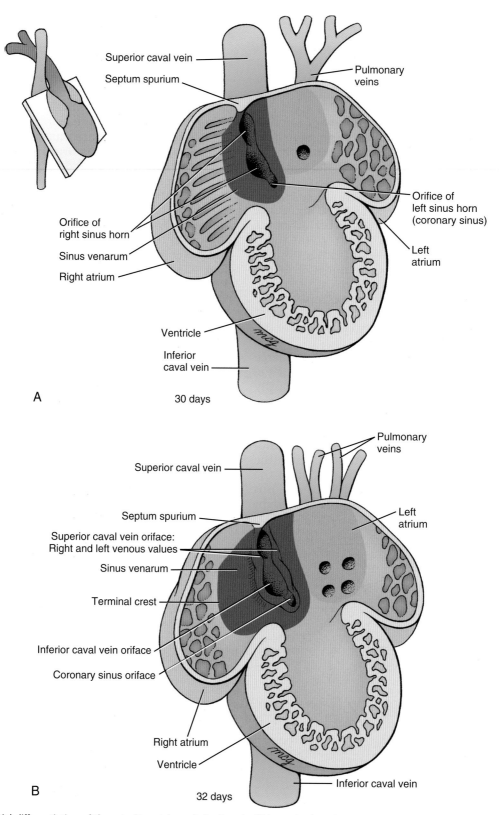

Figure 12-18. Initial differentiation of the primitive atrium. *A*, During the fifth week, the primitive atrial tissue on the left and right sides is displaced ventrally and laterally to form the trabeculated portion of the atria and auricles of the mature heart. On the right side, the right sinus horn is incorporated into the dorsal wall of the right side of the atrium as the smooth-walled sinus venarum. Meanwhile, a single pulmonary vein develops in the left side of the primitive atrium and then branches twice to produce two right and two left pulmonary veins. The sinus venarum continues to expand within the dorsal wall of the future right atrium. *B*, Further differentiation of the atrium. Later in the fifth week, the pulmonary vein system begins to undergo intussusception into the left dorsal wall of the primitive atrium. The first four pulmonary branches are incorporated into the dorsal wall of the left side of the primitive atrium, completing the formation of the smooth-walled part of the future left atrium.

the **atrioventricular node** using several preferred pathways.

While the right atrium is being remodeled during the fourth and fifth weeks, the left atrium undergoes a somewhat similar process. During the fourth week, the **pulmonary vein** originates as a midline structure within the caudal **dorsal mesocardium**, which connects the lung rudiments to the dorsal wall of the developing common atrium. From its initial midline position, the pulmonary vein shifts to the left (see Figs. 12-17, 12-18A) as a result of asymmetrical growth of a projection of second heart field mesenchymal cells called the **dorsal mesenchymal protrusion** or **spina vestibuli**. The pulmonary vein promptly splits into right and left pulmonary branches, which bifurcate again to produce a total of four pulmonary veins. These veins then grow toward the lungs, where they anastomose with veins developing within the mesoderm investing the bronchial buds (covered in Chapter 11). As a result of intussusception, the pulmonary venous system opens into the left atrium initially through a single orifice and eventually through four orifices forming the definitive pulmonary veins (see Fig. 12-18A, B), where they form the smooth wall of the definitive left atrium. The trabeculated left side of the primitive atrium is also displaced ventrally and to the left, where it forms a **left atrial appendage** (the **left auricle**).

SEPTATION OF HEART

 Animation 12-4: Partitioning of AV Canal.
Animations are available online at StudentConsult.

Structural and functional partitioning of the heart into four chambers is accomplished through the process called **valvuloseptal morphogenesis**, which encompasses septation (formation of septal structures) and valvulogenesis (formation of valves). Major events for cardiac septation occur between days twenty-eight and thirty-seven of gestation. Two basic processes play key roles in generating septa. Differential growth and remodeling are mainly responsible for generating the muscular ventricular and atrial septa, but these processes alone never fully partition the heart chambers. For that, endocardium-derived and neural crest cell–derived cushion tissue is required. In the atrioventricular and outflow tract regions, while cardiac looping continues, extracellular matrix is secreted between endocardium and myocardium, chiefly by the myocardial layer (Fig. 12-19A). This essentially causes the endocardial layer to balloon into the lumen of these two regions. Near the completion of cardiac looping, some of the endocardial cells in the atrioventricular and outflow tract regions undergo an **epithelial-to-mesenchymal transformation** (EMT), generating endocardium-derived mesenchyme that invades this extracellular matrix, proliferates, and differentiates into connective tissue. These mesenchyme-filled bulges (in the atrioventricular region) and ridges (along the length of the outflow tract) are often referred to as **cushion tissues** (Figs. 12-19B, 12-20).

After the initial formation of the endocardium-derived atrioventricular cushions, **epicardium-derived mesenchymal cells** also populate the atrioventricular cushions. As covered later in the chapter, not only does the cushion tissue of the outflow tract contain endocardium-derived cells, but these ridges are also invaded by neural crest cells. Thus, the cushion tissue of the outflow tract consists of both mesoderm-derived mesenchymal cells **(endocardium-derived cushion tissue)** and ectoderm-derived mesenchymal cells **(neural crest cell–derived cushion tissue)** (Fig. 12-19B). Proper development of atrioventricular and outflow tract cushion tissues is essential for completing septation. Two major atrioventricular cushions fuse and contribute to the separation of the atria and ventricles, generate the membranous (or fibrous) portion of the ventricular and atrial septa, and, together with lateral cushions, are involved in the formation of atrioventricular valves (see Fig. 12-19B). The outflow tract cushions are involved in separation of the aorta from the pulmonary artery, ventricular septation, and in formation of the semilunar valves.

In the Research Lab

EPITHELIAL-TO-MESENCHYMAL TRANSFORMATION DURING ENDOCARDIAL CUSHION CELL FORMATION

The epithelial-to-mesenchymal transformation (EMT) of the endocardium can be separated into two major steps: activation (signaling) of the event, which includes induction and cell-cell separation of a subpopulation of endocardial cells; and (2) delamination and invasion of endocardium-derived cells into underlying extracellular matrix. Once populating the extracellular matrix, these cells proliferate and differentiate into various connective tissue cell types.

What triggers the EMT of the endocardium, and why does this process occur only in the atrioventricular and outflow tract regions of the heart? The answer to this fundamental question is still unclear. Early studies using chick embryos and three-dimensional tissue culture models show that only the atrioventricular and outflow tract myocardium is competent to induce EMT of the endocardium, and that only atrioventricular and outflow tract endocardium is capable of responding. The inducing factor(s) is (are) released into the extracellular matrix by the myocardium, but the precise nature of this signal is still unclear. One possibility is a multicomponent aggregate referred to as the ES (EDTA soluble) complex. Expression of this complex within the heart is restricted to the atrioventricular and outflow tract regions, and antibodies directed against this complex block EMT.

One of the earliest signs of endocardial activation is that a subset of endocardial cells hypertrophy (in this case, the rough endoplasmic reticulum enlarges and the Golgi apparatus becomes more prevalent). Soon, this is followed by morphological signs of cell-cell separation in a subset of endocardial cells and is accompanied by downregulation of cell-cell adhesion molecules, including N-Cam (neural cell adhesion molecule), VE-cadherin (vascular endothelial-cadherin), and Pe-Cam-1 (platelet endothelial cell adhesion molecule-1). If these cell-cell adhesion molecules are not downregulated, EMT fails.

Endocardial EMT recapitulates many of the same steps as the EMT responsible for gastrulation and neural crest cell formation (covered in Chapters 3 and 4, respectively). In chick embryos,

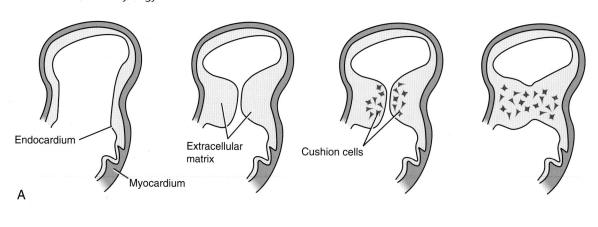

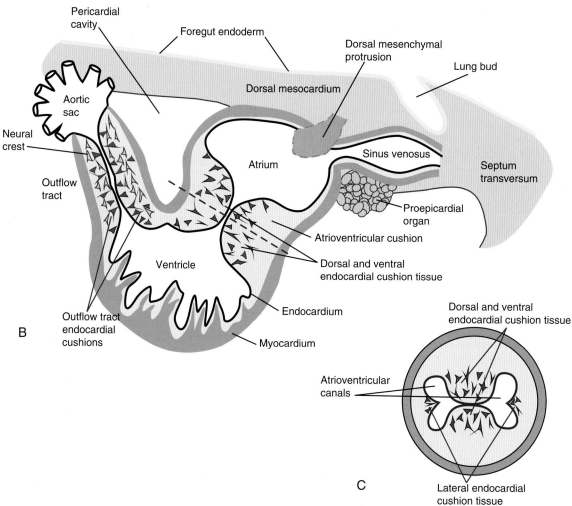

Figure 12-19. Cushion tissue formation. *A,* Steps in the formation of endocardium-derived cushion tissue. The myocardium deposits a unique extracellular matrix between the endocardium and itself at a specific stage in development. This induces an epithelial-to-mesenchymal transformation of the endocardium, resulting in the generation of migrating endocardial cushion cells necessary for cardiac septation. *B,* Sites of cushion tissue formation in the heart. Endocardium-derived cushion tissue forms in the atrioventricular region and the outflow tract region (which is also populated by invading neural crest cells). Eventual fusion of opposing cushion tissues forms the atrioventricular canals, outlets of both ventricles, the aorta and pulmonary trunk, and membranous portions of the interatrial and interventricular septa. Dashed line represents the level of the cross section illustrated in *C* and shows the atrioventricular cushion tissue and canals and the small lateral cushion tissue.

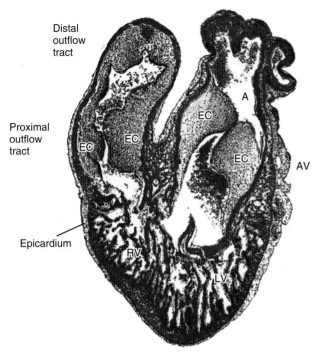

Figure 12-20. Photomicrograph of a sagittal section through a chick embryo heart showing endocardial cushion (EC) tissue surrounding the atrioventricular canal and within the outflow tract. A, Atrium; AV, atrioventricular region; RV and LV, right and left ventricles, respectively.

expression of snail2 (a zinc finger transcription factor) is upregulated in endocardial cells before EMT and during early migration of cushion cells, and blocking Snail2 expression prevents EMT of the endocardium in tissue culture. Notch1 and several of its ligands (covered in Chapter 5) are expressed in mouse endocardium at the time of EMT initiation, and notch1 null mice exhibit impaired EMT and develop hypoplastic endocardial cushion tissue. This impaired EMT correlates with reduced expression of snail and failure to downregulate VE-cadherin. Once activated, endocardial cells begin to extend filopodia into the extracellular matrix and to upregulate invasive cell markers (e.g., matrix metalloproteinases, serine proteases, hyaluronate synthetases, rho-associated kinases). This is soon followed by the transformation of this endocardial subset into mesenchymal cells that migrate and invade the extracellular matrix between endocardium and myocardium.

There are several growth factors, growth factor receptors, and transcription factors whose expression is required for the initial phase of EMT. Members of the Tgfβ family have important roles in initiating endocardial EMT. Blocking Tgfβ2 expression or neutralizing its activity using antibodies in the chick embryo inhibits both cell-cell separation and the invasive steps leading to EMT, whereas blocking Tgfβ3 inhibits EMT only after the cell-cell separation step has occurred. An important role for Tgfβs in EMT is supported by mouse Tgfβ knockout mutants, which exhibit atrioventricular valve defects, semilunar valve defects, and atrial septal defects. At least five different Bmps (another member of the Tgfβ family) are also expressed by atrioventricular and outflow tract myocardium. In mice, Bmp2 and Bmp4 are expressed in the myocardium beneath the atrioventricular and outflow tract endocardium. Using the chick tissue culture model, knocking down Bmp2 expression significantly reduces endocardial cushion cell migration; in mouse atrioventricular endocardial cultures, Bmp2 can substitute for the myocardium. These studies show that Bmp2 expressed by the myocardium has both autocrine and paracrine effects,

upregulating the expression of Tgfβ2 in both myocardium and endocardium, resulting in induction of endocardial EMT.

Both the growth factor, Vegf, and the transcription factor family, Nfatc (nuclear factor of activated T cells isoform c), play important roles in endocardial EMT and subsequent valve development. Vegf signaling activity is dose dependent and is dynamically controlled within a narrow spatial and developmental window during cushion and valve development. In mice at the onset of EMT, Vegf expression occurs in both endocardium and myocardium. If Vegf signaling is too high or too low, EMT does not occur. Specific isoforms of Nfatc (c2, c3, and c4) expressed in the myocardium are responsible for reducing Vegf signaling to levels necessary for initiating EMT. Once initiated, myocardial expression of Vegf begins to increase, and this increase is thought to play a role in terminating endocardial EMT. Both Vegf signaling and activity of the Nfatc1 isoform within the endocardium are also required for subsequent valve remodeling. Hence, proper spatial/temporal Vegf signaling and Nfatc transcriptional activity are required for EMT and valve differentiation and, if atypical, lead to abnormal heart development.

A myriad of other growth factors and growth factor receptors have been implicated or shown to have important roles in signaling endocardial EMT, including Egfs, Fgfs, and ephrins. Several other transcription factors are also important for proper cushion formation and valve development, many of which have been implicated in EMTs and mesenchymal tissue development elsewhere in the embryo, including Msx1 and Msx2, Prx1 and Prx2, Id, and Sox4.

EFFECTS OF HYPERGLYCEMIA AND HYPOXIA ON CUSHION TISSUE FORMATION

Neonates born to diabetic mothers have an almost three-fold increased risk of having congenital heart defects. Because the risk can be reduced by strict maternal glycemic control, hyperglycemia seems to be the teratogenic agent. In mice, hyperglycemic conditions inhibit the EMT required for cushion development. Hyperglycemia inhibits the release of Vegf from the myocardium, leading to retention of Pe-Cam-1 in endocardial cells. As mentioned earlier, endocardial cushion tissue formation requires proper levels of Vegf signaling and turnover of cell-cell adhesion molecules before the EMT. The effects of hyperglycemia on endocardial EMT in mice are mimicked by blocking the bioavailability of endogenous Vegf, and this is reversed by adding back appropriate levels of Vegf. Hypoxia increases the release of Vegf and, likewise, inhibits endocardial cushion formation. Thus, the negative effects of hyperglycemia and hypoxia on endocardial EMT are likely due to failure in maintaining proper Vegf signaling.

SEPTATION OF ATRIA AND DIVISION OF ATRIOVENTRICULAR CANAL

Animation 12-5: Partitioning of Atrium.
Animations are available online at StudentConsult.

A required step in separation of the systemic and pulmonary circulations consists of partial separation of the definitive atria and division of the common atrioventricular canal into right and left canals. The mature atrial septum is formed by the fusion of two embryonic partial muscular septa: the **septum primum** and the **septum secundum**. Both of these septa have openings that allow right-to-left shunting of blood throughout gestation. This shunting is required for normal development and expansion of the left atrium and left ventricle, and it permits oxygenated blood from the umbilicus to bypass the developing pulmonary system and enter the systemic circulation.

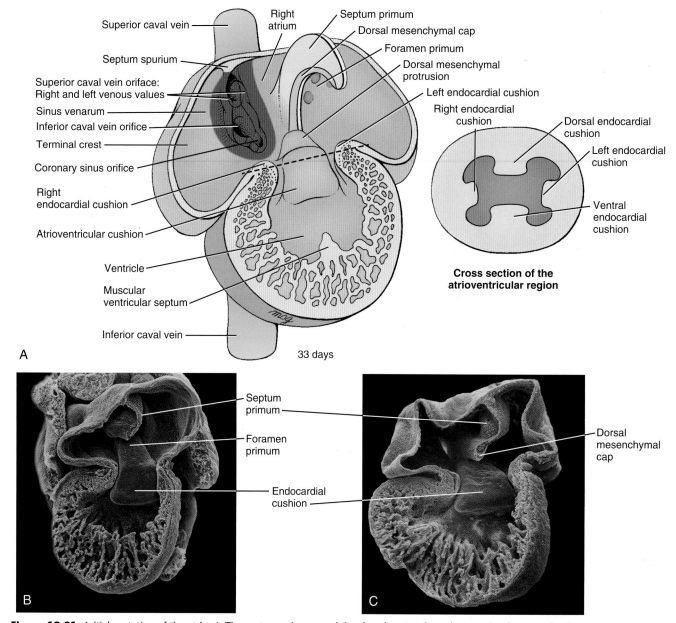

Figure 12-21. Initial septation of the atria. *A,* The septum primum and the dorsal mesenchymal protrusion form on the dorsal roof of the atrial chamber during the fifth week and grow together toward the atrioventricular canal. A ridge of endocardium-derived mesenchymal cells, called the dorsal mesenchymal cap, develops along the rim of the septum primum. Simultaneously, the atrioventricular canal is divided into right and left atrioventricular orifices by the growing dorsal and ventral endocardial cushions. Dashed line represents the level of the cross section through the atrioventricular canal region. *B, C,* Scanning electron micrographs show foramen primum and the developing septum primum and its dorsal mesenchymal cap.

On about day twenty-six, while atrial remodeling is ongoing, the roof of the atrium develops a depression along the midline at the site beneath the overlying outflow tract. On day twenty-eight, this deepening depression results in a crescent-shaped myocardial wedge, called the septum primum, which extends into the atrium from the cranial-dorsal wall as the primitive atrial chamber expands (Fig. 12-21*A*). On the leading edge of the septum primum, a mesenchyme-filled ridge called the **dorsal mesenchymal cap** is found, which, like the atrioventricular and outflow tract cushions, contains endocardially derived mesenchyme (Fig. 12-21*A-C*). Meanwhile at the venous pole, second heart field–derived cells project

into the atrium using the dorsal mesocardium as a port-of-entry (see Fig. 12-19*B*). This cell population, called the **dorsal mesenchymal protrusion** (or **spina vestibuli**), is contiguous with the dorsal mesenchymal cap on the septum primum and the dorsal atrioventricular cushion (Figs. 12-21*A*, 12-22*A*).

As the septum primum elongates by differential growth, the dorsal and ventral atrioventricular cushions fuse to form the **atrioventricular septum** (or **septum intermedium**), thereby dividing the common atrioventricular orifice into separate **right** and **left atrioventricular canals** (see Fig. 12-22*A*). The dorsal mesenchymal cap, dorsal mesenchymal protrusion, and atrioventricular

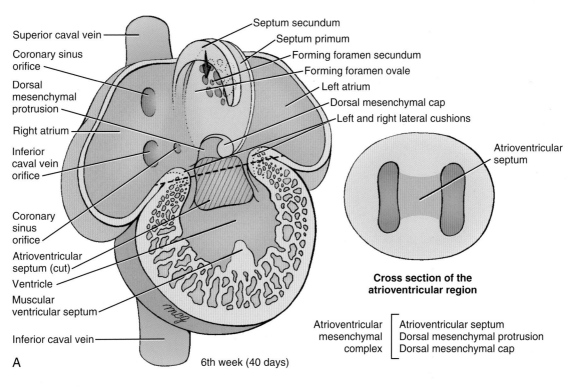

Superior caval vein
Coronary sinus orifice
Dorsal mesenchymal protrusion
Right atrium
Inferior caval vein orifice
Coronary sinus orifice
Atrioventricular septum (cut)
Ventricle
Muscular ventricular septum
Inferior caval vein

Septum secundum
Septum primum
Forming foramen secundum
Forming foramen ovale
Left atrium
Dorsal mesenchymal cap
Left and right lateral cushions

Atrioventricular septum

Cross section of the atrioventricular region

Atrioventricular mesenchymal complex
[Atrioventricular septum
Dorsal mesenchymal protrusion
Dorsal mesenchymal cap]

A   6th week (40 days)

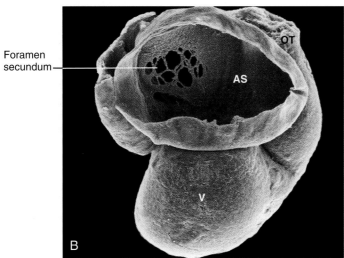

Foramen secundum

OT
AS
V

B

Mid 6th week (38 days)

Figure 12-22. Further septation of the atria. *A,* During the sixth week, the thick septum secundum grows from the roof of the right atrium, and the septum primum, its dorsal mesenchymal cap, and the dorsal mesenchymal protrusion fuse with the atrioventricular cushion to fill the foramen primum. However, before the foramen primum is obliterated, the foramen secundum forms by the coalescence of small ruptures in the septum primum. Dashed line represents the level of the cross section through the atrioventricular canal region. *B,* Scanning electron micrograph showing the development of the foramen secundum. AS, Atrial septum; OT, outflow tract; V, ventricle.

septum then fuse to form the **atrioventricular mesenchymal complex**, filling the remaining interatrial connection **(foramen primum** or **ostium primum)** (see Figs. 12-21, 12-22*A*, 12-23). As the atrioventricular mesenchymal complex closes the foramen primum, programmed cell death in the dorsal region of the septum primum creates small perforations that coalesce to form a new foramen, the **foramen secundum** (or **ostium secundum**) (see Fig. 12-22*A, B*). Thus, a new channel for right-to-left shunting between atrial chambers opens before the old one closes.

While the septum primum is lengthening, a second crescent-shaped ridge of tissue forms on the ceiling of the right atrium, just adjacent to and to the right of the septum primum (see Fig. 12-22*A*). This **septum secundum** is thick and muscular, in contrast to the thin septum primum. The edge of the septum secundum grows cranial-caudally and dorsal-ventrally, but it halts before it reaches the atrioventricular mesenchymal complex, leaving an opening called the **foramen ovale** near the floor of the right atrium (see Figs. 12-22*A*, 12-23). Therefore, throughout the rest of fetal

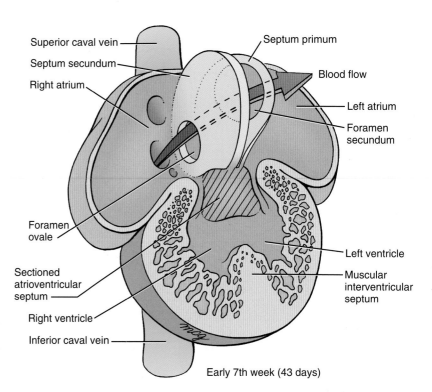

Superior caval vein
Septum secundum
Right atrium
Foramen ovale
Sectioned atrioventricular septum
Right ventricle
Inferior caval vein

Septum primum
Blood flow
Left atrium
Foramen secundum
Left ventricle
Muscular interventricular septum

Early 7th week (43 days)

Figure 12-23. Definitive fetal septation of the atria. The septum secundum does not completely close, leaving an opening in this septum called the foramen ovale. During embryonic and fetal life, much of the blood entering the right atrium passes to the left atrium via the foramen ovale and the foramen secundum.

development, blood shunts from the right atrium to the left atrium and passes through the two staggered openings. This arrangement allows blood to flow from the right atrium to the left atrium, but not in the reverse direction, as the thin septum primum collapses against the stiff septum secundum, effectively blocking blood flow back into the right atrium. This shunt closes at birth because abrupt dilation of the pulmonary vasculature combined with cessation of umbilical flow reverses the pressure difference between the atria and pushes the flexible septum primum against the more rigid septum secundum, even during atrial diastole (see "Dramatic Changes Occur in Circulatory System at Birth," in Chapter 13).

REALIGNMENT OF PRIMITIVE CHAMBERS

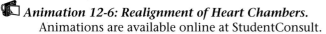 *Animation 12-6: Realignment of Heart Chambers.*
Animations are available online at StudentConsult.

Even after cardiac looping is nearly finished, the atrioventricular canal provides a direct pathway only between the primitive atrium and the primitive left ventricle (Fig. 12-24A). Moreover, the proximal end of the primitive right ventricle, but not the primitive left ventricle, is initially continuous with the outflow tract, which will give rise to both aortic and pulmonary outflow vessels. Proper cardiac tube looping, chamber expansion, and realignment must occur to bring the developing atrioventricular canal into alignment with the right atrium and the right ventricle, and to provide the left ventricle with a direct path to the outflow tract. This process is illustrated in Figure 12-24.

The atrioventricular canal initially lies mainly between the primitive atrium and the primitive left

ventricle. The mechanism by which the right and left atrioventricular canals come into alignment with the future right and left ventricles is unclear. However, this change may be accomplished by active remodeling of the **primary muscular fold**. Beneath the right (tricuspid) portion of the atrioventricular canal, a small slit forms in the myocardium of the **muscular ventricular septum**. This slit expands to form a proper right ventricular inflow tract, enabling the tricuspid orifice to become positioned above the right ventricle (Fig. 12-24C). At the same time, the left part of the common outflow tract becomes more associated with the left ventricle. Meanwhile, the dorsal and ventral atrioventricular cushions are growing, and by the time the common atrioventricular canal has split into right and left canals, the latter are correctly aligned with their respective atria and ventricles (see Fig. 12-24C).

Once the atrioventricular canals, ventricles, and cardiac outflow tract are all correctly aligned, the stage is set for the remaining phases of heart morphogenesis: completion of atrial septation, septation of the ventricles, septation of the outflow tract into ascending aorta and pulmonary trunk, and development of heart valves, coronary vasculature, and conduction system.

INITIATION OF SEPTATION OF VENTRICLES

Animation 12-7: Partitioning of Ventricle.
Animations are available online at StudentConsult.

At the end of the fourth week, the **muscular ventricular septum**, located between the presumptive right and left ventricular chambers, begins to become a more prominent structure as the ventricles are in the

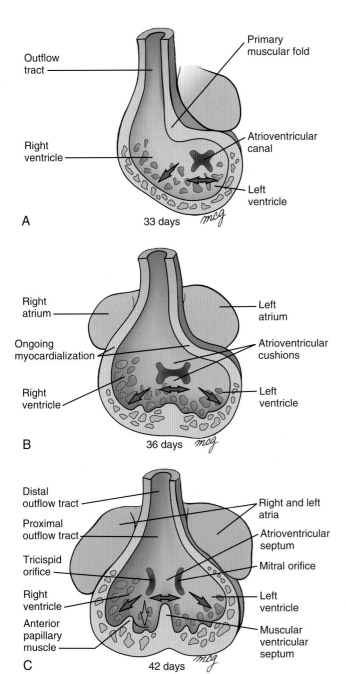

Outflow tract

Primary muscular fold

Right ventricle

Atrioventricular canal

Left ventricle

A 33 days

Right atrium

Left atrium

Ongoing myocardialization

Atrioventricular cushions

Right ventricle

Left ventricle

B 36 days

Distal outflow tract

Right and left atria

Proximal outflow tract

Atrioventricular septum

Tricispid orifice

Mitral orifice

Right ventricle

Left ventricle

Anterior papillary muscle

Muscular ventricular septum

C 42 days

Figure 12-24. *A-C,* Realignment of the heart. As the atrioventricular septum forms during the fifth and sixth weeks, the heart is remodeled to align the developing left atrioventricular canal with the left atrium and ventricle, and the right atrioventricular canal with the right atrium and ventricle. Red arrows indicate the direction of realignment of the atrioventricular canal and outflow tract and formation of the muscular interventricular septum. The blue arrow in *C* indicates formation of an enlarging slit carved out of the muscular ventricular septum; this is responsible in part for repositioning of the tricuspid orifice to the right, as well as for formation of the moderator band.

process of expanding (Fig. 12-25; see also Fig. 12-24). Although the muscular ventricular septum continues to grow, closure of the **interventricular foramen (primary ventricular foramen)** does not occur until the eighth week of development. If fusion of the

muscular ventricular septum with the atrioventricular mesenchymal complex would occur too soon, the left ventricle would be shut off from the ventricular outflow tract.

At the same time that the muscular ventricular septum is forming, the myocardium begins to thicken and myocardial ridges or **trabeculae** develop on the inner wall of both ventricles. Trabeculation begins at about the fourth week of development, with projections or ridges first forming in the outer curvature of the heart. These trabecular ridges are transformed into fenestrated trabecular sheets while the outer cardiomyocytes adjacent to the epicardium rapidly proliferate, forming an outer compact layer of myocardium (Figs. 12-25, 12-26).

On the right wall of the muscular ventricular septum, a prominent trabeculation called the **septomarginal trabeculation (moderator band)** develops. Owing to expansion of the right ventricular chamber inlet, the septomarginal trabeculation crosses the right lateral wall, extending toward the developing anterior papillary muscle of the tricuspid valve (see Fig. 12-24C). Expansion of the right ventricular chamber inlet drives formation of a large part of the mature right ventricular chamber. If expansion of this area is insufficient, the developing tricuspid portion of the atrioventricular canal can remain associated with the primary ventricular foramen, leading to tricuspid atresia and other valve anomalies.

In the Research Lab

MYOCARDIUM DEVELOPS TWO LAYERS

As mentioned earlier, the myocardial wall develops two basic layers: an inner **trabecular layer** of myocardium and an outer **compact layer** of myocardium. The trabecular layer contributes to cardiac contraction and increases the inner surface area, thereby facilitating nutritional and gaseous exchange while the coronary vasculature is developing. Trabeculae grow from clonal expansion of myocardial cells, leading to the formation of these myocardial infoldings (see Figs. 12-25, 12-26). In mice, the Egf receptors ErbB2 and ErbB3 (expressed in the myocardium) and one of their ligands, neuregulin (expressed in the endocardium), are required for trabecular development, as well as for gestational survival. In humans, overproduction of trabeculae at the expense of the compact myocardial layer leads to **isolated ventricular non-compaction**, a condition that can cause sudden heart failure. Formation of the outer compact layer of myocardium requires an interaction with the developing epicardium. A thin compact layer of myocardium can be the result of deficiencies in the interaction between epicardium-derived cells and outer myocardial wall. For example, in mice null for the retinoic acid receptor, RXRα, proliferation of myocardial cells in the compact layer fails and the mice die early in utero. Retinoic acid receptors are expressed in epicardial cells; in response to retinoic acid, the epicardium releases Fgfs that stimulate myocardial cell proliferation. In the absence of retinoic acid signaling, cardiomyocytes prematurely differentiate and hypertrophy rather than proliferate first. These mice exhibit dilated cardiomyopathy at birth.

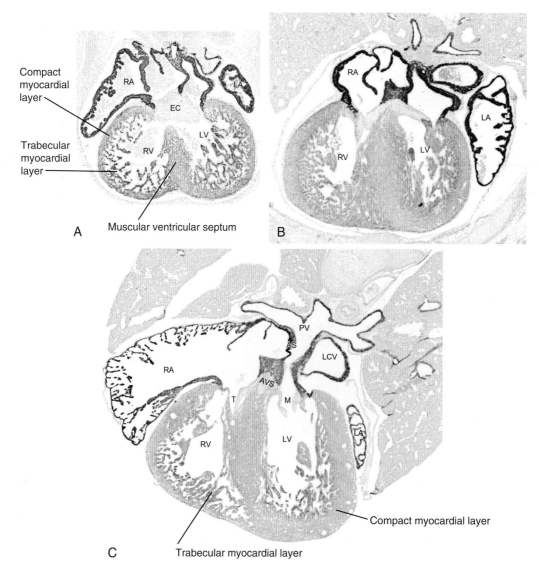

Figure 12-25. Photomicrographs showing the development of the atrioventricular valve, the muscular ventricular septum, and the trabecular and compact layers of myocardium in the developing mouse embryo. *A-C,* Tissue samples were immunostained with an antibody recognizing, a light chain atrial form of myosin expressed in both atria and ventricles at this stage of development. AS, Atrial septum; AVS, atrioventricular septum; EC, endocardial cushion tissues; LCV, left coronary vein; M and T, developing mitral and tricuspid valves, respectively; PV, pulmonary vein; RA and LA, right and left atria, respectively; RV and LV, right and left ventricles, respectively; VS, muscular ventricular septum.

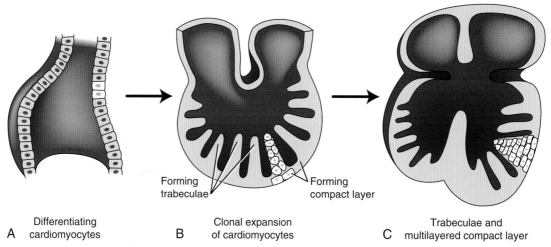

Figure 12-26. Formation of cardiac trabeculae. *A-C,* Myocardial trabeculae develop from clonal expansion of cardiomyocytes within the myocardial wall and are subsequently remodeled as the heart increases in size. Clonal expansion of the compact layer into a multilayered myocardium requires tissue-tissue interactions with the developing epicardium.

DEVELOPMENT OF ATRIOVENTRICULAR VALVES

Animation 12-8: Formation of AV Valves.
Animations are available online at StudentConsult.

The atrioventricular valves begin to form between the fifth and eighth weeks. These **valve leaflets** are firmly rooted in connective tissue (the **fibrous annulus**) surrounding the right and left atrioventricular canals and are thought to arise from proliferation and differentiation of the adjacent endocardial cushion tissues. How the mature valves are formed is not fully understood. Morphological and lineage tracing studies in several animal models show that the bulk of the leaflet cells are derived from endocardial cushion tissue with some contribution of cells coming from the epicardium (Fig. 12-27*A*, *B*). The leaflets are freed from the myocardial wall by remodeling and erosion of the ventricular myocardial wall. This leads to the formation of ventricular outpockets beneath the valve primordia and leaves thin strands of cells that form the **chordae tendineae** and small hillocks of myocardium called **papillary muscles** (Fig. 12-27*B*, *C*). The valve leaflets are designed so that they fold back to allow blood to enter the ventricles from the atria during diastole but shut to prevent backflow when the ventricles contract during systole. The left atrioventricular valve has only anterior and posterior leaflets and is called the **mitral (bicuspid) valve** The right atrioventricular valve usually (but not always) develops a third, small **septal cusp** during the third month; therefore, it is called the **tricuspid valve** (see Fig. 12-27*C*).

SEPTATION OF OUTFLOW TRACT AND COMPLETION OF VENTRICULAR SEPTATION

Animation 12-9: Partitioning of Outflow Tract.
Animations are available online at StudentConsult.

Animation 12-10: Formation of Membranous Interventricular Septum.
Animations are available online at StudentConsult.

When the muscular ventricular septum ceases to grow, the two ventricles still communicate with each other through the interventricular foramen (Fig. 12-28*A-C*). Separation of the outflow tract and ventricles must be coordinated with realignment of the outflow tract relative to the ventricles if the heart is to function properly. It is not surprising to note that a large proportion of cardiac

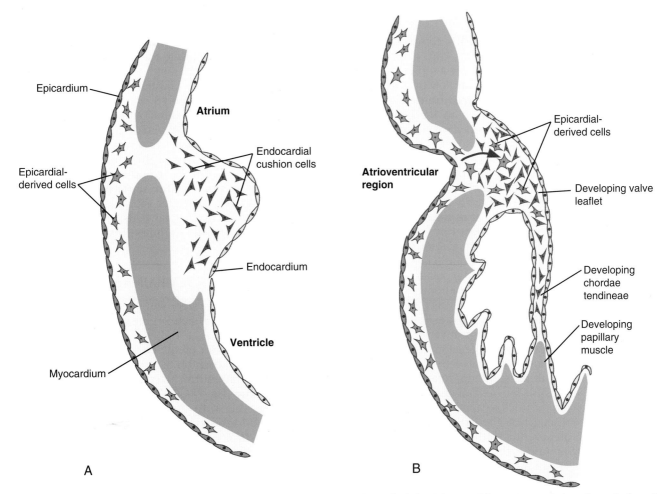

A

B

Figure 12-27. Development of the atrioventricular valves. *A, B,* Portion of the wall of the right ventricle at two stages in atrioventicular valve development. The structures composing the atrioventricular valves, including the papillary muscles, chordae tendineae, and cusps, are sculpted from the muscular walls of the ventricles. Valve leaflets are derived from endocardial cushion tissue, with some contribution from epicardium-derived cells entering along the margin of the atrioventricular region. Arrow in *B* indicates the direction of migration of these cells.

Continued

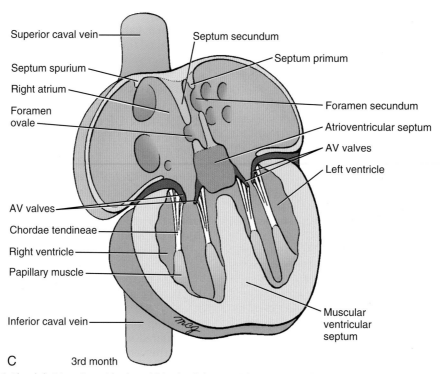

Superior caval vein
Septum secundum
Septum spurium
Septum primum
Right atrium
Foramen secundum
Foramen ovale
Atrioventricular septum
AV valves
Left ventricle
AV valves
Chordae tendineae
Right ventricle
Papillary muscle
Muscular ventricular septum
Inferior caval vein

C   3rd month

Figure 12-27, cont'd *C,* The definitive tricuspid valve within the right ventricle is not completely formed until the development of a septal cusp in the third month.

defects are the result of errors in this complex process (discussed later in the chapter).

Division of the cardiac outflow tract is complex and is not completely understood. The cardiac outflow tract is divided by the formation of a pair of **endocardium-derived outflow tract cushions** that develop in the lengthening outflow tract as second heart field–derived myocardium is added. These endocardial cushions can be discerned into proximal (conal) and distal (truncal) parts. The proximal cushions fuse to form the outflow septum and the wall of the conus portion of both ventricles. The proximal outflow tract septum (conal septum) eventually becomes muscularized through a process referred to as **myocardialization**, whereby the cushion cells are replaced by invading myocardial cells. In trisomy 16 mice (a model for **Down syndrome** in humans), this myocardialization fails, increasing the incidence of outflow tract–related septal defects, which are common in patients with Down syndrome.

The rotation process of the outflow tract and its cushion tissue is necessary for proper alignment of the aorta and pulmonary trunk with their respective ventricles. This realignment has been proposed to develop from the asymmetric addition of second heart field–derived myocardium at the arterial end, resulting in anterior rotation of the pulmonary orifice and trunk in front of the aorta with the aortic orifice remaining in close apposition with the left AV canal. As a consequence, the left and right ventricular outflow tracts and eventually the aorta and pulmonary trunk are twisted around each other in a helical arrangement (Fig. 12-28*D*)—an arrangement that is still obvious in the adult. In addition to the outflow tract septum, a mesenchymal wedge of tissue develops between the fourth and sixth aortic arch vessels (separating the future systemic and pulmonary circuits) in the roof of the aortic sac. This condensed wedge of neural crest–derived mesenchymal

tissue forms the **aorticopulmonary septum** (Fig. 12-29), which extends toward the developing outflow tract cushion swellings and fuses with them. Subsequent fusion of the paired outflow tract cushions then proceeds proximally (upstream of the blood flow), partitioning the distal part first and then the proximal outflow tract portion.

Separation of the right and left ventricles is completed when the muscular ventricular septum fuses with the outflow tract septum and the ventricular side of the atrioventricular septum. Development of this **membranous** part of the **ventricular septum** normally occurs between weeks five and eight. Failure of complete fusion results in a ventricular septal defect (see the following "In the Clinic" entitled "Common Heart Malformations: Ventricular Septal Defects").

DEVELOPMENT OF SEMILUNAR VALVES

Animation 12-11: Development of Semilunar Valves.
Animations are available online at StudentConsult.

During the formation of the outflow tract septum, two additional smaller cushion tissues form in opposite quadrants of the distal outflow tract called the **intercalated cushion tissue** (Fig. 12-30). The two major outflow tract cushions together with the lateral intercalated cushions are excavated to form cavities at the origin of the future ascending aorta and pulmonary artery. These cavities and the intervening tissue serve as the primordia for the **semilunar valves** and **semilunar sinuses**. Recent studies in mice show that semilunar valve leaflets are mainly of endocardium-derived cushion tissue origin, with some contribution by neural crest cells and possibly epicardial cells. Development of the semilunar valves is complete by nine weeks in humans.

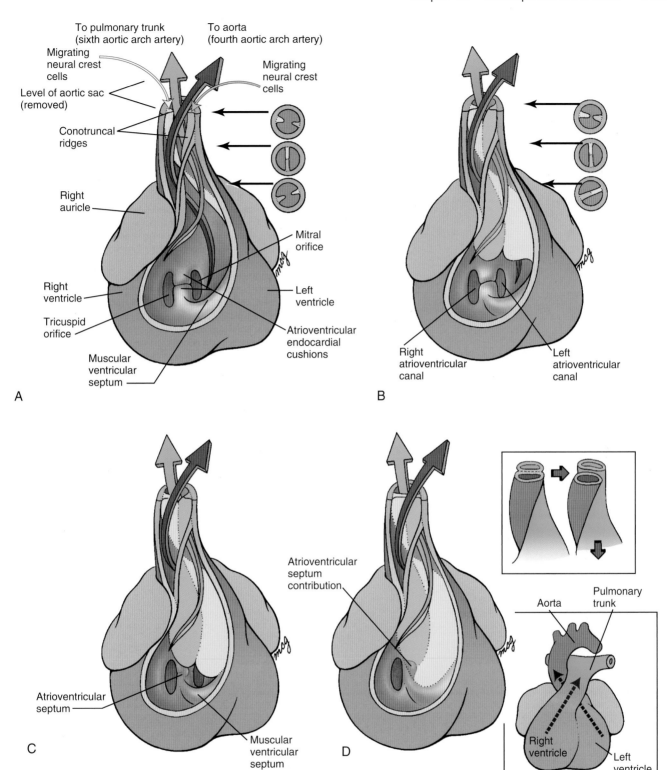

Figure 12-28. Septation of the cardiac outflow tract and completion of ventricular separation. Right oblique view. The cranial-lateral wall of the right ventricle has been removed to show the interior of the right ventricular chamber and the presumptive outflow tracts of both ventricles. *A, B,* Starting in the fifth week, the right and left conotruncal ridges grow out from the walls of the common outflow tract. These swellings are populated by endocardial and neural crest cell–derived cushion cells and develop in a spiraling configuration. They fuse with one another in a cranial-to-caudal direction, forming the conotruncal septum, which separates the aortic and pulmonary outflow tracts. The circular structures to the right of the developing outflow tract illustrate drawings of cross sections at three proximodistal levels. *C, D,* By the ninth week, the caudal end of the conotruncal septum has reached the level of the muscular portion of the ventricular septum and the atrioventricular septum. Here it fuses with these others to complete the ventricular septum.

In the Research Lab

NEURAL CREST CELL CONTRIBUTION TO OUTFLOW TRACT SEPTATION

The importance of neural crest cells in septation of the heart was first shown in ablation studies performed in chick embryos about thirty years ago. If the progenitors of cardiac neural crest cells are removed from embryos before neural crest cells begin to migrate, cardiac looping is abnormal and outflow tract septation is incomplete. Ablation of cardiac neural crest cells causes

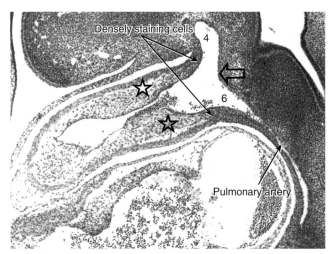

Figure 12-29. Division of the outflow tract in the human embryo. The developing aorticopulmonary septum (indicated by the open arrow) develops between the fourth (labeled 4) and sixth (labeled 6) aortic arch vessels in the roof of the aortic sac and extends toward the fusing outflow tract cushions (indicated by the stars). The densely stained cells include migrating neural crest cells.

persistent truncus arteriosus, tricuspid stenosis, ventricular septal defects, transposition of the great arteries, double-outlet right ventricle, and tetralogy of Fallot (see the following "In the Clinic" entitled "Common Heart Malformations: Tetralogy of Fallot"). Moreover, many structural cardiovascular congenital defects involve anomalies of the cardiac neural crest lineage. Further evidence for a role of neural crest cells in heart development is found in the frequent association of these cardiac anomalies with defects in development of the pharyngeal arch structures—through which the cardiac neural crest cells normally migrate. Birth defects in humans involving both the outflow tract and pharyngeal arches include **CHARGE syndrome** (coloboma of the eye, heart defects, atresia of the choanae, retarded growth and development, genital and urinary anomalies, and ear anomalies and hearing loss), **fetal alcohol syndrome**, and **22q11.2 deletion syndrome** (also known as **DiGeorge** or **velocardiofacial syndrome**; these syndromes are covered later and in Chapter 17).

Neural crest cells contributing to the outflow tract and the aorticopulmonary septum are derived from a specific level of the future rhombencephalon and are often referred to as **cardiac neural crest cells** (Fig. 12-31). Both cell-tracing studies using quail-chick transplantation chimeras and transgenic reporter mice (both experimental approaches are covered in Chapter 5) have revealed that not only do neural crest cells invade the outflow tract endocardial cushions, but a subset invade and localize adjacent to the ventricular septum and atrioventricular canal, with some also entering the venous inflow tract. Moreover, evidence suggests that after a time, these neural crest cells undergo apoptosis. What their role is in these regions is unclear, but it may relate to the remodeling that is required to realign the atrioventricular canal and the myocardialization processes in the proximal outflow tract region and in the inflow region. In addition to contributing to the connective tissue and smooth muscle of the distal outflow tract, aorticopulmonary septum, and wall of the aorta and pulmonary trunk, neural crest cells give rise to the parasympathetic postganglionic neurons of the heart (the cardiac ganglia).

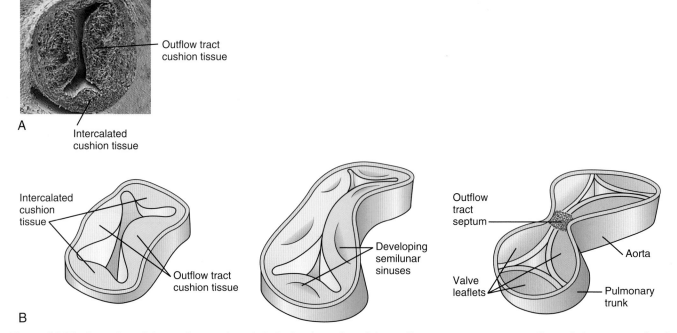

Figure 12-30. Formation of the semilunar valves. *A, B,* During formation of the outflow tract septum, two smaller and shorter intercalated cushion tissues form in the opposite quadrants. At the site of the aortic and pulmonary ostia, this new cushion tissue is excavated and remodeled within the wall of each new vessel to form three cavities. These cavities and the intervening tissue are subsequently remodeled to form the valve sinuses and semilunar valves.

As mentioned earlier, the loss of neural crest cell–derived mesenchymal cells in the outflow tract leads directly to cardiovascular defects. Loss of neural crest cell–derived mesenchyme in the heart can stem from faulty neural crest cell formation, migration, or proliferation. Perturbation of neural crest cell formation, migration, and differentiation results in hypoplasia of the neural crest and an inadequate number of neural crest–derived mesenchymal cells reaching the heart. Several genes have been shown to play important roles in maintaining proper cardiac neural crest cell number and migration. Splotch mice, characterized by a mutation of Pax3, have a reduced number of neural crest cells reaching the pharyngeal arches and entering the outflow tract. The phenotype of these mice resembles that of embryos in which neural crest cells are ablated, including persistent truncus arteriosus and ventricular septal defects. These heart defects, but not the axial defects associated with Splotch mice, are rescued using promoters and enhancers that drive initial neural crest cell–specific Pax3 expression in transgenic Splotch mice.

Double retinoic acid receptor knockout animals (e.g., RARα1 and all RARβ1-3) display intrinsic defects of the myocardium, but they also exhibit anomalies of heart development similar to those produced by ablation of neural crest cells. Lineage-tracing studies of neural crest cells in RARα1/RARβ-deficient mice suggest that neural crest cells themselves do not respond directly to retinoic acid, but rather that the effects on cardiac neural crest cells is indirect. Other important molecules for directing or enabling cardiac neural crest cell migration are semaphorins, a family of secreted molecules important in guiding axons, as well as in directing neural crest cell migration. Sema3C and their receptors, complexes of plexins and neuropilins, are important in targeting cardiac neural crest cells into the pharyngeal arches and outflow tract, as mice lacking Sema3C and neuropilin exhibit persistent truncus arteriosus and great vessel defects.

Endothelins and their converting enzymes and receptors also have important roles in cardiac neural crest development. Knocking out endothelin receptors or their converting enzymes in mice leads to several neural crest cell–related defects, including ventricular septal defects, defects resembling DiGeorge syndrome, pharyngeal arch artery anomalies (covered in Chapter 13), and enteric nervous system defects (covered in Chapter 14), which may be a consequence of neural crest hypoplasia rather than a defect in neural crest migration. In mice in which the Tgfβ type II receptor is knocked out specifically in neural crest cells, cardiovascular defects occur that resemble those seen in DiGeorge syndrome. In this case, migration of neural crest cells into the outflow tract seems normal. However, their subsequent differentiation into smooth muscle cells and connective tissue fails, resulting in persistent truncus arteriosus and ventricular septal defects.

SOME HEART DEFECTS MAY BE RELATED TO INTERACTIONS BETWEEN SECOND HEART FIELD AND NEURAL CREST CELLS

As stated earlier, if cardiac neural crest cells are removed from experimental animals before they migrate, several outflow tract and septal defects occur. However, these embryos exhibit other signs of abnormal cardiac development, including cardiac looping defects and early contractility defects, well before the stage when neural crest cells begin to invade the heart. As mentioned earlier, point mutations in Tbx1 lead to heart defects, such as persistent truncus arteriosus and tetralogy of Fallot. Tbx1 is expressed in the endoderm and mesoderm of the second heart field at the arterial pole, and Tbx1 deficiency leads to decreased levels of Fgf8 at that region. Recent studies in chick and mouse embryos suggest that specific levels of Fgf8 are required for proper second heart field cell proliferation. Ablation of neural crest cells increases Fgf8 levels in the second heart field, resulting in outflow tract defects that can be rectified by adding Fgf8 blocking antibodies in chick embryos. Notch signaling also plays a critical role, as loss of notch signaling results in abnormal neural crest migration, alters Fgf8 signaling in the second heart field, and causes outflow tract and great vessel defects. Therefore, it seems that neural crest cells are required for maintaining specific levels of Fgf8 within the second heart field—levels necessary for proper outflow tract lengthening, cardiac looping, and realignment. Neural crest cells may also regulate the expression of several other genes within the second heart field, including goosecoid, Dlx2 and Dlx3, and Hand2. Therefore, abnormal development of cardiac neural crest cells can lead to aberrant heart development by means other than loss of neural crest cell–derived cushion cells within the heart.

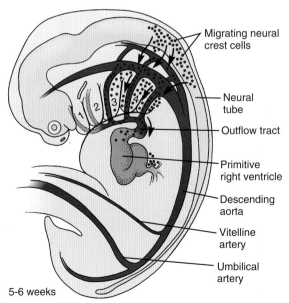

Figure 12-31. Source and migration route of cardiac neural crest cells. Neural crest cells migrate from the hindbrain through pharyngeal arches three, four, and six and then invade the outflow tract and contribute mesenchymal cells to the outflow tract septum. Some neural crest cells also enter the venous inflow region.

Labels in figure: Migrating neural crest cells; Neural tube; Outflow tract; Primitive right ventricle; Descending aorta; Vitelline artery; Umbilical artery; 5-6 weeks

DEVELOPMENT OF PACEMAKER AND CONDUCTION SYSTEM

The heart is one of the few organs that has to function almost as soon as it forms. The rhythmic waves of electrical depolarization (action potentials) that trigger the myocardium to contract arise spontaneously in the cardiac muscle itself and spread from cell to cell. The sympathetic and parasympathetic neural input to the heart that arises later in development modifies the heart rate but does not initiate contraction. Cardiomyocytes removed from the primary heart tube and grown in tissue culture will begin to beat in unison if they become connected to one another, and studies with voltage-sensitive dyes indicate that cardiomyocytes may begin to produce rhythmic electrical activity even before the two early endocardial tubes have fused.

Regulation of calcium levels and excitation-contraction coupling are essential for contraction of the first heartbeat. In mouse embryos lacking the sodium-calcium exchanger, Ncx1, the primary heart tube fails to beat, and the embryos are nonviable. In a normally functioning mature heart, the beat is initiated in the **sinoatrial (SA) node** (the **pacemaker**), which has a faster rate of spontaneous depolarization than the rest of the myocardium. Moreover, depolarization spreads from the SA node to the rest of the heart along specialized **conduction pathways** that control the timing of contraction of various regions of the myocardium, ensuring that the chambers contract efficiently and in the right sequence.

In the primary heart tube, the cardiomyocytes begin to contract asynchronously. Pacemaker activity starts from a transient left SA nodal region that is repositioned to a right SA node, found at the borderline of the entrance to the right common cardinal vein. These cells, derived from the posterior part of the second heart field, eventually differentiate to form the contractile, pacemaking component of the distinct ovoid SA node located at the transition of the superior caval vein and right atrium.

Soon after development of the SA node, cells within the atrioventricular junction adjacent to the endocardial cushion begin to form a secondary pacemaker center, the **atrioventricular (AV) node**, which regulates conduction of impulses from the atrium to the ventricles and coordinates the contraction of the two ventricles. The main conduction pathway between the SA node and the AV node runs through the terminal crest, although controversy continues regarding what internodal pathways do exist. Development of the AV node is accompanied by the formation of a bundle of specialized conducting cells, the **bundle of His**, which sends one branch (the left bundle branch) over the surface of the left side of the ventricular septum and another branch (the right bundle) along the right ventricular septal surface and into the moderator band. This conduction pathway must be carefully avoided during the repair of ventricular septal defects. Branches of **Purkinje fibers** spreading out from the right and left bundle branches then deliver the depolarization signal to the rest of the ventricular myocardium.

The detailed ontogeny of the cardiac conduction system is unclear. However, most of the conduction pathway arises from cardiogenic mesoderm and cardiomyocytes. The myocardial cells of the conducting system are in principle contractile, but they differentiate into cells specialized for generating and conducting action potentials responsible for mediating rhythmic and wave-like contraction of the heart. Expression of Tbx2 and Tbx3, important in patterning of non-chamber myocardium (e.g., atrioventricular canal and outflow tract myocardium) is required for proper development of the conduction system (Fig. 12-32). Subsequent expression of endothelin and neuregulin signaling from the overlying endocardium and coronary endothelium plays a major role in mediating the differentiation of cells constituting the central conducting and Purkinje system. Nkx2.5 expression levels increase during the development of the conducting system and mediate the expression of gap junctional proteins essential for coupling the specialized cardiomyocytes. Mice haploinsufficient for Nkx2.5 exhibit severe hypoplasia of the conducting system. In humans, mutations in NKX2.5 are associated with structural anomalies of the conduction system and progressive disease of the atrioventricular conduction system. Understanding development of this network is important, as many adults experience arrhythmias, with some anomalies being associated with mutations in developmental control genes having key roles in heart development. A better understanding of the embryonic development of the conducting system may shed light on the etiological basis of congenital arrhythmias.

DEVELOPMENT OF EPICARDIUM AND CORONARY VASCULATURE

The progenitor of the epicardium, the **proepicardial organ**, consists of a special group of splanchnic mesodermal cells formed at the caudal dorsal mesocardium/septum

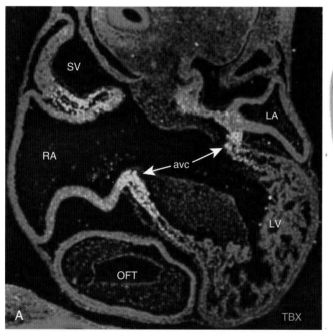
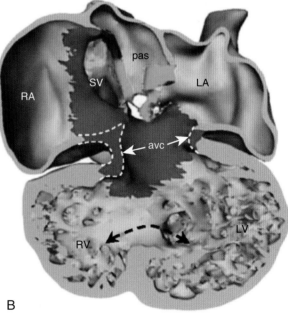

Figure 12-32. Expression pattern of TBX3 in the heart of a five-week-old human embryo. *A,* Localization of TBX3 mRNA expression in the atrioventricular region and sinus venous by situ hybridization. *B,* Three-dimensional reconstruction of TBX3 expression showing predominant expression in regions where the pacemaker and the conducting system develop. Dashed arrow indicates the location of the interventricular foramen. avc, Atrioventricular cushion; LA, left atrium; LV, left ventricle; OFT, outflow tract; pas, primary atrial septum (septum primum); RA, right atrium; RV, right ventricle; SV, sinus venosus.

transversum junction (Fig. 12-33A; see also Fig. 12-19B). Proepicardial cells express both Wilm's tumor protein-1 (Wt1) and Tbx18. With the exception of epicardial precursor cells migrating from the cranial dorsal mesocardium to cover a portion of the outflow tract, proepicardial organ cells migrate as an epithelial sheet of cells over the entire myocardial surface (Fig. 12-33B). Once covering the surface of the myocardium, the epicardial epithelium deposits and assembles an extracellular matrix between the epicardial epithelium and myocardium. This is followed by an

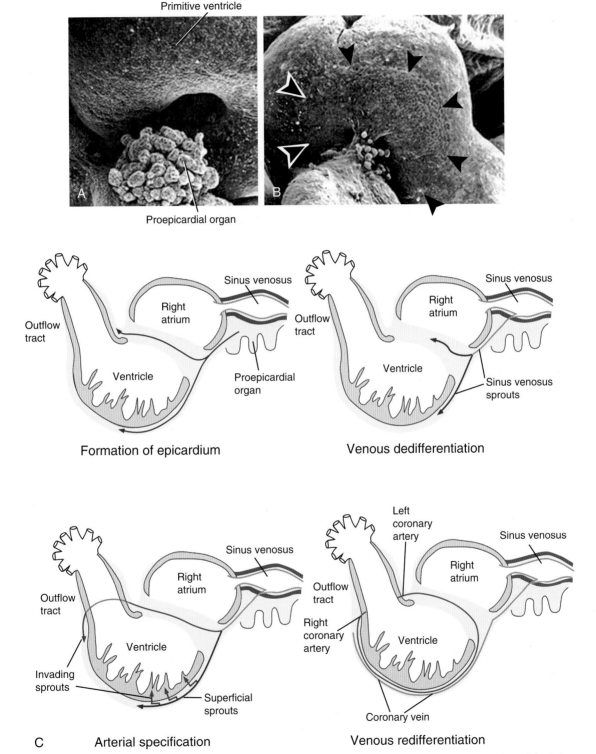

Figure 12-33. Formation of the epicardium and coronary vessels. *A, B,* The epicardium is formed from migrating cells derived from the proepicardial organ found in the region of the sinus venosus. As indicated in these scanning electron micrographs, these cells migrate over and cover the entire myocardium (arrowheads), eventually forming the epicardium. *C,* The endothelial precursors for the coronary vessels arise from sprouts of the sinus venosus. These sprouts lose their venous phenotype, migrate through the epicardium, and also invade the myocardium. The invading sprouts form endothelial cells expressing arterial markers and eventually form the right and left coronary arterial endothelia. The superficial sprouts form the coronary venous endothelium. Epicardium-derived cells form the coronary vascular smooth muscle and cardiac fibroblasts, and a subset also differentiate into cardiomyocytes.

epithelial-to-mesenchymal transformation of the epicardial epithelium, generating a mesenchymal cell population that invades the subepicardial extracellular matrix in much the same way that endocardium-derived cushion tissue is generated. Recent studies suggest that these **epicardium-derived mesenchymal cells** not only form cardiac fibroblasts and coronary vascular smooth muscle, but that they also differentiate into functional cardiomyocytes that contribute to the muscular ventricular septum and atria, with smaller numbers scattered throughout the ventricles.

Until recently, epicardium-derived mesenchymal cells were thought to provide the progenitor cells for the coronary endothelium. However, studies in mice show that coronary endothelial cells actually arise from angiogenesis (sprouting from preexisting blood vessels; covered in Chapter 13) of the sinus venosus (Fig 12-33C). Venous endothelial precursor cells of the sinus venosus dedifferentiate (lose venous markers) and migrate over and invade the myocardium. These cells differentiate into coronary endothelial cells of arteries and capillaries (express arterial markers), with only a minor contribution of endothelial cells coming from the endocardial lining. The endothelial precursor cells remaining on the surface of the heart redifferentiate into venous endothelial cells. The angiogenic processes leading to formation of the coronary vascular network involve many of the same signaling molecules and regulatory events as occur during blood vessel formation elsewhere in the embryo (covered in Chapter 13). The connection of the developing coronary vasculature to the aorta occurs by invasion of the developing coronary arteries through the wall of the (ascending) aorta. Why normally only two coronary artery trunks form and how they find their way to the future site of the aortic sinuses are still unclear.

In the Research Lab

MICRORNAS AS REGULATORS OF CARDIAC DEVELOPMENT

Studies suggest that microRNAs (miRNAs) play important roles in regulating cardiovascular development and disease. Genomically encoded, miRNAs are transcribed and processed by the nuclear enzymes drosha and dicer to yield mature miRNAs. miRNAs leave the nucleus and are incorporated into the RNA-inducing silencing complex, where they bind to their sequenced-matched target mRNAs and initiate the destruction or inhibit the translation of their target genes. Mice null for dicer in Nkx2.5-expressing cells develop a hypoplastic ventricular myocardium and die of cardiac failure while in utero. Mouse embryos with cardiac targeted loss or overexpression of specific miRNAs develop ventricular septal defects and conduction defects and exhibit abnormal expression of several transcription factors required for normal cardiomyocyte proliferation and development. Deletion of dicer from neural crest cells causes ventricular septal defects, double-outlet right ventricle, and aortic arch defects, as well as loss or hypoplasia of many neural crest–derived structures.

In humans, more than 600 miRNAs have been identified. Recent studies show that coding sequences for several miRNAs are located on chromosome 21. Individuals with Down syndrome overexpress several miRNAs and show corresponding decreases in expression of several target genes thought to be responsible for the Down syndrome phenotype, including congenital craniofacial and cardiac defects. Hence, a better understanding

of the regulation of miRNA expression, identification of their targets, and functional consequences of their expression will be necessary for elucidating the etiological mechanisms behind many congenital defects.

In the Clinic

FREQUENCY AND ETIOLOGY OF CARDIOVASCULAR MALFORMATIONS

Congenital cardiovascular malformations account for about 20% of all congenital defects observed in live-born infants. They occur in about 5 to 8 of every 1000 live births, and the percentage in stillborn infants is probably even higher. In addition, the recurrence risk in siblings with isolated heart malformations is 2% to 5%, indicating that heart defects include a genetic contribution.

Neither the cause nor the pathogenesis of most heart defects is completely understood. In fact, it is still unclear what genes and cellular process initiate the heartbeat and how the myriad of extracardiac cell lineages is integrated to give rise to a mature fully functional four-chambered heart. However, progressively more of these defects are being associated with specific genetic errors or environmental teratogens. Overall, about 4% of cardiovascular defects can be ascribed to single-gene mutations, another 6% to chromosomal aberrations such as trisomies, monosomies, or deletions, and 5% to exposure to specific teratogens. The teratogens known to induce heart defects include not only chemicals such as lithium, alcohol, and retinoic acid but also factors associated with certain maternal diseases such as diabetes and rubella (German measles). The etiology of most of the remaining cardiac abnormalities (about 80% to 85%) seems to be **multifactorial**—that is, they stem from the interaction of environmental or outside influences **(epigenetic)** with a poorly defined constellation of the individual's own genetic determinants. Thus, individuals may show very different genetic susceptibilities to the action of a given teratogen. Blood pressure and blood flow, factors unique to the developing cardiovascular system, play important roles in the development of the heart such that perturbations in pressure relationships among the heart chambers and outflow tracts cause malformations. Such perturbations may be brought about by several kinds of primary defects—by abnormal compliance or deformability of the atrial, ventricular, or outflow tract walls or by abnormal expansion or constriction of semilunar valves, ductus arteriosus, and great arteries (covered in Chapter 13). For example, if ejection of blood from the right ventricle is prevented by pulmonary valve atresia, the right ventricle becomes **hypoplastic** and the pulmonary arteries are underdeveloped. If blood flow into the right ventricle from the right atrium is prevented by tricuspid atresia, the right ventricle becomes **hypoplastic** while the left ventricle **hypertrophies** because of the extra workload placed on it to drive blood into the pulmonary circulation through a ventricular septal defect. Excessive interatrial flow can cause a septum secundum defect by enlarging the foramen ovale and eroding septal structures. The resulting increased inflow through the left side of the heart may interfere with the normal formation of the outflow tract septum and prevent development of the membranous ventricular septum.

COMMON HEART MALFORMATIONS

Atrial Septal Defects

In about 6 of 10,000 live-born infants, the septum secundum is too short to cover the foramen secundum completely (or the foramen secundum is too large), so that an **atrial septal defect** persists after the septum primum and septum secundum are pressed together at birth (Fig. 12-34). Atrial septal defects cause shunting of blood from the left atrium to the right atrium. Infants with this abnormality are generally asymptomatic, but the persistent increase in flow to the right atrium may lead to enlargement of the right atrium and ventricle, resulting in debilitating atrial arrhythmias later in life. Excessive pulmonary blood flow also causes pulmonary hypertension over time, leading to heart failure. Atrial septal defects are most often detected by echocardiography in childhood, and they may warrant closure surgically or by an occluding device to prevent the onset of cardiac hypertrophy and pulmonary hypertension. An atrial septal defect is associated with almost all documented autosomal and sex chromosome aberrations, and it is a common accompaniment of several partial and complete trisomies, including trisomy 21 (Down syndrome).

Persistent Atrioventricular Canal

Persistent atrioventricular canal or **atrioventricular septal defect** arises from failure of the dorsal and ventral endocardial cushions to fuse. Failure of the dorsal and ventral endocardial cushions to fuse can lead to a variety of secondary abnormalities, including atrial septal defects, ventricular septal defects, and malformation of the atrioventricular valves. One physiological consequence of the defect is persistent left-to-right shunting of blood after birth, the magnitude of which depends on the severity of the defect. Pulmonary hypertension and congestive heart failure in infancy are likely if the defect is severe. Atrial septal defects, malformed atrioventricular valves, and absence of a ventricular septum can be corrected surgically.

Ventricular Septal Defects

Ventricular septal defects are some of the most common of all congenital heart malformations, accounting for 25% of all cardiac abnormalities documented in live-born infants and occurring as isolated defects in 12 of 10,000 births (Fig. 12-35). The prevalence of this defect seems to be increasing—a statistic that may represent an actual increase in incidence or may reflect the application of better diagnostic methods. A ventricular septal defect can arise from several causes: (1) deficient development of the proximal outflow tract cushions, (2) failure of the muscular and membranous ventricular septal components to fuse, (3) failure of the dorsal and ventral endocardial cushions to fuse (atrioventricular septal defect), (4) insufficient development of the muscular ventricular septum, and (5) altered hemodynamics. Whatever the origin of a ventricular septal defect, its most serious consequence is the left-to-right shunting of blood and the consequent increased blood flow to the pulmonary circulation. In some cases, a ventricular septal defect closes spontaneously during infancy. If it persists and causes a hemodynamic problem, it can be repaired surgically or percutaneously with a device.

Atrioventricular Valve Defects

Atrioventricular valve defects arise from errors in the remodeling necessary for the formation of valve leaflets, chordae tendineae, and papillary muscles from the endocardial cushion tissue and ventricular myocardium. The pathogenesis of **atrioventricular valve atresia**, in which the valve orifice is completely obliterated, is not understood. In **tricuspid valve atresia**, the right atrium is cut off from the right ventricle as the result of abnormal development of the tricuspid valve. Tricuspid valve atresia could be due to an abnormal expansion of the right side of the atrioventricular canal so that a normal inflow tract of the right ventricle is not established. Alternatively, the tricuspid orifice may be only partly connected to the right ventricle, resulting in a straddling tricuspid valve with chordae attached to both ventricles. If the tricuspid orifice remains in its entirety above the left ventricle, a **double-inlet left ventricle** forms. Regardless, the result is that right atrial blood must be shunted to the left atrium through a **persistent foramen ovale**. Moreover, most of the blood reaching the pulmonary arteries does so by taking a roundabout route through a ventricular septal defect and/or via the aorta and a **patent (persistent) ductus arteriosus**. The ductus arteriosus is a connection between the aorta and the pulmonary trunk that normally closes soon after birth (covered in Chapter 13). As a consequence, the heart is functionally a univentricular heart, as the circulation is driven solely by the left ventricle. Hence, the right ventricle is **hypoplastic** while the left ventricle enlarges (i.e., **hypertrophies**). Over time, this leads to cardiac failure.

Malalignment of the outflow tract may lead to a ventricle having a double outlet (having both the aorta and the pulmonary artery). In **double-outlet right ventricle**, both aortic and pulmonary outflow tracts connect to the right ventricle, and this malformation is almost always accompanied by a ventricular septal defect. All arterial blood flow leaves from the right ventricle, and oxygenated blood is mixed with deoxygenated blood within the right ventricle. Symptoms show up within days after birth and include **cyanosis** (due to inadequate oxygenation of the blood), heart **murmur**,

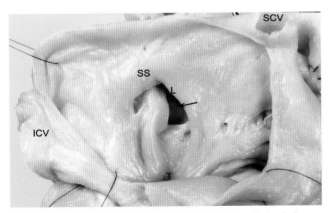

Figure 12-34. Heart with an atrial septal defect (arrow) from a human infant. The foramen secundum and foramen ovale in this heart overlap abnormally; therefore, the foramen ovale could not close at birth, resulting in continued mixing of right and left atrial blood after birth. ICV, Inferior caval vein; L, limbus of the foramen ovale; SCV, superior caval vein; SS, septum secundum; T, tricuspid orifice.

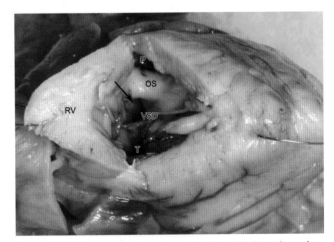

Figure 12-35. Typical ventricular septal defect (VSD) in a heart from a human infant. Failure of the membranous ventricular septum to fuse with the upper ridge of the muscular ventricular septum in this heart has resulted in a ventricular septal defect (arrow). OS, Outflow tract septum; P, pulmonary outlet; RV, right ventricle; T tricuspid orifice.

breathlessness, and (later) poor weight gain. The incidence of this malformation is approximately 1 in 3000 births, and it can be corrected surgically.

Semilunar Valve Stenosis

Semilunar valve stenosis involves stenosis of the aortic or pulmonary valve. **Aortic valve stenosis** leads to **hypertrophy** of the left ventricle, pulmonary hypertension, and eventually cardiac failure. It can be congenital (usually the case if symptoms appear before age 30), the result of an infection (such as rheumatic fever), or degenerative (a consequence of aging). Collectively, the incidence is 1% to 2% of the population, with greater frequency in males (4:1 male-to-female ratio). Congenital valve stenosis is likely

caused by an error in cavitation and remodeling within the distal outflow tract cushion tissue responsible for forming the aortic and pulmonary semilunar valves. This can lead to a **bicommissural aortic valve** (having two rather than three leaflets). A bicommissural valve can be asymptomatic or stenotic from infancy or may become stenotic over time, often as the result of calcification.

Septation Defects of Outflow Tract

A variety of malformations resulting from errors in septation of the outflow tract may be caused by abnormal neural crest cell development. In about 1 of 10,000 live-born infants, the outflow tract septa do not form at all, resulting in a **persistent truncus arteriosus** (Fig. 12-36A, B). This malformation necessarily includes a **ventricular septal defect**. The result is

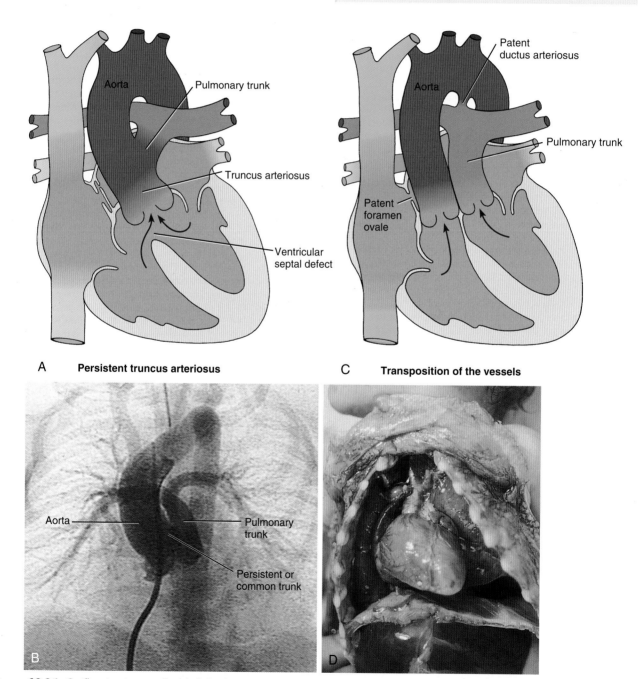

A **Persistent truncus arteriosus**

C **Transposition of the vessels**

Figure 12-36. Outflow tract anomalies. *A, B,* Persistent truncus arteriosus (shown in an angiogram in *B*). Incomplete separation of aortic and pulmonary outflow tracts accompanies a ventricular septal defect when the outflow tract septum fails to form. *C, D,* Transposition of the great arteries occurs when the ventricular outflow vessels run in parallel and do not connect to their proper outflow vessel.

that blood from the two sides of the heart mixes in the common outflow tract, mainly in left-to-right shunting toward the pulmonary side, leading to pulmonary hypertension. Left untreated, infants with this defect usually die within the first 2 years. Surgical correction is possible and involves repairing the ventricular septal defect and implanting a valved prosthetic shunt between the right ventricle and the pulmonary arteries.

In about 5 of 10,000 live-born infants, the outflow tract septa develop but the vessels are positioned in parallel and do not connect to the proper outflow vessel. New data suggest that this results from a disturbance in the contribution of the second heart field to the outflow tract myocardium. The result is **transposition of the great vessels**, in which the left ventricle pumps blood into the pulmonary circulation and the right ventricle empties into the systemic circulation (Fig. 12-36C, D). Transposition of the great vessels is often fatal unless the ductus arteriosus remains patent, or it is accompanied by intrinsic atrial or ventricular septal defects or by defects introduced surgically (to establish an interatrial communication), allowing the deoxygenated systemic and the newly oxygenated pulmonary blood to mix. Transposition can be surgically corrected with a favorable prognosis. Nevertheless, it is the leading cause of death in infants with cyanotic heart disease younger than 1 year of age.

Tetralogy of Fallot

Many cardiac defects occur together more often than in isolation. In some cases, such associated defects are actually components of the same malformation—as, for example, a ventricular septal defect is a necessary consequence of persistent truncus arteriosus. In other cases, a primary malformation sets off a cascade of effects that lead to other malformations. An example is the pathogenesis of **tetralogy of Fallot**, a syndrome referred to as *maladie bleue* by Etienne-Louis Arthur Fallot in 1888 (Fig. 12-37). Fallot used the term *tetralogy* to refer to the four classic malformations in this syndrome: (1) **pulmonary trunk stenosis**, (2) **ventricular septal defect**, (3) rightward displacement of the aorta (sometimes called **overriding aorta**), and (4) **right ventricular hypertrophy**. The primary defect is unequal division of the outflow tract, favoring the aorta, with malalignment of the outlet septum with respect to the right and left ventricles. All of these defects conspire to raise the

blood pressure in the right ventricle, resulting in progressive right ventricular hypertrophy. Tetralogy of Fallot is the most common cyanotic congenital heart malformation, occurring in approximately 1 of 1000 live-born infants. The condition may be corrected surgically by relieving the obstruction of the pulmonary trunk and repairing the ventricular septal defect.

KNOWN GENETIC CAUSES OF HEART MALFORMATIONS

Based on genetic studies in families, many cardiac malformations have been ascribed to single-gene mutations, with continuing progress in identifying more through animal studies and human genetic linkage studies. However, to date only a few have been found that are non–syndrome-associated gene mutations occurring in so-called isolated heart defects. One of the earliest acting of these mutations occurs in NKX2.5. This gene plays an important role in specification of the early cardiogenic field, but it is also involved in several subsequent cardiac morphogenic events. Mutations in NKX2.5 in humans are associated with atrial septal defects and defects in the conduction system. Mutations in GATA4 have also been found in the human population. These mutations alter the transcriptional activity of GATA4 and its interaction with other gene products important in cardiac development, including NKX2.5 and TBX5. Mutations in GATA4 have been linked to atrial septal defects and pulmonary valve stenosis. Mutations in TBX20, a transcription factor important in chamber specification (covered earlier), are linked to atrial and ventricular septal defects, valve defects, and abnormal chamber growth. Mutations in CYSTEINE-RICH PROTEIN WITH EGF-LIKE DOMAINS (CRELD1; a cell adhesion molecule) have been found in patients with atrioventricular septal defects.

A number of specific gene mutations have also been identified in syndromes that contain heart defects as a consistent finding. Mutations have been found in various genes causing laterality and cardiac looping defects. Mutations in genes encoding axonemal DYNEINS are found in patients with **Kartagener syndrome** (covered in Chapters 3 and 11). **Randomized laterality** and **visceroatrial heterotaxy** occur in patients with mutations in NODAL, LEFTY1, LEFTY2, CRYPTIC, and ACVR2B (an ACTIVIN receptor). Patients with **LEOPARD syndrome** or **Noonan syndrome** exhibit pulmonary trunk stenosis, atrioventricular septal defects, and conduction anomalies, as well as over-

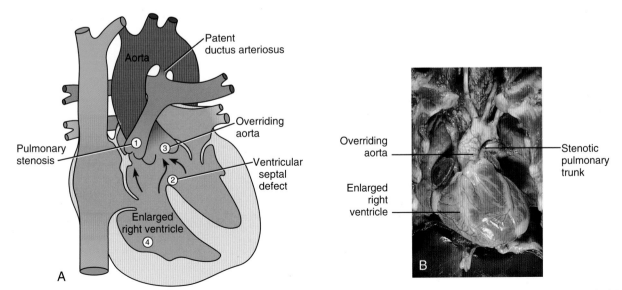

Figure 12-37. Tetralogy of Fallot. *A,* Classically, tetralogy of Fallot is characterized by (1) stenosis (narrowing) of the pulmonary trunk, (2) ventricular septal defect, (3) overriding aorta, and (4) an enlarged right ventricle. A patent ductus arteriosus is also present. *B,* The enlarged right ventricle and overriding aorta are obvious in this case of tetralogy of Fallot in a heart from a human infant.

lapping craniofacial and skeletal anomalies that can be caused by different mutations in the PTPN11 gene. This gene encodes an SHP2 protein, a non-receptor tyrosine phosphatase involved in intracellular signal transduction (Noonan syndrome is also covered in Chapter 13). Deletion or mutations in the JAGGED1 gene (a gene encoding a ligand for NOTCH signaling) or NOTCH1/NOTCH2 (genes encoding for NOTCH receptors) is responsible for **Alagille syndrome** (covered in Chapter 3, 5, 13, and 14), and 70% to 95% of these patients exhibit heart defects, including stenosis of the pulmonary and aortic arteries or valves, septal defects, and tetralogy of Fallot. However, it is unclear whether Alagille syndrome is caused by abnormalities in epithelial-to-mesenchymal transformation of the endocardium or in later valve development. Mutations of the CHD7 (CHROMODOMAIN HELICASE DNA-BINDING PROTEIN 7) gene on human chromosome 8 have been found in 60% of patients with **CHARGE syndrome** (incidence 1 of 9000 to 10,000; also covered in Chapters 4 and 17), and 75% of these patients exhibit heart defects. Studies in human embryos show that neural crest cell–derived mesenchyme is one of the primary tissues expressing this gene.

Most of the 250,000 individuals who suffer sudden death each year in the United States die of **cardiac arrhythmias**. One inborn cause of arrhythmias is **long QT syndrome**, characterized by prolongation of depolarization (Q) and repolarization (T) intervals diagnosed by electrocardiogram (ECG or EKG). Long QT syndrome predisposes affected individuals to **syncope** (loss of consciousness) and sudden death. It is no surprise that genetic disruptions underlying this autosomal dominant disease include mutations in KVLQT1, HERG, SCN5A, and other genes that encode **cardiac ion channels**.

22Q11.2 DELETIONS AND HEART MALFORMATIONS

Patients with **22q11.2 deletion syndrome** (also known as **DiGeorge** and **velocardiofacial syndromes**) exhibit congenital anomalies that place them within the neurocristopathy family of defects (covered in Chapter 4; 22q11.2 deletion syndrome is also covered in Chapters 13 and 17). These defects involve at least one element of abnormal neural crest cell development and manifest congenital heart defects as part of the pathology. These patients have microdeletions within the 22q11.2 region, which occur in 1 of 10,000 to 20,000 live births. Common heart defects are tetralogy of Fallot, interrupted aortic arch (covered in Chapter 13), ventricular septal defects, persistent truncus arteriosus, and vascular rings (covered in Chapter 13). Therefore, presentation of these types of defects should alert the physician to look for the possibility of 22q11.2 deletions and other pathologic conditions that may arise from such deletions. Examination of the genes in this region is underway to determine which may be responsible for the symptoms of these deletions. Links to several genes have been identified, of which TBX1, expressed in the second heart field and adjacent pharyngeal pouch endoderm, is the most likely one. Others include UFD1 (UBIQUITIN FUSION DEGRADATION-1, a gene regulated by HAND2) and HIRA (a gene encoding for a protein that interacts with PAX3). In the case of TBX1, rare mutations have been found in patients with DiGeorge phenotype but lacking a 22q11.2 deletion, suggesting that in some cases, a single gene can cause DiGeorge syndrome. However, in the vast majority of patients, loss of multiple linked 22q11.2 genes is likely responsible.

Embryology in Practice

CAUGHT IN THE MIDDLE

A previously healthy twenty-year-old man suddenly collapses while running during the final leg of a triathlon. Fortunately,

the triathlon emergency medical staff witnesses the event and rushes to his aid. They find him pulseless, and one begins CPR while the other retrieves the automatic cardiac defibrillator (ACD). After several shocks, the man is returned to a normal sinus rhythm and is transferred to the hospital by ambulance.

In the emergency department, the man is conscious, and after some time he is able to answer questions. When asked about his medical history, he states that he "has none," having "never been to a doctor." He describes himself as very healthy and states that he was a competitive runner in school. He denies previous fainting spells, chest pain, palpitations, or shortness of breath. An electrocardiogram shows ST segment changes and elevated cardiac troponins, indicating acute myocardial ischemia.

A cardiac catheterization shows no evidence of atherosclerotic narrowing of his coronary arteries and instead reveals an anomalous **left coronary artery** (LCA) originating from the *right* sinus of Valsalva (i.e., **aortic sinus**) and passing between the pulmonary and aortic trunks, where it is vulnerable to compression during systole, with subsequent reduced myocardial perfusion (Fig. 12-38). This situation can be exacerbated by exercise, the first symptom of which can be sudden cardiac death. The patient is taken to the operating room, where the surgeon is able to reimplant the LCA to the left sinus of Valsalva. He makes a full recovery.

Similar to other vascular structures, the coronary arterial system shows considerable plasticity. In contrast to variation seen in the systemic arteries, variation in the coronary arteries can have serious consequences for the heart muscle. A related condition, anomalous origin of the left coronary artery arising from the pulmonary artery (ALCAPA), can present in infancy, as the LCA in this instance is supplied by poorly oxygenated blood from the right side of the heart and is often hypoperfused as the result of pulmonary steal to the lower-pressure lung vasculature.

The pathogenesis of these conditions is not clearly known, but they might result from abnormal partitioning of the truncus arteriosus or from agenesis or regression of one of the coronary arterial buds.

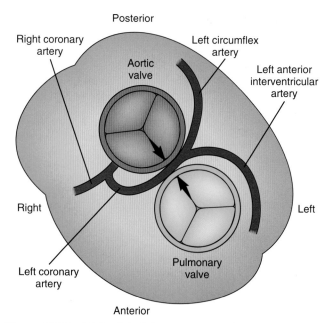

Figure 12-38. Origin of the left coronary artery from the right aortic sinus. Arrows indicate compression of the left coronary artery during systole. The outline of the heart at the level of the aortic and pulmonary valves is indicated.

SUGGESTED READINGS

Bruneau BG. 2008. The developmental genetics of congenital heart disease. Nature 451:943–948.

Cai CL, Martin JC, Sun Y, et al. 2008. A myocardial lineage derives from Tbx18 epicardial cells. Nature 454:104–108.

Chakraborty S, Combs MD, Yutzey KE. 2010. Transcriptional regulation of heart valve progenitor cells. Pediatr Cardiol 31:414–421.

Combs MD, Yutzey KE. 2009. Heart valve development: regulatory networks in development and disease. Circ Res 105:408–421.

Dunwoodie SL. 2007. Combinatorial signaling in the heart orchestrates cardiac induction, lineage specification and chamber formation. Semin Cell Dev Biol 18:54–66.

Dyer LA, Kirby ML. 2009. The role of secondary heart field in cardiac development. Dev Biol 336:137–144.

Gessert S, Kuhl M. 2010. The multiple phases and faces of wnt signaling during cardiac differentiation and development. Circ Res 107:186–199.

Harris IS, Black BL. 2010. Development of the endocardium. Pediatr Cardiol 31:391–399.

High FA, Epstein JA. 2008. The multifaceted role of Notch in cardiac development and disease. Nat Rev Genet 9:49–61.

Jain R, Rentschler S, Epstein JA. 2010. Notch and cardiac outflow tract development. Ann N Y Acad Sci 1188:184–190.

Liu N, Olson EN. 2010. MicroRNA regulatory networks in cardiovascular development. Dev Cell 18:510–525.

Mikawa T, Hurtado R. 2007. Development of the cardiac conduction system. Semin Cell Dev Biol 18:90–100.

Perez-Pomares JM, Gonzalez-Rosa JM, Munoz-Chapuli R. 2009. Building the vertebrate heart—an evolutionary approach to cardiac development. Int J Dev Biol 53:1427–1443.

Red-Horse K, Ueno H, Weissman IL, Krasnow MA. 2010. Coronary arteries form by developmental reprogramming of venous cells. Nature 464:549–553.

Rochais F, Mesbah K, Kelly RG. 2009. Signaling pathways controlling second heart field development. Circ Res 104:933–942.

Singh R, Kispert A. 2010. Tbx20, Smads, and the atrioventricular canal. Trends Cardiovasc Med 20:109–114.

Sizarov A, Ya J, de Boer BA, et al. 2011. Formation of the building plan of the human heart: morphogenesis, growth, and differentiation. Circulation 123:1125–1135.

Snarr BS, Kern CB, Wessels A. 2008. Origin and fate of cardiac mesenchyme. Dev Dyn 237:2804–2819.

Stankunas K, Ma GK, Kuhnert FJ, et al. 2010. VEGF signaling has distinct spatiotemporal roles during heart valve development. Dev Biol 347:325–336.

Taber LA, Voronov DA, Ramasubramanian A. 2010. The role of mechanical forces in the torsional component of cardiac looping. Ann N Y Acad Sci 1188:103–110.

van Wijk B, Moorman AF, van den Hoff MJ. 2007. Role of bone morphogenetic proteins in cardiac differentiation. Cardiovasc Res 74:244–255.

Watanabe Y, Buckingham ME. 2010. The formation of the embryonic mouse heart. Heart fields and myocardial cell lineages. Ann N Y Acad Sci 1188:15–24.

Chapter 13

Development of the Vasculature

SUMMARY

Starting on day seventeen, vessels begin to arise in the splanchnic mesoderm of the yolk sac wall from aggregations of cells called **hemangioblasts**. From these aggregates, two cell lineages arise: primitive **hematopoietic progenitor cells** and **endothelial precursor cells**. **Vasculogenesis** (de novo blood vessel formation) commences in the splanchnic mesoderm of the embryonic disc and continues later in the paraxial mesoderm. In the embryonic disc, endothelial cell precursors differentiate into endothelial cells and organize into networks of small vessels that coalesce, grow, and invade other tissues to form the primary embryonic vasculature. This primitive vasculature is expanded and remodeled by **angiogenesis** (budding and sprouting of existing blood vessels). Hematopoiesis begins in the yolk sac extraembryonic mesoderm. It is later shifted to the liver, where the embryonic hematopoietic cells are joined by a source of **definitive hematopoietic stem cells (HSCs)** arising from intraembryonic splanchnic mesoderm of the dorsal **aorta-gonad-mesonephros (AGM)** region, the vitelline and umbilical arteries, and most likely the placenta. Definitive HSCs are programmed from hemogenic endothelium, colonize the liver where they are expanded, and later relocate to the bone marrow and other lymphatic organs.

As body folding carries the developing primitive heart tube into the ventral thorax during the fourth week, the paired dorsal aortae attached to the cranial ends of the tubes are pulled ventrally to form a pair of dorsoventral loops, the **first aortic arch arteries**. During the fourth and fifth weeks, additional pairs of aortic arch arteries develop in craniocaudal succession, connecting the aortic sac at the distal end of the outflow tract to the dorsal aortae. This aortic arch artery system is subsequently remodeled to form the system of great arteries in the upper thorax and neck.

The paired dorsal aortae remain separate in the region of the aortic arch arteries but eventually fuse below the level of the fourth thoracic segment to form a single median dorsal aorta. The dorsal aorta develops three sets of branches: (1) a series of ventral branches, which supply the gut and gut derivatives; (2) lateral branches, which supply retroperitoneal structures such as the suprarenal glands, kidneys, and gonads; and (3) dorsolateral intersegmental branches called **intersegmental arteries**, which penetrate between the somite derivatives and give rise to part of the vasculature of the head, neck, body wall, limbs, and vertebral column. The ventral branches supplying the gastrointestinal tract are derived from remnants of a network of **vitelline arteries**, which develop in the yolk sac and vitelline duct and anastomose with the paired dorsal aortae. The paired dorsal aortae become connected to the **umbilical arteries** that develop in the connecting stalk and carry blood to the placenta. Hematopoietic cells may also arise in these arteries.

The primitive venous system consists of three major components, all of which are at first bilaterally symmetrical: the **cardinal system**, which drains the head, neck, body wall, and limbs; the **vitelline veins**, which initially drain the yolk sac; and the **umbilical veins**, which develop in the connecting stalk and carry oxygenated blood from the placenta to the embryo. All three systems initially drain into both sinus horns, but all three undergo extensive modification during development as the systemic venous return is shifted to the right atrium.

The cardinal system initially consists of paired **anterior (cranial)** and **posterior (caudal) cardinal veins**, which meet to form short **common cardinal veins** draining into the right and left sinus horns. However, the posterior cardinals are supplemented and later replaced by two subsidiary venous systems—the **subcardinal** and **supracardinal** systems, which grow caudally from the base of the posterior cardinals in the medial dorsal body wall. All three of these cardinal systems, along with a small region of the right vitelline vein, contribute to the inferior caval vein and its major branches. The supracardinals also form the azygos and hemiazygos systems draining the thoracic body wall. The vitelline venous system gives rise to the liver sinusoids and to the portal system, which carries venous blood from the gastrointestinal tract to the liver. Within the substance of the liver, the **vitelline system** also forms the **ductus venosus**, a channel shunting blood from the umbilical vein directly to the inferior caval vein during gestation.

All three venous systems undergo extensive modification during development. In the cardinal and vitelline systems, the longitudinal veins on the left side of the body tend to regress, whereas those on the right side persist and give rise to the great veins. Thus, a bilateral system that drains into both sinus horns becomes a right-sided system that drains into the right atrium. In contrast, the right umbilical vein disappears and the left umbilical vein persists. However, the left umbilical vein loses its original connection to the left sinus horn and secondarily empties into the ductus venosus within the developing liver.

A dramatic and rapid change in the pattern of circulation occurs at birth as the newborn begins to breathe, the pulmonary vasculature expands, and circulation from the placenta to the fetus stops. Much of the development described in this chapter is focused on the problem of producing a circulation that will effectively distribute the oxygenated blood arriving from the placenta via the umbilical vein to the tissues of the embryo and fetus, yet will be able to convert rapidly at birth to the adult pattern of circulation required by the air-breathing infant.

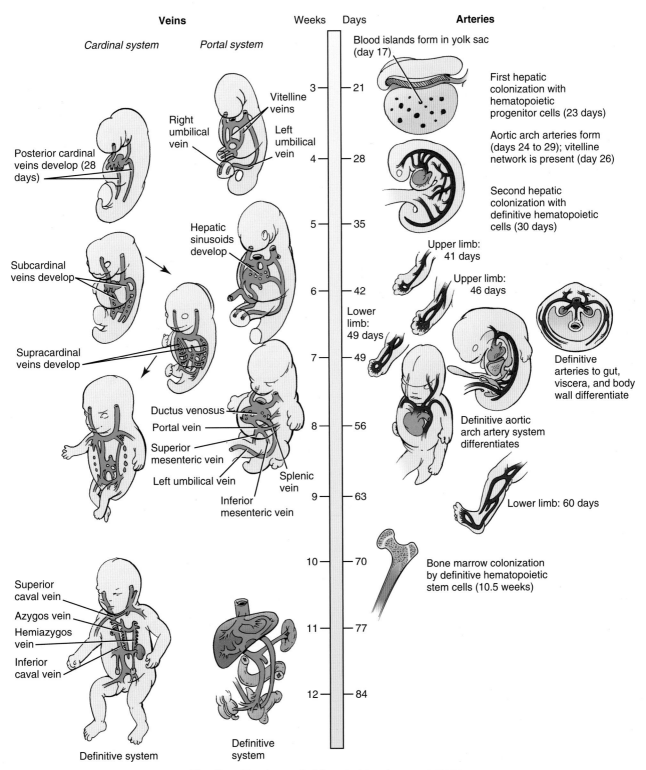

Time line. Development of the arterial and venous systems.

Clinical Taster

While examining a 14-year-old girl with a history of severe recurrent epistaxis (nosebleeds), an otolaryngologist—ear, nose, and throat (or ENT) specialist—notes several small dilated blood vessels on the mucosa of the nasal passages and mouth. The girl's nosebleeds started at age 11. Recently they have become more frequent and now occur two or three times a week. The bleeding has been severe enough to cause mild anemia despite treatment with iron.

In addition to nosebleeds, the patient has significant dyspnea (shortness of breath) during exercise that is out of proportion to her degree of anemia. She also has increased heart rate and subtle clubbing of the fingers. A pulse oximeter reading shows a blood oxygen saturation of 88%. The ENT makes a presumptive diagnosis of **hereditary hemorrhagic telangiectasia (HHT)**, also known as **Osler-Weber-Rendu disease**.

The girl is referred for an air-contrast **echocardiogram** that shows air bubbles passing from the right side of the heart to the left, indicating a pulmonary arterial-venous shunt. A CT (computed tomography) angiogram verifies the presence of a right-sided **pulmonary arterial-venous malformation** measuring 7 mm in diameter. Interventional radiology is consulted, and the shunt is corrected using coil embolization (inserting a small coil to clot off the vessel). Following the procedure, the girl's oxygen saturation increases to normal, and her exercise tolerance gradually improves. Genetic testing reveals an inactivating mutation in the **ENDOGLIN** gene.

HHT is an autosomal dominant condition characterized by abnormal connections between arteries and veins without intervening capillaries. When small, these abnormalities are called **telangiectases** and occur on the mucosal surfaces of the nose, mouth, and gastrointestinal tract, as well as on the fingers. These thin-walled lesions are near the surface and bleed easily. Larger telangiectases, or arterial-venous malformations (AVMs), can occur in the lungs, liver, or brain. Besides the morbidity associated with shunting of blood, a variety of other life-threatening complications are associated with AVMs, including stroke, abscess, and bleeding in the brain. HHT is caused by mutations in the genes encoding either the Tgfβ-binding protein ENDOGLIN or one type of Tgfβ receptor (ACTIVIN A RECEPTOR, TYPE II-LIKE KINASE 1). Both of these proteins are involved in cell signaling during the development of vascular endothelial cells.

FORMATION OF BLOOD AND VASCULATURE BEGINS EARLY IN THIRD WEEK

Animation 13-1: Formation of Blood Islands and Primitive Vessels.

Animations are available online at StudentConsult.

Hematopoietic cells and **endothelial cells** are among the first and earliest cell types to differentiate into a functional phenotype in the embryo. In humans, the earliest evidence for blood and blood vessel formation is seen in the extraembryonic splanchnic mesoderm of the **yolk sac** at about day seventeen in the form of clusters of **hemangioblast cells** developing adjacent to the endoderm (Fig. 13-1). In mice, the earliest marker

for these cell clusters is vascular endothelial growth factor receptor-2 (Vegfr2 or Flk1), also known as KDR in humans. These clusters arise from a subset of brachyury-positive cells within the primitive streak that migrate into the yolk sac. Several cell lineages arise from within these clusters of hemangioblasts, including **hematopoietic cell progenitors** and **endothelial precursor cells (EPCs)**. Endothelial cells will later surround aggregates of blood cells, forming what are often referred to as **blood islands** (see Fig. 13-1). Blood cells that form in the yolk sac blood islands are primarily **primitive erythrocytes**. Megakaryocytes and macrophages also form in the yolk sac wall, but the precise location of their precursor is not known. Some of the yolk sac endothelial cells arise from **hemangioblasts**, but most differentiate from proliferating EPCs. The differentiating endothelial cells organize into small capillary vessels through a process called **vasculogenesis** (described in the following section). These small capillaries lengthen and interconnect, establishing an initial primary vascular network. By the end of the third week, this network completely vascularizes the yolk sac, connecting stalk, and chorionic villi.

The yolk sac is the first supplier of blood cells to the embryonic circulation. The cells supplied are predominantly nucleated erythrocytes containing embryonic hemoglobin (primitive erythrocytes). By day sixty, the yolk sac no longer serves as an erythropoietic organ. Rather, the task of supplying erythrocytes and other lineages of mature blood cells to the circulation is transferred to intraembryonic organs, including the liver, spleen, thymus, and bone marrow. With the onset of the functional circulatory system, these organs are seeded with hematopoietic progenitors and **definitive hematopoietic stem cells (HSCs)** generated in the extraembryonic and/or intraembryonic mesoderm. The first organ to be colonized is the liver. This organ remains the main hematopoietic organ of the embryo and fetus until initiation of **bone marrow hematopoiesis** near parturition (birth). Colonization of the liver primordia by hematopoietic cells occurs in at least two waves, the first beginning at about day twenty-three and containing primitive hematopoietic cells and progenitors, and the second beginning about day thirty and containing the definitive HSCs (Fig. 13-2). These hematopoietic cells arise from at least two different sources (discussed in the following "In the Research Lab" entitled "Second Source of Hematopoietic Cells" and "Intraembryonic Hematopoietic cells, a Source of Adult Bone Marrow Hematopoietic Stem Cells"). The shift from generating primitive nucleated erythroblasts to enucleated erythrocytes synthesizing fetal hemoglobin (**definitive erythrocytes**) occurs by five weeks of gestation. This shift occurs at the time when the liver is colonized with HSCs, cells that have the potential to generate all the hematopoietic cell lineages of the adult including erythroid, myeloid, and lymphoid cells. HSCs colonize the bone marrow and contribute blood cells as early as ten and one-half weeks, but the bulk of the hematopoietic burden is still carried by the liver until birth. Thus, the extraembryonic, primitive hematopoietic cells serve mainly to provide an early, but necessary, blood supply for the developing embryo until the intraembryonic hematopoietic organs containing HSCs can assume the task.

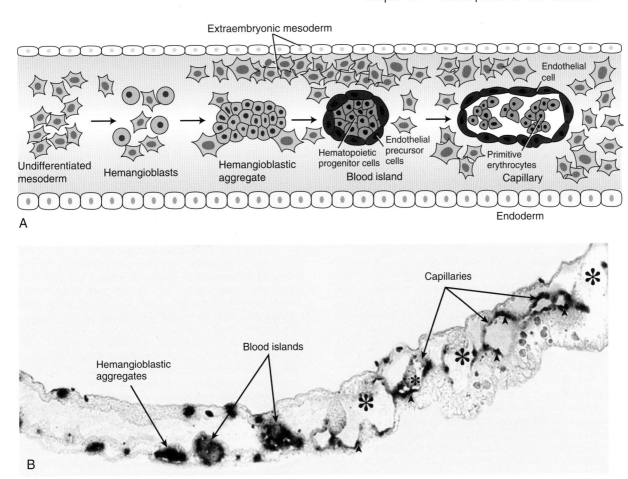

Figure 13-1. Hematopoiesis and blood vessel formation begin within the yolk sac wall with the formation of clusters of hemangioblasts. *A,* Drawing illustrating the formation of clusters of hemangioblasts and their differentiation into hematopoietic progenitor and endothelial precursor cells. Blood cells are surrounded by differentiating endothelial precursor cells forming blood islands. *B,* Expression of Vegfr2 mRNA, an early marker for the hemangioblasts within the yolk sac wall of a fifteen-somite avian embryo. As the blood islands develop, endothelial cells retain Vegfr2 expression, whereas hematopoietic progenitor cells progressively lose it. Asterisks indicate developing blood vessels.

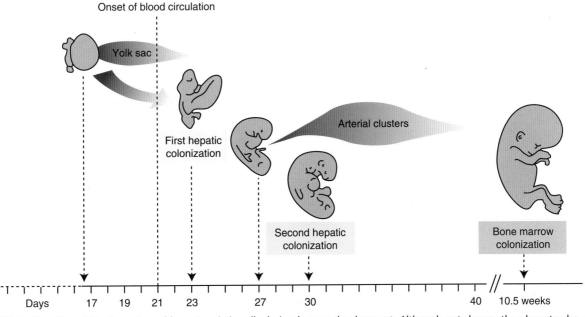

Figure 13-2. Time line of the formation of hematopoietic cells during human development. Although not shown, the placenta also contains hematopoietic cells.

In the Research Lab

SECOND SOURCE OF HEMATOPOIETIC CELLS

Although hematopoietic cells colonizing the developing liver initially arise from the yolk sac mesoderm, hematopoietic cells with greater potential and longevity eventually colonize the fetal liver from a separate intraembryonic source. Evidence for this second source of hematopoietic cells came from the use of quail-chick transplantation chimeras (technique covered in Chapter 5). In a remarkable experiment, the entire body of a two-day embryonic chick was removed from the blastoderm, leaving just the yolk sac, and replaced with the entire body of a quail embryo. When examined after a couple of days of incubation, all blood lineages in the chimera were of chicken yolk sac origin, with quail cells providing the stromal (connective tissue) cells. However, within five days of grafting, a mixture of quail- and chick-derived blood cells was found circulating within the embryo, and eventually all blood cells were quail derived. Thus, this experiment showed clearly that (1) the yolk sac gives rise to transient embryonic hematopoietic cells; and (2) cells generated in the embryo body eventually replaced these cells, producing the long-lived definitive hematopoietic system. Consequently, for the first time it was shown that by closely following yolk sac hematopoiesis, there had to be a potent second source, an intraembryonic source of hematopoietic cells.

Microscopic analysis of bird, amphibian, mouse, and human embryos at equivalent developmental times identified densely packed clusters of hematopoietic cells adhering to the ventral endothelium of the dorsal aorta in the **aorta-gonad-mesonephros (AGM) region** and to the endothelium of the vitelline and umbilical arteries. The appearance of the hematopoietic clusters corresponds with the onset of the second wave of hematopoiesis. In humans, hematopoietic clusters appear within the aorta of the AGM region at twenty-seven days of development as small groups of two or three cells, but by day thirty-five, they increase to thousands of cells that extend into vessels adjacent to the umbilical cord region. These cells express transcription factors and cell surface markers associated with early blood progenitors and HSCs (e.g., Gata2, c-Kit, Cd34, Cd41, Cd45). Although mammalian intraembryonic hematopoietic cluster cells could be derived from colonizing yolk sac hematopoietic cells, evidence suggests that they are of separate origin (covered later).

INTRAEMBRYONIC HEMATOPOIETIC CELLS, A SOURCE OF ADULT BONE MARROW HEMATOPOIETIC STEM CELLS

Studies in mice show that the yolk sac mesoderm forms hematopoietic progenitors capable of generating primitive erythrocytes, macrophages, and megakaryocytes. These primitive erythrocytes likely serve as a quickly forming stopgap population of blood cells that fulfill the oxygen needs of the rapidly developing embryo. Progenitors capable of generating definitive myeloid cells (definitive erythrocytes, macrophages, and granulocytes) appear later within the yolk sac. However, studies suggest that these cells must first colonize and interact with the developing liver to acquire long-term myeloid cell–generating capacity.

Definitive HSCs are defined by their ability for long-term, multilineage repopulation of the entire hematopoietic system (erythroid, myeloid, and lymphoid). Studies of mouse embryos show, by in vivo adult transplantation experiments, that the first functional HSCs are generated in the intraembryonic AGM region (Figs. 13-3, 13-4) before their appearance in the liver. One day following HSC generation in the AGM region, HSCs are detected in the liver, suggesting that AGM HSCs migrate to the liver in a second wave of colonization. In fact, live imaging of the mouse midgestation aorta has documented the generation of hematopoietic cells directly from endothelial cells lining the ventral wall of the aorta. Hence, the cellular source of the second wave of hematopoietic cell generation is the **hemogenic endothelial cell**. Similar multipotent in vivo adult hematopoietic repopulating cells were found in four- to five-week human AGM regions (by xenotransplantations of human cells into immunodeficient mice).

In humans, the liver primordia is colonized first by primitive hematopoietic cells from the yolk sac, possibly as early as day twenty-three to twenty-four, and then by a second wave containing HSCs from day thirty onward. In vitro assays of human tissue explants of both yolk sac and AGM mesoderm show that both explants can make myeloid cells. However, only the AGM mesodermal tissue gives rise to multipotent hematopoietic cells (that make myeloid and T- and B-lymphocytes). Collectively, these studies suggest that the yolk sac extraembryonic mesoderm generates primitive hematopoietic cells necessary for supporting the early cardiovascular needs of the embryo. The definitive HSCs that sustain lifelong adult hematopoiesis are derived from the intraembryonic AGM region (and possibly from hematopoietic clusters in the vitelline and umbilical arteries) and constitute the second wave of cells colonizing the fetal

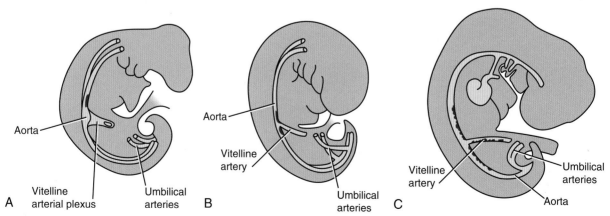

Figure 13-3. A source of hematopoietic cells arises within the splanchnic mesoderm of the aorta-gonad-mesonephros (AGM) region. These cells appear as clusters and emerge from the ventral floor of the dorsal aorta in this region. *A,* In humans at about day twenty-seven, a small number of hematopoietic clusters (in red) first appear in the dorsal aorta near the junction with the vitelline artery. *B,* By day thirty, the number of hematopoietic clusters is increased. *C,* By day thirty-six, clusters extend along the entire length of the aorta in the AGM region and into the vitelline artery. By day forty, hematopoietic cell clusters are no longer detected in the dorsal aorta.

liver before subsequently colonizing the lymphatic organs and bone marrow. The second wave occurs for only a short window of developmental time, ending by day forty of gestation.

Following the generation of HSCs in the embryo, their survival and proliferation depends on a trophic factor called stem cell factor (Scf, or c-Kit ligand) and its receptor, c-Kit receptor. Mouse mutants completely devoid of the c-Kit receptor or

its ligand die in utero of anemia between days fourteen and sixteen of gestation and contain reduced numbers of erythroid progenitors in the fetal liver. In humans, the C-KIT RECEPTOR protein is expressed in the yolk sac, AGM splanchnic mesoderm, and liver HSCs during all stages of liver hematopoietic development. However, the expression of its ligand, SCF, is temporally regulated. SCF protein is expressed in the AGM region at low levels between days twenty-five and thirty-four. It is well expressed in human liver by day thirty-four, before levels drop off in late-stage liver development (i.e., by forty-five days). Only weak expression of SCF mRNA is detected in the yolk sac (by quantitative RT-PCR) at thirty-two days of development. Hence, C-KIT RECEPTOR signaling by SCF in HSCs coincides with the generation of AGM HSCs and with HSC colonization of liver and the appearance of definitive, long-term HSCs. This supports the idea that SCF/c-KIT signaling is involved in survival, differentiation, and proliferation of AGM-derived HSCs in the liver.

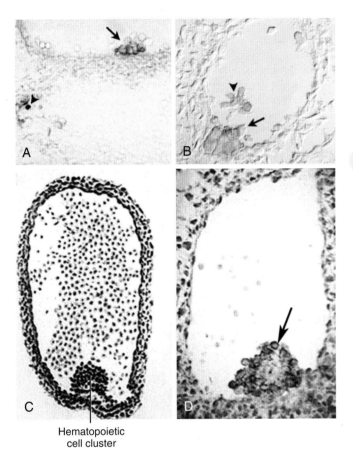

Hematopoietic cell cluster

Figure 13-4. Hematopoietic cell clusters on the ventral floor of the dorsal aorta in the AGM region of various vertebrates. A, Day three chick embryo showing Cd41-positive cells (arrow), a marker for hematopoietic progenitor cells. B, Day ten mouse embryo immunostained with Cd41 antibody (arrow and arrowhead). C, Six- to fifteen-mm pig embryo dorsal aorta in the AGM region showing hematopoietic clusters. D, Day thirty-five human embryo immunostained with an antibody to Cd45 (arrow), another hematopoietic cell marker.

VASCULOGENESIS AND ANGIOGENESIS

On day eighteen, blood vessels begin to develop in the intraembryonic splanchnic mesoderm. Unlike blood vessel formation in the extraembryonic mesoderm, blood vessel formation within intraembryonic mesoderm, with the exception of the AGM region (covered in the preceding "In the Research Lab" entitled "Second Source of Hematopoietic Cells" and "Intraembryonic Hematopoietic Cells, a Source of Adult Bone Marrow Hematopoietic Stem Cells"), is not coupled with hematopoiesis. Inducing substances secreted by the underlying endoderm cause some cells of the splanchnic mesoderm to differentiate into EPCs (or **angioblasts**) that develop into flattened endothelial cells and join together to form small vesicular structures. These vesicular structures, in turn, coalesce into long tubes or vessels (Fig. 13-5). This process is referred to as **vasculogenesis**. These cords develop throughout the intraembryonic mesoderm and coalesce to form a pervasive network of vessels that establishes the initial configuration of the circulatory system of the embryo. This network grows and spreads throughout the embryo by four main processes: (1) continued formation, migration, and coalescence of EPCs; (2) **angiogenesis**, the budding and sprouting of new vessels from existing endothelial cords; (3) **vascular intussusception** (non-sprouting angiogenesis), in which existing vessels are split to generate additional vessels; and (4) intercalation of new EPCs into the walls of existing vessels.

Vasculogenesis

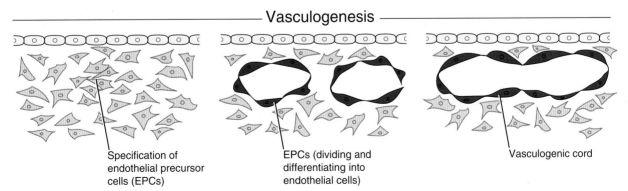

Specification of endothelial precursor cells (EPCs)

EPCs (dividing and differentiating into endothelial cells)

Vasculogenic cord

Figure 13-5. Vasculogenesis begins with the specification of the endothelial precursor cell lineage within the extraembryonic splanchnic mesoderm of the yolk sac and, later, within the intraembryonic splanchnic mesoderm. Endothelial precursor cells differentiate into endothelial cells and organize into small vascular cords that coalesce to form a primitive embryonic vascular plexus.

Because blood vessels form in the yolk sac on about day seventeen, but not in the embryonic disc until day eighteen, it was originally thought that intraembryonic vessels arose mainly because of centripetal extension of the yolk sac vasculature into the embryo proper. However, quail chick transplantation studies provide evidence that almost all of the intraembryonic splanchnic mesoderm has the ability to form blood vessels via vasculogenesis. Furthermore, these experiments show that the characteristic branching pattern of the blood vessels in each region is determined by cues from the underlying endoderm and its extracellular matrix. Although it is clear that the intraembryonic splanchnic mesoderm has the capacity to generate EPCs and to undergo vasculogenesis, the intraembryonic somatic lateral plate mesoderm may not be capable. Studies in avian and zebrafish embryos show that much of this vasculature develops from migrating EPCs derived from the paraxial mesoderm that subsequently forms via vasculogenesis (Fig. 13-6).

Once a primary vascular plexus is formed in the embryo, it must be remodeled to accommodate growth of the embryo and develop into a system of arteries and veins. Completion and continual remodeling of blood vessels require **angiogenesis**. Often, the term *angiogenesis* is inappropriately used interchangeably with *vasculogenesis*. However, angiogenesis is a different process. Angiogenesis is the expansion and remodeling of the vascular system using existing endothelial cells and vessels generated by vasculogenesis (Fig. 13-7). Expansion by angiogenesis occurs by **sprouting** or vascular **intussusception**, a splitting or fusion of existing blood vessels (see Fig. 13-7).

Organization of endothelial cells into recognizable blood vessels usually occurs at the site of EPC specification during vasculogenesis. However, evidence shows that EPCs can also migrate into and proliferate at distant secondary sites before organizing into blood vessels, in a process distinct from angiogenesis (see Fig. 13-6). Vessels that form through this modified form of vasculogenesis include (in the avian embryo) the posterior cardinal vein and perineural vascular plexus and (in the Xenopus embryo) the bulk of the dorsal aorta and intersegmental vessels.

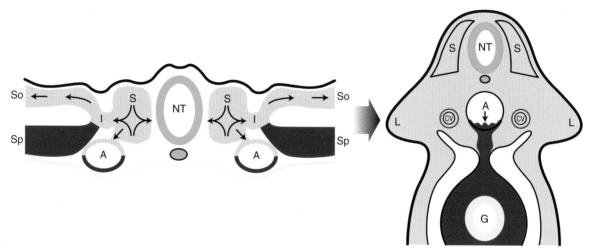

Figure 13-6. Vasculogenesis also occurs in the paraxial mesoderm. In avian embryos, in addition to vasculogenesis in the yolk sac wall and splanchnic mesoderm, the endothelial precursor cell lineage is specified within the paraxial mesoderm. Paraxially derived endothelial precursor cells migrate into distant sites (arrows), differentiate into endothelial cells, and organize a primitive vascular plexus throughout the light red areas. The primitive vasculature derived from endothelial precursor cells of splanchnic mesoderm origin is shown in dark red. The dorsal aorta is a mixture of both endothelial precursor cell lineages. A, Aorta; CV, cardinal vein; G, gut; I, intermediate mesoderm; L, limb bud; NT, neural tube; S, somite; So, somatopleuric mesoderm; Sp, splanchnic mesoderm.

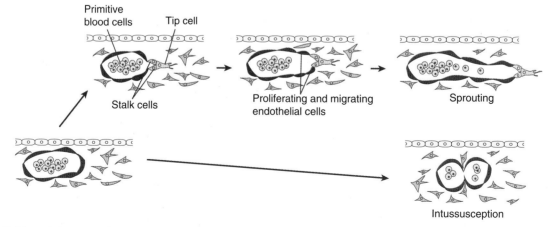

Figure 13-7. The primitive vascular network established through vasculogenesis is expanded and remodeled by angiogenesis. Expansion by angiogenesis occurs by sprouting from existing vessels or by intussusception, a splitting of existing vessels.

It was once thought that EPCs were present only in the embryo and fetus. However, evidence suggests that EPCs exist in adult bone marrow and peripheral blood. Vascular endothelial growth factor (Vegf), granulocyte-monocyte colony-stimulating factor, fibroblast growth factor-2 (Fgf2), and insulin growth factor-1 (Igf1) all stimulate EPC mobilization and differentiation. The decision of circulating endothelial cells to integrate into blood vessel walls is complex and may involve interactions with cytokine and cytokine receptors, binding to denuded endothelial regions, or localizing to areas of platelet aggregates.

In the Research Lab

WHAT INITIATES AND CONTROLS VASCULOGENESIS?

As covered in Chapter 12, in chick embryos, endodermally derived Bmps in the absence of Wnts induce the cardiogenic cell lineage, whereas Bmps in the presence of Wnts enables blood vessel formation in the splanchnic mesoderm. Moreover, Bmp/Tgfβ signals emanating from extraembryonic endoderm and Wnt signaling in mesoderm prime the extraembryonic mesoderm adjacent to the yolk sac endoderm to form blood islands. In mice, visceral endoderm provides inductive signals (e.g., Bmp, Vegf, Indian hedgehog) that are necessary for inducing the expression of blood island markers in this mesoderm. However, the precise trigger for forming hemangioblasts in vivo, and eventually the hematopoietic and EPC lineages, is still unclear. Both hematopoietic precursors and EPCs share many of the same early expression markers, so they are closely tied to one another with regard to cell lineage specification.

What is known is that Vegf signaling through the vascular endothelial growth factor receptor-2 (Vegfr2) is essential. Knockout mice for Vegfr2 have complete absence of hematopoietic progenitors and EPC lineages and die in utero. Moreover, homozygote knockout mice for vascular endothelial growth factor-A (VegfA) die as the result of lack of blood island formation. Mice lacking vascular endothelial growth factor receptor-1 (Vegfr1) also die, but the defect seems to be a consequence of abnormal EPC proliferation resulting in a disorganized vasculature. Vegf is a powerful promoter of vasculogenesis: injecting Vegf into embryos at the outset of vasculogenesis can vascularize normally avascular areas (e.g., cartilage-forming areas and cornea). **Hypervascularization** is also observed in transient transgenic gain-of-function quail embryos in which Vegf is overexpressed.

One group of transcription factors that seem to play a key role in endothelial cell specification is the Ets protein family. At least twelve different Ets factors are expressed in endothelial cells, with overlapping functions that work in combination to specify the endothelial cell lineage. One, Etv2, seems especially important, as it regulates expression of several early endothelial genes, and mice null for Etv2 lack endothelial cells, exhibit defects in hematopoiesis, and die early in development.

ANGIOGENESIS EXPANDS AND REMODELS INITIAL VASCULAR COMPLEX

As in vasculogenesis, Vegfs and their receptors play a major role in mediating angiogenesis. In response to VegfA, Vegfr2-expressing endothelial cells, called **tip cells**, produce long, dynamic filopodia that probe the environment for directional cues (see Fig. 13-7). Adjacent endothelial cells called **stalk cells** proliferate in response to VegfA and express cell adhesion molecules necessary for forming a lumen and maintaining the integrity of the new sprout. So why doesn't the entire endothelium develop tip cells in response to VegfA? Why do some become stalk cells? The answer involves notch signaling. Notch proteins (notch1-4) are cell-surface receptors for the membrane-bound ligands delta-like 1 (Dll-1), Dll-3, Dll-4, Jag1, and Jag2, which are important in cell fate decision (covered in Chapter 5).

Mouse embryos deficient in notch1 or notch2 form a normal initial capillary plexus but fail to properly remodel this vasculature. So notch signaling seems to be required for remodeling of the primitive capillary plexus rather than for its initial development.

During angiogenesis, the notch ligand, Dll-4, is predominantly expressed in tip cells, with the strongest notch signaling occurring in the stalk cells. Notch signaling represses sprouting, whereas blocking notch signaling causes excessive tip cell formation. Hence, a tip cell phenotype seems to be the default in the absence of notch signaling, whereas notch signaling promotes the stalk cell phenotype and stabilization of the sprout. In response to VegfA, it is thought that endothelial cells compete via bilateral Dll-4/notch signaling, eventually generating differences between the endothelial cell population of endothelial cells. Those receiving lower levels of notch signaling are specified as tip cells and those receiving higher levels are specified as stalk cells that then downregulate their expression of Vegf receptor. As a consequence, these differences in notch signaling alter their subsequent responses to VegfA signaling. This mechanism is consistent with studies showing that mice haploinsufficient for Dll-4 exhibit excessive numbers of tip cells and develop abnormally dense vascular networks.

Xenograph tumor transplant studies in which notch signaling is manipulated also suggest that notch may be an important mediator of tumor vascular patterning by mediating the proper balance in tip and stalk cell numbers. Collectively, these studies show that notch signaling plays a major role in angiogenesis and in remodeling of the primitive capillary plexus by mainly acting as a negative regulator of sprouting.

Another group of receptors and ligands that act in parallel to promote proper angiogenesis are the Tie (tyrosine kinase with immunoglobulin-like and Egf-like domains) receptor/angiopoietin group. Angiopoietin-1 (Ang1) and tyrosine kinase with immunoglobulin-like and Egf-like domains-2 (Tie2) are clearly involved in regulating intussusception of the vasculature, whereas Ang2, in cooperation with the stimulatory effects of Vegf, stimulates sprouting. Mice lacking the Tie2 gene or its ligand Ang1 develop abnormally large and leaky vessels and die in utero. Moreover, these mice exhibit a decrease in endothelial cell number and angiogenic sprouting, as well as failure of vascular intussusception. Tie1 knockout mice develop vessels with holes, and the endothelial cells appear necrotic. These results show collectively that Tie/Ang signaling along with Vegf signaling is essential for expansion and normal remodeling of blood vessels after the initial primitive vasculature is established.

The Tgfβ family and Tgfβ receptor signaling components—Alk1, activin A receptor, type II-like kinase 5 protein (Alk5), Tgfβ receptor-II, and endoglin—play critical roles in vasculogenesis and angiogenesis. Knockout mice for the Tgfβ receptors, Alk1 and Alk5, and the Tgfβ-binding protein, endoglin, are defective in angiogenic remodeling as the result of impaired endothelial cell migration and proliferation. They develop abnormal arterial-venous connections, much like those discussed in the "Clinical Taster" for this chapter. Moreover, recruitment of vascular smooth muscle is deficient, leading to poor vascular integrity and vascular instability. Tgfβ exhibits both stimulatory and inhibitory effects on endothelial cells. Recent studies suggest that the decision as to whether to continue angiogenesis or mature into a vessel depends on an interplay between the stimulatory effect of Tgfβ/Alk1 signaling (promoted by endoglin) and the inhibitory effect of Tgfβ/Alk5 signaling.

One of the main driving forces for vascularization by angiogenesis is the need to counteract hypoxia. Low oxygen saturation leads to stabilization of the transcription factor, hypoxia-inducible factor-1α (Hif1α). Hif1α upregulates VegfA expression and nitric oxide synthase expression. Nitric oxide production dilates existing blood vessels, thereby increasing the permeability and **extravasation** of plasma proteins, leading to an increase in expression and activation of the proteases, matrix metalloproteinases and plasmin. Matrix metalloproteinases and plasmin play major roles in promoting proliferation and migration of endothelial cells by activating growth factors and receptors and increasing extracellular matrix turnover, which is necessary for sprouting. Proper vascular development also involves trimming away vessels that are no longer necessary or that would be detrimental should they remain. For example, in its early development, the retina initially forms excess vascularity that must be trimmed down later. Experimental **hyperoxia** (i.e., surplus oxygen) in rodents suppresses Vegf levels in the retina. Because Vegf acts as a survival factor for retinal endothelial cells, hyperoxia resulting from the excess blood supply may drive the pruning of excess vessels by decreasing Vegf levels (Fig. 13-8). Hence, the degree of vascularity (i.e., driven by the formation or pruning of vessels) of a tissue may be mediated by oxygen-dependent regulation of Vegf and nitric oxide levels.

ARTERIES VERSUS VEINS

Arteries and *veins* are terms used to describe vessels whose direction of blood flow is either away from heart (artery) or toward the heart (vein). In addition to these differences in direction of blood flow, arteries and veins are very different in their morphology and physiology. So how does a network of interconnecting vessels become designated as one type or the other? Flow dynamics and the physiological requirements for various loads placed on the vessels are some of the considerations thought to drive arterial or venous specification. Based on studies in the chick embryo, where visualization and ready access to the extraembryonic vasculature are possible, it seems that as perfusion of some capillary-sized vessels increases (arterial side), some downstream side branches are disconnected. These disconnected vessels are then remodeled to establish a second, parallel vasculature that connects to vessels leading to the venous pole of the developing heart. Once this occurs, the connection to the arterial side is reestablished. Recent studies suggest that endothelial cells in these capillary beds are not all identical; rather, some acquire an arterial or venous specification even before blood flow ensues (covered later). However, studies also suggest that endothelial cells remain somewhat plastic in their ability to integrate into arterial or venous endothelium based on cues present in their local environment.

In the Research Lab

FORMATION OF ARTERIES VERSUS VEINS

The factors that direct and guide vessel remodeling and identity are still unclear, but several ligands and receptors known to play roles in neuronal guidance (covered in Chapters 9 and 10) seem to be involved in this process. One such group includes the Eph receptors and their membrane-bound ligands, the ephrins. The binding of ephrins to EphB receptors stimulates transduction signals in the EphB-expressing cells, but this binding can also transduce a reverse signal into the ephrin-expressing cell. Such interactions and signaling events play important roles not only in the development of the nervous system but also in blood vessel remodeling and in the specification of the artery or vein phenotype. EphrinB2 is specifically expressed on the surface of arterial endothelial cells, whereas the EphB4 receptor is specifically expressed on venous endothelial cells (Fig 13-9). When either ephrinB2 or EphB4 is knocked out in mice, the remodeling of primary vascular plexus into arteries and veins fails. How ephrinB2 and EphB4 mediate these changes is unclear, but it has been suggested that during angiogenesis, differential expression of these two molecules may restrain cell migration and create tissue boundaries used to sort out the arterial and venous systems. What is responsible for mediating specific expression of ephrins and Eph receptors is unclear but may involve Tgfβ-mediated signaling, as ephrinB2 expression is absent in Alk1-deficient mice.

Notch signaling may also play a key role in establishing arterial or venous identity upstream of ephrins/Eph receptor signaling even before the formation of the initial vascular complex (see Fig. 13-9). In mice, notch1, notch3, and notch4 receptors and their ligands, Dll-4, Jag1, and Jag2, are expressed in arteries but not in veins. Studies in zebrafish show that inhibiting the notch signaling pathway decreases the expression of ephrinB2, resulting in the ectopic expression of venous markers in the dorsal aorta. In contrast, increasing notch signaling decreases the expression of venous markers and induces the expression of arterial markers, including ephrinB2. In mice, expression of the venous transcription factor chicken ovalbumin upstream promoter transcription factor 2 (Coup-tfII) (also known as Nr2f2) actively represses notch signaling and the expression of the arterial marker neuropilin-1 (Nrp1) and promotes the expression of the venous marker Nrp2. Loss of Coup-tfII expression in veins promotes the expression of the arterial marker, Nrp1. Both Nrp1 and Nrp2 are co-receptors for Vegf that bind specific splice variants of Vegf and may mediate differential responses

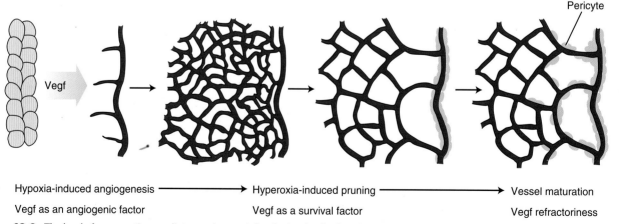

Hypoxia-induced angiogenesis ⟶ Hyperoxia-induced pruning ⟶ Vessel maturation

Vegf as an angiogenic factor   Vegf as a survival factor   Vegf refractoriness

Figure 13-8. The level of oxygenation mediates angiogenesis by altering levels of Vegf. Under hypoxic conditions, Vegf is released, thereby stimulating angiogenesis. Under hyperoxic conditions, Vegf levels decrease. Because endothelial cell survival during early angiogenesis requires Vegf, the capillaries are pruned or trimmed back under conditions of hyperoxia. Once a vessel matures and is stable, Vegf is no longer needed to maintain the vessel.

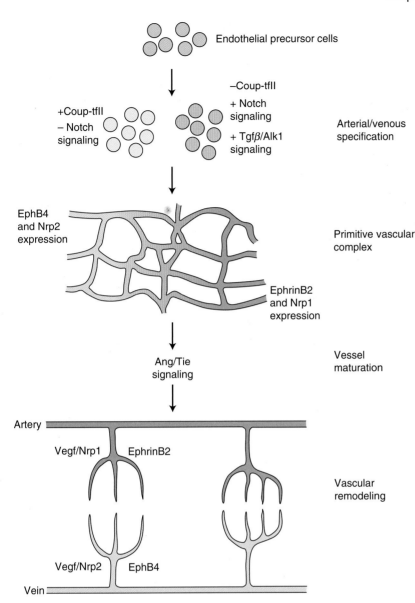

Figure 13-9. Hypothesized model for establishing arterial and venous identity and remodeling, leading to the formation of two separate types of vessels. Notch (by repressing the expression of the venous phenotype) and Tgfβ/Alk1 signaling promote the expression of arterial markers in endothelial precursor cells, while Coup-tfII expression, by suppressing notch signaling, promotes the venous phenotype. These combinations lead to the expression of ephrinB2 and Nrp1 in arterial cords and EphB4 and Nrp2 in the venous cords, which are ultimately responsible for segregating the two vessel groups. In this model, Ang/Tie signaling serves to stabilize these vessels and regulate their maturation. Angiogenic growth (mediated by Vegf/Nrp1 signaling in arterial beds and Vegf/Nrp2 signaling in venous beds) and remodeling then sculpts these vascular beds into their final configurations.

to Vegf signaling in endothelial cells. Therefore, notch signaling may have an important role in mediating not only vascular angiogenesis and remodeling but also arterial/venous specification of EPCs (see Fig. 13-9). Finally, notch signal plays an important role in mediating the diameter of developing blood vessels.

Several other ligands and receptors known to play roles in neuronal guidance are involved in guiding arterial and venous blood vessel formation and remodeling, including slit/robo, semaphorins/plexins, and netrins/Unc5b. This may not be too surprising given that vessels and peripheral nerves generally run in parallel with one another.

In the Clinic

ANGIOMAS

Blood and lymphatic vessels are stimulated by **angiogenic factors** to grow into developing organs. If vessel growth is not inhibited at the appropriate time, or if it is stimulated again later in life, blood or lymphatic vessels may proliferate until they form a tangled mass that may have clinical consequences. Excessive growth of small capillary networks is called a **capillary**

hemangioma or **nevus vascularis**; a proliferation of larger venous sinuses is called a **cavernous hemangioma. Hemangioma of infancy** is the most common benign tumor of childhood (incidence of about 2.5% in neonates and up to 10% to 12% in 1-year-olds; Fig. 13-10). These tumors grow rapidly and consist mainly of endothelial cells with or without lumens, multilayered basement membranes, and fibrous tissue. Hemangiomas differ from some vascular anomalies like **nevus flammeus**, which present at birth as **birthmarks** and grow proportionally with the growth of the child. Most cases of hemangioma of infancy pose no immediate or long-term danger. However, they can be potentially life threatening if they grow in vital organs (e.g., in the skull or vertebral canal, where they can lead to nervous system dysfunction, or in airways, where they can obstruct breathing) or are large enough to create a shunt of physiological significance leading to heart failure. In rare cases, a **hemangiosarcoma** (metastatic angioma) can develop.

Many hemangiomas seem to have a genetic basis to their origin, as they are associated with developmental syndromes resulting from chromosomal anomalies. In the case of hemangioma of infancy, some cases are linked to chromosome region 5q31-33. This region contains genes coding for FGF4, PDGFβ,

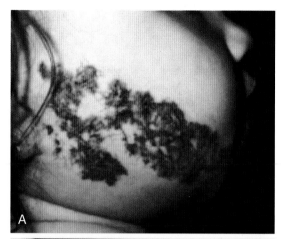

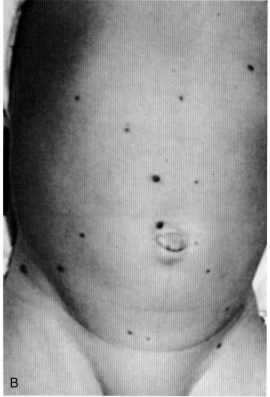

Figure 13-10. Hemangioma of human infancy. *A,* Hemangioma of infancy involving the region of the mandible and having airway involvement. This patient was treated with oral corticosteroids, which regresses these tumors in about a third of patients, thereby avoiding the need for surgical intervention for an otherwise progressing airway obstruction. *B,* Multifocal hemangiomas in an infant.

and FMS-RELATED TYROSINE KINASE—molecules important in blood vessel development. Some hemangiomas are also linked to dysregulation of the TIE/ANG signaling pathway and to VEGFR2 mutations. Multiple hemangioblastomas are associated with a rare, dominantly inherited, familial cancer syndrome called **von Hippel-Lindau disease** (incidence 1:36,000) characterized by mutations in a tumor suppressor gene located at chromosome 3p25-26. These individuals exhibit life-threatening multiple CNS, retinal, and liver hemangioblastomas, renal cell carcinomas, and visceral cysts. Studies show that stromal cells of these tumors produce high levels of VEGF and HIF1α, which could account for the excessive angiogenesis.

HEREDITARY HEMORRHAGIC TELANGIECTASIA

Mutations in ALK1 and ENDOGLIN have been linked to **hereditary hemorrhagic telangiectasia** (HHT). The most common manifestations of HHT (prevalence 1:5000 to 1:8000) are nosebleeds and small vascular anomalies called telangiectases; however, gastrointestinal bleeding and arterial-venous malformations in the lung, brain, and liver progressively develop. Mice heterozygous for mutations in Alk1 or endoglin exhibit very similar progressive pathologies, including the development of large arterial-venous shunts. Mutations in human ALK1 have also been linked to primary **pulmonary hypertension** involving abnormal remodeling of the pulmonary vasculature. Both HHT and some forms of pulmonary hypertension may stem from an improper balance between ALK1 and ALK5 signaling (covered earlier in the chapter). Endothelial cells from normal healthy patients form extensive, stable, and well-formed vessels in tissue culture, whereas endothelial cells from HHT patients are unable to do so. ENDOGLIN also interacts with the actin cytoskeleton. Endothelial cells from HHT patients exhibit a disorganized actin cytoskeleton, but normal actin organization can be restored if normal ENDOGLIN is overexpressed in these cells. Endothelial cells with a disorganized, abnormal cytoskeleton are more likely to form vessels prone to vascular instability, hemorrhaging, and vascular disarray.

DEVELOPMENT OF AORTIC ARCH ARTERIES

Animation 13-2: Development of Aortic Arch Arteries. Animations are available online at StudentConsult.

The respiratory apparatus of the jawless fish that gave rise to higher vertebrates consisted of a variable number of gill bars separated by gill slits (Fig. 13-11). Water flowed in through the mouth and out through the gill slits. Each of the gill bars, or **branchial arches**, was vascularized by an **aortic arch artery**, which arose as a branch of the dorsal and ventral aortae. Gas exchange took place in the gill capillaries, and the dorsal half of each aortic arch artery conveyed the oxygenated blood to the paired dorsal aortae.

In higher vertebrate and human embryos, four pairs of mesenchymal condensations develop on either side of the pharynx, corresponding to branchial arches one, two, three, four, and possibly six of the fish ancestor. The fifth arch never develops at all or forms briefly and then regresses, whereas evidence for the existence of a sixth arch is questioned. The mesodermal, ectodermal, and endodermal components of the arches have been modified through evolution, so that in humans they form the structures of the lower face and neck and derivatives of the pharyngeal foregut. Thus, these structures are more appropriately called **pharyngeal arches** rather than branchial arches. Development of the pharyngeal arches is detailed in Chapter 17; the following text is limited to development of the aortic arch arteries.

HUMAN AORTIC ARCH ARTERIES ARISE IN CRANIOCAUDAL SEQUENCE AND FORM BASKET OF ARTERIES AROUND PHARYNX

As covered in Chapter 12, the first pair of aortic arch arteries is formed between day twenty-two and day twenty-four. At this time in development, the process of

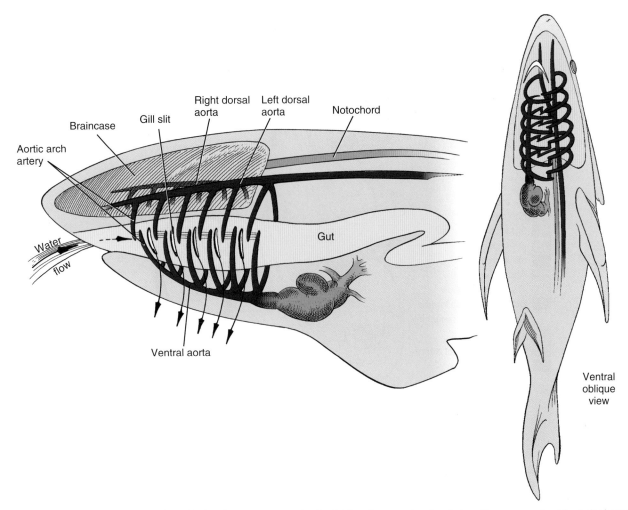

Figure 13-11. Schematic view of the branchial arch artery system of a shark. The pharyngeal arch arteries of humans evolved from the branchial arch arteries of protochordates and fishes. The branchial arch arteries occupy the gill bars and thus enclose the pharynx like a basket. The arteries supply blood to the gills, which extract oxygen from water flowing through the gill slits.

body folding, which carries the forming primitive heart tube into the future thorax, also draws the cranial ends of the attached aortae into a dorsoventral loop (see Fig. 12-4). The resulting first pair of aortic arch arteries lies in the thickened mesenchyme of the first pair of pharyngeal arches on either side of the developing pharynx. Ventrally, the aortic arch arteries arise from the **aortic sac**, an expansion at the distal end of the cardiac outflow tract (Fig. 13-12*A*). Dorsally, they connect to the left and right dorsal aortae. The bilateral dorsal aortae lie adjacent to the notochord. The dorsal aortae remain separate in the region of the aortic arches, but during the fourth week, they fuse together from the fourth thoracic segment to the fourth lumbar segment to form a midline **dorsal aorta**.

Studies in chick embryos suggest that the timely loss of chordin, released by the notochord along the cranial-caudal axis, along with the continued presence of vessel-promoting factors (e.g., Vegfs), promotes fusion of the dorsal aortae. How chordin expression is regulated along this axis is unknown.

Between days twenty-six and twenty-eight, aortic arch arteries two, three, and four develop by vasculogenesis and angiogenesis within their respective pharyngeal arches, incorporating EPCs that migrate in from the surrounding

mesoderm (see Figs. 13-12, 13-13). Neural crest–derived mesenchymal cells within the pharyngeal arches also play a significant role in the normal development of the arch arteries, although neural crest cells do not contribute to the endothelium of these vessels (see the following "In the Research Lab" entitled "Tissue Interactions Direct Aortic Arch Artery Remodeling"). A plexus of vessels also form from EPCs within the splanchnic mesoderm caudal to the fourth pharyngeal arch and eventually form a blood vessel channel between the dorsal aorta and the aortic sac by day twenty-nine. Classically, the literature refers to this blood vessel as a sixth aortic arch artery even though uncertainty exists as to whether a sixth pharyngeal arch exists in higher vertebrates. However, for ease of discussion, we will still refer to this vessel as a sixth aortic arch artery.

The first two arch arteries regress as the later arches form. The second arch artery arises in the second pharyngeal arch by day twenty-six and grows to connect the aortic sac to the dorsal aortae. Simultaneously, the first pair of aortic arch arteries begins to regress completely (except, possibly, for small remnants that may give rise to portions of the **maxillary arteries**) (Fig. 13-12*A*, *B*). On day twenty-eight, while the first arch is regressing, the

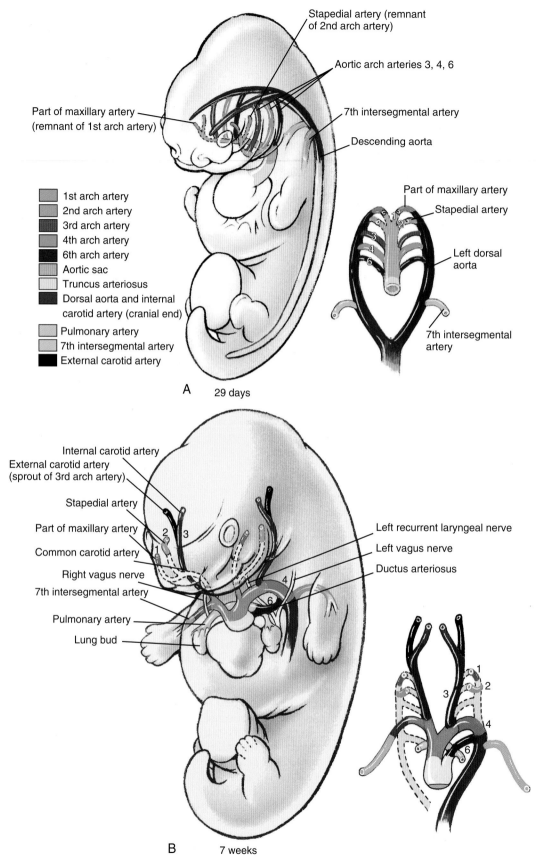

Figure 13-12. Development of the aortic system. *A,* Formation of the first arch is complete by day twenty-four but regresses as the second arch forms on day twenty-six. The third and fourth arches form on day twenty-eight; the second arch degenerates as the sixth aortic arch artery forms on day twenty-nine. *B,* Development of the arches in the second month. Note that the arteries arising from the first three pairs of aortic arch arteries are bilateral, whereas vessels derived from arches four and six develop asymmetrically.

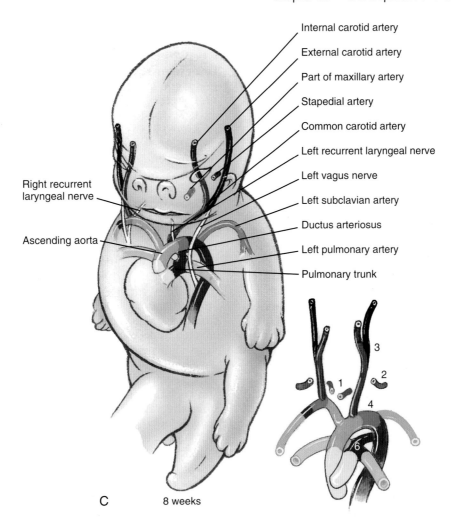

Internal carotid artery
External carotid artery
Part of maxillary artery
Stapedial artery
Common carotid artery
Left recurrent laryngeal nerve
Left vagus nerve
Left subclavian artery
Ductus arteriosus
Left pulmonary artery
Pulmonary trunk

Right recurrent laryngeal nerve

Ascending aorta

C   8 weeks

Figure 13-12, cont'd *C,* Eight weeks. Note the asymmetrical development of the recurrent laryngeal branches of the vagus nerve, which innervate the laryngeal muscles. As the larynx is displaced cranially relative to the arch system, the recurrent laryngeal nerves are caught under the most caudal remaining arch on each side. The right recurrent laryngeal nerve therefore loops under the right subclavian artery, whereas the left recurrent laryngeal nerve loops under the ductus arteriosus.

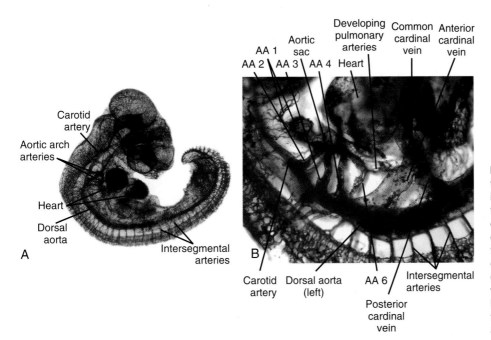

Carotid artery
Aortic arch arteries
Heart
Dorsal aorta
Intersegmental arteries

A

AA 1
AA 2
AA 3
AA 4
Aortic sac
Developing pulmonary arteries
Heart
Common cardinal vein
Anterior cardinal vein

B

Carotid artery
Dorsal aorta (left)
AA 6
Intersegmental arteries
Posterior cardinal vein

Figure 13-13. Chick embryo vasculature revealed by intravenous injection of ink into a living embryo, followed by fixation and clearing of the embryo. *A,* Vasculature of a three and one-half-day-old chick embryo. *B,* Higher magnification of the pharyngeal arch region in a similar embryo. Several of the aortic arch arteries (AAs) as well as other major arteries are visible. The common cardinal veins can be identified entering the venous pole of the heart. Note two branches: anterior and posterior cardinal veins.

third and fourth aortic arch arteries form. Finally, on day twenty-nine, the sixth arch arteries form, and the second arch arteries regress, except for a small remnant giving rise to part of the **stapedial artery** (Figs. 13-12*B, C;* 13-13) that supplies blood to the primordium of the stapes bone in the developing ear (development of the ear is covered in Chapter 18).

AORTIC ARCH ARTERIES GIVE RISE TO IMPORTANT VESSELS OF HEAD, NECK, AND UPPER THORAX

By day thirty-five, the segments of dorsal aorta connecting the third and fourth arch arteries disappear on both sides of the body, so that the cranial extensions of the dorsal aortae supplying the head receive blood entirely through the third aortic arches (see Fig. 13-12*B*). The third arch arteries give rise to the right and left **common carotid arteries** (Figs. 13-12*B, C*, 13-14*A*) and to the proximal portion of the right and left **internal carotid arteries**. The distal portion of the internal carotid arteries is derived from the cranial extensions of the dorsal aortae, and the right and left **external carotid arteries** sprout from the common carotids (see Fig. 13-12*B, C*).

By the seventh week, the right dorsal aorta loses its connections with both the fused midline dorsal aorta and the right sixth aortic arch artery, while remaining connected to the right fourth arch artery (see Fig. 13-12*B, C*). Meanwhile, it also acquires a branch, the **right seventh cervical intersegmental artery**, which develops within the right upper limb bud region. The definitive **right subclavian artery** supplying the upper limb is derived from (1) the right fourth arch, (2) a short segment of the right dorsal aorta, and (3) the right seventh intersegmental artery. The region of the aortic sac connected to the right fourth artery is modified to form the branch of the developing aorta called the **brachiocephalic artery** (see Fig. 13-12*C*).

The left fourth aortic arch artery retains its connection to the fused dorsal aorta, and, with a small segment of the aortic sac, it becomes the **aortic arch (arch of the aorta** or **ascending aorta)** and the most proximal

portion of the **descending aorta**. The remainder of the descending aorta, from the fourth thoracic level caudally, is derived from the fused dorsal aortae. The **left seventh intersegmental artery**, which forms in the paraxial mesoderm and limb region, gives rise to the **left subclavian artery** supplying the left upper extremity (see Fig. 13-12*B, C*). The development of the **coronary arteries** is covered in Chapter 12.

Both the right and left sixth arches arise from the proximal end of the aortic sac, but further development is then asymmetrical (see Figs. 13-12*B, C*, 13-13*B*, 13-14*B*). By the seventh week, the distal connection of the right sixth aortic arch artery to the right dorsal aorta disappears. In contrast, the left sixth aortic arch artery remains complete, and its distal portion forms the **ductus arteriosus**, which allows blood to shunt from the pulmonary trunk to the descending aorta throughout gestation (see Fig. 13-12*B, C*). This bypass closes at birth and is later transformed into the **ligamentum arteriosum**, which attaches the pulmonary trunk to the arch of the aorta. Changes in the circulation that take place at birth are covered in detail near the end of this chapter.

As shown in Figure 13-12*B* and *C*, the asymmetrical development of the left and right sixth aortic arch arteries is responsible for the curious asymmetry of the **left** and **right recurrent laryngeal nerves**, which branch from the vagus nerves. The laryngeal nerves originally arise below the level of the sixth aortic arch artery and cross under the right and left sixth aortic arch arteries to innervate intrinsic muscles of the larynx. During development, the larynx is translocated cranially relative to the aortic arch arteries. The left recurrent laryngeal nerve becomes caught under the sixth arch on the left side and remains looped under the future ligamentum arteriosum. Because the distal right sixth aortic arch artery disappears (and because a fifth aortic arch artery fails to develop), the right recurrent laryngeal nerve becomes caught under the fourth aortic arch artery, which forms part of the right subclavian artery.

Although the pulmonary arteries become connected to the sixth arch arteries and finally to the pulmonary trunk,

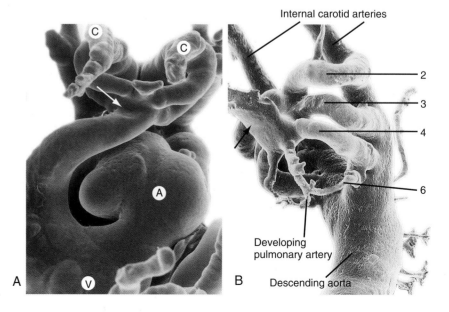

Figure 13-14. Vascular casts. *A,* Frontal view of a cast of the aortic arch arteries. The left and right common carotid arteries (C) are growing toward the viewer from the third arches. The third and fourth aortic arch arteries arise from the aortic sac (arrow). A, Primitive atrium; V, ventricle. *B,* Inferolateral view of a cast of the aortic arch arteries. Aortic arch arteries two, three, and four are fully developed, and the sixth pair is beginning to form. An arrow marks the distal outflow tract.

several classic observations, as well as more recent experiments, suggest that the pulmonary arteries develop as branches of the fourth aortic arch artery and then establish a secondary connection with the sixth aortic arch arteries before losing their connection with the fourth aortic arch arteries (see Figs. 13-13*B*, 13-14*B*). In the lungs, the distal ends of the pulmonary arteries then anastomose with the vasculature developing in the mesenchyme surrounding the bronchial buds (covered in Chapter 11).

In the Research Lab

TISSUE INTERACTIONS DIRECT AORTIC ARCH ARTERY REMODELING

As covered in Chapter 17, the mesoderm-derived and neural crest–derived mesenchyme of the pharyngeal arches is coated on the inside by endoderm and on the outside by ectoderm. Each pharyngeal arch is separated from adjacent ones by external indentations (pharyngeal ectodermal clefts or grooves) and internal foregut expansions (pharyngeal endodermal pouches), with the ventral floor region of the pharyngeal arches also serving as the site of the cranial second heart field (covered in Chapter 12). Within each of the pharyngeal arches, an aortic arch artery forms that is subsequently remodeled into the mature great vessels. Quail-chick transplantation experiments show that neural crest cells differentiate into the vascular smooth muscle and connective tissue cells forming the tunics of these great vessels. If neural crest cells are ablated or their migration from the neural tube into pharyngeal arches is perturbed, the initial aortic arch arteries still form, but regression and persistence of pharyngeal arch arteries is abnormal: the remaining mesoderm-derived mesenchyme is incompetent to sustain continued growth and development of the arteries after blood flow is initiated. Hence, neural crest cells not only provide the mesenchyme for tunics of these vessels, they also play an important role in patterning of pharyngeal arch arteries.

Based on recent avian and mouse studies, it is becoming clear that tissue-tissue interactions between neural crest–derived mesenchyme and the pharyngeal ectoderm and endoderm play key roles in mediating aortic arch artery development. As mentioned in Chapter 12, particular levels of Fgf8 signaling modulate proliferation, survival, and differentiation of cells in the second heart field. Fgf8 is specifically expressed in pharyngeal ectoderm and endoderm but not in pharyngeal arch mesoderm or neural crest–derived mesenchyme. Yet, it seems that neural crest cells somehow mediate Fgf8 signaling levels in this region. In addition to heart development being sensitive to Fgf8 signaling within the pharyngeal arches, pharyngeal vascular development is also dependent on Fgf8 signaling in both chick and mouse embryos. In mice, Fgf8 hypomorphs (an animal with a partial loss-of-function mutation, e.g., Fgf8 expression in the hypomorph is knocked down but is not eliminated completely) phenocopy many of the cardiac and aortic arch artery defects seen in **22q11.2 deletion syndrome** in humans (this syndrome is covered further in Chapters 4, 12, and 17), although FGF8 is located on human chromosome 10q25. If Fgf8 is specifically knocked out in pharyngeal arch ectoderm of developing mouse embryos, the fourth aortic arch artery is lost, leading to defects in aorta and subclavian artery development in the absence of cardiac defects. In contrast, loss of Fgf8 expression in third and fourth pharyngeal arch endoderm leads to defects in both glandular development (e.g., thyroid, parathyroid, and thymus; development of these organs is covered in Chapter 17) and aortic semilunar valve formation. Notch signaling in the neural crest seems to mediate Fgf8 signaling. Loss of notch

signaling in the cardiac neural crest not only perturbs outflow tract development but also causes aortic arch artery defects.

Mutations in humans in TBX1 (a transcription factor encoded within the affected 22q11.2 region) can also cause aortic arch artery defects that phenocopy the full deletion syndrome, including aortic arch artery anomalies, particularly those involving the fourth aortic arch artery (e.g., interrupted aortic arch, aberrant origin of the right subclavian artery, and aberrant origin of the right aortic arch). In mice, Tbx1 is highly expressed in the endoderm of the fourth pouch and mesoderm of the fourth pharyngeal arch. As covered in Chapter 12, loss of Tbx1 expression in this region leads to decreased Fgf8 levels, and its heterozygotic inactivation in mice causes the same spectrum of defects as seen in humans with TBX1 deletion. Hence, alterations in Tbx1 activity and subsequent changes in Fgf8 signaling could be partly responsible for the defects seen in patients with TBX1 mutations. Complete loss of several different genes expressed in pharyngeal arches causes similar defects, but Fgf8 and Tbx1 are the only genes identified to date that do this with a heterozygotic loss.

Endothelins represent a group of peptides important in blood pressure regulation in adults. During embryonic development, endothelins and their receptors have an important role in mediating neural crest cell development. Knockout mice for the endothelin receptor, Eta, or the converting enzyme that proteolytically generates active endothelins, endothelin-converting enzyme-1 (Ece1), have neural crest cell–related defects in cardiac development, pharyngeal arch artery development, and development of enteric ganglia. In the pharyngeal arches, endothelin-1 (Et1) is expressed by pharyngeal arch ectoderm and endoderm, but not by neural crest cells; Eta receptor is expressed only by neural crest cells in the pharyngeal arches. Knocking out Ece1 or the Eta receptor in mice leads to the formation of an interrupted aortic arch or an absence of the right subclavian artery. These knockout mice also show altered expression of other genes important in pharyngeal arch development, including Dlx2, Dlx3, EphA3, MsxE, and Hand2. These and other studies suggest that even with loss of Eta signaling, neural crest cells still migrate into the pharyngeal arches and that the normal developmental patterning of the initial aortic arch arteries still occurs. However, there seems to be a decrease in the number of neural crest cells within the pharyngeal arches, resulting in hypoplasia and abnormal aortic arch artery remodeling.

Obviously, aortic arch artery development is asymmetrical. Therefore, it is likely under the influence of gene expression responsible for determining sidedness. In mice, Pitx2c (an isoform of Pitx2) is expressed more prevalently in the left aortic sac and second heart field than in the right. Knockout mice for Pitx2c exhibit defects in remodeling of the aortic arch arteries, as well as cardiac defects that might be predicted from a perturbation of second heart field sidedness (covered in Chapter 12). About 30% of these mice have a right aortic arch, about 14% have double aortic arches, and some exhibit double-outlet right ventricles. Again, neural crest cell migration seems normal in these mice, and the pharyngeal arch arteries initially have similar amounts of mesenchyme surrounding their endothelia. How Pitx2c might mediate asymmetrical remodeling of the aortic arch artery is not known, but it has been suggested that Pitx2c may somehow sustain or recruit aortic arch artery supportive cells to the left side.

Cranial nerve innervation of the pharyngeal arches may also have a role in aortic arch artery development. Knockout mice for Tgfβ2 exhibit abnormal increases in apoptosis of fourth aortic arch artery mesenchyme, and they develop an interrupted fourth aortic arch and aberrant right subclavian vessels. Although neural crest cell migration and differentiation into vascular smooth muscle seem normal in these mice, defects coincide with loss of fourth pharyngeal arch innervation.

In summary, pharyngeal arch neural crest–derived mesenchyme plays an important role in maintaining the integrity of particular aortic arch arteries rather than in the initial formation of the early pharyngeal arch vasculature. Subsequent remodeling events seem to involve complex paracrine interactions between pharyngeal neural crest cells; pharyngeal arch endoderm, ectoderm, and mesoderm; and aortic arch artery endothelium. These interactions are still not fully understood.

DORSAL AORTA DEVELOPS VENTRAL, LATERAL, AND POSTEROLATERAL BRANCHES

VITELLINE ARTERIES GIVE RISE TO ARTERIAL SUPPLY OF GASTROINTESTINAL TRACT

The blood vessels that arise in the yolk sac wall differentiate to form the arteries and veins of the **vitelline system**. As the yolk sac shrinks relative to the folding embryo, the right and left vitelline plexuses coalesce to form a number of major arteries that anastomose both with the vascular plexuses of the future gut and with the ventral surface of the dorsal aorta (Fig. 13-15A). These vessels eventually lose their connection with the yolk sac, becoming the arteries that supply blood from the dorsal aorta to the gastrointestinal tract.

Cranial to the diaphragm, about five pairs of these arteries usually develop and anastomose with the dorsal aorta at variable levels to supply the thoracic esophagus. Caudal to the diaphragm, three pairs of major arteries develop to supply specific regions of the developing abdominal gut (Fig. 13-15B). The fields of vascularization of these three arteries constitute the basis for dividing the abdominal gastrointestinal tract into three embryologic regions: **abdominal foregut, midgut**, and **hindgut**.

The most superior of the three abdominal vitelline arteries, the **celiac artery**, initially joins the dorsal aorta at the seventh cervical level. This connection subsequently descends to the twelfth thoracic level. There the celiac artery develops branches that vascularize not only the abdominal part of the foregut, from the abdominal esophagus to the descending segment of the duodenum, but also the several embryological outgrowths of the foregut—liver, pancreas, and gallbladder. The celiac artery also produces a large branch that vascularizes the spleen, which develops within the mesoderm of the dorsal mesogastrium (covered in Chapter 14; the dorsal mesogastrium is the portion of the dorsal mesentery that suspends the stomach).

The second abdominal vitelline artery, the **superior mesenteric artery**, initially joins the dorsal aorta at the second thoracic level; this connection later migrates to the first lumbar level. This artery supplies the developing midgut—the intestine that reaches from the descending segment of the duodenum to a region of the transverse colon near the left colic flexure.

The third and final abdominal vitelline artery, the **inferior mesenteric artery**, initially joins the dorsal aorta at the twelfth thoracic level and later descends to the third lumbar level. It supplies the hindgut: the distal portion of the transverse colon, the descending and

sigmoid colon, and the superior rectum. As covered in Chapter 14, the inferior end of the anorectal canal is vascularized by branches of the iliac arteries.

LATERAL BRANCHES OF DESCENDING AORTA VASCULARIZE SUPRARENAL GLANDS, GONADS, AND KIDNEYS

The suprarenal (adrenal) glands, gonads, and kidneys are vascularized by lateral branches of the descending aorta. However as illustrated in Figure 13-16, these three organs and their arteries have different developmental histories. The suprarenal glands form in the posterior body wall between the sixth and twelfth thoracic segments and become vascularized mainly by a pair of lateral aortic branches that arise at an upper lumbar level. The suprarenal glands also acquire branches from the renal artery and inferior phrenic artery, but the **suprarenal arteries** developing from these aortic branches remain the major supply to the glands. These glands and their aortic branches develop in place. The presumptive gonads become vascularized by **gonadal arteries** that arise initially at the tenth thoracic level. The gonads descend during development, but the origin of the gonadal arteries becomes fixed at the third or fourth lumbar level. As the gonads (especially the testes) descend farther, the gonadal arteries elongate. In contrast, the definitive kidneys arise in the sacral region and migrate upward to a lumbar site just below the suprarenal glands. As they migrate, they are vascularized by a succession of transient aortic branches that arise at progressively higher levels. These arteries do not elongate to follow the ascending kidneys but instead degenerate and are replaced. The final pair of arteries in this series forms in the upper lumbar region and becomes the definitive **renal arteries**. Occasionally, a more inferior pair of renal arteries persists as accessory renal arteries. Displacement of the suprarenal glands, gonads, and kidneys as they develop is covered further in Chapters 15 and 16.

INTERSEGMENTAL BRANCHES ARISE FROM PARAXIAL MESODERM AND JOIN DORSAL AORTA

At the end of the third week, small posterolateral branches arise by vasculogenesis between the developing somites at the cervical through sacral levels and connect to the dorsal aorta (see Fig. 13-13). In the **cervical, thoracic**, and **lumbar** regions, a dorsal branch of each of these intersegmental vessels vascularizes both the developing neural tube and the epimeres that will form the deep muscles of the neck and back (Fig. 13-17A; epimeres and hypomeres are covered in Chapter 8). Cutaneous branches of these arteries also supply the dorsal skin. The ventral branch of each intersegmental vessel supplies the developing hypomeric muscles and associated skin. In the **thoracic** region, these ventral branches become the **intercostal arteries** and their cutaneous branches; in the lumbar and sacral regions, they become the **lumbar** and **lateral sacral arteries**. The short continuation of the dorsal aorta beyond its bifurcation into the common iliac arteries is called the **median sacral artery**.

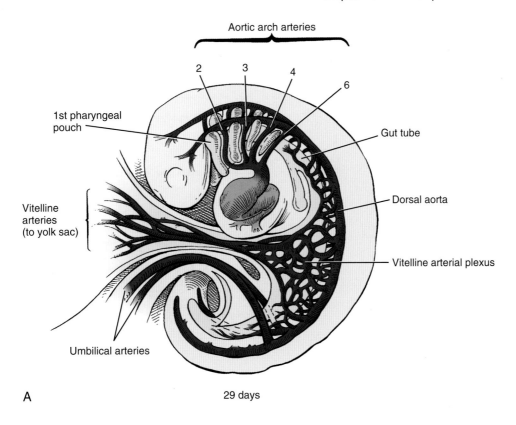

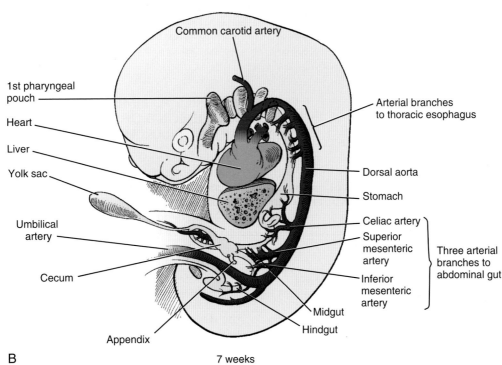

Figure 13-15. Development of the ventral aortic branches supplying the gut tube and derivatives. *A,* In the fourth week, a multitude of vitelline arteries emerge from the ventral surfaces of the dorsal aortae to supply the yolk sac. *B,* After the paired dorsal aortae fuse at the end of the fourth week, many of the vitelline channels disappear, reducing the final number to about five in the thoracic region and to three (the celiac, superior mesenteric, and inferior mesenteric arteries) in the abdominal region.

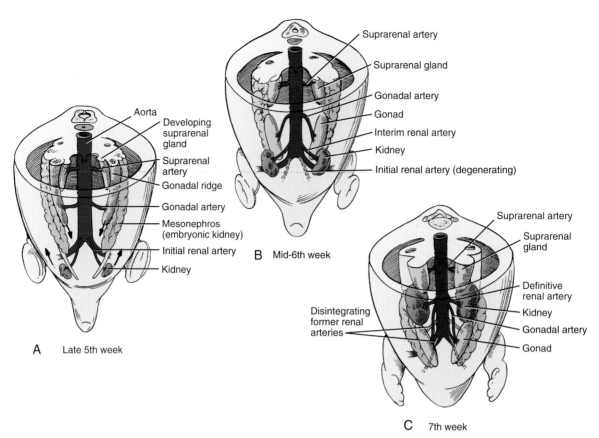

Figure 13-16. Development of the lateral branches of the abdominal aorta. *A,* Lateral sprouts of the dorsal aorta vascularize the suprarenal glands, gonads, and kidneys. During the sixth week, the gonads begin to descend, whereas the kidneys ascend (arrows). *B, C,* The gonadal artery lengthens during the migration of the gonad, but the ascending kidney is vascularized by a succession of new, more cranial aortic sprouts. The suprarenal arteries remain in place.

In the cervical region, the intersegmental branches anastomose with each other to form a more complex pattern of vascularization (Fig. 13-17*B-D*). The paired **vertebral arteries** arise from longitudinal branches that link together to form a longitudinal vessel, and they secondarily lose their intersegmental connections to the aorta. The **deep cervical, ascending cervical, superior intercostal, internal thoracic,** and **superior** and **inferior epigastric arteries** also develop from anastomoses of intersegmental arteries.

UMBILICAL ARTERIES INITIALLY JOIN DORSAL AORTAE BUT SHIFT THEIR ORIGIN TO INTERNAL ILIAC ARTERIES

The right and left **umbilical arteries** develop in the connecting stalk early in the fourth week and are thus among the earliest embryonic arteries to arise. These arteries form an initial connection with the paired dorsal aortae in the sacral region (see Fig. 13-15*A*). However, during the fifth week, these connections are obliterated as the umbilical arteries develop a new connection with the fifth pair of lumbar intersegmental artery branches called the **internal iliac arteries**. The internal iliac arteries vascularize pelvic organs and (initially) the lower extremity limb bud. As covered later, the fifth lumber intersegmental arteries also give rise to the **external iliac arteries**. Proximal to these branches, the root of the fifth intersegmental artery is called the **common iliac artery** (Fig. 13-18).

ARTERIES TO LIMBS ARE FORMED BY REMODELING OF INTERSEGMENTAL ARTERY BRANCHES

As indicated above, the arteries to the developing upper and lower limbs are derived mainly from the seventh cervical intersegmental artery and the fifth lumbar intersegmental artery, respectively. These arteries initially supply each limb bud by joining an **axial** or **axis artery** that develops along the central axis of the limb bud (see Figs. 13-18, 13-19). In the upper limb, the axis artery develops into the **brachial artery** of the upper arm and the **anterior interosseous artery** of the forearm and thus continues to be the main source of blood for the limb (Fig.13-19). In the hand, a small portion of the axis artery persists as the **deep palmar arch**. The other arteries of the upper limb, including the **radial, median,** and **ulnar arteries**, develop partly as sprouts of the axis artery.

In contrast, in the lower limb, the axis artery—which arises as the distal continuation of the internal iliac artery—largely degenerates, and the definitive supply is provided almost entirely by the **external iliac artery**, which, as mentioned above, arises as a new branch of the fifth lumbar intersegmental artery (see Fig. 13-18). The axis artery persists as three remnants: the small **sciatic (ischiadic) artery**, which serves the sciatic nerve in the posterior thigh; a segment of the **popliteal artery**; and a section of the **fibular (peroneal) artery** in the leg. Virtually all other arteries of the lower limb develop as sprouts of the external iliac artery.

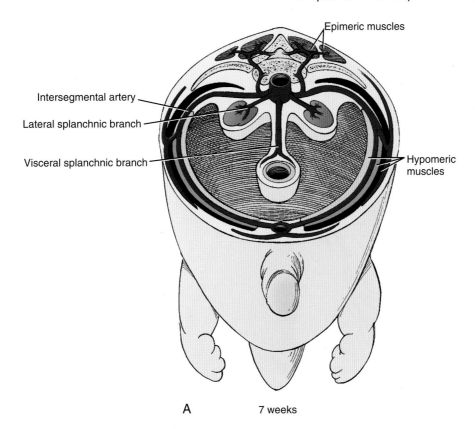

A   7 weeks

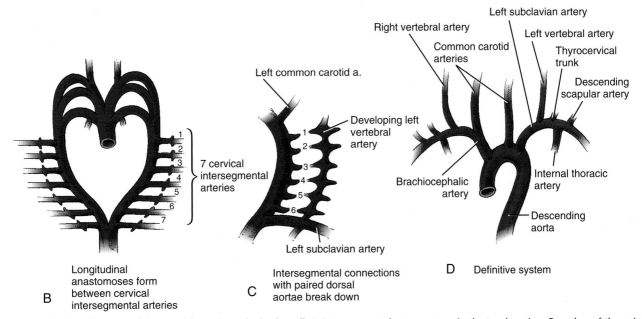

B   Longitudinal anastomoses form between cervical intersegmental arteries

C   Intersegmental connections with paired dorsal aortae break down

D   Definitive system

Figure 13-17. Development of the arterial supply to the body wall. *A,* Intersegmental artery system in the trunk region. Branches of the paired intersegmental arteries supply the posterior, lateral, and anterior body wall and musculature, the vertebral column, and the spinal cord. *B-D,* The vertebral artery is formed from longitudinal anastomoses of the first through seventh cervical intersegmental arteries.

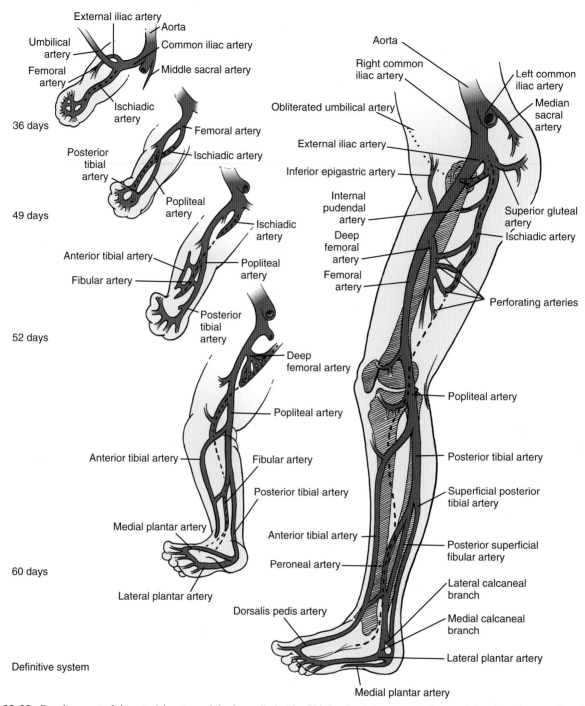

Figure 13-18. Development of the arterial system of the lower limb. The fifth lumbar intersegmental artery joins the axis artery forming in the lower extremity. The only remnants of the axis artery in the lower limb of the adult are the ischiadic artery, a small portion of the popliteal artery, and the peroneal artery.

In the Clinic

VASCULAR ANOMALIES ARISING FROM ERRORS IN REMODELING OF GREAT VESSELS

The bilaterally symmetrical vascular system of the early embryo undergoes an intricate sequence of regressions, remodeling, and anastomoses to produce the adult pattern of great veins and arteries. Regression affects mainly the left side of the venous system (covered later in this chapter; see also Chapter 12) and, conversely, the right side of the aortic arch arteries. As a result, systemic venous return is channeled to the right atrium, whereas the original left fourth aortic arch artery becomes the arch of the definitive aorta. Congenital vascular malformations can arise at many stages during this process. Vascular malformations can result

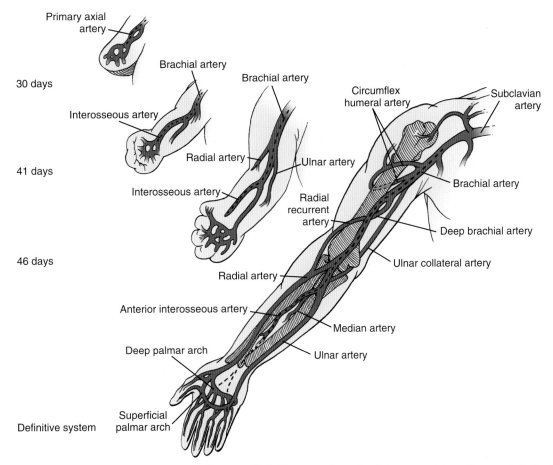

Primary axial artery

30 days

Brachial artery

Interosseous artery

41 days

Brachial artery

Radial artery

Ulnar artery

Circumflex humeral artery

Subclavian artery

Radial recurrent artery

Brachial artery

Deep brachial artery

Ulnar collateral artery

Interosseous artery

46 days

Radial artery

Anterior interosseous artery

Median artery

Deep palmar arch

Ulnar artery

Superficial palmar arch

Definitive system

Figure 13-19. Development of the arterial system of the upper limb. The seventh cervical intersegmental arteries grow into the limb buds to join the axis arteries of the developing upper limbs. The axis artery gives rise to the subclavian, axillary, brachial, and anterior interosseous arteries and to the deep palmar arch. Other arteries of the upper extremity develop as sprouts of the axis artery.

from the failure of some primitive element to undergo regression, or, alternatively, from inappropriate regression of an element.

FORMATION OF "VASCULAR RINGS" THAT CONSTRICT ESOPHAGUS AND TRACHEA

The aortic arch arteries and dorsal aorta initially form a vascular basket that completely encircles the pharyngeal foregut (see Figs. 13-13, 13-14, 13-15A). In normal development, the regression of the right dorsal aorta opens this basket on the right side, so that the esophagus is not encircled by aortic arch artery derivatives. However, occasionally the right dorsal aorta persists and maintains its connection with the dorsal aorta, resulting in a **double aortic arch** forming a **vascular ring** that encloses the trachea and esophagus (Fig. 13-20). This ring may constrict the trachea and esophagus, interfering with both breathing and swallowing.

Another malformation that can cause difficulties in swallowing (**dysphagia**) and possibly **dyspnea** (difficulty in breathing) results from the abnormal disappearance of the right fourth aortic arch artery. If the right fourth arch regresses, the seventh intersegmental artery (future right subclavian artery), which normally connects to the right fourth aortic arch artery, forms a connection with the descending aorta instead (Fig. 13-21). Therefore, the seventh intersegmental crosses over the midline, usually posterior to the esophagus, forming an **aberrant right subclavian artery** (seen in almost 1% of the general population and almost 40% of **Down syndrome** patients having congenital heart defects). After the great arteries mature, the esophagus may be pinched between the arch of the aorta and the abnormal right subclavian artery. Often this is asymptomatic.

However, in some individuals, the aberrant right subclavian artery compresses the esophagus, causing dysphagia, and the esophagus may reciprocally compress the right subclavian artery, reducing blood pressure in the right upper extremity.

Another common aortic arch artery defect is a **right-sided (right) aortic arch**. In this anomaly, the right dorsal aorta segment between the future right subclavian artery and future thoracic aorta (i.e., the right eighth dorsal aortic segment) is retained, whereas the left fourth aortic is lost (Fig. 13-22A). This anomaly is seen in 13% to 35% of patients with tetralogy of Fallot and in about 8% of patients with transposition of the great vessels. In cases of right-sided aortic arch, the ductus arteriosus (ligamentum arteriosum after its postnatal closure) stretches toward the right side in front or behind the esophagus and trachea. If it passes behind the esophagus, it can constrict the esophagus and trachea, causing dysphagia and/or dyspnea.

An **interrupted aortic arch** arises when both right and left fourth aortic arch arteries are obliterated while the distal right dorsal aorta is retained (Fig. 13-22B). After birth, the aorta supplies the head, upper limbs, and body, but the lower body and limbs are supplied by the pulmonary trunk (poorly oxygenated blood) via a **patent ductus arteriosus**.

COARCTATION OF AORTA

Coarctation of the aorta is a congenital malformation in which an abnormal thickening of the aortic wall severely constricts the aorta in the region of the ductus arteriosus. This malformation occurs in approximately 0.3% of all live-born infants. It is more common in males than females and is the

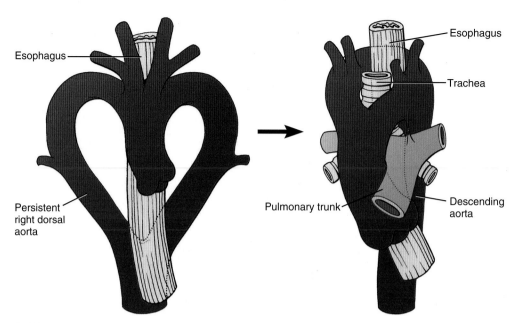

Figure 13-20. A double aortic arch results from failure of the right dorsal aorta to regress in the region of the heart. Both the esophagus and the trachea are enclosed in the resulting double arch.

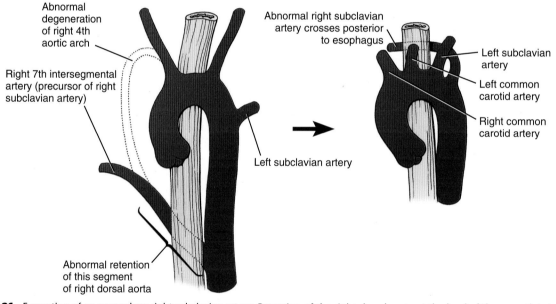

Figure 13-21. Formation of an anomalous right subclavian artery. Retention of the right dorsal aorta at the level of the seventh intersegmental artery coupled with abnormal regression of the right fourth aortic arch artery may result in an anomalous right subclavian artery that passes posterior to the esophagus.

most common cardiovascular anomaly in **Turner syndrome**. The pathogenesis of aortic coarctation is not understood, although the malformation may be triggered by genetic factors or by teratogens. Two ideas have been proposed to explain coarctation: (1) abnormal migration of cells into the aortic wall near the ductus arteriosus, and (2) abnormal hemodynamics resulting in abnormal growth of the left fourth aortic arch artery.

Aortic coarctation occurs most commonly in a juxtaductal position (i.e., adjacent to the ductus arteriosus) but may also occur more proximally (preductal; i.e., upstream) or distally (postductal; i.e., downstream) (Fig. 13-23A, B). **Postductal coarctation** may be asymptomatic in newborn infants if collateral circulation is established from the subclavian, internal thoracic, transverse cervical, suprascapular, superior epigastric, intercostal, and lumbar arteries during the embryonic and fetal periods (Fig. 13-23C, D).

However, with **preductal coarctation**, collateral circulation does not develop because sufficient oxygen- and nutrient-enriched blood from the placenta reaches the lower portion of the body via the **ductus arteriosus**. These infants typically develop problems after birth when the ductus arteriosus closes. This leads to **differential cyanosis**, where the upper part of the body and the head are well perfused but the lower part of the body is cyanotic. The clinical effects of coarctation are variable and depend on the degree of narrowing. Typically, coarctation requires surgical repair in the neonatal period.

As mentioned in Chapters 3, 5, 12, and 14, patients with **Alagille syndrome** exhibit a characteristic facial appearance, paucity of bile ducts, heart defects, vertebral defects, and arterial stenosis (usually pulmonary trunk/artery stenosis but sometimes including abdominal aortic coarctation). Mutations in JAGGED1

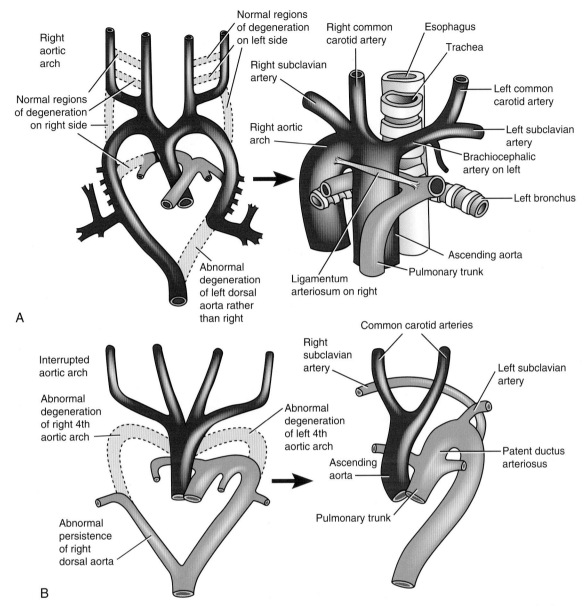

Figure 13-22. *A,* Right aortic arch. The left dorsal aorta downstream from the origin of the left subclavian artery is obliterated, whereas the right-side counterpart is retained. Symptoms may occur depending on whether the ligamentum arteriosum passes ventral or dorsal to the esophagus and trachea. *B,* Interrupted aortic arch. Both the right and left fourth aortic arch arteries degenerate, with the distal right dorsal aorta being retained. After birth, the ascending aorta supplies the head, upper limbs, and body, but the lower body and limbs are supplied by the pulmonary trunk (poorly oxygenated blood) via a patent ductus arteriosus.

and NOTCH2 have been identified in most of these patients. Hey2 (or Herp) is a basic HLH transcription factor important for mediating notch signaling. In zebrafish, mutants of the Hey2 homolog, gridlock, have defects in the aorta resembling human coarctation. However, in mice, Hey2 knockouts do not develop coarctation of the aorta. Rather, they develop other cardiac anomalies (such as ventricular septal defects). About 10% of patients with **Noonan syndrome** (also covered in Chapter 12) have coarctation of the aorta, a syndrome linked to mutations in the PTPN11 (a gene encoding a non-receptor TYROSINE PHOS-PHATASE involved in intracellular signal transduction; covered in Chapter 12). However, in a study of 157 humans with coarctation of the aorta (that excluded Noonan patients), a PTPN11 mutation was found in only a single patient, suggesting that mutations in PTPN11 are not the major cause of isolated coarctation.

PRIMITIVE EMBRYONIC VENOUS SYSTEM IS DIVIDED INTO VITELLINE, UMBILICAL, AND CARDINAL SYSTEMS

Animation 13-3: Remodeling of Vitelline and Umbilical Veins.
Animations are available online at StudentConsult.

The embryo has three major venous systems that fulfill different functions. The **vitelline system** drains the gastrointestinal tract and gut derivatives; the **umbilical system** carries oxygenated blood from the placenta; and the **cardinal system** drains the head, neck, and body wall. All three systems are initially bilaterally symmetrical

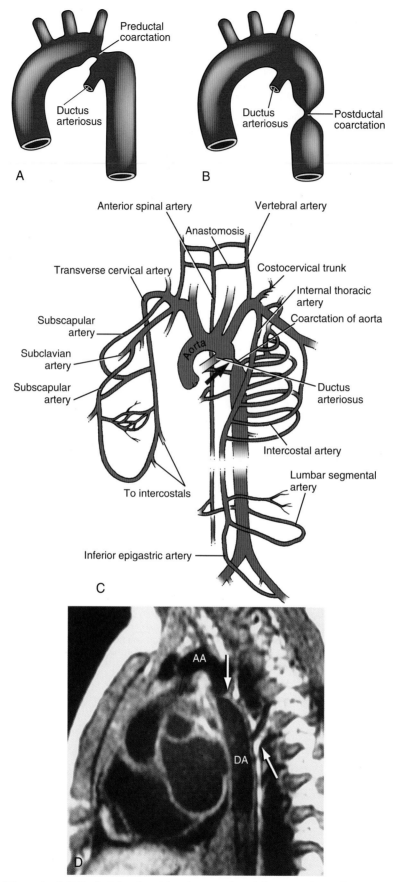

Figure 13-23. Coarctation of the aorta. *A, B,* Preductal and postductal coarctation of the aorta. *C,* Development of collateral circulation in post-ductal coarctation of the aorta. The aortic constriction (arrow) partly or completely blocks the flow of blood into the descending aorta. The trunk and lower extremities receive blood through enlarged collaterals that develop in response to the block. Collateral circulation established before birth may utilize internal thoracic arteries or the thyrocervical trunk to deliver blood to the descending aorta via segmental arteries of the trunk. *D,* Sagittal magnetic resonance imaging scan in lateral view showing the site of postductal coarctation (top arrow) and a major collateral entering the descending aorta (lower arrow). AA, Arch of the aorta; DA, descending aorta.

and converge on the right and left sinus horns of the sinus venosus (Figs. 13-24A, 13-25; see also Fig. 12-17). However, the shift of the systemic venous return to the right atrium (covered in Chapter 12) initiates a radical remodeling that reshapes these systems to yield the adult patterns.

VITELLINE SYSTEM GIVES RISE TO LIVER SINUSOIDS, PORTAL SYSTEM, AND A PORTION OF INFERIOR CAVAL VEIN

Like the vitelline arteries, the vitelline veins arise from the capillary plexuses of the yolk sac wall and form part

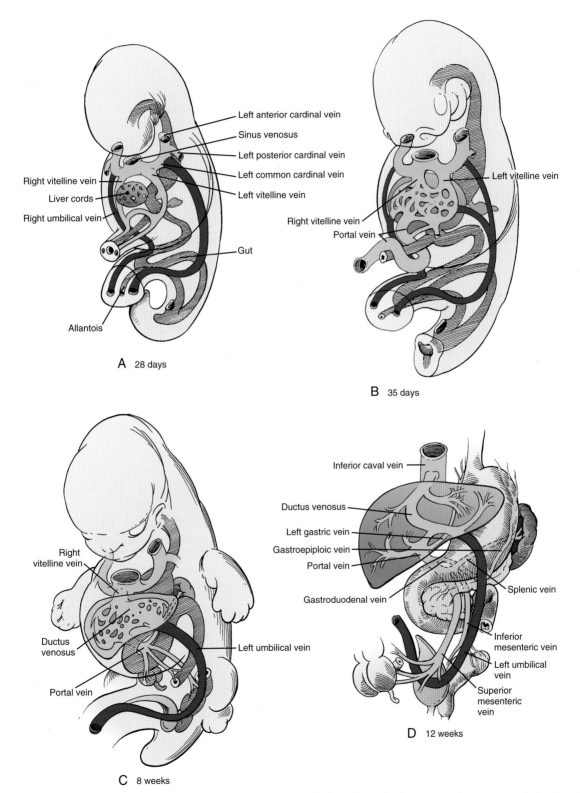

Figure 13-24. Fate of the vitelline and umbilical veins. *A-D,* The right and left vitelline veins form a portal system that drains blood from the abdominal foregut, the midgut, and the upper part of the anorectal canal. The right umbilical vein disappears, but the left umbilical vein anastomoses with the ductus venosus in the liver, thus shunting oxygenated placental blood into the inferior caval vein and to the right side of the heart.

of the vasculature of the developing gut and gut derivatives. Initially, the vitelline system empties into the sinus horns of the heart via a pair of symmetrical **vitelline veins** (see Fig. 13-24*A*). Right and left vitelline plexuses also develop in the septum transversum and connect to the vitelline veins. The vessels of these plexuses become surrounded by the growing liver cords and give rise to the **liver sinusoids**, a dense network of anastomosing venous spaces (see Fig. 13-24*A, B*). As the left sinus horn regresses to form the coronary sinus, the left vitelline vein also diminishes. By the third month, the left vitelline vein has completely disappeared in the region of the sinus venosus. The blood from the left side of the abdominal viscera now drains across to the right vitelline vein via a series of transverse anastomoses that have formed both within the substance of the liver and around the abdominal portion of the foregut (see Fig. 13-24*C*).

After the left vitelline vein loses its connection with the heart, the blood from the entire vitelline system drains into the heart via the enlarged right vitelline vein (see Fig. 13-24*C*). The cranial portion of this vein (the portion between the liver and the heart) becomes the **terminal portion of the inferior caval vein** (see Fig. 13-24*C*; see also 13-25*D, E*). Meanwhile, a single oblique channel among the hepatic anastomoses becomes dominant and drains directly into the nascent inferior caval vein. As described below, this channel, the **ductus venosus**, is crucial during fetal life because it receives oxygenated blood from the umbilical system and shunts it directly to the right vitelline vein and, hence, the right atrium.

The vitelline veins caudal to the liver regress during the second and third months, with the exception of the portion of the right vitelline vein just caudal to the developing liver and a few of the proximal ventral left-to-right vitelline anastomoses (see Fig. 13-24*B, C*). These veins become the main channels of the **portal system**, which drain blood from the gastrointestinal tract to the liver sinusoids. The segment of the right vitelline vein caudal to the liver becomes the **portal vein** and the **superior mesenteric vein** (see Fig. 13-24*C, D*). Persisting branches collect blood from the abdominal foregut (including the abdominal esophagus, stomach, gallbladder, duodenum, and pancreas) and the midgut. Prominent left-to-right vitelline anastomoses are remodeled to deliver blood to the distal end of the portal vein through two veins: the **splenic vein**, which drains the spleen, part of the stomach, and the greater omentum (covered in Chapter 14), and the **inferior mesenteric vein**, which drains the hindgut.

RIGHT UMBILICAL VEIN DISAPPEARS AND LEFT UMBILICAL VEIN ANASTOMOSES WITH DUCTUS VENOSUS

In contrast to the vitelline veins, in which the left regresses and the right persists, during the second month the right umbilical vein becomes completely obliterated and the left umbilical vein persists (see Fig. 13-24). Concurrently, with formation of the liver and remodeling of vessels in that area, the left umbilical vein loses its connection with the left sinus horn and forms a new anastomosis with the ductus venosus. Oxygenated blood from the placenta thus reaches the heart via the single umbilical vein and the ductus venosus. As covered at the end of this chapter,

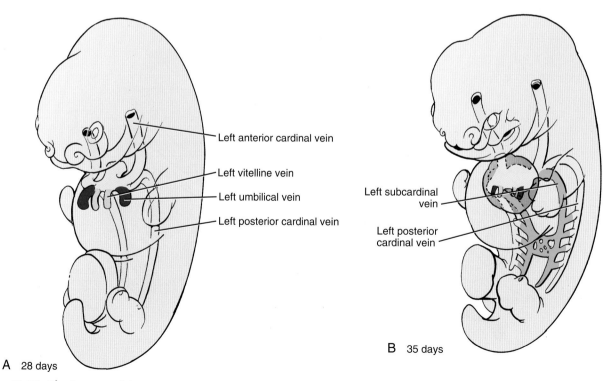

Figure 13-25. Development of the systemic venous system from the four bilaterally symmetrical cardinal vein systems. *A-E*, These systems are remodeled to drain blood from both sides of the head, neck, and body into the right atrium. The head and neck are initially drained by an anterior cardinal system, and the trunk is drained by a posterior cardinal system. The posterior cardinals are replaced by a set of subcardinal veins and a set of supracardinal veins.

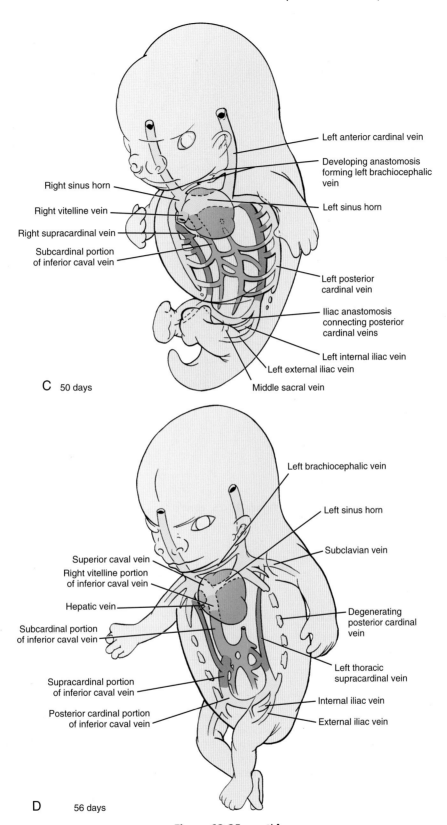

C 50 days

D 56 days

Figure 13-25, cont'd

Continued

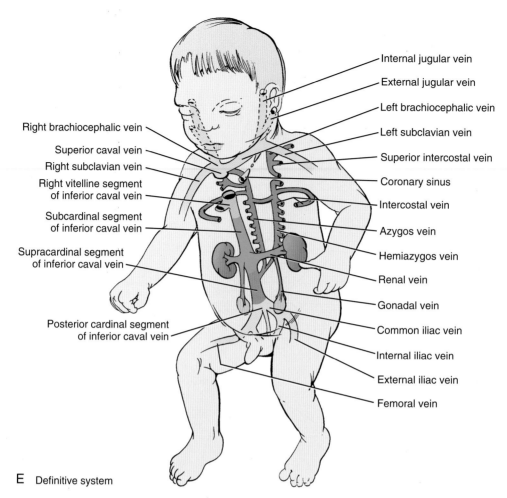

E   Definitive system

Figure 13-25, cont'd

the ductus venosus constricts shortly after birth, eliminating this venous shunt through the liver.

POSTERIOR CARDINAL SYSTEM IS AUGMENTED AND THEN SUPERSEDED BY PAIRED SUBCARDINAL AND SUPRACARDINAL VEINS

 Animation 13-4: Remodeling of Cardinal Veins and Formation of Inferior Caval Vein.
Animations are available online at StudentConsult.

As shown in Figure 13-25A, the bilaterally symmetrical cardinal vein system that develops in the third and fourth weeks to drain the head, neck, and body wall initially consists of paired **posterior (caudal)** and **anterior (cranial) cardinal veins**, which join near the heart to form the short **common cardinals** that empty into the sinus horns. The posterior cardinal veins are supplemented and later largely replaced by two additional pairs of veins, the **subcardinal** and **supracardinal** veins, which develop in the body wall medial to the posterior cardinal veins. Like the posterior and anterior cardinals, these two systems are bilaterally symmetrical at first but undergo extensive remodeling during development.

The left and right subcardinal veins sprout from the base of the posterior cardinals by the end of the sixth week

and grow caudally in the medial part of the dorsal body wall (see Fig. 13-25B). By the seventh and eighth weeks, these subcardinal veins become connected to each other by numerous median anastomoses and form some lateral anastomoses with the posterior cardinals. However, the longitudinal segments of the left subcardinal vein soon regress, so that by the ninth week, the structures on the left side of the body served by the subcardinal system drain solely through transverse anastomotic channels to the right subcardinal vein. Meanwhile, the right subcardinal vein loses its original connection with the posterior cardinal vein and develops a new anastomosis with the segment of the right vitelline vein just inferior to the heart to form the portion of the inferior caval vein between the liver and the kidneys (see Fig. 13-25C-E). Through this remodeling process, blood from the organs originally drained by the right and left subcardinal veins now returns to the right atrium via the ICV.

While the subcardinal system is being remodeled, a new pair of veins, the supracardinal veins, sprouts from the base of the posterior cardinals and grows caudally and just medial to the posterior cardinal veins (see Fig. 13-25C). These veins drain the body wall via the segmental **intercostal veins**, thus taking over the function of the posterior cardinals. The abdominal and thoracic portions of the supracardinal veins give rise to separate venous components in the adult and, therefore, will be described separately.

While the supracardinals are developing, the posterior cardinals become obliterated over most of their length (see Fig. 13-25C, D). The most caudal portions of the posterior cardinals (including a large median anastomosis) do persist but lose their original connection to the heart and form a new anastomosis with the supracardinal veins. This caudal remnant of the posterior cardinals develops into the common iliac veins and the caudalmost, sacral portion of the ICV. The common iliac veins in turn sprout the internal and external iliac veins, which grow to drain the lower extremities and pelvic organs.

In the abdominal region, remodeling of the supracardinal system commences with the obliteration of the inferior portion of the left supracardinal vein (see Fig. 13-25D, E). The remaining abdominal segment of the right supracardinal vein then anastomoses with the right subcardinal vein to form a segment of the ICV just inferior to the kidneys.

The thoracic part of the supracardinal system drains the thoracic body wall via a series of **intercostal veins**. The thoracic portions of the supracardinals originally empty into the left and right posterior cardinals and are connected to each other by median anastomoses (see Fig. 13-25C). However, the left thoracic supracardinal vein, called the **hemiazygos vein**, soon loses its connection with the left posterior cardinal vein and left sinus horn and subsequently drains into the right supracardinal system. The remaining portion of the inferior right supracardinal vein also loses its original connection with the posterior cardinal vein and makes a new anastomosis with the segment of the **superior caval vein** derived from the anterior cardinal vein. The latter, in turn, drains into the heart via a segment representing a small remnant of the right common cardinal vein. The right supracardinal vein is then called the **azygos vein**. The hemiazygos and azygos veins drain into the right atrium via the superior caval vein (see Fig. 13-25D, E).

Figure 13-25E shows the sources of the four portions of the ICV. From superior to inferior, (1) the right vitelline vein gives rise to the terminal segment of the ICV, (2) the right subcardinal vein gives rise to a segment between the liver and the kidneys, (3) the right supracardinal vein gives rise to an abdominal segment inferior to the kidneys, and (4) the right and left posterior cardinal veins plus the median anastomosis connecting them give rise to the sacral segment of the ICV.

BLOOD IS DRAINED FROM HEAD AND NECK BY ANTERIOR CARDINAL VEINS

The left and right anterior cardinal veins originally drain blood into the sinus horns via the left and right common cardinal veins (Fig. 13-25A-D). However, the proximal connection of the left anterior cardinal vein with the left sinus horn soon regresses (Fig. 13-25E), leaving only a small remnant, called the **oblique vein of the left atrium**, lying directly on the heart (see Fig. 12-17). This small remnant collects blood from the left atrial region of the heart and returns it directly to the coronary sinus, which is a vestige of the left sinus horn.

The cranial portions of the anterior cardinal veins in the developing cervical region give rise to the **internal jugular veins**; capillary plexuses in the face become connected with these vessels to form the **external jugular veins**. Simultaneously, a median anastomosis

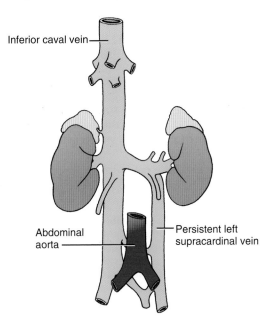

A   Double inferior caval vein

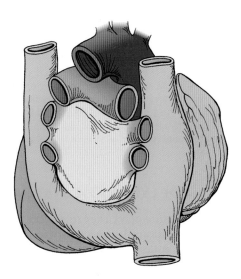

B   Double superior caval vein

Figure 13-26. Venous anomalies caused by failure of cardinal veins on the left to undergo normal regression. A, Preservation of the left supracardinal vein inferior to the kidney may result in double inferior caval vein. B, Preservation of the left anterior cardinal at the level of the heart may result in double superior caval veins (posterior view). The anomalous left superior caval vein empties into the coronary sinus.

connecting the left and right anterior cardinals develops (see Fig. 13-25C-E). Once the left anterior cardinal vein loses its connection with the heart, all blood from the left side of the head and neck shunts over to the right anterior cardinal through this anastomosis. The **subclavian vein**, which coalesces from the venous plexus of the left upper limb bud, also empties into the proximal left anterior cardinal vein. The intercardinal anastomosis thus carries blood from the left upper limb as well as from the left side of the head and is called the **left brachiocephalic vein** (see Fig. 13-25C-E). The left brachiocephalic vein enters the right anterior cardinal at its junction with the **right brachiocephalic vein**, draining the right upper limb bud and head. The small segment of right anterior cardinal vein between the junction of the right and left brachiocephalic veins and the right atrium becomes the superior caval vein (see Fig 13-25E). Thus, by the end of the eighth week, the definitive superior caval vein drains blood from (1) both sides of the head, (2) both upper limbs, and (3) the thoracic body wall (via the azygos vein).

In the Clinic

CAVAL VEIN ANOMALIES

A relatively rare anomaly called **double inferior caval vein** arises when the caudal portion of the left supracardinal system fails to regress, giving rise to an abnormal left ICV (see Fig. 13-26A). The blood entering this vessel ultimately drains into the right ICV via the left renal vein or into the hemiazygos vein arising from the thoracic part of the supracardinal system.

Occasionally the left anterior cardinal vein persists and maintains its connection with the left sinus venosus (incidence, 0.3% to 0.5% of the general population), resulting in a **persistent left (double) superior caval vein** (see Fig. 13-26B) or a **single left superior caval vein**. In 65% of these cases, the left brachiocephalic vein is also missing or is very small. With a persistent left superior caval vein, blood from the left side of the head and neck and from the left upper extremity drains through the abnormal left superior caval vein into the coronary sinus. A single left superior caval vein develops when the left anterior cardinal vein persists and the right is obliterated. In this case, the left anterior cardinal vein gives rise to a superior caval vein draining the blood from the entire head and neck, both upper extremities, and the azygos system, directing it into the coronary sinus and right atrium. However in a small subset of double and left superior caval veins, the left-sided superior caval vein empties directly into the left atrium (more common in cases of heterotaxy).

DEVELOPMENT OF LYMPHATIC SYSTEM

The lymphatic vasculature plays a key role in both normal and pathological conditions. It is necessary for maintaining proper fluid homeostasis and tissue fluid levels, it provides a pathway for immune cells and antigen-presenting cells to lymphatic organs, and it transports fats and nutrients for the digestive tract and serves other functions too numerous to list here.

Lymphatic channels arise by vasculogenesis and angiogenesis from venous precursor cells. In humans, **lymphangiogenesis** begins with the formation of bilateral sprouts from the anterior cardinal veins at about day forty-two of development. These sprouts eventually form a pair of enlargements, the **jugular lymphatic sacs**, which will collect fluid from the lymphatic vessels of the upper limbs, upper trunk, head, and neck (Fig. 13-27). In the sixth week, four additional lymphatic sacs develop to collect lymph from the trunk and lower extremities: the **retroperitoneal lymphatic sac, cisterna chyli**, and paired **posterior lymphatic sacs** associated with the junctions of the external and internal iliac veins.

The cisterna chyli initially drains into a symmetrical pair of thoracic lymphatic ducts that empty into the venous circulation at the junctions of the internal jugular and subclavian veins. However during development,

portions of both of these ducts are obliterated, and the definitive **thoracic duct** is derived from the caudal portion of the right duct, the cranial portion of the left duct, and a median anastomosis.

In the Research Lab

MOLECULAR MECHANISMS OF LYMPHATIC DEVELOPMENT

Despite knowledge of the existence of the lymphatic system for several centuries, the embryological origin of this important system is only now becoming clear. In mice, a subset of venous endothelial cells belonging to the cardinal veins migrates out and forms the initial lymphatic vessels. These migrating lymphatic endothelial cell precursors express the transcription factor, prospero-related homeobox-1 (Prox1), homologs of which have been found in humans, chicks, newts, frogs, Drosophila, and zebrafish. Initially, all cardinal vein endothelial cells seem to have lymphatic competency. However, only a subset of these endothelial cells are induced to begin to express Prox1, forming the rudimentary lymphatic sacs, and to begin to express more specific lymphatic markers. Recent studies suggest that expression of Sox18 (an SRY-related transcription factor) in combination with Coup-tfII activates Prox1 expression in a subset of endothelial cells, and Prox1 is responsible for lymphatic specification in these cells (Fig. 13-28). When Sox18 or Prox1 is knocked out in mice, the resulting embryos are unable to develop a lymphatic system. In Prox1-deficient mice, migration of these endothelial cells still occurs. However, they never go on to express lymphatic determination markers (e.g., Nrp2 and podoplanin; the latter is a transmembrane mucoprotein specific to the lymphatic system). Rather, they retain blood vessel endothelial markers such as Cd34 and laminin. Therefore, Sox18 and Prox1 are required for lymphatic cell specification in mice, and their expression may represent the master switch in programming lymphatic endothelial cell fate. In fact, ectopic expression of Prox1 in blood vascular endothelium can redirect vascular endothelial cells into a lymphatic lineage.

In the Clinic

LYMPHEDEMA MAY RESULT FROM LYMPHATIC HYPOPLASIA

A major hereditary congenital disorder of the lymphatic system is **hereditary lymphedema** (or primary lymphedema, a swelling of the lymphatic vasculature) caused by hypoplasia of the lymphatic system. This condition may or may not be associated with other abnormalities. Swelling generally occurs in the legs, but, in the case of lymphedema associated with **Turner syndrome**, blockage of lymphatic ducts in the neck and upper trunk may also result in the development of lymph-filled cysts (cystic hygromas). These cysts may disappear if lymphatic drainage improves during subsequent development. **Milroy disease**, a primary lymphedema syndrome, has been linked to mutations in the VEGFR3 gene. Other, more rare forms of lymphedema have been linked to the FOXC2 gene, a member of the forkhead family of transcription factors. Mutations in SOX18 have also been associated with dominant and recessive inherited forms of lymphedema. Several other potential genes identified from mouse models that when lost or mutated develop lymphedema include Ang2, Nrp2, Met (a proto-oncogene), podoplanin, and Syk (a tyrosine kinase).

DRAMATIC CHANGES OCCUR IN CIRCULATORY SYSTEM AT BIRTH

Animation 13-5: Fetal and Neonatal Circulation.
Animations are available online at StudentConsult.

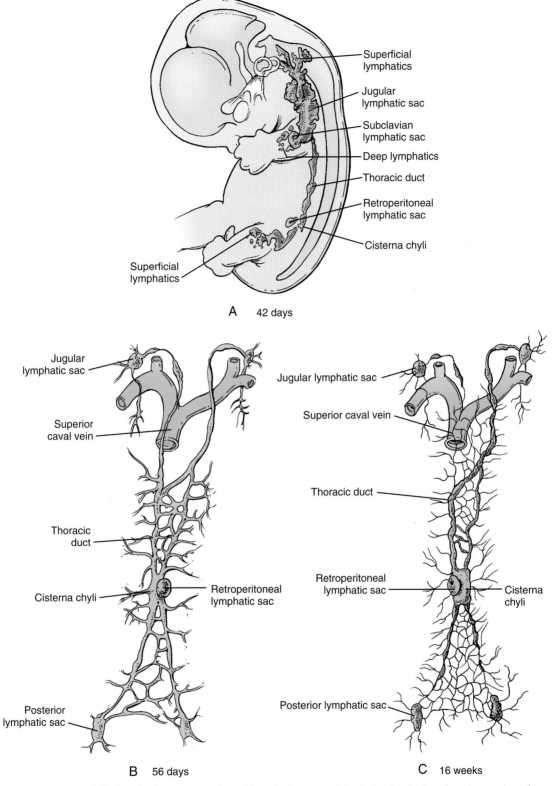

A   42 days

B   56 days

C   16 weeks

Figure 13-27. Development of the lymphatic system. *A,* Several lymphatic sacs and ducts develop by lymphangiogenesis and eventually drain fluid from tissue spaces throughout the entire body. *B-D,* The single thoracic duct that drains the cisterna chyli and the posterior thoracic wall is derived from parts of the right and left thoracic ducts and their anastomoses.

Continued

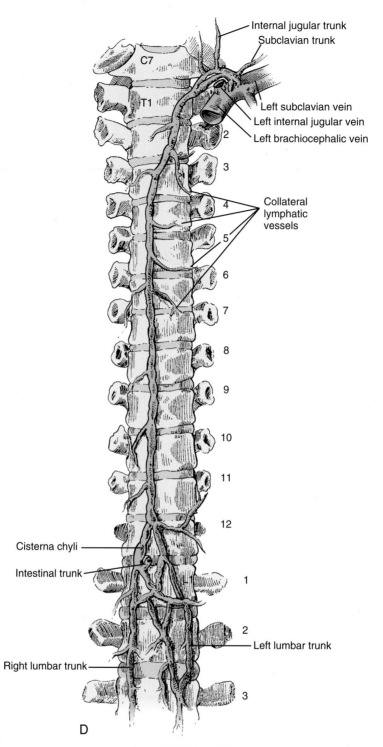

Figure 13-27, cont'd

Starting at birth, the systemic and pulmonary circulations are wholly separate and are arranged in series. This arrangement would have been impractical in the fetus because oxygenated blood enters the fetus via the umbilical vein, and little blood can flow through the collapsed lungs. Therefore, the fetal heart chambers and outflow tracts contain foramina and ducts that shunt the oxygenated blood entering the right atrium to the left ventricle and aortic arch, thus largely bypassing the developing pulmonary circulation. These shunts close at birth, abruptly separating the two circulations.

The transition from fetal dependence on maternal support via the placenta to the relatively independent existence of the infant in the outside world at birth brings about dramatic changes in the pattern of blood circulation within the newborn. In the fetal circulation (Fig. 13-29A), oxygenated blood enters the body through the left umbilical vein. In the **ductus venosus**, this

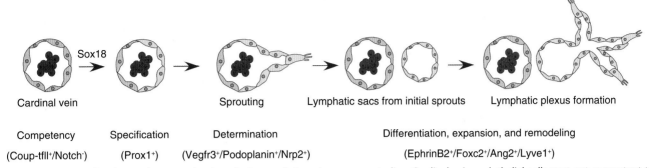

Figure 13-28. Postulated steps in generating lymphatic vessels based on mouse studies. Cardinal vein endothelial cells start out competent to form lymphatic vessels (i.e., they express Coup-tII and lack notch signaling). Expression of Sox18 in combination with Coup-tII activates Prox1 expression in a subset of endothelial cells responsible for lymphatic specification in these cells and then determination (i.e., they begin to express Vegfr3, podoplanin, and Nrp2). These lymphatic endothelial cells then migrate, form lymphatic sacs, undergo expansion and remodeling, and eventually express other lymphatic markers (e.g., Lyve1+).

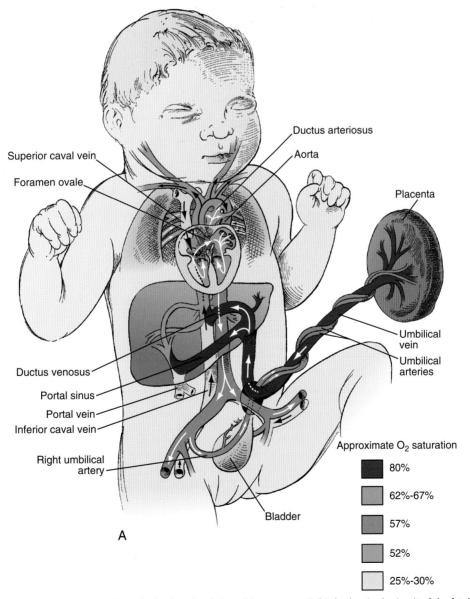

Figure 13-29. Conversion of the circulation from the fetal to the air-breathing pattern. At birth, the single circuit of the fetal circulation is rapidly converted to two circuits (pulmonary and systemic) arranged in a series. *A,* Pattern of blood flow in the fetus and placenta before birth.

Continued

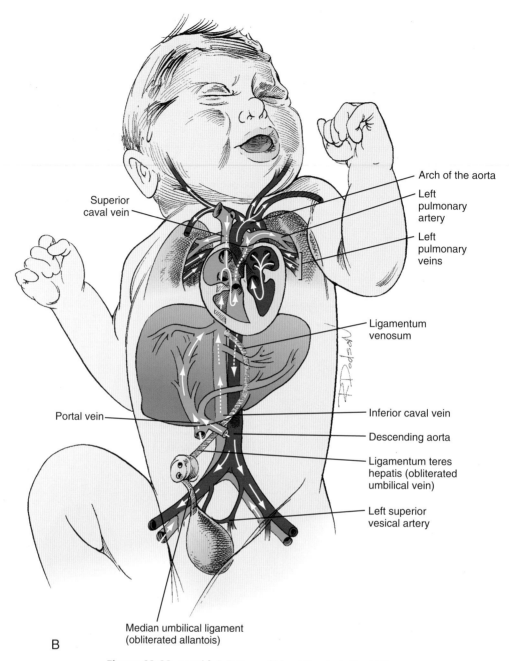

Superior
caval vein

Arch of the aorta

Left
pulmonary
artery

Left
pulmonary
veins

Ligamentum
venosum

Portal vein

Inferior caval vein

Descending aorta

Ligamentum teres
hepatis (obliterated
umbilical vein)

Left superior
vesical artery

Median umbilical ligament
(obliterated allantois)

B

Figure 13-29, cont'd *B,* Pattern of blood flow just after birth.

blood mixes with a small volume of deoxygenated portal blood and then enters the ICV, where it mixes with deoxygenated blood returning from the trunk and legs. In the right atrium, this stream of blood, still highly oxygenated, is largely shunted through the foramen ovale to the left atrium. The oxygenated blood entering the fetal right atrium from the ICV and the deoxygenated blood entering from the superior caval vein form hemodynamically distinct streams and undergo very little mixing in the atrium. This separation of streams is accomplished partly by the shape and placement of the valve of the ICV.

In the left atrium, oxygenated blood from the right atrium mixes with the very small amount of blood returning from the lungs via the pulmonary veins. Little blood flows through the pulmonary circulation during fetal life because the vascular resistance of the collapsed fetal lungs is very high. The oxygenated blood in the left ventricle is then propelled into the aorta for distribution first to the head, neck, and arms, and then, via the descending aorta, to the trunk and limbs. As blood enters the descending aorta, it mixes with less oxygenated blood shunted through the ductus arteriosus. This blood consists mainly of the blood entering the right atrium from the superior caval vein and expelled via the right ventricle and pulmonary trunk. Thus, the blood delivered to the head, neck, and arms by the fetal circulation is more highly oxygenated than the blood delivered to the trunk and lower limbs. After the descending aorta has distributed blood to the trunk and lower limbs, the remaining blood enters the umbilical arteries and returns to the placenta for oxygenation.

The fetal circulatory pattern functions throughout the birth process. However, as soon as the newborn infant takes its first breath, major changes convert the circulation to the adult configuration, in which the pulmonary and systemic circuits are separate (Fig. 13-29B). As the alveoli fill with air, the constricted pulmonary vessels open, and resistance of the pulmonary vasculature drops precipitously. In mammalian animal models, nitric oxide synthase levels drastically increase in the pulmonary vasculature at the time of birth, increasing the potential to generate **nitric oxide** and dilate these vessels. Opening of the pulmonary vessels is thought to be a direct response to oxygen, because hypoxia in newborns can cause pulmonary vessels to constrict. At the same time, spontaneous constriction (or obstetrical clamping) of the umbilical vessels cuts off the flow from the placenta.

The opening of the pulmonary circulation and the cessation of umbilical flow create changes in pressure and flow that cause the ductus arteriosus to constrict and the **foramen ovale** to close. When the pulmonary circulation opens, the resulting drop in pressure in the pulmonary trunk is thought to cause a slight reversed flow of oxygenated aortic blood through the **ductus arteriosus**. This increase in local oxygen tension apparently induces the vascular smooth muscle of the ductus arteriosus to contract and restrict blood flow through this vessel. The precise mechanism by which changes in oxygen tension initiate contraction of these cells is still unclear (covered further in the following "In the Clinic" entitled "Patent Ductus Arteriosus Leads to Heart Failure if Not Corrected"), but constriction of the ductus arteriosus normally occurs within a day after birth in infants born at term.

In contrast to the ductus arteriosus, the initial closing of the **foramen ovale** is mainly a mechanical effect of the reversal in pressure between the two atria. The opening of the pulmonary vasculature and the cessation of umbilical flow reduce the pressure in the right atrium, whereas the sudden increase in pulmonary venous return raises the pressure in the left atrium. The resulting pressure change forces the flexible septum primum against the more rigid septum secundum, functionally closing the foramen ovale. The septum primum and the septum secundum normally fuse by about three months after birth.

The **ductus venosus** also closes soon after birth. However, rapid constriction of the ductus venosus is not essential for the infant, because blood is no longer flowing through the umbilical vein. **Prostaglandins** (hormones with dilator effects on vascular smooth muscle) seem to play a role in maintaining the patency of the ductus venosus during fetal life, but the signal that brings about the apparently active constriction of this channel after birth is not fully understood. Nevertheless, a normal portal circulation within a few days of birth supplants the hepatic blood flow from the placenta.

In the Clinic

PATENT DUCTUS ARTERIOSUS LEADS TO HEART FAILURE IF NOT CORRECTED

In term infants, the ductus arteriosus constricts in response to a rise in oxygen tension. However during fetal life, the ductus is kept patent, in part by circulating prostaglandins. Studies in mice show that prostaglandin E_2 receptor subtype-4 is expressed in vascular smooth muscle of the ductus arteriosus. When this receptor is knocked out, mice develop **patent ductus arteriosus**. Animal models show that increases in oxygen levels decrease circulating levels of prostaglandins, signal the release of endothelins (vasoconstrictors released by endothelial cells), alter K^+ ion channel activity in vascular smooth muscle, and increase intracellular calcium ion levels, all of which promote contraction of vascular smooth muscle in the ductus arteriosus. The importance of increasing oxygen tension in closure of the ductus arteriosus is supported by the observation that patent ductus arteriosus is more prevalent in patients living under hypoxic conditions (i.e., at high altitudes). For reasons that are unclear, the incidence of patent ductus arteriosus is also higher in cases of **maternal rubella infection**.

Recent studies suggest that vasoconstriction alone is insufficient for complete closure. In addition, closure requires the formation of a platelet plug, likely in response to endothelial damage caused by the luminal constriction and ischemic hypoxia. In fact, preterm infants born with low platelet counts have over a ten times greater risk of a patent ductus than those with normal counts. Although counterintuitive, recent studies suggest that low levels of prostaglandins can be antithrombotic in vivo by mediating the sensitivity of platelets to their activators. Therefore, decreasing prostaglandin levels at birth would promote both vasoconstriction and formation of a platelet plug in the ductus arteriosus.

Infants who have cardiovascular malformations in which a patent ductus arteriosus is essential to life (see "Clinical Taster" of Chapter 12) may be treated with an infusion of prostaglandins to keep the ductus open until the malformation can be corrected surgically. Conversely, premature infants in whom the ductus arteriosus does not constrict spontaneously are sometimes treated with prostaglandin inhibitors, such as indomethacin and ibuprofen, to promote closure. In newborns having a large patent ductus arteriosus, about one third to one half of the blood is shunted from the aorta back into the pulmonary circulation. This means that on its return to the heart from the lungs, the same blood must be pumped back out again by the left ventricle (increasing its workload two to three times). If not corrected, this leads to progressive pulmonary vasculature obstructive disease, pulmonary hypertension, left atrial dilation and ventricular hypertrophy, and eventual heart failure. This abnormal blood flow pattern also increases the risk of bacterial **endocarditis**.

Embryology in Practice

RED SPOTS

A teenage boy and his mother meet with a pediatrician to discuss their concerns about the presence of multiple, small, red spots on his face, extremities, and trunk. During previous visits, his mother mentioned these spots to the doctor in passing, but now the spots are more troublesome to the boy as he is becoming conscious of his appearance. The mother is also concerned after reading online that spots like these, along with the frequent nosebleeds, which the boy also has had, can be caused by something called "HHT."

In the past, the doctor dismissed the nosebleeds as "very common" and "normal kids' stuff" caused by the dry local air and by "digital manipulation," and he recommended treating the nasal passages with Vaseline. Discussion at this visit continues to suggest benign nosebleeds that occur less than weekly and mostly in the winter. However, the doctor's curiosity is piqued when he learns that the boy's father has similar red spots but without other signs or symptoms.

The doctor examines the boy while listening to this story and sees multiple, red, blanchable (that is, they lose redness when pressed) lesions mostly on the boy's extremities and trunk. Further examination fails to find lesions on the boy's oral mucosa or nail beds. The review of systems does not uncover any additional concerning symptoms such as breathlessness or fatigue. The doctor also performs a hematocrit and a pulse oximetry in the office, both of which are normal.

He tells the mother and the boy that he is reassured by the benign history of epistaxis (nose bleeds) and the lack of other cutaneous or systemic symptoms and that the likely diagnosis is **hereditary benign telangiectasia**. He explains that this condition involves red spots on the skin that run in families, but it lacks the serious nose bleeds and systemic blood vessel abnormalities, called arteriovenous malformations (AVMs), that are seen in the more serious hereditary hemorrhagic telangiectasia (HHT). He adds that tests can be done to rule out HHT, including genetic testing, if other symptoms arise.

As opposed to HHT, which was described in the "Clinical Taster" in this chapter in a 14-year-old girl who also presented with telangiectases and nosebleeds, hereditary benign telangiectasia lacks the additional findings of mucosal telangiectases or symptoms associated with systemic AVMs, such as fatigue and shortness of breath.

Suggested Readings

Adams RH, Alitalo K. 2007. Molecular regulation of angiogenesis and lymphangiogenesis. Nat Rev Mol Cell Biol 8:464–478.

Adams RH, Eichmann A. 2010. Axon guidance molecules in vascular patterning. Cold Spring Harb Perspect Biol 2:a001875.

Augustin HG, Koh GY, Thurston G, Alitalo K. 2009. Control of vascular morphogenesis and homeostasis through the angiopoietin-tie system. Nat Rev Mol Cell Biol 10:165–177.

Boisset JC, van Cappellen W, Andrieu-Soler C, et al. 2010. In vivo imaging of haematopoietic cells emerging from the mouse aortic endothelium. Nat 464:116–120.

Brouillard P, Vikkula M. 2007. Genetic causes of vascular malformations. Hum Mol Genet 16 Spec. No. 2:R140–R149.

Coultas L, Chawengsaksophak K, Rossant J. 2005. Endothelial cells and VEGF in vascular development. Nature 438. 937–495.

De Val S, Black B. 2009. Transcriptional control of endothelial cell development. Dev Cell 16:180–195.

Dejana E. 2010. The role of wnt signaling in physiological and pathological angiogenesis. Circ Res 107:943–952.

Dzierzak E, Speck N. 2008. Of lineage and legacy: the development of mammalian hematopoietic stem cells. Nat Immunol 9:129–136.

Echtler K, Stark K, Lorenz M, et al. 2010. Platelets contribute to postnatal occlusion of the ductus arteriosus. Nat Med 16:75–82.

Fraisl P, Mazzone M, Schmidt T, Carmeliet P. 2009. Regulation of angiogenesis by oxygen and metabolism. Dev Cell 16:167–179.

Gaengel K, Genove G, Armulik A, Betsholtz C. 2009. Endothelial-mural cell signaling in vascular development and angiogenesis. Arterioscler Thromb Vasc Biol 29:630–638.

High F, Epstein J. 2008. The multifaceted role of Notch in cardiac development and disease. Nat Rev Genet 9:49–61.

Jain R, Rentschler S, Epstein J. 2010. Notch and cardiac outflow tract development. Ann N Y Acad Sci 1188:184–190.

Lohela M, Bry M, Tammela T, Alitalo K. 2009. VEGFs and receptors involved in angiogenesis versus lymphangiogenesis. Curr Opin Cell Biol 21:154–165.

Oliver G, Srinivasan R. 2010. Endothelial cell plasticity: how to become and remain a lymphatic endothelial cell. Development 137:363–372.

Phng L, Gerhardt H. 2009. Angiogenesis: a team effort coordinated by notch. Dev Cell 16:196–208.

Rentschler S, Jain R, Epstein J. 2010. Tissue-tissue interactions during morphogenesis of the outflow tract. Pediatr Cardiol 31:408–413.

Tavian M, Biasch K, Sinka L, et al. 2010. Embryonic origin of human hematopoiesis. Int J Dev Biol 54:1061–1065.

You LR, Lin F, Lee C, et al. 2005. Suppression of Notch signalling by the COUP-TFII transcription factor regulates vein identity. Nature 435:98–104.

Chapter 14

Development of the Gastrointestinal Tract

SUMMARY

The endodermal gut tube created by body folding during the fourth week (covered in Chapter 4) consists of a blind-ended cranial **foregut,** a blind-ended caudal **hindgut,** and a **midgut** open to the yolk sac through the vitelline duct. As covered in Chapter 13, the arterial supply to the gut develops through consolidation and reduction of the ventral branches of the dorsal aortae that anastomose with the vessel plexuses originally supplying blood to the yolk sac. About five of these vitelline artery derivatives vascularize the thoracic foregut, and three—the **celiac, superior mesenteric,** and **inferior mesenteric arteries**—vascularize the abdominal gut. By anatomical convention, the boundaries of the foregut, midgut, and hindgut portions of the abdominal gut tube are determined by the respective territories of these three arteries. However, these regions and the site of some gastrointestinal organs are already demarcated by specific gene expression patterns before this vasculature is established and are refined by subsequent reciprocal endodermal-mesodermal interactions.

By the fifth week, the thoracic and abdominal portion of the foregut is visibly divided into the **pharynx, esophagus, stomach,** and proximal **duodenum.** The stomach is initially fusiform, and differential growth of its dorsal and ventral walls produces the **greater** and **lesser curvatures.** Meanwhile, **hepatic, cystic,** and **dorsal** and **ventral pancreatic diverticula** bud from the caudal duodenum into the **mesogastrium** and give rise, respectively, to the **liver, gallbladder** and **cystic duct,** and **pancreas.** In addition, the **spleen** condenses from mesenchyme in the dorsal mesogastrium.

During the sixth and seventh weeks, the stomach rotates around longitudinal and dorsoventral axes so that the greater curvature is finally directed to the left and slightly caudal. This rotation shifts the liver to the right in the abdominal cavity and brings the duodenum and pancreas into contact with the posterior body wall, where they become fixed (i.e., **secondarily retroperitoneal**). This event converts the space dorsal to the rotated stomach and dorsal mesogastrium into a recess called the **lesser sac of the peritoneum.**

The pouch of dorsal mesogastrium forming the left lateral boundary of the lesser sac subsequently undergoes voluminous expansion, giving rise to the curtain-like **greater omentum,** which drapes over the inferior abdominal viscera.

The midgut forms the distal **duodenum, jejunum, ileum, cecum, ascending colon,** and proximal two thirds of the **transverse colon.** The future ileum elongates more rapidly than can be accommodated by the early peritoneal cavity so that by the fifth week the midgut is thrown into an anteroposterior hairpin fold, the **primary intestinal loop,** which herniates into the umbilicus during the sixth week. As the primary intestinal loop herniates, it rotates around its long axis by 90 degrees counterclockwise (as viewed from the ventral side) so that the future ileum lies in the right abdomen and the future large intestine lies in the left abdomen. Meanwhile, the cecum and appendix differentiate, and the jejunum and ileum continue to elongate. During the tenth through twelfth weeks, the intestinal loop is retracted into the abdominal cavity and rotates through an additional 180 degrees counterclockwise to produce the definitive configuration of the small and large intestines.

The hindgut forms the distal third of the **transverse colon,** the **descending** and **sigmoid colon,** and the upper two thirds of the **anorectal canal.** Just superior to the cloacal membrane, the primitive gut tube forms an expansion called the **cloaca.** During the fourth to sixth weeks, a coronal **urorectal septum** partitions the cloaca into the **urogenital sinus,** which will give rise to urogenital structures, and a **dorsal anorectal canal.**

Between the sixth and eighth weeks, the epithelium of the gut tube becomes thickened, forms intraepithelial lumens that eventually open into the gut lumen, and, together with the formation of mesodermal extensions that project into the lumen, forms the **villi** of the intestines. Cytodifferentiation of the gut epithelium depends on interactions with the underlying mesoderm and is regionally specified based on the cranial-caudal axis and the radial axis (lumen to outer tunic) of the gut. Migrating neural crest cells form the **enteric nervous system.**

341

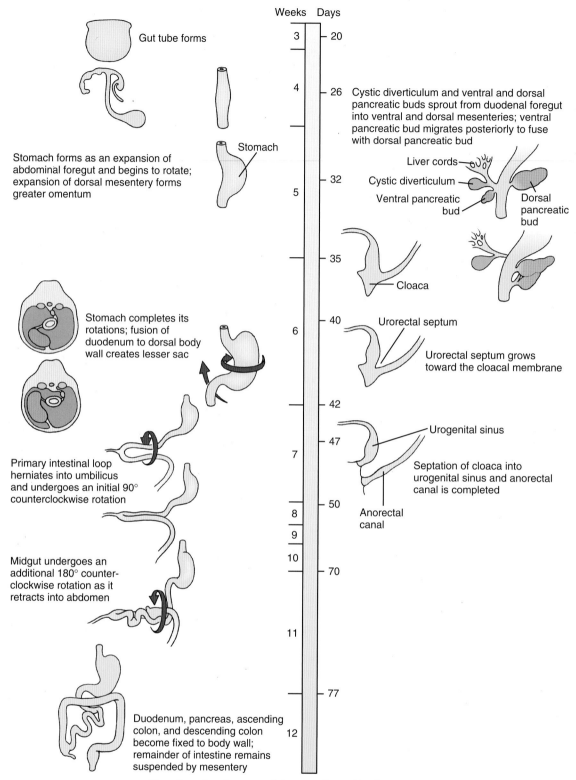

Weeks Days

3 — 20 Gut tube forms

Stomach forms as an expansion of abdominal foregut and begins to rotate; expansion of dorsal mesentery forms greater omentum

4 — 26 Cystic diverticulum and ventral and dorsal pancreatic buds sprout from duodenal foregut into ventral and dorsal mesenteries; ventral pancreatic bud migrates posteriorly to fuse with dorsal pancreatic bud

Stomach

Liver cords

32 Cystic diverticulum

Ventral pancreatic bud

Dorsal pancreatic bud

5

35 Cloaca

Stomach completes its rotations; fusion of duodenum to dorsal body wall creates lesser sac

6 — 40 Urorectal septum

Urorectal septum grows toward the cloacal membrane

42

Primary intestinal loop herniates into umbilicus and undergoes an initial 90° counterclockwise rotation

7 — 47 Urogenital sinus

Septation of cloaca into urogenital sinus and anorectal canal is completed

50

8

9

Anorectal canal

Midgut undergoes an additional 180° counter-clockwise rotation as it retracts into abdomen

10 — 70

11

77

Duodenum, pancreas, ascending colon, and descending colon become fixed to body wall; remainder of intestine remains suspended by mesentery

12

Time line. Development of the gut tube and its derivatives.

Clinical Taster

A one-week-old infant male is seen in a community health clinic. His mother says that the boy has not been eating well for two days and has been irritable, especially after feeds. Then, beginning last night, he started vomiting a dark greenish liquid consistent with bile. On examination, the infant cries inconsolably and is weak. His heart rate is elevated and his extremities are cool: symptoms of dehydration. His abdomen is somewhat distended. Sips of hydration fluid are returned with bilious vomit.

Intravenous hydration is begun and a nasogastric tube is placed to decompress the abdomen. The infant is transferred by ambulance to the children's hospital, where an upper gastrointestinal tract (upper GI) series is ordered (i.e., sequential X-rays

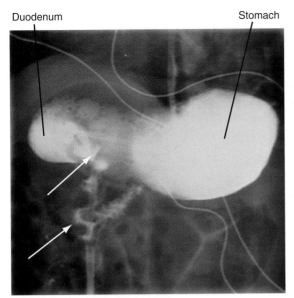

Duodenum   Stomach

Figure 14-1. Malrotation of the gut in a child. Barium contrast X-ray showing a dilated stomach and proximal duodenum, with a volvulus more distally. Note the delayed filling of the affected bowel (arrows).

done after ingestion of barium, a radio-opaque liquid used to coat the inside of the digestive system). This study shows markedly delayed gastric emptying and dilation of the duodenum with delayed filling of the jejunum. As the jejunum fills with barium, it takes on an "apple peel" appearance (Fig. 14-1). A subsequent X-ray shows partial filling of the small intestine, which lies predominantly in the right abdomen. The diagnosis of intestinal malrotation with intestinal obstruction is made, and emergency surgery is performed. In the operating room, the surgeons find a midgut volvulus (torsion of the small intestine) with ischemic bowel twisted around a narrow mesenteric pedicle. They untwist the bowel and return it to the abdomen. One day later, they re-examine the bowel and remove a 20-cm necrotic portion. Later, the small intestines are reconnected and the bowel fixed in place so that twisting cannot recur.

Intestinal malrotation occurs when the midgut fails to complete its rotation during the tenth through twelfth week of development as it returns to the peritoneal cavity from the umbilical herniation. This leaves the small intestine in the right side of the abdomen tethered to the mesenteric vasculature by a narrowed mesentery. The small bowel can twist around this narrow tether, causing intestinal obstruction and cutting off its circulation, resulting in necrosis. This usually presents in infancy, but cases presenting as late as young adulthood have been reported. The cause of intestinal malrotation is unknown.

BODY FOLDING

Animation 14-1: Formation of Gut Tube.
Animations are available online at StudentConsult.

As covered in Chapter 4, the longitudinal and transverse folding of the embryo in the third and fourth weeks converts the flat trilaminar embryonic disc into a trilaminar, elongated cylinder (Fig. 14-2). Because of cranial and caudal body folding, cranial and caudal endodermal pockets form (see Fig. 14-2A-F). As the cranial and caudal pockets elongate with lengthening of the embryo, the lateral

body folds meet in the ventral midline and fuse to generate the elongated body cylinder (see Fig. 14-2G-H). The outer layer is the ectoderm (the future epidermis), which now covers the entire outer surface of the embryo except in the umbilical region, where the yolk sac and the connecting stalk emerge. The innermost layer is the endodermal **primary gut tube**. Separating these two layers is a layer of mesoderm that contains the coelom. Thus, the three germ layers bear the same fundamental topologic relation to each other after folding as they did in the flat embryonic disc.

Body folding plays an essential role in internalizing the endoderm, as mutations in genes involved in body folding exhibit not only body folding defects but also endodermal tube defects. By the time body folding is nearly complete, the gut tube consists of cranial and caudal blind-ending tubes, the presumptive **foregut** and **hindgut**, and a central **midgut**, which still opens ventrally to the yolk sac. Cranially, the foregut terminates at the **oropharyngeal membrane** (or buccopharyngeal membrane); caudally, the hindgut terminates at the **cloacal membrane**. Because the embryo and gut tube lengthen relative to the yolk sac, and folding continues to convert the open midgut into a tube, the neck of the yolk sac narrows until it becomes the slender vitelline duct. The **vitelline duct** (or **yolk stalk**) and yolk sac are eventually incorporated into the umbilical cord. Table 14-1 lists the organs and structures that are ultimately derived from the three portions of the gut tube.

During the process of lateral body folding, the endodermal lining of the gut tube remains covered by a wall of lateral plate splanchnic mesoderm (see Fig. 14-2G-H). This mesoderm condenses and differentiates into the lamina propria, submucosa, muscular walls, vascular elements, and connective tissue of the gastrointestinal tract and organs. Once the basic gut tube regions are formed, various organs develop within specific regions that are delineated by restricted gene expression and tissue-tissue interactions.

DORSAL MESENTERY INITIALLY SUSPENDS ABDOMINAL GUT TUBE

When the coelom first forms, the gut is broadly attached to the dorsal body wall by mesoderm (Fig. 14-3A). However, in the region of the future abdominal viscera (from the abdominal esophagus to the most proximal part of the future rectum), the mesenchyme within this region of attachment gradually disperses during the fourth week, resulting in formation of a thin, bilayered **dorsal mesentery** that suspends the abdominal viscera in the coelomic cavity (Fig. 14-3B). Because the abdominal gut tube and its derivatives are suspended within this part of the intraembryonic coelom that later becomes the **peritoneal cavity**, they are referred to as **intraperitoneal** viscera.

In contrast to the intraperitoneal location of most of the gut tube and its derivatives, some of the visceral organs develop within the body wall and are separated from the coelom by a covering of serous membrane (Fig. 14-3C). These organs are said to be **retroperitoneal**. It

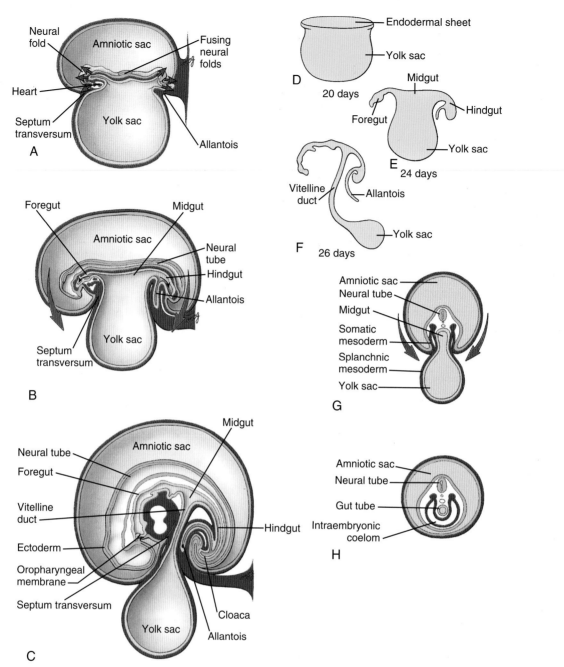

Figure 14-2. Gut formation by body folding. The foregut, midgut, and hindgut of the primitive gut tube are formed by the combined action of differential growth and lateral and craniocaudal folding, transforming the embryo from a flat disc to a three-dimensional vertebrate body form. As folding occurs, the embryo grows more rapidly than the yolk sac, the cavity of which remains continuous with the developing gut tube through the narrowing vitelline duct. The septum transversum forms cranial to the cardiogenic area in the germ disc (*A*) and is translocated to the future lower thoracic region through folding of the cranial end of the embryo (*B, C*). The foregut and hindgut are blind-ending tubes that terminate at the oropharyngeal and cloacal membranes, respectively. The midgut is at first completely open to the cavity of the yolk sac (*D, E*). However, as folding proceeds, this connection is constricted to form the narrow vitelline duct (*E-G*). Fusion of the ectoderm, mesoderm, future coelomic cavities, and endoderm from opposite sides is prevented in the immediate vicinity of the vitelline duct (*G*), but not in the more cranial and caudal regions (*H*).

is important to realize that the designation *retroperitoneal* means that an organ is located behind the peritoneum from a viewpoint inside the peritoneal cavity—not that it is necessarily located in the *posterior* body wall. Thus, the kidneys are retroperitoneal, but so is the bladder, which develops in the anterior body wall (see Fig. 14-3*C*).

Further complicating the intraperitoneal/retroperitoneal distinction is that some parts of the gut tube that are

initially suspended by mesentery later become fused to the body wall, thus taking on the appearance of retroperitoneal organs (Fig. 14-3*D*). These organs, which include the ascending and descending colon, duodenum, and pancreas, are said to be **secondarily retroperitoneal**.

At the end of the fourth week, almost the entire abdominal gut tube—the portion within the peritoneal cavity from the abdominal esophagus to the superior end

TABLE 14-1 DERIVATIVES OF PRIMITIVE GUT TUBE

Regions of Differentiated Gut Tube	Accessory Organs Derived from Gut Tube Endoderm
Foregut	
Pharynx	Pharyngeal pouch derivatives (see Chapter 17)
Thoracic esophagus	Lungs (see Chapter 11)
Abdominal esophagus	
Stomach	
Proximal half of duodenum (superior to ampulla of pancreatic duct)	Liver parenchyma and hepatic duct epithelium
	Gallbladder, cystic duct, and common bile duct
	Dorsal and ventral pancreas
Midgut	
Distal half of duodenum	
Jejunum	
Ileum	
Cecum	
Appendix	
Ascending colon	
Right two thirds of transverse colon	
Hindgut	
Left one third of transverse colon	
Descending colon	
Sigmoid colon	
Rectum	Urogenital sinus and derivatives (see Chapters 15 and 16)

of the developing cloaca—hangs suspended by the dorsal mesentery. Except in the region of the developing stomach, the coelomic cavities in the lateral plate mesoderm on either side of the embryonic disc coalesce during folding to form a single, continuous peritoneal cavity. In the stomach region, the gut tube remains connected to the ventral body wall by the thick septum transversum. By the fifth week, the caudal portion of the septum transversum thins to form the **ventral mesentery** connecting the stomach and developing liver to the ventral body wall (Fig. 14-4).

THREE REGIONS OF PRIMITIVE GUT

By convention, the terms *foregut*, *midgut*, and *hindgut* correspond to the territories of the three arteries supplying the abdominal gut tube. As covered in Chapter 13, the gut tube and its derivatives are vascularized by unpaired ventral branches of the descending aorta. These branches develop by a process of consolidation and reduction from the left and right vitelline artery plexuses that arise on the yolk sac, spread to vascularize the gut tube, and anastomose with the dorsal aortae

(see Fig. 13-15). About five definitive aortic branches supply the thoracic part of the foregut (the pharynx and thoracic esophagus; development of the pharyngeal part of the foregut is covered in Chapter 17). Three arteries serve the remainder of the gut tube: the **celiac trunk**, which supplies the abdominal foregut (the abdominal esophagus, stomach, and cranial half of the duodenum and its derivatives); the **superior mesenteric trunk**, which supplies the midgut; and the **inferior mesenteric artery**, which supplies the hindgut. The terms *foregut* and *hindgut* are also used to describe the endodermal regions cranial and caudal to the anterior and posterior intestinal portals, respectively.

Molecular studies show that different endodermal segments are marked by specific patterns of segmental and homeotic gene expression within the developing gut well before formation of the three arteries that supply the gut and are used by convention to subdivide it into foregut, midgut, and hindgut regions (Fig. 14-5). For instance, during late-stage mouse gastrulation, Lhx1 (Lim homeobox-1), Hesx1 (homeobox expressed in ES cells-1), and Cerl (cerberus-like) are expressed within the cranial definitive endoderm, whereas Cdx (caudal-type homeobox) expression demarcates the caudal endoderm.

In the Research Lab

REGIONALIZATION OF GUT TUBE DEMARCATES SITES OF ORGAN FORMATION

Regionalization of the gut plays an important role in demarcating sites of organ formation. Regional specification of endoderm and its interaction with mesoderm, neural crest cells, and ectoderm play important roles in mediating the development of the pharyngeal arches and pharyngeal vasculature, as well as in organ formation in the cranial region (covered in Chapters 13 and 17). The following text is limited to gastrointestinal development caudal to the pharyngeal arches.

How does the early endoderm obtain its cranial-caudal identity? Less is known regarding the regionalization of the early endoderm than is known regarding that of the ectoderm and mesoderm. The ectoderm and mesoderm acquire much of their regional identity during gastrulation through a variety of signaling molecules derived from the primitive streak and organizer (primitive node in humans) (covered in Chapter 3). These same signaling molecules are now known to be involved in the regionalization of the endoderm. One of the earliest known markers delineating regional differences of the definitive endoderm was discovered from work in Drosophila, where the gene caudal was identified and found to be required for gut formation (see Fig. 14-5). Caudal homologs in vertebrates include Cdx1, Cdx2, and Cdx4. In vertebrates, Cdx2 is expressed in the caudal endoderm, mesoderm, and ectoderm of primitive streak–stage embryos before the expression of most Hox genes (see Fig. 14-5). Loss of Cdx2 expression within the endoderm of mice transforms the distal hindgut endoderm into a foregut esophageal-like epithelium. Nodal expression in the primitive streak promotes anterior endodermal fate and expression of Hhex, an anterior endodermal gene. Mice null for Hhex fail to form a liver and die during embryogenesis. Caudal Wnt signaling is also required for early hindgut specification, as mice null for the Wnt downstream targets, Tcf4 and Tcf1, exhibit severe caudal truncations. Other genes important in early gut regionalization include Shh, Fgfs,

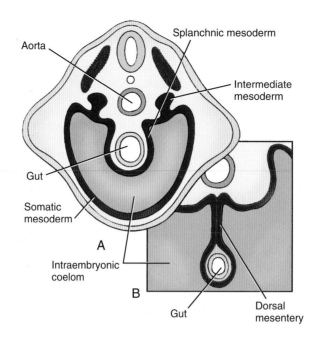
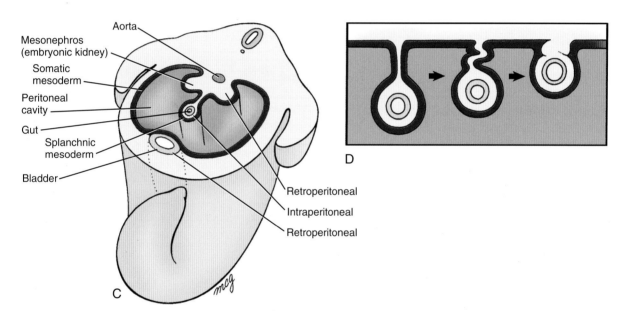

Figure 14-3. Formation of the dorsal mesentery. *A,* The primitive gut tube initially hangs from the posterior body wall by a broad bar of mesenchyme, but (*B*) in regions inferior to the septum transversum, this connection thins out to form a membranous dorsal mesentery composed of reflected peritoneum. *C,* Viscera suspended within the peritoneal cavity by a mesentery are called intraperitoneal, whereas organs embedded in the body wall and covered by peritoneum are called retroperitoneal. *D,* The mesentery suspending some intraperitoneal organs disappears as both the mesentery and the organ fuse with the body wall. These organs are then called secondarily retroperitoneal.

Bmps, and Wnt antagonists so that by the end of gastrulation, the endoderm is partitioned into broad regions along the cranial-caudal axis.

As indicated above, the process of regionalizing the gut tube into foregut, midgut, and hindgut is likely initiated by events that occur during gastrulation. However, regionalization of the endoderm is further refined by tissue-tissue interactions between the germ layers. The overlying ectoderm and mesoderm provide not only permissive influences but also inductive influences on the endoderm. For instance, in vitro, mouse cranial endoderm in presomitic embryos can be respecified to express caudal endodermal markers through interactions with caudal mesoderm. However, by the early somitic stage, the endoderm is more restricted in its developmental potential. Several transcription factors and morphogens involved in refining the regionalization of the gut have been identified, some of which are illustrated in Figures 14-5 and 14-6 and are covered briefly below.

After initiation of cranial body folding, the endoderm of the ventral foregut is situated adjacent to the caudal cardiogenic mesoderm. In fish, chick, and mouse embryos, cardiogenic mesoderm, by releasing Bmps and Fgfs, stimulates Shh

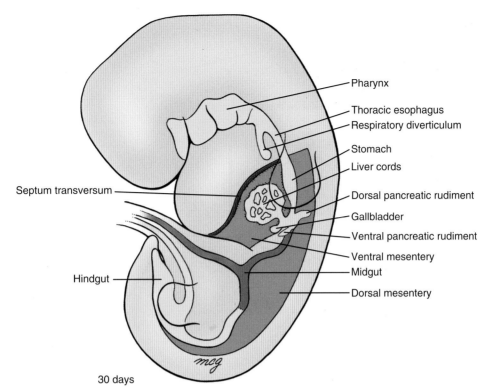

Pharynx
Thoracic esophagus
Respiratory diverticulum
Stomach
Liver cords
Dorsal pancreatic rudiment
Gallbladder
Ventral pancreatic rudiment
Ventral mesentery
Midgut
Dorsal mesentery

Septum transversum

Hindgut

30 days

Figure 14-4. Three subdivisions of the gut tube. The foregut consists of the pharynx, located cranial to the respiratory diverticulum, the thoracic esophagus, and the abdominal foregut. The abdominal foregut forms the abdominal esophagus, stomach, and half of the duodenum; it gives rise to the liver, gallbladder, pancreas, and their associated ducts. The midgut forms half of the duodenum, the jejunum and ileum, the ascending colon, and about two thirds of the transverse colon. The hindgut forms one third of the transverse colon, the descending colon, and the sigmoid colon and the upper two thirds of the anorectal canal. The abdominal esophagus, stomach, and superior part of the duodenum are suspended by dorsal and ventral mesenteries; the abdominal gut tube excluding the rectum is suspended in the abdominal cavity by a dorsal mesentery only.

expression in the ventral foregut endoderm, thereby promoting hepatic development (expression of hepatic markers, albumin, and alpha-fetoprotein) and repressing pancreatic development (see Fig 14-5). In regions where the ventral foregut endoderm is exposed to low levels of Fgf2, the endoderm begins expressing Pdx1 (pancreas and duodenal homeobox gene), which, in turn, represses Shh expression and supports pancreatic development. In the non-hepatic dorsal foregut endoderm, the expression of hepatic markers in the dorsal endoderm is repressed by the overlying dorsal axial mesoderm (possibly through Wnt and Fgf4 signaling). Thus, interactions between mesoderm and endoderm play crucial roles in dictating regional organ development.

The endoderm of the foregut forms many sections of the gastrointestinal tract including the esophagus, stomach, pancreas, and duodenum. Pdx1 is expressed in the early stomach and in the dorsal and ventral prepancreatic and preduodenal endoderm (see Fig. 14-5). In mice, Shh is expressed along the entire length of these endodermal regions, except at the site of pancreatic bud formation. Perturbation of Shh signaling within the Pdx1-expressing endoderm results in the ectopic expression of insulin in the stomach and duodenum, suggesting that Shh normally represses expression of pancreatic cell fate in all Pdx1-positive endoderm.

The dorsal endoderm of the gut tube is in contact with the notochord, and this interaction is required for proper dorsal pancreatic development. Studies in several species show that the notochord specifically represses Shh expression in the prepancreatic endoderm by releasing Fgf2 and activin β,

thereby removing its repressive effect on Pdx1 expression and promoting dorsal pancreas development (see Fig. 14-5). Induction of the dorsal pancreatic bud also requires retinoic acid signaling, which seems to regulate the expression boundaries of Pdx1 and Cdx and hence the position of the dorsal pancreas.

The notochord is eventually displaced from the pancreatic endoderm by the fusing dorsal aortae, and this places the pancreatic endoderm under the influence of endothelial cells. Recent in vivo and in vitro studies in Xenopus and mice show that Vegf released by the dorsal aortic endothelial cells promotes pancreatic endocrine cell fate specification.

Hox genes are also expressed within gut endoderm and play important roles in regional specification and development of the gut (see Fig. 14-5 and Fig. 14-6). In the chick, Hoxa3 gene expression is regionally restricted, demarcating the boundary between foregut and midgut, with Hoxd13 expression limited to the caudalmost hindgut mesoderm. Interactions between the hindgut endoderm and mesoderm seem to be responsible for restricting Hoxd13 expression. Hoxd13 instills caudal identity to the hindgut because when mis-expressed in more cranial mesoderm of chick embryos, the stomach endoderm can be transformed into intestinal endoderm. Hox genes also play a role in demarcating regions of the gastrointestinal tract, particularly specifying sites of sphincter formation that separate the gut segments (see Fig. 14-6). For instance, mice null for Hoxd12 or Hoxd13 have severe muscular defects in the anal sphincter, and mice null for the full Hoxd cluster between Hoxd4 and Hoxd13 lack ileocecal sphincters and form abnormal pyloric and anal sphincters.

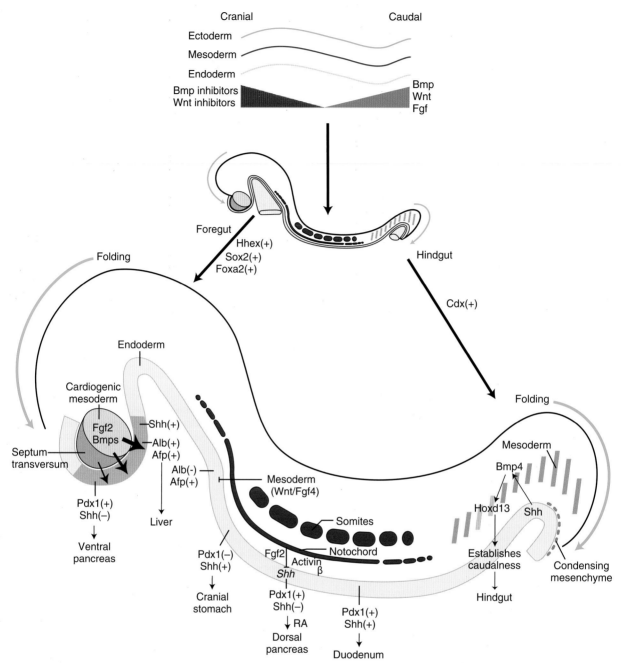

Figure 14-5. Signals and transcription factors important in establishing regional differences in the early developing gastrointestinal tract. The top drawing illustrates early cranial-caudal patterning of the endoderm during late gastrulation. Gradients of Wnt, Wnt antagonists, Bmps, and Fgfs establish expression patterns for foregut and hindgut transcription factors (e.g., Hhex, Cdx). Retinoic acid is thought to regulate the Pdx1 and Cdx expression boundary and to help establish the future position of the dorsal pancreas. The bottom two drawings represent an early mammalian embryo shortly after the initiation of embryonic folding and show some of the signaling events and transcription factors involved in liver, pancreas, and hindgut specification. After initiation of cranial body folding, the endoderm of the ventral foregut is situated adjacent to the caudal cardiogenic mesoderm and septum transversum. Tissue-tissue interactions between the cardiogenic mesoderm and the endoderm play a key role. Bmps and high levels of Fgf induce hepatocytic markers within the endoderm (e.g., albumin, alpha-fetoprotein) while suppressing ventral pancreatic development by upregulating Shh expression. Low levels of Fgfs permit the expression of the homeoprotein pancreatic/duodenal marker, Pdx1, promoting ventral pancreatic development. Much of the endoderm expresses Shh, but it is repressed by notochordal release of Fgf2 and activin β demarcating the future dorsal pancreatic region. Shh expression within the hindgut endoderm induces Bmp4 and Hoxd13 expression within the caudal mesoderm. Shh and Bmp4 induce only Hoxd13 expression in the caudal gut, possibly due to the caudal restriction of Cdx expression established during gastrulation. Hoxd13 instills a caudal identity to the hindgut. Afp, Alpha-fetoprotein; Alb, albumin; RA, retinoic acid.

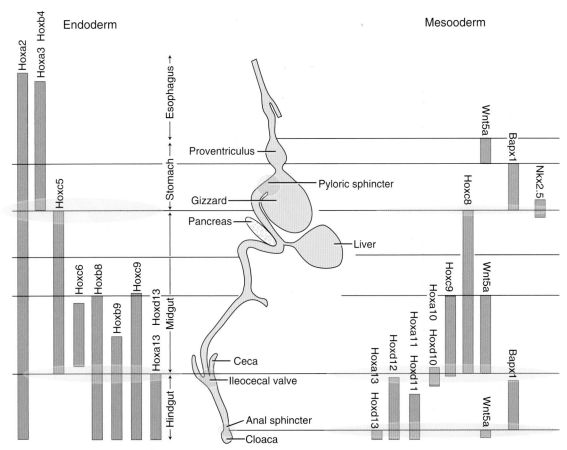

Figure 14-6. Hox gene expression boundaries in the endoderm and mesoderm during early chick gut development. Specific combinations of homeobox gene expression can be mapped to specific regions of the gastrointestinal tract, with some combinations demarcating the position of sphincters and organs. The regional expression patterns of mouse orthologs are similar.

DEVELOPMENT OF ABDOMINAL FOREGUT

 Animation 14-2: Development of Foregut.
Animations are available online at StudentConsult.

STOMACH FORMATION AND ROTATION

The stomach first becomes apparent during the early part of the fourth week, as the foregut just caudal to the septum transversum expands slightly. On about day twenty-six, the thoracic foregut begins to elongate rapidly. Over the next two days, the presumptive stomach, now much farther removed from the lung buds, expands further into a fusiform (Latin, "spindle-shaped") structure that is readily distinguished from adjacent regions of the gut tube (Fig. 14-7). During the fifth week, the dorsal wall of the stomach grows faster than the ventral wall, resulting in the formation of the **greater curvature of the stomach**. Concurrently, deformation of the ventral stomach wall forms the **lesser curvature of the stomach**. By the end of the seventh week, the continual differential expansion of the superior part of the greater curvature results in the formation of the **fundus** and **cardiac incisure**.

During the seventh and eighth weeks, the developing stomach undergoes a 90-degree rotation around its craniocaudal axis, so that the greater curvature lies to the left and the lesser curvature lies to the right (Fig. 14-7D). Cellular and structural changes in the **dorsal mesogastrium** (the portion of the dorsal mesentery attached to the stomach) are thought to play a role in this rotation (covered later in this chapter). The right and left vagus plexuses, which originally run through the mesoderm on either side of the gut tube, thus rotate to become posterior (dorsal) and anterior (ventral) vagal trunks in the region of the stomach. However, fibers of the left and right vagal plexuses mix to some degree and also connect with the celiac plexus, so that the caudal anterior and posterior vagal trunks contain fibers from each of the more cranial vagal plexuses. The stomach also rotates slightly around a ventrodorsal axis, so that the greater curvature faces slightly caudal and the lesser curvature slightly cranial (see Fig. 14-7D).

The rotations of the stomach bend the presumptive duodenum into a C shape and displace it to the right until it lies against the dorsal body wall, to which it adheres, thus becoming secondarily retroperitoneal. The rotation of the stomach and the fusion of the duodenum create an alcove dorsal to the stomach called the **lesser sac of the peritoneal cavity** (Fig. 14-8). The rest of the peritoneal cavity is now called the **greater sac**. The lesser sac

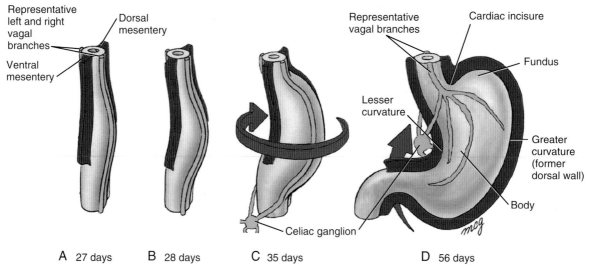

Figure 14-7. Rotation of the stomach. *A-C,* Oblique frontal views. *D,* Direct frontal view. The posterior wall of the stomach expands during the fourth and fifth weeks to form the greater curvature. During the seventh week, the stomach rotates clockwise on its longitudinal axis (when viewed from above). Arrows indicate directions of movement.

enlarges because of progressive expansion of the dorsal mesogastrium connecting the stomach to the posterior body wall. The resulting large, suspended fold of mesogastrium, called the **greater omentum**, hangs from the dorsal body wall and the greater curvature of the stomach and drapes over more inferior organs of the abdominal cavity (Fig. 14-8C). The portion of the lesser sac directly dorsal to the stomach is now called the **upper recess of the lesser sac**, and the cavity within the greater omentum is called the **lower recess of the lesser sac**. The lower recess is obliterated during fetal life as the anterior and posterior folds of the greater omentum fuse together.

LIVER AND GALLBLADDER DEVELOPMENT

On about day twenty-two, a small endodermal thickening, the **hepatic plate**, forms on the ventral side of the duodenum. Over the next few days, cells in this plate proliferate and form the **hepatic diverticulum**, which grows into the mesenchymal cells that give rise to the inferior region of the septum transversum (Fig. 14-9). The hepatic diverticulum gives rise to ramifying cords of **hepatoblasts** (the liver primordial cells). Under the influence of notch signaling and other regulatory proteins (covered in the following "In the Research Lab" entitled "Hepatoblast Specification and Fate"), hepatoblasts become **hepatocytes** (parenchyma), **bile canaliculi** of the liver, or **hepatic ducts**. In contrast, the mesoblastic **supporting stroma** of the liver develops from the septum transversum and splanchnic mesoderm originating near the stomach, as well as from endothelial precursor cells (that develop into the **sinusoidal endothelium** of the liver). Cardiogenic mesoderm, endothelium, and the septum transversum mesenchymal cells emit growth factor signals (including Vegfs, Bmps, and Fgfs) that are required for liver parenchymal development (covered in the following "In the Research Lab" entitled "Hepatoblast Specification and Fate").

As covered in Chapter 13, the liver is a major early **hematopoietic organ** of the embryo. Hematopoietic stem cells originating from the yolk sac wall (and later from the aortic, gonad, and mesonephric region) colonize the embryonic liver, expand their numbers, and diversify before populating other hematopoietic organs. Hepatic progenitors along with the hepatic stromal cells generate a hematopoietic microenvironment necessary for adult-type hematopoiesis. As the hematopoietic function is shifted to the peripheral organs, hepatocytes begin upregulating the expression of numerous genes related to mature liver function (e.g., those associated with amino acid metabolism and detoxification). Throughout embryonic and fetal development, hepatocytes proliferate (mainly mediated by autocrine mechanisms). This proliferation gradually slows and is arrested with postnatal development. From then on, migration and proliferation of hepatocytes require extraneous growth factors, including Egf and hepatocyte growth factor (Hgf).

By day twenty-six, a distinct endodermal thickening also forms on the ventral side of the duodenum just caudal to the base of the hepatic diverticulum and buds into the ventral mesentery (see Fig. 14-9). This **cystic diverticulum** will form the **gallbladder** and **cystic duct**. The gallbladder and cystic duct develop from histologically distinct populations of duodenal cells.

<table>
<tr><td>■</td><td>*In the Research Lab*</td></tr>
</table>

HEPATOBLAST SPECIFICATION AND FATE

As covered earlier in the chapter, cardiogenic mesoderm plays a significant role in specifying liver formation and hepatic gene expression within the foregut endoderm (see Fig. 14-5). However, additional signals promoting liver formation originate from the mesoderm of the septum transversum. As covered in earlier chapters, Bmp signaling has a major role in the development of lateral plate mesoderm, and this is true for the liver as well. Bmps

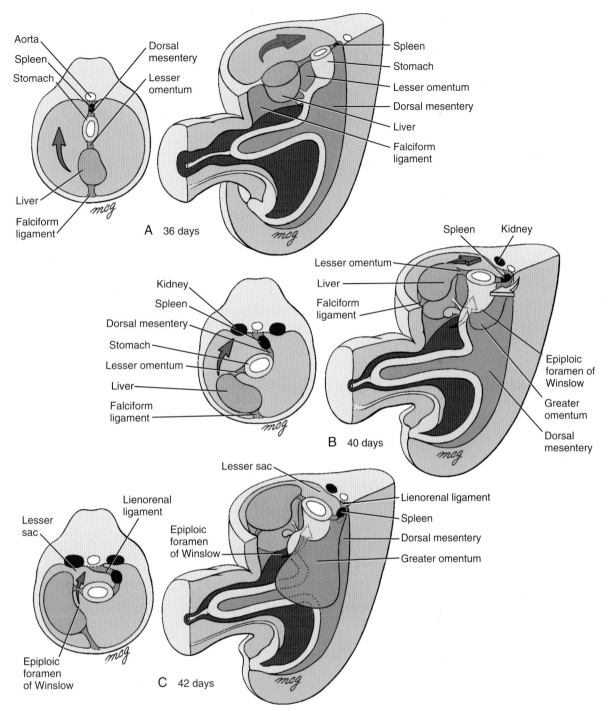

Figure 14-8. Development of the greater omentum and lesser sac. *A* and *B*, The rotation of the stomach and growth of the dorsal mesogastrium create a sac (the greater omentum) that dangles from the greater curvature of the stomach. *B* and *C*, When the duodenum swings to the right, it becomes secondarily fused to the body wall, enclosing the space posterior to the stomach and within the expanding cavity of the greater omentum. This space is the lesser sac of the peritoneal cavity. The remainder of the peritoneal cavity is now called the greater sac. The principal passageway between the greater and lesser sacs is the epiploic foramen of Winslow. Curved arrows indicate directions of movement; red coloring indicates the space surrounding the midgut intestinal loop as it initiates herniation into the umbilical cord.

are expressed in the septum transversum (see Fig. 14-5); in mice lacking Bmp4, the liver bud fails to grow or express albumin. As covered earlier in the chapter, Fgfs from the adjacent cardiogenic region stimulate albumin expression in the endodermal liver primordia. In explant cultures of the liver primordia, noggin (an antagonist of Bmps) inhibits this Fgf-induced albumin expression. Although Bmps alone are insufficient to induce hepatic development,

blocking of Bmp signaling with noggin increases the expression of the pancreatic marker Pdx1 in this endoderm. Therefore, Bmps contribute to Fgf-mediated endodermal patterning by promoting the liver phenotype and repressing the pancreatic phenotype. What downstream targets invoked by Fgfs and Bmps that induce hepatoblast lineage and growth remain unclear but may include Gata4, Hnf3 (hepatic nuclear factor-3), and C/EBP (CAAT-enhancer binding

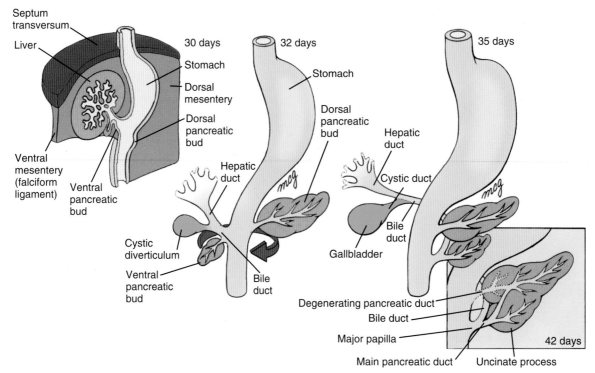

Figure 14-9. Development of the liver, gallbladder, pancreas, and their duct systems from endodermal diverticula of the duodenum. The liver bud sprouts during the fourth week and expands in the ventral mesentery. The cystic diverticulum and the ventral pancreatic bud also grow into the ventral mesentery, whereas the dorsal pancreatic bud grows into the dorsal mesentery. During the fifth week, the ventral pancreatic bud migrates around the posterior side (former right side) of the duodenum to fuse with the dorsal pancreatic bud. The main duct of the ventral bud ultimately becomes the major pancreatic duct, which drains the entire pancreas.

proteins). Wnt signaling has also been implicated in liver development and is required for bile duct lineage specification in mice.

Much more needs to be learned about how hepatoblasts acquire a hepatocytic or bile-ductal cell fate. A number of factors have been implicated in mediating cell determination of these two lineages. Like the segregation of neuronal and glial precursor cells from the neuroepithelium (covered in Chapter 9), notch signaling seems to have a role in mediating the decision as to whether a hepatoblast becomes a hepatocyte or bile duct lining cell (**cholangiocytes**). As covered in Chapters 3, 5, 12, and 13, mutations in the NOTCH ligand JAGGED1 (or in the receptor NOTCH2) are associated with autosomal dominant **Alagille syndrome**. These patients exhibit a paucity of bile ducts. Double heterozygotic mice for a jagged1 and notch2 null mutation lack intrahepatic bile ducts at birth and mimic Alagille syndrome. Recent studies in mice also show that jagged1 is expressed in cells adjacent to notch2-positive epithelium at the site of biliary differentiation, and that notch2 represses the hepatocyte lineage. Hence, jagged1/notch2 interactions likely have critical roles in hepatocyte/cholangiocyte determination.

A major change in liver functions occurs near birth as the burden of hematopoiesis is shifted away from the liver and the liver begins taking on the metabolic and detoxifying burdens. One group of transcription factors important in mediating these functions is the hepatocyte nuclear factor (Hnf) family. Hnfs activate specific liver genes. Mice with the Hnf4α gene deleted from the liver primordium using a cre-lox system (covered in Chapter 5) develop small livers that lack organized epithelia and fail to express almost all liver-specific genes. However, forced expression of Hnf4α in fibroblast cultures does not induce liver-specific gene expression, even though the fibroblasts take on an epithelial-like morphology. This suggests that other cell lineage–determining factors must be in place before Hnfs can initiate liver-specific gene expression.

Another transcription factor that activates several liver genes and is involved in the functional change to mature liver function is C/EBPα. C/EBPα-deficient mice die at birth because of hypoglycemia. Although the liver tissue appears normal, hepatocytes are deficient in their ability to store glycogen and lipids. Other molecules implicated in late fetal liver maturation are oncostatin M and glucocorticoids. Oncostatin M stimulates the expression of hepatic differentiation markers, promotes liver-like morphology, and induces liver-specific gene expression in liver progenitor explant cultures. Glucocorticoids alone are capable of inducing most of the cellular responses typical of the liver differentiation promoted by oncostatin M, suggesting that they work together to promote liver maturation. Other factors involved in liver maturation likely include Hgf (upregulated on hepatic injury and hepatic regeneration) and Tgfβ (which may inhibit hepatocyte proliferation and promote differentiation).

PANCREAS DEVELOPMENT

On day twenty-six, another duodenal bud begins to grow into the dorsal mesentery just opposite the hepatic diverticulum. This endodermal diverticulum is the **dorsal pancreatic bud** and will form the dorsal pancreas (see Fig. 14-9). As the dorsal pancreatic bud elongates into the dorsal mesentery, another endodermal diverticulum, the **ventral pancreatic bud**, sprouts into the ventral mesentery just caudal to the developing gallbladder. This bud will form the ventral pancreas as well as the bile duct (see Fig. 14-9).

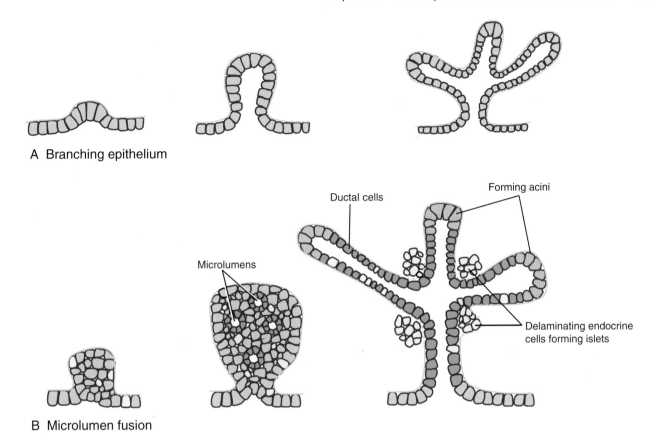

A Branching epithelium

B Microlumen fusion

Figure 14-10. Diagrammatic representation of basic branching mechanisms for the formation of tubular glands. *A,* Classic branching mechanism whereby the expanding epithelium is thrown into epithelial folds. *B,* Branching mechanism whereby a proliferating single-layered epithelium is converted into multiple layers and becomes stratified. This is followed by the formation of microlumens that coalesce within the epithelium to form branched lumens. Clusters of endocrine cells (yellow) delaminate from the epithelium to form islets lying peripheral to the developing ductal (green) and acinar (red) cells. The formation of the endocrine cell lineage within the early epithelium is indicated in yellow.

Once specified, the pancreatic endodermal bud thickens and continues to expand into the closely apposed mesoderm. Branching of this bud occurs differently from the classic branching of other organs, such as the developing lung (Fig. 14-10*A*). Rather than expanding and folding the epithelium, solid epithelial clusters form, followed by the formation of intraepithelial microlumens. These microlumens soon coalesce to generate continuous lumens, forming an epithelial tree draining exocrine products into the duodenum (Fig. 14-10*B*). The **pancreatic acinar cells** that produce digestive enzymes, the **pancreatic ductal cells** that transport the digestive enzymes, and the **pancreatic endocrine cells** in the **islets of Langerhans** that produce insulin, glucagon, somatostatin, pancreatic polypeptide, and ghrelin all differentiate from the endoderm of the pancreatic buds. The endocrine cell lineage proliferates within the endodermal epithelium, and soon these cells delaminate and subsequently aggregate into islets within the surrounding mesenchyme (see Fig. 14-10*B*), where they continue to proliferate throughout the embryonic period.

Interactions with the mesoderm play an essential role in growth and differentiation of the pancreas, and the expression of several growth-promoting transcription factors within the mesoderm is important in this.

Fgf10 is expressed in pancreatic mesoderm, and Fgf10 knockout mice have hypoplastic dorsal and ventral pancreatic buds. Isl1 (insulin gene enhancer protein-1) is expressed by mesoderm surrounding the pancreatic buds. If Isl1 is knocked out in mice, pancreatic mesenchyme is almost completely lost, and the expression of the pancreatic marker Pdx1 is greatly reduced. Mice lacking Pbx1 (pre–B-cell leukemia transcription factor-1), another transcriptional marker expressed in pancreatic endoderm and mesoderm that may act as a Pdx1 co-factor, exhibit severe hypoplasia of dorsal pancreas and loss of acinar development. This defect can be rescued in culture by wild-type mesoderm.

In humans, while the common bile duct is forming and the ventral pancreatic bud is branching, proliferating, and differentiating, the mouth of the common bile duct and the ventral pancreatic bud migrate posteriorly around the duodenum toward the dorsal mesentery (see Fig. 14-9). By the early sixth week, the ventral and dorsal pancreatic buds lie adjacent to one another in the plane of the dorsal mesentery. Late in the sixth week, the two pancreatic buds fuse to form the definitive pancreas. The dorsal pancreatic bud gives rise to the **head, body**, and **tail** of the pancreas, whereas the ventral pancreatic bud gives rise to the hook-like **uncinate process**. Like the duodenum, the pancreas fuses to the dorsal body wall and becomes secondarily retroperitoneal.

When the ventral and dorsal pancreatic buds fuse, their ductal systems also become interconnected (see Fig. 14-9). The proximal portion of the duct connecting the dorsal bud to the duodenum usually degenerates, leaving the ventral pancreatic duct, now called the **main pancreatic duct**, as the only conduit for both the ventral and dorsal pancreas into the duodenum. The main pancreatic duct and the common bile duct meet and empty their secretions into the duodenum at the **major duodenal papilla** or **ampulla of Vater**. However, in some individuals, the proximal dorsal pancreatic duct persists as an **accessory pancreatic duct** that empties into the duodenum at a **minor duodenal papilla**.

In the Clinic

ABNORMAL FORMATION AND ROTATION OF VENTRAL PANCREAS

Occasionally, the pancreas forms a complete ring encircling the duodenum, a condition known as **annular pancreas**. As shown in Figure 14-11, this abnormality probably arises when the two lobes of a bilobed ventral pancreatic bud (a normal variation) migrate in opposite directions around the duodenum to fuse with the dorsal pancreatic bud. An annular pancreas compresses the duodenum and may cause gastrointestinal obstruction (**duodenal stenosis**). Faulty hedgehog signaling may play a role in the development of annular pancreas. In mice, loss of Ihh (Indian hedgehog) signaling leads to ectopic branching of ventral pancreatic buds that then grow and wrap around the duodenum, forming an annular pancreas. Loss of Shh in some strains of mice also results in the development of an annular pancreas. Shh mutants exhibit duodenal stenosis and imperforated anus defects, both defects that are associated with annular pancreas in humans as well.

In the Research Lab

DETERMINATION OF PANCREATIC CELL LINEAGE

With expansion and branching of the pancreatic buds, the pancreatic epithelium consists of convoluted sheets of epithelium that uniformly express Pdx1. From this epithelium arise exocrine cells and endocrine cells. As in hepatic cell specification (covered earlier in this chapter "In the Research Lab" entitled "Hepatoblast Specification and Fate"), notch signaling plays an important role in mediating pancreatic cell specification, thereby determining which cells activate the endocrine lineage from a bipotential progenitor within the pancreatic epithelium. One downstream target of notch signaling in the pancreatic endoderm is Hes1 (hairy and enhancer-of-split-like-1). This transcription factor downregulates the proendocrine bHLH transcription factor neurogenin-3 (Neurog3), a member of the neurogenin/NeuroD family (Fig. 14-12). Neurog3 is expressed within scattered cells of the pancreatic endoderm and continues in endocrine progenitor cells throughout pancreatic development and even postnatally. Mice lacking Neurog3 not only fail to develop pancreatic endocrine cells but also lack intestinal enteroendocrine cells and gastric endocrine cells. Moreover, Pdx1 promoter-driven Neurog3 expression in mice generates massive quantities of glucagon-secreting endocrine cells in the gut. In the chick, ectopic Neurog3 expression induces the formation of glucagon-secreting cells within endoderm outside the pancreatic endoderm. Finally, introducing the expression of Neurog3 in cultured human pancreatic ductal cells induces endocrine marker expression. Hence, Neurog3 is a proendocrine transcription factor that, in the absence of notch signaling, is sufficient to initiate the endocrine pathway in pancreatic epithelium. However, recent evidence shows that activating notch signaling in Neurog3-positive progenitor cells can redirect early endocrine progenitors toward a ductal fate, suggesting that early pancreatic endocrine cells maintain a degree of developmental plasticity.

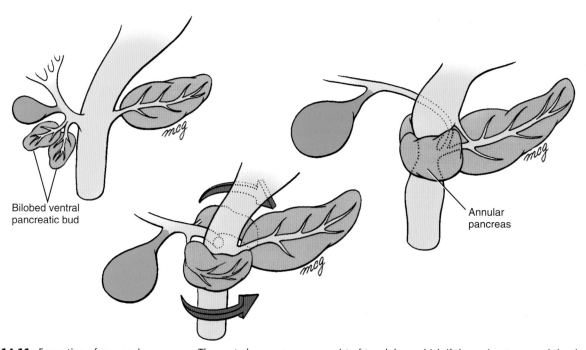

Bilobed ventral pancreatic bud

Annular pancreas

Figure 14-11. Formation of an annular pancreas. The ventral pancreas may consist of two lobes, which if they migrate around the duodenum in opposite directions to fuse with the dorsal pancreatic bud, form an annular pancreas.

Cells in which Neurog3 expression is repressed by notch signaling (i.e., via expression of Hes1) become part of the exocrine pancreas. The Ptf1 (pancreas specific transcription factor-1) complex is important for early pancreatic lineage specification and later for specifying the acinar pancreas (see Fig. 14-12). Mice lacking the Ptf1a (p48) component of the Ptf1 complex do not develop acini or ductal epithelia, whereas pancreatic islets still form within the adjacent mesenchyme. What controls early Ptf1a expression in the pancreatic primordia is still unclear but may involve factors released by the dorsal aorta and developing vessels.

Glucagon-synthesizing cells are the first endocrine cells to form within the endoderm, appearing early in the pancreatic bud stage. For a long time, it was thought that these cells were the precursors of both **alpha cells** (glucagon-producing) and **beta cells** (insulin-producing). Single-cell lineage tracing has shown that alpha and beta cells originate from different Neurog3-expressing endocrine cells. Specification of alpha and beta cells may depend on the relative amount of Pax4 and Arx (aristaless-related homeobox) expression. Recent studies suggest that higher levels of Pax4 expression relative to Arx expression promote beta/delta cell conversion, whereas higher levels of Arx expression promote alpha cell specification (see Fig 14-12). Hence the balance between Pax4 and Arx expression seems to be key in determining the beta or alpha cell lineage.

Nkx2.2 and Nkx6.1 act to promote beta cell specification (see Fig. 14-12). Knockout mice for Nkx2.2 generate equal numbers of endocrine precursor cells as compared to their wild-type littermates but fail to activate the insulin gene, suggesting that they have a deficiency in beta cell differentiation. Knockout mice for Nkx6.1, a transcription factor specifically expressed in adult beta islet cells, generate small numbers of insulin-producing cells but fail to maintain or increase their numbers during subsequent development.

NeuroD1, a transcription factor and direct transcriptional target of Neurog3, is expressed in all endocrine cells of the pancreas after their specification. NeuroD1 plays an important role in mediating the expression of differentiated endocrine products of the islet (e.g., insulin). Mice lacking the NeuroD1 gene develop the normal complement of islet cell types, but beta cell maturation is defective after birth. Mutations in NEUROD1 in humans are associated with **maturity-onset diabetes of the young**, where the beta cells become insensitive to blood glucose levels and/or are unable to synthesize adequate amounts of insulin. Mutations in NEUROD1 are also associated with human **type II diabetes**. Another transcription factor involved in beta cell specification is MafA (v-Maf musculoaponeurotic fibrosarcoma oncogene homolog A). MafA expression is limited to beta cells in the early pancreas. It is a strong activator of the insulin promoter and seems to function downstream of Nkx6.1.

The transcription factors and specification steps required for the development of PP and epsilon cells are still poorly understood.

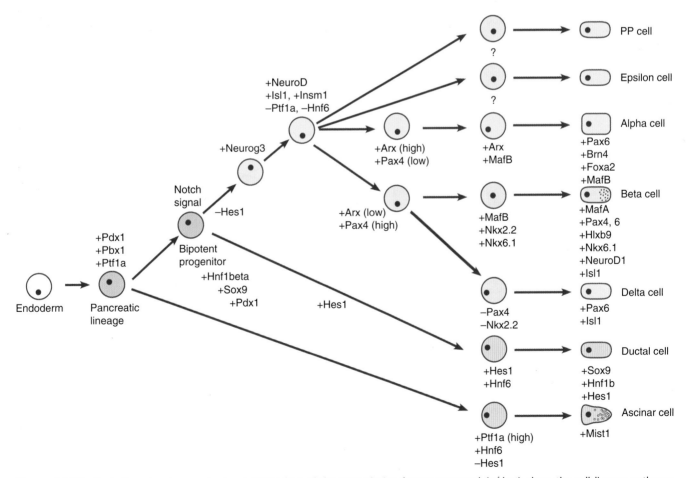

Figure 14-12. Illustration showing our basic understanding of the transcription factors expressed (or lost) along the cell lineage pathways responsible for specifying various cell types derived from pancreatic endoderm.

In the Clinic

REGULATION OF ISLET CELL NUMBER

The number of islet cells that develop in the pancreas is generally set during fetal life but can be influenced by such factors as **intrauterine growth restriction** (IUGR; covered in Chapter 6) due to vascular insufficiency, maternal diabetes, and fetal malnutrition. Embryonic and fetal islet cells, like those in the adult, respond to elevated blood glucose levels with compensatory hyperplasia. This fetal maladaptation is frequently seen in neonates born to diabetic mothers. Such hyperplasia, called **congenital hyperinsulinism** (sometimes referred to by the term *nesidioblastosis;* "nesidio" is Greek for islet), can occur locally or diffusely throughout the pancreas and lead to life-threatening decreases in blood glucose levels (i.e., **hypoglycemia**). Hyperinsulinemia is typically treated by diazoxide therapy until the hyperinsulinemia is resolved or by partial or near-total pancreatectomy. Some forms of congenital hyperinsulinism are associated with specific gene mutations or recessive disorders of the SULPHONYLUREA RECEPTOR, but a majority are non-familial and of unknown cause.

Before birth, islet cells are generated by the proliferation and differentiation of pancreatic progenitor cells. As just mentioned, the number of islets generated within the developing pancreas is amenable to the need to maintain proper glucose levels during the embryonic and fetal periods. However, the capacity to generate more islet cells after birth is greatly reduced. Nevertheless, the islet cell population still can increase after birth but does so very little after adolescence. Recent studies in adult mice show that new beta islet cells arise from preexisting beta cells rather than from unidentified resident pancreatic progenitor cells. Therefore, if human adult pancreatic beta cells share this proliferative capacity, the hope is that new therapeutic strategies for human **type I diabetes** (where beta cells have been destroyed or are non-functional) could be developed.

SPLEEN DEVELOPMENT

As the dorsal mesogastrium of the lesser sac begins its expansive growth at the end of the fourth week, a mesenchymal condensation develops within it near the body wall. This condensation differentiates during the fifth week to form the **spleen**, a vascular lymphatic organ (see Fig. 14-8). Smaller splenic condensations called **accessory spleens** may develop near the hilum of the primary spleen. It is important to remember that the spleen is a mesodermal derivative, not a product of the gut tube endoderm, like most of the intra-abdominal viscera. However, its mesenchyme shares a common origin with the pancreas. Rotation of the stomach and growth of the dorsal mesogastrium translocate the spleen to the left side of the abdominal cavity. The rotation of the dorsal mesogastrium also establishes a mesenteric connection called the **lienorenal ligament** between the spleen and the left kidney. The portion of the dorsal mesentery between the spleen and the stomach is called the **gastrosplenic ligament**.

VENTRAL MESENTERY DERIVATIVES

As the liver enlarges, the caudal portion of the septum transversum and the ventral mesentery are modified to form a number of membranous structures, including the serous coverings of the liver and the membranes that attach the liver to the stomach and to the ventral body wall. As covered in Chapter 11, the central tendon of the diaphragm forms from the **septum transversum**. By the sixth week, the enlarging liver makes contact with the septum transversum, and the portion of the ventral mesentery covering the liver begins to split apart (Fig. 14-13).

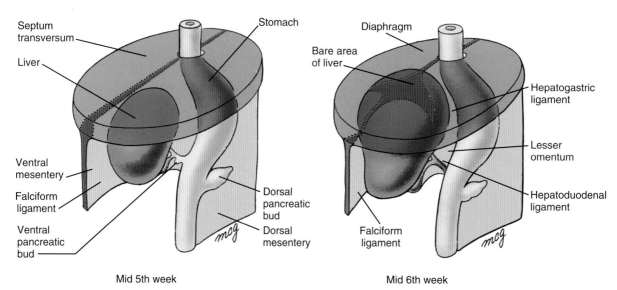

Mid 5th week   Mid 6th week

Figure 14-13. Formation of the liver and associated membranes. As the liver bud grows into the ventral mesentery, its expanding crown makes direct contact with the developing diaphragm. The ventral mesentery that encloses the growing liver bud differentiates into the visceral peritoneum of the liver, which is reflected onto the diaphragm. This zone of reflection, which encircles the area where the liver directly contacts the diaphragm (the bare area), becomes the coronary ligament. The remnant of ventral mesentery connecting the liver with the anterior body wall becomes the falciform ligament, whereas the ventral mesentery between the liver and lesser curvature of the stomach forms the lesser omentum.

The caudal portion of the ventral mesentery covering almost the entire surface of the liver becomes **visceral peritoneum**. However, at the cranial end, the liver tissue makes direct contact with the developing central tendon of the diaphragm and thus has no peritoneal covering. This zone becomes the **bare area of the liver** (see Fig. 14-13). Around the margins of the bare area, the peritoneum covering the inferior surface of the peripheral diaphragm makes a fold or reflection onto the surface of the liver. Because this reflection encircles the bare area like a crown, it is called the **coronary ligament**. Direct contact between the liver and the diaphragm in the bare area results in the formation of anastomoses between hepatic portal vessels and systemic veins of the diaphragm.

The narrow sickle-shaped flap of ventral mesentery attaching the liver to the ventral body wall differentiates into the membranous **falciform ligament** (see Fig. 14-13; also see Fig. 14-8). The free caudal margin of this membrane carries the umbilical vein from the body wall to the liver. The portion of the ventral mesentery between the liver and the stomach thins out to form a translucent membrane called the **lesser omentum**. The caudal border of the lesser omentum, connecting the liver to the developing duodenum, is called the **hepatoduodenal ligament** and contains the portal vein, the proper hepatic artery and its branches, and the hepatic, cystic, and common bile ducts. The region of the lesser omentum between the liver and the stomach is called the **hepatogastric ligament**.

When the stomach rotates to the left and the liver shifts into the right side of the peritoneal cavity, the lesser omentum rotates from a sagittal into a coronal (frontal) plane. This repositioning reduces the communication between the greater and lesser sacs of the peritoneal cavity to a narrow canal lying just posterior to the lesser omentum. This canal is called the **epiploic foramen of Winslow** (see Fig. 14-8).

MIDGUT DEVELOPMENT

 Animation 14-3: Development of Midgut.
Animations are available online at StudentConsult.

PRIMARY INTESTINAL LOOP

By the fifth week, the presumptive ileum, which can be distinguished from the presumptive colon by the presence of a cecal primordium at the junction between the two, begins to elongate rapidly. The growing ileum lengthens much more rapidly than the abdominal cavity itself, and the midgut is, therefore, thrown into a dorsoventral hairpin fold called the **primary intestinal loop** (Fig. 14-14A). The cranial limb of this loop will give rise to most of the ileum; the caudal limb will become the ascending colon and the transverse colon. At its apex, the primary intestinal loop is attached to the umbilicus by the vitelline duct, and the superior mesenteric artery runs down the long axis of the loop. By the early sixth week, the continuing elongation of the midgut, combined with pressure resulting from the dramatic growth

of other abdominal organs (particularly the liver), forces the primary intestinal loop to herniate into the umbilicus (Fig. 14-14B,C).

As the primary intestinal loop herniates into the umbilicus, it rotates around the axis of the superior mesenteric artery (i.e., around a dorsoventral axis) by 90 degrees counterclockwise as viewed from the anterior. Thus, the cranial limb moves caudally and to the embryo's right, and the caudal limb moves cranially and to the embryo's left (see Fig. 14-14B). This rotation is complete by the early eighth week. Meanwhile, the midgut continues to differentiate. The lengthening jejunum and ileum are thrown into a series of folds called the **jejunal-ileal loops**, and the expanding cecum sprouts a wormlike **vermiform appendix** (see Fig. 14-14C).

During the tenth week, the midgut retracts into the abdomen. The mechanism responsible for the rapid retraction of the midgut into the abdominal cavity during the tenth week is not understood but may involve an increase in the size of the abdominal cavity relative to the other abdominal organs. As the intestinal loop reenters the abdomen, it rotates counterclockwise through an additional 180 degrees so that now the retracting colon has traveled a 270-degree circuit relative to the posterior wall of the abdominal cavity (Fig. 14-14C-E). The cecum consequently rotates to a position just inferior to the liver in the region of the right iliac crest. The intestines have completely returned to the abdominal cavity by the eleventh week.

After the large intestine returns to the abdominal cavity, the dorsal mesenteries of the ascending colon and descending colon shorten and fold, bringing these organs into contact with the dorsal body wall, where they adhere and become secondarily retroperitoneal (see Fig. 14-3D). The cecum is suspended from the dorsal body wall by a shortened mesentery soon after it returns to the abdominal cavity. In the case of ascending and descending colons, shortening and folding of the mesenteries is probably related to the relative lengthening of the lumbar region of the dorsal body wall. The transverse colon does not become fixed to the body wall but remains an intraperitoneal organ suspended by mesentery. The most inferior portion of the colon, the sigmoid colon, also remains suspended by mesentery. Figure 14-15 summarizes the final disposition of the gastrointestinal organs with respect to the body wall.

In the Research Lab

CELLULAR AND MOLECULAR MECHANISMS OF GUT ROTATION

The gastrointestinal tract is a left-right asymmetrically patterned organ and undergoes an extensive and remarkable degree of lengthening, bending, and looping during its development. Although much is known about the early genes and signaling events involved in establishing left-right asymmetry (covered in Chapter 3), much less is known regarding how this is translated into the asymmetric morphology of endodermal organs. The earliest morphological sign of left-right asymmetry in the gut is the bulging of the foregut toward the left during the early development of the stomach, spleen, and pancreatic buds. The leftward growth may be driven by a structure derived from the surrounding splanchnic mesoderm called the **splanchnic mesodermal**

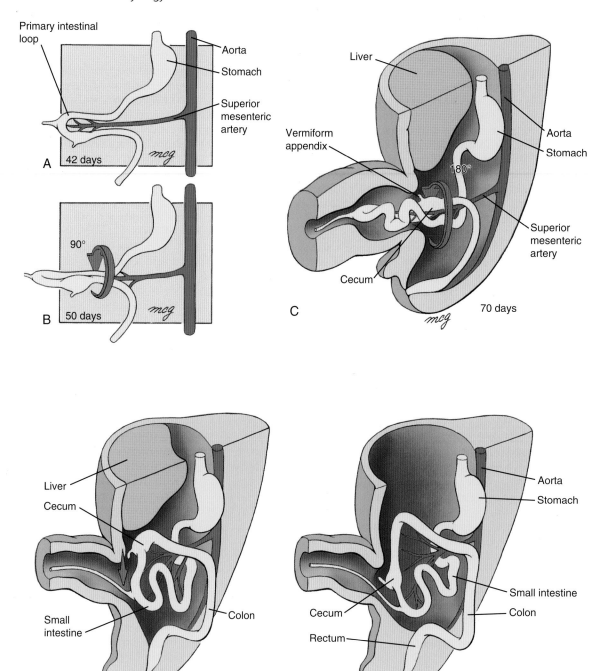

Figure 14-14. Herniation and rotation of the intestine. *A* and *B*, At the end of the sixth week, the primary intestinal loop herniates into the umbilicus, rotating through 90 degrees counterclockwise (in frontal view). *C*, The small intestine elongates to form jejunal-ileal loops, the cecum and appendix grow, and at the end of the tenth week, the primary intestinal loop retracts into the abdominal cavity, rotating an additional 180 degrees counterclockwise. *D* and *E*, During the eleventh week, the retracting midgut completes this rotation as the cecum is positioned just inferior to the liver. The cecum is then displaced inferiorly, pulling down the proximal hindgut to form the ascending colon. The descending colon is simultaneously fixed on the left side of the posterior abdominal wall. The jejunum, ileum, transverse colon, and sigmoid colon remain suspended by mesentery.

plate (SMP). This mesoderm exhibits a high degree of cell proliferation (driven by Nkx3.2-induced Fgf10 expression) on the left side, and this presumably drives leftward lateral growth, with the surface cells on the left maintaining a columnar epithelial morphology and those on the right becoming more flattened and mesenchyme-like (Fig. 14-16). This asymmetric growth

and epithelial change are dependent on earlier left-right signaling pathways, including nodal, lefty1, lefty2, and Pitx2 in the lateral plate mesoderm.

Asymmetric differences in cell adhesion, cell shape, and cell proliferation within the dorsal midgut and hindgut mesentery play a role in gut rotation. The earliest morphological evidence

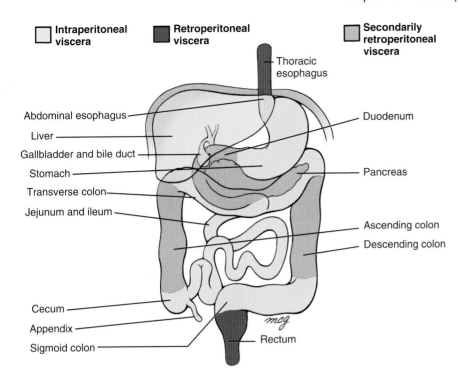

☐ **Intraperitoneal viscera**   ■ **Retroperitoneal viscera**   ☐ **Secondarily retroperitoneal viscera**

Thoracic esophagus

Abdominal esophagus

Liver

Gallbladder and bile duct

Stomach

Transverse colon

Jejunum and ileum

Cecum

Appendix

Sigmoid colon

Duodenum

Pancreas

Ascending colon

Descending colon

Rectum

Figure 14-15. Intraperitoneal, retroperitoneal, and secondarily retroperitoneal organs of the abdominal gastrointestinal tract.

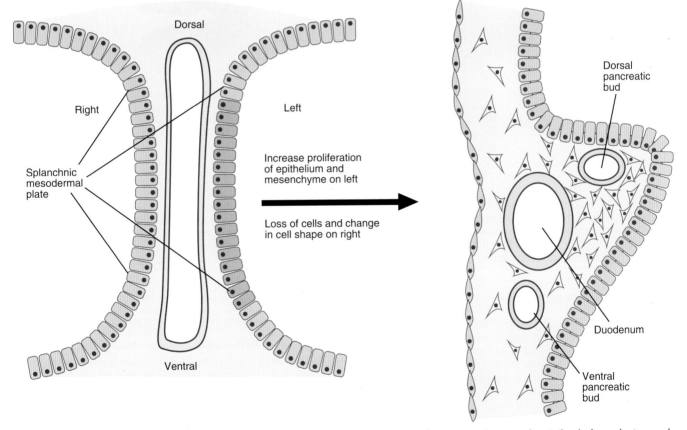

Dorsal

Right

Left

Splanchnic mesodermal plate

Increase proliferation of epithelium and mesenchyme on left

Loss of cells and change in cell shape on right

Ventral

Dorsal pancreatic bud

Duodenum

Ventral pancreatic bud

Figure 14-16. Proposed mechanisms driving asymmetric rotation of the foregut and midgut organs. Asymmetric rotation is dependent on early left-sided expression of nodal, lefty, and Pitx2. Leftward displacement of the stomach, spleen, duodenum, and pancreas is driven by differential growth and cell shape changes occurring within the splanchnic mesodermal plate (SMP) surrounding the gut tube. Left-sided Nkx3.2-induced Fgf10 expression (purple) increases mesenchymal cell proliferation and maintains an outer columnar epithelial morphology on the left side, whereas the epithelium on the right becomes flattened.

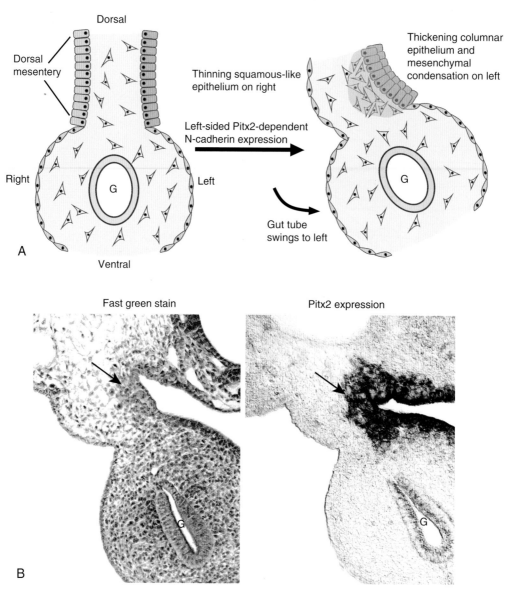

Figure 14-17. Proposed mechanisms driving asymmetric rotation of the dorsal mesentery of the midgut. *A,* Asymmetric rotation is dependent on early left-sided expression of Pitx2 (purple). Leftward movement and expansion of the midgut dorsal mesentery are driven by leftward expression of N-cadherin within the dorsal mesentery (shaded turquoise). As a result, subsequent changes in cell-cell adhesion, cell density, cell migration, and turnover of extracellular matrix components within the left mesentery generate mechanical forces responsible for the leftward movement of the dorsal mesentery. Arrows in *B* point to regions of increasing cell density and Pitx2 expression. G, Gut tube.

for asymmetry here can be seen in the leftward tilting of the dorsal mesentery (Fig. 14-17). In chick and mouse embryos, this leftward movement, unlike that in the SMP, is not dependent on differences in mesenchymal cell proliferation (albeit the proliferation of the left epithelial surface is greater than on the right) but rather is due to the exclusive left-sided expression of N-cadherin within the dorsal mesentery. As a result, subsequent changes in cell-cell adhesion, cell density, cell migration, and turnover of extracellular matrix components within the left mesentery generate mechanical forces thought to be responsible for the leftward movement of the dorsal mesentery. Again, these asymmetric changes are dependent on left-sided expression of nodal, lefty1, lefty2, and Pitx2 (Fig. 14-17B). Continued growth and lengthening of the gut tube in conjunction with the constraints of a lower growth rate in the dorsal mesentery also drives gut looping.

In the Clinic

ABNORMAL ROTATION AND FIXATION OF MIDGUT

As described in this chapter, the normal-handed asymmetry of the midgut is based on a relatively intricate series of rotations and fixations. Not surprisingly, errors in one or more of these steps lead to a varied spectrum of anomalies in humans.

Midgut Rotational Defects

The anomaly called **non-rotation of the midgut** arises when the primary intestinal loop fails to undergo the normal 180-degree counterclockwise rotation as it is retracted into the abdominal cavity (Fig. 14-18). The earlier 90-degree rotation may occur normally. The result of this error is that the original cranial limb of the primary intestinal loop (consisting of presumptive jejunum and ileum) ends up on the right side of the

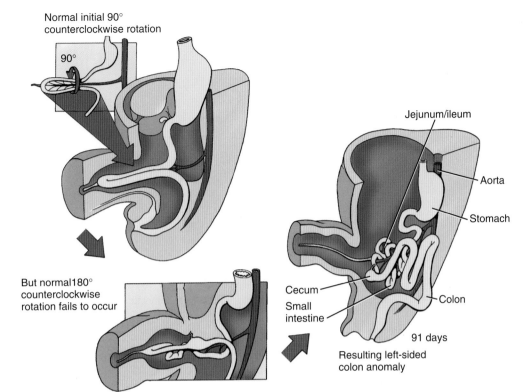

Normal initial 90°
counterclockwise rotation

90°

But normal 180°
counterclockwise
rotation fails to occur

Jejunum/ileum

Aorta

Stomach

Cecum

Small
intestine

Colon

91 days

Resulting left-sided
colon anomaly

Figure 14-18. Non-rotation of the gut (also called left-sided colon).

body, and the original caudal limb of the primary intestinal loop (consisting mainly of presumptive colon) ends up on the left side of the body. Therefore, this condition is sometimes called **left-sided colon**. The cecum and the most proximal region of the large intestine may or may not fuse to the dorsal body wall to become secondarily retroperitoneal.

In **reversed rotation of the midgut**, the primary intestinal loop undergoes the initial 90-degree counterclockwise rotation normally, but the second 180-degree rotation occurs *clockwise* instead of counterclockwise, so the net rotation of the midgut is 90 degrees clockwise (Fig. 14-19). This rotation brings the regions of the midgut and hindgut into their normal spatial relationships, with one important exception: the duodenum lies ventral to the transverse colon instead of dorsal to it. The duodenum thus does not become secondarily retroperitoneal, whereas the region of the transverse colon underlying it does.

In **mixed rotations of the midgut** (also called **malrotations**), only the cephalic limb of the primary intestinal loop undergoes the initial 90-degree rotation, whereas only the caudal limb undergoes the later 180-degree rotation (Fig. 14-20). The result of this mixed or uncoordinated behavior of the two limbs is that the distal end of the duodenum becomes fixed on the right side of the abdominal cavity, and the cecum becomes fixed near the midline just inferior to the pylorus of the stomach. This abnormal position of the cecum may cause the duodenum to be enclosed by a band of thickened peritoneum, thereby leaving the small intestines tethered on the right by a narrow mesentery, which increases the risk of an intestinal obstruction.

Intestinal Volvulus

Abnormal rotation or fixation of the midgut causes a significant fraction of the cases of intestinal obstruction. Specific regions of the intestine, such as the duodenum, may be pinned against the dorsal body wall by bands of abnormal mesentery (called **Ladd's bands**), resulting in constriction and obstruction. Alternatively,

malrotation may leave much of the midgut suspended from a single point of attachment on the dorsal body wall. Such freely suspended coils are prone to torsion or **volvulus**, which can lead to acute obstruction (Fig. 14-21). As covered in this chapter's "Clinical Taster," **bilious vomiting** is a common symptom of intestinal volvulus.

Intestinal volvulus may also compromise the arterial supply and venous drainage of the gut within the twisted mesentery. This may lead to ischemia or infarction due to hypoxia or, if only the venous side is affected, to **venous mucosal engorgement** and **gastrointestinal bleeding**.

The presence of a rotational abnormality is usually signaled during infancy or childhood by the sudden onset of acute abdominal pain, vomiting, or gastrointestinal bleeding, or by intermittent vomiting or failure to thrive. Occasionally, such an abnormality remains clinically silent until adulthood. Definitive diagnosis involves a barium swallow or barium enema in conjunction with X-rays. Volvulus must be treated surgically.

Umbilicus and Anterior Abdominal Wall Defects

Meckel's Diverticulum

The **vitelline duct** normally regresses between the fifth and eighth weeks (covered in Chapter 6), but in some cases of live-born infants, it persists as a remnant of variable length and location (Fig. 14-22). Most often, it is observed as a 1- to 5-cm intestinal diverticulum projecting from the mesenteric wall of the ileum within 100 cm of the cecum (Fig. 14-22A). This condition is known as **Meckel's diverticulum** in honor of J.F. Meckel, who first discussed the embryologic basis of the abnormality in the early nineteenth century. Meckel's diverticulum is seen in about 2% of the general population and is about twice as common in males as in females. In other cases, part of the vitelline duct within the abdominal wall persists, forming an open **omphalomesenteric fistula**, an **omphalomesenteric cyst** (or enterocyst), or an **omphalomesenteric ligament** (or

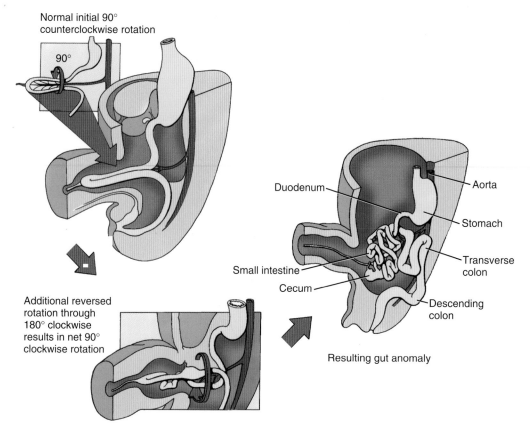

Figure 14-19. Reversed rotation of the gut. The net rotation is 90 degrees clockwise, so the midgut viscera are brought to their normal locations in the abdominal cavity, but the duodenum lies anterior to the transverse colon.

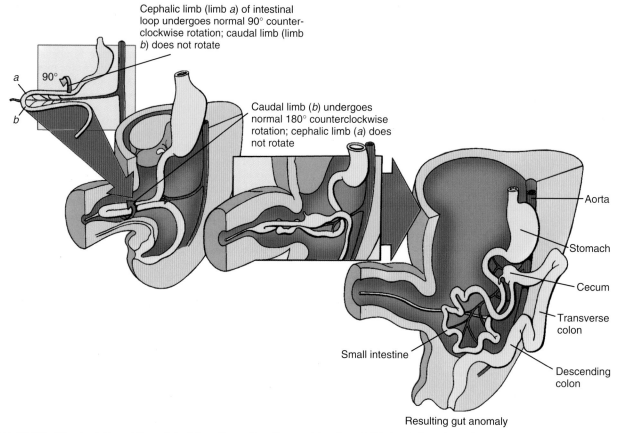

Figure 14-20. Mixed rotation of the gut. In this malformation, the cranial and caudal limbs of the primary intestinal loop rotate independently. As a result, the cecum becomes fixed near the midline just inferior to the pylorus of the stomach.

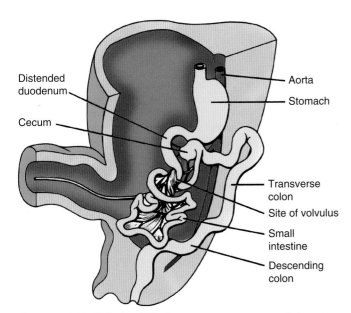

Figure 14-21. Volvulus. Volvulus may occur as suspended regions of the gut twist around themselves, constricting the intestine and/or compromising its blood supply.

fibrous band) connecting the small bowel to the umbilicus (Fig. 14-22B-D).

Most cases of Meckel's diverticulum are asymptomatic. However, 1% to 3% of individuals who have Meckel's diverticulum develop symptoms of intestinal obstruction, gastrointestinal bleeding, or peritonitis. Meckel's diverticulum complications can manifest as a consequence of bowel obstruction caused by trapping of part of the small bowel by a fibrous band representing a remnant of the vitelline vessels connecting the diverticulum to the umbilicus. Symptoms may closely mimic appendicitis, involving periumbilical pain that later localizes to the right lower quadrant. Up to 60% of Meckel's diverticula harbor abnormal tissue, usually pancreatic or gastric. In the latter case, patients may develop bleeding ulceration of the gut.

The facts about Meckel's diverticulum can be remembered using the "rule of two's": it occurs in 2% of the population and is 2 times more common in males; about 2% of individuals with Meckel's diverticulum have medical symptoms, usually by 2 years of age; it is usually present 2 feet proximal to the terminal ileum and is usually 2 inches long; and it contains 2 types of abnormal lining.

Umbilical Hernia, Omphalocele, and Gastroschisis

The terms used to describe defects of the anterior abdominal wall in which the abdominal contents protrude are often used inconsistently in the literature. Here, they are divided into three groups: **umbilical hernia, omphalocele,** and **gastroschisis.**

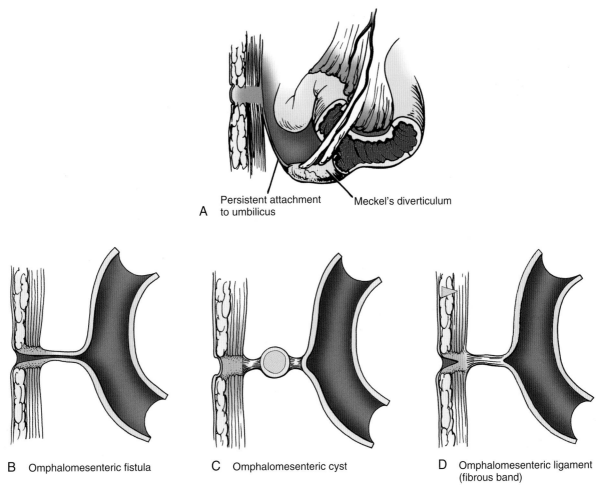

Figure 14-22. Meckel's diverticulum. *A,* A typical Meckel's diverticulum is a finger-like projection of the ileum. A Meckel's diverticulum may form: *B,* a patent fistula connecting the umbilicus with the ileum; *C,* an isolated cyst suspended by ligaments; or *D,* a fibrous band connecting the ileum and anterior body wall at the level of the umbilicus.

An **umbilical hernia** consists of a small protrusion of bowel through the **umbilical ring**, which is covered by skin. It is often more apparent when the infant cries or strains. More than 95% of umbilical hernias close spontaneously by five years of age.

Omphalocele (covered in Chapter 4; see Fig. 4-4) also involves herniation of bowel or other viscera through the **umbilical ring**, which is covered by a thin avascular membrane that may rupture. In contrast to an umbilical hernia, in extreme cases, an omphalocele can involve a large herniation consisting of the entire bowel and liver, with the umbilical cord inserting into the apex of the omphalocele. Omphalocele occurs in about 1:5000 births, and it is often associated with chromosome abnormalities or other malformation syndromes. Several possible explanations for omphalocele exist. Recall that during the sixth to tenth weeks of development, the midgut undergoes a physiologic herniation into the developing umbilical cord. One possibility is that the herniated bowel does not fully retract into the abdominal cavity during the tenth week and thus remains herniated. Another possibility is that lateral body folding and fusion fail to occur properly during the fourth to eighth week, creating a body wall weakness that allows the bowel to later herniate as it grows. A third possibility is failure of proper migration and differentiation of the mesoderm normally forming the connective tissue of the skin (covered in Chapter 7) and hypaxial musculature of the ventral body wall (covered in Chapter 8), again resulting in a body wall weakness.

Gastroschisis is a defect of the anterior abdominal wall in which bowel protrudes without a covering sac between the developing rectus muscles just lateral to, and almost invariably to the right of, the umbilicus (covered in Chapter 4; see Fig. 4-1). In gastroschisis, unlike in omphalocele, the **umbilical ring** closes, and herniation of the bowel occurs lateral to the ring rather than through it. The cause of gastroschisis, like that of omphalocele, is unclear, but the two defects likely share some of the same mechanisms postulated above. In addition, it has been proposed that premature obliteration of the right umbilical vein (normal obliteration of the right vein occurs during the second month of gestation, as covered in Chapter 13) and its draining vessels may create a localized right-sided body wall weakness owing to localized ischemia and infarct; subsequently, pressure generated by the growing intestines breeches the weakened body wall, resulting in intestinal herniation. The incidence of gastroschisis is about 1:3000 births, and this incidence is increasing in North America and Europe for unknown reasons. Gastroschisis also differs from omphalocele in that it is usually isolated and has no known associated chromosomal anomalies.

Other defects of the anterior body wall include ectopia cordis, isolated protrusion of the heart through the body wall; **cloacal** or **bladder exstrophy** (covered later in this chapter); and a constellation of five defects called **pentalogy of Cantrell** (supraumbilical abdominal wall defect, diaphragmatic hernia [covered in Chapter 11], pericardial defect, sternal cleft, and intracardiac anomaly).

CYTODIFFERENTIATION OF GUT ENDODERMAL EPITHELIUM

The gastrointestinal tract is composed of the endoderm forming the epithelial lining of the lumen, the splanchnic mesoderm forming the smooth muscle and connective tissue tunics, and the ectoderm. The latter forms the most cranial and caudal luminal linings (the oral cavity is covered in Chapter 17 and the anal opening is covered later in this chapter) and the enteric nervous system (derived from neural crest cells; also covered later in this chapter). As evident from the previous description, the orientations cranial-caudal, dorsal-ventral, and right-left (manifested mainly by the turning and looping of the gut and positioning of the stomach) reflect the final regionalization of organs and orientation of the adult intestinal tract. Superimposed on the cranial-caudal axis is another axis, the **radial axis**, with establishment of the glandular epithelium of the gastrointestinal tract. Early in development, much of the endodermal lining of the gastrointestinal tract remains uniform in morphology until epithelial-mesenchymal interactions, dictated by regionalization signals, direct endodermal differentiation. Many of the major morphologic changes and cytodifferentiation events occur during the midgestation (fetal) period.

Initially, the gastrointestinal epithelium is a simple epithelium, but it becomes pseudostratified and thickens to the point that the lumen is nearly occluded. Convergent extension of cells within the pseudostratified epithelium, much like what occurs during gastrulation and neurulation (covered in Chapters 3 and 4), is thought to be responsible for the formation of secondary lumens within the epithelial layer (Fig. 14-23). These lumens eventually merge and open into the primary lumen. Before and during formation of lumens, Shh and Ihh are expressed within the epithelium; however, Shh expression eventually becomes restricted to the intervillus endoderm. Shh increases Bmp expression in the underlying mesoderm, and Bmps mediate mesenchymal proliferation and condensation necessary for the formation of nascent villi (see Fig 14-23). Conversion to a simple columnar epithelium and formation of villi occur in a wave, beginning at the stomach and progressing toward the colon, with the length of the villi forming dependent upon their cranial-caudal position in the gut tube. In the stomach, villi do not form, but the endoderm does invaginate into the mesoderm, forming pits (future gastric glands). In the intestines, formation of villi is accompanied by endodermal invagination into the mesoderm, forming crypts.

Cytodifferentiation of the endodermal epithelium along the radial axis (i.e., base of the pit/crypts to the tip of the villi) depends on interactions with the underlying mesoderm and occurs late in development. As epithelial cells of the gastrointestinal tract undergo rapid turnover during our lifetime, they must be replaced by the activity of stem cells. These stem cells produce progenitors for **enterocytes** (absorptive cells), **enteroendocrine cells** (regulatory peptide-secreting cells), **Paneth cells** (antimicrobial peptide-secreting cells), and **goblet** or **mucus cells** (Fig. 14-24). Current evidence suggest that the self-renewing stem cells are located at the base of the intestinal crypts, nestled between Paneth cells, and express the surface marker Lgr5 (leucine-rich-repeat-containing G-protein-coupled receptor-5). These stem cells generate dividing progenitors for all epithelial cell types of the stomach, small intestines, and colon. In the small intestines, enterocytic, goblet, and enteroendocrine cells differentiate and mature while migrating up the villus to the tip, where they are eventually extruded into the lumen (a three- to six-day journey in humans). Paneth cells differentiate and remain in the base of the crypt (for about three weeks before dying and being removed by phagocytosis). However, Paneth cells do not develop in the colon segment.

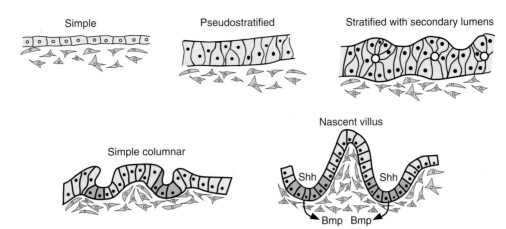

Figure 14-23. Morphogenesis of the intestinal endoderm and villus formation. Initially, the gastrointestinal epithelium is lined with a simple epithelium but becomes pseudostratified and thickens to the point that the gut lumen is nearly occluded. Convergent extension of cells within the pseudostratified epithelium results in the formation of secondary lumens within the epithelial layer. These lumens eventually merge with and open into the primary lumen. Shh expression becomes restricted to the intervillus endoderm and stimulates Bmp expression in the adjacent mesoderm. Bmp mediates the mesenchymal proliferation and condensation necessary for the formation of nascent villi.

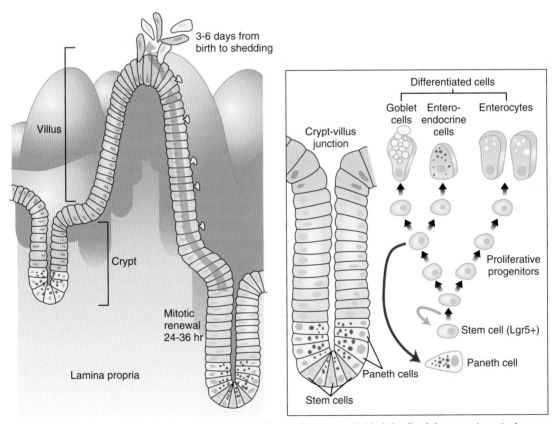

Figure 14-24. Cytodifferentiation of the endodermal epithelium of the small intestine. Epithelial cells of the gastrointestinal tract undergo rapid turnover and must be replaced by stem cells. In the small intestine, these stem cells produce the progenitors for enterocytes, enteroendocrine cells, Paneth cells, and goblet cells. Enterocytic, goblet, and enteroendocrine cells continue to proliferate, differentiate, and mature while migrating up the villus, where eventually they are shed into the lumen at the tip. Paneth cells reside at the base of the crypt. In the small intestine, the stem cells (Lgr5-expressing cells) reside within the base of the crypt between the Paneth cells. Committed progenitor cells differentiate near the crypt-villus border and migrate toward the villus tips (or in the case of Paneth cells, toward the bottom of the crypt).

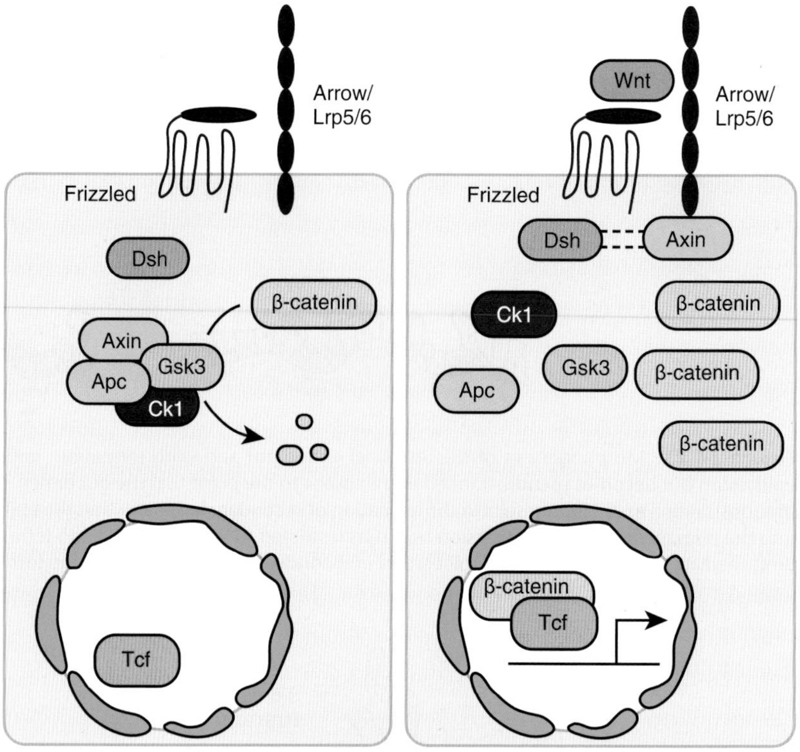

Figure 14-25. Diagram illustrating the Wnt canonical pathway. Wnt signaling is initiated by Wnt binding to the frizzled family of receptors and co-receptors, Lrp5 and Lrp6. In the absence of Wnt (cell on left), β-catenin is constantly degraded by a complex composed, in part, by Apc, axin, and Gsk3. However, in the presence of Wnt (cell on right), the action of this destruction complex is blocked, and as a consequence, β-catenin levels accumulate. As free β-catenin increases, it enters the nucleus and binds to the Tcf/Lef family of transcription factors, enabling the transcription of many other genes.

In the Research Lab

FAULTY WNT SIGNALING AND β-CATENIN TURNOVER ARE OFTEN A PRELUDE TO COLON CANCER

As covered in Chapter 5, Wnt signaling is initiated by binding to the frizzled family of receptors and the co-receptor Lrp5 or Lrp6. β-Catenin is constantly degraded by a complex containing adenomatous polyposis coli (Apc) protein, axin, and Gsk3 (Fig. 14-25). When bound to this complex, β-catenin becomes phosphorylated, which targets β-catenin for ubiquitination-mediated proteasomal destruction. However, in the presence of Wnt, the action of this destruction complex is blocked, and consequently β-catenin levels accumulate. With increasing levels of free cytoplasmic β-catenin, β-catenin enters the nucleus and binds to the Tcf4/Lef family of transcription factors, driving the transcription of many other genes (the so-called canonical pathway).

The Wnt/β-catenin/Tcf4 cascade is critical for maintaining the proliferative compartment within the gut epithelium and for patterning the glandular phenotype along the radial axis. The distribution pattern of β-catenin and Tcf4 within the gut epithelium coincides with the primary site of epithelial proliferation. Wnt signaling imposes continual proliferation (maintenance) of crypt epithelial cells, and in the absence of Wnt signaling, these cells go into cell cycle arrest and initiate differentiation. Thus, knockout mice for Tcf4 are unable to maintain an intestinal epithelial progenitor population. Therefore, Wnt signaling, through actions of the Tcf4/Lef family of transcription factors, mediates the switch between proliferation, maintenance, and differentiation of the epithelial cells. The switch itself depends on strict radial axis controls.

Familial adenomatous polyposis patients have one mutant copy of APC. Moreover, detectable APC mutations are found in about 80% of spontaneous cases of colorectal cancer, suggesting that APC is a key regulator of both forms of colorectal cancer (other cases of colorectal cancer are associated with mutations in β-CATENIN or AXIN). Any decrease in the functional levels of APC increases the level of β-catenin within the cytoplasm and nucleus, ultimately mimicking the effects of positive Wnt signaling. In the case of intestinal epithelial cells, this leads to inappropriate cell proliferation and malignant transformation. Candidate target genes for constitutive Wnt signaling associated with colorectal cancers include the cell cycle genes (e.g., C-MYC, CYCLIN D), matrix metalloproteinases, growth factors, and angiogenic factors. APC can also function as a nuclear-cytoplasmic shuttle; hence, mutations in APC might alter β-catenin entry into the nucleus.

DIFFERENTIATION OF GASTROINTESTINAL TRACT EPITHELIUM

The position of cells along the radial axis is one of the important factors mediating cellular differentiation. As covered in Chapters 5, 9, and 13, ephrins and their receptors play essential roles in mediating cell migration and establishing boundaries. These ligands and receptors are also expressed within the intestinal epithelium. EphB2 and EphB3 receptors and their ligands, ephrinB1 and ephrinB2, are expressed in an inverse gradient along the radial axis, with the ephrins most concentrated in the villus and villus/crypt border, and their receptors more prominent within the proliferating region (Fig. 14-26). This spatial relationship suggests a role for mediating the migration of epithelial cells along the radial axis: EphB2/EphB3 double knockout mice lose the proliferative/differentiation boundary, and ectopic proliferating epithelial cells can be found along the entire villus. In normal adults, EphB3 receptor expression is restricted to the columnar cells found in the base of the crypt, where Paneth cells usually reside. However, in EphB3 null mice, Paneth cells are found distributed throughout the crypt/villus unit. Experiments further suggest that expression patterns of ephrins and ephrin receptors within the gut are regulated by β-catenin/Tcf transcriptional activity. Thus, a Wnt signaling gradient may control gut epithelial cell positioning along the radial axis by mediating ephrin signaling.

What particular Wnts might drive gut epithelial proliferation and migration and what their sources might be remain unclear. Several different Wnts are expressed within the intestinal epithelium and mesoderm along the cranial-caudal axis, including Wnt4,

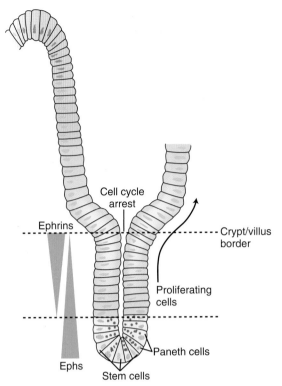

Figure 14-26. Ephrins and their receptors are expressed in an inverse gradient along the radial axis, with ephrins most concentrated in the crypt-villus border, and their receptors, EphB2 and EphB3, more prominent within the proliferating region and base of the crypt. This spatial relationship is important in mediating the migration of epithelial cells along the radial (crypt-to-villus) axis. Arrow indicates the direction of cell migration.

Wnt5a, and Wnt11. What regulates the levels of these Wnts or their signaling along the radial axis is unknown, but Shh and Ihh have been suggested as possible mediators of Wnt signaling.

As covered in an earlier "In the Research Lab" entitled "Determination of Pancreatic Cell Lineage," notch signaling increases Hes1 expression, thereby repressing the specification of the endocrine lineage in the *pancreatic* endoderm. Hes1 is also expressed within the *intestinal* precursor population, where it functions similarly in the specification of intestinal cell fate. Hes1 null mice have an increase in the number of secretory cells within the gut epithelium at the expense of enterocytes. In contrast, in mice null for Math1 (also called Atoh1), the intestinal epithelium is almost entirely composed of enterocytes. Because Hes1 represses the expression of Math1/Atoh1, these results suggest a model (Fig. 14-27) in which the balance between Hes1 and Math1/Atoh1, controlled by notch signaling, determines absorptive versus secretory cell specification in the intestinal epithelium. In the presence of Gfi1, a zinc-finger transcription factor that functions downstream of Math1/Atoh1, expression of neurog3 is suppressed, thereby promoting Paneth and goblet cell differentiation, but in the absence of Gfi1, endocrine cells form.

DEVELOPMENT OF OUTER INTESTINAL WALL AND ITS INNERVATION

As covered earlier in the chapter, the gut tube consists of an endodermally derived epithelium covered by splanchnopleuric mesoderm. The mesodermal component

develops into multiple layers, including lamina propria, muscularis mucosa, submucosa, circular and longitudinal muscular layers, and adventitia. These layers are innervated by neurons whose cell bodies lie within the gut wall (the **enteric nervous system**; also covered in Chapter 10), as well as by extrinsic neurons located in the sympathetic and parasympathetic ganglia (both vagal and pelvic ganglia) and sensory ganglia (nodose and dorsal root ganglia). Neurons of the enteric nervous system are clustered into ganglia that are located in two main layers, the inner **Meissner's** or **submucosal plexus** (within the submucosa adjacent to the circular muscle layer) and **Auerbach's** or the **myenteric plexus** (between the circular and longitudinal muscle layers). In humans, some neurons are located within the lamina propria.

Loss of both endodermal Ihh and Shh in mice results in failure of the gut mesoderm to grow. Studies suggest that Shh, in cooperation with Ihh, may mediate smooth muscle development of the gastrointestinal tract and indirectly mediate neuronal patterning via its effect on Bmp4 expression within the mesenchyme. In chick embryos, all gastrointestinal mesoderm has the potential to form smooth muscle. Shh emanating from the endoderm inhibits the expression of Smap (smooth muscle activating protein) in the adjacent mesoderm (Fig. 14-28), thereby restricting smooth muscle tunic formation to the outermost radial axis of the gut tube. Consequently, the mesoderm nearest the endoderm forms lamina propria and submucosa.

Hh signaling is also needed for proper enteric plexus colonization (by controlling Gdnf expression and, hence, vagal neural crest cell migration; covered below).

The **enteric nervous system**, which provides the intrinsic innervation of the gastrointestinal tract, consists of glia, interconnected afferent and efferent neurons, and interneurons. The enteric nervous system functions to regulate gut peristalsis, blood flow, secretion, absorption, and endocrine processes. It is also unique in the capacity to exhibit integrative neuronal activity in the absence of the central nervous system. Hence, it is sometimes referred to as "the brain" of the gastrointestinal tract, or "the second brain" of the body. Because of the complexity of the enteric nervous system, the frequency of gut motility disorders, and the side effects of many neuropharmaceutical drugs on the gastrointestinal tract physiology, the enteric nervous system is the subject of intense investigation.

Postganglionic sympathetic fibers originate from the sympathetic chain ganglia or paraortic ganglia and follow the gastrointestinal vascular supply to enter the wall of the gastrointestinal tract. The axons of parasympathetic preganglionic neurons in the brainstem project via the vagus nerve to innervate postganglionic neurons in the esophagus, stomach, and intestines. Postganglionic parasympathetic neurons in pelvic ganglia provide some innervation to the hindgut. Neural crest cells arising from the occipitocervical levels (somites one to seven) are the source of the vagal (parasympathetic) neurons and glia and begin colonizing the cranial end by about week four and eventually populate the gut's entire length by week seven (Fig. 14-29). Studies in chick and mouse embryos show that sacral enteric ganglionic neurons and

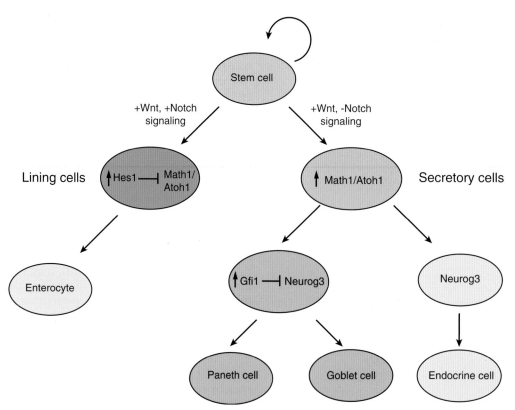

Figure 14-27. The role of Wnt and notch signaling in cell lineage specification of intestinal epithelial cells. In the presence of notch signaling, the expression of Hes1 is increased, which in turn represses the expression of Math1/Atoh1. These cells then take on an enterocyte lineage. In the absence of notch signaling, Hes1 expression fails to occur, and the expression of Math1/Atoh1 is not repressed. Whether these cells become Paneth cells, goblet cells, or endocrine cells depends on the presence of Gfi1, which suppresses Neurog3.

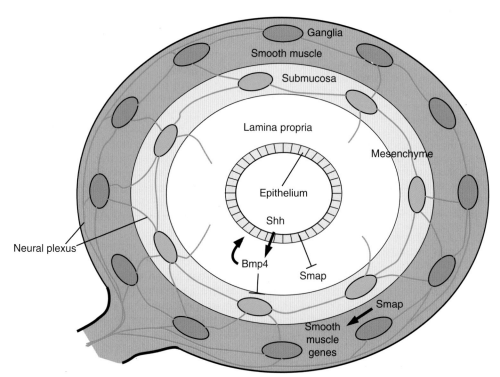

Figure 14-28. Schematic representation of the differentiation of the gut wall along the radial axis. Studies suggest that Shh emanating from the endoderm inhibits the expression of Smap (smooth muscle activating protein) in the adjacent mesoderm, thereby restricting smooth muscle tunic formation to the outermost radial axis of the gut tube. As a consequence, the mesoderm nearest the endoderm forms lamina propria and submucosa. Bmp4, induced by Shh within the lamina propria and submucosa, limits enteric neuronal cell differentiation to the outer region of the gut wall. Hedgehog signaling is also needed for proper enteric plexus colonization (by controlling Gdnf expression and, hence, vagal neural crest cell migration). Reciprocal signaling to the epithelium from mesodermal Bmps also plays an important role in villus formation (see text).

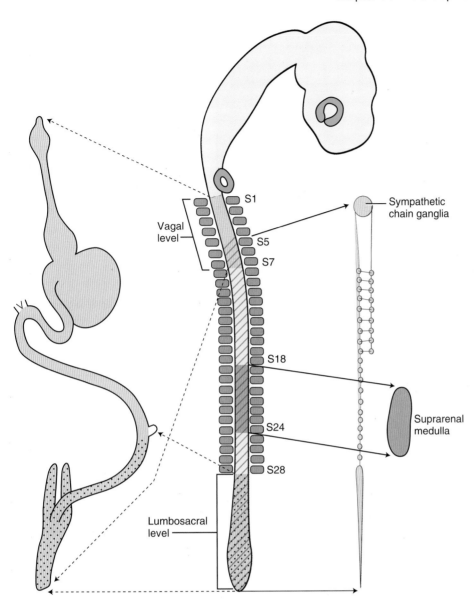

S1
Vagal
level
S5
S7
Sympathetic
chain ganglia
S18
Suprarenal
medulla
S24
S28
Lumbosacral
level

Figure 14-29. The origin of neural crest cells forming the enteric nervous system in the chick embryo. Postganglionic sympathetic fibers innervating the enteric nervous system are derived from neurons located within the sympathetic chain. These neurons and glia originate from neural crest cells arising from the dorsal neural tube at axial levels beginning at somite level five and extending into the sacrum (hatched). The origin of neural crest cells forming the suprarenal medulla is shown in purple. Vagal postganglionic neurons and glia are derived from neural crest cells arising at somite levels one to seven (tan, no stippling), whereas sacral enteric ganglionic neurons and glia arise from neural crest cells caudal to somite pair twenty-eight in chickens (tan, stippled).

glia arise from neural crest cells formed caudal to somite pair twenty-eight in birds and somite pair twenty-four in mice, and that this subset of cells colonizes the hindgut after the arrival of vagal neural crest cells. Although neural crest cells derived from the lumbosacral region align themselves with the vagal nerve plexus, experiments show that migration and differentiation of lumbosacral neural crest cell is normal when vagal neural crest cells are ablated. Hence, lumbosacral neural crest cells can innervate the hindgut independent of vagal innervation.

Interstitial cells of Cajal, located within the gut wall, play a major role in integrating signaling between the enteric nervous system and smooth muscle cells of the gut. These cells are regarded as the pacemakers of the gastrointestinal tract (driving peristalsis), and their dysfunction has been implicated in several gut motility disorders. Their origin is still unclear, but studies in mice suggest that they share a common mesodermal precursor with smooth muscle cells and are not derived from neural crest cells.

In the Clinic

HIRSCHSPRUNG DISEASE

Disorders of the **enteric nervous system** in humans can be divided into two major groups: those characterized by an abnormal number of ganglia (Hirschsprung) and those characterized by abnormal neuronal differentiation (intestinal neuronal dysplasia). In **Hirschsprung disease** (1 in 5000 live births), complete or partial obstruction of the intestine is due to total absence of both **myenteric** and **submucosa ganglia** in the most distal regions of the bowel. As enteric neurons are essential for propulsion of gut contents, this leads to abnormal dilation or distention of a variable length of the colon, and increased wall thickness due to muscular hypertrophy in the intestine proximal to the aganglionic segment. The enlarged bowel (i.e., megacolon) in patients with Hirschsprung disease is essentially a secondary symptom caused by obstruction and lack of peristalsis in the colon segment distal to the dilation (Fig. 14-30). Removal of the constricted distal segment remains the only effective treatment for the disease, and refinement of surgical approaches to Hirschsprung disease has led to decreased mortality.

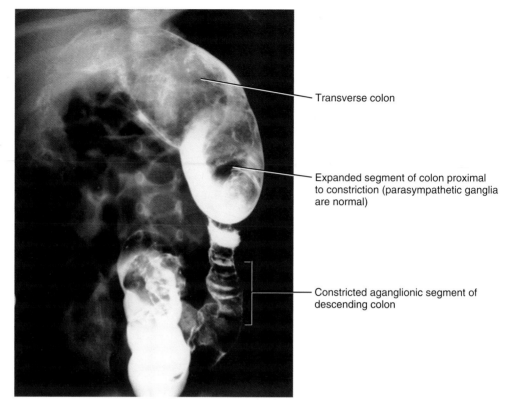

Transverse colon

Expanded segment of colon proximal to constriction (parasympathetic ganglia are normal)

Constricted aganglionic segment of descending colon

Figure 14-30. Radiograph after a barium enema showing the constricted distal gastrointestinal tract of an individual with Hirschsprung disease. The adjacent, more proximal, region of the tract with normal autonomic innervation is distended.

The first sign of Hirschsprung disease is usually a delay in the passage of meconium (usually meconium is passed within two days), the material filling the lower bowel of newborn infants. This may be accompanied by other symptoms such as constipation, vomiting, abdominal pain, and distention. These patients are at risk for life-threatening complications such as intestinal infection (enterocolitis) or rupture of the cecum. Most individuals with Hirschsprung disease are diagnosed during their first year of life. Barium enema examinations show that the non-peristaltic segment usually involves the sigmoid colon and rectum, although it may vary in length from a small portion of the rectum to the entire large intestine and part of the ileum. Diagnosis of Hirschsprung disease is made by biopsy of the mucosa, with histopathology demonstrating absence of enteric ganglia.

Hirschsprung disease occurs as an isolated, sporadic defect or in the context of a syndrome, and can be inherited as a familial trait or as part of a chromosomal anomaly. The latter is seen in about 12% of Hirschsprung disease patients, with trisomy 21 the most common. A family history of Hirschsprung disease is positive in about 7% of cases, and about 15% of Hirschsprung disease cases are associated with at least one other congenital anomaly. The genetic causes of Hirschsprung disease are heterogeneous and involve multiple factors, with evidence for both low penetrance and sex dependence, which vary with regard to the length of the aganglionic segment. The male-to-female ratio of Hirschsprung disease is 4:1 for short segmental ganglionic agenesis but is more equal in frequency between the sexes as the segment involved becomes longer. Hirschsprung disease (also covered in the following "In the Research Lab" entitled "Hirschsprung Disease and Neural Crest Cell Defects") is associated with multiple gene mutations and occurs as part of at least ten syndromes.

INFANTILE HYPERTROPHIC PYLORIC STENOSIS

Infantile hypertrophic pyloric stenosis (1 in 500 live births) is characterized by the development of pyloric hypertrophy and a gastric outlet obstruction, which classically present with projectile vomiting in the first two months postnatally. Abnormal thickening of the pyloric circular muscle can often be palpated on physical examination (described as the "olive"). The cause of stenosis may be an abnormal innervation of the pylorus. Some studies suggest that neurons in this region fail to express nitric oxide synthase, as mice null for the gene coding this enzyme exhibit pyloric stenosis and an enlarged stomach. In addition, Bmps have been implicated in mediating smooth muscle cell proliferation and differentiation here, as altering levels of Bmp4 signaling in this region alters the thickness of the muscular tunic as well as development of the enteric nervous system in chick embryos.

In the Research Lab

HIRSCHSPRUNG DISEASE AND NEURAL CREST CELL DEFECTS

The absence of enteric ganglia within the gut is recognized as the main cause of Hirschsprung disease and is generally attributed to failure of neural crest cell migration, proliferation, and differentiation, either before or after arrival within the gut wall. Defects in any of the developmental mechanisms required for neural crest cell morphogenesis could, therefore, result in congenital megacolon. Several studies in chick, mice, and humans support this hypothesis.

Many Hirschsprung-related mutations in humans are found in the gene coding for RET. The RET proto-oncogene, which has been mapped to human chromosome 10q11.2, encodes a TYROSINE KINASE that serves as a receptor for members of the GLIAL CELL–DERIVED NEUROTROPHIC FACTOR (GDNF) ligand family. During embryogenesis of vertebrates, Ret is expressed in the developing renal system and in all cell lineages of the peripheral nervous system. Vagal and sacral neural crest cells begin to express Ret just before their entry into the gut, and this is required for the survival, proliferation, migration, and differentiation of enteric neuron precursors in zebrafish, mice, and humans. Ret-positive neural crest cells, when injected into the stomach of mice having aganglionic intestines, colonize and reconstitute the enteric nervous system. In vitro, the ligand for Ret, Gdnf, is a chemoattractant for vagal neural crest cells. Studies suggest that Gdnf gradients within the gut direct vagal neural crest cell migration in a cranial-to-caudal direction and promote directional neurite outgrowth.

RET mutations have been identified in 50% of familial and 15% to 20% of sporadic Hirschsprung disease cases, including large deletions, microdeletions, insertions, and nonsense, missense, and splicing mutations. Haploinsufficiency is the most likely mechanism in Hirschsprung disease. This contrasts with **multiple endocrine neoplasia type 2**, in which RET mutations lead to constitutive dimerization and activation of RET and, therefore, to malignant transformation. Although RET mutations may lead to phenotypic expression with haploinsufficiency, hypomorphic RET mutations (i.e., partial loss-of-function mutations) may require a mutation in an additional pertinent gene (e.g., endothelin; covered below).

The lethal spotted and piebald lethal mouse mutants are characterized by mutations of the endothelin-3 gene (Et3) and the gene encoding its G protein–coupled receptor, the endothelin-B receptor (Etb). These mice lack enteric ganglia in the distal colon and exhibit Hirschsprung disease. Mice null for the Et3 or Etb gene also exhibit aganglionosis of the distal colon, and in these mice, neural crest migration along the gut is delayed, suggesting that Et3/Etb signaling promotes the migration of enteric neural crest cells. In contrast, the lack of ganglia in lethal spotted mice is thought to be due to a premature exit from the cell cycle and premature differentiation of enteric neural crest cells, resulting in an inability to generate enough progenitors to colonize the gut.

Mutations in ETB, which maps to human chromosome 13q22, have been found in about 5% of cases of isolated Hirschsprung disease in humans (i.e., in the absence of other congenital anomalies). Patients with **Waardenburg type 4 syndrome** have **Hirschsprung disease**, accompanied by pigmentary anomalies and sensorineural deafness. Patients with homozygous mutations in ET3 or ETB present with complete Waardenburg type 4 phenotype, including Hirschsprung disease, whereas heterozygotes for ET3 or ETB may have only isolated Hirschsprung disease.

Studies suggest that interactions between the independent gene loci of RET and ETB are necessary for normal formation of the enteric nervous system in humans and mice. Individuals carrying a RET mutation have a significantly higher risk of developing Hirschsprung disease if they also have a hypomorphic mutation in ETB. Mice heterozygotic for Ret and having a loss-of-function mutation for Etb develop Hirschsprung disease without exhibiting defects in renal development or pigmentation that otherwise are often seen in isolated Ret and Et3/Etb mutations. Thus, a balance between Ret and Et3/Etb signaling pathways seems to be required for normal colonization of the gut.

Splotch mutant mice harbor mutations of Pax3, a transcription factor that plays an important role in neural tube and musculoskeletal development. In addition to the neural tube defects that form in these mice, homozygotes of several well-described Pax3 mutations exhibit severe defects of neural crest cell migration and/or differentiation, including cardiovascular defects (covered in Chapter 12), hearing loss, pigmentation defects, and Hirschsprung disease. Among these, mutations arising from chromosomal deletions are most severe. In humans, deletions or mutations in PAX3 cause **Waardenburg type 1 syndrome**.

These patients have pigmentation and auditory system defects but lack Hirschsprung disease, suggesting that there is redundancy of PAX3 function in development of the enteric nervous system in humans that is not present in mice.

Other genes implicated in the development of neural crest cells and the enteric nervous system include netrin and netrin receptors; semaphorin3a; neurotrophin-3 and its receptor, TrkC (promoting survival and differentiation of enteric neurons and glia needed for formation of myenteric and submucosal plexuses); Bmp signaling molecules (mediating neurotrophin-3 signaling and Gdnf-driven expansion of the enteric precursor pool, and promoting intrinsic primary afferent enteric neuron development); Mash1 (a bHLH transcription factor required for forming enteric neurons containing serotonin and nitric oxide synthase); Phox2a and Phox2b (paired box homeodomain transcription factors; Phox2b when knocked out leads to loss of all peripheral autonomic nerves); Hand2 (necessary for differentiation of enteric neurons); Sox10 (required for Ret expression, cell survival, and glial differentiation); L1 cell adhesion molecule (influences migration by promoting cell-cell contact); β1-integrin (mediates interactions with the ECM); and Smad interacting protein-1.

Evidence from mouse studies suggests that environmental factors might also contribute to the penetrance and severity of Hirschsprung's disease. Studies show that retinoic acid is required to maintain intracellular signals necessary for enteric neural crest cell migration and that Ret heterozygosity increases the incidence of aganglionosis in conditions of vitamin A deficiency.

HINDGUT DEVELOPMENT

Animation 14-4: Development of Hindgut.
Animations are available online at StudentConsult.

The large intestines are designed mainly for the reuptake of water and ions and to protect the epithelium from increasingly hardening waste. A portion of the hindgut forms the large intestine, and although similar to the organization of the small intestine, it does not form villi, and it contains different cell types. The portion of the primitive hindgut tube lying just deep to the cloacal membrane forms an expansion called the **cloaca**. A slim diverticulum of the cloaca called the **allantois** extends into the connecting stalk (see Fig. 14-2). Between the fourth and sixth weeks, the cloaca is partitioned into a dorsal **anorectal canal** and a ventral **urogenital sinus** by the formation of a coronal partition called the **urorectal septum** (Fig. 14-31). The urogenital sinus gives rise to the presumptive bladder (although recent studies in humans suggest that the bladder develops from an expansion of the lower allantois), a narrow urethral portion forming the **membranous** and **prostatic urethra** in males and the **membranous urethra** in females, and a lower expansion, the phallic segment. As covered in Chapter 16, the phallic segment contributes in males to the **penile urethra** and in females to the **vestibule of the vagina**. All of these urogenital structures are thus lined with an epithelium derived from endoderm.

The urorectal septum is often described as forming from two integrated mesodermal septal systems: a cranial fold (called the Tourneux fold), growing toward the cloacal membrane, and a pair of lateral folds (called the

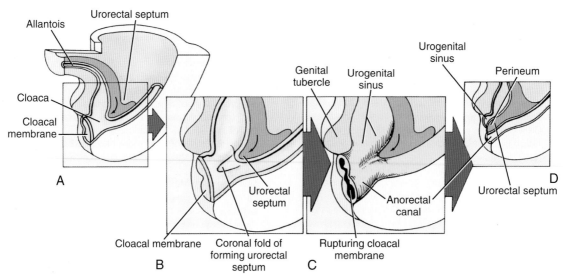

Figure 14-31. Progressives steps between four and six weeks in subdivision of the cloaca into a ventral primitive urogenital sinus and a dorsal anorectal canal (*A-D*). The urorectal septum is formed by the fusion of yolk sac extraembryonic mesoderm and allantois mesoderm, which produces a tissue wedge between the hindgut and urogenital sinus during craniocaudal folding of the embryo. As the tip of the urorectal septum approaches the cloacal membrane dividing the cloaca into the urogenital sinus and anorectal canal, the cloacal membrane ruptures, thereby opening the urogenital sinus and dorsal anorectal canal to the exterior. The tip of urorectal septum forms the perineum. *A, B, D,* Sections through the cloacal and related endoderm-derived structures. *C,* Surface view of the caudal endoderm to better depict its three-dimensional shape. Curved arrows indicate the direction of growth of the developing urorectal septum.

Rathke folds), growing toward the midline of the cloaca. However, closer examination of mouse, rat, and human embryos suggests that the urorectal septum is created by the fusion of yolk sac extraembryonic mesoderm and allantois mesoderm forming a tissue wedge between the hindgut and urogenital sinus during cranial-caudal folding of the embryo (see Fig. 14-2C for the locations of the caudal yolk sac mesoderm and allantois mesoderm in the region of the hindgut as these regions are brought together during body folding and formation of the umbilical cord). As the human embryo grows, the distance between the urorectal septum and the cloacal membrane decreases. Whether the urorectal septum descends toward the cloacal membrane (composed of opposing ectoderm and endoderm) actively by growing or passively through changes in caudal body folding and increased pelvic organ volume is unclear. Regardless, the urorectal septum and cloacal membrane approach one another, but before they can fuse, the cloacal membrane ruptures (about week eight). This opens the urogenital sinus and the dorsal anorectal canal to the exterior, with the tip of the urorectal septum forming the future perineal area (Fig. 14-31C,D).

Studies in mice show that Shh expression is necessary for maintaining mesenchymal cell proliferation in the urorectal septum, as loss of Shh signaling results in failed division of the cloaca into the urogenital and anorectal sinuses. Mutations in hedgehog signaling pathways in humans have also been linked to anorectal defects.

As the cloacal membrane ruptures, mesoderm adjacent to the phallic segment of the urogenital sinus expands, generating the **genital tubercle**, which eventually forms the phallus. With the rupture of the cloacal membrane, much of the floor of the phallic segment is lost, whereas the roof of the phallic segment expands along the lower surface of the genital tubercle as the genital tubercle enlarges (Fig. 14-32). This endodermal extension forms the **urogenital plate** (Figs. 14-32, 14-33). As covered in Chapter 16, this plate forms part of the penile urethra in males and the vaginal vestibule in females. **Urogenital folds** (or **cloacal folds**) then form on either side of this plate through expansion of mesoderm underlying the ectoderm adjacent to the urogenital plate.

Soon after the formation of the anorectal orifice, the anorectal walls become opposed to one another and the lumen narrows. Whether an ectodermal plug (sometimes referred to as the anal membrane) temporarily obliterates the anal canal as the anorectal canal narrows in humans is unclear and controversial. Meanwhile, the mesenchyme surrounding the anal canal proliferates, forming a raised border adjacent to the anal opening, creating an **anal pit** or **proctodeum** (see Fig. 14-33). Hence, the cranial two thirds of the definitive anorectal canal is derived from the distal part of the hindgut (lined with endodermally derived epithelium); the inferior one third of the definitive anorectal canal is derived from the anal pit (lined with ectodermally derived epithelium). The location of this juncture is marked in the adult by an irregular folding of mucosa within the anorectal canal, called the **pectinate line**. The vasculature of the anorectal canal is consistent with this dual origin: superior to the pectinate line, the canal is supplied by branches of the inferior mesenteric arteries and veins serving the hindgut; inferior to the pectinate line, it is supplied by branches of the internal iliac arteries and veins. Anastomoses between tributaries of the superior rectal vein and tributaries of the inferior rectal vein within the mucosa of the anorectal canal may later swell, forming hemorrhoids if the normal portal blood flow into the inferior caval vein is restricted.

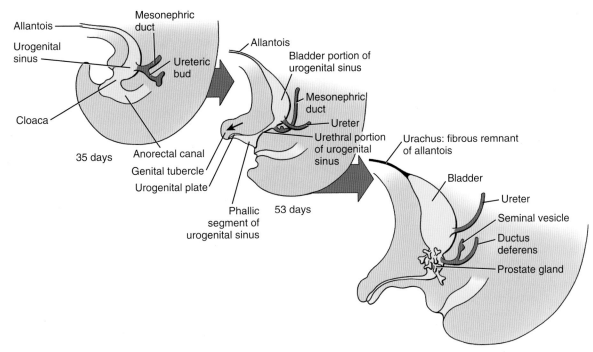

Figure 14-32. Fate of the allantois and urogenital sinus. The urogenital sinus is subdivided into a presumptive bladder, a narrow urethral region, and phallic segment. Normally, the allantois becomes occluded to form the urachus (or median umbilical ligament) of the adult. With the rupture of the cloacal membrane, the roof of the phallic segment forms a urogenital plate of endodermal cells that lengthens as the genital tubercle grows.

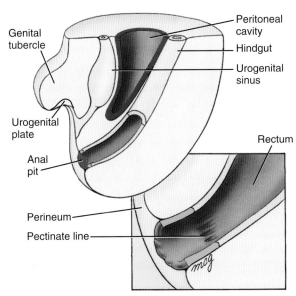

Figure 14-33. Development of the anus and rectum. After the formation of the anorectal orifice, the mesenchyme surrounding the anal canal proliferates, forming a raised border adjacent to the anal opening and establishing an anal pit. The cranial two thirds of the definitive anorectal canal is derived from the distal part of the hindgut (lined with endodermally derived epithelium, in green); the inferior one third of the definitive anorectal canal is derived from the anal pit (lined with ectodermally derived epithelium; green). The location of this juncture is demarcated in the adult as mucosal folds called the pectinate line.

In the Clinic

ANAL MALFORMATIONS

Abnormal development of the urorectal septum can cause the rectum to end blindly in the body wall (Fig. 14-34A). This condition is called **anal agenesis or atresia**. The rectum usually ends cranial to the pelvic diaphragm, which usually is accompanied by a fistula. Occasionally, the anorectal canal forms normally, but the anal membrane separating the ectodermal and endodermal portions of the anus is abnormally thick. This thickened anal membrane may fail to rupture or may rupture incompletely, resulting in an **imperforate anus** or **anal stenosis**, respectively (Fig. 14-34B).

Excessive dorsal fusion of urogenital folds may partly or completely cover the anus. This condition, called **covered anus**, usually occurs in males because the genital folds do not normally fuse at all in females. The resulting malformation is called **anocutaneous occlusion** if the anus is completely covered. In some cases, a defect in the perineal mesoderm just anterior to the anus results in the development of a displaced anterior anal opening, a condition called **anteriorly displaced anus** or **anterior ectopic anus**.

Embryology in Practice

TROUBLE WITH BUBBLES

A young couple expecting their first child has a twenty-week ultrasound at an outlying clinic. They are told that their baby has an abnormality of its intestine and that this defect could mean that their baby has Down syndrome.

Among the numerous "signs" and findings clinicians look for during mid-gestational ultrasound screening is the "double-

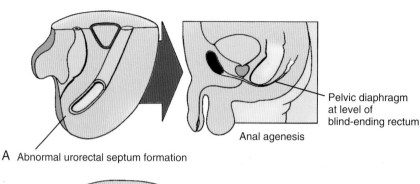

A Abnormal urorectal septum formation

Pelvic diaphragm at level of blind-ending rectum

Anal agenesis

Level of pelvic diaphragm

Imperforate anus

Abnormally thick anal membrane

B fails to perforate

Figure 14-34. Anomalies of the anus. *A,* Anal agenesis resulting from failure of proper urorectal septum formation. *B,* Imperforate anus may occur in cases where an abnormally thick anal membrane fails to rupture.

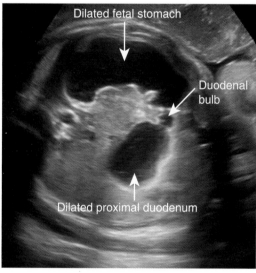

Dilated fetal stomach

Duodenal bulb

Dilated proximal duodenum

Figure 14-35. Sonogram at thirty-seven weeks of gestation showing the characteristic "double-bubble" sign, indicating the presence of a duodenal obstruction.

bubble" sign. The name describes a fluid distention of the stomach and proximal duodenum, which persists throughout pregnancy (Fig. 14-35); its cause is a duodenal obstruction. Ultrasonographers are often alerted to the double-bubble by accompanying polyhydramnios.

The causes of fetal duodenal obstruction may be intrinsic or extrinsic. Intrinsic causes include duodenal atresia, stenosis, and a duodenal web. Extrinsic causes include Ladd's bands (a stalk of peritoneum that attaches the intestine to the posterior wall of the abdomen and obstructs the intestine), gut malrotation or volvulus, and annular pancreas. Whatever the cause, duodenal obstruction can be treated surgically in the newborn period.

However, added concern accompanies the double-bubble sign because of the association of duodenal atresia with other fetal abnormalities. Approximately half of the time, the double-bubble is a harbinger of other conditions or malformations. Best known of these is the association of duodenal atresia with trisomy 21 (Down syndrome).

In the case of the couple described, further examination of the fetus reveals none of the associated concerns for trisomy 21 (e.g., congenital heart defects, nuchal thickening), and the maternal serum screen had previously been given a low risk (1:3800) of trisomy 21. Regardless, the anxious couple elects to have a chromosome study via amniocentesis.

Suggested Readings

Burn SF, Hill RE. 2009. Left-right asymmetry in gut development: what happens next? BioEssays 31:1026–1037.

Gittes GK. 2009. Developmental biology of the pancreas: a comprehensive review. Dev Biol 326:4–35.

Heanue TA, Pachnis V. 2007. Enteric nervous system development and Hirschsprung's disease: advances in genetic and stem cell studies. Nat Rev Neurosci 8:466–479.

Pan FC, Wright C. 2011. Pancreas organogenesis: from bud to plexus to gland. Dev Dyn 240:530–565.

Si-Tayeb K, Lemaigre FP, Duncan SA. 2010. Organogenesis and development of the liver. Dev Cell 18:175–189.

Spence JR, Lauf R, Shroyer NF. 2011. Vertebrate intestinal endoderm development. Dev Dyn 240:501–520.

van den Brink GR. 2007. Hedgehog signaling in development and homeostasis of the gastrointestinal tract. Physiol Rev 87:1343–1375.

van der Flier LG, Clevers H. 2009. Stem cells, self-renewal, and differentiation in the intestinal epithelium. Annu Rev Physiol 71:241–260.

van der Putte SC. 2005. The development of the perineum in the human. A comprehensive histological study with a special reference to the role of the stromal components. Adv Anat Embryol Cell Biol 177:1–131.

Zorn AM, Wells JM. 2009. Vertebrate endoderm development and organ formation. Annu Rev Cell Dev Biol 25:221–251.

Chapter 15
Development of the Urinary System

SUMMARY

The **urinary system** maintains the electrolyte and water balance of the body fluids that bathe the tissues in a salty, aqueous environment. The development of this system involves the transient formation and subsequent regression or remodeling of vestigial primitive systems, thereby providing a glimpse of evolutionary history (another glimpse is provided by the development of the pharyngeal apparatus, covered in Chapter 17). The development of the reproductive system is closely integrated with the primitive urinary organs in both males and females, as they share similar common tubular structures enabling both uresis and gamete transport. Therefore, this chapter has some overlap with Chapter 16, which covers the development of the reproductive system.

The **intermediate mesoderm** on either side of the dorsal body wall gives rise to three successive nephric structures of increasingly advanced design. The intermediate mesoderm, also known as the **nephrotome**, forms a segmental series of epithelial buds. In the cervical region, these structures presumably represent a vestige of the **pronephroi**, or primitive kidneys, which develop in some lower vertebrates. As these cranial pronephroi regress in the fourth week, a pair of elongated mesonephroi succeeds them, developing in the thoracic and lumbar regions. The mesonephroi become the first kidneys to function in the embryo, having complete, although simple, **nephrons**. A pair of **mesonephric (Wolffian** or **nephric) ducts** drains the mesonephroi; these grow caudally to open into the posterior wall of the primitive urogenital sinus. By the fifth week, a pair of **ureteric buds** sprouts from the distal mesonephric ducts, and tissue-tissue interactions with the overlying sacral intermediate mesoderm and developing blood vessels and nerves collectively generate the **metanephroi**, or definitive kidneys.

As described in Chapter 14, the cloaca (the distal expansion of the hindgut) is partitioned into a dorsal anorectal canal and a ventral urogenital sinus. The latter is continuous with the allantois, which projects toward the umbilical cord. The expanded superior portion of the urogenital sinus becomes the bladder, whereas its inferior portion gives rise, in males, to the **pelvic urethra (membranous and prostatic)** and **penile urethra** and, in females, to the **pelvic urethra (membranous)** and **vestibule of the vagina**. During this period, the openings of the mesonephric ducts are translocated down onto the pelvic urethra by a process that also emplaces the openings of ureters on the bladder wall. Several urachal anomalies, fistulas, and anorectal anomalies can occur as a result of abnormal urorectal septal and cloacal membrane development.

Clinical Taster

A pregnant woman is seen at twenty-weeks of gestation for her second transabdominal ultrasound. The imaging reveals a severe paucity of amniotic fluid (**oligohydramnios**) with no evidence of amniotic fluid leakage. Kidney profiles cannot be found within the renal fossae or in ectopic locations. She is referred to a high-risk perinatologist, and a two-week follow-up ultrasound confirms the suspected diagnosis of **bilateral renal agenesis** based on the absence of kidneys, ureters, and bladder and the accompanying severe oligohydramnios.

The perinatologist explains the diagnosis to the parents and that the condition is incompatible with extrauterine life. The parents are informed about their options. They can decide to terminate the pregnancy now or allow the pregnancy to proceed, knowing the neonate may be stillborn or will survive only several hours. Although it is not urgent to decide immediately, the ethical and legal difficulties of termination of pregnancy after twenty-four weeks are discussed.

The incidence of bilateral renal agenesis is approximately 1 in 4000 to 4500 births, and the condition is more common in males. Because the main source of amniotic fluid by sixteen weeks of gestation is urine production, the most prominent prenatal diagnostic feature of bilateral renal agenesis is reduced or absent amniotic fluid. As a consequence, neonates are characterized by a constellation of anomalies (**Potter sequence**), including a flat face, limb contractures, low-set ears, and dry, wrinkled skin. Neonatal mortality is due to the accompanying **pulmonary hypoplasia** caused by the altered dynamics of lung liquid movement during development. Bilateral renal agenesis is associated with other structural anomalies in more than 50% of cases, including an absent bladder, anal atresia, esophageal atresia, and genital anomalies.

Renal agenesis is often a component feature of syndromes caused by single gene mutations (e.g., EYA1, RET, GDNF, SIX1, WT1 genes) or is associated with chromosomal anomalies such as trisomy 13, 18, and 21 or the 22q11.2 deletion syndrome. About one third of cases are associated with non-syndromic, autosomal dominant inheritance having variable penetrance. It is estimated that 9% to 14% of first-degree relatives of neonates with bilateral renal agenesis or dysgenesis have renal anomalies themselves. Therefore, it is recommended that mothers be evaluated for possible renal defects at the time of the prenatal ultrasound and that both parents and siblings undergo genetic evaluation and counseling. The risk of recurrence in subsequent pregnancies is estimated to be 3% to 6%.

Potter sequence can have multiple causes. Other clinical scenarios that result in this syndrome are given in the "Embryology in Practice" for this chapter and in the "Clinical Taster" for Chapter 6.

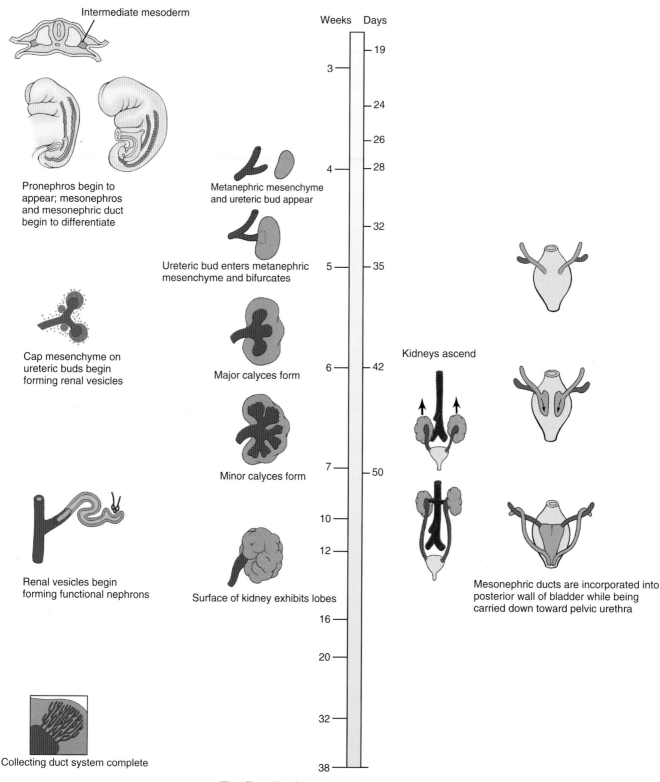

Intermediate mesoderm

Weeks | Days

Pronephros begin to appear; mesonephros and mesonephric duct begin to differentiate

Metanephric mesenchyme and ureteric bud appear

Ureteric bud enters metanephric mesenchyme and bifurcates

Cap mesenchyme on ureteric buds begin forming renal vesicles

Major calyces form

Kidneys ascend

Minor calyces form

Renal vesicles begin forming functional nephrons

Surface of kidney exhibits lobes

Mesonephric ducts are incorporated into posterior wall of bladder while being carried down toward pelvic urethra

Collecting duct system complete

Time line. Development of the urinary system.

THREE NEPHRIC SYSTEMS ARISE DURING DEVELOPMENT

 Animation 15-1: Development of Kidneys.
Animations are available online at StudentConsult.

As covered in Chapter 3, the intraembryonic mesoderm formed on either side of the midline during gastrulation differentiates into three subdivisions: paraxial mesoderm, **intermediate mesoderm** (also called the **nephrotome**), and lateral plate mesoderm (Fig. 15-1). The fates of the paraxial and lateral plate mesoderm are discussed in other chapters. The intermediate mesoderm gives rise to the nephric structures of the embryo, portions of the suprarenal glands, the gonads, and the genital duct system. During embryonic development,

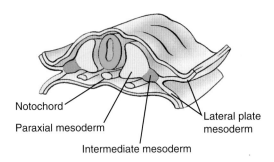

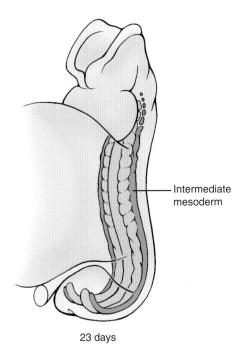

Figure 15-1. The intermediate mesoderm. The intermediate mesoderm gives rise to paired, segmentally organized buds from the cervical to the sacral region.

three sets of nephric systems develop in craniocaudal succession from the intermediate mesoderm. These are called **pronephros, mesonephros**, and **metanephros** (or definitive kidneys). Formation of the pronephric kidney (i.e., pronephros) lays the foundation for induction of the mesonephros, and it in turn lays the foundation for induction of the metanephros. Hence, formation of a pronephros is really the start of a developmental cascade leading to the formation of the definitive kidney.

FORMATION OF PRONEPHROS AND MESONEPHRIC DUCT

Early in the fourth week, intermediate mesoderm along the fifth to seventh cervical axial levels gives rise to a small duct generated by epithelialization of some of the intermediate mesoderm. This duct is called the **mesonephric duct (Wolffian** or **nephric duct)**. The mesonephric duct first appears as a solid longitudinal rod that condenses within the intermediate mesoderm beginning in the pronephric region (Figs. 15-2A-C, 15-3). These rods develop in a caudal direction, driven through inductive

mechanisms during ongoing mesenchymal-to-epithelial conversion of cells at their caudal tips. Meanwhile, intermediate mesoderm ventromedial and adjacent to the mesonephric duct condenses and reorganizes into a series of epithelial buds (see Fig. 15-2). These buds, which quickly become hollow, constitute the **pronephros** (plural, pronephroi; derived from the Greek for "first kidney") because they resemble the functional embryonic pronephroi of some lower vertebrates. In humans, these units do not differentiate into functional excretory structures but instead cease to develop and disappear by around day twenty-four or twenty-five.

As the mesonephric ducts develop and extend caudally, they induce the formation of **mesonephric buds** from mesenchyme in the more caudal intermediate mesoderm, thereby initiating mesonephros formation (see Fig. 15-2B, C). As the ducts grow into the lower lumbar region, they diverge from the intermediate mesodermal mesenchyme and grow toward and fuse with the ventrolateral walls of the cloaca on day twenty-six (see Figs. 15-2, 15-4A). This region of fusion will become a part of the posterior wall of the future bladder. As the rods fuse with the cloaca, they begin to cavitate at their caudal ends, forming a lumen, and this canalization progresses cranially. The caudal end of each mesonephric duct induces the evagination of a ureteric bud (Fig. 15-4).

DEVELOPMENT OF MESONEPHROS

Early in the fourth week, mesonephric tubules begin to develop within mesonephric buds adjacent to the mesonephric duct on either side of the vertebral column, from the upper thoracic region to the third lumbar level (see Fig. 15-2B-D). About forty **mesonephric tubules** are produced in craniocaudal succession within this mesonephric mesenchyme. Because the gonads begin to develop just medial to the mesonephric ridge, this region is sometimes collectively referred to as the **urogenital ridge**. As more caudal tubules differentiate, the more cranial ones regress, so there are never more than about thirty pairs in the mesonephroi. By the end of the fifth week, the cranial regions of the mesonephroi undergo massive regression, leaving only about twenty pairs of tubules occupying the first three lumbar levels. The mesonephric tubules differentiate into excretory units resembling an abbreviated version of the adult metanephric nephron (see Fig. 15-2D; discussed later) with the medial end of the tubule forming a cup-shaped sac, called **Bowman's capsule**, which wraps around a knot of capillaries, called a **glomerulus**, to form a **renal corpuscle**.

The lateral tips of the cranial six to seven mesonephric tubules fuse with the mesonephric duct, thus opening a passage from the excretory units to the cloaca. These mesonephric excretory units are functional between about the sixth and tenth weeks and produce small amounts of urine. After ten weeks, they cease to function; they regress in the female, whereas in the male, they are thought to give rise to the efferent ductules. As covered in Chapter 16, the mesonephric ducts also regress in the female. However, in the male, the mesonephric ducts persist and form important elements of the male genital duct system.

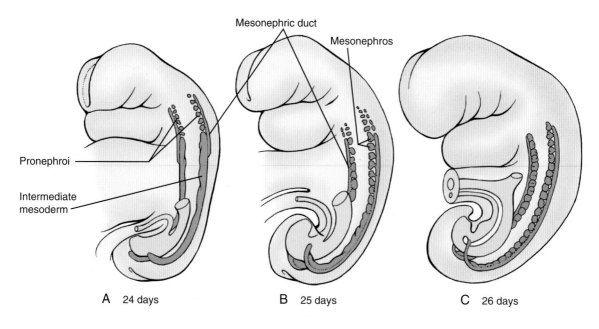

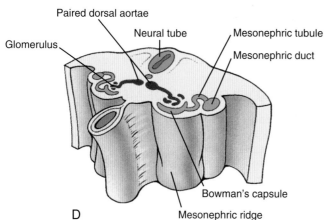

Figure 15-2. Development of the pronephros and mesonephros. *A,* A pair of pronephroi form along the fifth to seventh cervical segments, but these quickly degenerate during the fourth week. The mesonephric ducts first appear on day twenty-four. *B, C,* Mesonephric tubules form in a craniocaudal sequence throughout the thoracic and lumbar regions. The more cranial pairs regress as caudal pairs form, and the definitive mesonephroi contain about twenty pairs, confined to the first three lumbar segments. *D,* The mesonephroi contain functional nephric units consisting of glomeruli, Bowman's capsules, mesonephric tubules, and mesonephric ducts.

In the Research Lab

SPECIFICATION OF NEPHRIC LINEAGE

One of the earliest genes expressed in the nephrogenic intermediate mesoderm is Pax2. Mice deficient in Pax2 form a mesonephric duct in the pronephric and mesonephric regions, but the mesonephric duct fails to extend into the metanephric region. Therefore, the metanephros does not develop (because it is dependent on branching from the caudal mesonephric duct). When double knockout mice for Pax2 and Pax8 (another Pax family member expressed in the intermediate mesoderm) are generated, the intermediate mesoderm does not form any portion of the mesonephric duct nor express the nephric markers Lhx1 (Lim homeobox-1) and Ret (both required for subsequent metanephric kidney development). One downstream target of Pax2 and Pax8 activity is Gata3, which is necessary for Ret activation and specification of the nephric lineage. Pax2 is a particularly potent initiator of nephron development: ectopic

nephric structures can be induced almost anywhere within the intermediate mesoderm, including the gonadal ridge of chick embryos, when Pax2 is ectopically expressed by viral transfection of mesoderm at the mid-primitive streak stage.

The tissue interactions responsible for specifying the nephric lineage within intermediate mesoderm are unclear, but this lineage seems to depend on the developing somites because Pax2 and Lhx1 expression is lost in chick embryos if the intermediate mesoderm is separated from the somites. Moreover, one can induce ectopic pronephric tissue within the intermediate and lateral plate mesoderm by grafting somites into ectopic locations. Ectoderm may also have a role in specifying or maintaining nephric capacity within intermediate mesoderm, as removal of the overlying ectoderm decreases expression of Pax2 and Lhx1 within the intermediate mesoderm, and this mesoderm loses its nephrogenic capacity. Therefore, secreted factors from adjacent tissues are needed to induce and maintain nephrogenic mesoderm.

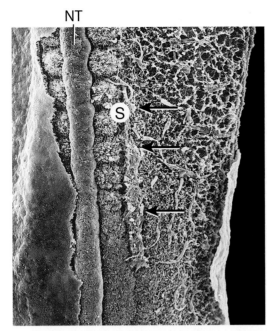

Figure 15-3. Formation of the mesonephric duct. Scanning electron micrograph show a growing mesonephric duct (arrows) just adjacent to the somites (S) on one side of a chick embryo. The duct is elongating in a cranial-to-caudal direction. The surface ectoderm has been removed to reveal the underlying mesoderm. NT, neural tube.

TABLE 15-1 **STRUCTURES COMPOSING THE COLLECTING AND EXCRETORY PORTIONS OF THE METANEPHROS**	
Collecting Portion (Ureteric Bud)	**Excretory Portion (or Nephron) (Metanephric Mesenchyme)**
Ureter	Bowman's capsule
Renal pelvis	Proximal convoluted tubule
Major and minor calyces	Loop of Henle
Collecting ducts	Distal convoluted tubule

DEVELOPMENT OF METANEPHROS

The definitive kidneys, or **metanephroi**, are composed of two functional components: the excretory portion and the collecting portion. These two portions are derived from different sources of intermediate mesoderm (Table 15-1). Development of the metanephros involves mesenchymal-to-epithelial conversion, epithelial tube formation and elongation, tubular branching, cell condensation, angiogenesis, and specification and differentiation of numerous specialized cell types.

Formation of the metanephros begins with the induction and formation of a pair of new structures, the **ureteric buds**, within the intermediate mesoderm of the sacral region. A ureteric bud sprouts from the caudal portion of each mesonephric duct on about day twenty-eight (Fig. 15-4). By day thirty-two, each ureteric bud penetrates a portion of the sacral intermediate mesoderm called the **metanephric mesenchyme**, and the bud begins to bifurcate (Figs. 15-4B, 15-5). As the ureteric bud branches, each new growing **ureteric tip (ureteric ampulla)** acquires a cap-like aggregate of metanephric mesenchymal tissue

referred to as **cap mesenchyme**. By the end of the sixteenth week, fourteen to sixteen lobes have formed, giving the metanephros a lobulated appearance.

The ureters and the collecting duct system of the kidneys differentiate from the ureteric bud; the **nephrons** (the definitive urine-forming units of the kidneys) differentiate from the metanephric mesenchyme. In the mature kidney, urine produced by the nephrons flows through a collecting system consisting of collecting ducts, minor calyces, major calyces, the renal pelvis, and, finally, the ureter. This system is entirely the product of the ureteric bud. The

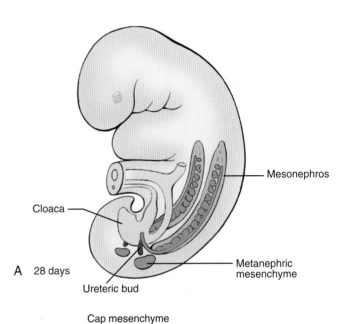

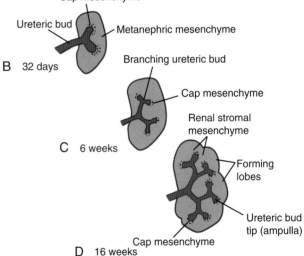

Figure 15-4. Origin of the metanephros. *A,* Metanephric mesenchyme develops from intermediate mesoderm on each side of the body axis early in the fifth week. Simultaneously, each mesonephric duct sprouts a ureteric bud that grows into the metanephric mesenchyme. *B-D,* By the fifth week, the ureteric bud bifurcates, and the two growing tips (ampullae) induce cranial and caudal lobes in the metanephros. As the ureteric bud tips grow and branch, each acquires a cap-like aggregation of metanephric mesenchyme. Cell-cell interactions between ureteric tip cells and cap mesenchymal cells drive continual branching of the ureteric buds and formation of renal lobules during the next ten weeks.

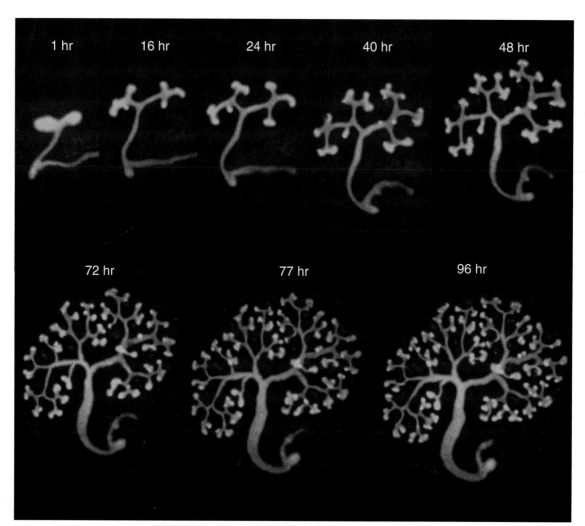

Figure 15-5. Time-lapse images of ureteric bud branching in the metanephric region isolated from a transgenic E11.5 mouse and placed in organ culture. Hoxb7-driven expression of a membrane-bound form of a fluorescent protein was used to visualize the ureteric epithelium.

ureteric bud undergoes an exact sequence of bifurcations (Fig. 15-6), and the expanded major and minor calyces arise through phases whereby previously formed branches coalesce. When the ureteric bud first expands into the metanephric mesenchyme, its tip expands to form an initial ampulla that will give rise to the **renal pelvis**. During the sixth week, the ureteric bud bifurcates four times, yielding sixteen branches. These branches then coalesce to form two to four **major calyces** extending from the renal pelvis. By the seventh week, the next four generations of branches also coalesce, forming the **minor calyces**. By thirty-two weeks, approximately eleven additional generations of bifurcation have formed one to three million branches, which will become the future **collecting ducts** of the kidney (Fig. 15-6F). The definitive morphology of the collecting ducts is created by variations in the pattern of branching and by a tendency for distal branches to elongate.

Like the nephrons and mesonephric duct of the mesonephric kidney, the differentiation of metanephric nephrons depends on inductive signals between the ureteric bud and the cap mesenchyme (see the following "In the Research Lab" entitled "Factors Expressed in Metanephric Mesoderm Regulate Induction and Branching of Ureteric Bud"). As the buds continue to grow into the future

renal cortex, some of the cap mesenchymal cells come to lie adjacent to the **ureteric stalk** (the portion of the ureteric bud found immediately adjacent to the ureteric tip; Fig. 15-7A, B), where the cells condense and undergo mesenchymal-to-epithelial conversion to form a **renal vesicle**. Several hours of direct contact between the ureteric stalk and the forming renal vesicle are required to induce subsequent nephron differentiation within the renal vesicle. If the ureteric bud is abnormal or missing, the nephron does not develop. Conversely, **reciprocal inductive signals** from the cap mesenchyme regulate the orderly branching and growth of the bifurcating tips of the ureteric buds. The number of nephrons formed ultimately depends on growth and branching of the ureteric bud and cap mesenchyme proliferation, as well as renal vesicle formation and conversion into epithelial tubules.

Each nephron originates from a renal vesicle derived from proliferating cap mesenchyme. Formation of a nephron from this vesicle involves several stages. First, the nephric vesicle develops into a comma-shaped structure, which then forms an S-shaped tubule (Fig. 15-7C, D). The S-shaped tubule fuses with the ureteric stalk, and eventually the two lumens become continuous, forming a **uriniferous tubule**. Meanwhile, the future renal

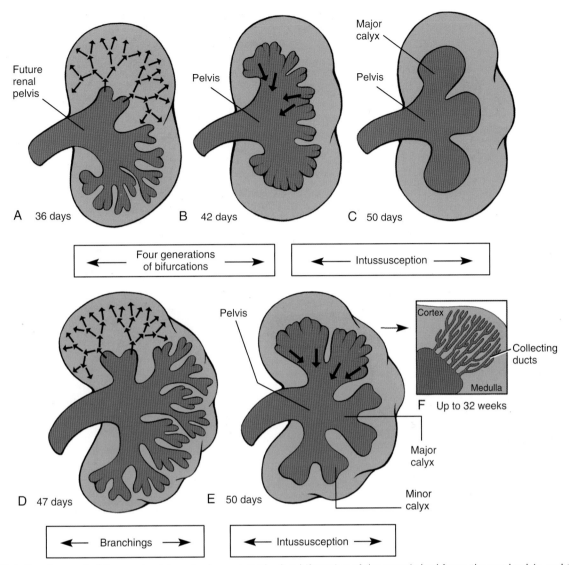

Figure 15-6. Development of the renal pelvis and calyces. *A-C,* The first bifurcation of the ureteric bud forms the renal pelvis, and the coalescence of the next four generations of bifurcations produces the major calyces. *D, E,* The next four generations of bifurcation coalesce to form the minor calyces of the renal collecting system. *F,* The ureteric buds continue to bifurcate until week thirty-two, producing one- to three-million collecting ducts.

corpuscle segment (proximal portion) of the S-shaped tubule forms the outer (parietal) layer of Bowman's capsule and the glomerular epithelial cells (**podocytes**) that surround the glomerular tuft of capillaries developing within the adjacent stroma. While the renal corpuscle is forming, the lengthening uriniferous tubule forms the remaining elements of the nephron: the proximal convoluted tubule, descending and ascending limbs of the loop of Henle, and the distal convoluted tubule (Fig. 15-7E). The medulla of the kidney also begins to take shape as the growing nephron tubules and interstitial tissue develop. **Nephrogenesis** is complete by birth in humans.

Morphogenesis of the renal vascular supply during development of the nephron and collecting systems is poorly understood. Organ cultures and interspecies grafting experiments show that angiogenesis is likely the major mechanism responsible for the development of the renal

vasculature, including the glomerular capillaries. However, the prevascular metanephric mesenchyme expresses vasculogenic markers (e.g., Vegf, Vegfr, Tie2), and if fetal mouse kidney tissue is grafted into the mouse anterior eye chamber (an area devoid of blood vessels), grafted tissue can form capillaries, suggesting that it has intrinsic vasculogenic capacity.

During the tenth week, the metanephroi become functional. Blood plasma from the glomerular capillaries is filtered within the renal corpuscle to produce a dilute glomerular filtrate, which is concentrated and converted to urine by the activities of the convoluted tubules and the loop of Henle. The urine passes down the collecting system into the ureters and thence into the bladder. Even though the fetal kidneys produce urine throughout the remainder of gestation, their main function is not to clear waste products out of the

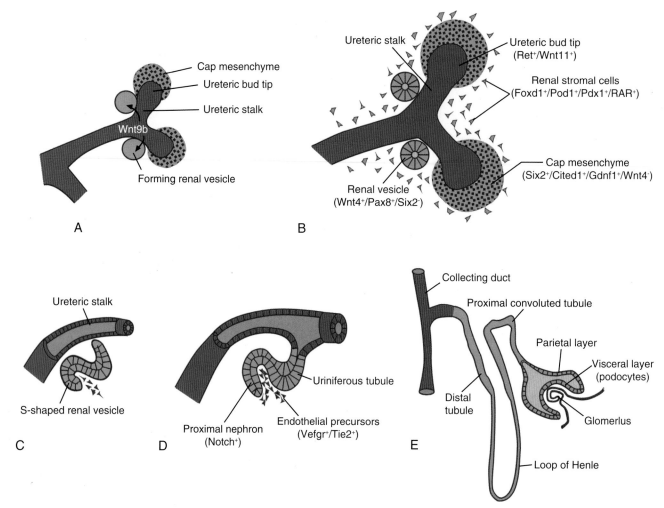

Figure 15-7. Development of renal vesicle and nephrons. *A, B,* Reciprocal inductive interactions between the ureteric bud tip and the cap mesenchyme regulate orderly branching and growth of the buds and continued proliferation of the cap stem mesenchymal cells. Wnt9b, expressed by ureteric stalk, promotes Wnt4 expression within the cap mesenchymal cells lying adjacent to ureteric stalk, and these cells undergo mesenchymal-to-epithelial conversion, forming a renal vesicle; Wnt4 is necessary for maintaining the survival of this mesenchyme and for subsequent nephron differentiation. Stromal cells express Foxd1, Pod1, and Pdx1 and the retinoic acid receptors, Rarα and Rarβ2, all of which are necessary for balancing stromal and nephron progenitor specification and survival. *C-E,* The renal vesicle develops into an S-shaped tubule, fuses with the ureteric stalk, and forms the nephron. Notch signaling within the S-shaped tubule delineates the proximal portion of the nephron, including the proximal and visceral layers of Bowman's capsule, the proximal and distal convoluted tubules, and the loops of Henle. Functional nephric units (of the type shown in *E*) first appear in distal regions of the metanephros at ten weeks.

blood; that task is handled principally by the placenta. Instead, the production of fetal urine is important because urine contributes to the amniotic fluid. Fetuses with **bilateral renal agenesis** (complete absence of both kidneys) do not have enough amniotic fluid (**oligohydramnios**) and hence are confined to an abnormally small amniotic space. This leads to a condition called **Potter sequence** (covered in the following "In the Clinic" entitled "Renal Agenesis and Dysplasia," and in the "Clinical Taster" and "Embryology in Practice" for this chapter, as well as in the "Clinical Taster" for Chapter 6).

Figure 15-8 shows the general structure of the definitive fetal kidney. This architecture reflects the events of the first ten weeks of renal development, that is, weeks five to fifteen of intrauterine development. The kidney is divided into an inner medulla and an outer cortex. The cortical

tissue contains the nephrons and collecting ducts, whereas the medulla contains the collecting ducts and loops of Henle. Each minor calyx drains a tree of collecting ducts within a **renal pyramid**; the collecting ducts converge to form the **renal papilla**. Zones of nephron-containing cortical tissue called renal columns separate the renal pyramids of the kidney. Thus, in the definitive kidney, the cortical tissue not only makes up the peripheral layer of the kidney, it also forms piers projecting toward the pelvis. Nevertheless, all nephrons in the cortical tissue arise from cortical regions of the metanephric mesenchyme.

The autonomic nervous system of the kidney, which regulates blood flow and secretory function, arises from neural crest cells that invade the metanephroi early in their development. Further aspects of development of the autonomic nervous system of the abdomen and pelvis are covered in Chapter 10.

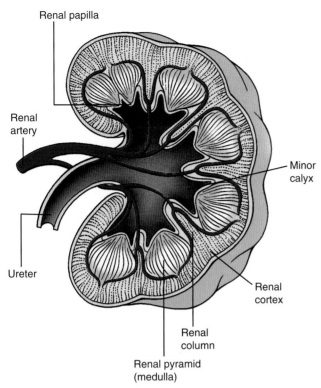

Figure 15-8. The definitive renal architecture of the metanephros is apparent by the tenth week.

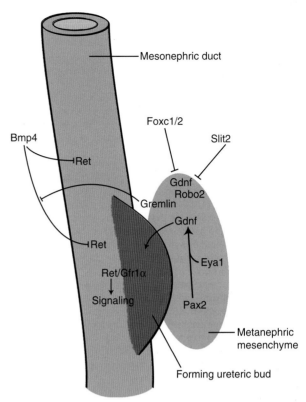

Figure 15-9. Positioning of ureteric bud formation is mediated by Ret signaling. Expression of Ret within the mesonephric duct epithelium is restricted to caudal portions of the duct by Bmp4 released from cranial urogenital ridge mesenchyme and by gremlin, a Bmp inhibitor expressed by the metanephric mesenchyme. Mesenchymal expression of the Ret ligand, Gdnf, requires Pax2 expression in the urogenital ridge but is restricted to the metanephric region by the cranial expression of Foxc1, Foxc2, and Slit2 in the mesenchyme. Robo2, the receptor for Slit2, is expressed in the urogenital ridge mesenchyme.

In the Research Lab

FACTORS EXPRESSED IN METANEPHRIC MESODERM REGULATE INDUCTION AND BRANCHING OF URETERIC BUD

What induces the formation of the ureteric bud and specifies its location along the mesonephric duct? It seems that the induction and location of the ureteric bud largely depend on the nephrogenic mesenchyme of the intermediate mesoderm. Formation of the ureteric bud from the mesonephric duct is induced by signals emanating from the adjacent mesoderm and involves the Ret receptor, its co-receptor, Gfr1α, and its ligand, Gdnf. Ret and Gfr1α are expressed within the mesonephric duct, whereas the ligand, Gdnf (and also Gfr1α), is expressed within the metanephric mesenchyme (Fig. 15-9). Misexpression of Gdnf elsewhere within the intermediate mesoderm is sufficient to induce ectopic ureteric buds, and mice deficient in Ret or Gdnf exhibit bilateral renal agenesis. Therefore, faults in tissue-tissue interactions between the metanephric mesoderm and the mesonephric duct mediated through Ret signaling may be responsible for the formation of duplex kidneys or for renal agenesis seen in humans. Among humans with renal agenesis, approximately 40% have RET mutations and 5% to 10% have mutations in GDNF.

Experiments suggest that the cranial-caudal positioning of ureteric bud formation may be the result of repression of nephrogenic determinants within the more cranial regions of the intermediate mesoderm. Forkhead genes make up one group of transcription factors that seem to be involved. Foxc1/2 expression is normally restricted to the cranial end of the nephrogenic mesoderm. When Foxc1 is knocked out in mice or Foxc1/2 null heterozygotes are generated, ectopic ureteric buds form over a broad span of the mesonephric duct. A similar phenotype is seen in mice deficient in Slit2, or its receptor, Robo2 (pathfinding signaling molecules; covered further in

Chapter 10). Foxc1/2 and Slit2/Robo2 may repress Gdnf expression in the more cranial regions, because Slit2 expression occurs in a cranial-caudal gradient within the mesenchyme that is the inverse of Gdnf expression.

Bmp4 is another extracellular signaling molecule implicated in restricting ureteric bud development. Bmp4-deficient mice develop ectopic ureteric buds and double ureters. Bmp4 is normally expressed in the mesoderm surrounding the mesonephric duct and ureteric buds but not in the mesonephric duct itself. Experiments suggest that Bmp4 inhibits Ret signaling within the mesonephric duct (see Fig. 15-9), rather than altering Gdnf levels released from the mesoderm, because Bmp4 can block the effect of ectopic Gdnf on ureteric bud formation in metanephric organ cultures. Metanephric mesenchyme also produces gremlin a Bmp inhibitor, thereby blocking any potential Bmp inhibition of Ret signaling in this region.

Other factors important in the formation and budding of the ureteric bud are Eya1 (eyes absent 1) and the Hox11 group of homeotic genes. Mutants deficient in these genes fail to turn on Gdnf and do not develop ureteric buds. Hence, the induction and position of the ureteric bud seems to depend on a balance between mesodermally mediated activation and negative regulation of Ret signaling within the mesonephric duct. Several malformations can arise if the ureteric buds sprout from incorrect sites along the mesonephric duct, as the resulting ureters will be incorrectly emplaced into the dorsal wall of the developing bladder.

URETERIC BUD INDUCES NEPHROGENIC MESODERM TO CONDENSE WHILE MESODERM DRIVES CONTINUAL URETERIC BRANCHING AND GROWTH

As the ureteric bud grows and branches into metanephric mesoderm, it induces the adjacent mesenchyme to condense around the tips of the ureteric branches. These condensations eventually serve as the primordia of the nephrons. However, reciprocal signaling from the metanephric mesenchyme is necessary for continual expansion and branching of ureteric buds to form the ureter, calyces, and collecting tubules and ducts.

One of the first genes identified as important in ureteric bud branching in humans was the **WT1 (WILMS TUMOR SUPPRESSOR 1)** gene (not to be confused with Wnt1, a wingless family member). WT1 is essential for normal urogenital development. WT1 is upregulated in the metanephric mesenchyme as it condenses, and it continues to be expressed during the mesenchymal-to-epithelial transition responsible for forming the nephric epithelial vesicles. Mice lacking the Wt1 gene fail to induce ureteric buds even though Gdnf is still expressed within the cap mesenchyme, suggesting that Wt1 operates independently of Gdnf signaling. Closer examination of Wt1 knockout mice reveals that waves of apoptosis occur within the metanephric mesenchyme, beginning about the time the mesenchyme begins to condense. Although the precise role for Wt1 in renal development is still unclear, it seems that Wt1 makes the mesenchymal population receptive to ureteric bud induction signals necessary for maintaining the mesenchymal population. Therefore, the inability to maintain a condensing cap mesenchyme adjacent to the ureteric buds may be the reason for failed ureteric bud growth and branching in these mice.

Cap mesenchyme can be subdivided into two groups: capping mesenchyme maintaining the "stem cell" cap population, and the induced mesenchyme that goes on to condense and generate the renal vesicle. Wt1, Six2 (sine oculis homeobox homolog-2), and Cited1 (Cbp/p300-interacting transactivator with Glu/Asp-rich carboxy-terminal domain 1) expression within the cap mesenchyme (see Fig. 15-7B) is required to maintain stemness of the proliferating cap mesenchyme, and loss of expression of these quickly depletes the cap mesenchymal cell population, thereby halting further ureteric branching and nephron formation. At birth, Six2 expression disappears in mice, thereby converting all remaining cap mesenchymal cells into nephrons. What triggers this loss of expression is unknown.

One of the first markers of the induced condensing cap mesenchyme is the expression of the wingless family member Wnt4. Wnt4 expression is required for the mesenchymal-to-epithelial transformation generating the renal vesicle because in its absence, no renal vesicles or nephrons form. Moreover, in organ cultures, Wnt4 can induce nephron formation in the absence of ureteric bud epithelium, and recent studies suggest Wnt4 induces the mesenchyme-to-epithelial conversion via a non-canonical calcium-dependent signaling pathway. So what does the ureteric bud epithelium release that mediates Wnt4 expression in the mesenchyme in vivo? Evidence suggests that it is Wnt9b (see Fig. 15-7A). In mice deficient in Wnt9b, the ureteric bud undergoes branching, but the mesenchyme fails to condense and undergo mesenchymal-to-epithelial transition, resulting in nephron agenesis. Wnt9b is expressed by the ureteric bud epithelium, and in explant cultures, Wnt9b can substitute for the ureteric epithelium in promoting nephrogenesis. Several frizzled family members (Wnt receptors) are also expressed in cap mesenchyme. However, their role in mediating Wnt signaling during renal development is still unclear.

Patterning of the kidney during development depends on interactions between the ureteric branches and condensing nephrogenic mesenchyme, but it also involves interactions with the interstitial stromal cells surrounding the condensing mesenchyme (see Fig. 15-7B). Fgf8 expression in the metanephric mesenchyme mediates branching by expanding the stromal compartment necessary for maintaining the cap mesenchymal population. Without Fgf8, few renal vesicles form and renal development is arrested. Six1 (sine oculis homeobox homolog-1) and Cited1 commit mesenchyme to the renal epithelial lineage, whereas stromal cells specifically express Foxd1, Pod1, and Pdx1. Mice with null mutations for Foxd1, Pod1, and Pdx1 genes develop small and dysmorphic kidneys with nephron and branching defects. All three types of knockout mice ectopically express Ret along the entire ureteric epithelium rather than just at the ureteric tips. This expanded Ret expression may be responsible for the branching defects seen in these mice, as similar defects are generated when Ret is misexpressed. Studies suggest that Foxd1, Pod1, and Pdx1 may also regulate the balance between stromal and nephron progenitor specifications. For instance in mouse metanephric explant cultures, the stromal-promoting growth factors Fgf2 and Bmp7 increase the number of Foxd1-positive cells at the expense of the nephron population.

Another stromal signaling factor important in kidney patterning is retinoic acid. The retinoic acid receptors, Rarα and Rarβ2, are expressed exclusively within the stromal compartment of the developing kidney (see Fig. 15-7B). In mouse embryos deficient in both Rarα and Rarβ2, the expression of Ret is not initiated in the ureteric buds, resulting in renal agenesis. Moreover, these receptor-deficient mice exhibit ectopic expression of Foxd1, Pod1, and Pbx1 within the ureteric epithelium. Normal renal development can be rescued if Ret expression is restored in these mice. Because Rarα, Rarβ2, Foxd1, Pod1, and Pdx1 are all normally expressed exclusively within the stromal compartment, these experiments imply that essential signals influencing ureteric bud Ret expression also emanate from the stroma.

FORMATION OF NEPHRON THROUGH MESENCHYMAL-TO-EPITHELIAL CONVERSION OF MESENCHYME

The mesenchyme adjacent to the tip of the branching ureteric stalk is surrounded by extracellular matrix that rapidly changes in composition in response to inductive influences of the ureteric stalk epithelium. Initially, the mesenchyme adjacent to the stalk is surrounded by extracellular matrix containing interstitial collagens (type I and type III), fibronectin, and syndecans. However with induction, collagen type I and type III are replaced by collagen type IV, fibronectin is replaced by laminin, and the mesenchyme begins expressing heparan sulfate proteoglycans. As the condensing mesenchyme forms, it increases its expression of Ncam cadherin-11, and syndecan-1 (as well as Wnt4), but these begin to disappear as R-cadherin, cadherin-6, and then E-cadherin levels increase and the mesenchyme begins to take on the organization of an epithelium. Upregulation of integrin α6 and α8 expression occurs concurrently with the changes leading to cell polarization and epithelial formation.

What is responsible for driving the conversion from a mesenchyme to an epithelium is unclear, but as discussed earlier, ureteric bud epithelium–induced expression of Wnt4 is required. During the condensation phase, Wnt4 expression increases and is maintained as the mesenchyme is converted into a comma-shaped epithelium and then an S-shaped epithelium. If Wnt4 is knocked out in mice, the mesenchyme begins condensing, but rather than organizing into an epithelium, it undergoes apoptosis.

Cadherin switching plays an important role in establishing epithelial cell polarity. Intracellularly, cadherins interact with the cytoskeleton through a network of α-, β-, and γ-catenins. As cells switch toward cadherin types associated with organizing an epithelium, β-catenin becomes localized to lateral cell surfaces. Therefore, in addition to mediating β-catenin transcriptional activity, Wnt signaling within the nephrogenic mesenchyme likely alters cadherin activity necessary for the mesenchymal-to-epithelial conversion.

Once formed, the S-shaped renal vesicle fuses with the ureteric bud stalk to form a continuous epithelial tube. As the renal vesicle extends, it must acquire proximal and distal regional designations to form proximal and distal segments. This proximodistal patterning of the S-shaped vesicle is dependent on notch signaling (Fig. 15-7C, D). Mice null for notch2 lack the entire proximal segment (i.e., visceral and parietal glomerular capsule, proximal convoluted tubules, and loop of Henle) but have normal ureteric branching and distal portions of the nephron. Moreover, forced activation of notch signaling in the distal portion of the S-shaped renal vesicle can transform this region to take on proximal fates.

In the Clinic

RENAL AGENESIS AND DYSPLASIA

Kidneys may fail to develop on one or both sides because of faulty tissue-tissue interactions between the ureteric bud and nephrogenic and stromal mesenchyme. Infants with **bilateral renal agenesis** are stillborn or die within a few days of birth. In contrast, infants with **unilateral renal agenesis** usually live because the remaining kidney undergoes compensatory hypertrophy. Although the relative frequencies of unilateral and bilateral renal agenesis are difficult to determine because unilateral renal agenesis often goes undetected, autopsy data suggest that unilateral renal agenesis is about four to eight times more common than bilateral renal agenesis.

Renal agenesis is typically associated with other congenital defects. The kidneys contribute to the amniotic fluid. Therefore, bilateral renal agenesis results in **oligohydramnios**, or insufficient amniotic fluid (also covered in Chapter 6). Oligohydramnios can result in a spectrum of abnormalities called **Potter sequence**. These include deformed limbs; wrinkly, dry skin; and an abnormal facies (in this context, *facies* means "facial appearance") consisting of wide-set eyes with infraorbital skin creases, beak-like nose, recessed chin, and low-set ears.

Renal agenesis is often associated with a spectrum of ipsilateral genitourinary abnormalities, including defects in structures derived from the mesonephric duct in males and paramesonephric (Müllerian) duct in females. Failure of the mesonephric duct to develop leads to absence of both the vas deferens and kidney because the kidney develops from an outgrowth of this duct, which in the male is also the progenitor of the vas deferens (covered in Chapter 16). This can occur bilaterally or unilaterally.

Abnormal kidneys may arise from abnormal inductive interactions. In some cases, subtle defects in the interaction between ureteric bud and metanephric mesenchyme result in hypoplasia or dysplasia of the developing kidney. A small number of nephrons in a hypoplastic kidney result either from inadequate branching of the ureteric bud or from an inadequate response by the metanephric cap tissue. In cases of renal dysplasia, the nephrons themselves develop abnormally and consist of primitive ducts lined by undifferentiated epithelium sheathed within thick layers of connective tissue. The genetic causes for some of these renal anomalies are beginning to be identified. Mutations in PAX2 are associated with dominant transmission of renal hypoplasia and dysplasia (seen in **renal-coloboma syndrome**). Mutations leading to haploinsufficiency of GATA3 are responsible

for **HDR (hypoparathyroidism-deafness-renal anomalies) syndrome**, in which patients exhibit multiple deficiencies, including renal dysplasia. Mutations in EYA1 (a transcription factor required for GDNF expression and, hence, ureteric bud development) and SIX1 (a transcription factor that interacts with EYA1) cause **BOR (branchio-oto-renal) syndrome** (covered in the "Clinical Taster" for Chapter 18). In addition to renal anomalies, EYA1 haploinsufficient individuals develop pharyngeal cleft cysts and have both outer and inner ear defects.

MUTATIONS CAUSING NEPHRON PATHOLOGIES

The glomerular and tubular systems of the nephron are composed of highly specialized cell types responsible for waste secretion. Initial filtration occurs between capillary and podocyte cells at the glomerulus. Defects in podocyte foot processes surrounding capillaries and defects in the basement membrane separating the two usually result in excessive protein loss into the urine (**proteinuria**).

In animal models, mutations in several genes and gene targets have been identified that are associated with deficient glomerular formation and function. Pdgfs and their receptors have an important role in renal corpuscle development. Initially, Pdgf and Pdgf receptors are expressed throughout the nephronic mesenchyme, stromal cells, and vascular cells but later become restricted to the intraglomerular **mesangial cells** (essential pericytes of glomerular capillaries). If either the Pdgfb ligand or Pdgfrβ receptor is knocked out in mice, the glomeruli lack mesangial cells and fail to form normal capillary tufts. Glomerular formation is initiated, and the endothelial and podocyte lineages are present; they just do not organize properly in the absence of mesangial cells.

Mice lacking the gene encoding integrin α3 exhibit severe kidney anomalies resulting in defects in the later stages of nephrogenesis. Although the number of nephrons formed is the same as in wild-type mice, the capillary beds surrounding the proximal convoluted tubules are abnormal, the glomerular basement membrane is disorganized, and the podocytes fail to form foot processes.

Mutations in WT1 are associated with several renal and gonadal malformations and are the most common cause (although rare) of children's kidney tumors. **Wilms tumors** (nephroblastoma) affect about 1:10,000 children. Inactivating mutations in the tumor suppressor gene, WT1, are responsible for 10% to 15% of these neoplasms. Tumors are typically diagnosed in children at 3 or 4 years of age and, fortunately, can be treated chemotherapeutically, with a cure rate of about 80% to 90%. WT1 is encoded on human chromosome 11p13, and mutations in WT1 lead to malformations of the urinary and genital systems.

Post-transcriptional modifications of WT1 mRNA lead to the production of up to 24 different isoforms of WT1 as a result of alternative mRNA splicing, the presence of multiple start codons, or RNA editing. Alterations in the ratio of two alternative splice variants of the WT1 gene—WT1(-Kts) and WT1(+Kts), each of which has a different DNA binding site and different transcriptional activity—can lead to abnormal glomerular development. For instance, a heterozygous point mutation causing a decrease in levels of WT1(+KTS) is associated with **Frasier syndrome**. These patients develop **renal mesangial sclerosis** (abnormal thickening of the glomerular basement membrane and mesangial extracellular matrix) with progressive renal failure and streaked gonads (WT1 has a key role in early gonadal development, as covered in Chapter 16; streaked, also called streak, gonads are undeveloped), in addition to Wilms tumors.

Heterozygous mutations in WT1 are also linked to **Denys-Drash syndrome**. These patients exhibit genitourinary malformations, including sexual ambiguity as well as podocytic underdevelopment and glomerular nephropathy caused by diffuse mesangial sclerosis leading to end-stage renal failure. In this case, the mutation is restricted to the WT1 locus, whereby a missense mutation results in the replacement of arginine for tryptophan at residue 394 in the zinc-finger domain of the WT1 protein. Other mutations occurring within this zinc-finger domain have also been identified in children with Denys-Drash syndrome. In adults, WT1 expression in the kidney is restricted to glomerular podocytes. WT1 regulates PODOCALYXIN, an integral membrane protein connected to the cytoskeleton of podocytes and thought to maintain podocyte three-dimensional shape. Mutations in the WT1 gene cause glomerulopathy-associated syndromes like Denys-Drash and Frasier, possibly by misregulating PODOCALYXIN expression.

Human mutations in the genes coding for NEPHRIN (NPHS1, a podocyte membrane slit protein) or PODOCIN (NPHS2) or the loss of COLLAGEN TYPE IV in the basement membrane (as seen in **Alport syndrome**) can all lead to defects in glomerular function in humans. In mice, the Kreisler gene (or MafB) mediates glomerular nephrin and podocin expression levels and is required for normal podocyte development. Kreisler mutant mice exhibit glomerular defects and proteinuria.

Approximately 40% to 50% of children with **Alagille syndrome**, an autosomal dominant disorder due to mutations in NOTCH2 or its ligand, JAG1, exhibit various forms of renal disease and dysplasia, including glomerulosclerosis, juvenile nephronophthisis, renal acidosis, and renal failure. Mutations in the LMX1B (LIM HOMEOBOX TRANSCRIPTION FACTOR 1 BETA) gene are responsible for **nail-patella syndrome**, which is characterized by skeletal anomalies and glomerular dysfunction.

LMX1B expression is involved in transcriptional regulation of COLLAGEN TYPE α3(IV) (or GOODPASTURE ANTIGEN), COLLAGEN TYPE α4(IV), and NPHS2 genes; it thus links together nail-patella syndrome, Alport, and congenital nephritic syndrome (caused by mutation in the NPHS1 gene).

CONGENITAL POLYCYSTIC KIDNEY DISEASE

Autosomal dominant polycystic kidney disease (ADPKD) is a common genetic disease associated with formation of cysts in the kidneys as well as in ductal epithelia in the liver, pancreas, testis, and ovary. Mutations in the genes encoding POLYCYSTIN1 (PDK1) and POLYCYSTIN2 (PDK2) account for 85% and 15% of ADPKD, respectively. The precise roles of the POLYCYSTIN1 and POLYCYSTIN2 proteins have not yet been elucidated. However, POLYCYSTIN1 seems to be required for normal elongation and maturation of tubular structures during renal development. It may also function as a mechanosensory channel in primary cilia. These functions may be related to the ability of PDK1 to modulate Wnt signaling by stabilizing endogenous β-catenin levels and altering β-catenin/Tcf-dependent gene expression.

Autosomal recessive polycystic kidney disease (AR-PKD) is associated with genes involved in mediating ciliary function. ARPKD is caused by mutations in the PKHD1 gene, which encodes the protein POLYDUCTIN (also called FIBROCYSTIN). This protein is necessary for the proper assembly and function of cilia. Patients in whom the gene is mutated slowly develop renal, hepatic, and biliary cysts. Mutations in HNFβ1 and TG737/POLARIS, two other genes with ties to ciliary assembly and function, are also associated with polycystic kidney disease. The role that cilia have in maintaining normal renal, hepatic, and biliary structures is unclear.

RELOCATION OF KIDNEYS

Between the sixth and ninth weeks, the kidneys relocate to a lumbar site just below the suprarenal glands, following a path just on either side of the dorsal aorta (Fig. 15-10). The mechanism responsible for this upward (cranial) relocation is not understood, although differential growth of the lumbar and sacral regions of the embryo may play a role. As covered in Chapter 13, the relocating kidney is progressively revascularized by a series of arterial sprouts from the dorsal aorta (see Fig. 13-16), and the original renal artery in the sacral region disappears. The right kidney usually does not rise as high as the left kidney because of the presence of the liver on the right side, although this is not always the case.

Several anomalies can arise from variations in this relocation process. Occasionally, one or more of the transient inferior renal arteries fail to regress, resulting in the

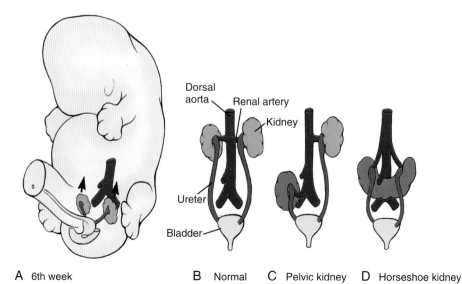

Figure 15-10. Normal and abnormal relocation of the kidneys. *A, B,* The metanephroi normally relocate from the sacral region to their definitive lumbar position between the sixth and ninth weeks. *C,* Infrequently, a kidney may fail to relocate, resulting in a pelvic kidney (colored blue). *D,* If the inferior poles of the metanephroi make contact and fuse before relocation, the resulting horseshoe kidney (colored blue) catches under the inferior mesenteric artery.

A 6th week

B Normal   C Pelvic kidney   D Horseshoe kidney

presence of **accessory renal arteries**. Rarely, a kidney completely fails to relocate, remaining as a **pelvic kidney** (Fig. 15-10C). The inferior poles of the two metanephroi may fuse during relocation, forming a U-shaped **horseshoe kidney** (prevalence in humans is approximately 1:1000). Horseshoe kidneys cross over the anterior (ventral) side of the aorta, and one long-standing theory is that during relocation, this kidney becomes caught under the inferior mesenteric artery and, therefore, does not reach its normal site (Fig. 15-10D). Recent studies in mice suggest Shh, released from the notochord, plays a key role in regulating correct mediolateral kidney positioning, as loss of axial Shh results in fusion of the two kidneys.

CONTRIBUTIONS OF HINDGUT ENDODERM TO URINARY TRACT

 Animation 15-2: Development of Urogenital Sinus. Animations are available online at StudentConsult.

As covered in Chapter 14, the cloacal region of the hindgut is partitioned by the urorectal septum into a ventral **urogenital sinus** and a dorsal **anorectal canal** (Fig. 15-11; see also Fig. 14-31). The urogenital sinus forms the presumptive **bladder** (however, as mentioned in Chapter 14, recent studies suggest that the bladder forms from an expansion of the lower allantois), a narrow neck that forms the **membranous** and **prostatic urethra** in males and membranous urethra in females, and a

phallic segment that expands beneath the growing **genital tubercle** (see Fig 15-11). In males, the phallic segment contributes to the **penile urethra**, and in females it contributes to the **vestibule of the vagina** (covered in Chapter 16).

Concurrently with the septation of the cloaca, the caudal ends of the mesonephric ducts and attached ureteric ducts become incorporated into the posterior wall of the presumptive bladder (Fig. 15-12). This process begins as the mouths of the mesonephric ducts flare into a pair of trumpet-shaped structures that begin to expand, flatten, and blend into the bladder wall. The cranial portion of this trumpet expands and flattens more rapidly than the caudal part so that the mouth of the narrow portion of the mesonephric duct appears to migrate caudally along the posterior bladder wall. This process incorporates the caudal end of the ureters into the wall of the bladder and causes the mouths of the narrow part of the mesonephric ducts to migrate caudally until they open into the pelvic urethra just below the neck of the bladder. This triangular area of the mesonephric duct on the posteroinferior wall of the bladder is called the **trigone** of the bladder. The mesodermal tissue of the trigone is later overgrown by endoderm from the surrounding bladder wall, but the structure remains visible in the adult bladder as a smooth triangular region lying between the openings of the ureters, laterally and superiorly, and the opening of the pelvic urethra, inferiorly. Splanchnic mesoderm associated with the hindgut forms the smooth muscle of the bladder wall in the twelfth week.

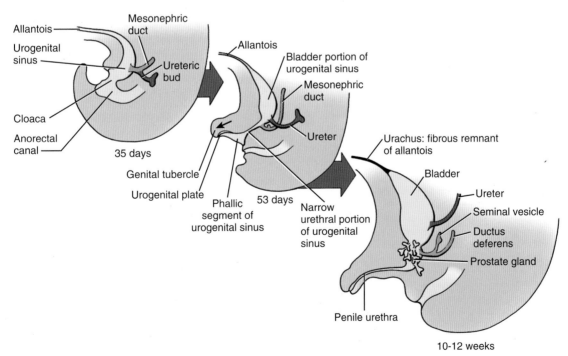

Figure 15-11. Development of the urogenital sinus. Between weeks four and six, the urorectal septum divides the cloaca into a ventral urogenital sinus and a dorsal anorectum. The urogenital sinus is subdivided into the presumptive bladder, a narrow urethral region, and a phallic segment. The narrow urethral portion at the base of the future bladder forms the membranous urethra in females, and the membranous and prostatic urethra in males. The phallic portion of the urogenital sinus forms the vestibule of the vagina in females, and the penile urethra in males. Normally, the allantois becomes occluded to form the urachus (or median umbilical ligament) of the adult.

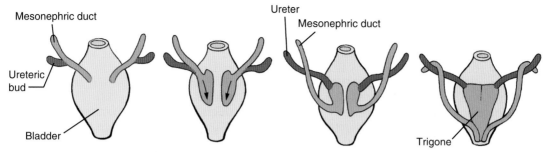

Figure 15-12. Incorporation of the mesonephric ducts and ureters into the bladder wall. Between weeks four and six, the root of the mesonephric duct is incorporated into the posterior wall of the developing bladder. This process brings the openings of the ureteric buds into the bladder wall, whereas the openings of the mesonephric duct are carried inferiorly to the level of the pelvic urethra. The triangular region of the incorporated mesonephric ducts into the posterior bladder wall forms the trigone of the bladder.

In the Clinic

URINARY TRACT ANOMALIES

About 1% of all newborns have a developmental abnormality of the urinary tract. Most of these anomalies do not cause clinical problems. However, about 45% of all cases of childhood renal failure result from anomalous development of the ureteric bud or metanephric mesenchyme. Development of each of these rudiments is dependent on inductive signals from the other. Thus, abnormalities in one rudiment often result in abnormal development of the other.

Duplicated Ureter

The ureteric bud normally does not bifurcate until it enters the substance of the metanephric mesenchyme. However, it occasionally bifurcates prematurely, resulting in a Y-shaped **bifid ureter** (Fig. 15-13). The undivided caudal end of the ureter attaches normally to the bladder. Typically, the branch attached to the kidney's caudal pole drains most of the kidney. One of the branches occasionally ends blindly. A bifid ureter is often, but not always, asymptomatic. Although the two branches of the Y arise from the same ureteric bud, the contractions of their muscular walls seem to be asynchronous. Therefore, urine may reflux from one branch into the other, resulting in stagnation of urine and predisposing the individual to infections of the ureter.

Occasionally, a mesonephric duct sprouts two ureteric buds, which penetrate the metanephric mesenchyme independently (Fig. 15-14). The more cranial bud induces formation of the cranial pole of the kidney, and the caudal bud induces formation of the caudal pole. As the mesonephric duct opens into the posterior wall of the bladder, the caudal ureteric bud is incorporated into the bladder wall in the normal manner. However, the cranial ureteric bud is carried caudally along with the descending mesonephric duct and may form its final connection with any derivative of the caudal mesonephric duct, pelvic urethra, or urogenital sinus (see Fig. 15-14). The caudal ureteric bud thus forms a normal, or **orthotopic**, ureter connected to the bladder, whereas the cranial bud forms a caudal **ectopic** ureter. Because the normal ureter drains the caudal pole of the kidney and the ectopic ureter drains the cranial pole, the two ureters cross each other. This crossing of the normal and ectopic ureters is called the **Weigert-Meyer rule**.

In males, an ectopic ureter may drain into the prostatic urethra, the ejaculatory duct, the vas deferens, or the seminal vesicle. These ectopic ureters thus always open superior to the sphincter urethra muscle and do not result in incontinence, although they may cause painful urination or recurrent infections. In females, ectopic ureters often connect to the vestibule, the vagina (see Fig. 15-14), or, less often, the uterus. These **extrasphincteric outlets** of the ectopic ureter result in con-

tinuous dribbling of urine unless surgically corrected. Anomalous insertion of the ureter within the bladder can also be a problem because the valve mechanism for preventing reflux of urine to the kidney fails to develop. Reflux predisposes individuals to urinary tract infection.

EXSTROPHY OF BLADDER AND ASSOCIATED ABDOMINAL WALL DEFECTS

In a series of abnormalities ranging from **epispadias** (the urethral opening is on the dorsum of the genital tubercle rather than on its ventral side; covered in Chapter 16) to **exstrophy of the bladder** or **cloaca**, hindgut structures can remain open to the anterior surface of the body through a defect in the anterior body wall. In exstrophy of the bladder, the bladder is revealed by an abdominal wall defect; in exstrophy of the cloaca, the lumens of both the bladder and the anorectal canal are exposed. The abdominal wall defect in these conditions may be a secondary effect of anomalous development of the cloacal membrane. According to one idea, the primary defect is that the cloacal membrane is abnormally large so that when it breaks down, it produces an opening too wide to permit normal midline fusion of the tissue layers on either side of it. An alternative theory posits an inability to reduce the size of the cloacal membrane at its superior and lateral sides because of insufficient tissue proliferation and migration in the infraumbilical region. Coupled with the membrane's subsequent rupture, this could also lead to exstrophy of the bladder, epispadias, or cloacal exstrophy depending on the degree and timing of the deficiencies. Epispadias may also arise if the genital tubercle develops from the urorectal septum rather than from mesoderm adjacent to the phallic segment of the urogenital sinus. Exstrophy of the bladder with epispadias is the most common anomaly of those discussed in this section, occurring in approximately 1 of 40,000 births. Exstrophy of the cloaca is much less frequent, occurring in about 1 of 200,000 births. All these malformations are about twice as common in males as in females.

URACHAL ANOMALIES

Normally, the allantois and the superior end of the presumptive bladder undergo regression between the fourth and sixth weeks, at the same time that the urorectal septum partitions the cloaca into the urogenital sinus and a dorsal anorectal canal. The allantois and the constricted bladder apex are transformed into a ligamentous band, the **urachus** or **median umbilical ligament**, which runs through the subperitoneal fat from the bladder to the umbilicus (see Fig. 15-11). This band is about 5 cm long and 1 cm wide in the adult.

In a very small number of individuals, part of or the entire allantois and bladder apex remains patent, resulting in a **patent urachus (urachal fistula), umbilical urachal sinus,**

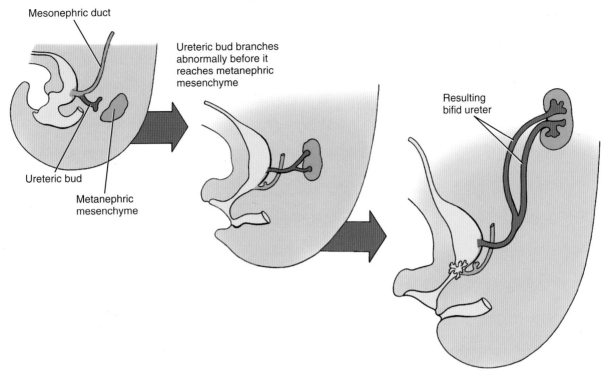

Figure 15-13. Formation of a bifid ureter. A bifid ureter forms when the ureteric bud bifurcates before entering the metanephric mesenchyme.

Labels: Mesonephric duct; Ureteric bud branches abnormally before it reaches metanephric mesenchyme; Ureteric bud; Metanephric mesenchyme; Resulting bifid ureter

vesicourachal diverticulum, or **urachal cyst** (Fig. 15-15). Symptoms include leakage of urine from the umbilicus, urinary tract infections, and peritonitis resulting from perforation of the patent urachus. These conditions may be life threatening. The initial symptoms of infection, as with Meckel's diverticulum, are easily confused with those of appendicitis.

DEFECTIVE PARTITIONING OF CLOACA

As covered in Chapter 14, partitioning of the cloaca by the urorectal septum into the urogenital sinus and anorectal canal is a complicated process that still is not well understood. In as many as 1 of 5000 infants, this partitioning is incomplete. Depending on the location and size of the defect, a wide range of malformations involving cloacal derivatives and their connections with the ureters and genital ducts may result. A few of the more common examples are described in the following text.

Fistulas and Anorectal Malformations

If the urorectal septum fails to separate the cloaca into a urogenital sinus and anorectal canal, or if the cloaca membrane is too small, the result may be development of various fistulas between the urethra and anorectal canal (Fig. 15-16). In males, these connections usually take the form of a narrow **rectoprostatic urethral fistula** connecting the rectum to the prostatic urethra (Fig. 15-16C) or a **rectourethral fistula** connecting the prostatic urethra to the lower anal canal (Fig 15-16D). In the latter situation, the penile urethra and the anal canal empty through their normal channels, but the penile urethra is frequently stenotic, causing urine to exit preferentially through a rectourethral fistula and out the anorectal canal. In females, the situation is complicated by the presence of the paramesonephric ducts. Most often, the paramesonephric ducts attach to the pelvic urethra just cranial to the rectourethral fistula. The caudal undivided region of the cloaca thus becomes a common outlet for the urethra, the vagina, and the rectum and is called a **rectocloacal canal** (Fig. 15-16E). Occasionally, the uterovaginal

canal incorporates the rectourethral fistula while moving to a more caudal position on the posterior wall of the cloaca. In these cases, the vagina and urethra open separately into the vestibule, but the rectum communicates with the vagina through a **rectovaginal fistula** (Fig. 15-16F). This fistula may be located high or low in the vagina. When the fistula is located low at the vaginal-cloacal junction, the resulting **rectovestibular fistula** opens into the vestibule of the vagina.

An abnormal communication between the rectum and bladder, called a **rectovesical fistula** (Fig. 15-17), can also form if development of the urorectal septum is insufficient. In females, this anomaly may interfere with the normal fusion of the inferior ends of the paramesonephric ducts, resulting in separate bilateral vaginas and uteri that empty directly into the bladder.

DEVELOPMENT OF SUPRARENAL GLAND

The **suprarenal (adrenal) gland** is a crucial component of the hypothalamic-pituitary-suprarenal axis that is responsible for coordinating mammalian stress response and metabolism. Initially, formation of the suprarenal gland is closely tied to that of the gonads, as both arise from a common region of intermediate mesoderm lying adjacent to the developing kidney. Segregation of the suprarenal and gonadal primordia occurs when primordial germ cells enter the gonadal region. By the ninth week, the suprarenal primordia are completely enclosed by a capsule. As might be expected, the specification of the suprarenal primordia depends on many of the same transcription factors and signaling molecules as those involved in kidney and gonadal development (e.g., Wt1, Wnt4).

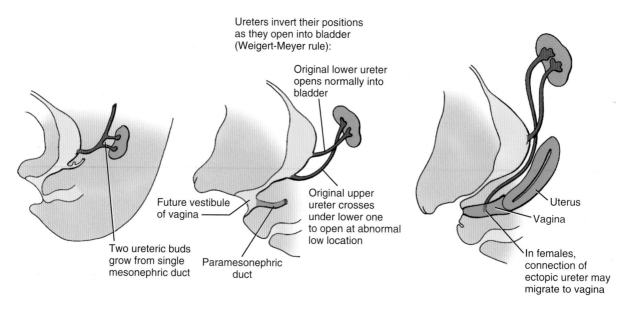

Figure 15-14. Formation of an ectopic ureter. An ectopic ureter forms from an anomalous "extra" ureteric bud. The mechanisms of formation of the trigone and placement of the vas deferens and ureters on the posterior wall of the primitive urogenital sinus were deduced largely from the Weigert-Meyer rule (see text).

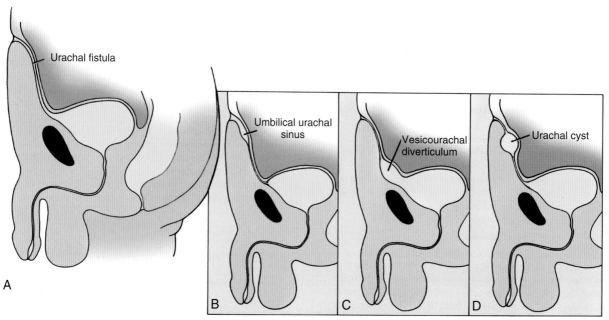

Figure 15-15. Fate of the allantois. Normally, the allantois becomes occluded to form the urachus or median umbilical ligament of the adult. Very rarely, parts of the allantois may remain patent, producing urachal fistula (*A*), umbilical urachal sinus (*B*), vesicourachal diverticulum (*C*), or urachal cyst (*D*).

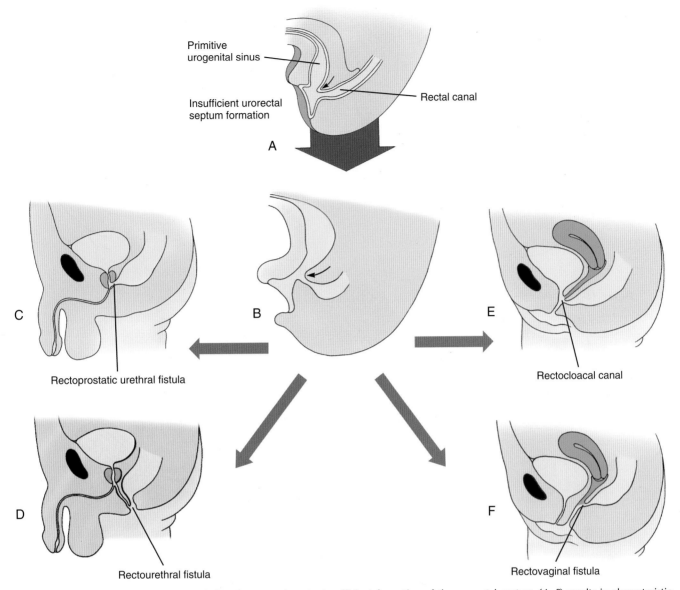

Figure 15-16. Anomalies of the urogenital and anorectal tracts. Insufficient formation of the urorectal septum (*A, B*) results in characteristic anomalous development in males and females: rectoprostatic urethral fistula (*C*), rectourethral fistula (*D*), rectocloacal fistula (*E*), rectovaginal fistula (*F*).

During the fifth week of development, the coelomic epithelium adjacent to the developing gonadal ridge proliferates, and a subset of these cells delaminates and enters the underlying mesoderm (Fig. 15-18). These delaminating cells differentiate into large acidophilic cells, forming the **fetal suprarenal cortical cells**. A second wave of delaminating cells subsequently migrates, proliferates, and forms a thinner **definitive cortex** that almost completely surrounds the fetal cortex. Ultrastructurally, cells of both fetal and definitive cortical layers exhibit cytologic characteristics of steroid-producing cells. During the second trimester, the fetal cortical layer grows rapidly in size and begins to secrete **dehydroepiandrosterone (DHEA)**, a hormone converted by the placenta to **estradiol**, which is essential for maintaining pregnancy.

Moreover, products from the fetal suprarenal cortex influence the maturation of the lungs, liver, and digestive tract and may regulate **parturition**. By the second postnatal month, much of the fetal cortex rapidly regresses and the remaining definitive cortical cells then organize into the **zona glomerulosa, zona fasciculata**, and **zona reticularis** layers seen in the adult suprarenal gland.

Before being cordoned off by formation of the suprarenal capsule, neural crest cells migrate into the suprarenal medullary region adjacent to the developing fetal cortex. These neural crest cells differentiate into **chromaffin cells**, which are specialized postganglionic sympathetic neurons innervated by preganglionic sympathetic fibers that release epinephrine and norepinephrine upon sympathetic stimulation.

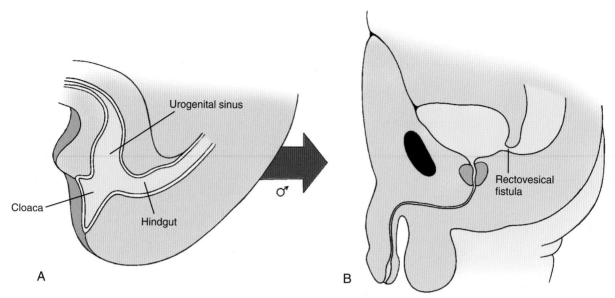

Figure 15-17. Development of a rectovesical fistula. *A, B,* The urorectal septum fails to descend toward the cloacal membrane.

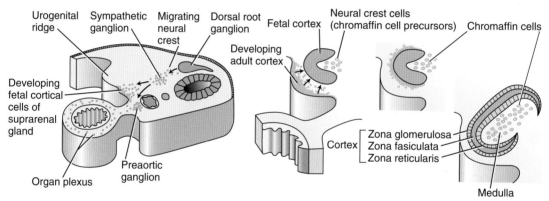

Figure 15-18. Suprarenal gland development. During the fifth week of development, the coelomic epithelium adjacent to the developing gonadal ridge proliferates, and a subset of cells delaminates and enters the underlying mesoderm, forming the fetal suprarenal cortical cells. A second wave of delaminating cells migrates and forms a thinner definitive cortex surrounding the fetal cortex. By the second postnatal month, much of the fetal cortex rapidly regresses and the remaining definitive cortical cells organize into the zona glomerulosa, zona fasciculata, and zona reticularis layers seen in the adult suprarenal gland. Before they are cordoned off by the forming suprarenal capsule, neural crest cells migrate into the medullary region and differentiate into chromaffin cells.

In the Clinic

CONGENITAL ADRENAL HYPERPLASIA

Congenital adrenal (suprarenal) hyperplasia (CAH) is usually caused by a genetically determined deficiency of the suprarenal cortical enzymes necessary for the synthesis of **glucocorticoids**. This deficiency leads to **adrenocorticotropic hormone**–driven hyperplasia of the suprarenal cortex. The most common form of CAH (an incidence of 1:15,000 live births) results from a deficiency in 21-HYDROXYLASE (encoded by the CYP21A2 gene). This deficiency causes a reduction in cortisol production by the suprarenal cortex, resulting in an accumulation of 17-hydroxyprogesterone that, in turn, results in suprarenal

hyperplasia and excess production of suprarenal androgens (these are negatively regulated by the presence of cortisol). Excessive levels of suprarenal androgens masculinize the external genitalia of XX individuals during their in utero development (covered in Chapter 16; see Fig. 6-16 in Chapter 6). During childhood, excessive levels of suprarenal androgens accelerate skeletal maturation. In the salt-wasting form of 21-HYDROXYLASE deficiency, insufficient aldosterone secretion can lead to life-threatening **hyponatremia** (low blood sodium).

Mutations in the DAX1 gene (covered in Chapter 16 with respect to gonadal development) can also lead to CAH. These patients (most often males) exhibit suprarenal insufficiency, skin hyperpigmentation, and delayed puberty.

Embryology in Practice

URINE TROUBLE

A child is born after a thirty-eight-week gestation and is found to have an **imperforate anus** and **ambiguous genitalia**. On physical examination, there is a phallus-like structure without clear urethral or vaginal openings, and there is a lack of scrotal or labial tissues. The umbilical cord is somewhat broad. The remainder of the examination is normal, including the appearance of the abdominal wall. The infant is admitted to the neonatal intensive care unit, and surgery to create an intestinal ostomy is planned for the following morning.

The diagnosis of **urorectal septum malformation sequence** is proposed, and concerns about the kidneys and lungs are raised. The argument is made that, although not obvious on examination, a urethral opening must be present, or else the infant would have been born with **oligohydramnios** and **lung hypoplasia (Potter sequence)**, but this infant is crying and stable on room air.

After twelve hours, the child still has not voided, and examination suggests that the bladder is becoming distended. The staff remains unable to identify a urethral opening, so a percutaneous bladder catheterization is performed, yielding a large volume of urine.

Further discussion among the delivery room staff reveals that a serous fluid appeared to be seeping out of the cord after it was clamped, and this was interpreted as cord edema. The cord was re-clamped nearer the abdominal wall, and the drainage subsided.

It becomes clear that this fluid was urine coming from a patent **urachus**. Cross clamping this omphalomesenteric remnant resulted in the observed bladder distention. If not for the percutaneous drainage of the bladder, this would have led, in turn, to renal dilation and eventually to permanent kidney damage.

Normally the urorectal septum divides the cloaca into urogenital and rectal cavities after the cloacal membrane breaks down, creating the rectal and urogenital openings. When this process fails or is incomplete, persistence of the cloaca with complete or partial persistence of the cloacal membrane results in imperforate anus, absent urethral or vaginal openings, and ambiguous genitalia. Children with these urorectal septum malformations usually succumb to lung hypoplasia and kidney dysfunction in the neonatal period. In the case of this rare survivor, a ruptured patent urachus allowed normal kidney and lung development.

A chromosome study showed a normal 46,XX karyotype. The girl had an excellent outcome after multiple surgeries to repair her urogenital anomalies.

Potter sequence can have multiple causes. Other clinical scenarios that result in this sequence are given in the "Clinical Taster" for this chapter and for Chapter 6.

SUGGESTED READINGS

Costantini F, Kopan R. 2010. Patterning a complex organ: branching morphogenesis and nephron segmentation in kidney development. Dev Cell 18:698–712.

Dressler GR. 2009. Advances in early kidney specification, development and patterning. Development 136:3863–3874.

Kluth D. 2010. Embryology of anorectal malformations. Semin Pediatr Surg 19:201–208.

Little MH, Brennan J, Georgas K, et al. 2007. A high-resolution anatomical ontology of the developing murine genitourinary tract. Gene Expr Patterns 7:680–699.

Uetani N, Bouchard M. 2009. Plumbing in the embryo: developmental defects of the urinary tracts. Clin Genet 75:307–317.

van der Putte SC. 2005. The development of the perineum in the human. A comprehensive histological study with a special reference to the role of the stromal components. Adv Anat Embryol Cell Biol 177:1–131.

Chapter 16

Development of the Reproductive System

SUMMARY

The development of the **reproductive system** is closely integrated with the primitive urinary organs in both males and females, as they share similar common tubular structures enabling both uresis and gamete transport. In addition to the nephric structures, the **intermediate mesoderm** on both sides of the dorsal body wall gives rise to a gonadal ridge. By the sixth week, the **germ cells** migrating from the yolk sac begin to arrive in the mesenchyme of the dorsal body wall. The arrival of germ cells in the area just medial to the mesonephroi at the tenth thoracic segment induces the coelomic epithelium to generate **somatic support cells** that invest the germ cells. Somatic support cells will differentiate into **Sertoli cells** in the male and **follicle cells** (or granulosa cells) in the female. During the same period, a new pair of ducts, the **paramesonephric (Müllerian) ducts**, form in the dorsal body wall from coelomic epithelium just lateral to the mesonephric ducts.

The sexual differentiation of genetic males begins at the end of the sixth week, when a specific gene on the Y chromosome (SRY) is expressed in the somatic support cells. Embryos in which this gene is not expressed develop as females. The product of this gene, called the **SRY protein**, initiates a developmental cascade that leads to formation of the testes, the male genital ducts and associated glands, the male external genitalia, and the entire constellation of male secondary sex characteristics. The SRY protein exerts autonomous control of somatic support cell development into **pre-Sertoli cells**. Pre-Sertoli cells then recruit mesenchymal cells into the gonadal ridge, and these cells give rise to **Leydig cells** and testicular endothelial cells. Differentiating Sertoli cells then envelop the germ cells and together with the myoepithelial cells organize into **testis cords** (future **seminiferous tubules**). The deepest portions of the somatic support cells in the developing gonad, which do not contain germ cells, differentiate into the **rete testis**. The rete testis connects with a limited number of mesonephric tubules and canalizes at puberty to form conduits connecting the seminiferous tubules to the mesonephric duct. These nephric tubules become the **efferent ductules** of the testes, and the mesonephric ducts become the **epididymides** (singular, **epididymis**) and **vasa deferentia** (singular, **vas deferens**). The paramesonephric ducts degenerate. During the third month, the distal vas deferens sprouts the **seminal vesicle**, and the **prostate** and **bulbourethral glands** grow from the adjacent pelvic urethra. Simultaneously, the indifferent external genitalia (consisting of paired **urogenital** and **labioscrotal folds** on either side of the **urogenital plate** and an anterior **genital tubercle**) differentiate into the **penis** and **scrotum**. Late in fetal development, the testes descend into the scrotum through the **inguinal canals**.

Because genetic females lack a Y chromosome, they do not produce SRY protein. Hence, the somatic support cells do not form Sertoli cells but rather differentiate into follicle cells that surround the germ cells to form **primordial follicles** of the ovary. The mesonephric ducts degenerate, and the paramesonephric ducts become the genital ducts. The proximal portions of the paramesonephric ducts become the **Fallopian tubes** (or **oviducts**). Fusion of the distal portions of the ducts gives rise to the **uterus** and the **vagina**. The indifferent external genitalia develop into the female external genitalia: the **clitoris** and the paired **labia majora** and **minora**.

Clinical Taster

A couple, expecting a boy based on prenatal ultrasound, is surprised when told by the delivery room nurse that they, instead, have a baby girl. Then some confusion seems to ensue among the caregivers. Later, a doctor from the nursery arrives and informs the family that their child has "ambiguous genitalia," with an enlarged clitoris that was likely confused with a penis on the ultrasound. She tells them that the genitals look more like a girl's than a boy's, with a separate urethra and vagina, but that there is partial fusion of the labia with what may be testes being palpable in the groin area. She explains that further testing will be needed to determine the infant's sex.

The family is visited by several doctors over the next two days, including specialists in urology, endocrinology, and genetics. They hear, variously, that the child should be "thought of as a girl," or that the child is "a boy but may need to be raised as a girl." They hear terms that are new to them, like "intersex" and "undervirilized." A battery of tests is done. These include laboratory tests on blood that show normal testosterone and luteinizing hormone levels and an ultrasound that shows no cervix, uterus, or Fallopian tubes. Gonads, likely testes, are found in the inguinal canal. Later in the week, they find out that their child has a "Y" chromosome (46,XY) and is, therefore, genetically, a boy. Further tests (such as measuring androgen response in skin fibroblasts) confirm the diagnosis of androgen insensitivity syndrome (AIS). Males with AIS (also known as testicular feminization) have mutations in the androgen receptor gene and are unable to respond appropriately to testosterone during development.

Options for sex assignment are presented to the baby's parents. One is male sex assignment. Although this choice

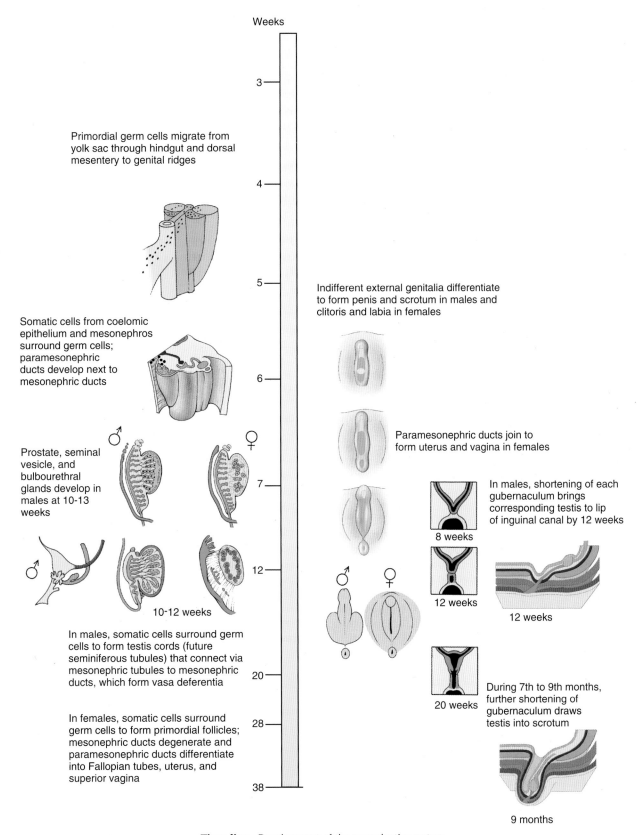

Weeks

Primordial germ cells migrate from yolk sac through hindgut and dorsal mesentery to genital ridges

Somatic cells from coelomic epithelium and mesonephros surround germ cells; paramesonephric ducts develop next to mesonephric ducts

Prostate, seminal vesicle, and bulbourethral glands develop in males at 10-13 weeks

10-12 weeks

In males, somatic cells surround germ cells to form testis cords (future seminiferous tubules) that connect via mesonephric tubules to mesonephric ducts, which form vasa deferentia

In females, somatic cells surround germ cells to form primordial follicles; mesonephric ducts degenerate and paramesonephric ducts differentiate into Fallopian tubes, uterus, and superior vagina

Indifferent external genitalia differentiate to form penis and scrotum in males and clitoris and labia in females

Paramesonephric ducts join to form uterus and vagina in females

8 weeks

12 weeks

20 weeks

In males, shortening of each gubernaculum brings corresponding testis to lip of inguinal canal by 12 weeks

12 weeks

During 7th to 9th months, further shortening of gubernaculum draws testis into scrotum

9 months

Time line. Development of the reproductive system.

would be consistent with the karyotype, it would involve multiple surgeries in childhood and adolescence, along with testosterone treatment (the response to androgens usually is not completely absent). Another would be female sex assignment, which involves estrogen therapy along with surgery in childhood or puberty to remove the gonads, enlarge the vaginal opening, and reduce the size of the clitoris. With either option, there is the risk that the child will be uncomfortable with gender identity later in life. Given all the uncertainties, the parents find it difficult to commit to a gender assignment and decide on a third option: to make a temporary assignment of female, but to wait to consider surgery until the child is old enough to make her own decisions.

REPRODUCTIVE SYSTEM ARISES WITH URINARY SYSTEM

Animation 16-1: Development of Gonadal Ridges.
Animations are available online at StudentConsult.

Sex determination and manifestation begin with genetic sex determination (i.e., 46,XX or 46,XY), which occurs at fertilization (covered in Chapter 1). The sexual genotype is responsible for directing gonadal development (i.e., testis versus ovary). This in turn directs reproductive tract (internal organs) and external genitalia development. Genotypic, gonadal, and phenotypic sex assignments may be discordant. Although steady progress has been made in our understanding of the molecular and developmental mechanisms responsible for sex determination and genital development, approximately 75% of the genetic alterations responsible for human sex reversal are still unresolved.

In individuals of both sexes, formation and differentiation of the gonads begin with the arrival of primordial germ cells in the intermediate mesoderm. As discussed in Chapter 1, primordial germ cells normally migrate from the yolk sac via the dorsal mesentery to populate the mesenchyme of the posterior body wall in an area near the tenth thoracic level during the fifth week (Fig. 16-1*A*). There, they move to the area adjacent to the coelomic epithelia, located just medial and ventral to the developing mesonephric kidneys. In response, the coelomic epithelia proliferate, thicken, and, together with the primordial germ cells, form a pair of **genital ridges** (Figs. 16-1, 16-2).

During the sixth week, cells derived from each coelomic epithelium form somatic supporting cells (Fig. 16-1*D*) that then completely invest the germ cells. **Somatic support cells** are essential for germ cell development within the gonad; if these cells do not invest the germ cells, the germ cells degenerate. After the sixth week, these somatic support cells pursue different fates in males and females.

Also during the sixth week, a new pair of ducts, the **paramesonephric ducts** (or **Müllerian ducts**), begin to form just lateral to the mesonephric ducts in both male and female embryos (see Fig. 16-1*B-D*). These ducts arise by the craniocaudal invagination of a ribbon of thickened proliferating coelomic epithelial cells extending from the third thoracic segment caudally to the posterior wall of the urogenital sinus. The caudal tips of the paramesonephric ducts then grow to connect with the developing pelvic urethra just medial to the openings of the right and left mesonephric ducts. The caudal tips of the two paramesonephric ducts adhere to each other just before they contact the developing pelvic urethra. The cranial ends of the paramesonephric ducts form funnel-shaped openings into the coelom. The further development of the paramesonephric ducts in the female is covered later in the chapter.

At the end of the sixth week, the male and female genital systems are indistinguishable in appearance, although subtle cellular differences may already be present. In both sexes, germ cells and somatic support cells are present in the presumptive gonads, and complete mesonephric and paramesonephric ducts lie side by side. The **ambisexual** or **bipotential phase** of genital development ends at this point. From the seventh week on, the male and female systems pursue diverging pathways. Table 16-1 lists the homologous male and female adult reproductive cells and organs derived from these embryonic progenitors.

IN PRESENCE OF Y CHROMOSOME, MALE DEVELOPMENT OCCURS

As detailed in Chapter 1, genetic females have two X sex chromosomes, whereas genetic males have an X and a Y sex chromosome. Although the pattern of sex chromosomes determines the choice between male and female developmental paths, the subsequent phases of sexual development are controlled not only by sex chromosome genes but also by hormones and other factors, most of which are encoded on **autosomes**.

A single sex-determining factor seems to control a cascade of events leading to male development. This sex-determining transcription factor is encoded by the **SRY (SEX-DETERMINING REGION OF THE Y CHROMOSOME)** gene. When this transcription factor is expressed in the somatic support cells of the indifferent presumptive gonad, male development is triggered. This step is called **primary sex determination**. If the factor is absent or defective, female development occurs (Fig. 16-3). Thus, femaleness has been described as the basic developmental path for the human embryo. However, it should be emphasized that claiming that ovarian development and femaleness is a passive (i.e., default), rather than active, process, is a gross oversimplification (covered later in the chapter).

MALE GENITAL DEVELOPMENT BEGINS WITH DIFFERENTIATION OF SERTOLI CELLS

Animation 16-2: Development of Testes.
Animations are available online at StudentConsult.

The first event in male genital development is the expression of SRY protein within the somatic support cells of the XY gonad (Figs. 16-3, 16-4). Under the influence of this factor, somatic support cells begin to differentiate into Sertoli cells and envelop the germ cells

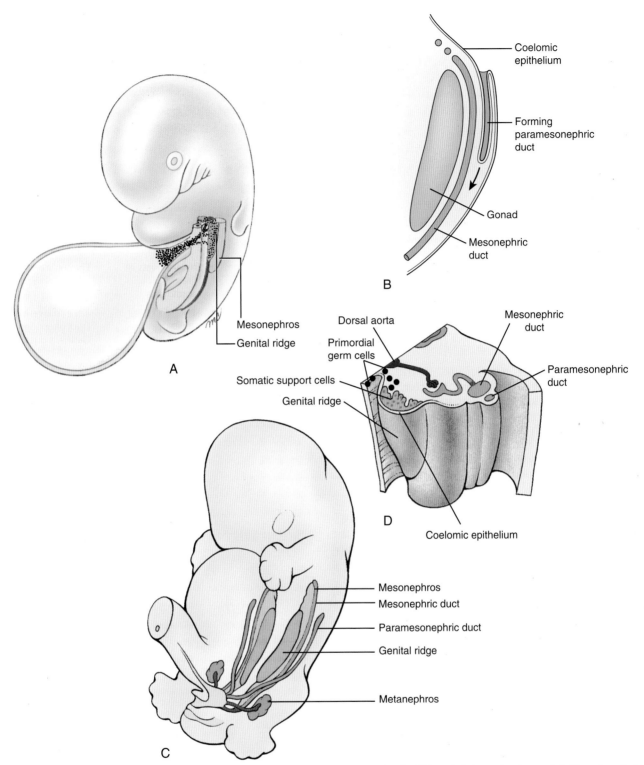

Figure 16-1. Formation of the genital ridges and paramesonephric ducts. *A, D,* During the fifth and sixth weeks, the genital ridges form in the posterior abdominal wall just medial to the developing mesonephroi in response to colonization by primordial germ cells (black dots) migrating from the yolk sac. *B,* Each paramesonephric duct develops from an invagination and proliferation of coelomic epithelial cells extending caudally (arrow) alongside and parallel to the mesonephric duct. *C,* The relationship of the mesonephric ducts and paramesonephric ducts to one another and to the developing gonads and kidneys. *D,* The primordial germ cells induce the coelomic epithelium lining the peritoneal cavity to proliferate and form the somatic support cells.

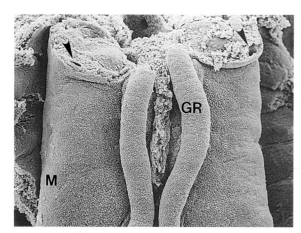

Figure 16-2. Scanning electron micrographs showing the relationship between the developing genital ridges (GR) and the mesonephroi (M). Arrowheads, mesonephric ducts seen in cross section.

TABLE 16-1 ADULT DERIVATIVES AND VESTIGIAL REMNANTS OF EMBRYONIC MALE AND FEMALE REPRODUCTIVE STRUCTURES

Presumptive Rudiments	Male Structure	Female Structure
Indifferent gonad	Testis	Ovary
Primordial germ cell	Spermatogonia	Oocytes
Somatic support cell	Sertoli cells	Follicle cells
Stromal cells	Leydig cells	Thecal cells
Gubernaculum	Gubernaculum testis	Round ligament of ovary Round ligament of uterus
Mesonephric tubules	Efferent ducts of testis Paradidymis	Epoöphoron-paroöphoron
Mesonephric duct	Appendix of epididymis Epididymis Vas deferens Seminal vesicle Ejaculatory duct	Appendix vesiculosa Duct of epoöphoron Gartner's duct
Paramesonephric ducts	Appendix of testis	Fallopian tubes Uterus Vagina
Urogenital sinus	Prostatic and membranous urethra Prostatic utricle Prostatic gland Bulbourethral glands	Membranous urethra Urethral/paraurethral glands Greater vestibular glands
Genital tubercle	Glans penis Corpus cavernosa of penis Corpus spongiosum of penis	Glans clitoris Corpus cavernosa of clitoris Bulbospongiosum of vestibule
Urogenital folds and urogenital and glans plate	Penile urethra/ventral part of penis	Labia minora
Labioscrotal folds	Scrotum	Labia majora

(Figs. 16-3, 16-5). If SRY is absent (i.e., in XX gonads), somatic support cells will differentiate into ovarian follicle cells that envelop the germ cells (see Figs. 16-3, 16-5).

SRY is a single-copy gene located on the Y chromosome. The SRY gene, a transcription factor, is activated only for a short period within gonadal somatic cells and likely upregulates testis-specific genes and represses ovarian genes (covered in the following "In the Research Lab" entitled "Sox9 Gene is Likely Target of SRY Expression"). SRY expression is first detected between days forty-one and forty-four postovulation and remains detectable there until day fifty-two.

During the seventh week, the differentiating Sertoli cells, together with interstitial cells of the gonad, organize to form **testis cords**, enclosing germ cells in the center of these cords (Figs. 16-3, 16-5, 16-6). The testis cords become canalized at puberty and differentiate into a system of **seminiferous tubules**. In the region adjacent to the mesonephros and devoid of germ cells, Sertoli cells organize into a set of thin-walled ducts called the **rete testis** (see Fig. 16-6). The rete testis, which connects the seminiferous tubules with a limited number of mesonephric tubules (future efferent ductules), canalizes at puberty to form a conduit connecting the seminiferous tubules to the mesonephric ducts. The mesonephric ducts later develop into the **epididymides** (singular, **epididymis**), **spermatic ducts** or **vasa deferentia** (singular, **vas deferens**), and **seminal vesicles** in the male (covered later).

During the seventh week, the testes begin to round up, reducing their area of contact with the mesonephros (see Figs. 16-3, 16-5, 16-6). As the testes continue to develop, the coelomic epithelium is separated from the testis cords by an intervening layer of connective tissue called the **tunica albuginea.**

DEVELOPMENT OF MALE GAMETES

Although the mechanism has not been elucidated, it is clear that direct cell-to-cell contact between Sertoli cells and primordial germ cells within the gonadal ridge plays a key role in the development of the male gametes. This interaction occurs shortly after the arrival of the primordial germ cells in the region of the presumptive genital ridge. It has the immediate effect of inhibiting further mitosis of the germ cells and preventing them from entering meiosis. No further development of the germ cells occurs until about three months postnatal, when they differentiate into type A spermatogonia. The remaining phases of male gametogenesis—further mitosis, differentiation into type B spermatogonia, meiosis, and spermatogenesis—are delayed until puberty (covered in Chapter 1).

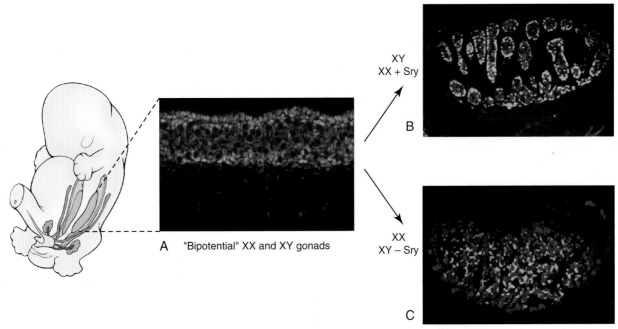

Figure 16-3. Primary sex determination of the bipotential gonads. *A,* Gonads are initially bipotent, but with expression of Sry, they take on a testis fate. *B,* In an XY mouse or XX mouse experimentally expressing Sry, the somatic support cells differentiate into Sertoli cells (green). Sertoli cells together with the germ cells (red) then organize testis cords. *C,* In the absence of Sry (XX or XY karyotype lacking the Sry gene), the somatic support cells differentiate into follicle cells (green) and surround oogonia (red) to form primordial follicles. The gonad then takes on an ovarian fate.

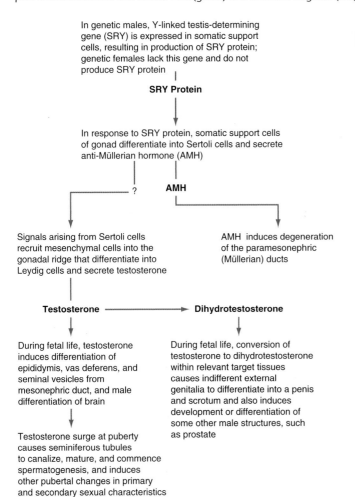

Figure 16-4. Summary of the differentiation cascade of male genital system development.

In the Research Lab

SOX9 GENE IS LIKELY PRIMARY TARGET OF SRY EXPRESSION

Much of what we have learned regarding the molecular and cellular mechanisms involved in gonad development stems from analyses of mouse mutants and **genotype-phenotype correlations** with humans who have disorders in sex development. Several genes are required for the early formation of the indifferent gonad, including Wt1, steroidogenic factor-1 (Sf1; also known as Nr5a1), Emx2, Lim homeobox protein-9 (Lhx9), and Gata-binding protein-4 (Gata4). Several of these genes, in addition to being necessary for initial formation of the indifferent gonad, are required for subsequent expression of Sry and Sry-targeted genes (Fig. 16-7). For instance, mutations in WT1 and SF1 in humans result in malformed gonads and ambiguous genitalia.

Although the Sry gene is instrumental in sex determination, Sry-specific target genes still have not been identified. The Sry protein binds to minor grooves in DNA via its HMG box motif, and this induces DNA bending and conformational changes that expose binding sites for several other transcriptional regulators. This makes it difficult to identify particular targets of Sry specifically involved in driving sex determination.

The Sox9 (Sry-related HMG box-9) gene seems to be one key target of Sry expression. In the indifferent gonad, Sox9 is weakly expressed in both XX and XY mouse embryos. In XY mice, Sox9 is upregulated just after the expression of Sry in pre-Sertoli cells (Figs. 16-7, 16-8*A*, 16-9). XY mice with a conditional knockout for Sox9 lack testis cords, do not form Sertoli cells, and express female-specific markers within the gonad. Upregulation of Sox9 expression in XX gonads can also lead to testicular development. Humans with heterozygotic mutations inactivating SOX9 develop **campomelic dysplasia** (a severe limb long-bone defect covered in Chapter 8; Sox9 has an important role in cartilage development, which is also covered in Chapter 8). Almost 75% of XY patients with campomelic

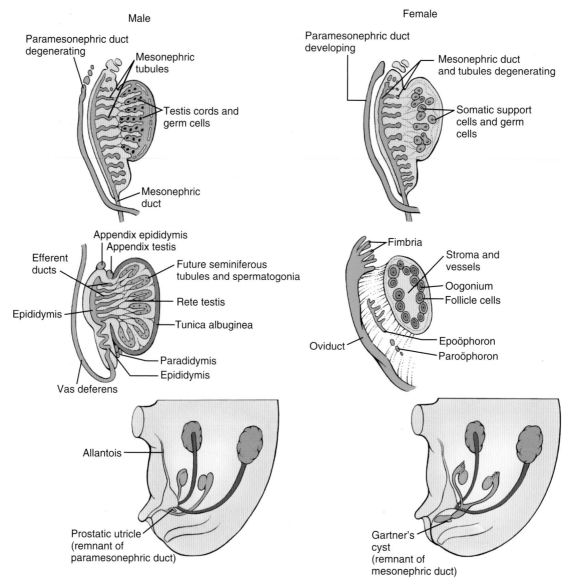

Figure 16-5. Comparison of human male and female gonadal development at the tissue level. The male and female genital systems are virtually identical through the seventh week. In the male, SRY protein causes the somatic support cells to differentiate into Sertoli cells. Sertoli cells, together with germ cells and myoepithelial precursor cells, then organize into testis cords and rete testis tubules. AMH produced by the Sertoli cells causes the paramesonephric ducts to regress. Leydig cells also develop, which in turn produce testosterone, the hormone that stimulates development of the male genital duct system. In the absence of SRY, the somatic support cells differentiate into follicle cells and surround the germ cells to form primordial follicles, Leydig cells do not develop, and the mesonephric duct degenerates, whereas the paramesonephric duct is retained, forming the female genital duct system.

dysplasia exhibit some degree of sex reversal (i.e., female development), whereas XX patients exhibiting campomelic dysplasia have normal gonads. Moreover, XX individuals with chromosomal duplications in the SOX9 gene develop as males. These observations strongly suggest that many SRY effects on sex determination are conveyed through activation of SOX9.

SERTOLI CELLS ARE MAIN ORGANIZERS OF TESTES

Primordial germ cells respond very differently to the gonadal environment depending on sex. Upon entering the gonad, primordial germ cells proliferate. In males, the primordial germ cells become surrounded by pre-Sertoli cells and enter mitotic arrest. In females, the primordial germ cells continue mitosis a bit longer and then enter meiosis and quickly arrest. These arrested meiotic germ cells apparently induce the differentiation of follicle cells because in their absence, follicle cells never form. Why germ

cells in males do not begin meiosis is unclear, but recent studies in mice suggest they are protected from the effects of retinoic acid generated within the mesonephros when surrounded by Sertoli cells (Sertoli cells express Cyp26b1, a gene coding for an enzyme that metabolizes retinoic acid). What directs male primordial germs cells into mitotic arrest is unknown but may include prostaglandin D2 (Pdg2) and the protein encoded by the Tdl gene (see Chapter 1).

Sertoli cells act as the main organizing center for testis development because they direct lineage specification and differentiation of other cells within the gonad. In mice, pre-Sertoli cells begin expressing Sry and are capable of initiating the recruitment of other non-Sry expressing cells into the Sertoli cell lineage. Pre-Sertoli cells produce Fgf9, which mediates Sertoli cell precursor proliferation and maintains Sox9 expression in these cells (covered later in the chapter), and Pgd2, which further

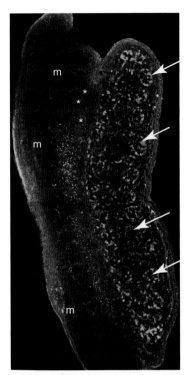

Figure 16-6. Development of the mouse testis showing morphogenesis of the testis cords. Developing testis cords (arrows) are demarcated by Sertoli cells (Sox9 expression in green) and outlined by basement membranes (red). Vascularization of the gonad (VE-cadherin, blue) also plays an important role in testis cord formation (see text). Basement membranes also demarcate the mesonephric duct (m) and mesonephric tubules (asterisks).

upregulates Sox9 expression; both of these reinforce male gonadal development through a positive autoregulatory feedback loop maintaining high Sox9 levels (see Figs. 16-7, 16-8).

What is the origin of the initial Sertoli cell population? Lineage-tracing studies in mice show that the earliest Sertoli cell precursors delaminate from the coelomic epithelium of the genital ridge, rather than arising from the mesonephric/gonadal ridge mesenchyme (although additional pre-Sertoli cells may be recruited from the mesonephros by pre-Sertoli cells within the gonadal ridge). Moreover, these experiments found that an unidentified interstitial cell population of unknown function also delaminates from the same epithelium. Studies suggest that these two epithelially derived lineages are set apart by differences in the degree of Sf1 expression. Sf1 encodes a nuclear hormone receptor protein and is expressed in the forming suprarenal gland and early somatic cells of both early XX and XY gonads. In XX mice, gonadal expression of Sf1 soon decreases, but in XY mice it is retained in early Sertoli and Leydig cells (where it promotes anti-Müllerian hormone production by Sertoli cells and testosterone production by Leydig cells). Studies in mice suggest that a proliferating, highly expressing Sf1 subset of coelomic epithelial cells delaminates first and that these cells give rise to pre-Sertoli cells (see Fig. 16-8A). In the absence of Sry, these delaminating cells do not differentiate into Sertoli cells but rather take on a follicle cell lineage (see Fig. 16-8B). Newly formed pre-Sertoli cells, now expressing Sry, Sox9, and Fgf9, then signal low Sf1-expressing coelomic epithelial cells to divide, delaminate, and generate interstitial cell precursors (see Fig. 16-8A). These results are consistent with observations showing that mutations in SF1 result in XY gonadal dysgenesis in humans and that

dose-dependent levels of Sf1 mediate temperature-dependent sex determination of the bipotential (indifferent) gonads in some vertebrates (e.g., in some reptiles and birds).

The coelomic epithelium is not the only source of cells within the developing gonad. Cells are recruited into the gonadal ridge from the mesonephros by signals emanating from Sf1-positive pre-Sertoli cells (the nature of which is unknown; see Figs. 16-7, 16-8A). These immigrating cells include endothelial cells and precursors for Leydig cells that are critical for gonadal development. At one time, precursors of myoepithelial cells were thought to be included in this immigrating group of cells, but recent studies show that they are not. Rather, myoepithelial precursor cells seem to be induced from within the testis stroma. However, organization of testis cords is dependent on endothelial cell immigration from the mesonephric mesenchyme, as perturbation of their migration and ability to form blood vessels blocks testis cord formation (see Fig. 16-9). The myoepithelial progenitors, together with the Sertoli cells and germ cells, then organize into epithelial testis cords.

ANTI-MÜLLERIAN HORMONE AND MALE GENITAL DEVELOPMENT

Animation 16-3: Development of Genital Ducts in Males.
Animations are available online at StudentConsult.

As pre-Sertoli cells begin their morphologic differentiation in response to Sry, they also begin secreting a glycoprotein hormone called **anti-Müllerian hormone (Amh)** or **Müllerian-inhibiting substance (Mis)**. Amh is a member of the Tgfβ family and is expressed specifically by Sertoli cells, beginning in humans at about week eight, causing the paramesonephric ducts to regress rapidly between the eighth and tenth weeks (see Figs. 16-4, 16-5, 16-8). Nevertheless, small paramesonephric duct remnants can be detected in the adult male, including a small cap of tissue associated with the testis, called the **appendix testis**, and an expansion of the prostatic urethra, called the **prostatic utricle** (see Fig. 16-5). In female embryos, as described later, the paramesonephric ducts do not regress.

In the Research Lab

PARAMESONEPHRIC DUCT REGRESSION REQUIRES MESENCHYMAL-EPITHELIAL INTERACTIONS

Amh signaling acts indirectly through interactions with the Amh receptor–type II receptor (Amhr-II; also known as Misr-II) on mesenchymal cells surrounding the paramesonephric duct, rather than directly on the epithelium of the duct (see Fig. 16-8A). Upon receptor activation, mesenchyme-to-epithelial signaling induces paramesonephric duct regression. Continual reciprocal epithelial-to-mesenchyme signaling is important for maintaining Amhr-II expression in the mesenchyme because, in the absence of Wnt7a expressing duct epithelium, Amhr-II expression is lost and paramesonephric derivatives are inappropriately retained in the male. AMH and AMHR-II gene mutations have been identified in human males and result in features typical of **persistent Müllerian duct syndrome** (covered below) including **cryptorchidism** (undescended testis) or ectopic testes with inguinal hernias.

Recently, another Amh receptor group, the Amh receptor–type I (Amhr-I) receptor group, has been identified based on Amh being a Tgfβ/Bmp family member. Studies have found Alk2,

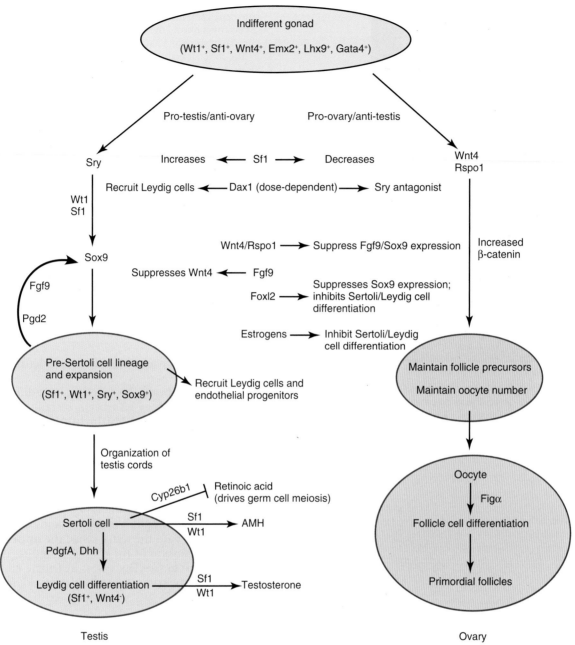

Figure 16-7. Comparison of male and female gonadal determination at the cellular and molecular levels. Expression of Sry gene in the indifferent gonad initiates a cascade of events that are "pro-testis," including initiating Sox9 and Fgf9 expression and increasing Sf1 expression. Female gonadal development is promoted by "pro-ovarian" and "anti-testes" factors, including Wnt4/Rspo1 and Foxl2. Dax1 expression can be "pro-testes" or "anti-testes" depending on dosage, but regardless, it is essential for normal testis development. Expression of the Sry gene results in Sertoli cell differentiation, and these cells then recruit other cells and organize the testis cords. In the absence of the Sry gene, the somatic support cells differentiate into follicle cells under the influence of the oocytes. Together with the oocytes, the follicle cells organize into primordial ovarian follicles.

Alk3 (or Bmpr1a), and Alk6 also serve as Amhr-I receptors. When these receptors are knocked out in male mice, or if their signaling is blocked within the paramesonephric duct mesenchyme, Amh-induced paramesonephric duct regression also no longer occurs.

What downstream targets of Amh signaling within the mesenchyme might be responsible for loss of the ductal epithelium? Few have been found, but one might be matrix metalloproteinase-type 2 (Mmp2), an extracellular protease (see Fig. 16-8A) that degrades several basement membrane components and releases bioactive peptides and growth factors from the extracellular matrix. Soon after Amh signaling occurs in the mesenchyme, cells of the paramesonephric duct begin

undergoing apoptosis, but only after there is evidence of basement membrane degradation. Increases in Mmp2 expression parallel the appearance of Amhr-II expression, and in Amh-deficient male mice, upregulation of Mmp2 does not occur. In addition, general synthetic inhibitors of Mmp enzymatic activity repress Amh-induced paramesonephric duct regression in vitro (however, specifically blocking Mmp2 expression using anti-sense technologies only partially represses regression, suggesting other Mmps are involved). Thus, by degrading basement membrane or releasing proapoptotic signals, Mmps (including Mmp2) may promote Amh-dependent regression of paramesonephric duct.

Time

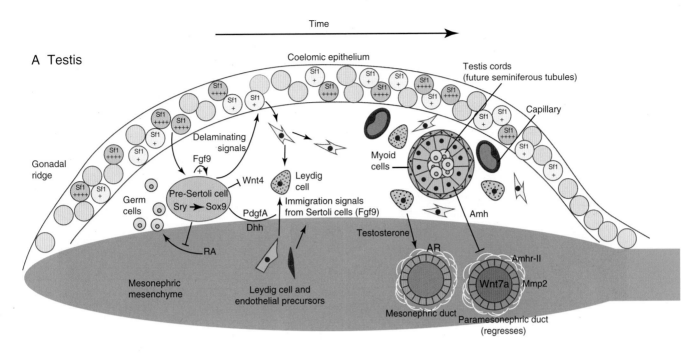

A Testis

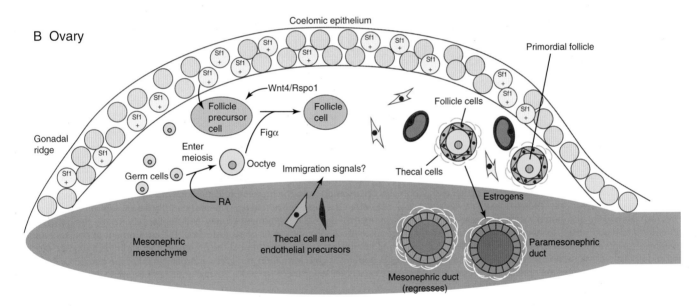

B Ovary

Figure 16-8. Overview of transcription factors, growth factors, and origin of various cell types responsible for forming the male (*A*) and female (*B*) gonads. Amh, anti-Müllerian hormone; AR, androgen receptor; RA, retinoic acid.

MUTATIONS IN AMH OR ITS RECEPTOR CAUSE PERSISTENT MÜLLERIAN DUCT SYNDROME IN XY INDIVIDUALS

Individuals who are 46,XY and have mutations in AMH or AMH RECEPTOR genes exhibit features typical of **persistent Müllerian duct syndrome** because the paramesonephric (müllerian) ducts fail to regress. These individuals develop structures that are derived from the paramesonephric duct, in addition to those derived from mesonephric duct (Fig. 16-10). Hence, a male with

persistent paramesonephric duct syndrome develops a vagina, cervix, uterus, and Fallopian tubes, as well as vasa deferentia and male external genitalia. The female organs are in their normal position, but the position of the testes varies. In 60% to 70% of cases, both testes lie in the normal position for the ovaries (i.e., within the broad ligament; Fig. 16-10A); about 20% to 30% of the time, one testis lies within the inguinal hernial sac (Fig. 16-10B); in other instances, both testes lie within the same inguinal hernial sac (Fig. 16-10C). In all cases, the vasa deferentia run along the lateral sides of the uterus.

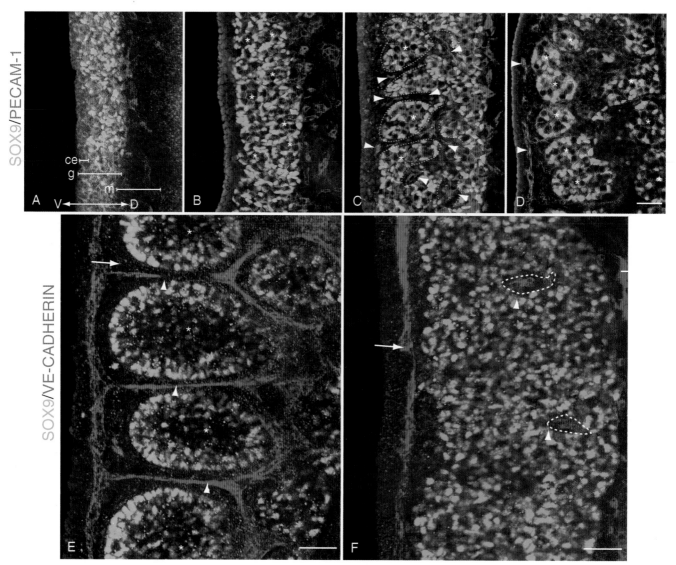

Figure 16-9. Time course of testis cord formation and endothelial cell invasion from the mesonephric mesenchyme in the mouse. *A,* Sertoli cells (Sox9, green) and germ cells (Pecam-1, red) are equally distributed within the bipotent gonad (g), whereas endothelial cells (also Pecam-1 positive, red) are equally distributed within the mesonephric mesenchyme (m). *B-D,* As development ensues, endothelial cells invade the gonad and organize into blood vessels (arrowheads), whereas Sertoli and germ cells organize into testis cords (asterisks). *E,* Development of control mouse gonadal explants cultured for 24 hr. *F,* Development of mouse gonadal explants cultured for 24 hr in the presence of VE-cadherin antibody. Blocking endothelial cell migration using VE-cadherin antibodies disrupts both testis cord formation and vascular organization of the gonad. Only a few endothelial cells (red) enter the gonad (arrowheads), but coelomic vessels are still present (arrows). Ce, coelomic epithelium; D dorsal; V, ventral. Bar represents 100 μm in *A-D* and 50 μm in *E, F.*

Differentiation of the Testis Leydig Cells

In the ninth or tenth week, **Leydig cells** differentiate from mesenchymal cells recruited by pre-Sertoli cells. Recent studies in mice suggest that these precursor cells are derived from both the mesonephric-gonad border and coelomic epithelium (see Figs. 16-7, 16-8). These endocrine cells produce the male sex steroid hormone, **testosterone**, which promotes survival of the mesonephric duct, necessary for development of the male reproductive tract and later for the development of secondary sexual characteristics. At this early stage of development (up to twelve weeks), testosterone secretion is regulated by the peptide hormone **chorionic gonadotropin**, secreted by the placenta. Later in development, pituitary gonadotropins of

the male fetus take over control of synthesizing the masculinizing sex steroids (androgens). Under control of the placental chorionic gonadotropin, both Leydig cell number and testosterone levels peak by fourteen to eighteen weeks of gestation. Luteinizing hormone receptors on Leydig cells begin appearing at twelve weeks, and there is a concomitant increase in expression of steroidogenic enzymes released by these cells at this time. But after sixteen weeks, the number of Leydig cells and levels of steroidogenic enzymes begin falling as gonadotropin control shifts to the pituitary. Pituitary gonadotropin release begins during the second and third trimesters. Mutations affecting Leydig cell differentiation and function, or in genes involved in testosterone synthesis, generally lead to 46, XY disorders of sex development (covered later in this chapter).

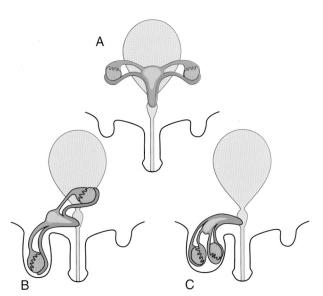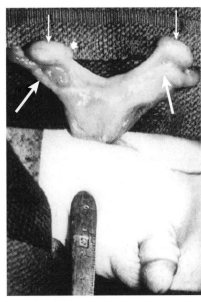

Figure 16-10. Persistent Müllerian duct syndrome. In 46,XY individuals with mutations in AMH or AMH RECEPTOR genes, the paramesonephric (Müllerian) ducts fail to regress. These individuals develop paramesonephric derivatives, in addition to those from the mesonephric duct. These individuals have a cervix, uterus, and Fallopian tubes, as well as vasa deferentia and male external genitalia. The phenotype varies in that the female organs are in their normal position, but the testes may lie in the normal position for ovaries (i.e., within the broad ligament, A), one testis may lie within the inguinal hernial sac (B), or both testes may lie within same inguinal sac (C). D, Phenotype typical of the scenario shown in A. The lower two arrows point to the Fallopian tubes, and the upper two arrows indicate the position of the testes within the broad ligament.

Two distinct populations of Leydig cells are responsible for androgen biosynthesis during fetal and postnatal life. Fetal Leydig cells generate testosterone necessary for stimulating male organ development (i.e., to make the epididymis, vas deferens, and seminal vesicles from the mesonephric duct). From testosterone, Leydig cell **5α-reductase** generates **dihydrotestosterone**, needed to induce male urethra, prostate, penis, and scrotum (covered later in the chapter) and for testicular descent into scrotum (see Fig. 16-4). However, fetal Leydig cells eventually regress and degenerate late in fetal and early postnatal life. At puberty, a new population of adult Leydig cells differentiates from Leydig progenitor cells residing within peritubular interstitium. Androgens produced by this set of Leydig cells play a major role in masculinizing the brain, mediating male sexual behavior, and initiating spermatogenesis.

In the Research Lab

DIFFERENTIATION OF LEYDIG CELLS

Once Leydig progenitors immigrate into the developing gonad, paracrine interactions between Leydig progenitors and Sertoli cells play a central role in fetal and adult Leydig cell differentiation. Both desert hedgehog (Dhh) and PdgfA are released by fetal Sertoli cells; their receptors, patched1 (Ptch1) and Pdgfrα, are expressed by fetal Leydig cells (see Figs. 16-7, 16-8). More than 90% of XY mice with null mutations for Dhh exhibit disorders of sex development, and mice deficient in Pdgfrα exhibit abnormal Leydig cell differentiation. Similar phenotypes (including blind vaginas and underdeveloped mesonephric duct derivatives and prostate glands) are found in XY humans with DHH mutations.

Less is known regarding the differentiation of adult Leydig cells. Although the growth factors Dhh and Pdgf seem to be involved as in fetal differentiation of Leydig cells, several hormones are also involved in adult Leydig cell differentiation. In addition, testicular macrophages are somehow required for adult Leydig cell development. If testicular macrophages are absent from the testicular interstitium, Leydig cells fail to develop, suggesting that these macrophages provide essential growth and differentiation factors for Leydig cells. However, the nature of these signals is still unclear.

Mesonephric Ducts and Accessory Glands of Male Urethra Differentiate in Response to Testosterone

Between eight and twelve weeks, the initial secretion of testosterone stimulates mesonephric ducts to transform into a system of organs—the epididymis, vas deferens, and seminal vesicle—that connect the testes with the urethra. These mesonephric derivatives are distinguishable by their morphologies and specific pattern of gene expression even though they are contiguous (see the following "In the Research Lab" entitled "Development of Epididymis, Vas Deferens, and Seminal Vesicles").

The bulk of the mesonephric duct differentiates into the spermatic duct called the **vas deferens** (see Fig. 16-5). The most cranial end of each mesonephric duct degenerates, leaving a small remnant called the **appendix epididymis**, and the region of the mesonephric duct adjacent to the presumptive testis differentiates into the convoluted **epididymis**. During the ninth week, five to twelve mesonephric tubules in the region of the epididymis make contact with the cords of the future rete testis. However, it is not until the third month that these

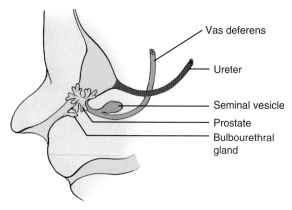

Figure 16-11. Development of the seminal vesicles, prostate, and bulbourethral glands. These glands are induced by androgens between the tenth and twelfth weeks.

epigenital mesonephric tubules actually unite with the presumptive rete testis. The epigenital mesonephric tubules are thereafter called the **efferent ductules**, and they will provide a pathway from the seminiferous tubules and rete testis to the epididymis. Meanwhile, the mesonephric tubules at the caudal pole of the developing testis (called the **paragenital mesonephric tubules**) degenerate, leaving a small remnant called the **paradidymis**.

The three accessory glands of the male genital system—the seminal vesicle, prostate, and bulbourethral gland—all develop near the junction between the mesonephric ducts and the urethra (Fig. 16-11). The glandular **seminal vesicles** sprout during the tenth week from the mesonephric ducts near their attachment to the urethra. The portion of the vas deferens (mesonephric duct) between each seminal vesicle and the urethra is thereafter called the **ejaculatory duct**.

The **prostate gland** also begins to develop in the tenth week as a cluster of endodermal evaginations that bud from the urethra. These presumptive prostatic outgrowths are induced by the surrounding mesenchyme, the inductive activity of which probably depends on the conversion of secreted testosterone to dihydrotestosterone. The prostatic outgrowths initially form at least five independent groups of solid prostatic cords. By eleven weeks, these cords develop a lumen and glandular acini, and by thirteen to fifteen weeks (just as testosterone concentrations reach a high level), the prostate begins its secretory activity. The mesenchyme surrounding the endodermally derived glandular portion of the prostate differentiates into the smooth muscle and connective tissue of the prostate.

As the prostate is developing, the paired **bulbourethral glands** (or **Cowper's glands**) sprout from the urethra just inferior to the prostate. As in the prostate, the mesenchyme surrounding the endodermal glandular tissue gives rise to the connective tissue and smooth muscle of this gland.

Eventually, the secretions of the seminal vesicles, prostate, and bulbourethral glands all contribute to the seminal fluid protecting and nourishing the spermatozoa after ejaculation. It should be noted that these secretions are not necessary for sperm function; spermatozoa removed directly from the epididymis can fertilize oocytes.

In the Research Lab

DEVELOPMENT OF EPIDIDYMIS, VAS DEFERENS, AND SEMINAL VESICLES

The mesonephric duct requires testosterone for retention and subsequent differentiation; otherwise, it regresses. Testosterone acts via paracrine interactions, rather than being delivered by the vasculature to the mesonephric duct, as unilateral castration in male rabbits results only in unilateral regression of the mesonephric duct (hence, testosterone from the gonad may be transported down the lumen of the mesonephric duct). Testosterone binds the androgen receptor (also known as the dihydrotestosterone receptor), which is expressed by the mesenchyme adjacent to the mesonephric duct. Mice lacking the androgen receptor exhibit agenesis of mesonephric duct derivatives and develop female external genitalia. Abnormal mesonephric duct development also occurs in humans having mutations in the ANDROGEN RECEPTOR that lead to 46,XY disorders of sex development (covered in the "Clinical Taster" for this chapter).

As mentioned earlier, the mesonephric duct forms different structures along its cranial-caudal length. Development of these mesonephric-derived structures depends on regionally specific epithelial-mesenchymal interactions that are initiated by the adjacent mesenchyme. For instance, in vitro studies show that the cranial mesonephric duct, which normally develops into the epididymis, can be redirected toward seminal vesicle development when recombined with seminal vesicle mesenchyme. Moreover, the continued growth of the surrounding mesenchyme also requires reciprocal interaction with the mesonephric duct epithelium. These interactions likely involve regional expression of several growth factors (Fig. 16-12). For instance, mice deficient in the growth factor Gdf7 (growth differentiation factor-7) or Fgf10 all exhibit defects in the epididymis and seminal vesicle development. In mice, mesonephric duct and tubule development is dependent on Fgf8 expression. In its absence, the cranial mesonephric duct degenerates, and the efferent ductules, epididymis, and cranial vas deferens do not form (Fig. 16-13). If loss of Fgf8 expression is restricted to developing mesonephric tubules growing out from the mesonephric duct, the mesonephric duct is retained and the epididymis and vas deferens form normally, but the efferent ductules are lost.

The cranial-caudal expression of Hox genes also plays an important role in the differentiation of the various segments of the mesonephric duct. In XY mice, Hoxa9 and Hoxd9 are expressed in the epididymis and vas deferens, Hoxa10 and Hoxd10 are mainly expressed in the caudal epididymis and throughout the vas deferens, Hoxa11 is expressed only in the vas deferens, and Hoxa13 and Hoxd13 are expressed in the caudal vas deferens and region of the developing seminal vesicle (see Fig. 16-12). Mutations or disruptions in the expression of these genes can lead to homeotic transformation. For example, if Hoxa11 expression is lost, the vas deferens is transformed into an epididymal-like cytoarchitecture; if Hoxa10 is lost, the distal epididymis and proximal vas deferens exhibit epididymal-like cytoarchitecture.

In the Clinic

CYSTIC FIBROSIS TRANSMEMBRANE CONDUCTANCE REGULATOR IS REQUIRED FOR VAS DEFERENS DEVELOPMENT

Disorders of mesonephric duct development are quite common. For example, the incidence of human **congenital bilateral aplasia of the vas deferens (CBAVD)** ranges from 1:1000 to 1:10,000, and CBAVD is responsible for 1% to 2% of male infertility and almost 10% of obstructive **azoospermia** (absence

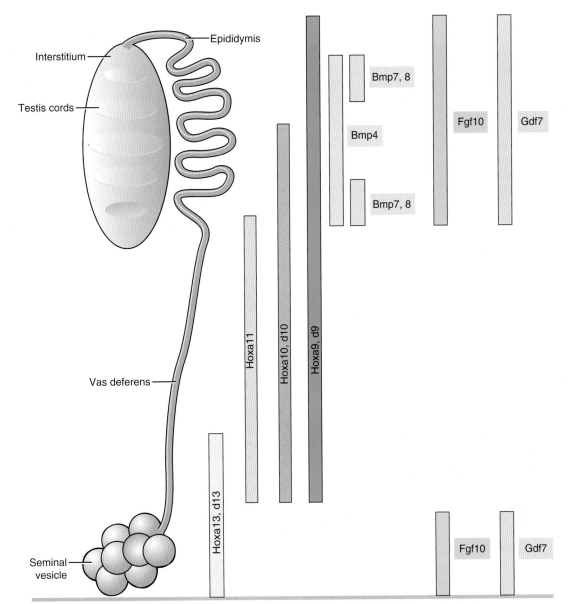

Figure 16-12. Male mesonephric duct differentiation. Under the influence of testosterone, the mesonephric duct forms different structures along its cranial-caudal length, the nature of which depends on regionally specific epithelial-mesenchymal interactions. In mice, restricted expression of several growth factors (including Bmps, Gdf7, and Fgf10) and Hox genes within the mesenchyme play major roles in mediating the regional characteristics taken by the mesonephric duct. Mutations or disruptions in the expression of these genes can lead to homeotic transformation of the mesonephric duct derivatives.

of spermatozoa in semen due to duct blockage, rather than to absence of spermatozoa production, which is called non-obstructive azoospermia). CBAVD is characterized by absence of the body and tail of the epididymis, vas deferens, and seminal vesicle. Mutations in both alleles of the **cystic fibrosis transmembrane conductance regulator** (CFTR; the gene that when mutated causes cystic fibrosis; covered further in Chapter 11) are found in approximately 80% of CBAVD cases. This ion transporter is required for vas deferens development: a high proportion of males suffering from cystic fibrosis also exhibit CBAVD and are infertile. Isolated CBAVD in some male patients, who do not exhibit the cystic fibrosis lung phenotype, is caused by abnormal splicing of the CFTR mRNA in the vas deferens but not in the lungs.

In the Research Lab

DEVELOPMENT OF PROSTATE GLAND

The prostate gland develops from the pelvic urethra. When testicular-generated androgens increase, they induce an outgrowth of solid endodermal buds from the urethral epithelium into the urogenital mesenchyme. Like the mesenchyme surrounding the mesonephric duct, androgen receptors are expressed within the surrounding urogenital mesenchyme, and it seems that an unknown substance is released by the mesenchyme that signals prostatic epithelial development. Not only are androgens required to initiate prostatic development, they maintain its growth and development during the embryonic, fetal, and neonatal periods. Prostatic development relies heavily on conversion

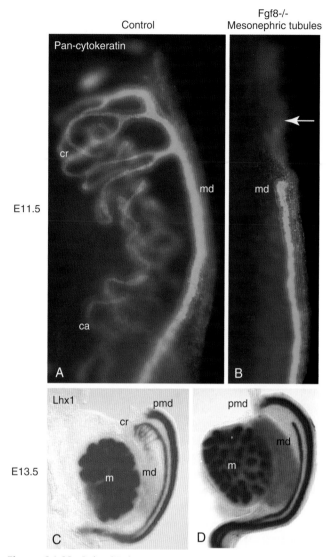

Figure 16-13. Role of Fgf8 expression in development of the mesonephric tubules and ducts. *A, C,* Fgf8 expression in the mesonephric tubules is required for maintaining cranial mesonephric tubules and ducts (both pan-cytokeratin positive and Lhx1-expressing structures) in the mouse. *B, D,* In its absence, massive apoptotic death results in failure of the efferent ductules, epididymis, and cranial mesonephric duct (md) to develop (arrow) in XY mice. ca, caudal mesonephric tubules; cr, cranial mesonephric tubules; m, metanephric kidney; pmd, paramesonephric duct.

of testosterone to 5α-dihydrotestosterone by the enzyme 5α-reductase, as it binds the androgen receptor more efficiently than does testosterone. Mice lacking androgen receptors do not develop a prostate and are feminized externally, although they do develop testes.

The nature of the factor, or factors, released by androgen-stimulated prostatic mesenchyme and responsible for initiating prostatic bud formation is unknown. However, studies in rat and mouse embryos show that once initiated, Shh released from the urethral epithelium increases the expression of Nkx3.1 in the epithelium, and Hoxa13 and Hoxd13 in the adjacent mesenchyme, all necessary for normal prostatic development (Fig. 16-14). Epithelial Fgfr2 signaling by Fgf7 and Fgf10 released from mesenchymal cells mediates continual growth and

elongation of the prostatic epithelium. This signaling maintains Shh expression and is essential for prostate gland development, as mice deficient in Fgf10 or having Fgfr2 signaling blocked fail to develop a prostate. The positive effects of Fgf on Shh expression are tempered by a negative feedback loop, as Shh released from the epithelium downregulates mesenchymal Fgf expression. Sox9 expression during prostate gland development is restricted to the early developing epithelial buds, and studies suggest it also has a role in regulating prostatic epithelial differentiation from the urogenital sinus epithelium, whereas the growth-inhibitory effect of Bmp4 and Bmp7 mediates branching of the ductal epithelium. Subsequent differentiation of the prostate epithelium occurs in a proximal-to-distal progression and is mediated by the expression of several transcription factors including p63 (a tumor suppressor gene with homology to p53) and Foxa1.

IN ABSENCE OF Y CHROMOSOME, FEMALE DEVELOPMENT OCCURS

The basic developmental pathway of the gonad results in ovarian development. Expression of SRY diverts the developmental pathway of the gonad toward the testis pathway by initiating the differentiation of Sertoli cells. In the female embryo, the XX **somatic support cells** do not contain a Y chromosome or the SRY gene. Therefore, they differentiate as **follicle cells** instead of Sertoli cells. Sertoli cells are responsible for the production of AMH and the differentiation of all other cell types in the testis. In their absence, neither AMH nor testosterone is produced. Therefore, male genital ducts and accessory sexual structures are not stimulated to develop. Instead, the paramesonephric ducts persist and are stimulated to differentiate into the Fallopian tube, uterus, and vagina (Fig. 16-15).

FORMATION OF OVARIAN PRIMORDIAL FOLLICLES

Animation 16-4: Development of Ovaries.
Animations are available online at StudentConsult.

In genetic females, the somatic support cells delaminating from the coelomic epithelium do not differentiate into Sertoli cells as they do in males but, rather, surround clusters of primordial germ cells. In the male, Sertoli cells inhibit further germ cell development before meiosis begins. In the female, the germ cells go on to differentiate into oogonia, proliferate, and enter the first meiotic division to form primary oocytes (see Figs. 16-15, 16-8B). These meiotic oocytes stimulate adjacent somatic support cells to differentiation into follicle cells (or granulosa cells) that then surround individual oocytes and form **primordial follicles** within the ovary. These follicles become generally localized to the cortical region of the ovary. The medullary region of the ovary is devoted to developing the vasculature, nerves, and connective tissue of the organ. Follicle cells then arrest further oocyte development until puberty, at which point a group of individual oocytes resumes gametogenesis each month (covered in Chapter 1).

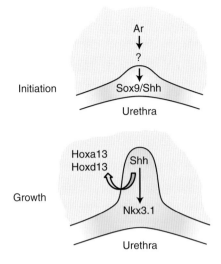

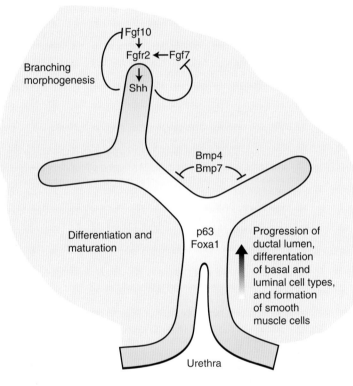

Figure 16-14. Prostatic gland development. When 5α-dihydrotestosterone binds androgen receptors (Ar), the prostatic mesenchyme releases unidentified signaling molecules that induce an outgrowth of endodermal prostatic buds into the urogenital mesenchyme. In rodent embryos, the prostatic bud releases Shh and Sox9. Shh increases epithelial Nkx3.1 and mesenchymal Hoxa13 and Hoxd13 expression. Fgf7 mediates continual growth and elongation of the prostatic epithelium. Fgf10 released from the mesenchyme and Fgf signaling within the epithelium maintain Shh expression (Fgf7 signaling through Fgfr2 is shown outside the epithelium due to space constraints within the epithelium of the figure). However, Shh expression is tempered by a negative feedback caused by mesenchymal Fgf expression. Inhibitory effects of Bmp4 and Bmp7 released by the mesenchyme mediate branching of the ductal epithelium. Subsequent differentiation of the prostate epithelium occurs in a proximal-to-distal progression and is mediated by the expression of several transcription factors including p63 and Foxa1.

In the Research Lab

FEMALE GONADOGENESIS IS NOT A SIMPLE MATTER OF DEFAULT

In the absence of SRY and thus pre-Sertoli cells, the primordial germ cells differentiate into oogonia that proliferate, cluster, and become surrounded by somatic support cells. Under the influence of retinoic acid from the mesonephric mesenchyme, the oocytes enter meiosis. Once oogonia enter their first meiotic division, they are committed to the oocyte lineage. These oocytes provide a key stimulus for the differentiation of follicle cells from somatic support cells generated by delamination of the coelomic epithelium (see Figs. 16-7, 16-8B). Somatic support cells surround individual oocytes breaking down the germ cell clusters to form primordial follicles. Recruitment and differentiation of these follicle cells are driven by and dependent on an oocyte-released factor called Figα (factor in germline alpha). Figα activates the **folliculogenesis** program

in the ovary. Without Figα, primordial follicles never form and oocytes regress soon after birth. Figα also stimulates formation of the **zona pellucida** in the primordial follicle.

Often development of the female gonad is described as the "default" path for the human embryo in the absence of the SRY gene. However, this is a great oversimplification. In fact, several "pro-ovarian" and "anti-testis" pathways and associated genes have been identified. As covered in Chapter 15, Wnt4 is essential for development of the mesonephric and metanephric kidneys, but studies in knockout mice also show that Wnt4 is crucial for normal female sexual development. Wnt4 is initially expressed in the mesonephric and genital ridge mesenchyme and is required for the initial formation of the paramesonephric duct in both sexes. Studies show that XX mice null for Wnt4 have less than 10% of the normal number of oocytes found in their wild-type and heterozygotic littermates. The loss of oocytes is not the result of failure of primordial germ cell migration into

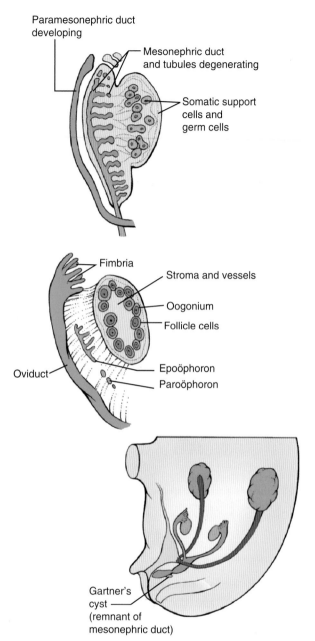

Female

Paramesonephric duct developing

Mesonephric duct and tubules degenerating

Somatic support cells and germ cells

Fimbria

Stroma and vessels

Oogonium

Follicle cells

Oviduct

Epoöphoron

Paroöphoron

Gartner's cyst (remnant of mesonephric duct)

Figure 16-15. Human female gonadal development at the tissue level. In the absence of SRY, the somatic support cells differentiate into follicle cells. These cells surround the oocytes to form primordial follicles, which tend to localize to the outer cortical region of the ovary. The mesonephric ducts and mesonephric tubules disappear except for remnants such as the epoöphoron, the paroöphoron, and Gartner's cysts. The paramesonephric ducts continue to develop to form the oviducts, uterus, and vagina. See Figure 16-5 for a comparison of female and male gonadal development.

the gonadal ridge. Rather, in the absence of Wnt4, the interstitial cell population of the gonad, including follicle cells, is compromised, leading to subsequent degeneration of the oocytes.

As the gonads develop in mice, Wnt4 is downregulated in the testis by pre-Sertoli cell expression of Fgf9 but is retained in the ovary by a synergistic effect of Wnt4 and Rspo1 (roof plate specific spondin-1) in activating β-catenin signaling in somatic support cells (see Fig. 16-7). Rspo1 codes for a secreted molecule activating

β-catenin signaling through frizzled/Lrp receptor complex. Duplication of either Wnt4 or Rspo1 loci in mice or stabilizing of β-catenin in somatic support cells (Fig. 16-16) has "pro-ovarian" activity capable of XY male-to-female sex reversal. Moreover, humans with mutations in WNT4 or RSPO1 exhibit female-to-male sex reversal.

In addition to "pro-ovarian" activities, Wnt4 and Rspo1 exhibit "anti-testis" activities. XX mice lacking Wnt4 or Rspo1 upregulate Fgf9 and Sox9 expression and develop ectopic Leydig-like cells and partially masculinized genitalia. In wild-type XY mice, Fgf9 suppresses Wnt4 expression, thereby promoting Sertoli cell differentiation in males (see Figs. 16-7, 16-8). However in Fgf9 null XY mice, even though Sry levels are normal, Wnt4 fosters ovarian development. This suggests that the fate of gonad differentiation depends on antagonism between Fgf9 and Wnt4/Rspo1 signaling, with expression of the Sry gene tipping the balance in favor of Fgf9 and, hence, development of a male gonad.

Another gene associated with "pro-ovarian/anti-testis" activity is Foxl2. Foxl2 is a member of the folkhead/winged helix transcription factors that is expressed in follicle cells during early stages of gonadal development. Foxl2 is essential for follicle cell differentiation, and its loss masculinizes the gonad as Sertoli cells and testis cords start appearing in XX mice. Foxl2 represses Sox9 expression and inhibits Sertoli cell and Leydig cell differentiation. When Foxl2 is conditionally deleted in adult mouse ovaries, follicle and thecal cells are transdifferentiated into testicular Sertoli and Leydig cells (Fig. 16-17). Thus, it seems that maintaining the female gonad phenotype during adulthood requires a constant suppression of Sox9 expression by Foxl2.

Dax1 (dosage-sensitive sex reversal, adrenal hypoplasia congenita critical region of the X chromosome, gene 1) is described as being an ovarian-promoting factor because it can act as an "anti-testis" factor. The human DAX1 gene is found on the X chromosome. When the DAX1-containing portion of the X chromosome is duplicated in XY individuals, DAX1 leads to sex reversal. In this case, DAX1 may antagonize SRY, because if both DAX1 expression and Sry expression are driven from the Sry promoter in XX mice, 100% of the offspring develop as females, whereas in XX transgenic mice expressing the Sry gene with the normal genetic complement of Dax1, the XX mice develop as males. These observations suggest that Dax1 acts as an "anti-testis" gene rather than as an ovarian-determining gene (see Fig. 16-7).

In XX mice, knocking out Dax1 has little effect on ovarian development, but in XY mice, it leads to testis dysgenesis. Closer examination of the phenotype in Dax1 knockout XY mice shows these mice exhibit abnormal testis cord development even though they have normal levels of Sry and have Sertoli and germ cells. However, these mice seem to have lower levels of Sox9 and fewer peritubular myoepithelial cells, and they exhibit compromised development of Leydig cells. This shows that Dax1 expression is also a "pro-testis" factor (see Fig. 16-7). How Dax1 operates as both a "pro-testis" and "anti-testis" factor is unclear, but it is speculated that particular levels of Dax1 are required within a narrow window of time for normal gonadogenesis to occur (Fig. 16-18). If Dax1 levels are higher than normal (e.g., through gene duplication) or lower than normal (e.g., as the result of an inactivating mutation) during this critical period, an ovary or abnormal testis would develop. Much more needs to be learned regarding the regulation of Dax1, its target genes, and its dosage-dependent effects to understand its precise role in sex determination and in the etiology of sex reversal.

Steroids and steroid receptors also play an important role in female gonadogenesis. Ovaries in mice lacking both estrogen receptors, Erα and Erβ, express Sertoli cell markers and develop what resemble seminiferous tubules and Sertoli cells within their gonads during postnatal development. XX mice lacking the gene coding for aromatase (a key enzyme in the conversion of androgens into estrogens) also begin expressing Sox9 and markers for Sertoli

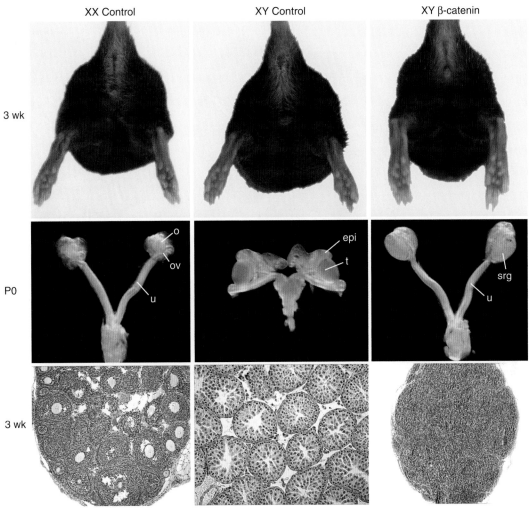

XX Control   XY Control   XY β-catenin

3 wk

P0

3 wk

Figure 16-16. Stabilization of β-catenin within somatic support cells in XY males causes sex reversal of gonads, ducts, and external genitalia in mice. At birth (P0) and three weeks postnatally, normal gonads, ducts, and external genitalia are present in both control XX and XY mice. However, in XY mice expressing a stabilized form of β-catenin in somatic support cells, reverse-sexed gonads form and male organs are lacking, whereas uteri and female external genitalia are present. epi, epididymis; o, ovary; ov, oviduct; srg, sex reversed gonad; t, testis; u, uterus.

and Leydig cells. Early postnatal treatment with 17β-estradiol in aromatase-deficient mice reduces the numbers of Sertoli and Leydig cells in these ovaries and increases folliculogenesis of the existing follicles (these mice still express estrogen receptors). Male mice lacking estrogen receptors also exhibit defects in testis development. The testes are reduced in size with few intact seminiferous tubules, and there is a reduction in the number of germ cells. Whether these effects represent a reversal of later steps in gonad formation (a regression) or are the result of abnormalities in initial gonadal development is unclear. However, what is clear is that the estrogenic environment plays a key role in gonadal development.

In the Clinic

OVOTESTICULAR DISORDERS OF SEX DEVELOPMENT

Ovotesticular disorders of sex development (DSD), previously referred to as true hermaphroditism (i.e., individuals having sex chromosomes, genitalia, and/or secondary sex characteristics that are a mixture of both male and female), may occur as chromosomal males (46,XY), chromosomal females (46,XX), or mosaics (e.g., 45,X/46,XY; 46,XX/47,XXY; or 46,XX/46,XY). The mosaic cases of ovotesticular DSD are the easiest to explain: in these individu-

als, ovarian tissue develops from cells without a Y chromosome, whereas testicular tissue develops from cells with a Y chromosome. Evidence suggests that individuals with DSD having a 46,XX karyotype may also be mosaics. Apparently, the X chromosome in some cells of these individuals carries a fragment of the short arm of the Y chromosome, including the SRY gene. This fragment was likely acquired by abnormal crossing over early in cleavage. Hence, random X-inactivation in cells would account for the mosaicism.

46,XY ovotesticular DSDs are more difficult to explain, as only 15% of these individuals have mutations in SRY. The cause may be mutations in other essential genes in the testis pathway (e.g., defects in androgen action) or misregulation of genes such as WNT4 or RSPO1.

The gonads of ovotesticular DSD individuals are usually streak-like, composite ovotestes containing both seminiferous tubules and follicles. However, in about 20% of cases, an individual has an ovary or ovotestis on one side and a testis on the other. A Fallopian tube and single uterine horn may develop on the side with the ovary. A few ovotesticular DSD individuals have ovulated and conceived, although none is known to have carried a fetus to term. A vas deferens always develops in conjunction with a testis. The testis is usually immature, but spermatogenesis is occasionally detectable. Most ovotesticular DSD individuals are reared as males because a phallus is usually present at birth.

Control adult XX gonad   Foxl2-ablated adult XX gonad

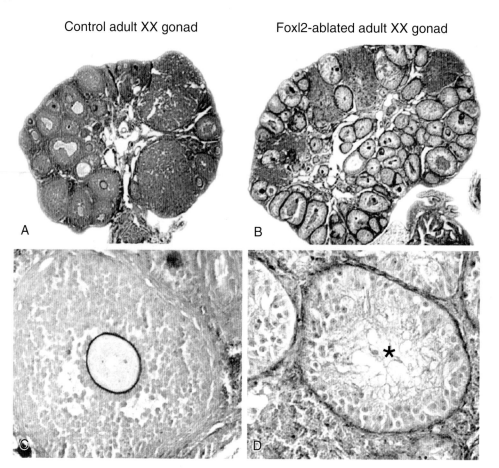

Figure 16-17. Ablation of Foxl2 in adult XX mice increases expression of Sox9 in the ovary, causing transdifferentiation into a testis within three weeks. Maintaining Foxl2 expression is necessary for continual "anti-testis" activity in adult female gonads. *A, C,* Ovary and ovarian follicle in control XX mouse gonad. *B, D,* Transdifferentiation into a testis in Foxl2-ablated XX mouse gonad. Seminiferous tubule (asterisk).

Figure 16-18. Window of DAX1 activity during gonadal determination. DAX1 has both "anti-testis" and "pro-testis" activities, but how it functions is unclear. Particular levels of DAX1 may be required within a narrow window of time for normal gonadogenesis to occur. For example, in an XY individual, the testes would be formed if the DAX1 dosage/activity was within a "window." If DAX1 levels were higher than normal (e.g., through gene duplication) or lower than normal (e.g., because of an inactivating mutation) during this critical period, an ovary or abnormal testis would develop. The male window is shown in blue and the female window is shown in pink. Abbreviations: ♀ represents a male phenotype; ♂ represents a female phenotype.

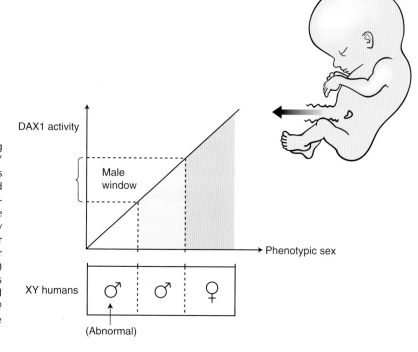

PARAMESONEPHRIC DUCTS GIVE RISE TO FALLOPIAN TUBES, UTERUS, AND VAGINA, WHEREAS MESONEPHRIC DUCTS DEGENERATE

 Animation 16-5: Development of Genital Ducts in Females.

Animations are available online at StudentConsult.

In the absence of Sry and subsequent expression of male pathway genes, the female gonads form primordial follicles and **thecal cells** (the Leydig cell homolog in females). The stromal thecal cells, which do have steroidogenesis activity, express only low levels of the genes necessary for synthesizing testosterone. Because mesonephric ducts and mesonephric tubules require testosterone for their development, they rapidly disappear in the female except for a few vestiges. Two remnants, the **epoöphoron** and **paroöphoron**, are found in the mesentery of the ovary, and a scattering of tiny remnants called **Gartner's cysts** cluster near the vagina (Fig. 16-19C; see also Fig. 16-15). The paramesonephric ducts, in contrast, develop uninhibited.

Recall that the caudal ends of the growing paramesonephric ducts adhere to each other just before they contact the posterior wall of the urethral portion of the urogenital sinus. The wall of the urethral segment at this point forms a slight thickening called the **sinusal tubercle** (Fig. 16-19A). As soon as the fused tips of the paramesonephric ducts connect with the sinusal tubercle, the paramesonephric ducts begin to fuse from their caudal tips cranially, forming a short tube with a single lumen (Fig. 16-19B, C). This tube, called the **uterovaginal canal** or **genital canal**, becomes the uterus and contributes to the vagina (the latter idea is controversial and is covered in the following paragraph). The unfused, cranial portions of the paramesonephric ducts become the Fallopian tubes (or oviducts or uterine tubes), and the funnel-shaped cranial openings of the paramesonephric ducts become the infundibula of the Fallopian tubes.

The formation of the vagina is poorly understood, and different hypotheses have been proposed. One longstanding proposal is that endodermal tissue of the sinusoidal tubercle thickens, forming a pair of evaginating swellings called the sinuvaginal bulbs that fuse to form a solid block of tissue called the **vaginal plate** (see Fig. 16-19). The vaginal plate is then thought to give rise to the inferior portion of the vagina, whereas the caudal region of the uterovaginal canal is thought to form the upper vagina. Subsequently, the vaginal plate is canalized by a process of **desquamation** (cell shedding), thereby forming the vaginal lumen.

Alternatively, it has been suggested that the vagina arises from downward growth of both mesonephric and paramesonephric ducts, and that the vaginal plate is really a derivative of persistent caudalmost segments of the mesonephric duct. However, increasing evidence showing the expression of specific molecular markers for select cell populations in mice and detailed morphological examination of human embryos suggests that the entire adult vagina arises solely from the distal caudal end of the fused paramesonephric ducts. Hence, in either of the alternative scenarios, the mucous membrane lining the vagina would be derived from the mesoderm rather than from the endodermal epithelium of the urogenital sinus.

Regardless of the origins of the vagina, the lower end of the developing vagina lengthens between the third and fourth months, and its junction with the urogenital sinus is translocated caudally until it comes to rest on the posterior wall of the urogenital sinus and opens separately from the urethra within the vestibule (see Fig. 16-19C). A membrane (either endodermally or mesodermally derived) temporarily separates the lumen of the vagina from the urogenital sinus (the latter forms the **vestibule of the vagina**). This barrier degenerates partially after the fifth month, but its remnant persists as the vaginal **hymen**.

In the Research Lab

PARAMESONEPHRIC DUCT DEVELOPMENT AND REGIONALIZED EXPRESSION OF HOX GENES

In females, the mesonephric duct regresses because of lack of male androgens. In contrast, the paramesonephric duct proliferates and differentiates in a cranial-caudal progression, forming the Fallopian tube, uterus, and vagina. During this time, the single-layered paramesonephric duct epithelium differentiates into distinct morphologies ranging from ciliated columnar epithelium in the Fallopian tube to stratified squamous epithelium in the vagina. It should not be surprising, given that the paramesonephric and mesonephric ducts share much of the same mesenchyme, that Hox gene expression plays a key role in mediating the regional characterization of structures found along the cranial-caudal axis of the female reproductive tract. Similar to those described for the mesonephric duct earlier in the chapter, Hox deficiencies can lead to homeotic transformations within paramesonephric ducts. For example, in mice, Hoxa10 deficiency transforms the cranial part of the uterus into Fallopian tube–like structures and reduces fertility.

Wnt7a expression is also important for proper Hox expression and radial axis patterning of paramesonephric ducts. Female mice deficient in Wnt7a show dramatic caudal transformation of the reproductive tract, whereby Fallopian tubes are absent and the uterus exhibits the cytoarchitecture of the vagina. Normal mesenchymal expression of Hoxa10 and Hoxa11 in these regions is lost in these mice, suggesting that Wnt7a is required for maintaining normal Hox expression in this region. In addition, Wnt7a-deficient mice exhibit abnormal myometrial patterning and lack uterine glands.

In the Clinic

ANOMALIES OF UTERUS

The incidence of paramesonephric duct anomalies has been difficult to assess but is thought to be about 1% of normal fertile women and about 3% of women with repeated miscarriages. Most women with paramesonephric duct anomalies can conceive, but they have higher rates of spontaneous abortion, premature delivery, and **dystocia** (difficult or abnormal delivery).

Many anomalies related to the development of the uterus and vagina are attributable to abnormal fusion or regression of the caudal portion of the paramesonephric duct (Fig. 16-20). At about nine weeks of development, the paramesonephric ducts fuse at their inferior (caudal) margin, forming a single-lumen uterovaginal canal. Incomplete fusion of the lower segments of the paramesonephric ducts leads to development of a duplicated uterus with or without a duplicated vagina. Failed regression of the uterine septum (a transient structure resulting from paramesonephric duct fusion) can lead to the development of a bicornuate uterus (two uterine bodies with a single cervical portion), a septated uterus (accounting for approximately 55%

of paramesonephric duct anomalies), or atresia of the cervix. A unicornuate uterus (approximately 20% of paramesonephric duct anomalies) results when one of the entire paramesonephric ducts regresses or when one fails to elongate during development. In cases of congenital absence of the vagina (incidence of 1 in 4000 to 5000 female births), the entire uterus may also be missing, as tissue-tissue interactions responsible for inducing the vagina and for uterine differentiation may be absent.

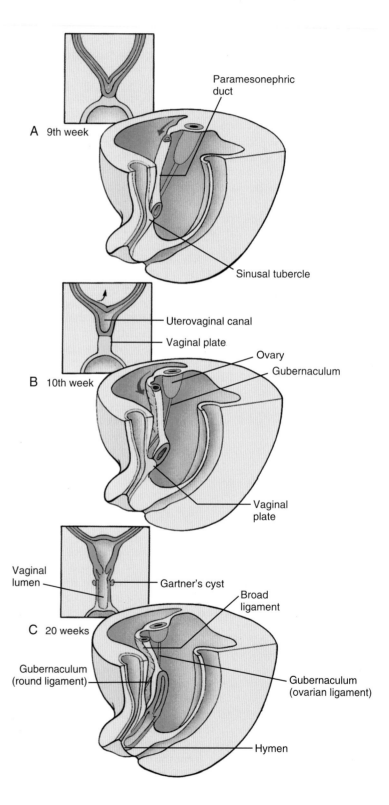

Figure 16-19. Formation of the uterus and vagina. *A*, The uterus and vagina begin to form as the paramesonephric ducts fuse together near their attachment to the posterior wall of the urogenital sinus. *B, C*, The ducts then zip together in a cranial direction between the third and fifth months. As the paramesonephric ducts are pulled away from the posterior body wall, they drag a fold of peritoneal membrane with them, forming the broad ligaments of the uterus. *A-C*, The entire vagina may form from the paramesonephric duct (see text).

DIETHYLSTILBESTROL CAUSES SEVERAL REPRODUCTIVE ANOMALIES

Diethylstilbestrol (DES) was the first synthetic estrogenic compound orally administered to pregnant women to prevent miscarriage (from years 1947 to 1971). It became evident that young women born of DES-treated mothers had significantly higher risks of developing **clear cell adenocarcinoma of the vagina**, a rare cancer usually found in women fifty years and older. In addition, in utero exposure to DES increased the risk of reproductive tract anomalies, including uterine anomalies and **vaginal adenosis** (transformation of stratified squamous epithelium to a columnar type—a possible precursor step toward development of adenocarcinoma), whereas males exposed to DES in utero exhibited such anomalies as cryptorchidism, hypospadias (condition where penile urethra opens on the ventral surface of the penis), and testicular hypoplasia.

DES binds to the estrogen receptor, Erα, with much higher affinity than its endogenous ligand, 17β-estradiol, and it seems to have a much longer half-life. Therefore, it is a strong estrogen. In mice, DES has similar teratogenic effects on female reproductive development as described in humans. These defects closely resemble those observed in Hox and Wnt7a mutants. In mice, DES treatment represses Hoxa10, Hoxa11, and Wnt7a expression during the critical period of uterine and vaginal development. Moreover, DES alters the expression pattern of the tumor suppressor gene p63 within the epithelium of these reproductive organs, providing a link for the increase in adenocarcinomas seen in DES-exposed women.

DEVELOPMENT OF EXTERNAL GENITALIA

 Animation 16-6: Development of External Genitalia. Animations are available online at StudentConsult.

Early development of the external genitalia is similar in males and females. As covered in Chapter 14, the urorectal septum separates the urogenital sinus and anorectal canal from one another. Meanwhile, mesoderm anterior and cranial to the **phallic segment** of the urogenital sinus expands, generating the **genital tubercle**, which eventually forms the **phallus** (Fig. 16-21A). With rupture of the cloacal membrane, much of the floor of the

phallic segment of the urogenital sinus is lost, whereas the roof of the phallic segment expands along the lower surface of the genital tubercle as the genital tubercle enlarges (Fig. 16-22A; see also Fig. 16-21). This endodermal extension forms the **urogenital plate** (or **urethral plate**). At its distal end, remnants of the cloacal membrane adjacent to the genital tubercle remain as the **glans plate**.

Early in the fifth week, a pair of swellings called **urogenital folds** (or **cloacal folds**) develops on either side of the urogenital plate through an expansion of mesoderm underlying the ectoderm (see Fig. 16-22A; see also Fig. 16-21C, D). Distally, these folds meet and join the genital tubercle. Similarly, there is an expansion of underlying mesoderm flanking the anal membrane forming the **anal folds**. A new pair of swellings, the **labioscrotal swellings**, then appear on either side of the urethral folds (see Fig. 16-22A).

The appearance of the external genitalia is similar in male and female embryos through the twelfth week, and embryos of this age are difficult to sex on the basis of their external appearance. See Table 16-1 for the adult derivatives of the embryonic external genital structures.

IN MALES, URETHRAL GROOVE BECOMES PENILE URETHRA AND LABIOSCROTAL SWELLINGS FORM SCROTUM

During the sixth week, a **urethral groove** forms along the ventral surface of the urogenital plate as the genital tubercle elongates (see Figs. 16-21, 16-22A, B). Initially, the urethral groove and urethral folds extend only part of the way along the shaft of the elongating phallus. Distally, the urethral groove and urogenital plate terminate at the solid glans plate (see Fig. 16-22B). As the phallus continues to elongate, the urethral folds grow toward one another and fuse in the midline, beginning proximally in the perineal region and extending distally toward the glans penis. This converts the urethral groove into a tubular **penile urethra**. Exactly how the human urethra forms within the glans penis is unclear,

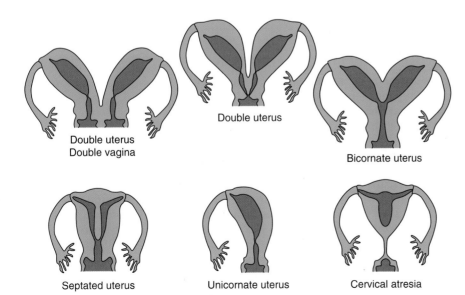

Figure 16-20. Anomalies of the uterus and vagina. Many anomalies related to development of the uterus and vagina are attributable to abnormal fusion or regression of the caudal portion of the paramesonephric duct.

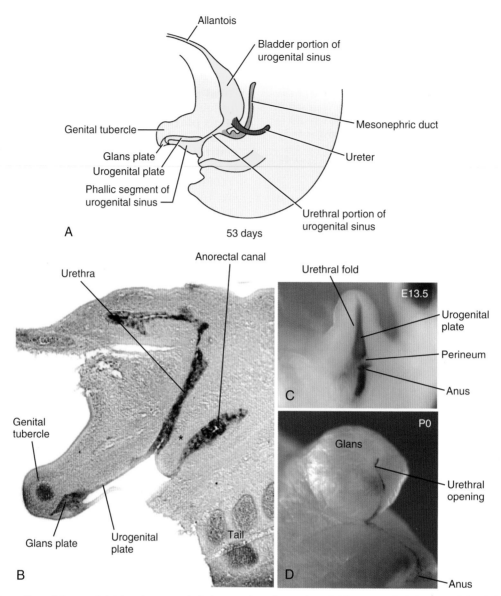

Figure 16-21. Formation of the genital tubercle, urogenital plate, and penile urethra. *A,* The urogenital sinus is subdivided into the bladder, urethral region, and phallic segment. With rupture of the cloacal membrane, the roof of the phallic segment forms a urogenital plate of endodermal cells that lengthens as the genital tubercle grows with a solid glans plate at its distal tip. *B-D,* Shh-driven expression of β-galactosidase (Lac-Z; blue) showing the endodermal origin of the penile urethra and glans plate in the mouse. The glans plate is subsequently canalized to form the glans urethra (*D*). *B,* Light micrograph of a sagittal section through the caudal region of a mouse embryo just after the initial rupture of the cloacal membrane. Note that the entire urethra is lined by endodermally derived epithelium (blue). *C, D,* External views of the genital region at two stages of development. Asterisk, urorectal septum.

but examination of human embryos suggests the solid glans plate canalizes and joins the developing penile urethra to form the **glans urethra** and **external penile meatus** (see Fig. 16-22*B*). Recent experimental studies in mice support this as well. **Hypospadias** (covered later in this chapter) is thought to result from failure of formation or fusion of the urethral folds (penile hypospadias) or abnormal canalization of the glans plate (glans hypospadias).

Starting in the fourth month, the effects of dihydrotestosterone on the male external genitalia become readily apparent. The perineal region separating the urogenital sinus from the anus begins to lengthen. The labioscrotal folds fuse at the midline to form the **scrotum**, and the urethral folds fuse to enclose the **penile**

urethra. The penile urethra is completely enclosed by fourteen weeks.

IN FEMALES, GENITAL TUBERCLE DOES NOT LENGTHEN AND LABIOSCROTAL AND URETHRAL FOLDS DO NOT FUSE

In the absence of dihydrotestosterone in female embryos, the genital tubercle does not lengthen, and the labioscrotal and urethral folds do not fuse across the midline (Fig. 16-22*C*). The phallus bends inferiorly, becoming the **clitoris**, and the phallic portion of the urogenital sinus becomes the **vestibule of the vagina**. The urethral folds become the **labia minora**, and the labioscrotal swellings become the **labia majora**.

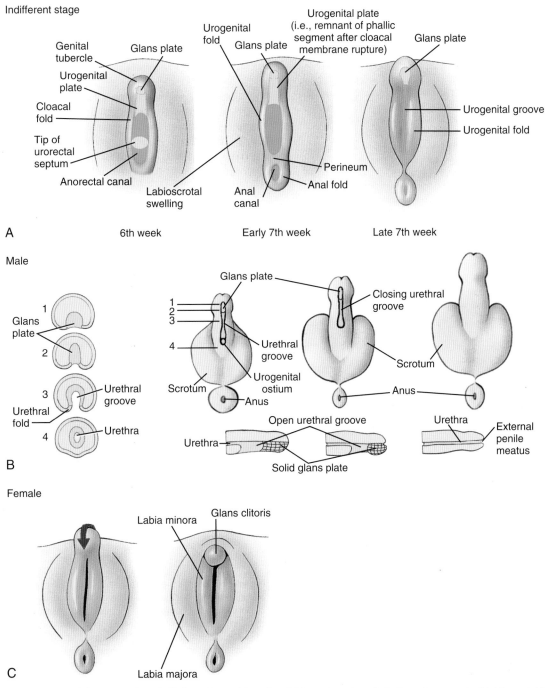

Figure 16-22. Formation of the external genitalia in males and females. *A,* The external genitalia form from a pair of labioscrotal folds, a pair of urogenital folds, and an anterior genital tubercle. Male and female genitalia are morphologically indistinguishable at this stage. *B,* In males, the urogenital folds fuse, and the genital tubercle elongates to form the shaft and glans of the penis. Fusion of the urethral folds encloses the phallic portion of the urogenital sinus to form the penile urethra. The glans urethra is formed by canalization of a solid endodermally derived glans plate. The labioscrotal folds fuse to form the scrotum. *C,* In females, the genital tubercle bends inferiorly to form the clitoris, and the urogenital folds remain separated to form the labia minora. The labioscrotal folds form the labia majora.

In the Research Lab

FORMATION OF EXTERNAL GENITALIA

The role of the distal end of the urogenital plate epithelium in promoting the outgrowth of the genital tubercle is in some ways akin to that of the apical epidermal ridge of the limb bud (covered in Chapter 20). In mice, if the distal urogenital plate is removed, the genital tubercle is hypoplastic. Shh is expressed in the endoderm of the cloacal membrane and developing urogenital plate. In Shh null mice, genital tubercle development is arrested at the initial outgrowth phase, as continual genital growth is dependent on Shh-mediated mesenchymal cell proliferation. Loss of Shh signaling in mice lengthens the G1 phase of the cell cycle in the genital tubercle mesenchymal cells, resulting in an almost 75% reduction of genital growth.

Bmp4, Bmp7, and Wnt5a are expressed within the genital tubercle, and their expression is required for genital outgrowth. Whereas loss of Shh expression in the cloacal epithelium does not prevent the initial expression of Bmp4, Bmp7, or Wnt5a in the genital tubercle, Shh is necessary for maintaining their continual expression during urogenital plate elongation and genital growth. Conditional knockouts of the Bmp4 receptor, Bmpr1a, or overexpression of the Bmp antagonist, noggin results in hypospadias. Human mutations in NOGGIN are associated with feminization of the external genitalia in XY individuals.

Shh from the urogenital plate also upregulates Hoxa13 and Hoxd13 expression within the genital tubercle mesenchyme. The expression of these two Hox genes is required for the development of the early cloaca and genital tubercle because these structures fail to develop in double knockout mice for these two genes (likely reflecting their importance in hindgut development). Hoxa13 also regulates urogenital plate and mesenchymal Bmp7 expression important for urogenital plate elongation and urethral closure. Deficits in human HOXA13 expression are seen in a dominant autosomal disorder causing **hand-foot-genital syndrome**, which is characterized by malformed distal limbs and hypospadias.

Hypospadias is a common defect, suggesting that closure of the urethral folds is very sensitive to perturbations. Shh is involved not only in early stages of genital tubercle development but also in formation of the penile urethra. Fgf10 null mice exhibit severe glans dysgenesis and urethral defects, whereas initial genital tubercle development seems normal (Fig. 16-23). Fgf10 is expressed in the urethral fold mesenchyme adjacent to the Shh-expressing urogenital plate, and antibodies directed against Shh can alter Fgf10 expression in the genital tubercle mesenchyme. This suggests that Shh has an important role not only in early genital tubercle development but also in regulation of Fgf10 expression during urogenital plate expansion and maintenance of epithelial integrity during subsequent urethral closure in males. In mice, Shh signaling within the ectoderm of the ventral phallic midline is also necessary to maintain the floor of the early forming penile urethra; otherwise hypospadias results. Ephrins and their receptors have also been implicated as playing a role in this process, as mice deficient in ephrinB2 and EphB2/EphB3 signaling exhibit faulty urethral closure.

Although both 5α-reductase and androgen receptors are expressed in females, females do not develop male external genitalia because of their low levels of testosterone. Even though the early steps of genital tubercle and urogenital plate formation occur in females, the lack of dihydrotestosterone means that the genital tubercle and urogenital plate do not lengthen and grow to any great extent, nor do the urethral folds fuse. Unfortunately, little is known regarding the molecular embryology of the later stages of female external genitalia development that are responsible for formation of the clitoris, labia, and vestibule.

SUSPENSION OF MESONEPHRIC-GONADAL COMPLEX WITHIN ABDOMEN

Animation 16-7: Repositioning of the Gonads.
Animations are available online at StudentConsult.

As the mesonephric-gonadal complex becomes more segregated from the adjacent intermediate mesoderm, it remains anchored by two ligaments, the **cranial suspensory ligament** and the **gubernaculum** (or **caudal genito-inguinal ligament**). The cranial suspensory ligament runs from the cranial portion of the mesonephric-gonadal complex to the diaphragm (Fig. 16-24). The gubernaculum was first described by John Hunter in 1762 and was given the name *gubernaculum* (Latin: rudder or helm), as "it connects the testis with the scrotum, and directs its course in its descent." The gubernaculum is attached to the caudal portion of the male and female

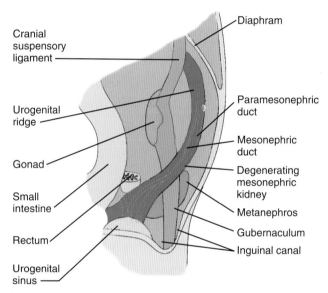

Figure 16-24. At the indifferent gonad stage, two ligaments, a cranial suspensory ligament and the gubernaculum, anchor each mesonephric-gonadal complex. The cranial suspensory ligament runs from the cranial portion of the mesonephric-gonadal complex to the diaphragm. The gubernaculum is attached to the caudal portion of the gonad and extends to the peritoneal floor, where it is attached to the fascia between the developing external and internal oblique abdominal muscles in the region of the labioscrotal swellings.

Figure 16-23. Scanning electron micrographs of external genitalia and urethral development in the mouse. Shh emanating from the urogenital plate also signals the adjacent bilateral mesenchyme to express Fgf10. Fgf10 expression must be maintained by Shh if the urethral folds are to fuse properly. *A*, Wild-type. *B*, Fgf10 gene mutation leads to severe defects in urethra formation.

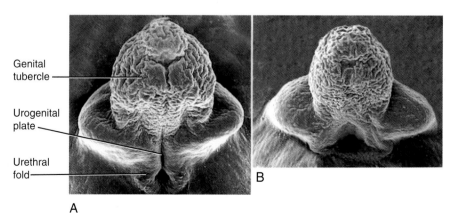

mesonephric-gonadal complex and extends to the peritoneal floor, where it is attached to the fascia between developing external and internal oblique abdominal muscles in the region of the labioscrotal swellings.

DEVELOPMENT OF INGUINAL CANALS

A slight evagination of the peritoneum, called the **vaginal process** or **processus vaginalis**, develops on three sides of each gubernaculum, forming a nearly annular,

blind-end cavity. The **inguinal canal** is a caudal evagination of the abdominal wall that forms when the vaginal process grows inferiorly, pushing out a sock-like evagination consisting of various layers of the abdominal wall (Figs. 16-25 , 16-27).

The first layer encountered by the vaginal process is the transversalis fascia, lying just deep to the transversus abdominis muscle. This layer will become the internal spermatic fascia of the spermatic cord. The vaginal process does not encounter the transversus abdominis muscle itself because this muscle has a large hiatus in

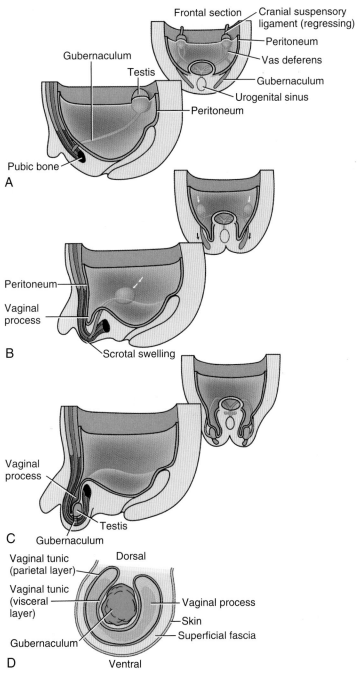

Figure 16-25. Descent of the testes. *A-C,* Between the seventh week and birth, shortening of the gubernacula causes the testes to descend from the tenth thoracic level into the scrotum. The testes pass through the inguinal canal in the anterior abdominal wall. *D,* Cross section of the gubernaculum showing the layers of the vaginal tunic and vaginal process at the level of the labioscrotal swelling.

Continued

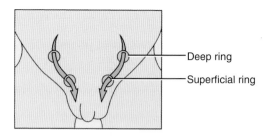

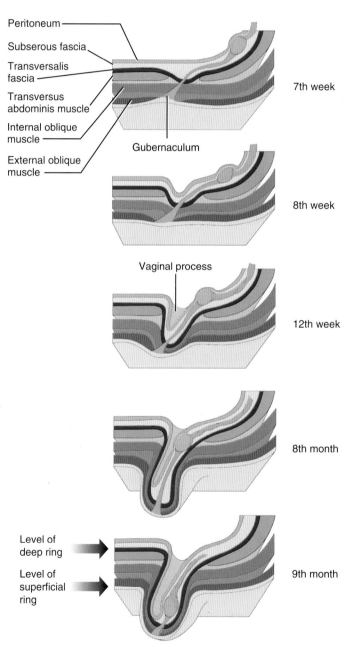

Figure 16-25, cont'd *E,* After the eighth week, a peritoneal evagination called the vaginal process forms just ventral to the gubernacula and pushes out sock-like extensions of the transversalis fascia, the internal oblique muscle, and the external oblique muscle, thus forming the inguinal canals. The inguinal canals extend from the base of the everted transversalis fascia (the deep ring) to the base of the everted external oblique muscle (the superficial ring). After the vaginal process has evaginated into the scrotum, the gubernacula shorten and pull the gonads through the canals. The gonads always remain within the plane of the subserous fascia even though they bulge into the abdominal cavity and later the vaginal process.

this region. Next, the vaginal process picks up the fibers and fascia of the internal oblique muscle. These become the cremasteric fascia of the spermatic cord. Finally, the vaginal process picks up a thin layer of external oblique muscle, which will become the external spermatic fascia. As the vaginal process elongates, it hollows out the inguinal canals and the labioscrotal swellings, providing a cavity into which the testes descend in the male. The superior ring of the canal is called the **deep ring of the inguinal canal** (Fig. 16-25E). The inferomedial rim of the canal formed by the point of eversion of the external oblique muscle is called the **superficial ring of the inguinal canal**. In females, the vaginal process remains rudimentary and normally degenerates during development.

DESCENT OF TESTES

During embryonic and fetal life, both the testes and the ovaries descend from their original position at the tenth thoracic level, although the testes ultimately descend much farther. In both sexes, the descent of the gonad depends on the ligamentous gubernaculum. The gubernaculum condenses during the seventh week within the subserous fascia of a longitudinal peritoneal fold on either side of the vertebral column. Between the seventh and twelfth weeks (the intra-abdominal phase), the extrainguinal portions of the gubernacula shorten and in males pull the testes down to the vicinity of the deep inguinal ring within the plane of the subserous fascia, while the cranial suspensory ligament regresses (see Fig. 16-25). The gubernacula shorten mainly by swelling at their base; this serves the secondary purpose of enlarging the inguinal canal.

The testes remain in the vicinity of the deep ring from the third to the seventh month but then enter the inguinal canal in response to renewed shortening and migration of the gubernacula (the inguinoscrotal phase). The testes remain within the subserous fascia of the **vaginal process**, through which they descend toward the scrotum (see Fig. 16-25). The increased abdominal pressure created by the growth of the abdominal viscera aids the movement of the testes through the canal. By the ninth month, just before normal term delivery, the testes have completely entered the scrotal sac and the gubernaculum is reduced to a small ligamentous band attaching the caudal pole of the testis to the scrotal floor. **Cryptorchidism** (undescended testes) is a common condition and is a risk factor for development of malignancy within the gonad (covered in the following "In the Clinic" entitled "Cryptorchidism").

Within the first year after birth, the cranial portion of the vaginal process is usually obliterated, leaving only a distal remnant sac, the **vaginal tunic** or **tunica vaginalis,** which lies ventral/anterior to the testis (Figs. 16-26A, 16-27). During infancy, this sac wraps around most of the testis. Its lumen is normally collapsed, but under pathologic conditions, it may fill with serous secretions, forming a **testicular hydrocele** (Fig. 16-26B, D).

As mentioned earlier, it is not rare for the entire vaginal process to remain patent, forming a connection between the abdominal cavity and the scrotal sac. During childhood, loops of intestine may herniate into the vaginal process, resulting in an **indirect inguinal hernia** (Fig. 16-26C). Repair of these hernias is one of the most common childhood operations.

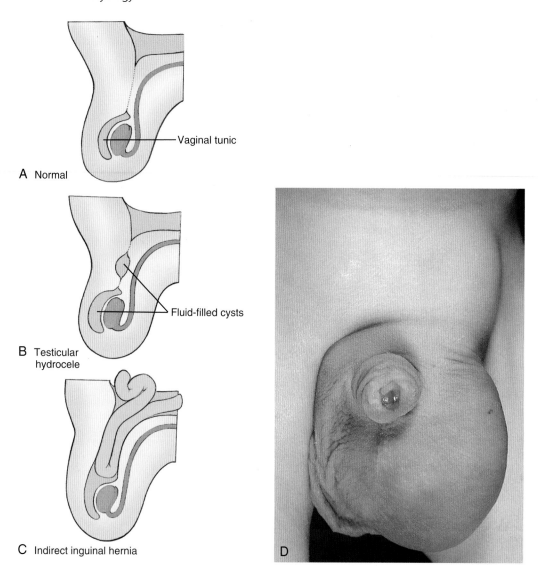

A Normal

Vaginal tunic

B Testicular hydrocele

Fluid-filled cysts

C Indirect inguinal hernia

D

Figure 16-26. Normal and abnormal development of the vaginal process. *A,* The proximal end of the vaginal process normally disintegrates during the first year after birth, leaving a distal remnant called the vaginal tunic. *B,* Some proximal remnants may remain, and these and the Vaginal tunic may fill with serous fluid, forming testicular hydroceles in pathologic conditions or subsequent to injury. *C,* If the proximal end of the vaginal process does not disintegrate, abdominal contents may herniate through the inguinal canal into the scrotum. This condition is called congenital inguinal hernia. *D,* Infant with a testicular hydrocele.

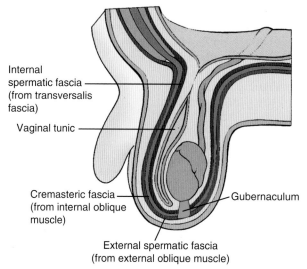

Internal spermatic fascia (from transversalis fascia)

Vaginal tunic

Cremasteric fascia (from internal oblique muscle)

Gubernaculum

External spermatic fascia (from external oblique muscle)

Figure 16-27. The three extruded layers of abdominal wall pushed into the scrotum by the evaginating vaginal process from three layers of spermatic fascia. These three layers enclose the vaginal tunic and the testis in a common compartment.

OVARIES BECOME SUSPENDED IN BROAD LIGAMENT OF UTERUS AND ARE HELD HIGH IN ABDOMINAL CAVITY BY CRANIAL SUSPENSORY LIGAMENTS

Like the male embryo, the female embryo develops a gubernaculum and a rudimentary inguinal canal (Fig. 16-28). In females, the gubernaculum does not swell or shorten. Nevertheless, it causes the ovaries to descend during the third month and to be swept out into a peritoneal fold called the **broad ligament of the uterus** (see Fig. 16-28; see also Fig. 16-19). This translocation occurs because during the seventh week, the gubernaculum becomes attached to the developing paramesonephric ducts, where these two structures cross each other on the posterior body wall. As the paramesonephric ducts zip together from their caudal ends to make the vagina and uterus, they sweep out the broad ligaments and simultaneously pull the ovaries into these peritoneal folds.

In the absence of male hormones, the female gubernaculum remains intact and grows in step with the rest of the body. The inferior gubernaculum becomes the **round ligament of the uterus**, connecting the fascia of the labia majora to the uterus, and the superior gubernaculum becomes the **round ligament of the ovary**, connecting the uterus to the ovary (see Fig. 16-28). Also, in the absence of androgens, the cranial suspensory ligament persists and anchors the ovary high in the abdomen.

As in males, the vaginal process of the inguinal canal is normally obliterated. However, it occasionally remains patent and may become the site of an **indirect inguinal hernia**.

In the Clinic

DISORDERS OF SEX DEVELOPMENT

Disorders of sex development (DSDs) are anomalies in which development of the chromosomal gonads or phenotypic sex is atypical and occurs with an estimated incidence of 1:5000 live births. Many congenital defects of sex development are caused by mutations or chromosomal anomalies affecting autosomes or sex chromosomes. It is no surprise that mutations of the sex-determining region of the Y chromosome have drastic effects, as do deletions or duplications of the sex chromosomes. However, most genital system malformations arise from alterations in autosomal genes.

An individual can have gonads and sex chromosomes that are discordant with secondary sex characteristics, including the genital tract and external genitalia. Given advances in our understanding of the molecular causes, genetic males (46,XY) with feminized genitalia, once referred to as male pseudohermaphrodites, are now classified as **46,XY DSD**s, and genetic females (46,XX) with virilized genitalia, once referred to as female pseudohermaphrodites, are now classified as **46,XX DSD**s. These DSDs are usually caused by abnormal levels of sex hormones or by anomalies in the sex hormone receptors.

46,XY DSD Individuals

In genetically male fetuses, any deficiency in androgen action will tend to allow autonomous female development to proceed, resulting in some degree of genital feminization. Which structures show feminization depends on which of the male sex steroids are affected by the deficiency.

Although not restricted to individuals with DSD, one common manifestation of 46,XY DSD is **hypospadias**, the condition in which the urethra opens onto the ventral surface of the penis. Hypospadias occurs in about 0.5% of all live births. In simple cases, a single anomalous opening is found on the underside of the glans or shaft (Fig. 16-29A, B). In more severe cases, the penile urethra has multiple openings or is not enclosed at all. Hypospadias of the glans is influenced by multiple factors, but its direct cause is probably defective canalization of the distal glans plate. Openings on the penile shaft represent failures of the urethral folds to fuse completely.

A more complex condition, **penoscrotal hypospadias**, results when the labioscrotal swellings as well as the urethral folds fail to fuse (Fig. 16-29C, D). If the labioscrotal folds fuse partially, the urethra will open through a hole between the base of the penis and the root of the scrotum. In the most severe form of the defect, the labioscrotal folds do not fuse at all, and the urethra opens into the bottom of a depression in the perineum. This condition is usually accompanied by restricted growth of the phallus, so that the genitals seem to be female at birth.

46,XY DSDs affecting the external genitals may be caused by 5α-REDUCTASE deficiency. Mutations that reduce or disable this enzyme have little consequence in females, but in males the resulting loss of dihydrotestosterone results in severe penoscrotal hypospadias and genitalia that seem to be female at birth. These individuals have normal testes located within the inguinal canals or inside the labioscrotal swellings. The testes produce AMH and testosterone at the appropriate times, so paramesonephric duct derivatives are absent, and the mesonephric ducts differentiate into vasa deferentia. In 46,XY DSDs of this type, the sudden rise of testosterone at puberty may cause dramatic differentiation of the external genitalia and accessory glands into typically male structures. The urethral folds and labioscrotal swellings may fuse completely, and the genital tubercle may differentiate into a penis. These former DSDs may be fertile and produce offspring. The normal testosterone levels during fetal life and after puberty are thought to result in normal male differentiation of the brain and, hence, a sense of male gender identity.

46,XY DSDs may be caused by **testosterone deficiency**. Mutations that affect enzymes required for the synthesis of testosterone—such as 20,22-DESMOLASE, 17-HYDROXYLASE, STEROID 17,20-DESMOLASE, and 17β-HYDROXYSTEROID DEHYDROGENASE—cause a deficiency or absence of testosterone. The resulting DSD affects all structures that depend on androgens for their differentiation. The mesonephric ducts do not differentiate, the testes do not descend, and both external genitalia and gender identity are female. Because testosterone levels do not rise at puberty, feminization is not reversed, and the individual may continue to resemble a normal female. However, because testes develop and produce AMH, the paramesonephric ducts degenerate.

If ANDROGEN RECEPTORS are disabled or absent, the male fetus may have normal or high levels of male steroid hormones, but the target tissues do not respond, and development proceeds as though androgens were absent. This condition is called **androgen insensitivity syndrome** (also called testicular feminization syndrome). As in cases of primary testosterone deficiency, testes are present and AMH is produced, so the paramesonephric ducts regress, although a blind-ending vagina may form. The phenotype is usually female but can range from a complete female genital morphology (Fig. 16-30) to an ambiguous type (covered in the "Clinical Taster" in this chapter) to a male phenotype with infertility. Mutations in the SRY DNA-binding domain of human SRY are found in cases of **Swyer syndrome**, where there is total gonadal dysgenesis (neither testes nor ovaries) in XY individuals. These individuals are phenotypically female and have a female reproductive tract, but they do not enter puberty. Individuals with Swyer syndrome are usually treated with estrogen and progesterone to facilitate development of secondary sexual characteristics and engender a menstrual cycle. The streaked gonads are removed because they have a tendency to develop cancer. Although these individuals cannot generate ova, they may be able to become pregnant by embryo transfer into the uterus.

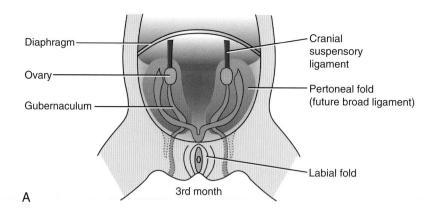

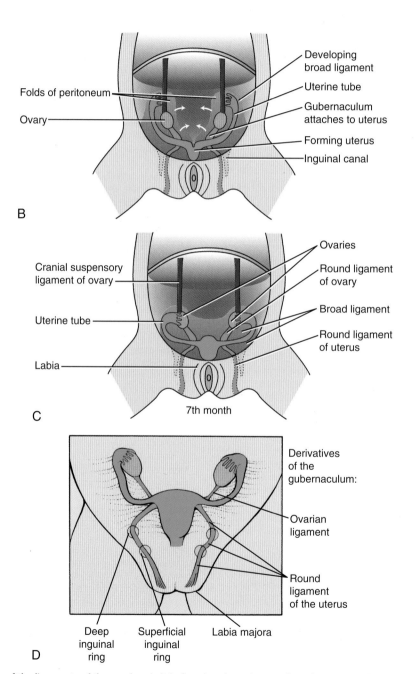

Figure 16-28. Formation of the ligaments of the ovaries. *A, B,* In females, the gubernaculum does not swell or shorten. Nevertheless, the ovaries still descend to some extent during the third month and are swept out into a peritoneal fold called the broad ligament of the uterus (see Fig. 16-19). This translocation occurs because the gubernaculum becomes attached to the developing paramesonephric ducts. As the paramesonephric ducts zip together from their caudal ends, they sweep out the broad ligaments and simultaneously pull the ovaries into these peritoneal folds. As a consequence, the remnant of the female gubernaculum connects the labia majora with the wall of the uterus and is then reflected laterally, attaching to the ovary. *C,* Completely formed broad ligament containing ovaries and ovarian round ligament. *D,* The round ligament of the uterus (remnant of the gubernaculum) exits the abdominal cavity via the deep and superficial inguinal rings and connects to the base of the labia majora.

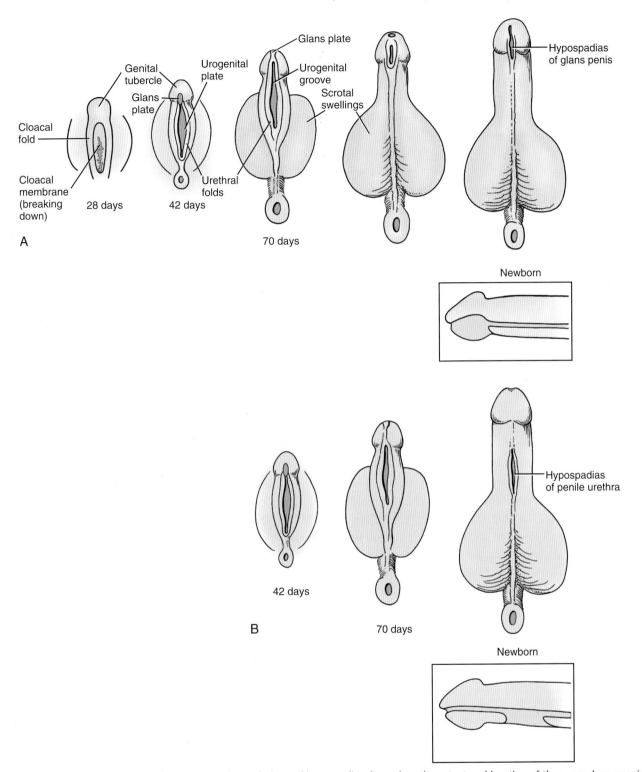

Figure 16-29. Hypospadias. *A-C,* The severity and morphology of hypospadias depend on the extent and location of the anomalous opening into the penile urethra. *D,* Infant with penoscrotal hypospadias.

Continued

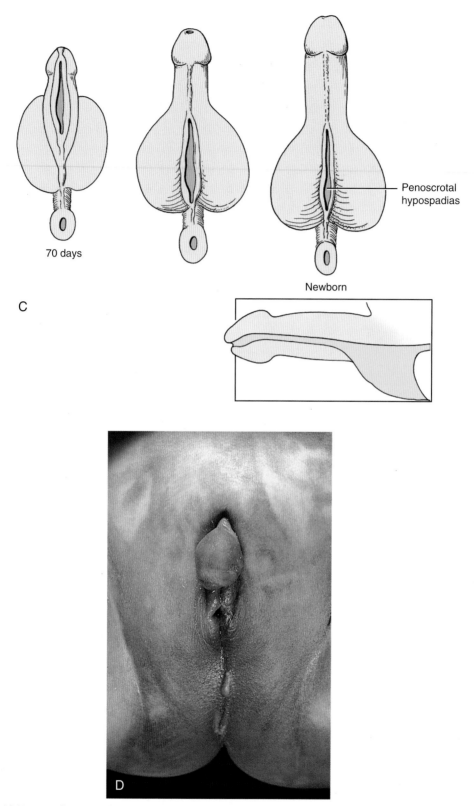

70 days

Penoscrotal
hypospadias

Newborn

C

D

Figure 16-29, cont'd Hypospadias. *A-C,* The severity and morphology of hypospadias depend on the extent and location of the anomalous opening into the penile urethra. *D,* Infant with penoscrotal hypospadias.

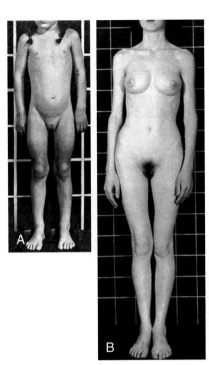

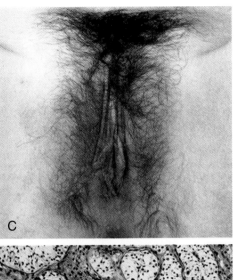

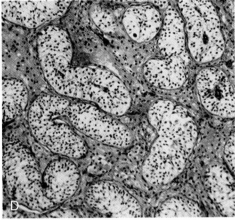

Figure 16-30. Patients with androgen insensitivity syndrome having 46,XY karyotypes and female external genitalia. *A*, Eleven-year-old patient. *B*, Seventeen-year-old patient. *C*, Photograph showing normal female external genitalia in patient in B. *D*, Photomicrograph of the cytoarchitecture of the testis removed from the inguinal canal of the patient in B showing Sertoli cell–lined seminiferous tubules. Germ cells are missing and the interstitial cells are hypoplastic.

46,XX DSD Individuals

46,XX DSD is seen in genetic females who possess ovaries but whose genitalia are virilized by exposure to abnormal levels of virilizing sex steroids during fetal development. In most cases, the virilizing androgens are produced as the result of **congenital adrenal (suprarenal) hyperplasia** (covered further in the "In the Clinic" entitled "Congenital Adrenal Hyperplasia" in Chapter 15). Some cases have seemingly been caused by the administration of virilizing progestin compounds to prevent spontaneous abortion. Whatever the cause, the external genitalia of 46,XX DSD individuals exhibit clitoral hypertrophy and fusion of the urethral and labioscrotal folds (see Fig. 6-16 in Chapter 6). However, because testes and AMH are absent, the vagina, uterus, and Fallopian tubes develop normally.

Failure to Enter Puberty

When an individual fails to undergo the developmental changes associated with puberty, the cause is usually a deficiency of the appropriate sex steroids normally secreted by the gonads—testosterone in males and estrogen in females. Increased levels of pituitary gonadotropic hormones stimulate the pubertal surge in sex steroid production. Hypogonadism may thus be caused by a defect in the gonads themselves or in the hypothalamus and pituitary.

In **primary hypogonadism**, the hypothalamus and pituitary are normal and produce high levels of circulating gonadotropins, but the gonad does not respond with increased production of sex steroids. Most cases of primary hypogonadism are associated with one of two major chromosomal anomalies, although a few cases are of unknown (idiopathic) origin.

In males, primary hypogonadism is usually a component of **Klinefelter syndrome**, which occurs in about 1 of 500 to 1000 live male births. Klinefelter syndrome is caused by a variety of sex chromosome anomalies involving the presence of an extra X chromosome. As discussed in Chapter 1, the extra X chromosome is acquired by nondisjunction during gametogenesis or early cleavage. The most common karyotype of Klinefelter syndrome is 47,XXY. Other individuals with Klinefelter syndrome are mosaics: either mosaics of cells with normal male karyotype (46,XY) and cells with an abnormal karyotype (e.g., 47,XXY; 48,XXYY; 45,X; and 47,XXY), or mosaics of cells with a female 46,XX karyotype and cells with an abnormal 47,XXY karyotype. In all cases, the primary defect is failure of the Leydig cells to produce sufficient quantities of male steroids, which results in small testes and **azoospermia** (lack of spermatogenesis) or **oligospermia** (low sperm count). Many of these individuals also exhibit **gynecomastia** (development of breasts in males) and **eunuchoidism** (slender habitus, elongated extremities, and sparse hair).

Primary hypogonadism in females is usually associated with **Turner syndrome**. This condition occurs in 1 of 5000 live female births. The cause is a 45,X karyotype or 45,X/46,XX or 45,X/46,XY mosaicism. In addition to failure of normal sex maturation at puberty, Turner syndrome is characterized by a range of anomalies, including short stature and webbed neck, coarctation of the aorta (covered in Chapter 13), and cervical lymphatic cysts.

Secondary hypogonadism is caused by defects of hypothalamus or anterior pituitary gland. Individuals with **secondary hypogonadism** have depressed levels of gonadotropins as well as depressed levels of sex steroids. Most often, the cause is an insufficient secretion of gonadotropin-releasing hormone by the hypothalamus, as in **Kallmann syndrome** (covered in Chapter 9) or the **fertile eunuch syndrome** in males. A variety of secondary hypogonadotropic disorders in males and females show autosomal recessive inheritance.

Embryology in Practice

SHORT STATURE

A seven-year-old girl is seen by a gastroenterologist for poor growth and gastrointestinal symptoms. A history of intermittent diarrhea and abdominal discomfort led the physician to suspect celiac disease, and the family returns to clinic to discuss the results of testing, which confirm that diagnosis. The family had suspected as much and came prepared to discuss gluten-free diet plans, food restrictions, and other celiac issues.

However, they are not prepared for the discussion that comes next. The physician states, "I'd also like to do a chromosome study to rule out Turner syndrome, which could explain your daughter's short stature and celiac disease." She goes on to add that the girl has a few of the outward features of Turner syndrome, including a broad neck and numerous moles.

After ten more days, chromosome testing shows a 45,X karyotype, confirming the diagnosis of Turner syndrome. No evidence of mosaicism is found (some girls with Turner syndrome are mosaic for other cell lines such as 46,XX or 46,XY).

The girl is referred to an endocrinologist for further discussion and management. An ultrasound of the abdomen shows normal kidneys (which can be abnormal in 30% of the girls with Turner syndrome) but shows no ovaries, consistent with the gonadal dysgenesis seen in Turner syndrome. Instead of the rapid proliferation of oocytes in the genital ridge that normally occurs during mid-gestation, the ovaries of 45,X females undergo accelerated loss of oocytes, resulting in few follicles and fibrous "streak ovaries" at birth.

The endocrinologist explains that most girls with Turner syndrome will never have normal menstrual cycles or unassisted pregnancies. The onset and adequacy of pubertal development are variable and may be assisted by hormone replacement therapy. The family is informed that this treatment will need to be coordinated with growth hormone therapy, which can be used to restore normal linear growth in girls with Turner syndrome if timed appropriately.

SUGGESTED READINGS

Cai Y. 2009. Revisiting old vaginal topics: conversion of the Müllerian vagina and origin of the "sinus" vagina. Int J Dev Biol 53:925–934.

Cool J, Capel B. 2009. Mixed signals: development of the testis. Semin Reprod Med 27:5–13.

DiNapoli L, Capel B. 2008. SRY and the standoff in sex determination. Mol Endocrinol 22:1–9.

Ewen KA, Koopman P. 2010. Mouse germ cell development: from specification to sex determination. Mol Cell Endocrinol 323:76–93.

Franco HL, Yao HH. 2011. Sex and hedgehog: roles of genes in the hedgehog signaling pathway in mammalian sexual differentiation. Chromosome Res 20:247–258.

Hughes IA, Houk C, Ahmed SF, Lee PA. 2006. Consensus statement on management of intersex disorders. J Pediatr Urol 2:148–162.

Joseph A, Yao H, Hinton BT. 2009. Development and morphogenesis of the Wolffian/epididymal duct, more twists and turns. Dev Biol 325:6–14.

Kousta E, Papathanasiou A, Skordis N. 2010. Sex determination and disorders of sex development according to the revised nomenclature and classification in 46,XX individuals. Hormones 9:218–231.

Liu CF, Liu C, Yao HH. 2010. Building pathways for ovary organogenesis in the mouse embryo. Curr Top Dev Biol 90:263–290.

Rey RA, Grinspon RP. 2011. Normal male sexual differentiation and aetiology of disorders of sex development. Best Pract Res Clin Endocrinol Metab 25:221–238.

Richardson BE, Lehmann R. 2010. Mechanisms guiding primordial germ cell migration: strategies from different organisms. Nat Rev Mol Cell Biol 11:37–49.

Schlessinger D, Garcia-Ortiz JE, Forabosco A, et al. 2010. Determination and stability of gonadal sex. J Androl 31:16–25.

van der Putte SC. 2005. The development of the perineum in the human. A comprehensive histological study with a special reference to the role of the stromal components. Adv Anat Embryol Cell Biol 177:1–131.

Chapter 17

Development of the Pharyngeal Apparatus and Face

SUMMARY

The skeleton of the head and pharynx is made up of the **neurocranium**—the bones that support and protect the brain and sensory organs (olfactory organs, eyes, and inner ears)—and the **viscerocranium**—the bones of the face and pharyngeal arches. The neurocranium can be subdivided into cranial base (the bones underlying the brain), cranial vault (the bones covering the brain), and sensory capsules (the bones encapsulating the sensory organs). There are two types of bone in the head. One type, **endochondral bone**, forms from a cartilaginous intermediate and ossifies through the process of **endochondral ossification**. The bones of the cranial base are formed by endochondral ossification and are collectively called the **chondrocranium**. The other type of bone develops from an ossification directly in the mesenchyme through the process of **intramembranous ossification**; this type of bone is known as **membrane** or **dermal bone**. The jaws and the skull vault are formed almost entirely of membrane bone. Many of the skeletal structures in the head are unusual in that they are formed from **neural crest cells** rather than from mesoderm, as they are in the rest of the body.

In humans, four pairs (numbered one through four in craniocaudal sequence) of **pharyngeal arches** (also called branchial arches, especially in the older literature) form on either side of the pharyngeal foregut, starting on day twenty-two. In addition, based on their evolutionary history from ancestors with six arches, a more caudal pair of arches, termed the sixth pharyngeal arches, have been proposed to also form in humans. Each pharyngeal arch, regardless of its craniocaudal position, has an outer covering of ectoderm, an inner lining of endoderm, and a core of mesenchyme derived from paraxial and lateral plate mesoderm and neural crest cell–derived **ectomesenchyme**. Each pharyngeal arch contains a cartilaginous supporting element, an aortic arch artery, and an arch-associated cranial nerve. The pharyngeal arches are separated externally by ectodermal-lined **pharyngeal clefts** (also called **grooves**) and internally by endodermal-lined **pharyngeal pouches**.

The skeletal elements in at least pharyngeal arches one through four (and perhaps six) are derived from neural crest cells, whereas the muscles and endothelial cells are derived from the mesoderm. The first pharyngeal arch (and more cranially associated mesenchyme) initially forms the transient **Meckel's** and **palatopterygoquadrate cartilages**, which ultimately give rise to the **malleus** and **incus** of the middle ear, respectively. The second pharyngeal arch initially forms **Reichert's** cartilage, and later the **stapes, stylohyoid**, the **lesser horns**, and part of the **body of the hyoid**. The third pharyngeal arch forms the **greater horns** and part of the **body of the hyoid**. The fourth and sixth pharyngeal arches form the **cartilages of the larynx.**

The mesoderm of the first pharyngeal arch forms the **muscles of mastication**, and the mesoderm of the second pharyngeal arch forms the **muscles of facial expression**. The mesoderm in pharyngeal arches three, four, and six forms the intrinsic muscles of the larynx. The muscles derived from each pharyngeal arch are innervated by a corresponding cranial nerve (first, second, third, and fourth and sixth arches are innervated by cranial nerves V, VII, IX, and X, respectively). The extraocular muscles form from the most rostral paraxial mesoderm and prechordal plate mesoderm. These are innervated by the oculomotor (III), trochlear (IV), and abducens (VI) nerves.

The human face is formed between the fourth and tenth weeks by the fusion of five **facial prominences: the frontonasal prominence**, a pair of **maxillary prominences**, and a pair of **mandibular prominences**. During week five, a pair of thickened ectodermal **nasal (olfactory) placodes** develops on the frontonasal prominence and then invaginates to form the nasal pits and simultaneously divide part of the frontonasal prominence into the **medial** and **lateral nasal processes**. The facial primordia join to form the **face**; failure to do so results in **facial clefts**. During normal development, the medial nasal processes merge to generate the bridge of the **nose**, the **philtrum**, and the **primary palate;** the lateral nasal processes give rise to the side of the nose; and the maxillary processes generate much of the cheeks. The **secondary palate** is formed from shelves that grow out from the maxillary swellings and fuse across the midline. The mandibular processes form the lower jaw.

Each of the pharyngeal pouches forms an adult structure. The first pouch forms most of the **tympanic cavity** and all of the **auditory (Eustachian) tube**. The second pouch gives rise to the **palatine tonsils**. The third pouch forms the **thymus gland** and **inferior parathyroid glands**, and the fourth pouch forms the **superior parathyroid glands**. The fifth pouch forms the **ultimobranchial body**. The thymus, ultimobranchial glands, and parathyroid glands migrate to their final position in the neck.

The **thyroid gland** forms as a midline, ventral endodermal evagination of the pharynx; its point of

429

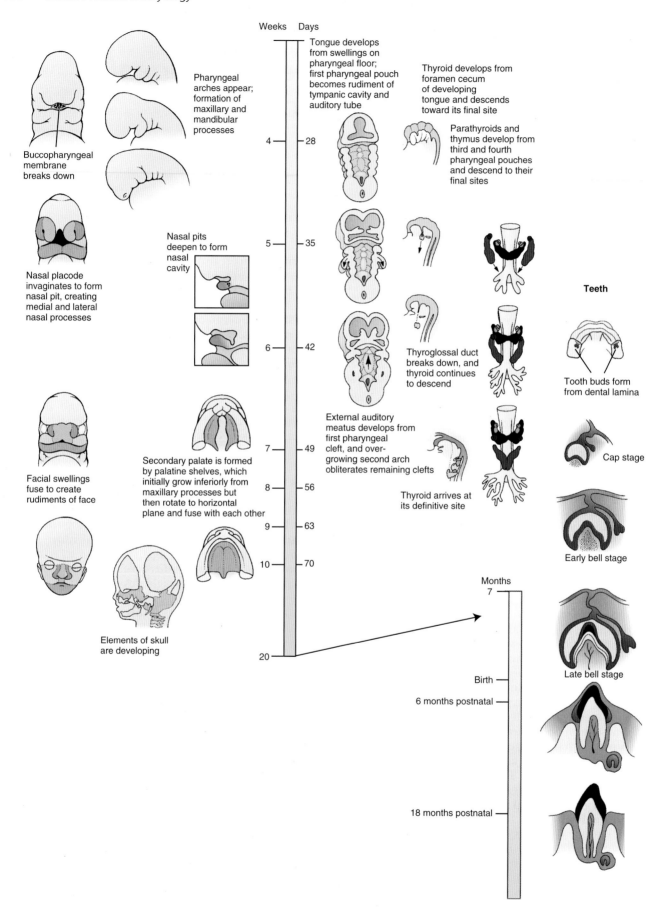

Weeks   Days

Buccopharyngeal membrane breaks down

Pharyngeal arches appear; formation of maxillary and mandibular processes

Nasal placode invaginates to form nasal pit, creating medial and lateral nasal processes

Nasal pits deepen to form nasal cavity

Facial swellings fuse to create rudiments of face

Secondary palate is formed by palatine shelves, which initially grow inferiorly from maxillary processes but then rotate to horizontal plane and fuse with each other

Elements of skull are developing

Tongue develops from swellings on pharyngeal floor; first pharyngeal pouch becomes rudiment of tympanic cavity and auditory tube

Thyroid develops from foramen cecum of developing tongue and descends toward its final site

Parathyroids and thymus develop from third and fourth pharyngeal pouches and descend to their final sites

Thyroglossal duct breaks down, and thyroid continues to descend

External auditory meatus develops from first pharyngeal cleft, and overgrowing second arch obliterates remaining clefts

Thyroid arrives at its definitive site

Teeth

Tooth buds form from dental lamina

Cap stage

Early bell stage

Late bell stage

Months

7

Birth

6 months postnatal

18 months postnatal

Time line. Development of the head, neck, and pharyngeal apparatus.

evagination is marked in the adult by the **foramen cecum** on the upper surface of the tongue. This primordium of the thyroid gland elongates after its evagination, detaches from the pharyngeal endoderm, and finally migrates to its definitive location just inferior and ventral to the larynx. Cells from the ultimobranchial body become incorporated into the thyroid gland to form the calcitonin producing **C-cells.**

The **tongue** develops from endodermal-covered swellings on the floor of the pharynx. The anterior two thirds of the tongue mucosa is derived from first-pharyngeal arch swellings, whereas the posterior one third receives contributions from the third and fourth pharyngeal arches. In contrast, most tongue muscles are formed from myocytes arising from **occipital** somites and are innervated by the **hypoglossal nerve.** For this reason, the motor and sensory nerve fibers of the tongue are contained within separate sets of cranial nerves.

With the exception of the first pharyngeal cleft (the cleft separating the first and second pharyngeal arches), which forms the **external auditory meatus,** all other pharyngeal clefts are obliterated by overgrowth of the second pharyngeal arch, although they occasionally persist as abnormal cervical cysts or fistulae.

Teeth arise from ectoderm and neural crest–derived mesenchyme. The first sign of tooth development is the formation of a U-shaped epidermal ridge, called the **dental lamina,** along the crest of the upper and lower jaws. Twenty dental lamina downgrowths, which induce condensation of the underlying neural crest cell–derived mesenchyme, together form the **tooth buds** of the primary (deciduous) teeth. The secondary, permanent teeth are formed by secondary tooth buds that sprout from the primary buds. Soon after each tooth bud forms, its mesenchymal component forms a hillock-like **dental papilla** that indents the epithelial **enamel organ** formed from the bud. This stage of dental development is called the **cap stage** because the enamel organ sits on the papilla like a cap. By the tenth week, the dental lamina becomes a bell-shaped structure that completely covers the dental papilla. At the late **bell stage,** the cells of the enamel organ differentiate into enamel-producing **ameloblasts,** which begin to secrete organic matrix that mineralizes to form radially arranged prisms of enamel between themselves and the underlying papilla. The outermost cells of the papilla differentiate into **odontoblasts,** which secrete the dentine of the tooth. The inner cells of the dental papilla give rise to the tooth pulp. Nerves and blood vessels gain access to the pulp through the tips of the tooth roots.

Clinical Taster

An 18-year-old woman was taken to the emergency room complaining of a "heart attack." She was noticeably sweaty, out of breath, and experiencing chest pain. The symptoms began an hour earlier, while she was jogging. She became especially alarmed when her jogging mate said, "I can see your heart beating in your neck!"

A normal ECG, normal laboratory tests, and improvement without therapy ruled out a heart attack. Physical findings of costochondritis (inflammation of the rib joints) provided a likely cause for the chest pain, which, in turn, led to a panic attack. However, the ER physician continued to hear inspiratory stridor (a sound made by partial obstruction of a large airway) well after the panic attack had subsided. This, combined with visible arterial pulsations at the base of the patient's neck, suggested a vascular anomaly. The doctor also noticed that the woman had minor craniofacial anomalies, including low-set, abnormally shaped ears, retrognathia (a setback jaw), a short philtrum (the structure between the upper lip and nose), and a broad nasal tip. In addition, the patient had a bifid uvula and hypernasal speech, suggestive of palatal dysfunction.

Magnetic resonance angiography (MRA) done one week later revealed a **cervical aortic arch** (CAA) that was impinging on, and partially obstructing, the trachea, causing stridor during deep inhalation. CAA results from abnormal development of the aortic arches, with regression of the left fourth aortic arch and enlargement of the left third aortic arch. Normally, as covered in Chapter 13, the left fourth aortic arch persists and contributes to the arch of the aorta. CAA and related vascular anomalies, especially when accompanied by craniofacial defects and velopharyngeal insufficiency (dysfunction of the palate and pharynx; "velo" refers to palate), commonly occur in chromosome **22q11.2 deletion syndrome** (also known as **velocardiofacial** or **DiGeorge syndrome**). Genetic testing confirmed this deletion. 22q11.2 deletion syndrome is characterized by a wide range of abnormalities, often subtle in infancy (Fig. 17-1), affecting the craniofacial and pharyngeal arch neural crest cell derivatives.

ORIGIN OF SKULL

In humans, the bones of the head can be divided into the **neurocranium** and **viscerocranium.** These bones arise from more than one-hundred ossification centers that consolidate to form forty-five bones in the neonatal skull. Fusion of these bones postnatally reduces this number to twenty-two bones in the adult skull. The **neurocranium** encompasses the bones surrounding and protecting the brain and sensory organs: the bones of the cranial base, sensory organs, and skull vault (Fig. 17-2*A*). The **viscerocranium** encompasses the bones of the face and pharyngeal arches (see Fig. 17-2*A*). The neurocranium and viscerocranium consist of two types of bones: those formed through ossification of a cartilaginous intermediate are known as **endochondral bones,** and those formed through direct ossification in the mesenchyme are known as **membrane** or **dermal bones** (covered in Chapter 8). In humans, dermal bones, with the exception of part of the **clavicle,** are found only in the head.

The presence of these two types of bones in the head was conserved during evolution. The cranial skeleton of fishes is composed of (1) the **chondrocranium,** which encloses and protects the brain and helps to form the **sensory capsules** that support and protect the olfactory organs, eyes, and inner ears; (2) an external armor of **membrane (dermal) bones,** which overlie the chondrocranium; and (3) the **visceral skeleton** or **viscerocranium,** which supports the gill bars and jaws (Fig. 17-2*B*). The bones of the chondrocranium (as the name indicates) are preformed in cartilage. These three components of the cranial skeleton of fishes can still be

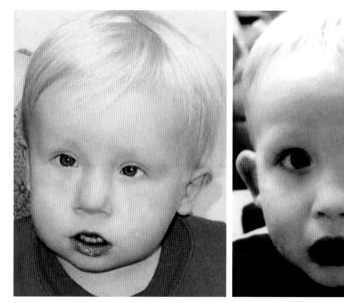

Figure 17-1. Two unrelated children with the characteristic, but subtle, facial appearance of 22q11.2 deletion syndrome, including prominent nose with rounded tip and hypoplastic alae nasi, reduced midface, small mouth and chin, unusually shaped ears, and small palpebral fissures (eye openings).

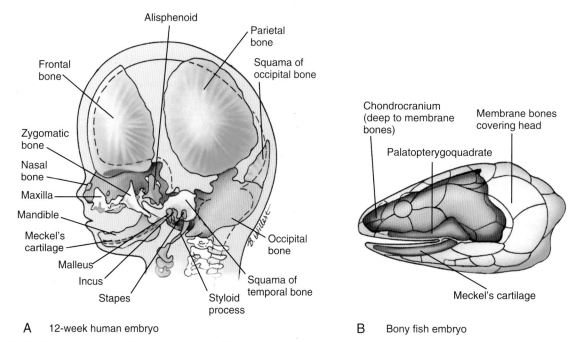

A   12-week human embryo

B   Bony fish embryo

Figure 17-2. The evolutionary origin of the human skull from the pharyngeal arch skeleton, braincase, and dermal bones of primitive vertebrates. *A,* In humans, the chondrocranium (purple) forms the cranial base, whereas the skull vault is formed by membrane bones (blue). Membrane bones also form a large part of the highly modified facial skeleton of humans. The cartilaginous viscerocranium is shown in green. *B,* The expanding brain in the line of fishes leading to humans was housed in a cranium formed partly by the chondrocranium (purple) and partly by membrane bones (blue). The pharyngeal arches in fish give rise to a series of cartilaginous bones (green), shown here by Meckel's and the palatopterygoquadrate bones derived from the first pharyngeal arch.

distinguished in the development of the human skull (compare Figs. 17-2*A, B*). However, during evolution, with establishment of the novel temporomandibular joint, the pharyngeal arch cartilages (i.e., the viscerocranium) were modified to form the cartilages of the larynx and bones of the middle ear. Also, as the brain expanded, the chondrocranium came to underlie, rather than surround, the developing brain, forming the cranial base, whereas the dermal bones expanded to form the cranial vault.

In humans, the **chondrocranium** is also defined as that portion of the neurocranium formed by endochondral ossification. The chondrocranium, in part, develops from three pairs of cartilaginous precursors that were also present in our early ancestors—**prechordal cartilages (trabeculae cranii), hypophyseal cartilages**, and **parachordal cartilages** (Fig. 17-3*A*). These cartilages contribute to the cranial base and, together with the cartilage from the occipital somites (see next paragraph) and the cartilaginous elements that develop around the eye, otic pits, and nasal pits, form the chondrocranium, which helps to protect the brain and sensory organs.

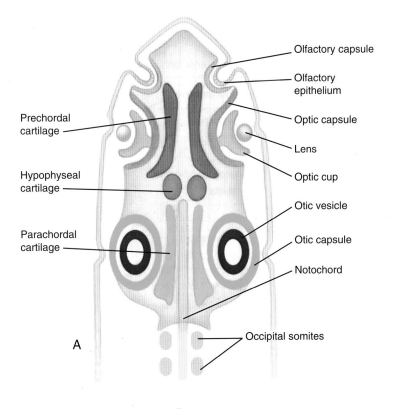

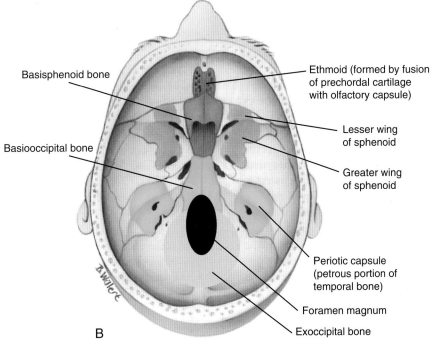

Figure 17-3. Origin of the human skull from primitive ancestors. *A,* Three pairs of cartilaginous plates formed in early ancestors: the prechordal, hypophyseal, and parachordal cartilages. The sensory organs are protected by sensory capsules. The "optic capsule" consists of the alisphenoid, hypochiasmatic, and orbitosphenoid cartilages. *B,* The base of the skull in humans, including the basisphenoid and basioccipital, is derived from the three pairs of cartilaginous plates formed in early ancestors. The most posterior element contributing to the skull base, the exoccipital bone, is derived from the primitive occipital somites of early ancestors.

The most caudal pair of elements that contributes to the chondrocranium, the **parachordal cartilages**, is derived from unsegmented paraxial mesoderm and is the first pair of elements to develop. The two cartilages will fuse across the midline to form the base of the occipital bone (i.e., the **basioccipital bone;** Fig. 17-3*B*). The **occipital somites** (see Fig. 17-3*A*) form the **exoccipital bone** (see Fig. 17-3*B*), which is, therefore, a modified vertebral element derived from segmented paraxial mesoderm (covered in Chapter 8).

The **periotic capsules** are derived from the primitive **otic capsule** ossification centers (see Fig. 17-3*A*) which will eventually form the petrous and mastoid regions of the temporal bone (see Fig. 17-3*B*). The basioccipital, exoccipital, and periotic capsule derivatives will eventually unite to form the **occipital bone** encircling the **foramen magnum** (see Fig. 17-3*B*).

The **hypophyseal cartilages**, the middle cartilages that contribute to the cranial base, fuse to form the **body of the sphenoid bone** (i.e., the **basisphenoid** bone; see Fig. 17-3*B*). Similarly, the posterior region of the **prechordal cartilages**, the most anterior pair of elements that contributes to the chondrocranium, forms the **presphenoid bone** (Fig. 17-4*A*). These bones will unite with three cartilages that develop around the eye: the **alisphenoid (ala temporalis) cartilage** (see Fig. 17-2*A*), the **hypochiasmatic cartilage** (see Fig. 17-4*A*), and the **orbitosphenoid (ala orbitalis) cartilage**. The alisphenoid cartilage will ultimately contribute to the **greater wing of the sphenoid bone,** whereas the **orbitosphenoid** and **hypochiasmatic cartilages** contribute to the **lesser wing of the sphenoid** bone (see Fig. 17-3*B*). In addition, the **prechordal cartilages** form the **ethmoid bone**, which, together with the **nasal** and **turbinate bones**, encapsulates the **nasal cavity** (see Figs. 17-2*A*, 17-3).

By birth, most of the cranial base has ossified, but two key regions of cartilage persist that are important for postnatal growth: **nasal septum** and **spheno-occipital synchondrosis (SOS)** (see Fig. 17-4*A*). The nasal septum is important for growth of the upper face until the age of seven, whereas the SOS contributes to growth along the anterior-posterior axis of the cranial base until age thirteen to fifteen in girls and age fifteen to seventeen in boys. The SOS consists of a modified epiphyseal growth plate that grows in two directions (see Chapter 8).

Defects in development of the chondrocranium are rare, although a mutation in a factor that controls endochondral bone formation will also affect development of the cranial base (see Chapter 8 for additional coverage of endochondral bone formation). As the cranial base is linked to the upper jaw, this will have a secondary consequence on upper jaw development, resulting in malocclusion of the upper molars. This is illustrated in Chapter 8 (Fig. 8-1), which shows a girl with achondroplasia. In addition to shortening of the long bones, a defect in development of the cranial base results in **midface hypoplasia**.

The membrane-bone armor that covered the skull of our piscine ancestors (bony fishes) is represented in humans by the membrane bones of the skull, consisting of the flat bones of the **cranial vault**, or **calvaria**, as well as many bones of the face (Fig. 17-5, also see Fig. 17-2). The mesenchyme from which they develop is derived from both neural crest cells and mesoderm (see the following "In the Research Lab" entitled "Origin of Vertebrate Head").

The bones of the cranial vault do not complete their growth during fetal life. The soft, fibrous sutures that join them at birth permit the skull vault to deform as it passes through the birth canal and allow it to continue to grow throughout infancy and childhood. Six such membranous sutures or **fontanelles** occupy the areas between the corners of cranial vault bones at birth (see Fig. 17-5). The **posterior** and **anterolateral fontanelles**, the smaller of the fontanelles, close by three months after birth, whereas the **anterior** and **posterolateral fontanelles**, which are larger, normally close during the second year. Palpation of the anterior fontanelle can be used to detect elevated intracranial pressure or premature closure of the skull sutures.

In the Research Lab

ORIGIN OF VERTEBRATE HEAD

The "new head hypothesis" proposed that the vertebrate head evolved by adding structures, derived from neural crest cells, cranial to the notochord. Cell lineage tracing, for example, using genetically modified mice to label neural crest–derived and mesoderm-derived structures, has confirmed this hypothesis. In the cranial base, the structures that develop around and caudal to the cranial tip of the notochord (i.e., the occipital bone) are derived from the mesoderm (yellow; see Fig. 17-4*A*). Structures that form rostral to the notochord (i.e., the sphenoid and ethmoid bones) are derived from the neural crest (tan; see Fig. 17-4*A*). Therefore, the neural crest–mesoderm boundary lies at the sphenoid-occipital interface, with one exception—the **hypochiasmatic cartilage**, which provides the attachment for the extraocular muscles, contributes to the sphenoid bone, and is derived from mesoderm, even though it lies rostral to the notochord (yellow islands; see Fig. 17-4*A*).

These lineage-tracing studies have revealed the contributions of neural crest and mesoderm to the mammalian cranial vault and pharyngeal arches. Neural crest–derived cells contribute to the **frontal bone** and to a portion of the **interparietal bones** in the cranial vault, whereas the mesoderm forms the **parietal bones** and the lateral part of the **interparietal bones** (see Fig. 17-4*B, C*). Neural crest cells are also found between paired parietal bones. Therefore, two sutures (**coronal** and **sagittal sutures**) are formed at a neural crest–mesoderm interface. This is significant, as mutations affecting formation of these boundaries result in craniosynostosis (see the following "In the Clinic" entitled "Craniosynostosis"). Neural crest cells also give rise to pharyngeal arch cartilages.

The chondrocranium is induced to form in response to signals from surrounding tissues. In the trunk, the notochord, which expresses Shh, is essential for formation of the axial skeleton (see Chapter 8). However, the structures of the anterior cranial base develop cranial to the notochord. Therefore, they must form in response to signaling from different tissues. Shh signaling from the developing brain and/or facial ectoderm is required for development of the midline structures of the cranial base, whereas FGF signals from the otic and nasal epithelium induce the formation of the otic and nasal capsules, respectively. Consequently, treatment of zebrafish embryos with cyclopamine (a chemical inhibitor of hedgehog signaling) results in loss of the trabecular bones. Similarly, ablation of the hedgehog receptor, smoothened, in the cranial neural crest in mice results in loss of the structures of the anterior cranial base. Therefore, it seems that the brain and ectoderm induce formation of the cranial base, and that similar signaling networks control development of the trunk and cranial axial structures.

In the Clinic

CRANIOSYNOSTOSIS

Craniosynostosis, the premature closure of sutures, affects approximately 1 in 2500 children. Sutures, which occur where two membrane bones meet, contain the progenitor cells that will give rise to new bone cells, the osteoblasts. These are the sites where growth of membrane bone occurs. Craniosynostosis can be caused by gene mutations or chromosomal abnormalities and occurs in many syndromes, including **Crouzon, Apert, Pfeiffer, Muenke,** and **Saethre-Chotzen syndromes**. Craniosynostosis can also be a consequence of environmental

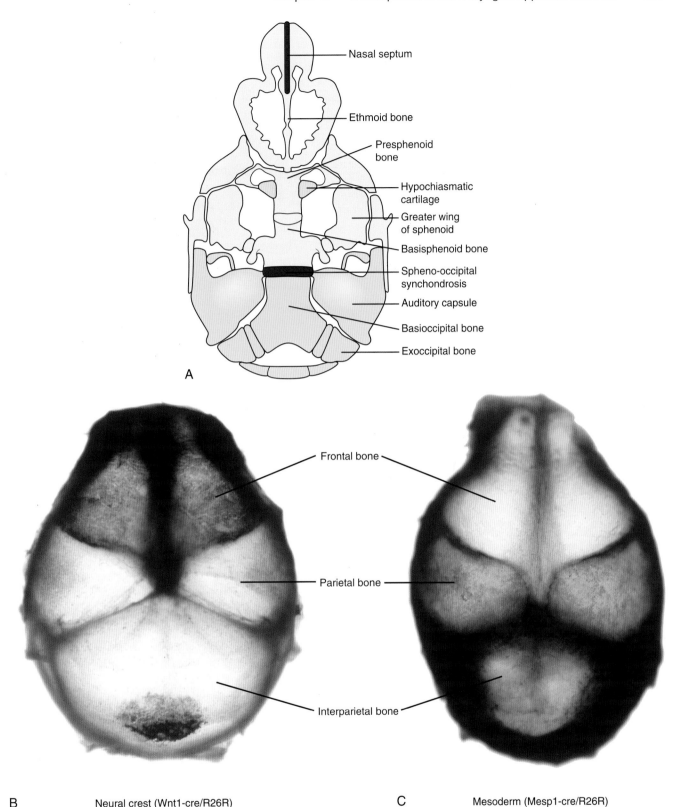

Figure 17-4. Developmental origins of the bones of the skull. *A,* Sketch showing the contributions of neural crest (tan) and mesoderm (yellow) to the cranial base. Regions of cartilage that persist postnatally to contribute to growth are shown in red. *B, C,* Dorsal views of the skull showing the contributions (blue staining) of neural crest (Wnt1-cre/R26R) and mesodermal cells (Mesp1-cre/R26R) to the cranial vault. As compared to the human, the interparietal bone in the mouse occupies a much larger proportion of the cranial vault.

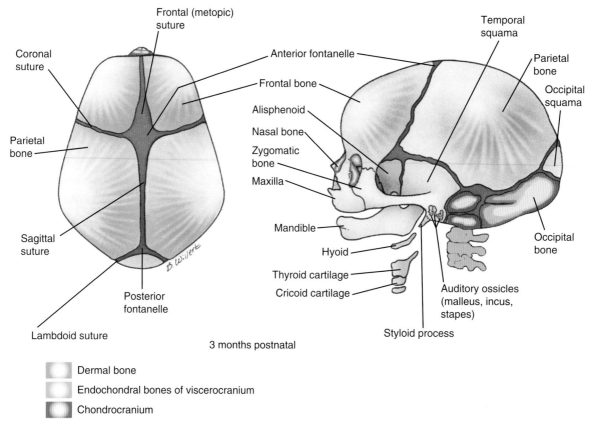

Dermal bone

Endochondral bones of viscerocranium

Chondrocranium

Figure 17-5. The brain in humans is mostly enclosed by the dermal bones of the cranial vault, which are separated by sutures and fontanelles. These bones do not fuse together until early childhood. The unfused sutures allow the cranium to deform during birth and to expand during childhood as the brain grows.

factors such as a restricted intrauterine environment or exposure to teratogens.

The sagittal and coronal sutures are most commonly affected. Closure at one suture causes increased growth at other sutures, thereby deforming the brain and skull, which develop a characteristic deformation depending on the suture(s) that is closed. This is shown in Figure 17-6A. Here, the coronal suture has closed, so that the head cannot grow in length, and now the developing brain forces growth along the other sutures. The result is a skull deformity, with possible changes in neurologic function, increased intracranial pressure, and inability to feed and close the eyes, together with respiratory and hearing abnormalities. **Dolichocephaly** and **scaphocephaly** are the terms used to describe long and narrow skulls. **Acrocephaly** describes a towered skull; **trigonocephaly** describes a skull that is triangular at the front; **brachycephaly** describes a skull that is broad and flattened; and **plagiocephaly** describes a skewed skull (Fig. 17-6B).

The most common genetic causes of **craniosynostosis syndromes** are mutations in (1) FGF RECEPTORS 2 (**Apert, Crouzon,** and **Pfeiffer syndromes**) and 3 (**Muenke** and **Crouzon syndromes** with **acanthosis nigricans**); (2) the transcription factor, TWIST (**Saethre-Chotzen syndrome**); and (3) a membrane-bound ligand, EPHRIN-B1 (EFNB1) (**craniofrontonasal syndrome**; Fig 17-7A). Pfeiffer syndrome is highly variable, but the most severe form is characterized by multiple synostoses (union of separate bones to form a single bone) that are associated with high mortality. Distinguishing characteristics of the hand and face can

be used to help with an initial diagnosis of the syndrome. For example, Pfeiffer syndrome is defined by a broad thumb and a big toe, Apert's syndrome by syndactyly, and craniofrontonasal syndrome by split nails (also see Chapter 20).

In the Research Lab

MOLECULAR MECHANISMS OF CRANIOSYNOSTOSIS

As was just covered, mutations in FGF RECEPTORS (FGFR1, 2, and 3) result in craniosynostosis. All of these mutations cause a gain of function in FGF signaling owing to the constitutive activation of receptors (i.e., these mutations result in an increase in FGF signaling). FGFs are expressed in the osteoblastic front of membrane bones (see Fig. 17-6C). Therefore, the highest levels of signaling are found in the cells adjacent to the bone, whereas lower levels are found in the sutural mesenchyme (see Fig 17-6C). The cognate receptors are expressed in the sutural mesenchyme (FGFR2) and in differentiating osteoblasts (FGFR1 and 3; see Fig. 17-6C).

Fgf signaling has two roles in suture development. Low levels of Fgfs in the sutural mesenchyme promote cell proliferation whereas high levels promote osteoblast differentiation. Therefore, the rate of osteogenesis is carefully controlled by balancing the level of Fgf signaling (see Fig. 17-6C). Increased Fgf signaling through constitutive activation of the receptors decreases cell proliferation and accelerates osteoblast differentiation, resulting in synostosis across the sutures (i.e., premature

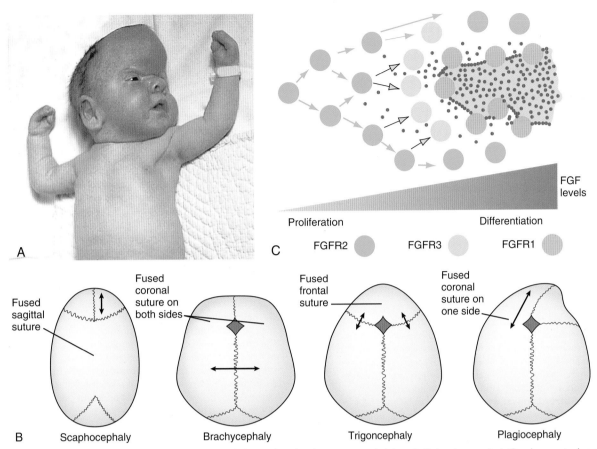

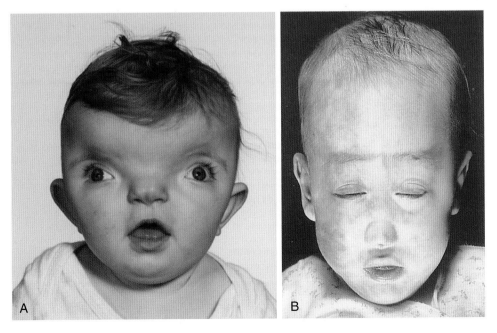

Figure 17-6. Abnormal development of the skull, and cellular and molecular events underlying skull development. *A,* Craniosynostosis occurring in Apert syndrome. In this infant, the coronal suture has fused prematurely. Therefore, the cranium has been forced to adopt a "tower skull" (acrocephalic) shape to accommodate the growing brain. *B,* Craniosynostosis results in different skull shapes, depending on which suture is affected. Following premature closure of each of the individual sutures, the arrows indicate the predominant direction of growth. *C,* Diagram showing expression of FGFs (purple dots) and FGFR1, 2, and 3 in a suture. FGF levels are highest at the bone interface, with lower levels in the sutural mesenchyme. Bone growth is controlled by balancing the level of FGF signaling with a low dose, increasing proliferation, and a high dose, promoting bone differentiation. Therefore, the increased FGF signaling that occurs in many craniosynostotic syndromes causes premature suture closure.

Figure 17-7. Infants with two types of craniofacial malformations. *A,* Craniofrontonasal dysplasia. In this infant there is hypertelorism, an expansion of the midline, and a central nasal groove. This syndrome is also characterized by bilateral or unilateral coronal craniosynostosis, as the neural crest–mesoderm boundary does not form at the coronal suture. *B,* An infant with holoprosencephaly. This spectrum of malformations ranges in severity from minor midfacial defects to extremely devastating malformations. In this infant, narrowing of the upper face and a single nostril can be seen.

closure of the fontanelles). In mouse models of craniosynostosis, administration of pharmacological inhibitors against the Fgf pathway during pregnancy and postnatally prevents premature suture closure. Such approaches may eventually allow non-surgical or reduced surgical intervention for the treatment of craniosynostosis in humans. Curiously, FGFR2 and 3 mutations are usually inherited as spontaneous new mutations through the paternal lineage, increasing in frequency with paternal age. One such mutation in FGFR2 (a mutation that causes **Apert syndrome**) increases the clonal expansion of mutant spermatogonia, thereby increasing the number of sperm carrying the mutation.

The EFNB1 and TWIST mutations specifically affect the coronal suture. Long-term lineage tracing studies in mice have shown that the coronal suture arises at a neural crest cell–mesoderm interface (see Fig. 17-4*B*, *C*). The frontal bone is derived from neural crest, whereas the adjacent parietal bone and the coronal sutural mesenchyme are derived from mesoderm. The neural crest–derived mesenchyme and the mesoderm have different cell adhesion properties and do not mix, thereby creating a sharp boundary. These distinct properties are controlled by the differential expression of ephrin ligands and their Eph receptors in the neural crest– and mesoderm-derived tissues (also see Fig. 8-5 in Chapter 8 and Fig. 20-29 in Chapter 20, as well as Chapters 9, 13, 14, for other examples of the differential expression of ephrin ligands and Eph receptors inhibiting cell mixing). Mutations in the ephrin signaling pathway and twist, which regulate ephrin expression, will affect the formation of this boundary.

Craniofrontonasal dysplasia, caused by an EFNB1 mutation, is an unusual X-linked syndrome in that heterozygote females show more severe phenotypes than hemizygous males. The ephrin ligand EFNB1 is specifically expressed in the neural crest and prevents mixing of neural crest–derived cells with mesodermal cells. In heterozygote females, the frontal bone will consist of a mixture of cells that either express one copy of the functional EFNB1 gene or express the mutated non-functional EFNB1 protein. Cells that express the normal EFNB1 gene have different cell adhesion and signaling properties than cells expressing the non-functional EFNB1 gene, such that the two populations will clump and segregate: the result is that some of these cells cross and abolish the sutural boundary. Additional features of craniofrontonasal dysplasia include severe hypertelorism (widely spaced eyes) and a bifid nasal tip in females (see Fig. 17-7*A*).

In the Clinic

HOLOPROSENCEPHALY

Holoprosencephaly (HPE) is the most common developmental defect of the forebrain, affecting 1 in 16,000 births and an estimated 1 in 250 fetuses. It results from a disturbance in early patterning of the forebrain (see Fig. 17-7*B*). The spectrum of phenotypes is wide and there is variable expressivity, which means that the same mutation can produce different phenotypic outcomes. This indicates the possibility of silent modifier genes and the fact that HPE should be viewed as a **multihit** or **digenic** disorder. It is estimated that approximately 30% of people with HPE mutations have no phenotype.

HPE can be classified into five forms: **alobar, lobar, semilobar, microform**, which are classical forms of HPE, and **MIH** (**middle interhemispheric form**; also known as **syntelencephaly**). In its most severe form, alobar HPE, only a single cerebral lobe forms (hence the name of the condition)

rather than paired right and left hemispheres. Defects of the olfactory nerves, olfactory bulbs, olfactory tracts, basal olfactory cortex, and associated structures including the limbic lobe, hippocampus, and mammillary bodies can also occur. The corpus callosum is sometimes affected; the hindbrain is usually normal. Patients with alobar HPE typically die within the first year. In the milder forms of HPE, semilobar and lobar HPE, partial separation of the single cerebral lobe is noted. In MIH, the anterior forebrain develops normally, but the hemispheres fail to separate in the posterior parietal and frontal regions.

Except for MIH, forebrain defects are accompanied by a spectrum of facial abnormalities that often, but not always, reflect the severity of the forebrain defect. Facial anomalies typical of holoprosencephaly include a flat nose, ocular **hypotelorism** (closely spaced eyes), deficient philtrum or cleft lip, high arched or cleft palate, and microcephaly (small skull) (see Fig. 17-7*B*). Particularly severe cases involve dramatic defects of the facial structures arising from the frontonasal prominence, most notably the nasal placodes (development of the face is covered in detail later in this chapter). Failure of the medial nasal processes to form results in agenesis of the intermaxillary process and reduction or absence of other midfacial structures such as the nasal bones, nasal septum, and ethmoid. The consequence may be **cebocephaly** (a single nostril; see Fig. 17-7*B*) and, at the most extreme, **cyclopia** (a single, midline eye). Mild cases of holoprosencephaly are characterized by relatively minimal midface anomalies and by **trigonocephaly**, a triangular skull shape that develops as a result of premature closure (synostosis) of the suture between the frontal bones and causes compression of the growing cerebral hemispheres (see Fig. 17-6*B*). Occasionally, the presence of a single, central incisor and the loss of the maxillary midline frenulum are the only indications of a holoprosencephalic phenotype. In **microform HPE**, mild facial abnormalities occur in the absence of forebrain defects.

At least twelve genetic loci have been implicated in holoprosencephaly in humans, and mutations in nine genes in these loci have been identified. Of these, four are components of the SONIC HEDGEHOG signaling pathway (SHH, PTC1, GLI2, and DISP1: DISPATCHED HOMOLOG 1). Mutations in SHH and in three transcription factors, ZIC2, SIX3, and TRANSFORMING GROWTH FACTOR INTERACTING FACTOR (TGIF), are the leading genetic causes of non-syndromic HPE.

Holoprosencephaly is also a feature of more than twenty-five syndromes and is seen in 5% of Smith-Lemli-Opitz syndrome patients. Smith-Lemli-Opitz syndrome affects about 1 in 9000 births (live and stillborn) and is the result of a mutation in the DHCR7 gene, which encodes 7-DEHYDROCHOLESTEROL REDUCTASE, an enzyme involved in the penultimate step of cholesterol synthesis. A cholesterol modification of Shh is necessary for full Shh activity (see Chapter 5); hence, it is believed that some Smith-Lemli-Opitz phenotypes are due to loss of hedgehog signaling.

Environmental agents associated with HPE include maternal exposure to **alcohol**, excess **vitamin A**, or **statins**, and **maternal diabetes**. Infants of diabetic mothers have a risk of holoprosencephaly that may be as high as 1%.

Conversely, some syndromes have **hypertelorism** (widely spaced eyes) as a component. This is seen in **craniofrontonasal dysplasia**, resulting from mutations in EFNB1 (EPHRIN-B1; see Fig. 17-7*A*); **Gorlin syndrome** resulting from mutations in PTC1; and **Greig cephalopolysyndactyly**, resulting from mutations in GLI3. As Gli3 and Ptc1 are components of the Shh pathway and can repress Shh signaling, it is believed that the hypertelorism observed in Gorlin and Greig cephalopolysyndactyly is due to a gain in Shh signaling (see the following "In the Research Lab" entitled "Cranial Midline and HPE").

In the Research Lab

CRANIAL MIDLINE AND HPE

Establishment of the cranial midline involves three major steps during development (Fig. 17-8A): (1) formation of the prechordal plate during gastrulation; (2) signaling from the prechordal plate to the overlying forebrain, which initially consists of a single cerebral lobe (covered in Chapter 9), to divide the forebrain into two cerebral lobes; surgical ablation of the prechordal plate results in cyclopia, owing to loss of this signaling; and (3) signaling by the forebrain to the facial ectoderm in post-neurulation stages to induce and/or maintain gene expression in this area. Signaling by the facial ectoderm regulates the outgrowth of the frontonasal prominence during subsequent formation of the midline of the face (development of the face is covered later in this chapter).

The use of different animal models has revealed how genetic mutations result in HPE. In humans, SHH mutations are the leading genetic cause of non-syndromic HPE. In animal models, Shh is expressed, and is required, in the prechordal plate, forebrain,

and facial ectoderm to establish the midline (Fig. 17-8A). Clearly emphasizing the importance of the Shh pathway, Shh–/– mutant mice exhibit cyclopia and develop a proboscis (Fig 17-8B). The developing upper face normally consists of the medial nasal and lateral nasal processes (Fig. 17-8C; also see Fig. 17-18). In Shh mutants, a total collapse of the midline is shown by loss of the medial nasal processes (see Fig 17-8C). With loss of these processes, the lateral nasal processes become positioned at the midline of the upper face (see Fig. 17-8C). Loss of factors involved in Shh signaling, such as dispatched, which is needed for the transport of Shh out of the cell, and Sil, an intracellular factor needed to activate the Smo receptor, also results in holoprosencephalic phenotypes in mice.

During the establishment of the midline, Shh signaling is first required in the prechordal plate region to divide the single midline eye primordium in the forebrain into eye (Pax6 expressing) and non-eye (non-Pax6 expressing) territories (see Fig. 17-8A). Shh expression also maintains cell survival of the prechordal plate and activates Shh expression in the developing

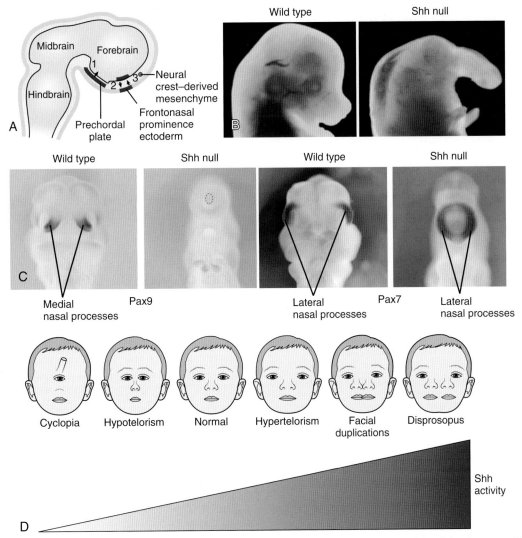

Figure 17-8. The role of Shh during establishment of the midline. *A*, Shh is required at three stages of facial development (Shh expression is shown in red and arrows indicate the directions of signaling; see text for details). *B, C*, Lateral (*B*) and frontal (*C*) views of the head of wild-type mice and Shh mutants. In the Shh mutant, the facial structures are not well defined and there is a proboscis, the medial nasal processes (shown by Pax9 expression) are not present, and the lateral nasal processes (shown by Pax7 expression) meet at the midline. *D*, Levels of Shh signaling control the spectrum of midline patterning abnormalities. Absence of Shh signaling results in cyclopia and alobar HPE, whereas increased Shh signaling may result in diprosopus.

diencephalon (see Fig. 17-8A). As the prechordal plate also expresses other factors necessary for midline patterning, such as the Wnt antagonist, Dkk1, and the Bmp antagonist, noggin, loss of Shh signaling results in the loss of additional factors required for midline development. Subsequently, Shh signaling from the diencephalon activates the expression of Shh in the ectoderm of the frontonasal prominence and creates a unique zone called the frontonasal ectodermal zone (FEZ; see later "In the Research Lab" entitled "Patterning of Facial Prominences"), which is required for proximodistal outgrowth and dorsoventral patterning of the upper face (see Fig. 17-8A). Induction of Shh in the facial ectoderm requires the presence of neural crest cells that migrate into the upper facial prominence. Application of Shh-blocking antibodies in the diencephalon or frontonasal prominence of developing chick embryos results in hypotelorism, showing that both domains of Shh expression are needed for appropriate midline development.

Treatment of developing chick embryos with cyclopamine, an inhibitor of hedgehog signaling, has shown that loss of Shh function earlier in development (e.g., in the prechordal plate) has a more severe effect than loss of Shh function later in development (e.g., in the facial ectoderm). As HPE is due to haploinsufficiency (i.e., the presence of one mutated gene and one wild-type allele), this could, in part, explain the spectrum of phenotypes observed as a result of Shh mutations. An environmental insult, such as in utero exposure to alcohol or retinoic acid, would downregulate the expression of the wild-type allele of Shh, further decreasing the levels of Shh. An early environmental insult would have the most severe consequences, as this would affect both the forebrain and subsequently the facial prominence, whereas later insults would affect only the facial structures, thereby resulting in milder forms of HPE.

Mutations in silent modifier genes may also determine the phenotypic spectrum of particular Shh mutations. The severity of the HPE defect would be dependent on when and where these silent modifier genes are expressed. Modifier genes would include components or regulators of the Shh pathway, such as the cell-surface molecules Gas1 and Cdo, which are expressed at sites distant to the source of Shh and are thought to increase levels of Shh signaling.

Conversely, gain of function of Shh signaling results in expansion of the midline. Misexpression of Shh in the diencephalon or the ectoderm of the frontonasal prominence in chicken embryos results in an expansion of the midline. Hence, it is believed that the levels of Shh signaling may define a spectrum of facial disorders from cyclopia to diprosopus—the duplication of facial structures (see Fig. 17-8D).

Mutations in TGIF, ZIC2, and SIX3 also result in loss of Shh signaling, explaining why their loss of function causes HPE. TGIF and ZIC2 are required for development of the prechordal plate. Therefore, mutations in these factors results in early loss of Shh signaling. Six3 directly regulates Shh expression in the forebrain and, hence, affects later stages of midline patterning.

The MIH form of HPE is caused by a hypomorphic variant of ZIC2. Zic2 induces the formation of the roof plate of the neural tube, which expresses Bmps important for patterning the dorsoventral axis of the developing brain (see Chapters 4 and 9).

DEVELOPMENT OF PHARYNGEAL ARCHES

 Animation 17-1: Development of Pharyngeal Apparatus.
Animations are available online at StudentConsult.

The pharyngeal arches evolved from the gill arches of jawless fish and have been evolutionarily conserved.

These arches form during the embryogenesis of all vertebrates. In jawed vertebrates, the first arch gives rise to the lower jaw and part of the upper jaw. The remaining arches form the gills in modern fish and many structures of the face and neck in humans.

PHARYNGEAL APPARATUS

Human embryos include four pairs of well-defined pharyngeal arches numbered one, two, three, and four. Arch five either never forms in humans or forms as a short-lived rudiment and promptly regresses, and evidence for the presence of a true sixth arch is questioned. Arches four and six cannot be readily seen externally (Fig. 17-9). Like so many other structures in the body, the pharyngeal arches form in craniocaudal succession: the first arch forms on day twenty-two; the second and third arches form sequentially on day twenty-four; and the fourth and sixth arches form sequentially on day twenty-nine.

Pharyngeal arches consist of a mesenchymal core (mesoderm and neural crest cells) that is covered on the outside with ectoderm and lined on the inside with endoderm (Fig. 17-9D, E). Each arch contains (1) a central cartilaginous skeletal element (derived from neural crest cells); (2) striated muscle rudiments (derived from head mesoderm) innervated by an arch-specific cranial nerve; and (3) an aortic arch artery (covered in Chapter 13).

The pharyngeal arches of human embryos initially resemble the gill arches of fish, except that they never become perforated to form gill slits. Instead, the external **pharyngeal clefts** or **grooves** between the arches remain separated from the apposed, internal **pharyngeal pouches** by thin **pharyngeal membranes**. These membranes are **initially** two-layered, consisting of ectoderm and endoderm; they are later infiltrated by mesenchymal cells.

PHARYNGEAL ARCH CARTILAGES AND ORIGIN OF SKELETAL ELEMENTS

The cartilages that form within the pharyngeal arches develop from neural crest cells originating from the midbrain and hindbrain regions. As covered in Chapter 4, neural crest cells arise from the neural folds and migrate ventrolaterally. In the trunk region, their migration occurs mainly by active neural crest cell movement. In the head, migration also involves active neural crest cell movement. But in contrast to trunk neural crest cells, migration of head neural crest cells also involves a passive component in which ventral displacement of the surrounding tissue translocates neural crest cells ventrally.

Figure 17-10 and Table 17-1 illustrate and summarize, respectively, the skeletal elements derived from the pharyngeal arch cartilages.

The first pharyngeal arch has two pairs of prominences associated with it: the **mandibular** and **maxillary prominences** (or **swellings**; see Fig. 17-9A-C), which give rise to the lower jaw and part of the upper jaw, respectively. Although the maxillary prominences were long thought to develop from branching of the first pharyngeal arches, it is now known that the maxillary prominences arise from mesenchyme cranial to the

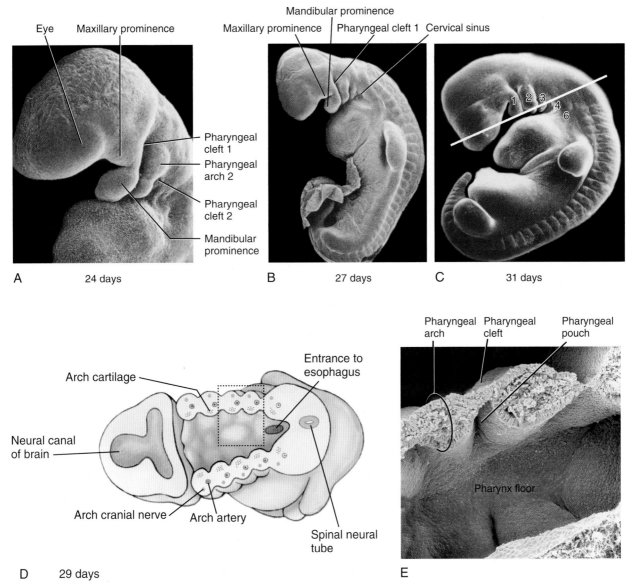

Figure 17-9. Formation of the pharyngeal arches. The pharyngeal arches form in craniocaudal sequence during the fourth and fifth weeks. *A,* By day twenty-four, the first two arches have formed, as have the maxillary and mandibular prominences. *B,* By day twenty-seven, the first three arches have formed. *C,* By the early fifth week, all five arches have formed. The line indicates the plane of the section shown (at a slightly earlier stage) in part *D. D,* Schematic cross section through the pharyngeal arches, showing the cartilage, artery, and cranial nerve in each arch. The box indicates the region enlarged in *E. E,* Scanning electron micrograph of a section similar to that shown in *D.*

first arch. Each pair of maxillary and mandibular prominences contains a transient central cartilaginous element. The central cartilage of each maxillary prominence is the **palatopterygoquadrate bar**, and the central cartilage of each mandibular prominence is **Meckel's cartilage** (see Fig. 17-10). These cartilages arise between days forty-one and forty-five. Both the maxillary and mandibular prominences are formed largely from neural crest cells that migrate from the neural folds of the midbrain (mesencephalon) and the cranial hindbrain (metencephalon) (covered later in this chapter).

Most of **Meckel's cartilage** disappears, being resorbed or becoming encapsulated by the developing mandibular bone. However, the proximal part forms the **malleus, sphenomandibular ligament**, and **anterior ligament of the malleus** (see Fig. 17-10).

The maxillary cartilage (palatopterygoquadrate bar) forms the **incus** and a small bone, called the **alisphenoid,** located in the orbital wall (see Fig. 17-10; see also Figs. 17-2A, 17-5). These derivatives become surrounded by the maxilla, zygomatic, and squamous portions of the temporal bones, which together with the mandible are all membrane bones. Therefore, most of the facial skeletal structures are derived from bones of dermal origin.

The second pharyngeal arch cartilage forms from neural crest cells that migrate from neural folds at the level of rhombomere 4 of the hindbrain (rhombomeres are covered further in Chapter 9; see Fig. 17-14). After the jaws evolved, the second-arch cartilages were recruited as bracing elements to help support the jaws and attach them to the neurocranium. The human second-arch cartilage, which is called **Reichert's cartilage,** arises between

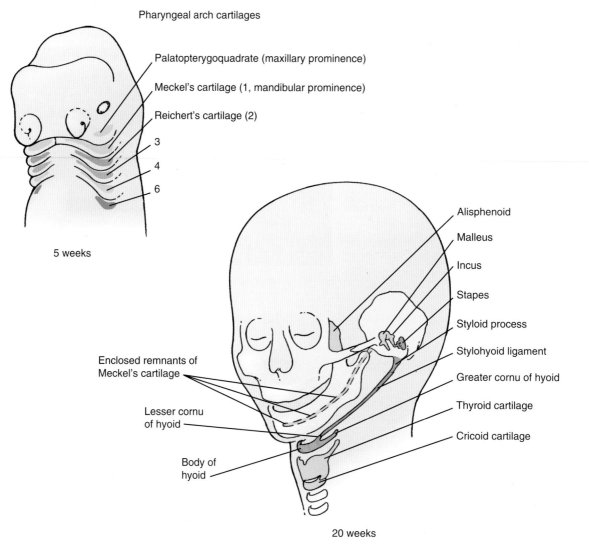

Pharyngeal arch cartilages

Palatopterygoquadrate (maxillary prominence)

Meckel's cartilage (1, mandibular prominence)

Reichert's cartilage (2)

3

4

6

5 weeks

Alisphenoid

Malleus

Incus

Stapes

Styloid process

Stylohyoid ligament

Greater cornu of hyoid

Thyroid cartilage

Cricoid cartilage

Enclosed remnants of Meckel's cartilage

Lesser cornu of hyoid

Body of hyoid

20 weeks

Figure 17-10. Fate of the pharyngeal arch cartilages. These cartilages give rise to the alisphenoid (a small bone of the orbit), elements of the jaw skeleton, three auditory ossicles, and the hyoid and laryngeal skeleton.

days forty-five and forty-eight. This arch will ultimately form the **stapes** of the middle ear, the **styloid process** of the temporal bone, the fibrous **stylohyoid ligament**, and the **lesser horns** (**cornua**) and part of the **body of the hyoid** bone (its midline and the regions that articulate with the greater horns; see Fig. 17-10). The hyoid bone is stabilized by muscle attachments to the styloid process and mandible; through its muscular attachments to the larynx and the tongue, it functions in both swallowing and vocalization.

The third pharyngeal arch cartilage is formed from neural crest cells that migrate from the caudal hindbrain (myelencephalon). Ossification of this cartilage occurs endochondrally to form the **greater horns** (cornua) and part of the **body of the hyoid** bone (see Fig. 17-10).

The fourth and sixth pharyngeal arches give rise to the **larynx**, consisting of the **thyroid, cuneiform, corniculate, arytenoid,** and **cricoid cartilages** (see Fig. 17-10). The thyroid cartilage is derived from the fourth-arch neural crest. The **epiglottal cartilages** do not form until the fifth month, long after the other pharyngeal arch cartilages have formed. These cartilages

also arise from the fourth-arch neural crest. Whether the remaining cartilages of the larynx arise from neural crest or mesoderm is uncertain.

DEVELOPMENT OF TEMPOROMANDIBULAR JOINT

In all jawed vertebrates except mammals, the jaw joint is formed from endochondral bones that develop from the maxillary and mandibular cartilages, even though other portions of the jaw may be formed from membrane bones. However, among the immediate ancestors of mammals, a second, novel jaw articulation developed between two membrane bones: the temporal and mandible. As this new **temporomandibular joint (TMJ)** became dominant, the bones of the ancient endochondral jaw articulation shifted into the adjacent middle ear and joined with the preexisting stapes to form the unique three-ossicle auditory mechanism of mammals.

The components and cavities of the TMJ are established by week fourteen of gestation. The TMJ consists of a synovial joint between the **mandibular condyle** and

TABLE 17-1   DERIVATIVES OF THE PHARYNGEAL ARCHES AND THEIR TISSUES OF ORIGIN

Pharyngeal Arch	Arch Artery[a]	Skeletal Elements	Muscles	Cranial Nerve[b]
1	Terminal branch of maxillary artery	Derived from arch cartilages (originating from neural crest cells): from maxillary cartilage: alisphenoid, incus. From Meckel's cartilage: malleus. Derived by direct ossification from arch dermal mesenchyme: maxilla, zygomatic, squamous portion of temporal bone, mandible (originate from neural crest cells)	Muscles of mastication (temporalis, masseter, medial and lateral pterygoids), mylohyoid, anterior belly of the digastric, tensor tympani, tensor veli palatini (originate from head mesoderm)	Maxillary and mandibular divisions of trigeminal nerve (V)
2	Stapedial artery (embryonic), caroticotympanic artery (adult)	Stapes, styloid process, lesser horns and part of body of hyoid (derived from the second-arch [Reichert's] cartilage; originate from neural crest cells)	Muscles of facial expression (orbicularis oculi, orbicularis oris, risorius, platysma, auricularis, frontalis, and buccinator), posterior belly of the digastric, stylohyoid, stapedius (originate from head mesoderm)	Facial nerve (VII)
3	Common carotid artery, root of internal carotid	Lower rim and part of body of hyoid (derived from the third-arch cartilage; originate from neural crest)	Stylopharyngeus (originates from head mesoderm)	Glossopharyngeal nerve (IX)
4	Arch of aorta (left side), right subclavian artery (right side); original sprouts of pulmonary arteries	Thyroid and epiglottal laryngeal cartilages (derived from the fourth-arch cartilage; originate from neural crest cells)	Constrictors of pharynx, cricothyroid, levator veli palatini (originate from occipital somites)	Superior laryngeal branch of vagus nerve (X)
6	Ductus arteriosus; roots of definitive pulmonary arteries	Remaining laryngeal cartilages (derived from the sixth-arch cartilage; uncertain whether they originate from neural crest or mesoderm)	Intrinsic muscles of larynx (except the cricothyroid; originate from occipital somites)	Recurrent laryngeal branch of vagus nerve (X)

[a]Aortic arch artery development is covered in Chapter 13.
[b]Cranial nerve development is covered in Chapter 10.

the **glenoid blastema** (associated with the temporal bone), which are separated by an **interarticular disc**. The joint forms from week nine, starting with development of the condylar process on the mandible. One week later, the condylar cartilage has formed and the blastema of the temporal bones has started to develop. At this time, the condylar cartilage and temporal bone are separated by the condensation of the interarticular disc. Cavitation starts at week ten in two waves: first between the condylar process and interarticular disc, forming the **inferior joint space;** and then (one week later) between the disc and temporal bone, forming the **superior joint space**.

The condylar cartilage is distinct from endochondral cartilages in that it arises within the periosteum of a membrane bone. It is one of several cartilages, termed **secondary cartilages**, to develop in this way during facial growth. Secondary cartilages have unique properties, including that they grow in response to mechanical stimulation. Unlike the other facial secondary cartilages, the condylar cartilage persists postnatally and plays a significant role in postnatal growth of the lower jaw.

ORIGIN OF VASCULAR SUPPLY

As covered in detail in Chapter 13, the aortic arch artery system initially takes the form of a basket-like arrangement of five pairs of arteries that arise from the expansion at the end of the outflow tract called the **aortic sac.** These arteries connect the paired ventral aortae with the paired dorsal aortae (Fig. 17-11). This system is remodeled to produce the great arteries of the thorax and the branches that supply the head and neck (illustrated in Figure 17-11 and summarized in Table 17-1; see Chapter 13 for details of this remodeling).

As covered in Chapter 13, arterial blood reaches the head via paired vertebral arteries that form from anastomoses among intersegmental arteries and via the **common carotid arteries**. The common carotid arteries branch to form the **internal** and **external carotid arteries**. The internal carotid and vertebral arteries supply the brain, and the external carotid arteries supply the face. The common carotids and the roots of the internal carotids are derived from the third-arch arteries, whereas distal portions of the internal carotids are derived from

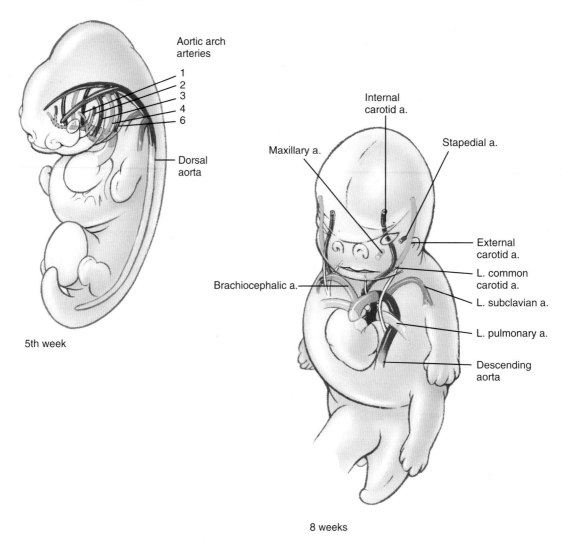

Figure 17-11. Fate of the pharyngeal arch arteries. These arteries are modified to form definitive arteries of the upper thorax, neck, and head (covered in Chapter 13).

the cranial extensions of the paired dorsal aortae. The external carotid arteries sprout de novo from the common carotids. The endothelium of the head vasculature and aortic arch arteries is derived from mesoderm.

ORIGIN AND INNERVATION OF MUSCULATURE

The musculature of the pharyngeal arches is derived from the cranial head mesoderm. This includes the first five (so-called occipital) somites, which form the muscles in arches four and six, and the unsegmented mesoderm located rostral to these somites (paraxial mesoderm), which forms the musculature in arches one through three. Myoblasts for each pharyngeal arch, along with the precursors of the extraocular muscles, arise at discrete locations within this unsegmented mesoderm. The muscles that form in each pharyngeal arch are innervated by a cranial nerve branch that is specific to that arch, and they maintain their relationship in the adult. This close relationship has been conserved since the evolution of jawed fish; along with the pharyngeal pouches, it defines a conserved segmental organization for the pharyngeal arch

system. Figure 17-12 shows the muscles derived from the pharyngeal arches, and Figure 17-13 shows the innervation of these muscles; Table 17-1 summarizes the muscles formed in each pharyngeal arch and their innervation.

In the first arch, paraxial mesoderm originating beside the metencephalon (rhombomeres 1 and 2) gives rise to the **muscles of mastication** (the **temporalis, masseter,** and **medial** and **lateral pterygoids**), as well as to the **mylohyoid, anterior belly of the digastric, tensor tympani,** and **tensor veli palatini** muscles. Branches of the **trigeminal (V) nerve** innervate all of these muscles.

In the second arch, paraxial mesoderm gives rise to the muscles of facial expression, including the **orbicularis oculi, orbicularis oris, risorius, platysma, auricularis, frontalis,** and **buccinator** muscles, as well as to the **posterior belly of the digastric, stylohyoid,** and **stapedius** muscles. The muscle primordia of this arch migrate to their final position in the head and are innervated by the **facial (VII) nerve.**

In the third arch, paraxial mesoderm gives rise to a single muscle: the long, slender **stylopharyngeus,** which originates on the styloid process and inserts into the wall of the pharynx. This muscle raises the pharynx during

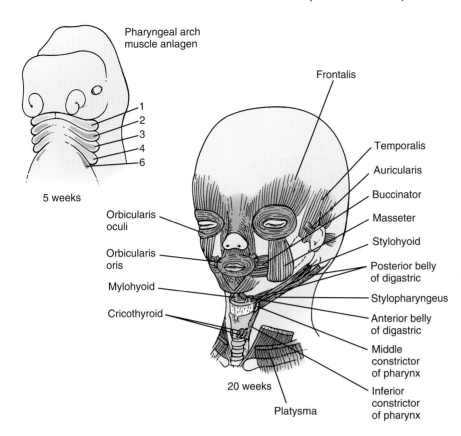

Pharyngeal arch muscle anlagen

1
2
3
4
6

5 weeks

Frontalis

Temporalis

Auricularis

Buccinator

Masseter

Stylohyoid

Posterior belly of digastric

Stylopharyngeus

Anterior belly of digastric

Middle constrictor of pharynx

Inferior constrictor of pharynx

Orbicularis oculi

Orbicularis oris

Mylohyoid

Cricothyroid

20 weeks

Platysma

Figure 17-12. Fate of the pharyngeal arch musculature. The pharyngeal arch muscles develop from cranial paraxial mesoderm and occipital somites. The myoblasts of the sixth arch become the intrinsic laryngeal muscles (not shown).

vocalization and swallowing, and it is innervated by the **glossopharyngeal (IX) nerve**.

Muscles originating in the fourth and sixth arches arise from the occipital somites and are the **superior, middle**, and **inferior constrictors** of the pharynx, the **cricothyroid**, and the **levator veli palatini**, which function in vocalization and swallowing. These muscles are innervated by the **vagus (X) nerve**.

In addition, myoblasts from the myotomes of the occipital somites coalesce beside somite four and extend ventrally as an elongated column, the **hypoglossal cord**, eventually becoming located ventral to the caudal region of the pharynx. Some of these myoblasts shift dorsally to form the **intrinsic laryngeal musculature** (i.e., the lateral **cricoarytenoids, thyroarytenoids**, and **vocalis** muscles), which is mainly devoted to vocalization. Like the muscles of the fourth and sixth arches, which also arise from the occipital somites, these muscles are innervated by the **vagus nerve**. However, most of the myoblasts of the hypoglossal cord remain ventral and shift cranially. These will form the **intrinsic** and **extrinsic musculature** of the tongue. All of these muscles except one (the palatoglossus, which is innervated by the **vagus nerve**; covered later in the chapter in the section on development of the tongue) are innervated by the **hypoglossal (XII) nerve**.

To summarize, four of the cranial nerves arising in the hindbrain supply branches to the pharyngeal arches and their derivatives (see Fig. 17-13; the cranial nerves are covered in detail in Chapter 10): (1) the maxillary and mandibular prominences (derivatives of the cranial mesenchyme and first arch) are innervated, respectively, by the **maxillary**

and **mandibular branches** of the **trigeminal nerve** (cranial nerve V); (2) the second arch is innervated by the **facial nerve** (cranial nerve VII); (3) the third arch is innervated by the **glossopharyngeal nerve** (cranial nerve IX); and (4) the fourth and sixth arches are innervated by the **superior laryngeal** and **recurrent laryngeal** branches of the **vagus nerve** (cranial nerve X). Most of the tongue muscles are innervated by the **hypoglossal nerve** (cranial nerve XII). Therefore, innervation of muscles in the adults reflects the embryonic origin of the muscles.

Additional Cranial Nerve Innervation

As covered in greater detail in Chapter 10, in addition to the cranial nerves just discussed, seven other cranial nerves innervate structures that develop in association with the pharyngeal apparatus. Six **extraocular muscles** (derived from mesoderm that migrates to surround the developing eyes) are innervated by cranial nerves: four muscles (**inferior oblique, medial rectus, superior rectus**, and **inferior rectus**) are innervated by the **oculomotor nerve** (cranial nerve III; originates from the mesencephalon); one muscle (**superior oblique**) is innervated by the **trochlear nerve** (cranial nerve IV; originates from the hindbrain); and one muscle (**lateral rectus**) is innervated by the **abducens nerve** (cranial nerve VI; originates from the hindbrain). The **accessory nerve** (cranial nerve XI) innervates another group of muscles including two important neck muscles (**sternocleidomastoid, trapezius**).

Three **sensory organs** are innervated by cranial nerves: (1) the **olfactory nerve** (cranial nerve I; originates from the nasal placode and is associated with the

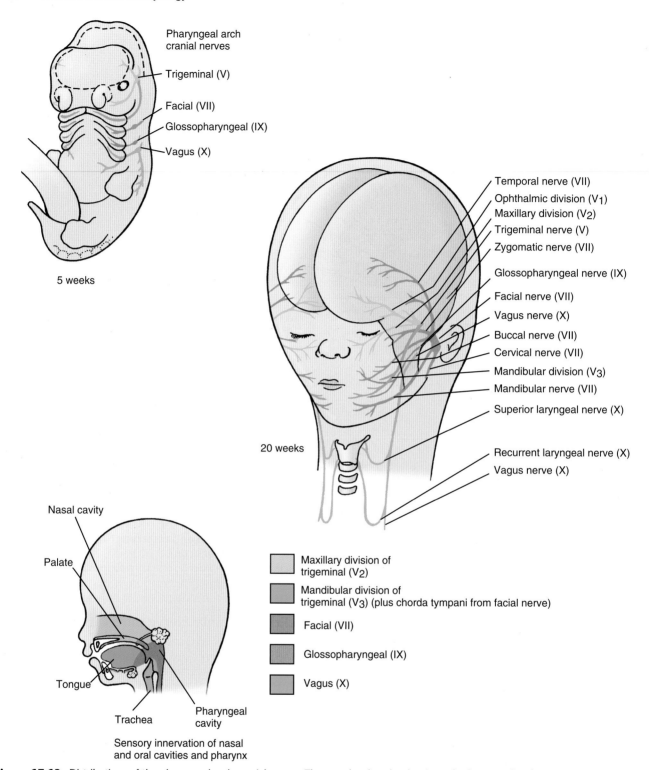

Figure 17-13. Distributions of the pharyngeal arch cranial nerves. The muscles that develop in each pharyngeal arch are served by the cranial nerve that originally innervates that arch. The sensory innervation of the nasal and oral cavities and pharynx is also diagrammed.

telencephalon) innervates the olfactory epithelium of the developing nasal cavities; (2) the **optic nerve** (cranial nerve II; originates from the sensory layer of the optic cup and is associated with the diencephalon) innervates the developing retina of the eye; and (3) the **vestibulocochlear nerve** (cranial nerve VIII; originates from the otic placode and is associated with the hindbrain) innervates the developing inner ear.

MANY CRANIAL NERVES ARE MIXED NERVES

As covered in Chapter 10, the various cranial nerves carry different combinations of somatic motor, autonomic, and sensory fibers. In the trunk, nerves are mixed, but in the head, cranial nerves can be mixed (V, VII, IX, and X), predominantly sensory (I, II, and VIII), or motor (III, IV, VI, XI, and XII). However, in all cases, the somatic motoneurons have their cell bodies in the brain, whereas the cell bodies of the sensory neurons are located in cranial nerve ganglia. In the trunk, the sensory neurons are always derived from neural crest cells, but in the head, some sensory neurons (V, VII, VIII, IX, and X) are derived from two populations—neural crest cells, as in the trunk, and special areas of ectoderm known as **neurogenic ectodermal placodes**. These placodes are covered in detail in Chapter 10.

The sensory innervation of the face is provided by the ophthalmic, maxillary, and mandibular divisions of the trigeminal nerve, as would be expected from the fact that the dermis in this region develops from neural crest cells that migrate into the first pharyngeal arch and frontonasal prominence of the face (see Fig. 17-13). The sensory innervation of the dorsal side of the head and neck is provided by the second and third cervical spinal nerves. The sensory innervation of the mouth, pharynx, and larynx is provided by cranial nerves V, VII, IX, and X, as illustrated in Figure 17-13.

In the Research Lab

HINDBRAIN IS SEGMENTED

As covered in Chapter 9, the developing brain is initially subdivided into the prosencephalon, mesencephalon, and rhombencephalon, and the latter is transiently subdivided into distinct segments called rhombomeres (r). Each rhombomere expresses a unique combination of transcription factors. Of particular relevance are those of the Hox gene family, which, as in the trunk, are expressed in nested patterns along the cranial-caudal axis (see Chapter 8 for further coverage). In the hindbrain, their rostral limit of expression corresponds to a rhombomere boundary (Fig. 17-14A). Members of the Hox gene family, alone or in combination, specify the identity of the individual rhombomeres. For example, Hoxa1 is necessary for the development of r4 and 5, as both are severely reduced or absent in mice in which Hoxa1 is inactivated. Hoxb1 is specifically expressed in r4. Genetic inactivation of Hoxb1 in mice and zebrafish results in the transformation of r4 to r2. Conversely, when Hoxb1 is misexpressed in r2 in chick, r2 acquires r4 characteristics. As the neural crest cells typically express the Hox genes from the rhombomeres they arise from, this in turn helps specify the identity of the neural crest derivatives.

One important aspect of hindbrain segmentation is that it provides the framework for establishing neuronal patterning within the developing pharyngeal arches: the motor nuclei of cranial nerves V, VII, and IX arise in a two-segment (i.e., rhombomere) periodicity, with each of their nerves innervating one pharyngeal arch (see Fig. 17-14A). Thus, cranial nerve V innervates pharyngeal arch one, cranial nerve VII innervates pharyngeal arch two, and cranial nerve IX innervates pharyngeal arch three (cranial nerves X and XII innervate pharyngeal arches four and six). When Hoxb1 function is lost in mice, the motoneurons that arise from r4 behave like those that arise from r2, migrating in a pattern characteristic of r2 neurons. In a converse experiment in chick in which Hoxb1 is overexpressed in r2, r2 motoneurons migrate into the second arch instead of toward their usual first arch targets.

Hindbrain segmentation also plays a role in keeping different neural crest cell populations apart so that hindbrain neural crest cells migrate in register in three segmental streams: a stream derived from r1 and r2, a stream from r4, and a stream from r6, r7 (Fig. 17-14B; note that in addition to the three streams of hindbrain neural crest cells, a cranial stream of neural crest cells arises from the midbrain and caudal forebrain). Formation

of the three hindbrain streams is achieved in part by the fact that comparatively few neural crest cells originate from r3 and r5; those that do originate from r3 and r5 migrate cranially or caudally into adjacent neural crest cell streams (see Fig. 17-14B). In addition, mesodermal signals keep the distinct neural crest populations apart. Separation of these neural crest streams is important, as they express different combinations of Hox genes necessary for patterning of the pharyngeal arches. For example, the first (those from r1 and r2) and second (those from r4) hindbrain neural crest cell streams are characterized by the absence and presence, respectively, of Hoxa2 expression: specifically, r2 neural crest cell progeny downregulate Hoxa2 expression as they start to migrate, and Hoxa2 expression in the presumptive r1 neural crest cells is inhibited by Fgf8 signaling from the isthmus (a constricted zone consisting of the caudal midbrain and cranial hindbrain) (Fig. 17-15A). If Hoxa2 is mutated in mice, the second pharyngeal arch is homeotically transformed into the first pharyngeal arch. Thus, second arch derivatives, such as the stapes and styloid process, are absent and are replaced by an ectopic tympanic ring, malleus, and incus, usually derivatives of the first pharyngeal arch (Fig. 17-15B). Conversely, overexpression of Hoxa2 in the first pharyngeal arch in both chick and Xenopus transforms the first pharyngeal arch into a second pharyngeal arch. Hence, the absence or presence of Hoxa2 determines first versus second pharyngeal arch identity. Likewise, expression of Hoxa2 together with Hoxa3 and Hoxa4 patterns the third and fourth pharyngeal arches: in the absence of all three Hox genes, pharyngeal arches two, three, and four now all form structures characteristic of the first pharyngeal arch. This regulation of skeletal identity by Hox gene expression also occurs in the trunk axial skeleton (see Figs. 8-10, 8-11 in Chapter 8). The Hox genes not only are important for patterning the pharyngeal arch skeletal derivatives but are required for the development of pharyngeal arch endodermal structures. For example, Hoxa3 is required for development of the thymus and parathyroid, which arise from the third pharyngeal pouches (see development of pharyngeal pouches, covered later in this chapter).

RETINOIC ACID ACTS IN NORMAL AND ABNORMAL DEVELOPMENT OF HEAD AND NECK

Retinoic acid (RA), the biologically active derivative of vitamin A (retinol), is needed for development and segmentation of the caudal pharyngeal arches. But when it is given in excess, it acts as a potent craniofacial **teratogen**, especially affecting pharyngeal arches one and two, in which it causes hypoplasia. Isotretinoin (accutane or 13-cis-retinoic acid), a drug used to treat a severe form of acne, can cause such hypoplasia when embryos are exposed during gastrulation and early organogenesis (i.e., exposure during early pregnancy). The developmental sensitivity to RA is, in part, explained by the gradient of RA that forms across the hindbrain during development owing to the differential expression of RA-synthesizing enzymes, Raldh1-4, and RA-catabolizing cytochrome P450 enzymes (Cyp2A1, B1, and C1). Raldh2 is expressed in the mesoderm underlying the developing caudal hindbrain, whereas the catabolic enzyme Cyp26C1 is expressed in the mesoderm underlying the presumptive cranial hindbrain and midbrain (Fig. 17-16).

The gradient of RA patterns the hindbrain and pharyngeal arches. As covered in Chapter 5, RA acts by binding to the ligand-dependent transcription factors RAR and RXR, which act as heterodimers to activate RA-sensitive genes. Two RA target genes are Hoxa1 and Hoxb1, which contain retinoic acid response elements (RAREs) in their enhancers. Ectopic application of RA to developing chick embryos transforms rhombomeres 2/3 to rhombomeres 4/5. Conversely, loss of RA as in Raldh2 knockout mice or in vitamin A (VAD)-deficient quails results in cranialization of the hindbrain, such that the normal expression of Hoxa1 and Hoxa2 in the neuroepithelium caudal to

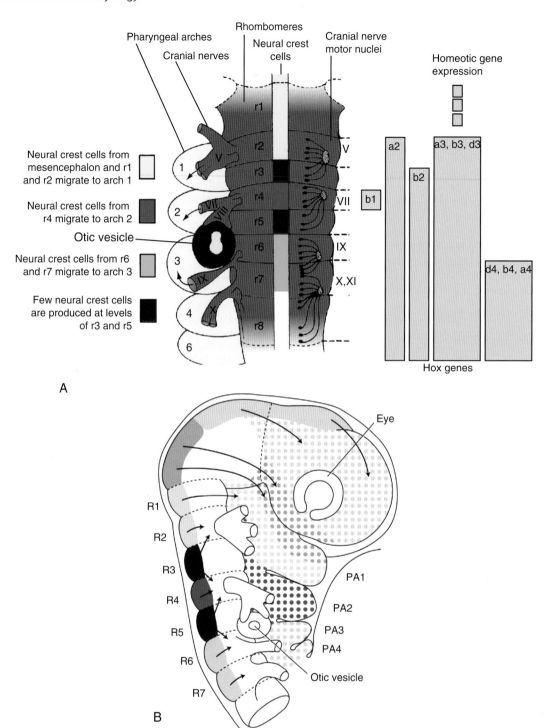

Figure 17-14. Diagrams showing the segmental nature of the hindbrain and craniofacial region. *A,* Sketch of the hindbrain region and pharyngeal arches showing segmentation and spatial relationships of the pharyngeal arches, cranial nerves, cranial nerve motor nuclei, rhombomeres, and rhombomere-specific neural crest cell derivatives. Rhombomeres are associated with the expression of specific combinations of Hox genes, which in most cases (see text for important exceptions) are also expressed by their neural crest cell derivatives. The Hox code expressed by each rhombomere is illustrated by the colored vertical bars on the right. *B,* Routes of migration of the head neural crest cells (arrows). PA1 to PA4, pharyngeal arches one to four; r1 to r7, rhombomeres one to seven.

r4 is abolished. RA regulation of Hox gene expression during somitogenesis is also covered in Chapter 8 (see Figs. 8-11 and 8-12 in Chapter 8).

The endoderm, which is required for pharyngeal arch segmentation, is also a direct target of RA signaling. Loss of RA signaling downregulates Tbx1, a transcription factor

implicated in **22q11.2 syndrome** (covered in the "Clinical Taster" in this chapter and in Chapters 4 and 12), Pax9 (another type of transcription factor), and Fgf8 expression. All of these are needed for normal pharyngeal arch development and patterning, and in the absence of RA, the third and fourth pharyngeal arches do not form.

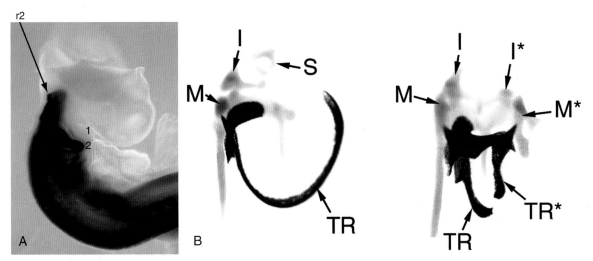

Figure 17-15. Hoxa2 determines second arch identity. *A,* Whole mount in situ hybridization showing the expression of Hoxa2 in a developing chick embryo. Hoxa2 is specifically expressed in the second (2) and more caudal pharyngeal arches, but not in the first (1) pharyngeal arch mesenchyme. r2 indicates the position of rhombomere two of the hindbrain. *B,* Loss of Hoxa2 function in mice (wild type on left; mutant on right) results in loss of the stapes (S), styloid process, and lateral horn of the hyoid—all derivatives of the second arch. In contrast, first arch structures—the malleus (M), incus (I), and tympanic ring (TR)—are duplicated (duplicated member indicated by asterisk).

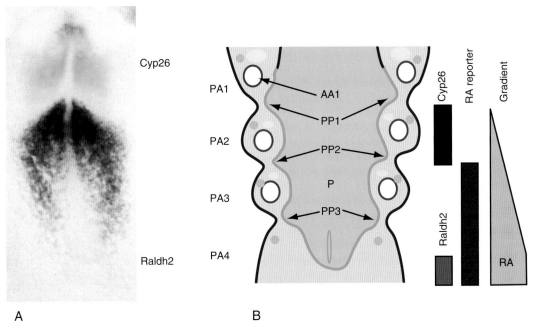

Figure 17-16. A gradient of retinoic acid patterns the hindbrain. *A,* Whole mount in situ hybridization showing the expression of Raldh2, a retinoic acid–producing enzyme, and Cyp26, a retinoic acid–degrading enzyme, in the early chick embryo. Raldh2 (dark blue) is expressed caudally, whereas Cyp26 (light blue) is expressed cranially. Thus there is a gradient of retinoic acid signaling across the cranial-caudal axis of the future hindbrain, which spans the transition between these two expression patterns. *B,* Sketch of a frontal section through the pharyngeal region illustrating the gradient of retinoic acid signaling (RA). AA1, aortic arch one; PP1-3, pharyngeal pouches one through three; P, pharynx; PA1-4, pharyngeal arches one through four. A cartilaginous bar (blue) and a cranial nerve (tan) are also shown in each arch.

DEVELOPMENT OF FACE

 Animation 17-2: Development of Face.
Animations are available online at StudentConsult.

The basic morphology of the face is established between the fourth and tenth weeks by the development and joining of five prominences: the **frontonasal prominence** overlying the forebrain, plus the two **maxillary prominences** and two **mandibular**

prominences associated with the first pharyngeal arches (Fig. 17-17). The mesenchyme in the frontonasal prominence arises from neural crest cells derived from the midbrain and forebrain, whereas the maxillary and mandibular prominences receive neural crest cell contributions from both the midbrain and hindbrain (see Fig. 17-14). The spectrum of congenital facial defects known as **facial clefts**—including cleft lip and cleft palate—result from failure of some of these facial processes to grow and join correctly. These relatively common

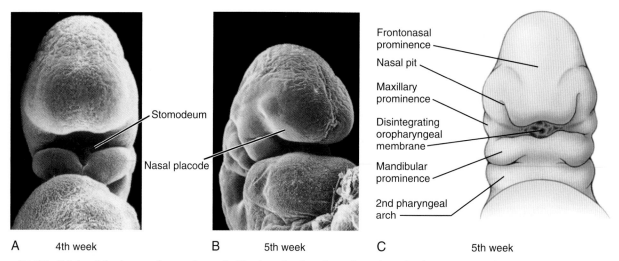

A   4th week   B   5th week   C   5th week

Figure 17-17. Origin of the human face and mouth. The face develops from five primordia that appear at the end of the fourth week: the frontonasal prominence, the two maxillary prominences, and the two mandibular prominences. Two nasal placodes, small circular ectodermal thickenings, develop on the frontonasal prominence. The oropharyngeal membrane breaks down in the fifth week to form the opening to the oral cavity. *A, C,* Ventral views. *B,* Oblique lateral view.

congenital anomalies are covered in the following "In the Clinic" entitled "Facial Clefting."

All five facial swellings form by the end of the fourth week. These initially surround the primitive oral cavity, the **stomodeum** (Fig. 17-17*A*), which is separated from the gastrointestinal tract by the **oropharyngeal (buccopharyngeal** or **oral) membrane** (Fig. 17-17*C*). During the fifth week, the paired maxillary prominences enlarge and grow ventrally and medially. Simultaneously, a pair of ectodermal thickenings, called the **nasal** or **olfactory placodes** (also called **nasal discs** or **nasal plates**) form on the frontonasal prominence and begin to enlarge (Fig. 17-17*B*). In the sixth week, the ectoderm at the center of each nasal placode invaginates to form an oval **nasal pit**, dividing the frontonasal prominence into the **lateral** and **medial nasal processes** (Fig. 17-18). The groove between the lateral nasal process and the adjacent maxillary prominence is called the **nasolacrimal groove (naso-optic furrow)** (see Fig. 17-18*C*). During the seventh week, the ectoderm at the floor of this groove invaginates into the underlying mesenchyme to form tubular structures called the **nasolacrimal duct** and **lacrimal sac**. The nasolacrimal duct is invested by bone during ossification of the maxilla. After birth, it functions to drain excess tears from the conjunctiva of the eye into the nasal cavity.

During the sixth week, the medial nasal processes approximate toward the midline and join to form the primordium of the bridge and septum of the nose (Fig. 17-18*A, B*). By the end of the seventh week, the inferior tips of the medial nasal processes expand laterally and inferiorly and join to form the **intermaxillary process** (Fig. 17-18*C, D*). The tips of the maxillary prominences grow to meet the intermaxillary process and fuse with it. The intermaxillary process gives rise to the **philtrum** (Fig. 17-18*E*) and the **primary palate** containing four incisor teeth.

Although the two mandibular prominences seem to be separated by a fissure midventrally (see Fig. 17-18*A*), they actually form in continuity with each other, like the rest

of the pharyngeal arches. The transient intermandibular depression is filled in during the fourth and fifth weeks by proliferation of mesenchyme (see Fig. 17-18*B-D*). Meanwhile, during the fifth week, rupture of the oropharyngeal membrane occurs to form a broad, slit-like embryonic mouth (see Fig. 17-18*C, D*). The mouth is reduced to its final width during the second month, as fusion of the lateral portions of the maxillary and mandibular swellings creates the cheeks (see Fig. 17-18*E*). Too little fusion results in **macrostomia** (a large mouth), whereas too much fusion results in **microstomia** (a small mouth).

In the Research Lab

PATTERNING OF FACIAL PROMINENCES

Facial development requires the integration of multiple reciprocal and changing tissue interactions among neural crest cells, mesoderm, ectoderm, and endoderm, with each tissue playing specific roles. Transplantation of neural crest cells between different species has shown that the characteristic species facial morphology is determined by the neural crest cell donor. Thus, if duck neural crest cells are transplanted into a quail host, or vice versa, the resulting structures are characteristic of the donor neural crest cells (Fig. 17-19*A, B*). The donor neural crest cells also establish the temporal pattern of gene expression in the overlying ectoderm and the development and patterning of ectodermal-derived structures such as feathers (Fig. 17-19*C*). The ectoderm then signals back to the mesenchyme to coordinate facial outgrowth. These epithelial-mesenchymal interactions control cell proliferation and cell survival and are mediated by Shh and members of the Fgf, Wnt, and Bmp family (see following "In the Research Lab" entitled "Environmental and Genetic Mechanisms of Orofacial Clefting").

The ectoderm also has patterning ability, illustrated by the fact that the odontogenic epithelium can induce tooth development in non-odontogenic mesenchyme (see later "In the Research Lab" entitled "Tooth Induction"), and that the **frontonasal ectodermal zone (FEZ)**, a region in the frontonasal prominence characterized by the juxtaposition of Shh and Fgf8

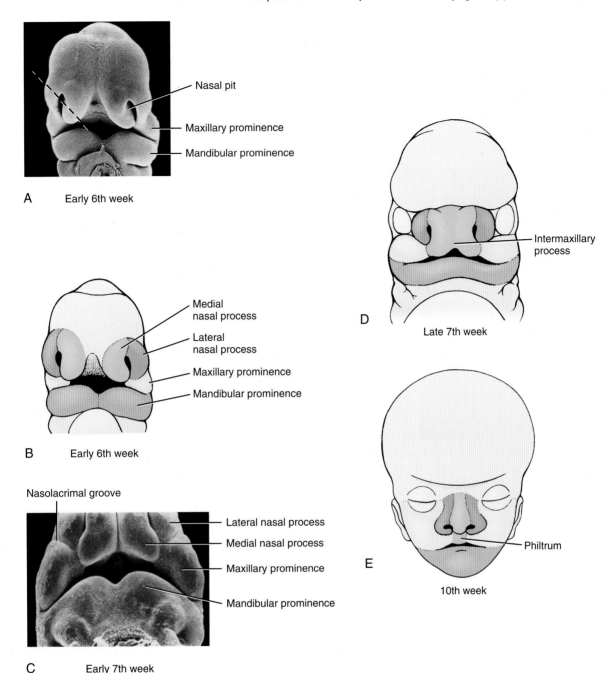

Figure 17-18. Development of the face. *A, B,* In the sixth week, the nasal placodes of the frontonasal prominence invaginate to form the nasal pits and the lateral and medial nasal processes. Dashed line in *A* indicates section level shown in Figure 17-21. *C, D,* In the seventh week, the medial nasal processes fuse at the midline to form the intermaxillary process. *E,* By the tenth week, the intermaxillary process forms the philtrum of the upper lip.

expression, can induce duplicated distal beak structures when transplanted ectopically. Finally, the endoderm is essential for facial development: ablation of endoderm results in loss of facial structures, whereas transplantation of endoderm causes the formation of ectopic facial structures. Strikingly, the identity and orientation of the skeletal structures is determined by the region of endoderm that is transplanted and its orientation in the host. Shh is one of the signals from the endoderm that controls patterning.

Studies of "Darwin's finches" from the Galapagos Islands have identified two candidate genes that may determine facial morphology. Expression of the growth factor Bmp4, which controls

mesenchymal cell proliferation and chondrogenesis, is highest in the finches with the broadest and deepest beaks, the ground finches. In contrast, the facial primordia of finches with long and slender beaks, the cactus finches, have higher levels of the intracellular signaling factor calmodulin kinase II, which promotes distal outgrowth.

FIRST PHARYNGEAL ARCH IS PATTERNED BY DLX CODE

In the caudal pharyngeal arches and the trunk, Hox genes control patterning of tissues, including skeletal structures (see the preceding "In the Research Lab" entitled "Hindbrain Is Segmented," and Chapters 8 and 9). Members of

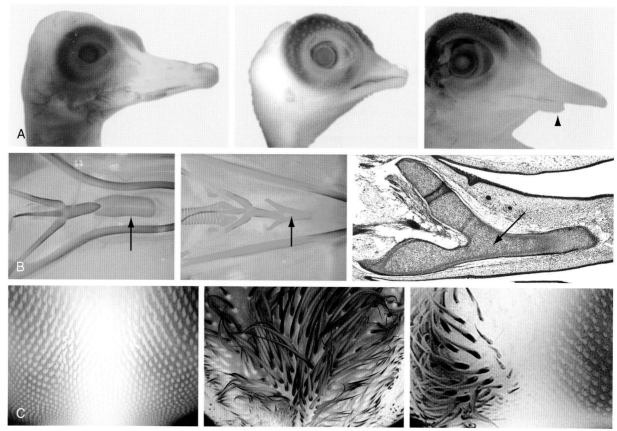

Figure 17-19. Neural crest cells control patterning of the facial primordia. *A,* Length and shape of the jaws in a duck (left), quail (center), and transplantation chimera in which neural crest cells that contribute to the lower jaw were transplanted from a quail to a duck (right). Note that the lower jaw length in the chimera mimics that of the quail (arrow head) and is shorter than that of the duck. *B,* Bones of the lower jaw stained to highlight cartilage in a duck (left) and quail (center). The entoglossum bone (arrows) is a supporting bone for the tongue. In the duck, this bone is broad and flat, whereas in the quail, it is spear shaped. In a duck embryo in which quail neural crest cells were transplanted (right), the entoglossum mimics the shape of the quail entoglossum (i.e., it is spear shaped, as seen in histological section; adjacent sections, not shown, revealed that the entoglossum was derived entirely from quail neural crest cells). *C,* Head skin patches show feathers in duck (left), quail (center), and chimeric embryos (right). The feathers, which are ectodermally derived, also develop according to the timetable and pattern of the donor neural crest cells, as shown in a duck embryo in which quail neural crest cells were transplanted on the left side of the figure showing the chimera (right panel). The difference in pigmentation between duck and quail feathers is due to the presence of neural crest cell–derived quail melanocytes.

the Hox gene family (A, B, C, D) are not expressed in the first pharyngeal arch or in ectomesenchyme cranial to it; therefore, Hox genes do not pattern the facial primordia. Rather, this patterning role is thought to be controlled by the related homeobox-containing genes Msx1, 2, Dlx1-6 (former Dlx7 is now called Dlx4), Gsc1, Lhx6/7, and Barx1, with the combinatorial expression of these factors determining facial structures. The Dlx family together with the transcription factor Hand2 has been shown to pattern the maxillary versus the mandibular prominence. Like the classic Hox cluster in more caudal regions of the body, members of the Dlx family are expressed in nested domains in the mandibular prominence (Fig. 17-20A). Dlx1 and 2 are also expressed in the maxillary prominence (see Fig. 17-20A). Loss of both Dlx5 and 6 in mouse results in a homeotic transformation such that part of the mandibular prominence is replaced with skeletal structures normally formed in the maxillary prominence. Specifically, the proximal part of the dentary bone is absent and is replaced with an ectopic maxilla, ala temporalis, jugal, squamosal, and palatine bones (Fig. 17-20B). These bones are mirror image duplications of their endogenous counterparts, suggesting that there is a signaling center controlling patterning of the surrounding

structures between the maxillary and mandibular prominences. This transformation is also associated with transformation of overlying structures: there is an additional set of vibrissae in the transformed mandibular prominence, and ectopic rugae also form in association with the ectopic palatine bone. This is consistent with the role of neural crest–derived mesenchyme in patterning overlying ectodermal structures (also see Fig. 17-19C).

Expression of Dlx5 and 6 is controlled by the small peptide, endothelin-1 (Et1), which is expressed in the mesoderm and ectoderm. Expression of Dlx5 and 6, in turn, regulates the expression of Hand2 (heart- and neural crest derivatives-expressed protein 2, a basic helix-loop-helix transcription factor; formerly called dHand) in the mesenchyme. Genetic inactivation of Et1, its receptor, or the enzyme involved in its activation (Ece1) or inactivation of Hand2 also results in transformation of the mandibular arch. Crucially, misexpression of Hand2 or Et-1 in the maxillary prominence transforms it to that of the mandibular prominence. This reveals a signaling network, Et-1 to Dlx5/6 to Hand2, which is necessary for mandibular development and is sufficient to transform the maxillary prominence into that of the mandibular arch.

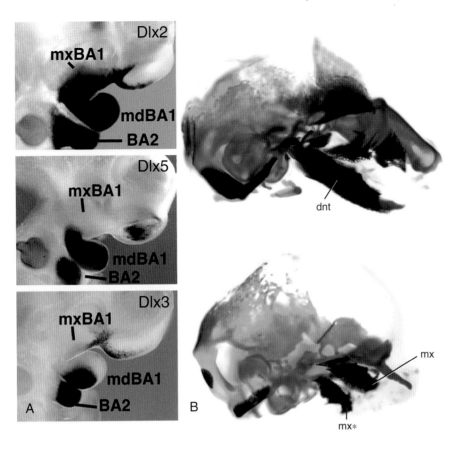

Figure 17-20. Dlx code patterns the first branchial arch. *A,* Whole mount in situ hybridization showing the nested expression of members of the Dlx family in the mandibular (mdBA1) and maxillary prominences (mxBA1). *B,* The loss of both Dlx5 and 6 in mice results in derivatives of the mandibular prominence being transformed into derivatives of the maxillary prominence (top = wild-type; bottom = double knockout). Namely, Meckel's cartilage and the dentary bone (dnt) are replaced by an ectopic maxilla (mx*) and other maxillary derived bones (not shown). mx, position of normal maxilla.

The identity of the frontonasal versus the maxillary prominences is controlled by Bmp and RA signaling. The frontonasal prominence is characterized by high levels of RA from the forebrain and nasal epithelium, whereas the maxillary prominence is characterized by higher levels of Bmp signaling. Thus, application of RA, together with the Bmp antagonist, noggin, into the maxillary prominence of a developing chick embryo transforms the derivatives of the maxillary prominence into structures that are normally derived from the frontonasal prominence (i.e., the palatine bone is lost and is replaced with the nasal septum).

DEVELOPMENT OF NASAL AND ORAL CAVITIES

 Animation 17-3: Development of Palate.
Animations are available online at StudentConsult.

Figure 17-21 illustrates the process by which the nasal pits give rise to the nasal passages. The nasal pits deepen by invagination and growth of the nasal epithelium with simultaneous forward growth of the frontonasal prominence (indicated by arrows in Fig. 17-21*A*). At the end of the sixth week, the medial nasal processes start to merge, bringing together the dorsal region of the deepening nasal pits, which join to form a single, enlarged ectodermal nasal sac lying superoposterior to the intermaxillary process (Fig. 17-21*A, B*). From the end of the sixth week to the beginning of the seventh week, the

floor and posterior wall of the nasal sac proliferate to form a thickened, plate-like fin, or keel, of ectoderm separating the nasal sac from the oral cavity. This structure is called the **nasal fin** (see Fig. 17-21*B*). Vacuoles develop in the nasal fin and fuse with the nasal sac, thus enlarging the sac and thinning the fin to a thin membrane called the **oronasal membrane**, which separates the sac from the oral cavity (Fig. 17-21*C*). This membrane ruptures during the seventh week to form an opening called the **primitive choana** (Fig. 17-21*D, E*). The floor of the nasal cavity at this stage is formed by a posterior extension of the intermaxillary process called the **primary palate** (see Fig. 17-21*E*).

At this point the nasal and oral cavities are continuous, but these will be separated during the seventh and eighth weeks by formation of the palatal shelves, formed as a pair of thin extensions from the medial walls of the maxillary prominences (Figs. 17-22*A, B*). At first, these shelves grow downward, parallel to the lateral surfaces of the tongue. However, at the end of the seventh week, they rotate rapidly upward into a horizontal position and then fuse with each other and with the primary palate to form the secondary palate (Fig. 17-22*C, D*). Rotation of the palatal shelves has been ascribed to the rapid synthesis and hydration of hyaluronic acid within the extracellular matrix of the shelves, and alignment of the elevated shelves in a horizontal plane may be determined by the orientation of collagen and mesenchymal cells. Fusion occurs near the middle of the palatal shelves and continues both anteriorly and posteriorly. During fusion, the medial epithelial seam disappears, and a continuous

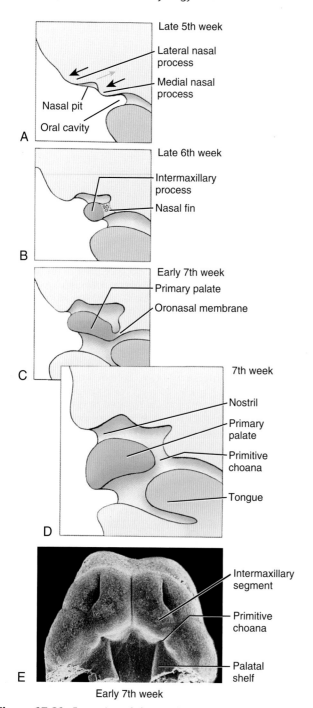

Late 5th week
Lateral nasal process
Medial nasal process
Nasal pit
Oral cavity
A

Late 6th week
Intermaxillary process
Nasal fin
B

Early 7th week
Primary palate
Oronasal membrane
C

7th week
Nostril
Primary palate
Primitive choana
Tongue
D

Intermaxillary segment
Primitive choana
Palatal shelf
E
Early 7th week

Figure 17-21. Formation of the nasal cavity and primitive choana (see Fig. 17-18A for orientation of the sections). A, B, The nasal pits invaginate to form a single nasal cavity separated from the oral cavity by a thick partition called the nasal fin. C-E, The nasal fin thins to form the oronasal membrane, which breaks down completely to form the primitive choana. The posterior extension of the intermaxillary process forms the primary palate.

mesenchymal bridge is formed between the two palatal shelves (see Fig. 17-22D). The central region, where the primary palate and the secondary palate meet, is marked by the incisive foramen (see Fig. 17-22D). Growth and lowering of the mandibular primordium are also important for palatal shelf elevation, as they lower the tongue, which initially fills the oral cavity (see Fig. 17-22A, B).

Therefore, cleft palate can be secondarily associated with defects in lower jaw development (see the following "In the Clinic" entitled "Facial Clefting").

Intramembranous condensations within the mesenchyme in the anterior portion of the secondary palate form the bony **hard palate**. Defects in bone development result in a **submucosal cleft palate**. In the posterior portion of the secondary palate, myogenic mesenchyme condenses to give rise to the musculature of the soft palate, which is innervated by the vagus and trigeminal (V$_3$) nerves. At birth, the soft palate and epiglottis are in contact. Therefore, newborns are obligate nasal breathers. Consequently, nasal obstruction such as **choanal atresia** (obstruction at the back of the nasal passage) will affect the baby's ability to breathe. However, by the age of six months, growth of the larynx separates the epiglottis and soft palate.

While the secondary palate is forming, ectoderm and mesenchyme of the frontonasal prominence and the medial nasal processes proliferate to form a midline **nasal septum** that grows down from the roof of the nasal cavity to fuse with the upper surface of the primary and secondary palates along the midline (see Fig. 17-22). The nasal cavity is now divided into two **nasal passages** that open into the pharynx behind the secondary palate through an opening called the **definitive choana** (see Fig. 17-22D).

In the Clinic

FACIAL CLEFTING

As covered earlier in this chapter, the face is created by the growth and fusion of five facial swellings. Complete or partial failure of fusion between any of these swellings results in a **facial cleft**, which may be unilateral or bilateral, and is a component of more than three-hundred syndromes. However, most orofacial clefts are non-syndromic. Facial clefts can affect feeding, speech, hearing, and social integration. The two most common types of facial cleft are **cleft lip** (Figs. 17-23, 17-24) and **cleft palate** (see Fig. 17-24). Cleft lip usually results from failure of the maxillary prominence and medial nasal processes to join together, whereas cleft palate results from failure of the two palatal shelves to fuse with each other along the midline. Median cleft lip resulting from failure of the two medial nasal processes to merge is much more rare (see Fig. 4-12A in Chapter 4). Although cleft lip and cleft palate often occur together, the two defects differ in their distribution with respect to sex, familial association, race, and geography. Therefore, they probably have different etiologies. Cleft lip occurs more frequently on the left-hand side and is more prevalent in males, whereas isolated cleft palate occurs more frequently in females. The latter is attributable to the one-week delay in palatal shelf elevation in females, which occurs at week eight as compared with week seven in males.

The etiology of orofacial clefts is generally multifactorial, and a number of common drugs—including the anticonvulsant phenytoin (Dilantin), vitamin A, some vitamin A analogs, particularly isotretinoin, and some corticosteroid anti-inflammatory drugs—have been shown to induce cleft lip in experimental animals. Vitamin A and its analogs are notorious for their ability to cause facial defects. Other environmental factors include smoking, alcohol, viral infection, and poor nutrition. The multifactorial etiology is emphasized by the incomplete

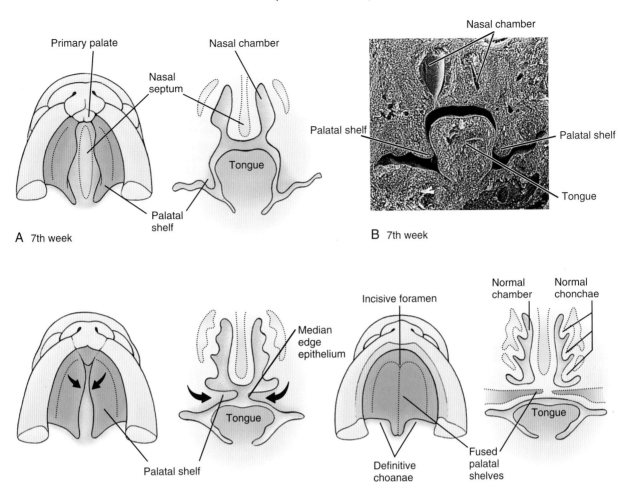

Figure 17-22. Formation of the secondary palate and nasal septum. The secondary palate forms from palatal shelves that grow medially from the maxillary swellings. During the same period, growth of the nasal septum separates the left and right nasal passages. The palatal shelves at first grow inferiorly on either side of the tongue (A, B) but then rapidly rotate upward to meet in the midline (C), where they fuse with each other and with the inferior edge of the nasal septum (D).

(i.e., less than 100%) concordance of cleft lip and palate in identical twins (25%). Mutations in a number of susceptibility genes have been identified, which, together with specific environmental factors, significantly increase the risk of clefts (e.g., TGFβ3 mutations with steroids or mutations in the GABA RECEPTOR B3 with anticonvulsants). Long-term studies have shown that the parents, mainly the mother, of children with orofacial clefts are at increased risk of cancer because they are carrying genetic mutations and/or have been exposed to teratogens/mutagens. Likewise, affected children also show increased rates of cancer, particularly of the lung and breast—it is unclear whether this increase reflects underlying genetic mutations or differences in lifestyles/environmental factors.

Cleft lip has been ascribed to underdevelopment of the mesenchyme of the maxillary prominence and medial nasal process, which would result in their inadequate contact. The resulting cleft may range in length from a minor notch in the vermilion border of the lip, just lateral to the philtrum, to a cleft that completely separates the lateral lip from the nasal cavity. The depth of clefting also varies: some clefts involve just the soft tissue of the lip; others divide the lateral portion of the maxillary bone from the premaxillary portion (the portion bearing the incisors) of the primary palate.

Clefts of this type often result in deformed, absent, or supernumerary teeth. Asians and Native Americans are most susceptible to cleft lip (1/500 live births), whereas African populations show the lowest incidence of cleft lip (1/2000). The rate of cleft lip in Caucasians is intermediate at approximately 1/1000. Clefts may also occur between the lateral nasal process and the maxillary prominence (**oblique cleft**) exposing the nasolacrimal duct or between the maxillary and mandibular primordia (**lateral clefts**). Although extremely rare, clefts can also form along the midline of the two mandibular prominences (**median mandibular cleft**). As the facial prominences fuse, the apposing epithelium disintegrates. Remnants of these epithelial seams may result in cyst formation.

Any of several pathogenetic factors might account for clefting. These include inadequate migration or proliferation of neural crest cell ectomesenchyme and excessive cell death. Cleft palate may also occur as the result of failure of the shelves to elevate at the correct time, defects in muscle development, an excessively wide head, failure of the shelves to fuse, and secondary rupture after fusion. Cleft palate can also be a secondary consequence of mandibular dysplasias. During normal development, the mandibular primordium grows, thereby lowering the tongue relative to the palatal shelves and allowing them to elevate. If the first

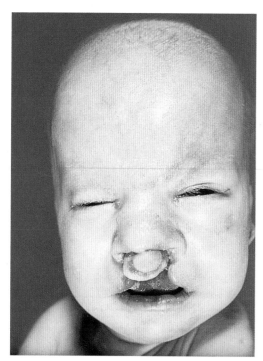

Figure 17-23. Bilateral cleft lip. This malformation results from failure of the medial nasal processes to fuse with the maxillary swellings.

pharyngeal arch does not develop appropriately, the tongue will not be lowered and will physically obstruct palatal shelf elevation. This secondary cleft palate resulting from a smaller lower jaw (**micrognathia**) and occurring with **glossoptosis** (backward displacement of the tongue) is referred to as **Pierre Robin sequence** and is often seen as part of syndromes like **Stickler** and **Treacher Collins syndromes** (see a later "In the Research Lab" entitled "Developmental Basis of Treacher Collins Syndrome").

Several mutations in humans have now been linked to syndromic cleft lip and palate. These include mutations in the transcription factors MSX1, TP63, INTERFERON REGULATORY FACTOR 6 (IRF6), and TBX22 and the cell adhesion molecule POLIO VIRUS RECEPTOR RELATED-1 (PVR1, NECTIN-1). Mutations in IRF6 are responsible for **van der Woude syndrome**, the most common combined cleft lip and palate syndrome. Mutations in TBX22 (**cleft palate plus ankyloglossia**) are the most common cause of cleft palate. Isolated Pierre Robin sequence has now been attributed to deregulation of the expression of SOX9, a transcription factor essential for chondrogenesis, whereas Stickler syndrome, which also shows the Pierre Robin triad of defects, can be caused by dominant mutations in collagens that are expressed by chondrocytes (see Chapter 8 for additional coverage of chondrocyte differentiation). These mutations affect the development of Meckel's cartilage within the first pharyngeal arch, impacting normal growth and lowering of the lower jaw.

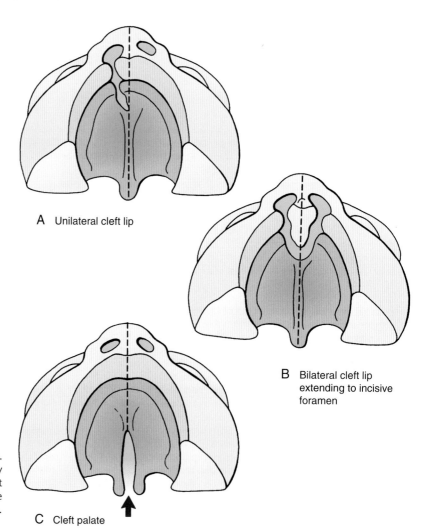

A   Unilateral cleft lip

B   Bilateral cleft lip extending to incisive foramen

C   Cleft palate

Figure 17-24. Cleft lip and cleft palate. *A, B,* Cleft lip. The cleft may involve the lip only or may extend dorsally along one or both edges of the primary palate. *C,* Cleft palate results from failure of the palatal shelves to fuse properly during development of the secondary palate. Arrow indicates the palatal gap.

ENVIRONMENTAL AND GENETIC MECHANISMS OF OROFACIAL CLEFTING

Outgrowth of the facial primordia is controlled by epithelial-mesenchymal interactions; thus, if the epithelium is removed, the facial prominences are truncated. These interactions are mediated by growth factors that commonly signal elsewhere (e.g., Shh and members of the Bmp, Fgf, and Wnt families). Therefore, it is not surprising that mutations in components of these pathways and their downstream targets have been linked to cleft lip and palate. For example, mutations in BMP4, FGFR1, FGFR2, WNT3, WNT7A, GLI2, PTC1, and MSX1 have all been linked to orofacial clefts.

Bmp4, Fgf8, Wnt3, and Shh are expressed in the facial epithelium. These factors signal to the underlying mesenchyme to control homeobox gene expression, cell proliferation, and/or cell survival. For example, Bmp4 controls the expression of Msx1 in the underlying mesenchyme. Loss of function of Bmps, Fgfs, Wnts, or Shh results in cleft lip. Curiously, in Bmp4 mutants, the cleft lip is able to spontaneously heal itself during development. Thus, at E12.5, 100% of embryos have cleft lip, whereas at E14.5, this percentage is reduced to 12.5%, suggesting that other Bmp members may be able to compensate for the loss of Bmp4. This may explain, in part, the microform cleft lip (a defect in the orbicularis oris muscle) that is observed in humans with a mutation in BMP4.

The same signaling pathways control palatal shelf development, where they also regulate homeobox gene expression, cell proliferation, and survival. For example, Fgf10 signaling from the palatal shelf mesenchyme controls Shh expression in the palatal shelf epithelium (Fig. 17-25). Shh in turn activates Bmp2 expression in the palatal mesenchyme, which then induces Msx1 expression. Bmp signaling also controls p63 expression in the epithelium. Finally, Msx1 signals back to Bmp2 to maintain its expression. Therefore, a complex signaling network between the ectoderm and mesenchyme coordinates palatal shelf development.

Wnt5a has a novel role during palatal shelf morphogenesis in controlling directed cell movement during growth of the palatal shelves. The homeobox gene, Stab2, also controls patterning and cell growth in the developing palatal shelves, and in Stab2 mouse mutants, the palatal shelves do not form the correct shape and elevate on time.

Fusion of the facial primordia requires removal of the epithelium to generate a seamless body of mesenchyme. First, the periderm is sloughed off. Second, the epithelial cells extend filopodia toward the epithelium on the adjacent primordium to bridge the gap. Third, cell adhesion increases, and epithelial cell intercalation, matrix degradation, and ultimately epithelial cell

death ensue. TGFβ3 and TGFα, factors linked to cleft palate susceptibility in humans, are essential for this process. Tgfβ3 and Tgfα are expressed in the medial edge epithelium (MEE) of the palatal shelves, and in their absence, the epithelial cells fail to adhere. Emphasizing the key role of cell apoptosis, loss of function of Apaf1 in mice (apoptotic protease activation factor 1, which is expressed in the MEE) results in cleft palate. Other epithelial factors essential for proliferation, survival, and differentiation of the epithelium include TP63 (see Chapter 7), its downstream target IRF6, and PVR1. Mutations in all of these factors result in cleft lip/cleft palate in humans.

Additional understanding of how environmental factors increase the risk of clefting has been obtained. For example, in humans, mutations in genes involved in the detoxification pathways significantly increase the risk of orofacial clefts in mothers who smoke during pregnancy. In addition, several transcription factors implicated in cleft lip and palate (e.g., MSX1, TBX22, TP63, STAB2) have been shown to require post-translational modification by the Sumo (small ubiquitin-like modifier) pathway. Addition of the Sumo moiety is thought to regulate nuclear localization and transcriptional activity. Mutations in SUMO1, a key enzyme in this pathway, result in cleft palate in humans, demonstrating the key role of sumoylation during palatal shelf development. Environmental factors such as free radicals, hypoxia, and viral infection affect the sumoylation of proteins. Therefore, genetic mutation in a susceptibility gene(s) together with defects in sumoylation due to environmental factors will have additive effects, enhancing the risk of clefting.

DEVELOPMENT OF SINUSES

At birth, the ratio of the volume of the facial skeleton to the volume of the cranial vault is about 1:7. During infancy and childhood, this ratio steadily decreases, mainly as a result of the development of teeth and viscerocranium, together with the growth of four pairs of **paranasal sinuses: maxillary, ethmoid, sphenoid**, and **frontal sinuses** (Fig. 17-26). The maxillary, ethmoid, and frontal sinuses develop from invaginations of the nasal cavity that extend into the bones, whereas the sphenoid sinus forms by closure of the sphenoid-ethmoidal recess. The maxillary sinus, the largest of the paranasal sinuses, forms during the third fetal month as invaginations of the nasal sac that slowly expand within the maxillary bones. The resulting cavities are very small at birth (pea-size) but continue to expand throughout

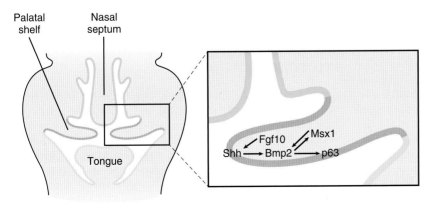

Figure 17-25. Factors expressed within the mesenchyme and epithelium of the palatal shelves act in a regulatory network to control palatal shelf outgrowth and elevation. Drawing of a coronal section through the oral-nasal level of an embryo and an enlargement of a palatal shelf (from boxed area in lower power illustration).

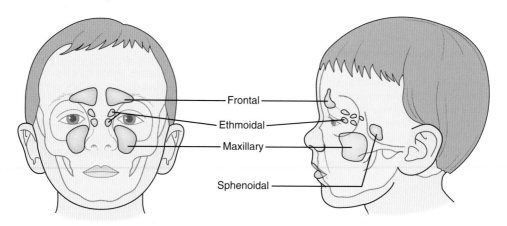

Figure 17-26. Locations of the four paired paranasal sinuses.

childhood. The initial invagination of the sinus is called **primary pneumatization**, whereas the expansion is known as **secondary pneumatization**. The sphenoid and frontal sinuses initiate development during the fourth fetal month and undergo secondary pneumatization (i.e., expansion) during infancy. The frontal sinuses are not radiographically visible until the fifth or sixth postnatal year. Each frontal sinus actually consists of two independent spaces that develop from different sources. One forms by expansion of the ethmoid sinus into the frontal bone, and the other develops from an independent invagination of the middle meatus of the nasal passage (the space underlying the middle nasal concha). Because these cavities never coalesce, they drain independently. The ethmoid sinuses form during the fifth fetal month as invaginations of the middle meatus of the nasal passages and grow into the ethmoid bone postnatally. Growth of the sinuses continues until adulthood.

FATE OF PHARYNGEAL CLEFTS

As described earlier, the pharyngeal arches are separated by pharyngeal clefts externally and by pharyngeal pouches internally (Fig. 17-27A; see also Fig. 17-9D, E). The first pharyngeal cleft and pouch, located between the first and second pharyngeal arches, participate in the formation of the ear: the first cleft becomes the **external acoustic meatus** and the **external part of the tympanic membrane**. The first pouch expands to contribute to a cavity called the **tubotympanic recess**, which differentiates to become the **tympanic cavity** of the middle ear and the **auditory (Eustachian) tube**. The development of these structures is covered in greater detail in Chapter 18.

The remaining three pharyngeal clefts are normally obliterated during development. During the fourth and fifth weeks, the rapidly expanding second pharyngeal arch overgrows these clefts and fuses caudally with the cardiac eminence, enclosing the clefts in a transient, ectoderm-lined **lateral cervical sinus** (Fig. 17-27B, C). This space normally disappears rapidly and completely.

However, the lateral cervical sinus occasionally persists on one or both sides in the form of a **cervical cyst** located just anterior to the sternocleidomastoid muscle (see sites 2 and 3 in Fig. 17-27F). A completely enclosed cyst may expand to form a palpable lump as its epithelial lining desquamates or if it becomes infected. Occasionally, the cyst communicates with the skin via an **external cervical fistula** or with the pharynx via an **internal cervical fistula** (see Fig. 17-27D, E). Internal cervical fistulae most commonly open into the embryonic derivative of the second pouch, the **palatine tonsil**. Less often, they communicate with derivatives of the third pouch. Rarely, a cervical cyst has both internal and external fistulae (see Fig. 17-27E). Cysts of this type may be diagnosed by the drainage of mucus through the small opening of the external fistula on the neck on the anterior border of the sternocleidomastoid muscle (Fig. 17-27F). Cervical cysts are usually of minor clinical importance but may require resection if they become seriously infected.

Infrequently, duplication of the first pharyngeal cleft results in formation of an ectoderm-lined **first-cleft sinus** or **cervical aural fistula** located in the tissues anterior to the external acoustic meatus (the so-called preauricular area; see site 1 in Fig. 17-27F). A fully enclosed first-cleft sinus may become apparent as a swelling just anterior to the auricle or external ear. Alternatively, it may drain to the exterior through a cervical aural fistula, which usually opens into the external auditory canal. Depending on its position, a first-cleft cyst or fistula may threaten the facial nerve if it becomes infected and may require resection. **Periauricular** (or preauricular) pits, sinuses, or fistulae may also arise as the result of defects in fusion of the periauricular hillocks during formation of the outer ear (see Chapter 18).

PHARYNGEAL ARCHES GIVE RISE TO TONGUE

At the end of the fourth week, the floor of the pharynx consists of the five pharyngeal arches and the intervening pharyngeal pouches. The development of the tongue begins late in the fourth week, when the first arch forms a median swelling called the **median tongue bud** or **tuberculum impar** (Fig. 17-28A). An additional pair of lateral swellings, the **distal tongue buds** (also called **lateral lingual swellings**), develop on the first arch

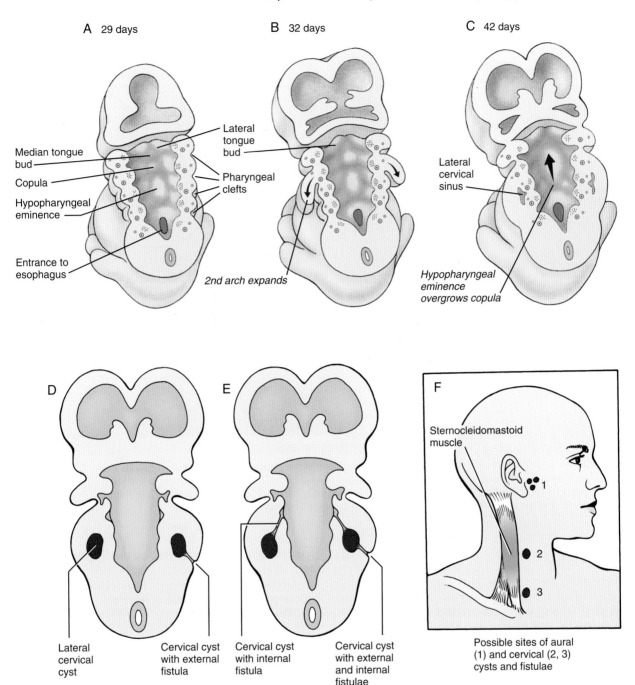

Figure 17-27. Normal and abnormal fates of the pharyngeal clefts. *A-C,* Three stages in normal development. The first pharyngeal cleft forms the external auditory meatus. The second pharyngeal arch expands and fuses with the cardiac eminence to cover the remaining pharyngeal clefts, which form the transient lateral cervical sinus. *D-F,* Formation of cysts. *D, E,* Sections through the pharynx and pharyngeal arches show that cervical cysts may be isolated or may connect to the skin of the neck by an external cervical fistula, or to the pharynx by an internal fistula, or both. *F,* Lateral cervical cysts (2, 3) are located just medial to the anterior border of the sternocleidomastoid muscle. Anomalous derivatives of the first pharyngeal cleft, known as aural (or preauricular) cysts, may form anterior to the ear (1).

early in the fifth week and rapidly expand to overgrow the median tongue bud (Fig. 17-28*A-D*). These swellings continue to grow throughout embryonic and fetal life and form the anterior two thirds of the tongue.

Late in the fourth week, the second arch develops a midline swelling called the **copula** (see Fig. 17-28*A*). This swelling is rapidly overgrown during the fifth and sixth weeks by a midline swelling of the third and fourth arches called the **hypopharyngeal eminence**, which

gives rise to the posterior one third of the tongue (see Fig. 17-28*A*). The **epiglottis** develops just posterior to the hypopharyngeal eminence (see Fig. 17-28*A, B, D*). The hypopharyngeal eminence expands mainly by the growth of third-arch endoderm, whereas the fourth arch contributes only a small region on the most posterior aspect of the tongue (Fig. 17-28*D*). Thus, the bulk of the tongue mucosa is formed by the first and third arches. During its development, the ventral surface of

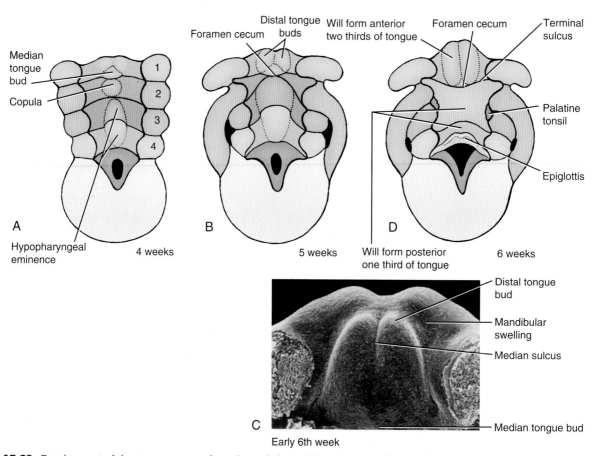

Figure 17-28. Development of the tongue mucosa from the endoderm of the pharyngeal floor. *A, B, D,* Drawings showing that the mucosa of the anterior two thirds of the tongue develops mainly from the distal tongue buds (lateral lingual swellings) of the first pharyngeal arch, whereas the mucosal lining of the posterior one third of the tongue is formed by the hypopharyngeal eminence of the third and fourth arches, which overgrows the copula of the second arch. *C,* Scanning electron micrograph of the developing tongue.

the tongue is initially attached to the floor of the mouth (Fig. 17-28*C*). This attachment eventually regresses in the anterior region, thereby freeing the anterior part of the tongue, but more posteriorly it persists as the **frenulum**. If regression fails to occur, the resulting defect is called **ankyloglossia** (tongue-tied). Table 17-2 summarizes the developmental origins of the parts of the tongue.

The surface features of the definitive tongue reflect its embryonic origins. The boundary between the first-arch and third-arch contributions—roughly, the boundary between the anterior two thirds and posterior one third of the tongue—is marked by a transverse groove called the **terminal sulcus** (see Fig. 17-28*D*). The line of fusion between the right and left distal tongue buds is marked by a midline groove, the **median sulcus**, on the anterior two thirds of the tongue. A depression called the **foramen cecum** is visible where the median sulcus intersects the terminal sulcus (see Fig. 17-28*B, D*). As covered in the next section, this depression is the site of origin of the thyroid gland.

All muscles of the tongue except the **palatoglossus** are formed by mesoderm derived from the myotomes of the occipital somites, and the proliferation of this mesoderm is responsible for most of the growth of the tongue primordia. The innervation of the tongue muscles is consonant with their origin: all muscles except the

palatoglossus are innervated by the **hypoglossal nerve**, which is the cranial nerve associated with the occipital somites; the palatoglossus is innervated by the **pharyngeal plexus of the vagus nerve**.

The mucosal covering of the tongue is derived from pharyngeal arch endoderm and is innervated by sensory branches of the corresponding four cranial nerves (V, VII, IX, and X; see Table 17-2 and Fig. 17-13). Thus, the tongue mucosa is innervated by different nerves from those of the tongue musculature (most of the tongue musculature, as stated in the previous paragraph, is innervated by cranial nerve XII). The general sensory receptors on the anterior two thirds of the tongue are supplied by a branch of the mandibular nerve (cranial nerve V_3) called the **lingual nerve**. The taste buds of the anterior two thirds of the tongue are supplied by a special branch of the facial nerve (cranial nerve VII) called the **chorda tympani**. In contrast, the vallate papillae (a row of large taste buds flanking the terminal sulcus) and the general sensory endings over most of the posterior one third of the tongue are supplied by the **glossopharyngeal nerve** (cranial nerve IX). The small area on the most posterior aspect of the tongue that is derived from the fourth pharyngeal arch and the epiglottis receives sensory innervation from the **superior laryngeal** branch of the vagus nerve (cranial nerve X).

TABLE 17-2 DEVELOPMENT OF THE TONGUE FROM PHARYNGEAL ARCHES ONE THROUGH FOUR AND THE OCCIPITAL SOMITES

Embryonic Precursor	Intermediate Structure	Adult Structure	Innervation
Pharyngeal arch 1	Median tongue bud	Overgrown by lateral lingual swellings	Lingual branch (sensory) of mandibular division of trigeminal nerve (V)
	Lateral lingual swellings	Mucosa of anterior two thirds of tongue	Chorda tympani from facial nerve (VII; innervating arch 2) (innervates all taste buds except vallate papillae)
Pharyngeal arch 2	Copula	Overgrown by other structures	
Pharyngeal arch 3	Large, ventral part of hypopharyngeal eminence	Mucosa of most of posterior one third of tongue	Sensory branch of glossopharyngeal nerve (IX) (also supplies vallate papillae)
Pharyngeal arch 4	Small, dorsal part of hypopharyngeal eminence	Mucosa of small region on dorsal side of posterior one third of tongue	Sensory fibers of superior laryngeal branch of vagus nerve (X)
Occipital somites	Myoblasts	Intrinsic muscles of tongue	Hypoglossal nerve (XII)
Head mesoderm	Myoblasts	Palatoglossus muscle	Pharyngeal plexus of vagus nerve (X)

In the Research Lab

TASTE BUDS DEVELOP FROM PLACODES, AND THEIR DEVELOPMENT REQUIRES INNERVATION

Like other epithelial derivatives (covered in Chapter 7), taste buds develop from an epithelial placode, the papilla placode, which undergoes epithelial-mesenchymal interactions to form the final papilla. Following placode formation, the placode initially evaginates and then differentiates to form the specialized cells of the papilla (i.e., gustatory or sensory cells, supporting cells, and basal cells). There are three types of papillae: **fungiform**, **circumvallate**, and **foliate**.

Development of the fungiform papilla, like other epithelial-derived structures, requires Wnt and Bmp signaling (see Chapter 7 for further coverage). Wnt signaling is required for the initiation of placode development, and the development of fungiform papilla is blocked in the absence of canonical Wnt signaling. The fungiform papillae are arranged in an ordered array across the anterior region of the tongue (Fig. 17-29). As for the hair follicles (covered in Chapter 7), this spatial pattern is generated by Bmp signaling from the taste bud placode, which inhibits development of the placode in neighboring cells. The placode also expresses the Bmp antagonist, noggin, which ensures that only the surrounding epithelial cells receive the Bmp signal.

The papillae express brain-derived neurotrophic factor (Bdnf), which promotes the migration of the sensory nerves toward the papillae (see Fig. 17-29): loss of papillae is linked to a decrease in the number of sensory neurons, whereas the formation of an excess number of papillae, for example, by increased Wnt signaling, is associated with increased innervation. Although the patterning of the fungiform papillae seems to be intrinsic to the endoderm, innervation is essential for later stages of taste bud development and maintenance. Taste buds are regenerated throughout life.

DEVELOPMENT OF THYROID GLAND

Figure 17-30 illustrates the embryogenesis of the **thyroid gland**. The gland primordium first forms late in the fourth week and appears as a small, solid mass of endoderm proliferating at the apex of the foramen cecum on the developing tongue. The thyroid primordium descends through the tissues of the neck at the end of a slender **thyroglossal duct**. The thyroglossal duct breaks down by the end of the fifth week, and the isolated thyroid, now consisting of lateral lobes connected by a well-defined isthmus, continues to descend, reaching its final position just inferior to the cricoid cartilage by the seventh week. Studies of the ability of the embryonic thyroid to incorporate iodine into thyroid hormones and to secrete these hormones into the circulation show that this gland begins to function as early as the tenth to the twelfth week in human embryos. The developing thyroid gland becomes invested with neural crest cells as well as cells from the ultimobranchial bodies. The ultimobranchial bodies form the parafollicular cells, the **C-cells**, which produce **calcitonin**.

Thyroid function is necessary for development of the brain. Hypothyroidism is characterized by mental retardation, deafness, muscle hypertonia, and dwarfism. Iodine deficiency is a leading cause of mental retardation. **Congenital hypothyroidism** is the most common disorder of the endocrine system, affecting approximately 1 in 3500 children. Congenital hypothyroidism may be due to **athyreosis** (absence of the thyroid gland), **thyroid ectopia** (mal-positioned thyroid gland), **thyroid hypoplasia**, or **dyshormonogenesis** (failure to make thyroid hormones due to mutations in the genes required for thyroxine production). In **DiGeorge** syndrome (also called 22q11.2 deletion syndrome), a defect in development of the caudal pharyngeal arches affects normal development of the thyroid (covered in a following "In the Research Lab" entitled "Developmental Basis of DiGeorge Syndrome"). Mutations in NKX2.1, PAX8, FOXC1, and HHEX in humans also result in thyroid hypoplasia/athyreosis. These transcription factors are required for thyroid bud formation and function in later stages of thyroid development.

Normally, the only remnant of the thyroglossal duct is the foramen cecum itself. However, occasionally, a portion of the duct persists as an enclosed **thyroglossal cyst** or as a **thyroglossal sinus**, which opens on

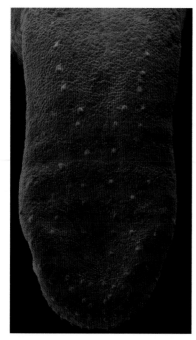

Figure 17-29. Developing taste buds. Scanning electron micrograph showing developing taste buds and their sensory innervation (red). Signals from the developing taste bud guide the migration of the sensory nerves.

the surface of the neck. Rarely, a fragment of the thyroid becomes detached during the descent of the gland and forms a patch of ectopic thyroid tissue (**thyroid ectopia**), which may be located anywhere along the route of descent. Commonly (i.e., in about 50% of the population), additional thyroid tissue may form on or near the superior surface of the thyroid, forming the so-called **pyramidal lobe**.

DEVELOPMENT OF PHARYNGEAL POUCHES

Figures 17-31 and 17-32 summarize the origin and migration of structures that arise from the pharyngeal pouches. The fate of the first pharyngeal pouch, which differentiates into the tympanic cavity and auditory tube, is covered in Chapter 18.

The palatine tonsils arise from the endoderm lining the second pharyngeal pouch (located between the second and third arches). Development of these tonsils begins early in the third month as the epithelium of the second pouch proliferates to form solid endodermal buds, or ledges, growing into the underlying mesenchyme, which will give rise to the tonsillar stroma. The central cells of the buds later die and slough, converting the solid buds into hollow **tonsillar crypts** infiltrated by lymphoid tissue. However, the definitive lymph follicles of the tonsil do not form until the last three months of prenatal life.

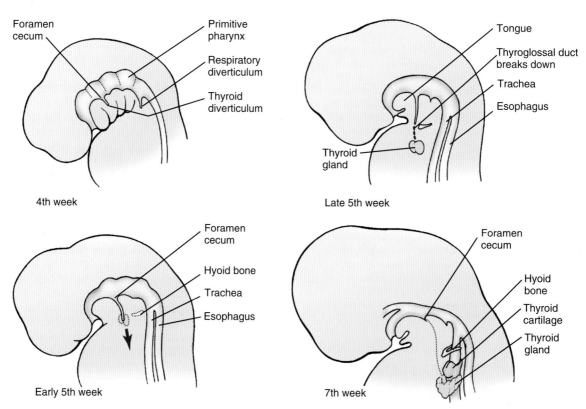

Figure 17-30. The thyroid originates as an endodermal proliferation at the tip of the foramen cecum of the developing tongue and migrates inferiorly to its final site anterior and inferior to the larynx. Until the fifth week, the thyroid remains connected to the foramen cecum by the thyroglossal duct. The gland reaches its final site in the seventh week. Arrow indicates the direction of migration of the developing thyroid gland.

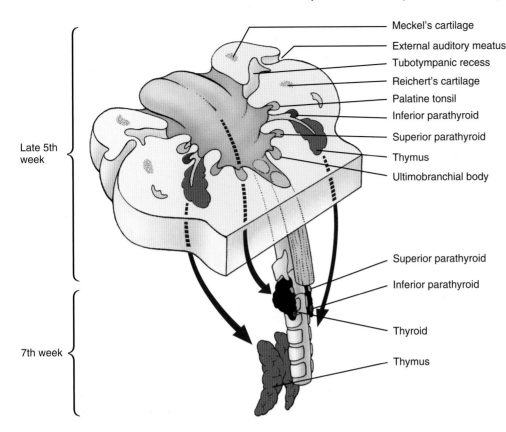

Meckel's cartilage
External auditory meatus
Tubotympanic recess
Reichert's cartilage
Palatine tonsil
Inferior parathyroid
Superior parathyroid
Thymus
Ultimobranchial body

Late 5th week

Superior parathyroid
Inferior parathyroid

Thyroid

Thymus

7th week

Figure 17-31. Development of the pharyngeal pouch derivatives. All of the pharyngeal pouches give rise to adult structures. These are the tubotympanic recess (pouch one), the palatine tonsils (pouch two), the inferior parathyroid glands and thymus (pouch three), the superior parathyroid glands (pouch four), and the ultimobranchial (telopharyngeal) body (inferior part of pouch four or a hypothetical pouch five). The parathyroids, thymus primordia, and ultimobranchial bodies separate from the lining of the pharynx and migrate to their definitive locations within the neck and thorax.

Similar lymphatic tonsils, called **pharyngeal tonsils**, develop in association with mucous glands of the pharynx. The major pharyngeal tonsils are the **adenoids, tubal tonsils** (associated with the auditory tubes), and **lingual tonsils** (associated with the posterior regions of the tongue). Minor intervening patches of lymphoid tissue also form.

The third pharyngeal pouch gives rise to the thymus and inferior parathyroid glands. The two thymic primordia arise at the end of the fourth week in the form of endodermal proliferations at the end of ventral elongations of the third pharyngeal pouches. These endodermal proliferations form hollow tubes that invade the underlying mesenchyme and later transform into solid, branching cords. These cords are the primordia of the polyhedral thymic lobules.

Between the fourth and seventh weeks, the thymus glands lose their connections with the pharynx and migrate caudally and medially to their definitive location inferior and ventral to the developing thyroid and just dorsal to the sternum. There they are joined via connective tissue to form a single, bilobate thymus gland. At this point, the thymus is still epithelial but it quickly becomes infiltrated by neural crest cells to form septa and the capsule. During the third month, lymphocytes and dendritic cells infiltrate the thymus, and by twelve weeks, each thymic lobule is 0.5 to 2 mm in diameter and has a well-defined cortex and medulla. The whorl-like **Hassall's corpuscles** in the medulla are thought to arise from the ectodermal cells of the third pharyngeal cleft. Hassall's corpuscles produce signals necessary for the development of regulatory T cells. The loosely

organized **epithelial reticulum** is thought to be of endodermal origin.

The thymus is highly active during the perinatal period and continues to grow throughout childhood, reaching its maximum size at puberty. After puberty, the gland involutes rapidly and is represented only by insignificant fibrofatty vestiges in the adult.

The rudiments of the **inferior parathyroid glands (parathyroids III)** form in the dorsal portion of the third pouch, and the rudiments of the **superior parathyroid glands (parathyroids IV)** form in the fourth pouch early in the fifth week. They detach from the pharyngeal wall and migrate inferiorly and medially, coming to rest by the seventh week. The inferior parathyroid glands lie on the dorsal side of the inferior end of the thyroid lobes, whereas the superior parathyroid glands are in a position slightly superior to the inferior parathyroid glands. Thus, the superior parathyroids arise more inferiorly on the pharynx than the inferior parathyroids, and the two glands switch position during their descent; their names reflect their final relative positions.

During the fifth week, a minor invagination forms just caudal to each fourth pharyngeal pouch. This pair of invaginations has been described by many embryologists as the **fifth pharyngeal pouches**. Almost immediately after they appear, these invaginations become populated by cells that form the rudiments of the paired **ultimobranchial bodies**. These rudiments immediately detach from the pharyngeal wall and migrate medially and caudally to implant into the dorsal wall of the thyroid gland, where they become dispersed within the thyroid. The ultimobranchial bodies form the

Parathyroid III (inferior)
Parathyroid IV (superior)
Ultimobranchial body
Thymus
Thyroid

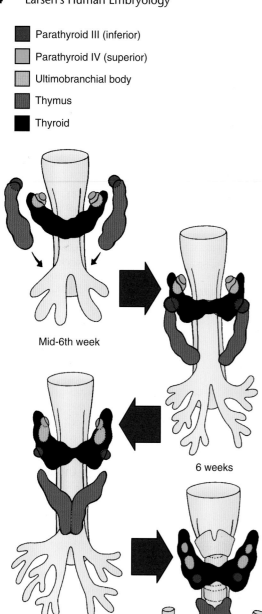

Mid-6th week

6 weeks

7 weeks

Definitive condition

Figure 17-32. Migration of pharyngeal pouch derivatives. The parathyroid glands and the ultimobranchial bodies migrate inferiorly to become embedded in the posterior wall of the thyroid gland. The two parathyroids exchange position as they migrate: parathyroid III becomes the inferior parathyroid, whereas parathyroid IV becomes the superior parathyroid.

calcitonin-producing **C-cells (parafollicular cells)** of the thyroid.

As with the thyroid gland, defects in migration of the parathyroid and thymus glands may occur, with ectopic fragments left along the migratory pathway. When the abnormality is asymmetric, the defect almost always occurs on the left side of the neck.

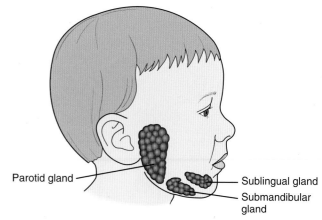

Parotid gland — Sublingual gland
Submandibular gland

Figure 17-33. Locations of the salivary glands.

DEVELOPMENT OF SALIVARY GLANDS

Three pairs of major salivary glands develop in humans: the **parotid, submandibular**, and **sublingual glands** (Fig. 17-33). Small salivary glands are also found in the inside of the cheeks, lips, tongue, hard palate, and floor of mouth. The salivary glands produce serous (watery) or mucous (viscous) secretions required for lubrication, digestion, and taste. These secretions constitute the saliva; it contains water, electrolytes, mucus, enzymes, and antibacterial compounds. The saliva is important for oral health, and defects in salivary gland formation and the subsequent production of saliva can result in periodontal disease, dental caries, ulcers, and problems with swallowing, as well as **xerostomia**: dry mouth. Decrease in salivary gland function occurs as a natural consequence of aging.

The parotid gland develops from a groove-like invagination of ectoderm that forms in the crease between the maxillary and mandibular swellings during week six. This groove differentiates into a tubular duct that sinks into the underlying mesenchyme toward the ear. The invaginating duct maintains a ventral opening at the angle of the primitive mouth. As the cheek portions of the maxillary and mandibular swellings fuse, this opening is transferred to the inner surface of the cheek. The blind end of the tube differentiates to form the parotid gland, whereas the stem of the tube becomes the **parotid** or **Stensen's duct**. Similar invaginations of the endoderm in the floor of the oral cavity and in the paralingual sulci on either side of the tongue give rise to the submandibular and sublingual salivary glands, respectively.

As for other epithelial-derived organs, development of the salivary glands involves a number of stages: prebud, bud, pseudoglandular, canalicular, and terminal bud. Specialized clusters of cells called **acini,** which produce the saliva, are formed during the terminal bud stage. Development and branching of the salivary glands are dependent on epithelial-mesenchymal interactions. Therefore, it is not surprising that some syndromes, such as autosomal dominant **lacrimoauriculodentodigital (LADD) syndrome** (the result of a mutation in FGF10), encompass both the salivary glands and other tissues dependent on epithelial-mesenchymal interactions for their development (i.e., lacrimal glands, distal limb, teeth, and ears).

In the Clinic

CAUSES OF CRANIOFACIAL ANOMALIES

It has been estimated that the various kinds of **craniofacial anomalies**—including malformations of the frontonasal process, clefting defects, calvarial malformations, and anomalies of the pharyngeal arch derivatives—account for approximately one third of all congenital defects. Most craniofacial anomalies have a multifactorial etiology, although in some types, a clear genetic basis can be demonstrated, as, for example, in **Treacher Collins syndrome** (covered in the next section of this "In the Clinic" entitled "Craniofacial Syndromes" and in the following "In the Research Lab" entitled "Developmental Basis of Treacher Collins Syndrome"), which is inherited as an autosomal dominant trait. A number of teratogens are also known to cause craniofacial malformations. Probably the most clinically significant craniofacial teratogen is **alcohol**. Drugs such as the anticonvulsant **hydantoin** and the oral antiacne drug **isotretinoin** (Fig. 17-34) can also cause craniofacial anomalies in humans, as can **toluene**, **cigarette smoking**, **ionizing radiation**, and **hyperthermia**. Finally, many craniofacial abnormalities are associated with cardiac abnormalities that are, in part, explained by the migration of cranial neural crest cells through the fourth and sixth pharyngeal arches to form the aorticopulmonary septum and the requirement for cranial neural crest cells in remodeling of the aortic arches. The secondary heart field, which contributes to the outflow tract and other regions of the heart, also arises from the cranial mesoderm (covered in Chapter 12). Recent studies have illustrated a common role of the endoderm in development of the face and aortic arches (see Chapter 13 and a following "In the Research Lab" entitled "Developmental Basis of DiGeorge Syndrome").

CRANIOFACIAL SYNDROMES

It is not surprising that errors in development of the numerous pharyngeal arch and pouch elements that contribute to the human head and face can cause various malformations. After cleft lip and cleft palate, the most common facial malformations are defects caused by underdevelopment of the first and second arches. A **lateral facial cleft** is an example: incomplete fusion of the maxillary and mandibular prominences in the cheek region results in a cleft extending from the corner of the mouth to, occasionally, as far as the tragus of the auricle.

Lateral clefting can occur as part of a group of more extensive deformities collectively known as **hemifacial microsomia** (*microsomia* is from the Greek for "small body"). In this condition, the lateral cleft of the face usually is not large, but the posterior portion of the mandible, the temporomandibular joint, the muscles of mastication, and the outer and middle ear may all be underdeveloped. As the name indicates, only one side of the face is affected. This is attributed to a vascular insult on one side of the face as remodeling of the pharyngeal arches occurs during weeks six through eight. **Goldenhar syndrome** is a particularly severe member of this group, including defects of the eye (scleral dermoids and colobomata of the eyelids) and vertebral column. This entire group of disorders is also referred to as **oculoauriculovertebral spectrum** (**OAVS**).

Another group of syndromes is classified as **mandibulofacial dysostosis** and involves generalized underdevelopment of the first pharyngeal arch, resulting in defects of the eye, ear, midface, palate, and jaw. The autosomal-dominant **Treacher Collins syndrome** is a member of this group. Treacher Collins syndrome affects approximately 1 in 50,000 people, and 60% of cases arise as new mutations. The gene for Treacher Collins syndrome, TCOF1, has been identified. It encodes a nucleolar phosphoprotein called Treacle (see the following "In the Research Lab" entitled "Developmental Basis of Treacher Collins Syndrome" for additional coverage).

In addition, craniofacial defects can extend into the pharyngeal arch derivatives and encompass abnormalities of the neck, heart, thymus, thyroid, and parathyroid glands. The complex of congenital malformations known as **DiGeorge syndrome** falls into this group and is characterized by a triad of malformations: (1) minor craniofacial defects, including **micrognathia** (small jaw), low-set ears, auricular abnormalities, cleft palate, and hypertelorism (see Fig. 17-1); (2) total or partial agenesis of the derivatives of the third and fourth pharyngeal arches (the thymus, thyroid, and parathyroid glands); and (3) cardiovascular anomalies, including persistent truncus arteriosus and interrupted aortic arch. DiGeorge syndrome is seen in **22q11.2 deletion syndrome**, which encompasses more than thirty-five genes and is the most common chromosomal deletion.

In the Research Lab

DEVELOPMENTAL BASIS OF TREACHER COLLINS SYNDROME

Treacher Collins syndrome is due to a mutation in TCOF1, which encodes the protein **TREACLE.** Genetic inactivation of treacle in mice has shown that this syndrome is due to a defect in the development of neural crest cells that will give rise to the first pharyngeal arch. As for other gene mutations, the genetic background can affect the phenotypic penetrance of the syndrome. Treacle is expressed in the neural folds as neural crest cells are forming and migrating, and later in the neural crest–derived mesenchyme of the first and second pharyngeal arches. Analysis of treacle mutant mice has shown increased apoptosis and decreased proliferation of the neural crest precursors and progeny. Neural crest migratory defects have not been observed. Treacle is required for the synthesis of ribosomal RNAs and hence is needed for protein synthesis in the rapidly proliferating neuroepithelial and neural crest cells. In addition, treacle may regulate microtubule dynamics. Microarray studies have shown that the tumor suppressor, p53, is upregulated as part of the cellular stress response to the reduction in levels of treacle. Moreover, pharmacological inhibition of p53 rescues the defects observed in treacle mutants. Although this is encouraging and shows a potential therapeutic strategy for Treacher Collins syndrome, this approach could not be used clinically, as most cases arise by spontaneous mutation and the defect arises before week three, when the genetic status of an embryo could not be determined. p53 is also a tumor suppressor, raising serious concerns about the consequences of inhibiting its function.

Mutations in TCOF1 account for 80% to 90% of Treacher Collins syndrome patients. However, recently, mutations in two additional genes, POLR1D and POLR1C, which also control ribosomal RNA transcription, have been identified. Therefore, Treacher Collins syndrome can be classified as **ribosomopathy**.

DEVELOPMENTAL BASIS OF DIGEORGE SYNDROME

DiGeorge syndrome or **22q11.2 deletion syndrome** occurs in approximately 1/4000 live births and is predominantly a disorder of the endoderm and mesoderm, which secondarily affects the development of neural crest cells. Indeed, the syndrome is phenocopied by loss of neural crest cells, and it was originally thought that the primary defect in 22q11.2 deletion syndrome was intrinsic to neural crest cells. However, genetic studies characterizing the function of each gene that is deleted in the crucial 22q11.2 chromosomal region do not support this original view. These studies have shown that TBX1, a T-box transcription factor, is the key player in the syndrome. Tbx1 is expressed in the pharyngeal endoderm and mesoderm including the secondary heart field, but not in neural crest cells. These studies have also revealed a crucial role of the endoderm in patterning the pharyngeal arches.

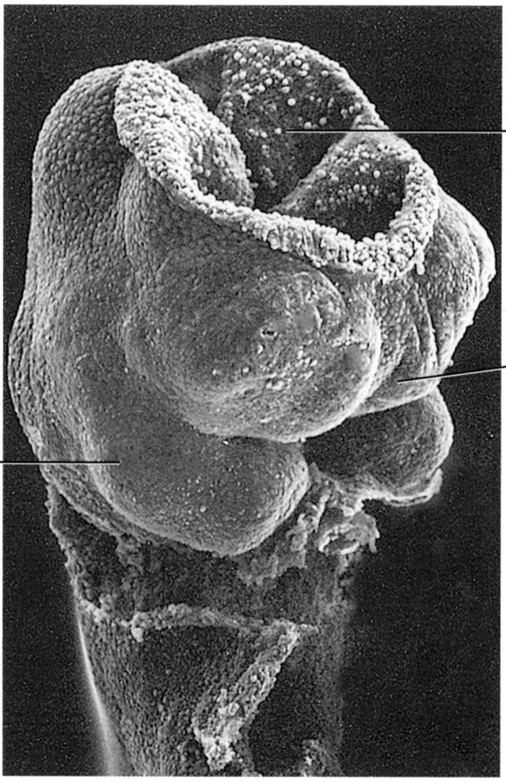

Figure 17-34. Mouse embryo treated with the teratogen isotretinoin (an analog of vitamin A) exhibiting a neural tube defect and first pharyngeal arch and frontonasal prominence abnormalities. Isotretinoin has been implicated in malformations of the skull, face, central nervous system, lungs, cardiovascular system, and limbs of human infants born to mothers ingesting it during the first three months of pregnancy.

Heterozygous deletion of Tbx1 in mouse recapitulates the main features of DiGeorge syndrome: fourth arch aortic arch remodeling defects, parathyroid and thyroid hypoplasia, and behavioral abnormalities. Homozygous deletion of Tbx1 in mouse recapitulates all features of the DiGeorge spectrum of cardiac and cranial defects. In Tbx1 mutants, development of the pharyngeal arches is affected with a craniocaudal gradient of severity: the first pharyngeal arch is slightly hypoplastic, and the third through sixth pharyngeal arches do not form. Timed deletion studies have identified when Tbx1 function is required for the development of the different cranial and cardiac derivatives. For example, aortic arch abnormalities are due to the requirement of Tbx1 during formation of the fourth pharyngeal arches, whereas thymus development requires Tbx1 function during both the formation of the third pharyngeal pouches and later thymus morphogenesis. Studies in which the Tbx1 gene has been conditionally inactivated in the mesoderm or endoderm show that Tbx1 is needed in both tissues. Tbx1 regulates cell proliferation, and loss of Tbx1 function results in decreased Fgf signaling together with increased Bmp and retinoic acid signaling. Retinoic acid (RA) decreases Tbx1 expression. As discussed above, RA is a potent teratogen that induces craniofacial malformations overlapping with those observed in DiGeorge patients, and the downregulation of Tbx1 function could be one mechanism of RA-induced pathogenesis.

Recent studies have shown that in addition to Tbx1, other genes contained within the 22q11.2 deletion are involved in DiGeorge syndrome. One such gene is CRKL, which encodes an adaptor protein needed for Fgf signaling. If one copy of Tbx1 and one copy of Crkl are deleted in mice, then the resultant phenotype encompasses those seen in the face and pharyngeal arch derivatives of 22q11.2 deletion syndrome patients. This shows that 22q11.2 deletion syndrome is a **contiguous gene syndrome** (i.e., requires deletion of multiple, contiguous genes to manifest the phenotype).

DEVELOPMENT OF TEETH

Teeth are composed of three types of hard tissues: **enamel**, **dentine**, and **cementum**. Enamel is the hardest substance in the body, with a low protein and a high mineral content of highly organized tightly packed calcium hydroxyapatite crystals. Dentine is harder than bone and cementum, but softer than enamel. Dentine forms the bulk of the tooth, with the crown covered by enamel and the root by cementum. Dentine consists of hydroxyapatite crystals, collagen type I, and dentine sialophosphoprotein, which is cleaved into three protein products: dentine glycoprotein, dentine sialoprotein, and dentine phosphoprotein. Teeth have three tissue origins: (1) ectoderm gives rise to ameloblasts that form the enamel; (2) neural crest cells give rise to odontoblasts and cementoblasts that form the dentine and cementum, respectively, as well as all connective tissues of the teeth; and (3) mesoderm contributes to the endothelial cells of the developing blood vessels.

In the sixth week of gestation, a U-shaped ridge of epidermis called the **dental lamina** forms on the upper and lower jaws (Figs. 17-35A, 17-36A, E). In the seventh week, ten centers of epidermal cell proliferation develop at intervals on each dental lamina and grow down into the underlying mesenchyme. A condensation of mesenchyme, derived from neural crest cells, forms under and around each of these twenty ingrowths. The composite structure consisting of the invaginating dental lamina and the underlying mesenchymal condensation is called a **tooth bud** (see Figs. 17-35A, 17-36B, F; see also Chapter 7).

During the ninth week, instructive influences from the epidermis cause the mesenchymal condensation to coalesce beneath the invaginating dental lamina,

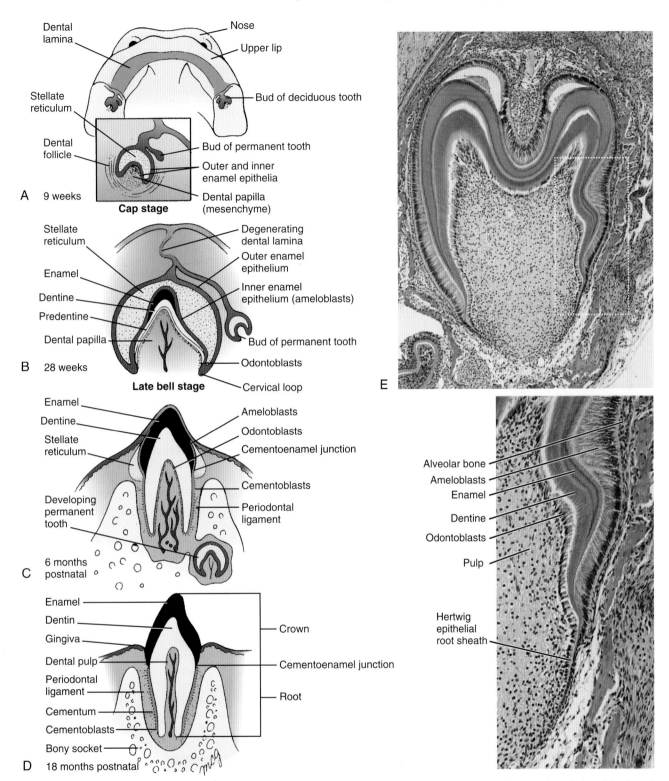

Figure 17-35. Development and eruption of the primary dentition. *A-D,* Drawings of sequential stages. The ectodermal dental lamina gives rise to the enamel organ, which secretes the enamel of the tooth, whereas the neural crest cells that initially form the dental papilla differentiate into the odontoblasts, which secrete dentine. *E,* Histological section and enlargement (boxed area in lower power micrograph) through a fully developed, unerupted tooth showing the different tissue layers.

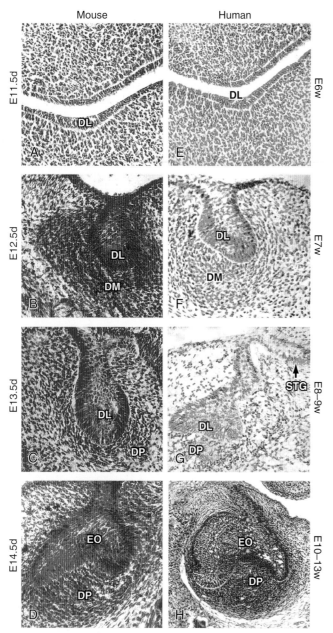

Mouse   Human

E11.5d · E12.5d · E13.5d · E14.5d

E6w · E7w · E8–9w · E10–13w

DL · DL · DM · DL · DM · STG · DL · DP · DP · EO · DP · EO · DP

Figure 17-36. Early stages in molar tooth development. *A-D,* Development in the mouse embryo from day 11.5 through 14.5. *E-H,* Development in the human embryo from week 6 through 10 to 13. In both mice and humans, development of the tooth begins with formation of the dental lamina (DL; panels *A, E*); its expansion to form the tooth bud, which consists of the thickened and folded dental lamina and underlying dental mesenchyme (DM; panels *B, F*); invagination of the dental lamina by growth of the condensed dental mesenchyme called the dental papilla (DP) at the cap stage (*C, G*), with formation of the secondary tooth germ (STG); and development of the enamel organ (EO; panels *D, H*) at the bell stage.

forming a hillock-shaped mesenchymal **dental papilla** (see Figs. 17-35*A*, 17-36*C, G*). This stage of tooth development is called the **cap stage** because the dental lamina invests the top of the papilla like a cap. At the cap stage, the dental lamina differentiates to form the **enamel organ**, which will produce the **enamel layer** of the tooth. First, the dental lamina becomes a three-layered structure, consisting of an **inner enamel epithelium** overlying the

dental papilla; a central layer, the **stellate reticulum** composed of star-shaped cells dispersed in an extracellular matrix; and an **outer enamel epithelium** (see Fig. 17-35*A*). The mesenchyme surrounding the papilla and its dental lamina cap condenses to form an enclosure called the **dental follicle**. By fourteen weeks, the dental papilla is enclosed by the dental lamina and constitutes the core of the developing tooth. This is called the **bell stage** of tooth development because the dental lamina looks like a bell resting over the dental papilla (see Fig. 17-36*D, H*; also see Fig. 17-35*B*).

During the bell stage, the cusps start to form and the size of the crown of the tooth increases. The outermost cells of the dental papilla, adjacent to the inner enamel epithelium, become organized into a distinct layer. In the late bell stage, these cells differentiate into **odontoblasts**, which will produce the **dentine** of the teeth (see Fig. 17-35*B, E*).

Dentine production starts around the third month in utero when the odontoblasts begin to secrete the non-mineralized matrix of the dentine, called **predentine**, which later progressively calcifies to form **dentine**. Production of predentine is induced by signals from the inner enamel epithelium and begins at the apex of the tooth and moves downward toward the coronal margin (see Fig. 17-35*B*). As the odontoblasts migrate downward, they leave long cell processes (**odontoblastic processes**) that extend through the thickness of the dentine behind them (see Fig. 17-35*E*). The inner mesenchyme of the dental papilla becomes the tooth pulp (see Fig. 17-35*E*). Odontoblasts persist after tooth eruption and dentine forms throughout life, narrowing the pulp cavity. This dentine is known as secondary dentine. Tertiary dentine is produced in response to certain stimuli, such as tooth damage, and may be produced by odontoblasts or progenitor pulp cells (i.e., non-odontoblast cells).

As soon as the first predentine is laid down, the cells of the inner epithelium are induced to differentiate into enamel-producing **ameloblasts**, which begin by secreting a thin layer of prismless enamel between themselves and the underlying dentine (see Fig. 17-35*B, C*). The ameloblasts then migrate coronally as they continue to secrete enamel, forming an enamel-surrounded projection that can be seen histologically, called a Tomes process. Once enamel has been laid down, a period of maturation takes place during which the mineral content of the enamel increases significantly. Ameloblasts die once enamel formation is complete. Therefore, enamel, unlike bone and dentine, cannot be remodeled and is not made after tooth eruption. The crowns of all primary teeth are partially mineralized by birth and are completely mineralized by twelve months of age. Crown formation in the secondary dentition, with the exception of the third molars, begins between three months and three years of age and is complete by around eight years of age.

The developing blood vessel network for the tooth enters the dental papilla from the early bell stage, with the nerves arriving much later, at the end of the bell stage (see Fig. 17-35*B*).

The roots of the primary teeth begin to form at the late bell stage after odontoblast differentiation in the cervical region of the tooth germ during late fetal and early postnatal life. At the junction of the inner and outer enamel epithelia, the **cervical loop**, the cells proliferate and elongate to form the double-layered **Hertwig's epithelial root sheath** (see Fig. 17-35*B, E*). The mesenchyme just internal to the epithelial sheath differentiates into odontoblasts, which produce dentine. Each root contains a narrow canal of dental pulp, through which nerves and blood vessels enter the tooth (see Fig. 17-35*C, D*).

The tooth roots are enclosed by extensions of the mesenchymal dental follicle. The inner cells of the follicle differentiate into **cementoblasts**, which secrete a layer of **cementum** to cover the dentine of the root. The epithelial root sheath breaks down to form the **cell rests of Malassez,** allowing intermingling of odontoblasts and cementoblasts and the formation of a strong union between cementum and dentine. At the neck of the tooth root, the cementum meets the enamel at the **cementoenamel junction** (see Fig. 17-35*C, D*). The outermost cells of the dental follicle participate in bone formation as the jaws ossify and also form the **periodontal ligament** that holds the tooth in its bony socket, or **alveolus**. The cementum, periodontal ligament, alveolar bone, and gingivae are supporting structures of the teeth, known as the periodontium. Root formation is usually completed two to three years after eruption. A histological section of a fully formed but not yet erupted tooth is shown in Figure 17-35*E*.

The initial twenty tooth buds give rise directly to the **primary** (**deciduous** or **milk**) **teeth**, consisting in each half-jaw of two incisors, one canine, and two molars. However, early in the cap stage, the dental lamina superficial to each of these buds produces a small diverticulum that extends to the base of the primary tooth bud and is known as the **successional lamina** (see Fig. 17-35*A,* 17-36*G*). This produces the bud of the **secondary** (**permanent**) successional tooth that will replace the first tooth (see Fig. 17-35*B, C,* 17-36*G*). These secondary teeth develop to the bell stage and arrest until about six years of age. Then, they start to develop secondarily, destroying the root of the primary tooth in the process.

The buds of the permanent molars, which do not have a deciduous precursor, arise during postnatal life from a pencil-like extension of the dental lamina that burrows back into the posterior jaw from the hindmost primary tooth buds. The full human dentition consists of thirty-two teeth, including three molars, but the third molars (wisdom teeth) often fail to develop or to erupt.

The primary teeth start to erupt at about six months after birth. Mandibular teeth usually erupt earlier than the corresponding maxillary teeth. The primary dentition is usually fully erupted by two and one-half years. Between approximately age six and eight years, the primary teeth begin to be shed and are replaced by the permanent teeth.

In the Research Lab

TOOTH INDUCTION

Experiments in which dental epithelial and mesenchymal components have been cultured with and without each other have shown that tooth development requires both components. Initially, the instructive signal is present in the epithelium, and if early odontogenic epithelium is recombined with non-odontogenic mesenchyme, teeth will

develop. Crucially, the non-odontogenic mesenchyme must be derived from neural crest cells, as teeth will not form when odontogenic epithelium is recombined with trunk-derived mesenchyme. Later, during tooth development, the neural crest–derived mesenchyme becomes instructive, that is, it can specify tooth development in non-odontogenic or naïve epithelium. This "transfer" of inducing ability correlates with a switch in Bmp4 expression from the epithelium to the underlying mesenchyme.

Odontogenic development starts with specification of the odontogenic field marked by Pax9 expression. This is achieved by antagonistic interactions between Fgf8 and Bmp4 signaling in the oral epithelium: Fgf8 promotes Pax9 expression, whereas Bmp2/4 inhibits it. The dental lamina also expresses the transcription factors Pitx2 and p63, which are required for early development of the teeth (see next "In the Clinic" entitled "Tooth Anomalies" and Chapter 7). Subsequent development requires multiple factors, including Shh, Bmps, Fgfs, Wnts, and downstream targets such as Msx1. Loss of these signals results in the arrest of tooth development at the bud stage or earlier. Shh, which is expressed in the odontogenic epithelium, is mitogenic, as it is in hair follicles (see Chapter 7). Enamel knots—transient, nonproliferative structures in the enamel organ that express a number of signaling molecules (Shh; Bmp2, 4, 7; Fgf4, 9)—are thought to act as signaling centers, promoting proliferation and folding of the adjacent epithelium (Fig. 17-37*A*). Thus, they specify the number of cusps that a tooth will form. The primary enamel knot forms at the center of the inner enamel epithelium during the late bud to early cap stage. In molar teeth, secondary enamel knots develop at the bell stage. Enamel knots are later removed by apoptosis. Aberrant enamel knot formation and morphogenesis, for example, following loss of Eda signaling or loss of the Bmp antagonist ectodin, are associated with changes in cusp number and morphology (see Fig. 17-37*B, C*; also see Fig. 7-10 in Chapter 7).

Patterning of different types of teeth is thought to occur by the differential expression of homeobox genes in the cranial mesenchyme: for example, the homeobox gene Barx1 and Dlx family members have been proposed to specify molars, whereas early expression of Msx1/2 expression has been proposed to specify incisors. Definitive evidence for this proposal is lacking, although the transformation of skeletal structures following loss of Dlx5/6 in the developing face (see Fig. 17-20) makes this proposal likely.

In the Clinic

TOOTH ANOMALIES

Malformations in teeth can arise from patterning defects or from abnormalities in differentiation. For example, the presence of a single maxillary incisor at the mild end of the holoprosencephaly spectrum is due to failure to specify (i.e., pattern) the embryonic midline. In contrast, defective development of enamel or dentine, as occurs in **amelogenesis imperfecta** (e.g., DLX3 mutations) and **dentinogenesis imperfecta** (DENTINE SIALOPHOSPHOPROTEIN mutations), involves faulty differentiation. To a discerning dentist, dental abnormalities may be the first indication of a more widespread syndrome. For example, the first indications of the **familial adenomatous polyposis** variant, **Gardner syndrome**, can be the formation of extra teeth and osteomas in the jaw, which can occur before the formation of colorectal polyps that predispose the individual to colon cancer. In the bone disorder, **hypophosphatasia adult form**, premature loss of primary teeth occurs before the age of four as the result of a deficiency in cellular and acellular cementum. This syndrome, also characterized by bone disorders and calcification of the ligaments, is caused by mutations in alkaline phosphatase, which normally hydrolyzes pyrophosphate. Excessive levels of pyrophosphate inhibit cementum deposition.

Enamel production occurs in two discrete steps, a secretory and mineralization phase. Defects in either of these processes results in **amelogenesis imperfecta (AI)**, which can be classified into three types (Fig. 17-38A). Hypoplastic AI is characterized by hard enamel that is deficient in quantity: it can be thin, grooved, or pitted. This is due to a defect in the secretory phase and can result from mutations in **ENAMELIN**, a component of the early enamel. Hypocalcified AI is due to a defect in the mineralization, whereas hypomaturation AI is the result of a defect in removal of the organic matrix and/or maturation of the crystals. Hypomaturation AI can be caused by mutations in enzymes (**ENAMELYSIN**, also known as MMP20) and **KALLIKREIN**, also known as KLK4) that cleave the enamel proteins to remove the organic components of the enamel. In hypocalcified and hypomaturation AI, the enamel is of normal thickness but is softer. Enamel defects can also be caused by **vitamin A deficiency** or diseases such as measles, or the enamel may be discolored following exposure to antibiotics such as **tetracyclines** or environmental factors such as **fluoride**.

Dentinogenesis imperfecta (DGI) can be caused by COLLAGEN TYPE I or DENTINE SIALOPHOSPHOPROTEIN mutations (Fig. 17-38B). Collagen type I mutations may also cause osteogenesis imperfecta (see Chapter 8). DGI will often be associated with enamel fractures, as the dentine is not hard enough to support the enamel.

Alternatively, there may be too few teeth (**hypodontia**; or **oligodontia**, when more than six teeth are absent; Fig. 17-38C). **Anodontia** is the complete lack of primary and/or secondary dentition. Hypodontia is slightly more prevalent in females than males, affects up to 20% of the population, and typically affects the secondary dentition. If primary teeth are affected, the secondary teeth will always be affected, as these arise from the lingual extension of primary teeth. The second mandibular and maxillary premolars and the lateral maxillary incisor are the most frequently affected teeth (see Fig. 17-38C). The consequences of missing teeth include malocclusion, caused by inappropriate positioning of the teeth, depletion of alveolar bone around the missing tooth, and drifting of adjacent teeth.

Non-syndromic hypodontia can be the result of mutations in the transcription factor PAX9 or MSX1. MSX1 mutations typically affect the premolars and third molars of the secondary dentition, whereas PAX9 mutations typically affect the molars. These defects presumably reflect a requirement for these genes in bud formation (see preceding "In the Research Lab" entitled "Tooth Induction").

Syndromes that include congenital absence of teeth include Down syndrome, HPE, and ectodermal dysplasias (e.g., EDA/EDAR, p63 mutations; see Chapter 7). PITX2 mutations (Axenfeld-Rieger syndrome) affect both deciduous and permanent dentition. In Pitx2 mouse mutants, a decrease in Fgf8 expression and an expansion of Bmp4 expression result in a smaller dental field. AXIN2 mutations (**oligodontia-colorectal cancer syndrome**) can result in the loss of eight to twenty-seven permanent teeth. Axin2 is a component of the Wnt signaling pathway, and this mutation may reflect loss of Wnt signaling, which is essential for tooth development.

Hyperdontia in the primary dentition occurs in 0.2% to 0.9% of the population (Fig. 17-38D). For the secondary dentition, this figure increases to 1% to 4%. The frequency of hyperdontia is slightly greater in males. Supernumerary teeth can be classified in various ways: **supplemental** teeth have normal morphology, **conical** teeth have a conical peg shape, **tuberculate** teeth are multicusped teeth with a large barrel shape, and **odontomas** are a mass of distinct or disorganized dental tissues. The most commonly occurring supernumerary tooth is a mesioden that forms in the primary palate between the maxillary central incisors. Supernumerary teeth may have no consequence, but they may affect development of the adjacent permanent teeth, causing delayed or retained eruption, displacement or damage such as root resorption, and periodontal lesions.

It is thought that some supernumerary teeth may arise by over-proliferation and/or survival of the dental lamina. In mouse models, Wnt signaling has been shown to promote the budding of teeth from the oral epithelium and primary tooth germs. This may explain the supernumerary teeth that are observed following mutation in APC, a negative regulator of the Wnt/β-catenin pathway, in **familial adenomatous polyposis syndrome**. Supernumerary teeth may also arise as the result of cleft lip. During development, dental placodes in the medial nasal process and maxillary process fuse to form a single progenitor of the deciduous lateral incisor. Failure of these placodes to fuse as a result of clefting can result in the development of two lateral incisors. The supernumerary teeth that occur in **cleidocranial dysplasia** are thought to represent a third dentition, as their development is delayed relative to the permanent dentition. In mice, loss of Runx2, the gene that is mutated in cleidocranial dysplasia (see Chapter 8),

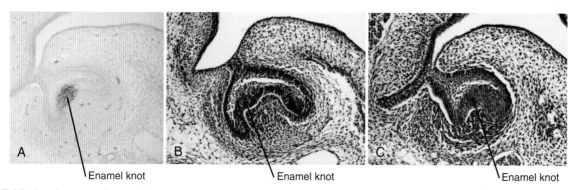

Enamel knot   Enamel knot   Enamel knot

Figure 17-37. Development of enamel knots. *A*, Expression of Shh in the developing enamel knot of a bell stage tooth bud. *B, C*, Development of the enamel knot in a wild-type (*B*) and a crinkled (part of the Eda/Edar pathway) mutant (*C*) tooth bud. In the crinkled mutant, the enamel knot and the tooth bud are abnormally shaped.

results in a larger lingual extension of the cap stage teeth and an upregulation of Shh. It is proposed that loss of Runx2 prolongs Shh expression and hence proliferation of the dental lamina, promoting the formation of successional teeth.

Tooth size and shape may also be affected. Teeth may be too small (**microdontia**; Fig. 17-38*E*) or too large (**megadontia**; Fig. 17-38*F*). Shape changes (Fig. 17-38*G*) may reflect abnormal formation of the enamel knot (see preceding "In the Research Lab" entitled "Tooth Induction"). There may also be fusions between different teeth (Fig. 17-38*H*).

Finally, adult **stem cell niches** have been found in the dental pulp of deciduous and permanent teeth, raising the possibility that they may be used to regenerate teeth and for the repair of other tissues.

Embryology in Practice

CLOSED EARLY

A couple brings their infant son to the doctor because of his irregular head shape. They had noticed some time ago that instead of a round head, their son had a more elongated head, bulging in the front and back (Fig. 17-39*A*). They had searched the Web, doing research on their own, and learned that treatment with a "helmet" could fix the irregular head shape as long as it was done early enough.

After examining their son, the doctor states that he is concerned about a more serious issue with the skull bones called **craniosynostosis** and recommends that the child be seen by a neurosurgeon. Besides the unusual head shape that he refers

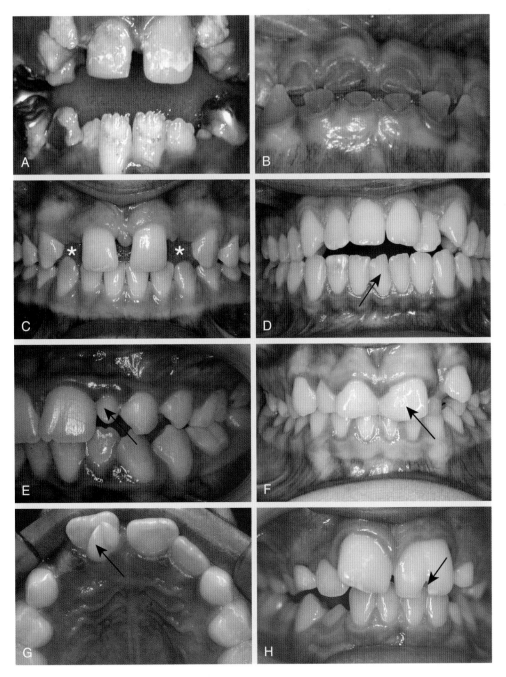

Figure 17-38. Inherited disorders of dental development. *A, B,* Hard tissue formation: *A,* Amelogenesis imperfecta in the mixed dentition; *B,* dentinogenesis imperfecta in the primary dentition. *C, D,* Tooth number: *C,* Agenesis of the maxillary permanent lateral incisor teeth (*); *D,* supplemental mandibular permanent incisor tooth (arrow). *E, F,* Tooth size: *E,* Microdont maxillary permanent lateral incisor tooth (arrow); *F,* megadont maxillary permanent central incisor tooth (arrow). *G, H,* Tooth shape: *G,* Talon cusp affecting a maxillary permanent central incisor tooth (arrow); *H,* fused maxillary permanent central and lateral incisor teeth (arrow).

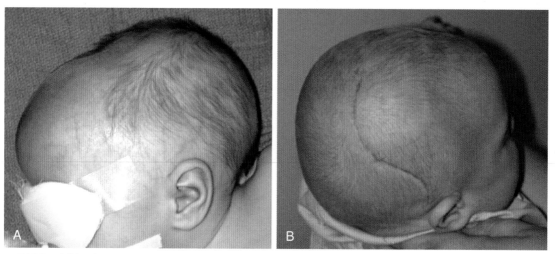

Figure 17-39. Child with craniosynostosis. *A,* Preoperative photo at three months of age. *B,* Postoperative photo six weeks later.

to as **scaphocephaly**, he points out the smaller than usual "soft spot" and the raised ridges on the top of their son's head. He reassures them that their son's head circumference is normal, indicating that brain growth is proceeding appropriately.

In this case, scaphocephaly (meaning boat-shaped head) is caused by premature fusion of the sagittal suture, a defect that can occur by biomechanical or genetic factors. This limits the ability of the skull to grow *wider*, so it grows *longer* instead. Premature fusion of the sagittal suture is the most common craniosynostosis, accounting for more than half of cases. It is more common in boys, at an incidence between 0.2 and 1 per 1000 births.

Although increased pressure on the brain can rarely result, this usually occurs only with synostosis of multiple sutures. For most children with sagittal craniosynostosis, surgical correction is performed for cosmetic and psychosocial reasons. The best cosmetic results are achieved if calvarial reconstruction is performed between three and six months of age.

The couple took their son to two separate neurosurgeons (who presented both open and endoscopic treatment options) before their son had an open cranial vault remodeling through a "zig-zag" coronal incision with excellent results (Fig. 17-39*B*).

Suggested Readings

Bailleul-Forestier I, Berdal A, Vinckier F, et al. 2008. The genetic basis of inherited anomalies of the teeth. Part 2: syndromes with significant dental involvement. Eur J Med Genet 51:383–408.

Bailleul-Forestier I, Molla M, Verloes A, Berdal A. 2008. The genetic basis of inherited anomalies of the teeth. Part 1: clinical and molecular aspects of non-syndromic dental disorders. Eur J Med Genet 51:273–291.

Cobourne MT, Sharpe PT. 2010. Making up the numbers: the molecular control of mammalian dental formula. Semin Cell Dev Biol 21:314–324.

Dixon MJ, Marazita ML, Beaty TH, Murray JC. 2011. Cleft lip and palate: understanding genetic and environmental influences. Nat Rev Genet 12:167–178.

Fagman H, Nilsson M. 2010. Morphogenesis of the thyroid gland. Mol Cell Endocrinol 323:35–54.

Goldberg M, Kulkarni AB, Young M, Boskey A. 2011. Dentin: structure, composition and mineralization. Front Biosci (Elite Ed) 3:711–735.

Grevellec A, Tucker AS. 2010. The pharyngeal pouches and clefts: development, evolution, structure and derivatives. Semin Cell Dev Biol 21:325–332.

Harunaga J, Hsu JC, Yamada KM. 2011. Dynamics of salivary gland morphogenesis. J Dent Res 90:1070–1077.

Johnson D, Wilkie AO. 2011. Craniosynostosis. Eur J Hum Genet 19:369–376.

Levi B, Wan DC, Wong VW, et al. 2012. Cranial suture biology: from pathways to patient care. J Craniofac Surg 23:13–19.

Melville H, Wang Y, Taub PJ, Jabs EW. 2010. Genetic basis of potential therapeutic strategies for craniosynostosis. Am J Med Genet A 152A:3007–3015.

Minoux M, Rijli FM. 2010. Molecular mechanisms of cranial neural crest cell migration and patterning in craniofacial development. Development 137:2605–2621.

Passos-Bueno MR, Ornelas CC, Fanganiello RD. 2009. Syndromes of the first and second pharyngeal arches: a review. Am J Med Genet A 149A:1853–1859.

Roessler E, Muenke M. 2010. The molecular genetics of holoprosencephaly. Am J Med Genet C Semin Med Genet 154C:52–61.

Sambasivan R, Kuratani S, Tajbakhsh S. 2011. An eye on the head: the development and evolution of craniofacial muscles. Development 138:2401–2415.

Simmer JP, Papagerakis P, Smith CE, et al. 2010. Regulation of dental enamel shape and hardness. J Dent Res 89:1024–1038.

Trainor PA. 2010. Craniofacial birth defects: the role of neural crest cells in the etiology and pathogenesis of Treacher Collins syndrome and the potential for prevention. Am J Med Genet A 152A:2984–2994.

Tzahor E. 2009. Heart and craniofacial muscle development: a new developmental theme of distinct myogenic fields. Dev Biol 327:273–279.

Chapter 18
Development of the Ears

SUMMARY

The ear is a composite structure with multiple embryonic origins. The external and middle ears arise from the first and second pharyngeal arches and the intervening pharyngeal cleft, membrane, and pouch. The inner ear, in contrast, develops from an ectodermal otic placode that appears on either side of the neural tube at the level of the future caudal hindbrain. At the end of the third week, this **otic placode** invaginates and then pinches off to form an **otic vesicle (otocyst)** within the head mesenchyme. The otic vesicle rapidly differentiates into three subdivisions: a slender **endolymphatic duct**, the expanded **pars superior**, and a tapered **pars inferior**. From the fourth to seventh weeks, the pars superior differentiates to form the three **semicircular canals** and the **utricle**. The pars inferior elongates and coils to form the **cochlear duct** distally and the **saccule** proximally. All of these otic vesicle derivatives collectively constitute the **membranous labyrinth**. The otic placode also gives rise to the sensory ganglia of the **vestibulocochlear (statoacoustic) nerve** (cranial nerve VIII). In addition, neural crest cells contribute to the vestibulocochlear nerve and its glial cells, as well as to melanocytes, which invade the cochlear duct. From weeks nine to twenty-three, the mesenchymal condensation that surrounds the membranous labyrinth, called the **otic capsule**, first chondrifies and then ossifies to form a **bony labyrinth** within the petrous part of the temporal bone.

The first pharyngeal pouch lengthens to form the **tubotympanic recess**, which differentiates into the **auditory (Eustachian) tube** and contributes to the tympanic cavity of the middle ear. Three auditory ossicles, the **malleus, incus**, and **stapes**, develop in the mesenchyme adjacent to the tympanic cavity. The malleus and incus are formed from the first pharyngeal arch mesenchyme, whereas the stapes is a second arch derivative. In the last month of gestation, the mesenchyme surrounding the ossicles regresses and the tympanic cavity expands to enclose the ossicles.

The **auricle (pinna)** of the external ear develops from six **auricular hillocks**, which appear during the sixth week on the lateral edges of the first and second pharyngeal arches. The first pharyngeal cleft lengthens to form the primordium of the **external auditory canal**. The ectoderm lining the canal subsequently proliferates to form a **meatal plug** that completely fills the inner portion of the canal. The definitive canal is formed by recanalization of this plug during the twenty-sixth week. The tympanic membrane is derived from the pharyngeal membrane that separates the first pharyngeal pouch and cleft. It develops as a three-layered structure, consisting of an external layer of ectoderm, a middle layer of ectoderm derived from **neural crest cells**, and an inner layer of endoderm. The definitive tympanic membrane is formed during recanalization of the external auditory meatus.

▍ *Clinical Taster*

A 2-year-old boy with **profound hearing loss** is admitted to the pediatric service for fever and vomiting. Urinalysis showed leukocytes and bacteria. He is diagnosed with pyelonephritis (urinary tract infection with kidney involvement) and started on intravenous antibiotics.

The boy's hearing loss was detected by a local Department of Health newborn hearing screening program and verified with a sedated brainstem auditory evoked response (BAER). His hearing loss was determined to be both **conductive** (caused by abnormalities of the external or middle ear) and **sensorineural** (caused by defects of the cochlea or cranial nerve VIII). He had been using hearing aids since four months of age.

A renal ultrasound done on admission showed small, dysplastic kidneys and hydronephrosis (dilation of the ureter and renal pelvis) on the right side. Later that night, while researching the differential diagnosis of hearing loss and kidney abnormalities, the medical student on call finds the description of **branchio-oto-renal (BOR)** syndrome. Intrigued by this possibility, the student returns to the patient's bedside and finds that the boy has cup-shaped ears, preauricular pits, and small cysts over the sternocleidomastoid muscle (Fig. 18-1A). These cysts are later determined to be pharyngeal (branchial) cysts (persisting rudiments of the pharyngeal apparatus, as covered in Chapter 17). During his hospital stay, the patient has a thin-cut CT (computed tomography) of the temporal bone that shows malformations of the middle ear bones and hypoplastic cochlea.

As suspected by the medical student, the combination of pharyngeal (branchial) arch, otic (ear), and renal (kidney) abnormalities seen in the patient suggests the diagnosis of BOR. Also known as Melnick-Frasier syndrome, BOR is most often caused by mutations in the EYES ABSENT HOMOLOG 1 (EYA1) gene. As the name suggests, mutations in the Drosophila homolog of this gene (Eya) affect the eyes (Fig. 18-1B). Humans with EYA1 mutations rarely have abnormalities of the eyes, likely because of functional redundancy of multiple EYA genes (four EYA homologs are present in humans) during eye development.

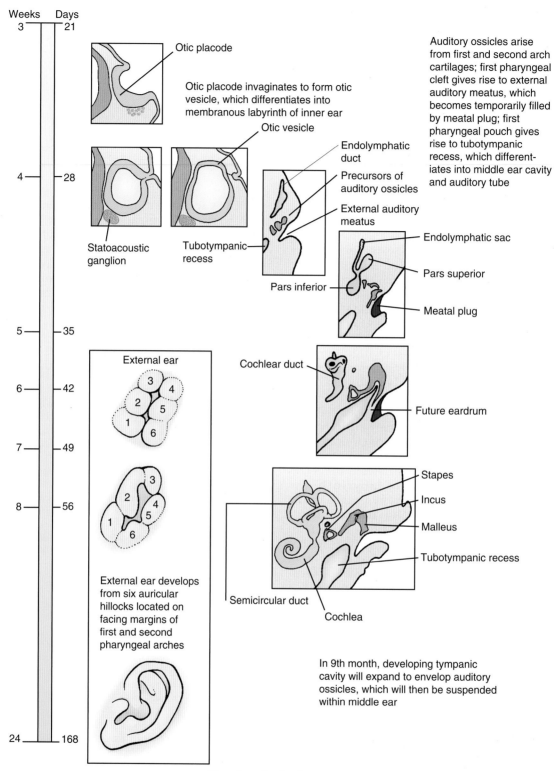

Weeks Days

Otic placode

Otic placode invaginates to form otic vesicle, which differentiates into membranous labyrinth of inner ear

Otic vesicle

Endolymphatic duct

Precursors of auditory ossicles

External auditory meatus

Statoacoustic ganglion

Tubotympanic recess

Endolymphatic sac

Pars superior

Meatal plug

Pars inferior

Auditory ossicles arise from first and second arch cartilages; first pharyngeal cleft gives rise to external auditory meatus, which becomes temporarily filled by meatal plug; first pharyngeal pouch gives rise to tubotympanic recess, which differentiates into middle ear cavity and auditory tube

External ear

Cochlear duct

Future eardrum

External ear develops from six auricular hillocks located on facing margins of first and second pharyngeal arches

Stapes

Incus

Malleus

Tubotympanic recess

Semicircular duct

Cochlea

In 9th month, developing tympanic cavity will expand to envelop auditory ossicles, which will then be suspended within middle ear

Time line. Ear development.

EAR CONSISTS OF THREE INDIVIDUAL COMPONENTS

 Animation 18-1: Development of the Ears.
Animations are available online at StudentConsult.

The ear can be divided into three parts, the external, middle, and inner ear, each of which has distinct tissue

origins. The external ear consists of the **pinna** (or **auricle**) and **external auditory canal** (ear canal). The middle ear contains the auditory ossicles—the **malleus, incus,** and **stapes**—arranged in a chain in the **tympanic cavity.** The external and middle ear capture and carry the sound waves to the inner ear. The inner ear consists of the **cochlea** and **vestibular apparatus.** The three **semicircular canals,** the **utricle,** and the **saccule**

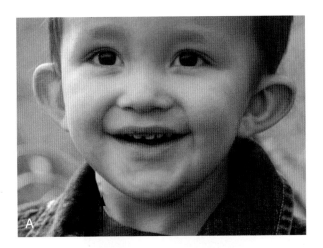

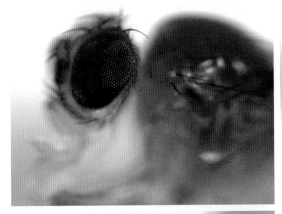

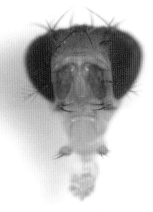

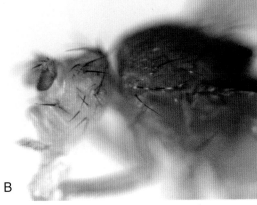

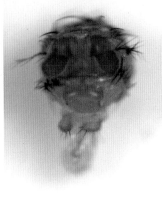

Figure 18-1. The role of Eya1 in embryonic development. *A,* Boy with branchio-oto-renal syndrome (mutation in the EYA1 gene). Note the cup-shaped ears and branchial cysts (arrow). Preauricular pits and tags (not shown in this case) sometimes accompany the syndrome. *B,* Wild-type Drosophila adult (top) and Eya1 mutant (bottom) showing the head in lateral (left) and on-front (right) views. Note the total absence of the eyes in the mutant (large reddish-orange structures in the wild-type Drosophila).

comprise the vestibular apparatus. The cochlea perceives sound waves, whereas the vestibular apparatus perceives orientation, movement, and gravity and is necessary for balance. The derivatives of the inner ear are collectively known as the **membranous labyrinth**. Innervated by the **vestibulocochlear nerve** (cranial nerve VIII), the inner ear receives contributions from neural crest cells in the form of melanocytes and Schwann cells.

DEVELOPMENT OF INNER EAR

All of the inner ear derivatives arise from ectoderm. Late in the third week, a thickening of the surface ectoderm called the **otic placode** or **otic disc** appears next to the hindbrain (Fig. 18-2A, B). During the third and fourth weeks, the otic placode gradually invaginates to first form an **otic pit** and then a closed, hollow **otic vesicle** or **otocyst** (Fig. 18-2C-G), which is connected briefly to the surface by a stem of ectoderm (Fig. 18-2E, F). Young neurons delaminate from the ventral otocyst to form the **statoacoustic (vestibulocochlear) ganglion** (see Fig. 18-2C).

By day twenty-eight, the dorsomedial region of the otic vesicle begins to elongate, forming an **endolymphatic appendage** (Fig. 18-3A; see Fig. 18-2G). Shortly thereafter, the rest of the otic vesicle differentiates into an expanded **pars superior** and an initially tapered **pars inferior** (Fig. 18-3B, C). The endolymphatic appendage

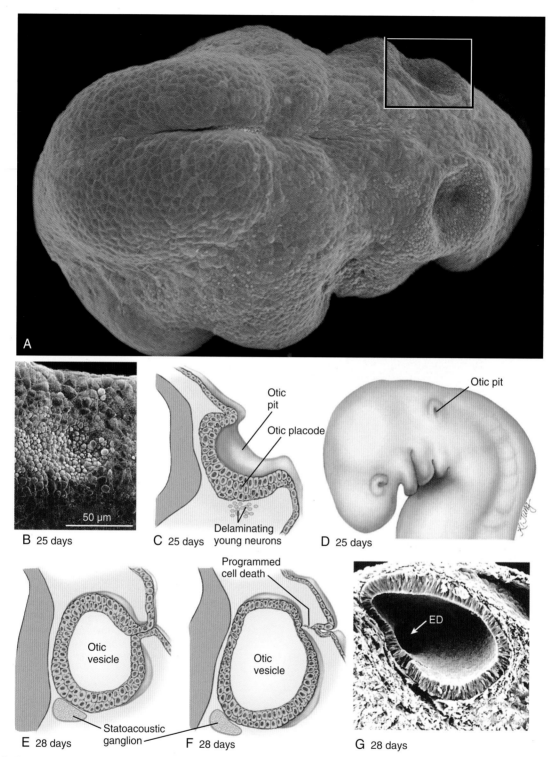

Figure 18-2. Formation of the otic vesicle. *A,* Head of an embryo showing the otic pits adjacent to the rhombencephalon. The box shows the otic pit and the orientation of the image in part *B. B,* The otic placode appears in the surface ectoderm late in the third week. *C, D,* By day 25, the placode invaginates to form the otic pit. *E-G,* By the end of the fourth week, continued invagination forms the otic vesicle, which quickly detaches from the surface ectoderm. ED, endolymphatic duct.

elongates over the following week, and its distal portion expands to form an **endolymphatic sac**, which is connected to the pars superior by a slender **endolymphatic duct** (see Fig. 18-3*C*).

During the fifth week, the ventral tip of the pars inferior begins to elongate and coil, forming the **cochlear duct**, which is the primordium of the cochlea (Fig. 18-3*D, E*). The pars inferior also gives rise to the saccule, which is connected to the cochlea by a narrow channel called the **ductus reuniens**. During the seventh week, cells of the cochlear duct differentiate to form the **spiral organ of Corti** (the structure that contains the sensory

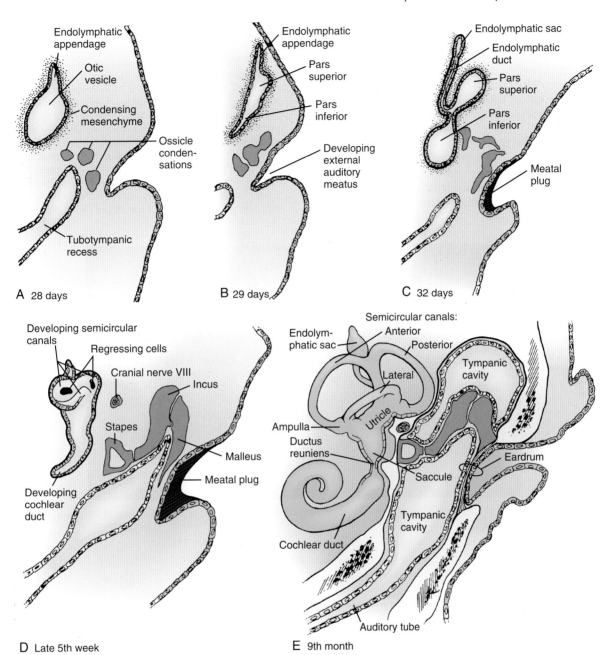

Figure 18-3. Development of the ear. The components of the inner, middle, and external ears arise in coordination from several embryonic structures. The otic vesicle gives rise to the membranous labyrinth of the inner ear and to the ganglia of cranial nerve VIII. *A, B,* The superior end of the otic vesicle forms an endolymphatic appendage, and the body of the vesicle then differentiates into pars superior and pars inferior regions. *C-E,* The endolymphatic appendage elongates to form the endolymphatic sac and duct; the pars superior gives rise to the three semicircular canals and the utricle; and the pars inferior gives rise to the saccule and coils to form the cochlear duct. Simultaneously, the three auditory ossicles arise from mesenchymal condensations formed by the first and second pharyngeal arches, the first pharyngeal pouch enlarges to form the tubotympanic recess (forms the future auditory tube and contributes to the middle ear cavity), and the first pharyngeal cleft (the future external auditory meatus) becomes filled with a transient meatal plug of ectodermal cells. Finally, in the ninth month, the tubotympanic cavity expands to enclose the auditory ossicles, contributing to the functional middle ear cavity (the most superior region of this cavity was recently shown to be derived from neural crest cells). The definitive eardrum is derived from the first pharyngeal membrane and is thus composed of pharyngeal cleft ectoderm and pharyngeal pouch endoderm, plus neural crest cells (ectoderm) that infiltrate the space between the cleft ectoderm and the pouch endoderm. Therefore, the definitive eardrum is a three-layered structure derived from two germ layers.

hair cells responsible for transducing sound vibrations into electrical impulses; see Fig. 18-5B). The sensory hair cells in the different regions of the cochlea are activated by different frequencies of sound waves.

Beginning late in the fifth week, flattened bilayered discs grow dorsally and laterally from the pars superior

(see Fig. 18-3D). In the center of the discs, the epithelial walls meet, and in these regions the epithelium regresses, leaving the rudiments of the semicircular canals. The semicircular canals are oriented perpendicularly to each other and consist of **anterior, posterior**, and **lateral semicircular canals** (see Fig. 18-3D, E). A small expansion called the **ampulla**, which houses the sensory cells, forms at one end of each semicircular canal (see Fig. 18-3*E*; see also Fig. 18-5*A, B*).

The morphogenesis of the mouse inner ear closely resembles that of the human inner ear. Figure 18-4 shows the morphogenesis of the mouse inner ear over a seven-day period of embryogenesis, using an injection procedure in which the cavity of the otocyst is filled with an opaque paint and the head of the embryo is cleared. This approach provides a more three-dimensional view of the developing inner ear. Because the embryo can be turned and photographed in various orientations, the relationships of the three semicircular canals can be readily understood (Fig. 18-5*A*).

In the Research Lab

DEVELOPMENT OF PLACODES

The placodes (otic, epibranchial, trigeminal, olfactory, adenohypophyseal, and lens; see Fig. 4-21 in Chapter 4) arise from a horseshoe-shaped domain surrounding the anterior neural plate, called the preplacodal region (see Fig. 3-11*D*). The preplacodal region is initially multipotent, is competent to form all of the placodal derivatives, and is characterized by the expression of the Six and Eya families of transcription factors (specifically, Six1, Six4, Eya1, and Eya2) throughout the preplacodal domain. This domain, together with neural crest progenitors, is established by Fgf signaling and intermediate levels of Bmp signaling (low levels of Bmps specify the neural plate, and high

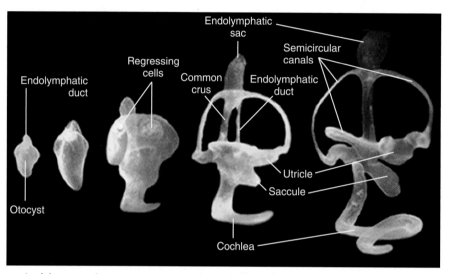

Figure 18-4. Morphogenesis of the mouse inner ear over a seven-day period in embryogenesis, revealed by filling of the cavity of the developing otocyst with opaque paint.

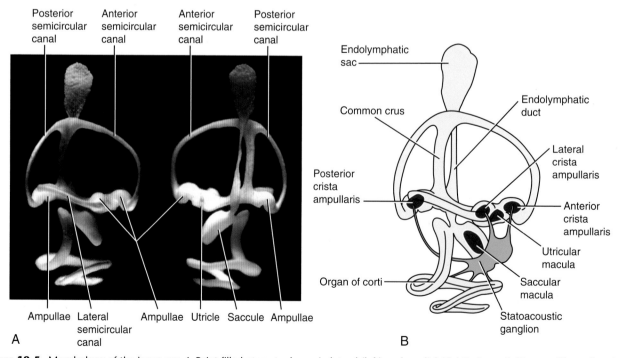

Figure 18-5. Morphology of the inner ear. *A,* Paint-filled otocysts shown in lateral (left) and medial (right) views. *B,* Diagram illustrating the six prosensory regions (red) in the developing inner ear.

levels the ectoderm; see Chapter 4 for further coverage). The preplacodal region progressively becomes regionalized to form the precursors for the distinct placodes. For example, following formation of the preplacodal region, the presumptive olfactory and lens placodes are initially characterized by the expression of Pax6, whereas the presumptive otic and epibranchial placodes express Pax2. Later, Pax6 is specifically expressed in the developing lens, whereas the developing olfactory placode switches off Pax6 expression and is now distinguished by Dlx5 expression. Differential and combinatorial signaling of Shh, Fgfs, Bmps, and Wnts from the surrounding tissues gradually restricts the developmental competence of the preplacodal region. These factors act to promote or inhibit the development of specific placodes. Fgf signaling from the mesoderm, endoderm, and anterior neural ridge (the cranial U-shaped junction between the ectoderm of the neural plate and the non-neural, or

surface, ectoderm) is initially required for olfactory, trigeminal, otic, and epibranchial placode development but is inhibitory for lens induction. Signals (Tgfβ) from neural crest cells also inhibit lens development; hence, the lens develops only in the ectoderm in contact with the optic cup, where neural crest cells are excluded. Ablation of neural crest cells in chicks and amphibians results in ectopic lens development. Canonical Wnt signaling from the hindbrain is also needed for otic induction, whereas sustained Fgf signaling, together with Bmps from the pharyngeal pouches, is required for formation of the epibranchial placodes. Shh from the prechordal mesoderm (see Chapter 17 for coverage of other roles of Shh signaling in the head mesoderm) is required for development of the adenohypophyseal placode. In the absence of Shh signaling, the adenohypophyseal placode fails to develop and the lens placode expands.

INDUCTION AND PATTERNING OF RUDIMENTS OF INNER EAR

The otic placode is induced by Fgf signaling from the mesoderm, together with signals such as Wnts and Fgfs from the hindbrain. Overexpression of Fgfs is sufficient to induce formation of ectopic otic vesicles in chick embryos, whereas in the double Fgf3/Fgf10 mouse mutant, the otic placode does not form. Fgf8 (expressed by the endoderm in chick and by all three germ layers in mouse) induces the expression of other Fgfs in the mesoderm. The epibranchial placode arises adjacent to the otic placode and, as stated above, also requires Wnt and Fgf signaling. Otic versus epibranchial fate is determined by the duration and level of exposure to Fgf and Wnt signals.

Once the placode has formed, it invaginates to form the otic vesicle or otocyst, which now must become specified into its different regions (i.e., vestibular structures and the cochlea). The ventral otic vesicle forms the cochlea and saccule, whereas the dorsal otic vesicle forms the remainder of the vestibular structures. This is achieved by the differential expression of homeobox genes. For example, Pax2 is expressed in the ventral otocyst and is essential for development of the cochlea (Figs. 18-6, 18-7). In contrast, the homeobox genes Dlx5 and 6 are expressed in the dorsal otocyst and are required for development of the vestibular apparatus (see Figs. 18-6, 18-7). Loss of function of some

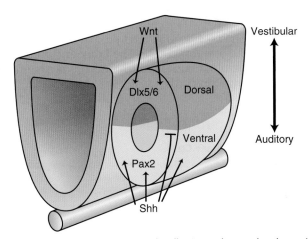

Figure 18-6. Signals from the hindbrain and notochord specify homeobox gene expression in the dorsal and ventral regions of the otic vesicle. The dorsal part of the hindbrain secretes Wnt and the notochord and floor plate secrete Shh.

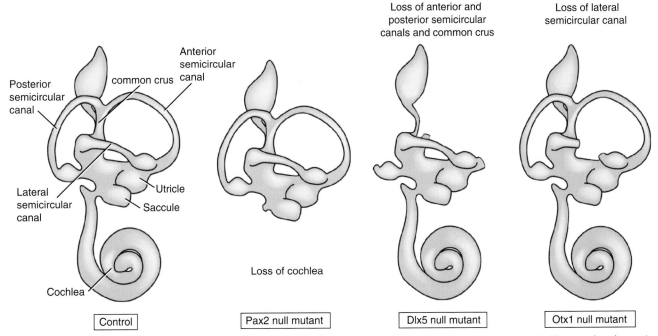

Figure 18-7. Development of the vestibular structures and cochlea is differentially controlled by homeobox genes, as revealed by using knockout mice.

homeobox genes (e.g., Otx1) leads to more limited defects, such as loss of the lateral canal (see Fig. 18-7).

Experimental manipulations in which the otocyst (or adjacent structures) has been rotated at different stages of development have shown that the cranial-caudal axis is specified first, followed by the dorsal-ventral axis. These analyses, together with analysis of knockout mice, have also shown that signals from the hindbrain and notochord control homeobox gene expression. Shh signaling from the notochord and floor plate controls Pax2 expression, whereas Wnt signaling from the dorsal neural tube controls expression of Dlx5 and 6 (see Fig. 18-6). In the absence of Shh, the cochlea duct and saccule do not form. Again emphasizing the importance of hindbrain signals, double knockout of Hoxa1 and Hoxb1, which results in the loss of rhombomere 5, affects the development and morphogenesis of the entire inner ear.

Inner ear hair cells, specialized mechanotransducers, arise in six prosensory regions within the developing otic vesicle (see Fig. 18-5B). In the cochlea, the prosensory region forms the **organ of Corti**. In the saccule and utricle, it forms the **maculae**, and in the semicircular canals, it forms the **cristae**. The maculae are responsible for detecting gravity and linear acceleration. The cristae detect angular acceleration. All of these sensory regions are innervated by the **statoacoustic ganglion** of the **vestibulocochlear nerve** (cranial nerve VIII). The vestibular structures are innervated by the **vestibular branch**, whereas the cochlea is innervated by the **spiral (cochlear) branch**. The latter branches synapse in the auditory nuclei, which develop in the alar plate of the brainstem (development of the brainstem is covered in Chapter 9).

Two types of hair cells are present in the organ of Corti, the **outer hair cells** and **inner hair cells**, which differ in their physiologic and morphologic properties. One row of inner hair cells and three rows of outer hair cells are noted (Fig. 18-8). About 95% of the sensory nerve fibers to the cochlea innervate the inner hair cells, which are, therefore, the primary transducers of signals to the brain. In contrast, outer hair cells receive about 80% of the motor input to the cochlea. The outer hair cells change their length with exceptional rapidity in response to sound (a process known as **electromotility**); this amplifies the sound waves, increasing sensitivity. This ability has been attributed to a unique membrane protein called prestin, and, in fact, non-syndromic deafness in humans can result from mutations in the gene encoding PRESTIN.

In the organ of Corti, the **stereocilia** (specialized microvilli) of the hair cells project into an acellular gelatinous matrix called the **tectorial membrane**, which is necessary for hair cell function (Fig. 18-8C). The tectorial membrane consists of collagens (types II, V, IX, and XI) and ear-specific non-collagenous proteins such as α- and β-tectorin. In both the maculae and the cristae, the hair cells are also overlain (i.e., capped) by an acellular matrix; this is called the **otoconial membranes** in the maculae and the **cupula** in the cristae. Hair cells are surrounded by endolymph. In the cochlea, the endolymph has a high K$^+$ concentration that is necessary for hair cell function. The vestibular sensory organs are functional at birth, but the organ of Corti does not become fully differentiated and hence fully functional until after birth.

Beginning in the ninth week of development, the mesenchyme surrounding the membranous labyrinth chondrifies to form a cartilage called the **otic capsule**. Transplantation experiments have shown that the otic vesicle induces chondrogenesis in this mesenchyme, and that the shape of the vesicle controls the morphogenesis of the capsule. During the third to fifth month, the layer of cartilage immediately surrounding the membranous labyrinth undergoes vacuolization to form a cavity called the **perilymphatic space**. The perilymphatic space is filled with a fluid called **perilymph**, which communicates with the cerebrospinal fluid via the **perilymphatic duct**. Around the cochlea, these spaces are known as the **scala vestibuli** and **scala tympani**; because it is positioned between the scala vestibule and scala tympani, the cavity of the cochlear duct is also known as the **scala media** (Fig. 18-8B). The otic capsule ossifies between sixteen and twenty-three weeks to form the **petrous portion** of the temporal bone (Fig. 18-9; covered in Chapter 17; see Fig. 17-3). Continued ossification later produces the **mastoid portion** of the temporal bone. The bony enclosure that houses the membranous labyrinth and the perilymph is called the **bony labyrinth**.

In the Research Lab

FORMATION OF SENSORY CELLS

The prosensory regions containing the presumptive hair cells express a number of factors, including Bmp4, Sox2, Islet1, Ids1, 2, and 3—inhibitors of differentiation genes—jagged 1, and Fgf10. The transcription factors Sox2 and jagged 1 are essential for development of the prosensory region, whereas the Ids inhibit hair cell differentiation by binding to basic helix-loop-helix (bHLH) proteins (bHLH proteins are covered in Chapter 5 in the context of notch signaling, Chapter 10 in the context of neuronal differentiation, and Chapter 14 in the context of intestine development) and preventing them from binding to DNA. The prosensory region contains bipotential precursors that will give rise to hair cells or to the supporting cells that surround them. The proneural gene Atoh (also known as Math1), a bHLH transcription factor, is essential for hair cell development, whereas Hes1 and 5 (the hairy and enhancer of split transcription factors) are required for the development of supporting cells. Consequently, in Atoh mutant mice, hair cells do not develop, whereas in Hes1 or 5 mouse mutants, an excess of hair cells is seen. In addition, overexpression of Atoh1 can induce the formation of ectopic hair cells. Specification of a hair cell versus a supporting cell from a common precursor is achieved by **lateral inhibition** (see Chapters 5 and 10 for further coverage). The presumptive hair cell expresses the notch ligands jagged 2 and delta 1, which activate notch signaling in adjacent cells (presumptive supporting cells). Notch activation results in the release of the intracellular notch fragment, N^{ICD}, which enters the nucleus to induce the expression of Hes1 and 5 (Fig. 18-10). The Hes proteins inhibit Atoh activity, thereby preventing hair cell differentiation and allowing cells to develop as supporting cells. Thus, following loss of notch signaling (e.g., as a result of loss of the notch receptor or the ligands that activate the receptor), excess hair cells are seen. This is strikingly illustrated in the **mind bomb** zebrafish mutant, which has defective notch signaling. In this mutant, all prosensory cells differentiate as hair cells, and supporting cells are totally absent.

Specialized microvilli called **stereocilia** develop on each hair cell. Stereocilia consist of parallel dense bundles of actin

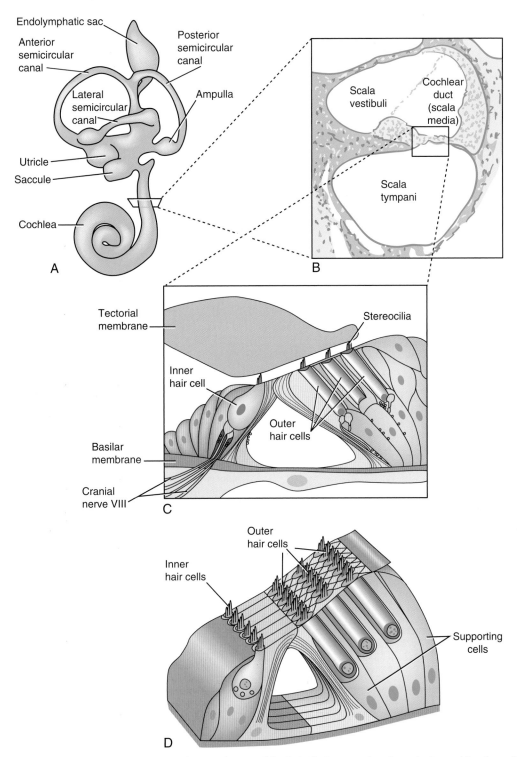

Figure 18-8. Development of the organ of Corti. *A,* The membranous labyrinth. *B,* Cross section through the cochlea (boxed in *A*). *C,* Details of the organ of Corti (boxed in *B*). *D,* The tectorial membrane has been removed to show a more three-dimensional view of the organ of Corti.

filaments and are the mechanosensors of the hair cell. Between 50 and 200 interconnected stereocilia are present on each hair cell. They are arranged in a "staircase" pattern at one edge of the cell, with stereocilia in adjacent rows of the "staircase" interconnected by fibrous **tip links** (Fig. 18-11*A*). In the cochlea, all stereocilia on different hair cells are oriented in the same direction. The ordered and repetitive pattern of stereocilia formation is essential for hearing and is achieved by signaling

via the **planar cell polarity (PCP) pathway**. As covered in Chapter 5, in Drosophila the PCP pathway is mediated by frizzled receptors and determines the aligned orientation of the sensory bristles in the thorax, hairs in the wings, and ommatidia in the developing eye. Such orientation of structures is also seen in vertebrates—for example, to ensure that all cilia in the respiratory tract or in the oviduct beat in the same orientation. However, the most striking and intricate example in vertebrates

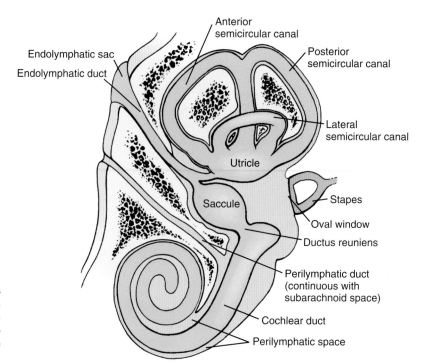

Figure 18-9. The definitive membranous labyrinth is suspended in the fluid-filled perilymphatic space within the bony labyrinth of the petrous portion of the temporal bone. The perilymphatic space is connected to the subarachnoid space by the perilymphatic duct. The membranous labyrinth itself is filled with endolymph.

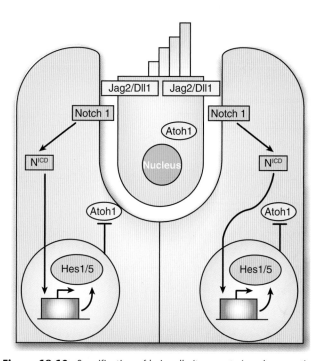

Figure 18-10. Specification of hair cells (top center) and supporting cells (bottom sides) is determined by lateral inhibition involving notch signaling.

is the precisely controlled orientation of the inner ear hair cell stereocilia. Many components of the Drosophila PCP pathway have been conserved in vertebrates. Therefore, the stereocilia are misoriented when components of the PCP pathway, such as the transmembrane proteins van Gogh–like 2 (Vangl2) or flamingo (Celsr1), are mutated in mice (Fig. 18-11*B, C*). Likewise, double gene inactivation of the frizzled 3 and 6 receptors results in defects in hair cell polarity.

In the Clinic

TYPES OF HEARING LOSS

Total or partial **hearing loss** occurs in more than 1 in 1000 live births and places a significant burden on health-care and special education programs. The prevalence of individuals who have hearing loss or who are **deaf** rises to 1 in 500 by adulthood. **Conductive hearing loss** is the result of malformations in the external and/or middle ear, whereas **sensorineural hearing loss** can arise from defects in the inner ear, **vestibulocochlear nerve** (cranial nerve VIII), or auditory regions of the brain. About half of all hearing loss has genetic causes, with the other half attributed to environmental factors. The latter include in utero viral infections (e.g., **cytomegalovirus, rubella**) and neonatal exposure to **aminoglycoside antibiotics** (e.g., **gentamicin, tobramycin**). Postnatal exposure to loud noise can also result in hearing loss.

Hearing loss and deafness due to genetic causes can be **non-syndromic**, that is, occurring as an isolated defect, or **syndromic**, that is, occurring in conjunction with other anomalies. To date, more than 150 chromosomal loci have been linked to non-syndromic hearing loss, and gene mutations have been identified in more than 50 of them. Mutations have been found in a variety of genes, including those that encode transcription factors, ion channels, membrane proteins, actin cytoskeletal components and transporters, and microRNAs. Although syndromic hearing loss is less common (constituting about 10% to 15% of all cases), more than 300 genetic syndromes have been described in which hearing loss occurs as a component finding. Whether caused by inherited or environmental factors, hearing loss may be present at birth or soon afterward (**congenital** or **prelingual** hearing loss, such as in **Usher syndrome type I**), or it may be associated with age-dependent or progressive loss of hearing (**postlingual**, as in the case of mutations in the transcription factors POU4F3 and EYA4). Prelingual hearing loss is associated with greater disturbances in the development of communication. In addition, hearing loss occurs naturally with aging—a condition called **presbycusis**.

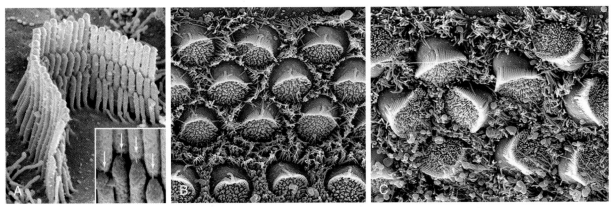

Figure 18-11. Hair cells of the inner ear. *A,* The "staircase" structure of the stereocilia on the inner ear hair cells. Inset shows the tip links (arrows) that interconnect stereocilia in adjacent rows of the "staircase" and act as mechanotranducers. *B, C,* The orientation of the hair cells is determined by the planar polarity pathway, as shown by randomization of hair cells in mice mutant for the Celsr1 gene (*C*), as compared with wild-type mice (*B*).

MALFORMATIONS OF INNER EAR: SENSORINEURAL HEARING LOSS

Sensorineural hearing loss and balance dysfunction can result from various structural malformations or improper functioning of inner ear structures, including the cochlea and vestibular system. These **vestibulocochlear dysplasias** range from complete absence of the membranous labyrinth (**labyrinthine aplasia**) to partial absence or underdevelopment of specific inner ear structures such as the cochlea (**cochlear hypoplasia**). In addition to relatively gross malformations of inner ear components, hearing loss can result from more subtle dysplasias that affect only a single cell type (e.g., disruption of stereocilia organization in individuals with mutations in cadherin 23, also known as otocadherin). A range of inner ear defects is discussed below.

An example of a syndrome characterized by vestibulocochlear dysplasias is **CHARGE syndrome** (coloboma of the eye, heart defects, atresia of the choanae, retarded growth and development, genital and urinary anomalies, and ear anomalies and hearing loss), often caused by mutations in CHD7 (chromodomain helicase DNA-binding protein; covered in Chapter 12). Inner ear defects commonly range from labyrinthine aplasia (sometimes called **Michel aplasia**) to reduction in the number of cochlear turns (fewer than 2.5 turns; having 2.5 to up to 3 turns is considered normal in humans) and/or semicircular canal defects (collectively often referred to as **Mondini dysplasia**). Hearing loss in CHARGE syndrome can also result from defects in development of the middle ear, and external ear abnormalities are a cardinal feature of the syndrome.

An inner ear dysplasia that enlarges the bony canal that transmits the endolymphatic duct (i.e., the vestibular aqueduct; Fig. 18-12) is a common cause of sensorineural hearing loss and vestibular anomalies. **Large vestibular aqueduct** (LVA; also called enlarged vestibular aqueduct, or EVA) can be diagnosed radiographically (i.e., thin-cut CT) and is associated with **Pendred syndrome**. The responsible gene encodes a protein called **PENDRIN**, a chloride-iodide transporter.

Hair cells play an essential role in both hearing and balance. Many genes affect the development and function of hair cells and, when mutated, result in hearing loss and vestibular dysfunction. These include genes that encode **stereocilia** cytoskeletal components (e.g., ACTIN, DIAPHANOUS 1, ESPIN, HARMONIN, SANS, WHIRLIN), intracellular motors that control actin assembly (e.g., MYO6, MYO7a, MYO15A), and cell adhesion components (e.g., CADHERIN 23, PROTOCADHERIN 15; Fig. 18-13). Alternatively, the gene may be necessary for hair cell survival (e.g., POU3F4).

The sensitivity of stereocilia to gene mutations is illustrated by **Usher syndrome type 1**, an autosomal recessive

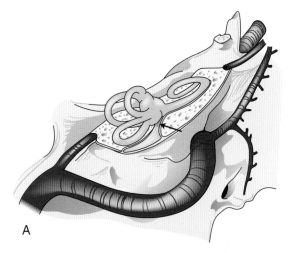

A

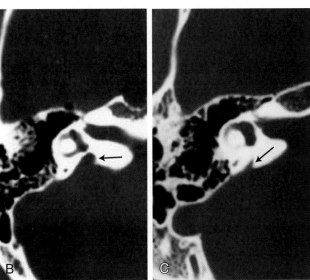

Figure 18-12. Large vestibular aqueduct. *A,* Normal inner ear anatomy showing the endolymphatic duct (arrow) that connects the endolymphatic sac to the vestibule, passing through the bony vestibular aqueduct. *B,* Large vestibular aqueduct (arrow) shown by axial CT of the temporal bone. *C,* Normal caliber of the bony aqueduct (arrow) is less than 1.5 mm. Bone appears as a white signal.

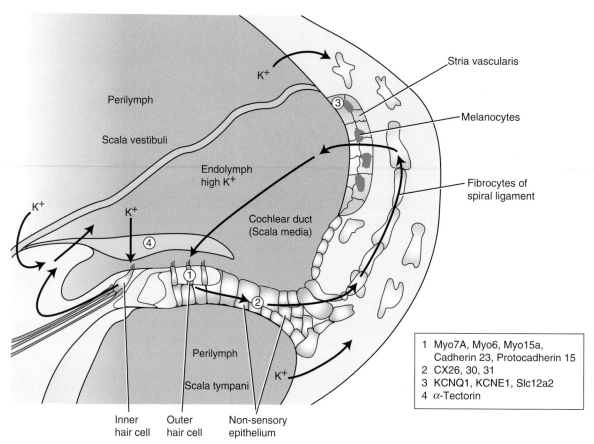

Figure 18-13. Hearing loss can result from mutations of the many different genes expressed in the inner ear.

disorder characterized by **sensorineural hearing loss** and **retinitis pigmentosa**. This syndrome can be caused by mutations in one of several of the genes listed in the preceding paragraph (i.e., MYO7A, HARMONIN, CADHERIN 23, SANS, PROTOCADHERIN 15). CADHERIN 23, HARMONIN, WHIRLIN, and PROTOCADHERIN 15 form a complex at the stereocilia tip links (see Fig. 18-11A), which contain the mechanotransduction channels. MYO7A transports PROTO-CADHERIN 23 and HARMONIN to the tip links. Analysis of the relevant mouse mutants, which also are all characterized by deafness, has shown that the stereocilia are disorganized and do not have the normal "staircase" pattern. Auditory hair cell function also requires contact of the stereocilia with the overlying **tectorial membrane**. Mutation in α-TECTORIN, a key constituent of this membrane (Fig. 18-13), results in an autosomal dominant non-syndromic hearing disorder, and analysis of α-tectorin mutant mice has shown that the tectorial membrane is not attached to the sensory hair cells.

Signaling through the **ion channels** in hair cells and maintenance of hair cell integrity require high K⁺ levels in the endolymphatic fluid. This is achieved by recycling the K⁺ that enters the activated hair cells via gap junctions to the **stria vascularis**. From here, K⁺ is transported back into the lymph by the channel proteins KCNQ1 and KCNE1 (see Fig. 18-13). Defects in K⁺ recycling can result in hearing loss. For example, mutations in several **connexin proteins** (CX26, CX30, CX31), which are components of **gap junctions**, have been identified in many patients with deafness. In fact,

mutations in the gene encoding CX26, which is expressed in the non-sensory epithelium between the organ of Corti and the stria vascularis (see Fig. 18-13), are responsible for between 20% and 30% of cases of prelingual non-syndromic deafness, making it the most common known cause of hereditary congenital deafness. Mutation in KCNQ1 can cause **Jervell and Lange-Nielsen syndrome**, characterized by prelingual sensorineural hearing loss and cardiac arrhythmia (**long QT syndrome**; also covered in Chapter 12); the latter can result in sudden death.

Auditory neuropathy is classified as a defect in auditory nerve function and can be due to mutations in VGLUT3, OTOFERLIN, PEJVAKIN, and DIAPHANOUS3. VGLUT3 is expressed in the inner hair cells and produces glutamate in synaptic vesicles, whereas OTOFERLIN is necessary for synaptic vesicle production and fusion of the synaptic vesicles in the ribbon synapses.

Finally, a number of deafness syndromes are the result of mutations affecting **mitochondrial** function and can be caused by mutations in mitochondrial DNA (which, because we inherit all our mitochondria from our mothers, are **maternally inherited**). One such condition is caused by mutations in the MTRNR1 gene that encodes the mitochondrial 12S ribosomal RNA and causes late-onset sensorineural hearing loss. However, hearing loss in individuals carrying MTRNR1 mutations may be precipitated suddenly by treatment with **aminoglycoside antibiotics** because of the increased sensitivity the mutation confers to the **ototoxic** effects of these drugs.

DEVELOPMENT OF MIDDLE EAR

As covered in Chapter 17, the first pharyngeal pouch elongates to form the **tubotympanic recess**, which subsequently differentiates to form most of the expanded **tympanic cavity** of the middle ear and all of the slender **auditory (Eustachian) tube**, which connects the tympanic cavity to the pharynx. Cartilaginous precursors of the three **auditory ossicles** condense in the mesenchyme near the tympanic cavity (see Fig. 18-3). The **malleus** and **incus** arise from the first pharyngeal arch, whereas the **stapes** arises from the second pharyngeal arch. The developing ossicles remain embedded in the mesenchyme adjacent to the tympanic cavity until the eighth month of gestation. During the ninth month of development, the mesenchyme surrounding the auditory ossicles is removed, and the tympanic cavity expands to enclose them (see Fig. 18-3E). Transient endodermal mesenteries suspend the ossicles in the cavity until their definitive supporting ligaments develop.

Two muscles are associated with the ossicles—the **tensor tympani** and the **stapedius**—both of which form in the ninth week from first- and second-pharyngeal arch mesoderm, respectively. Reflecting their developmental origin, the tensor tympani muscle is innervated by the **trigeminal nerve** (cranial nerve V), whereas the **stapedius** muscle is innervated by the **facial nerve** (cranial nerve VII).

Meanwhile, the pharyngeal membrane separating the tympanic cavity from the external auditory meatus (derived from the first pharyngeal cleft) develops into the **tympanic membrane** or **eardrum** (see Fig. 18-3E). The tympanic membrane is composed of an outer lining of ectoderm, an inner lining of endoderm, and an intervening layer called the **fibrous stratum**. The intervening layer is derived from infiltrating **neural crest cells**.

During the ninth month, the suspended auditory ossicles assume their functional relationships with each other and with associated structures of the external, middle, and inner ears. The ventral end of the malleus becomes attached to the eardrum, and the foot plate of the stapes becomes attached to the **oval window**, a small fenestra in the bony labyrinth (see Figs. 18-3E, 18-9). Sonic vibrations are transmitted from the eardrum to the oval window by the articulated chain of ossicles, and from the oval window to the cochlea by the fluid filling the perilymphatic space. The cochlea transduces these vibrations into neural impulses. The ossicles are not totally free to vibrate/move in response to sound until two months after birth.

During the ninth month, the tympanic cavity expands into the mastoid part of the temporal bone to form the **mastoid antrum**. The **mastoid air cells** in the mastoid portion of the temporal bone do not form until about two years of age, when the action of the sternocleidomastoid muscle on the mastoid part of the temporal bone induces the mastoid process to form.

DEVELOPMENT OF EXTERNAL EAR

The external ear consists of the funnel-shaped **external auditory meatus** and the **auricle (pinna)**. The precursor of the external auditory meatus develops by an invagination of the first pharyngeal cleft during the sixth week and requires the formation of the tympanic ring. The ectodermal lining of the deep portion of this tube later proliferates, producing a solid core of tissue called the **meatal plug**, which completely fills the medial end of the external auditory meatus by week twenty-six (see Fig. 18-3C, D). Canalization of this plug begins almost immediately and produces the medial two thirds of the definitive meatus (see Fig. 18-3E). The external ear is separated from the middle ear by the **tympanic membrane** (see above section on development of the middle ear). The definitive tympanic membrane is formed during recanalization of the external auditory meatus.

The auricle develops from six **auricular hillocks** that arise during the fifth week on the first and second pharyngeal arches (Fig. 18-14). From ventral to dorsal, the hillocks on the first pharyngeal arch are called the **tragus**, **helix**, and **cymba concha** (or one to three, respectively), and the hillocks on the second arch are called the **antitragus**, **antihelix**, and **concha** (or four to six, respectively). These names indicate which hillocks eventually form each part of the pinna. During the seventh week, the auricular hillocks begin to enlarge, differentiate, and fuse to produce the definitive form of the auricle. As the face develops, the auricle is gradually translocated from its original location low on the side of the neck to a more lateral and cranial site (covered in Chapter 17).

In the Clinic

CONDUCTIVE HEARING LOSS

As mentioned earlier in the chapter, hearing loss may be sensorineural or conductive. **Conductive hearing loss** is caused by structural abnormalities of the middle or external ear that impede conduction of sound to the inner ear. Besides having a potential impact on hearing, malformations of the external and middle ear have important clinical implications. These defects are common as a whole and may have a significant cosmetic impact on patients. In addition, they may be indicative of a more widespread syndrome.

MALFORMATIONS OF EXTERNAL AND MIDDLE EAR

Defects of the external ear (i.e., the **pinna** or **auricle**) result from abnormal growth and morphogenesis of one or more of the auricular hillocks derived from the first and second pharyngeal arches. Suppressed growth of all hillocks results in **microtia** (small auricle; Fig. 18-15A, B) or **anotia** (absence of the auricle; Fig. 18-15C). Overgrowth of the hillocks results in **macrotia** (large auricle). Accessory hillocks may also form, producing ectopic **preauricular tags**, which may or may not be accompanied by **preauricular pits** (Fig. 18-15D). Defects of the external auditory meatus include **atresia** and **stenosis**.

Significant malformations of the external ear should raise suspicions about potential abnormalities elsewhere in the body. From 20% to 40% of children with microtia/anotia will have additional defects that could suggest a syndrome. For example, microtia occurs in several single-gene disorders, including **branchio-oto-renal** (BOR; Fig. 18-15E; also covered in Chapter 15), **CHARGE** (also covered in Chapters 4 and 12), and **Treacher Collins syndromes** (also covered in Chapter 17), as well as in **trisomy 21** (also covered in Chapters 1, 5, 9, 12,

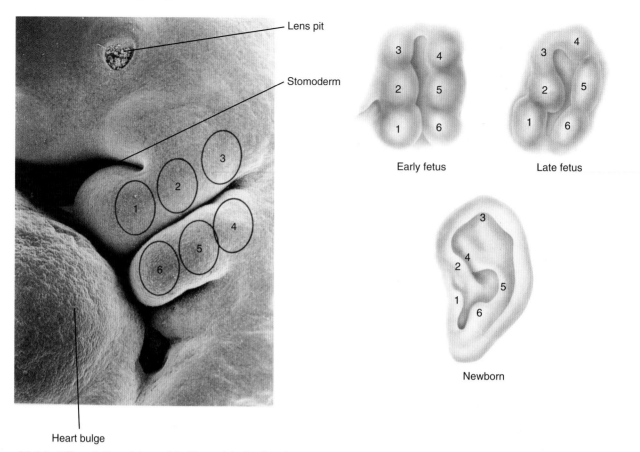

Figure 18-14. Differentiation of the auricle. The auricle develops from six auricular hillocks, which arise on the apposed surfaces of the first and second pharyngeal arches.

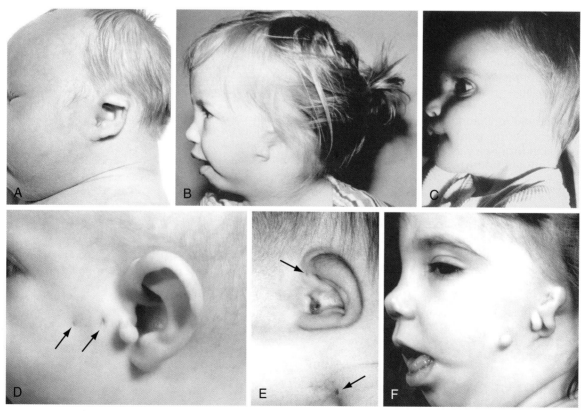

Figure 18-15. Anomalies of the external ear. *A, B,* Microtia, mild and moderately severe, respectively. *C,* Anotia. *D,* Preauricular pits (arrows) and tag. *E,* External ear of a boy with BOR syndrome. The upper arrow indicates a preauricular pit and the lower arrow indicates a cervical fistula. *F,* Girl with hemifacial microsomia showing preauricular tags.

and 17) and **18** (also covered in Chapters 8 and 9). Microtia can occur following prenatal exposure to **alcohol** or **isotretinoin**. Microtia and preauricular tags (and, more rarely, pits) occur in **oculoauriculovertebral spectrum** (**OAVS**) (Fig. 18-15F; also covered in Chapter 17). Macrotia can occur in **Fragile X syndrome**, the most common cause of mental retardation in males. This syndrome is caused by trinucleotide repeat expansions in the FMR1 (FRAGILE X MENTAL RETARDATION 1) gene. Atresia or stenosis of the external auditory meatus can suggest deletion of the long arm of chromosome 18.

Defects of the middle ear result from abnormal formation or ossification of the middle ear ossicles, malleus, incus, and stapes, derived from neural crest cells populating the first and second pharyngeal arches. Suppressed growth of these neural crest cells results in **ossicle hypoplasia** or **aplasia** and **fixation**. These defects occur in association with skeletal dysplasias, such as **achondroplasia** (FGFR3 mutation; covered in Chapters 5 and 8) and **osteogenesis imperfecta** (multiple COLLAGEN mutations), or in various syndromes, such as **BOR, Treacher Collins**, and **OAVS** (see Fig. 18-15).

Embryology in Practice

HOT OFF THE PRESS

A few years has passed since a boy was born without a right ear, actually, with grade 3 microtia; he has a shallow pillar of skin-covered cartilage and no external auditory canal on the right side. His parents meet with several plastic surgeons to review the timing and process of surgical reconstruction.

They are presented with multiple options that differ slightly in the timing and number of surgeries. The typical multistage surgical approach involves removing a significant amount of cartilage from the rib cage, shaping it, and implanting it along with skin grafts to create an ear. Usually the process begins around six years of age, when the chest circumference is large enough to allow removal of sufficient cartilage. Alternative techniques use artificial scaffolds that do not grow with the child.

The couple views with apprehension photos of other patients' ears as they went through the process and, later, discuss their concerns about the chest wall surgery and overall outcomes. While weighing the pros and cons of these several

traditional surgical approaches, the couple is struck by reports of a new technology, still in development, that could dramatically facilitate their son's surgical repair and potentially improve the long-term outcome.

The couple sees a story online describing how scientists have succeeded in creating a realistic human ear using 3D printing with biological materials. Combined with cultured cells from the recipient that grow and replace the scaffold, this technique could obviate the need for cartilage harvesting, resulting in a more natural appearing, better functioning ear.

Some degree of microtia occurs in up to 1 in 250 children. It more commonly affects the right ear and is more frequent in males. The defect can be isolated or part of a broader condition, such as oculoauriculovertebral spectrum (OAVS), and it can be genetic or may result from external conditions such as maternal diabetes.

With estimates for human trials using this new technique to start within the next three to five years, the couple adopted a "wait-and-see" stance on decisions about the type and timing of surgical reconstruction.

SUGGESTED READINGS

Chapman SC. 2011. Can you hear me now? Understanding vertebrate middle ear development. Front Biosci 16:1675–1692.

Driver EC, Kelley MW. 2009. Specification of cell fate in the mammalian cochlea. Birth Defects Res C Embryo Today 87:212–221.

Dror AA, Avraham KB. 2010. Hearing impairment: a panoply of genes and functions. Neuron 68:293–308.

Groves AK, Fekete DM. 2012. Shaping sound in space: the regulation of inner ear patterning. Development 139:245–257.

Kelly MC, Chen P. 2009. Development of form and function in the mammalian cochlea. Curr Opin Neurobiol 19:395–401.

Ladher RK, O'Neill P, Begbie J. 2010. From shared lineage to distinct functions: the development of the inner ear and epibranchial placodes. Development 137:1777–1785.

Ogino H, Ochi H, Reza HM, Yasuda K. 2012. Transcription factors involved in lens development from the preplacodal ectoderm. Dev Biol 363:333–347.

Okano T, Kelley MW. 2012. Stem cell therapy for the inner ear: recent advances and future directions. Trends Amplif 16:4–18.

Schwander M, Kachar B, Muller U. 2010. Review series: the cell biology of hearing. J Cell Biol 190:9–20.

Chapter 19
Development of the Eyes

SUMMARY

The eyes first appear early in the fourth week in the form of a pair of lateral grooves, the **optic sulci**, which evaginate from the forebrain neural groove to form the **optic vesicles**. As soon as the distal tip of the optic vesicle reaches the surface ectoderm, it invaginates, transforming the optic vesicle into a goblet-shaped **optic cup** that is attached to the forebrain by a narrower, hollow **optic stalk**. The adjacent surface ectoderm simultaneously thickens to form a **lens placode**, which invaginates and pinches off to become a hollow **lens vesicle**. Posterior cells of the lens vesicle form long, slender, anteroposteriorly oriented **primary lens fibers**. Anterior cells develop into a simple epithelium covering the face of the lens and give rise to the **secondary lens fibers**, which make up most of the mature lens.

The inner wall of the optic cup gives rise to the **neural retina**, whereas the outer wall gives rise to the thin, melanin-containing **pigmented epithelium**. Differentiation of the neural retina takes place between the sixth week and the eighth month. Six types of neuronal cells and one glial (Müller) cell are produced in the neural retina, which is proliferative, forming three layers in the mature retina: the **ganglion cell layer**; an **inner nuclear layer** containing the amacrine, horizontal, Müller, and bipolar cells; and an **outer nuclear layer** containing the rods and cone photoreceptors. Axons from the neural retina grow through the optic stalk to the brain, converting the optic stalk into the **optic nerve**.

Blood is supplied to the developing lens and retina by a terminal branch of the ophthalmic artery, the **hyaloid artery**, which enters the optic vesicle via a groove called the **optic fissure**. The portion of the artery that traverses the vitreous body to reach the lens degenerates during fetal life as the lens matures; the remainder of the artery becomes the **central artery of the retina**.

As the optic vesicle forms, it is enveloped by a sheath of mesenchyme that is derived from neural crest cells and head mesoderm. This sheath differentiates to form the two coverings of the optic cup: the thin inner vascular **choroid** and the fibrous outer **sclera**. The mesenchyme overlying the developing lens splits into two layers to enclose a new space called the **anterior chamber**. The inner wall of the anterior chamber, overlying the lens, is called the **pupillary membrane**, which is a transient vascular structure. Deep layers of this wall undergo vacuolization to create a new space, the **posterior chamber**, between the lens and the thin remaining pupillary membrane. Early in fetal life, the pupillary membrane breaks down completely to form the **pupil**. The rim of the optic cup differentiates to form the **iris** and **ciliary body**. Mesoderm adjacent to the optic cup differentiates in the fifth and sixth weeks to form the **extrinsic ocular muscles**. The connective tissue components of the extrinsic ocular muscles are derived from neural crest cells. The eyelids arise as folds of surface ectoderm and are fused from the eighth week to about the fifth month.

Clinical Taster

A boy born with bilateral **anophthalmia** (missing eyes) is seen at ten months of age by an endocrinologist. He was referred by his regular doctor because of underdevelopment of his penis (micropenis), undescended testicles (cryptorchidism), and poor linear growth. Although his weight had tracked along the fiftieth percentile, his height had lagged from the fiftieth percentile in the past to the tenth percentile now. These findings and the association of anophthalmia with pituitary abnormalities prompted the referral. A family history questionnaire does not uncover any relatives with birth defects, and both parents are in good health.

Although the boy had brain imaging in the newborn period that demonstrated a normal pituitary gland, testing reveals deficiency of several pituitary hormones (**hypopituitarism**). Hypogonadotropic hypogonadism due to reduced release of LH and FSH explains the small genitalia, and his parents are informed that testosterone replacement treatment will be required at the age of twelve to initiate puberty. His short stature is explained by reduced release of growth hormone, which can be managed in the future with growth hormone replacement. The rest of the endocrine workup is normal, but the family is warned that other hormone deficiencies can develop and regular follow-up visits with an endocrinologist are planned.

The family then asks a question that they have asked other doctors, but they have not yet received a conclusive answer, "Will this happen again in our next pregnancy?" To help the family define its recurrence risk and to address the need for other clinical evaluations, genetic testing is discussed.

The clinical picture supports screening of the SOX2 gene, a high mobility group (HMG) box transcription factor (SRY-related) important for development of the hypothalamo-pituitary axis, as well as the eye. Human SOX2 mutations are associated with bilateral anophthalmia or severe microphthalmia in association with pituitary endocrine deficits. Additional variable abnormalities include developmental delay, learning difficulties, esophageal atresia, sensorineural hearing loss, and genital abnormalities.

This patient is found to have a de novo SOX2 nonsense mutation that is predicted to result in a truncated protein with an incomplete transactivation domain and impaired transactivator activity. De novo SOX2 mutations are the most commonly identified cause of syndromic bilateral anophthalmia/microphthalmia and have low risk of recurrence in future pregnancies.

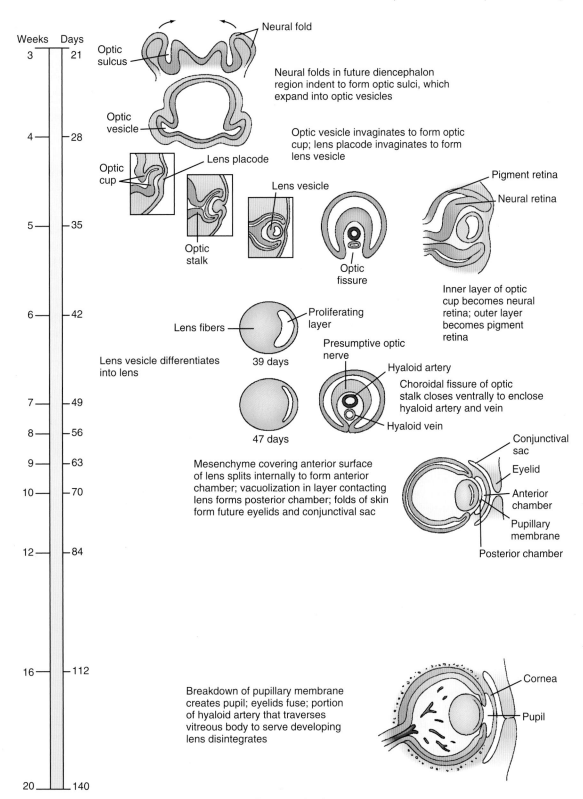

Time line. Eye development.

Weeks	Days
3	21
4	28
5	35
6	42
7	49
8	56
9	63
10	70
12	84
16	112
20	140

Neural fold

Optic sulcus

Neural folds in future diencephalon region indent to form optic sulci, which expand into optic vesicles

Optic vesicle

Optic vesicle invaginates to form optic cup; lens placode invaginates to form lens vesicle

Optic cup

Lens placode

Lens vesicle

Pigment retina

Neural retina

Optic stalk

Optic fissure

Inner layer of optic cup becomes neural retina; outer layer becomes pigment retina

Lens fibers

Proliferating layer

Lens vesicle differentiates into lens

39 days

Presumptive optic nerve

Hyaloid artery

Choroidal fissure of optic stalk closes ventrally to enclose hyaloid artery and vein

Hyaloid vein

47 days

Mesenchyme covering anterior surface of lens splits internally to form anterior chamber; vacuolization in layer contacting lens forms posterior chamber; folds of skin form future eyelids and conjunctival sac

Conjunctival sac

Eyelid

Anterior chamber

Pupillary membrane

Posterior chamber

Breakdown of pupillary membrane creates pupil; eyelids fuse; portion of hyaloid artery that traverses vitreous body to serve developing lens disintegrates

Cornea

Pupil

EYE ORIGINATES FROM SEVERAL EMBRYONIC TISSUES LAYERS

 Animation 19-1: Development of the Eyes.
Animations are available online at StudentConsult.

The eye develops from several embryonic tissue layers. The ectoderm gives rise to the lens and part of the cornea.

The neuroectoderm forms the pigmented epithelium and the neural retina, the non-neural ciliary body, and iris structures, including the smooth muscles. Neural crest cells contribute to the stroma of the cornea, the ciliary muscles, and the vascular choroid layer together with the fibrous sclera. The mesoderm contributes to the cornea and forms the angioblasts of the choroid layer.

DEVELOPMENT OF OPTIC CUP AND LENS

The first morphologic evidence of the eye is the formation of the **optic sulcus** in the future diencephalic region of the prosencephalic neural groove (forebrain) at twenty-two days (Fig. 19-1*A, B*). By the time that the cranial neuropore closes on day twenty-four, the **optic stalk** is evident (Fig. 19-1*C-E*), and the optic primordia have developed into lateral evaginations of the neural tube called **optic vesicles** (Fig. 19-1*D, E*). The walls of the optic vesicles are continuous with the neuroepithelium of the future brain, and the cavity or **ventricle** within the optic vesicle is continuous with the neural canal. As the optic vesicle forms, it becomes surrounded by a layer of mesenchyme derived from neural crest cells and head mesoderm. Fate mapping studies in birds and mice have revealed that this mesenchyme gives rise to many ocular tissues, such as the sclera, ocular muscles, connective tissue, and cartilage, together with vascular endothelial cells. The extraocular mesenchyme begins to form on day twenty-two and completely envelops the optic vesicle by day twenty-six. By day twenty-four, the distal part of the optic vesicle contacts the overlying surface ectoderm. At about this time, the optic cup becomes patterned along its planar axes (see below and the "In the Research Lab" of Chapter 9 entitled "Positional Information Patterns Neural Plate and Neural Tube").

On about day twenty-eight, the distal end of the optic vesicle invaginates, converting the optic vesicle into a goblet-shaped **optic cup** (Fig. 19-1*F-I*). Simultaneously, the ventral part of the optic stalk invaginates, and the dorsal optic cup folds around the invagination to form the **optic (choroidal) fissure**. Blood vessels later enter the optic cup through the optic fissure (Fig. 19-2), following which the two lips of the fissure fuse together (see Fig. 19-2*C*). Upon closing of the fissure, the primitive ciliary epithelium secretes aqueous fluid, establishing intraocular pressure.

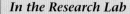

In the Research Lab

FORMATION OF EYE FIELD

Eye development starts with the formation of a single eye field in the cranial neural plate (i.e., the presumptive forebrain during gastrulation and neurulation). The transcription factor Otx2 is necessary for forebrain development. At the neural plate stage, the morphogen sonic hedgehog (Shh) is secreted by the underlying prechordal plate and is essential for separating the initially single eye field into two individual **optic primordia**; failure of Shh signaling results in the persistence of a single eye field and the formation of both **holoprosencephaly** (covered in Chapter 17 in the "In the Clinic" entitled "Holoprosencephaly") and **cyclopia** (single, midline eye). Furthermore, several transcription factors, which regulate normal eye development, are specifically expressed in the eye field and are necessary for eye field specification. Eye field transcription factors include Tbx3, Pax6, Six3, Six6 (also known as Optx2), Rx/Rax, and Lhx2. Their loss results in failure of eye development. For example, the homeobox gene Rx/Rax is expressed in the eye field in both mice and humans. When deleted in mice, it leads to arrest of eye development at the neural plate stage. This results in **anophthalmia** (absence of the eye) or **microphthalmia** (small eye). Moreover, ectopic expression of individual eye field transcription factors such as

Pax6, Six3, or Six6, which are expressed in the developing eyes of model organisms as diverse as Drosophila and mouse, results in the formation of ectopic eyes. These and other findings support the idea that progressive patterning of the neural plate, and subsequently of the eye field, is regulated by a feedback network of eye field transcription factors.

As soon as the optic vesicle contacts the surface ectoderm, the ectoderm apposed to it thickens to form a **lens placode** (Fig. 19-3*C*). Shortly thereafter, the lens placode invaginates to form a **lens pit** (Fig. 19-3*A, B, E*). By day thirty-three, the placode separates from the surface ectoderm, becoming a hollow **lens vesicle** surrounded by a basal lamina (lens capsule). Mesodermally derived mesenchymal cells migrate into the **lentiretinal space** between the lens vesicle and the inner wall of the expanding optic cup and secrete a gelatinous matrix called the **primary vitreous body** (Fig. 19-3*E, F*). Beginning on day thirty-three, the cells of the posterior (deep) wall of the lens vesicle differentiate to form long, anteroposteriorly oriented **primary lens fibers** that express crystallins (α, β, and γ) necessary for the transparency of the lens (Fig. 19-4). Elongation of these cells transforms the lens vesicle into a rounded **lens body**, obliterating the cavity of the lens vesicle by the seventh week. Anterior lens epithelial cells closest to the cornea remain proliferative throughout life. They migrate peripherally to the lens equator, giving rise to future secondary fetal and adult cortical lens fibers (lens bow). Secondary lens fibers start to be formed by the third month.

In the Research Lab

FORMATION AND MORPHOGENESIS OF LENS

Following lens induction (see the "In the Research Lab" of Chapter 18 entitled "Development of Placodes"), the optic cup influences growth, differentiation, and maintenance of the developing lens. If the portion of the optic cup in contact with the ectoderm is removed, the lens eventually degenerates. Studies using null mutations in mice have demonstrated that several genes are required for induction and maintenance of the lens placode, including Pax6, Bmp4, and Bmp7. Using conditional mutagenesis, Pax6 has been specifically knocked out in the lens ectoderm, resulting in absence of all lens structures and failure of the optic vesicle to invaginate properly. The latter result shows that signals from the lens are required for appropriate morphogenesis of the optic vesicle. This has also been demonstrated by experiments in which the lens ectoderm has been removed.

Several different growth factor families and transcription factors regulate differentiation of lens fibers. These include, respectively, Fgfs, Tgfβs, and Wnts, and Maf and Prox-1. For example, once the lens vesicle has formed, Fgf in the aqueous humor (produced by the retina) induces cells in the posterior region of the lens to differentiate. Lower levels of Fgf signaling from the vitreous humor, and notch signaling, maintain proliferation in the anterior lens epithelium. The homeobox gene FoxE3 also maintains proliferation, whereas Prox1, which is expressed at the equatorial zone of the lens, induces cell-cycle exit by switching on expression of the cell cycle inhibitors $p27^{kip1}$ and $p57^{kip2}$ and the crystallin genes.

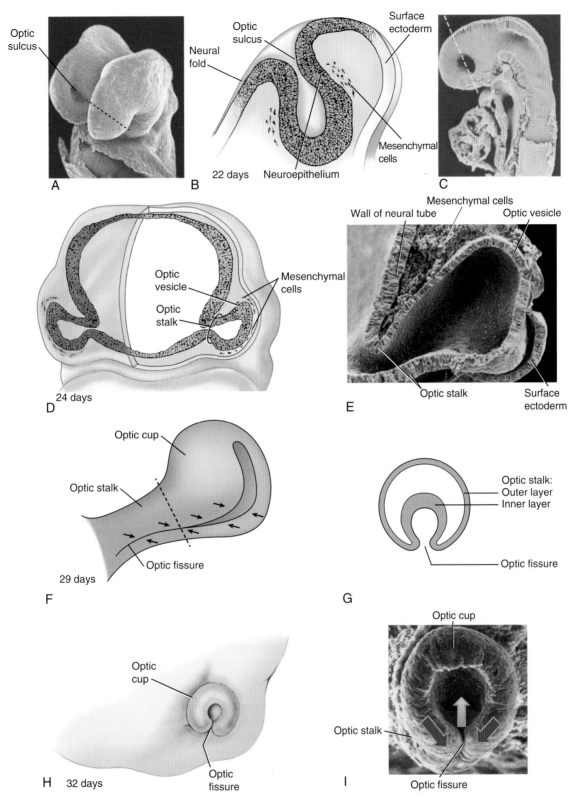

Figure 19-1. Formation of the optic sulcus, vesicle, and cup. *A, B,* Formation of the optic sulcus in the forming forebrain during neurulation. The dashed line in *A* (scanning electron micrograph of the anterior neuropore region of a mouse embryo) indicates the level of the section shown in *B. C-E,* Formation of the optic vesicles. The dashed line in *C* (scanning electron micrograph of a midsagittal section through the head of a mouse embryo after closure of the anterior neuropore) indicates the level of the section shown in *D;* the ectoderm (tan, with cut surface shown in light blue) has been removed on the right side of the drawing (left side of embryo). The scanning electron micrograph in *E* amplifies the information shown on the right side of the drawing in *D.* By day twenty-four, the optic vesicles lie adjacent to the surface ectoderm. *F, G,* Drawing of an optic cup and optic stalk with the invaginated optic fissure at 29 days and a section through the optic stalk (at the level indicated by the dashed line in *F*). Arrows indicate sites of fusion. *H, I,* End-on view of the optic cup during the fifth week in a drawing and in a scanning electron micrograph (the surface ectoderm and associated head mesenchyme have been removed in preparation of the micrograph). Arrows (*F, I*) indicate directions of movement.

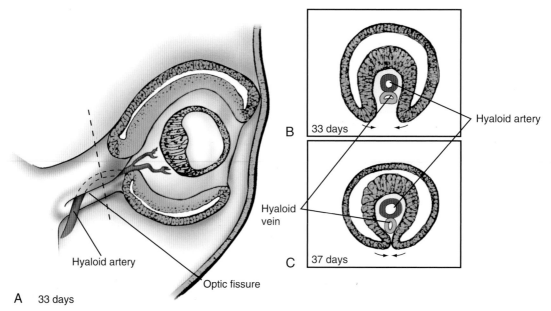

Figure 19-2. Vascularization of the lens and retina. *A,* As the lens vesicle detaches from the surface ectoderm, it becomes vascularized by the hyaloid vessels, which gain access to the lens through the optic fissure. *B, C,* During the seventh week, the edges of the optic fissure fuse together, enclosing the hyaloid artery and vein in the hyaloid canal. When the lens matures, the vessels serving it degenerate, and the hyaloid artery and vein become the central artery and vein of the retina (see Figure 19-7*D*). The dashed line in *A* indicates the level of the sections shown in *B* and *C.*

The non-canonical Wnt PCP pathway is necessary for fiber elongation (similar to the role of PCP signaling during elongation of muscle fibers in the myotome; see Chapter 8 for further coverage). Malformations of the anterior segment of the eye can include failure of the lens to undergo separation from the surface ectoderm, resulting in a persistent lens stalk and leading to an arrest of lens development (**aphakia**). Several genes regulating lens vesicle separation have been identified in mouse (e.g., FoxE3, Pitx3, Ap-2α). Lens defects are also associated with corneal and iris abnormalities, showing that signals from the lens are important for initiating differentiation of overlying ectoderm and mesenchyme. For example, Tgfβ signaling from the lens induces expression of Pitx2 and Foxc1 in the anterior mesenchyme, which is necessary for differentiation of the corneal epithelium and cornea. Conversely, corneal abnormalities can lead to secondary lens defects.

DEVELOPMENT OF NEURAL RETINA AND PIGMENTED EPITHELIUM

The two walls of the optic cup give rise to the two layers of the retina: the thick pseudostratified inner wall of the cup develops into the **neural retina**, which contains the light-receptive **rods** and **cones** plus associated neural processes, and the thin outer wall of the cup becomes the cuboidal melanin-containing **pigmented epithelium** (Fig. 19-5; see also Fig. 19-3*F*). These two walls are initially separated by a narrow **intraretinal space**. The intraretinal space between the neural retina and pigmented epithelium disappears by the seventh week. However, the two layers of the retina never fuse firmly, and various types of trauma—even a simple blow to the head—can cause **retinal detachment** (i.e., mechanical separation of these two layers).

Melanin first appears in the cells of the developing pigmented epithelium on day thirty-three. Soon afterward, the basal lamina of the pigmented epithelium, **Bruch's membrane**, develops. Differentiation of the neural retina begins at the end of the sixth week, as the layer of retinal progenitor cells adjacent to the intraretinal space (which is homologous to the proliferative neuroepithelium lining the neural tube; covered in Chapters 4 and 9) begins to produce waves of cells that migrate inward toward the vitreous body. By the sixth week, two cellular embryonic retinal layers are present: an **outer neuroblastic layer** and an **inner neuroblastic layer**. By the ninth week, two additional membranes develop to cover the two surfaces of the neural retina. An **external limiting membrane** is interposed between the pigmented epithelium and the proliferative zone of the neural retina, and the inner surface of the retina is sealed off by an **internal limiting membrane** (Fig. 19-5*B, C*).

The definitive cell layers of the mature neural retina arise from multipotent precursors that can give rise to all cell types within the pseudostratified neuroblastic layers (see Fig. 19-5*B*). The progenitors divide at the apical side of the neuroepithelium, and the differentiated cells then move into the appropriate layers. Six major cell classes of neurons and one glial cell type are produced in an evolutionary conserved order: **ganglion cells**, **cone photoreceptors**, and **horizontal cells** are born early; **amacrine cells** and **rod photoreceptors** are born next; and **bipolar cells** and **Müller glia** are born last. The axons of the ganglion cells form the definitive **fiber layer** that lines the inner surface of the retina and courses to the developing optic nerve (see Fig. 19-5*B, C*). By the sixteenth week, the developing neuropil (i.e., the network of neuronal processes within the wall of the neural retina) becomes organized into inner and outer plexiform layers between the nuclear layers (see Fig. 19-5*C*).

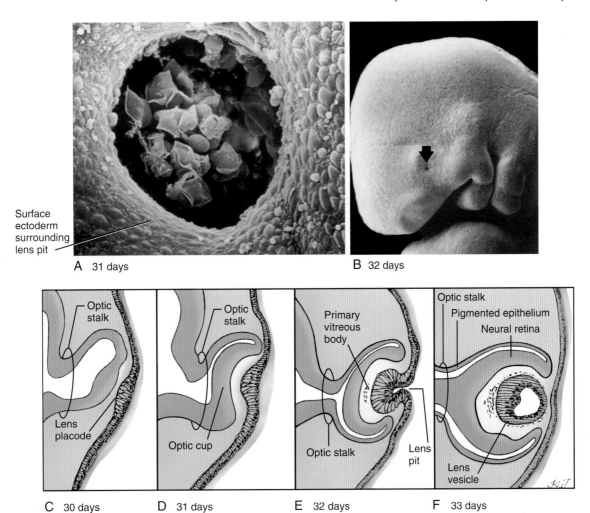

Surface
ectoderm
surrounding
lens pit

A 31 days

B 32 days

C 30 days   D 31 days   E 32 days   F 33 days

Figure 19-3. Formation of the lens placode and lens vesicle. Contact with the optic cup is necessary for maintenance and development of the lens placode, although other influences are more important in its induction. *A-F,* During the fifth week, the lens placode begins to invaginate to form the lens pit (arrow in *B;* both A and B show scanning electron micrographs). The invaginating lens placode eventually pinches off of the surface ectoderm to form a lens vesicle enclosed in the optic cup (*E, F*).

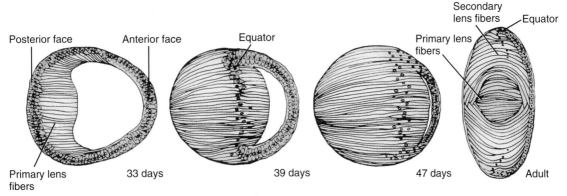

Figure 19-4. Differentiation of the lens. The lens develops rapidly in the fifth to seventh weeks as the cells of its posterior wall elongate and differentiate to form the primary lens fibers. Secondary lens fibers begin to form in the third month.

All cell layers of the definitive retina are apparent by the eighth month.

Cellular differentiation progresses in a wave from the central to peripheral retina. Macular differentiation occurs around the sixth month, when cone precursor cells and multiple rows of ganglion cells accumulate in the central macular area. At seven months, the central macular depression or **primitive fovea** forms. By several months postpartum, the **fovea centralis**, the region of the eye with the highest visual acuity, contains only a dense population of cone photoreceptors. This region is also avascular, reducing light scattering within the eye.

There are two types of photoreceptors: rods and cones. Rods are required for vision in low light; cones

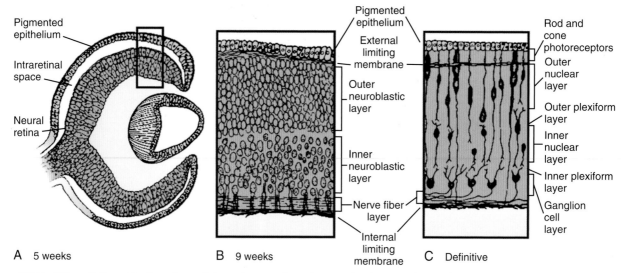

Figure 19-5. Differentiation of the inner layer of the optic cup to form the neural retina. *A*, At five weeks, the neural retina consists of a thickened pseudostratified columnar epithelium similar to that of the wall of the neural tube. *B*, By nine weeks, the neural retina is subdividing into outer and inner neuroblastic layers, a nerve fiber layer, and external and internal limiting membranes. *C*, Definitive layers of the neural retina develop during late fetal life.

function in daylight and are necessary for color vision. There are three types of cones; each expresses distinct pigments and responds to one of the three different color wavelengths. S-cones respond to short wavelengths (blue light), M-cones respond to medium wavelengths (green), and L-cones respond to longer wavelengths (red). **Color blindness** is due to the absence of one or more types of cones. **Protanopes** lack L-cones, **deuteranopes** lack M-cones, and **tritanopes** lack S-cones. The genes OPN1LW and OPN1MW encode photopigments. Color blindness occurs frequently in males (>2%), as these genes are located on the X chromosome. Achromatopsia (rod monochromatism, resulting in total color blindness) can be caused by mutations in CNGA3, CNGB3, and GNAT2.

In the Research Lab

PATTERNING OF EYE

As the optic cup forms, it becomes specified as the pigmented epithelium, neural retina, and optic stalk (Fig. 19-6; see Fig. 19-3F). These distinct regions are characterized by differential expression of transcription factors necessary for their specification (see Fig. 19-6). The neural retina expresses Vsx2 (previously called Chx10), Pax6, Six6, and Rax; the pigmented epithelium expresses Mitf and Otx2; and the optic stalk expresses Pax2 (Fig. 19-6C). Initially, all optic cup cells are equally competent to form the different regions of the eye; subsequent differentiation is induced by surrounding tissues (see Fig. 19-6C). Signaling from the surface ectoderm, possibly mediated by Fgfs, specifies the neural retina (e.g., induces Vsx2 expression), whereas signaling from the extraocular mesenchyme, such as the Tgfβ family member activin A, specifies the pigmented epithelium (i.e., induces Mitf expression). Shh signaling from the midline tissues specifies the optic stalk (i.e., induces Pax2 expression). In the absence of these signals, the eye will not differentiate appropriately. For example, if the ectoderm (the source of Fgfs)

is removed, the neural retina develops as pigmented epithelium. The posterior boundary between the optic stalk and neural retina is maintained by antagonistic interactions between Pax2 and Pax6, which repress the expression of each other. Likewise, the boundary between the neural retina and pigmented epithelium is maintained by antagonistic interactions between the Vsx2 and Mitf transcription factors. The neural retina is also patterned along the dorsoventral and nasotemporal axes, and this patterning guides appropriate axonal migration (see Chapter 9). As in the case of the neural tube (see Chapter 4 for further coverage), Shh and Bmps are two of the signals that specify the ventral axis and the dorsal axis, respectively.

DIFFERENTIATION OF PIGMENTED EPITHELIUM

The transcription factors Mitf and Otx2 are required for specification of pigmented epithelium in the optic cup. Both genes have been shown to activate melanogenic genes such as Trp1 and tyrosinase. Mitf is expressed specifically in the pigmented epithelium (see Fig. 19-6A). In Mitf and Otx1/2 mouse mutants, the pigmented epithelium is respecified to form an ectopic neural retina. Signals from the RPE are necessary for growth of the eye, differentiation of photoreceptors, and lamination of the retina. Therefore, loss of the RPE also results in microphthalmia.

REGULATION OF PROLIFERATION AND DIFFERENTIATION OF RETINAL PROGENITOR CELLS

Several signals that regulate proliferation of retinal progenitor cells have been identified. For example, the homeobox transcription factor Vsx2 is specifically expressed in the neural retina (see Fig.19-6B) and is required for retinal proliferation. This effect is mediated by regulators of the cell cycle (cyclin D1, p27). Other factors controlling proliferation are notch-delta signaling, Fgf, Igf, Wnt2b, Hes1, Hdac (histone deacetylase), Rax, and sonic hedgehog.

Lineage studies have shown that neural retinal cells are multipotent and in some instances can give rise to all cell types. However, at any one time, the competence of the progenitors is generally restricted to a few cell types. For example, early progenitors predominantly produce ganglion cells, whereas "older" progenitors mainly generate rod photoreceptors. This restricted

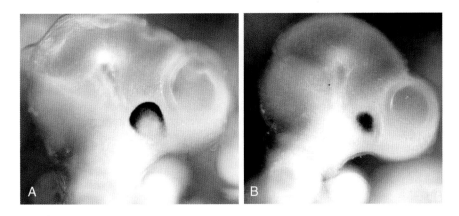

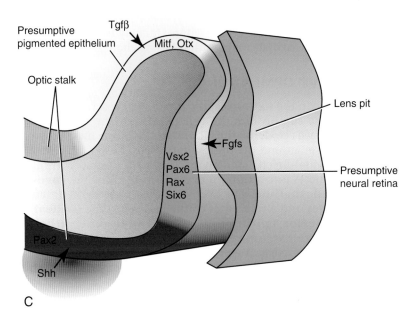

Figure 19-6. Gene expression in the mouse optic cup. *A*, The bHLH transcription factor Mitf is expressed in the pigmented epithelium. *B*, The homeobox transcription factor Vsx2 is expressed in the neural retina. *C*, Expression of transcription factors in different regions of the optic cup and stalk is regulated by growth factor signaling (arrows) from adjacent tissues.

competence is not determined by environmental signals and reflects an intrinsic behavior of the neural progenitors. If "older" progenitors are placed in a "younger" environment, they differentiate according to their original fate.

Differentiation starts centrally in the fovea and is induced by Fgf signals from the optic stalk. Subsequently, a wave of Fgf expression induces differentiation in the periphery. The balance of proliferation versus neuronal differentiation is controlled by various basic helix-loop-helix (bHLH) transcription factors. Hes1 and 5, components of the notch signaling pathway, function to maintain proliferation. Therefore, the activity of notch signaling favors production of the non-neuronal Müller glia cells (normally the last to be born). Hes1 expression is induced by Shh signaling. In contrast, other bHLH factors, such as Mash1, Ngn2, and Math5, are necessary for differentiation of the neuronal cell types. Math5 is required for ganglion cell development, and Mash1 together with Math3 is required for bipolar cell development. In contrast, NeuroD together with Math3 is required for formation of amacrine cells. Loss of one cell type (e.g., loss of ganglion cells in the Math5 mutant) is accompanied by an increase in another cell type (in this case, amacrine and cone cells). Differentiation is also controlled by homeobox genes. Pax6 is required for multipotency. Therefore,

in the absence of Pax6, many of the neuronal derivatives are affected, and only one cell type (amacrine cells) is generated. In contrast, the homeobox gene Vsx2 is required for bipolar cell development, whereas in Prox1 mutants, horizontal cells do not form. Although specific genes are required for the development of various neuronal subtypes, gain of function does not necessarily result in the converse effect. Furthermore, the expression of a particular gene (e.g., Math5) does not necessarily commit the progenitor to a particular cell lineage (e.g., in this case, ganglion cells). It is possible that the combination of homeobox gene and bHLH gene expression determines the progenitor fate.

Following differentiation, autoregulatory mechanisms control the number of each neuronal cell type. If amacrine cells are ablated in frogs or goldfish, they are replaced with new amacrine cells from retinal progenitors. Similarly, the number of retinal ganglion cells (RGCs) seems to be regulated by this autoregulatory feedback. RGCs express Shh after they have differentiated, and loss of function of Shh increases the number of RGCs. It is thought that high levels of Shh, for example, as produced by several RGCs, will inhibit further RGC differentiation, favoring the development of other cell types. In this way, development of one cell type (an RGC in this example) will promote the differentiation of the next cell type (cone, in this example).

DEVELOPMENT OF OPTIC NERVE

The nerve fibers that emerge from the retinal ganglion cells in the sixth week travel along the inner wall of the optic stalk to reach the brain. The lumen of the stalk is gradually obliterated by growth of these fibers, and by the eighth week, the hollow optic stalk is transformed into the solid **optic nerve** (cranial nerve II). Just before the two optic nerves enter the brain, they join to form an X-shaped structure called the **optic chiasm**. Within the chiasm, about half of the fibers from each optic nerve cross over to the contralateral (opposite) side of the brain. The resulting combined bundle of ipsilateral and contralateral fibers on each side then grows back to the lateral geniculate body of the thalamus (covered in Chapter 9), where the fibers synapse, starting in the eighth week. More than one million nerve fibers grow from each retina to the brain. The mechanism of axonal pathfinding that allows each of these axons to map to the correct point in the lateral geniculate body is covered in Chapter 9. The astrocytes around the optic nerve arise from the inner layer of the optic stalk, which is of neuroectodermal origin. Oligodendrocytes enter the nerve at the chiasm from the brain. Myelinization of the optic nerve begins at the optic chiasm around seven months and continues toward the eye.

VASCULARIZATION OF OPTIC CUP AND LENS

There are two sources of vascularization to the eye: the **choroid** layer around the eye (see the next section of this chapter) and the transient **hyaloid artery**. The hyaloid artery develops from a branch of the ophthalmic artery and gains access to the lentiretinal space via the optic fissure on the ventral surface of the optic stalk. The hyaloid artery vascularizes the developing retina and initially also vascularizes the lens vesicle (see Fig. 19-2). Branches of the hyaloid artery extend over the lens and are known as the **tunica vasculosa lentis**. The lips of the optic fissure fuse by day thirty-seven, enclosing the hyaloid artery and its accompanying vein in a canal within the ventral wall of the optic stalk (see Fig. 19-2B, C). The hyaloid vasculature is maximally developed at approximately ten weeks of gestation. When the lens matures during fetal life and ceases to need a blood supply, the portion of the hyaloid artery that crosses the vitreous body degenerates and is removed by macrophages (end of fourth month; Fig. 19-7D). However, even in the adult, the course of this former artery is marked by a conduit through the vitreous body called the **hyaloid canal**. The proximal portion of the hyaloid artery becomes the **central artery of the retina**, which supplies blood to the retina. Vascularization of the retina starts as the hyaloid artery is regressing and is predominant during the final trimester. Formation of this vascular plexus begins at the optic head and extends into the periphery following the wave of neuronal differentiation.

DEVELOPMENT OF CHOROID, SCLERA, AND ANTERIOR CHAMBER

During weeks six and seven, the mesenchymal capsule that surrounds the optic cup differentiates into two layers: an inner, pigmented, vascular layer called the **choroid**, and an outer, fibrous layer called the **sclera** (Fig. 19-7A, D). The choroid layer is homologous in origin with the pia mater and arachnoid membranes investing the brain (the leptomeninges), and the sclera is homologous with the dura mater. The choroid is pigmented and develops from neural crest cell–derived mesenchyme (stromal cells, melanocytes, and pericytes) and mesoderm (endothelial cells). The primitive blood vessels/spaces give rise to the embryonic choriocapillaris (i.e., the capillaries forming the inner vascular layer of the choroid) at around two months of gestation and supply blood to the retinal epithelium and photoreceptors.

The tough sclera supports and protects the delicate inner structures of the eye. The anterior sclera begins as a condensation of mesenchymal tissue that is continuous with the cornea. By approximately twelve weeks, the mesenchymal condensation has reached the optic nerve.

DEVELOPMENT OF CORNEA

Late in the sixth week, the mesenchyme surrounding the optic cup invades the region between the lens and the surface ectoderm, thus forming a complete mesenchymal jacket around the optic cup (see Fig. 19-7A). The mesenchyme directly underlying the surface ectoderm differentiates into a thin inner epithelium called the **corneal endothelium**. The overlying surface ectoderm differentiates into a thin outer epithelium called the **corneal** or **anterior epithelium**. An **acellular postepithelial layer** or **stroma** forms between the corneal epithelium and the corneal endothelium, and by the eighth week, these layers are apparent. The stroma consists of a matrix of collagen fibers, hyaluronic acid (which binds water, causing the matrix to swell), and glycosaminoglycans. Mesenchymal cells rapidly invade the stroma and convert it to a cellular **stromal layer (substantia propria)**. Hyaluronidase removes the hyaluronic acid, reducing the matrix volume. Thyroxine (circulated from the thyroid gland) also induces dehydration of the stroma, and the transparent cornea is formed. Recent fate mapping studies have shown that both neural crest cells and head mesoderm contribute to corneal endothelial and stromal layers, together with the trabecular meshwork. Thus, the cornea has three tissue origins: mesodermal and neural crest cells form the mesothelium and the substantia propria, whereas the outer corneal epithelium is derived from the overlying surface ectoderm.

DEVELOPMENT OF PUPILLARY MEMBRANE

By the ninth week, the mesenchyme overlying the lens splits into two layers that enclose a new cavity called the **anterior chamber of the eye** (see Fig. 19-7C). The anterior (superficial) wall of this chamber is continuous with the sclera, and the posterior (deep) wall is continuous with the choroid. The thick posterior wall of the anterior chamber rests directly against the lens. The deep layers of this wall subsequently break down by a process of vacuolization to create a new space, the **posterior chamber**, between the lens and the thin remaining layer of the wall (see Fig. 19-7C). This thin remaining layer,

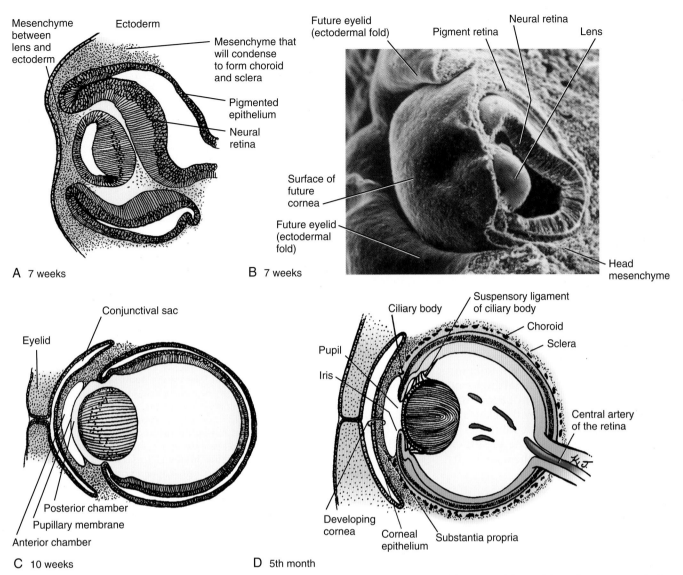

Figure 19-7. Development of the anterior and posterior chambers, eyelids, and coverings of the optic globe. *A,* Mesenchyme surrounds the developing eyeball (optic globe) between the fifth and seventh weeks to form the choroid and sclera. *B,* Scanning electron micrograph showing that at seven weeks the eyelids start to form. *C, D,* Vacuolization within the anterior mesenchyme in the seventh week forms the anterior chamber. Shortly thereafter, vacuolization in the layer of mesenchyme immediately anterior to the lens forms the posterior chamber. The pupillary membrane, which initially separates the anterior and posterior chambers, breaks down in early fetal life. Extension of the rim of the optic cup gives rise to the ciliary body and part of the iris. The upper and lower eyelids form as folds of surface ectoderm. They fuse together by the end of the eighth week and separate again between the fifth and seventh months.

called the **pupillary membrane**, regresses early in the fetal period (between the sixth and eighth months) to form the opening called the **pupil**, through which the anterior and posterior chambers communicate. On rare occasions, the pupillary membrane fails to break down completely, leaving strands that traverse the pupil. The posterior chamber eventually underlies the iris and part of the ciliary body (covered in next paragraph).

DEVELOPMENT OF IRIS AND CILIARY BODY

At the end of the third month, the anterior rim of the optic cup expands to form a thin ring that projects between the anterior and posterior chambers and overlaps the lens. This ring differentiates into the **iris** of the

eye (see Fig. 19-7*D*). The iris stroma develops from mesenchymal tissue of both neural crest cell and mesodermal origin. The posterior iris epithelium and the circumferentially arranged smooth muscle bundles of the **pupillary muscles (sphincter pupillae and dilator pupillae)** in the iris originate from the neuroepithelium of the optic cup. These muscles act as a diaphragm, controlling the diameter of the pupil and thus the amount of light that enters the eye.

Just posterior to the developing iris, the optic cup differentiates and folds to form the **ciliary body** (see Fig. 19-7*D*). The lens is suspended from the ciliary body by a radial network of elastic fibers called the **suspensory ligament** of the lens (lens zonules). Around the insertions of these fibers, the optic cup epithelia of the ciliary body proliferate to form a ring of highly vascularized, feathery elaborations that are specialized to secrete the aqueous humor of the eye. Mesenchymal cells that invade the choroid of the ciliary body differentiate to form the smooth muscle bundles of the **ciliary muscle**, which controls the shape and hence the focusing power (accommodation), of the lens. Contraction of this muscle reduces the diameter of the ciliary ring from which the lens is suspended, thus allowing the lens to relax toward its natural spherical shape and providing the greater focusing power needed for near vision.

DEVELOPMENT OF EYELIDS

By the sixth week, small folds of surface ectoderm with a mesenchymal core appear just cranial and caudal to the developing cornea (see Fig. 19-7*B*). These upper (fronto-nasal process) and lower (maxillary process) eyelid primordia rapidly grow toward each other, meeting and fusing by the eighth week. The space between the fused eyelids and the cornea is called the **conjunctival sac**. The eyelids separate again between the fifth and seventh months. The eyelid muscles (orbicularis and levator) are derived from mesoderm.

The **lacrimal glands** form from invaginations of the ectoderm at the superolateral angles of the conjunctival sacs but do not mature until about six weeks after birth. The tear fluid produced by the glands is excreted into the conjunctival sac, where it lubricates the cornea. Excess tear fluid drains through the **nasolacrimal duct** (covered in Chapter 17) into the nasal cavity.

In the Clinic

ABNORMALITIES OF EYE

Congenital eye defects can arise at any stage of eye morphogenesis and differentiation. The scope of defects depends on the timing of the embryologic insult. Eye malformations can be widespread or can affect specific regions or specific cell types. Eye defects can be isolated but are often part of other genetic syndromes. Because of the close relationship between eye and brain development, malformations of the eye often suggest the presence of underlying abnormalities of the brain.

Abnormalities occurring in the very earliest stages of eye development can disrupt formation of the optic field, as in the case of **anophthalmia**, in which the eyes are absent. Defects occurring at later stages of development can result in small eyes (**microphthalmia**) or abnormalities of various components of the eye. For example, a **coloboma** results when the optic fissure fails to fuse, leaving a gap in eye structures. A complete coloboma extends throughout the entire eye (from optic nerve to iris), whereas more localized colobomata may occur, as in coloboma of the iris (Fig. 19-8). Anophthalmia/microphthalmia can be caused by mutations in genes that act at various stages of eye development, including OTX2, BMP4, VSX2, and RAX, whereas coloboma can be caused by mutations in PAX2 (which is expressed in the optic stalk, as discussed in the preceding "In the Research Lab" entitled "Patterning of Eye"). The most common genetic cause of anophthalmia/microphthalmia is haploinsufficiency of the SOX2 transcription factor. Analysis of Sox2 mouse mutants has shown that Sox2 regulates notch expression, which is required for proliferation and differentiation of the optic cup.

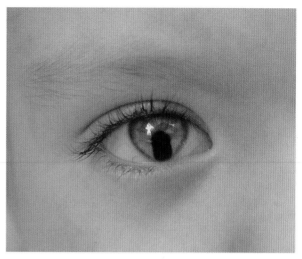

Figure 19-8. Coloboma of the iris.

Various defects of the anterior part of the eye can occur. Abnormalities of the most anterior eye structures, the eyelids and the sclera, are common. Many types of eyelid anomalies occur. Folds of skin that cover the inner corner (i.e., canthus) of the eye, **epicanthal folds**, are a characteristic feature of **Down syndrome**, but they are also normally present in many ethnic groups. The fissure that separates upper and lower eyelids (i.e., the palpebral fissure) can fail to form properly, resulting in fusion of the eyelids. In **cryptophthalmos**, fusion is complete, whereas in **blepharophimosis**, the lids are partially fused. Other anomalies of the eyelids include **ptosis** (drooping eyelids) and **epicanthus inversus** (folds curving down and laterally from the inner canthus). Tumorous growth of the sclera, called **epibulbar dermoids**, is one of the cardinal findings in **Goldenhar syndrome** (part of the **OAVS spectrum** covered earlier in the chapter and in Chapter 17). Ocular **telangiectasia** (permanent dilation of capillaries of the sclera) is seen in **ataxia-telangiectasia** (also mentioned in Chapter 9) and is associated with cerebellar degeneration (resulting in ataxia) and immunodeficiency.

Anterior segment ocular dysgenesis (ASOD) involves defects of the cornea, iris, lens, and ciliary body. It can affect vision and increase the risk of high-tension glaucoma due to alterations in Schlemm's canal and the trabeculae that drain the aqueous fluid. Specific defects include iris hypoplasia or rupture (**corectopia**), corneal opacity (**leukoma**), ectopic pupils (**polycoria**), adhesion between the lens or iris and cornea, and **sclerocornea** (peripheral scleralization of the cornea). These defects are etiologically related, being caused by an overlapping set of genes (the result, for example, of mutations in the FOXC1, FOXE3, PITX2, and PAX6 transcription factors). Mutations in PAX6 can specifically result in **aniridia** (absence of the iris, as in **WAGR association**—Wilms' tumor, aniridia, genitourinary anomalies, mental retardation), or more widespread ocular defects affecting the cornea, lens, retina, and optic nerve, reflecting its early role in specification of the eye field. Persistence of the **pupillary membrane** may occur as part of the above anomalies or may occur as an isolated defect. The presence of nodules on the iris, called **Lisch nodules**, can be a clue to the diagnosis of neurofibromatosis type 1 (covered in Chapter 10).

Congenital cataracts (lens opacities) can result from genetic or environmental factors. Genetic factors involve a large number of mutations in diverse genes ranging from structural components of the lens, such as mutations in CRYSTALLIN or gap junction proteins, to transcription factors such as MAF or HEAT SHOCK TRANSCRIPTION FACTOR 4 (HSF4). Cataracts may also develop as the result of metabolic disorders such as **galactosemia** (a defect in galactose metabolism) or from congenital infections such as **rubella**.

Strabismus, or misalignment of gaze, can be caused by abnormalities of the extraocular muscles or their innervation. **Duane anomaly** is a rare cause of strabismus characterized by abnormal abduction/adduction, narrowing of the eye fissure, and retraction of the globe with adduction; it is caused by abnormal development of the **abducens nerve** (cranial nerve VI), which innervates the **lateral rectus** eye muscle. Duane anomaly, accompanied by abnormalities of the hands and/or kidneys, is caused by mutations in the gene encoding the SAL4 transcription factor. If left untreated, strabismus can lead to **amblyopia**, permanent loss of vision resulting from changes in the visual cortex. Injury to the lateral rectus muscle and/or its innervation (the abducens nerve) sometimes results from forceps-assisted deliveries. This injury typically resolves itself within a few weeks after birth.

Defects of the **retina** are common. **Retinitis pigmentosa** affects 1 in 4000 worldwide and is caused by defects in photoreceptors or the RPE, which is required for photoreceptor survival. Retinitis pigmentosa can be caused by mutations in more than forty genes, including RHODOPSIN and RPE65 the enzyme that converts 11-*cis* retinaldehyde to its all-*trans* form following activation of the photoreceptor. Crucially, the photoreceptors eventually die and cannot regenerate. Therefore, stem cells are used to provide neurotrophic factors to enable photoreceptor survival or to replace the damaged photoreceptors. The eye is particularly amenable to these approaches, as cells can be grafted into the intraretinal space. Recent work has shown that rod progenitors derived from embryonic stem (ES) cells can integrate and differentiate appropriately, rescuing impaired vision in mouse models and in human clinical trials. It has also been shown that with addition of the correct factors, dissociated human and mouse ES cells can be induced to form an optic cup complete with the laminated arrangement of the neural retina, showing that it is possible to recapitulate both differentiation and morphogenesis in vitro. Within the eye, stem cells are found in the ciliary body and in the limbus at the junction of the corneal epithelium and conjunctiva. Müller glia can re-enter the cell cycle in response to damage. Gene therapy approaches are also being used. For example, adenoviral delivery of RPE65 has been shown to be of clinical benefit in dogs and humans.

Wnt signaling plays an important role in eye development, including development of the retina. **Norrie disease**, characterized by **retinal dysplasia** and abnormal vascularization (and sensorineural hearing loss), arises from mutations in a novel ligand for the WNT pathway, NORRIN. Moreover, mutations in the WNT (and NORRIN) RECEPTOR FRIZZLED4 cause **familial exudative vitreoretinopathy**, another syndrome characterized in part by incomplete vascularization of the retina (the retinal blood vessels do not reach the periphery of the retina). Abnormal vascularization also occurs in **osteoporosis-pseudoglioma syndrome**, which is the result of a mutation in the WNT coreceptor LRP5. However, in this case the hyaloid artery persists, rather than regressing as it normally does, increasing the risk of retinal detachment.

The retina has one of the highest requirements for oxygen in the body, utilizing more oxygen/unit weight than any other tissue. Therefore, the eye is exceptionally sensitive to defects in vascularization. During development, angiogenesis is controlled by local regions of hypoxia generated by the newly differentiated retinal cells. Hypoxia induces the astrocyte and Müller cells to express the angiogenic factor Vegf, promoting further vascularization. Increases in oxygen levels (e.g., during oxygen support for premature babies) prevent angiogenesis. The neovascularization that follows from this can lead to hemorrhage and fibrosis—a condition known as **retinopathy of prematurity**, which is a major cause of infantile blindness.

Hypoplasia of the optic nerve occurs in a wide array of syndromes. In **septo-optic dysplasia** (also called **De Morsier syndrome**), which can be caused by mutations in the HESX1 gene, optic nerve hypoplasia occurs in conjunction with pituitary hypoplasia and midline brain abnormalities. Children with this syndrome are short as the result of growth hormone deficiency. Some forms of optic nerve hypoplasia are segmental, and in **superior segmental optic nerve hypoplasia**, there are inferior visual defects. This may sometimes occur in children born to diabetic mothers.

Embryology in Practice

BORN EARLY

After more than three months of intensive care, a former twenty-five week preterm infant is nearing discharge from the neonatal intensive care unit (NICU). The parents of this girl, who is now age adjusted to thirty-seven weeks gestation (nearing full term), review her medical issues and future care needs with the staff.

She weighed one pound two ounces at birth and has gained almost four pounds over the course of three months. She had experienced the effects of multiple medical issues, including hypoglycemia, anemia, jaundice, sepsis, chronic lung disease, and intraventricular (brain) bleeding. Follow-up for these medical issues will involve a list of specialist caregivers.

On the list of follow-up appointments is a visit with an ophthalmologist. The staff reviews with the parents what has been an ongoing concern: the degree to which their daughter will have vision loss due to problems with the blood vessels in her retinas.

The retinal vasculature begins development at three months and continues until birth. This development can be disrupted by preterm birth or influenced by factors in the subsequent care of these preterm infants, resulting in a disease process called **retinopathy of prematurity** (ROP).

An example of a factor that may affect the onset of ROP is the oxygen concentration used to ventilate infants with chronic lung disease. Concern that excessive use of oxygen could worsen retinal vessel hyperproliferation has led to tighter control of oxygen concentrations, but the effect of oxygen concentration on the incidence of ROP is not completely clear.

ROP is still a problem with undergrowth or overgrowth of the vessels and with retinal bleeding. Despite steady improvement in survival for preterm infants, rates of related health issues and disabilities, especially for infants born before twenty-six weeks of gestation, have been stubbornly stable.

This patient had multiple risk factors for ROP and was found during ophthalmology screening in the NICU to have bilateral stage three ROP. She had laser surgery in the NICU to ablate the peripheral portion of the retinas. Plans to follow the patient frequently with the possible need for retreatment are reviewed. Her parents are reassured that, although there is a risk for some impact on her vision, only a small minority of patients with stage three ROP go on to have severe visual impairment or blindness.

SUGGESTED READINGS

Andreazzoli M. 2009. Molecular regulation of vertebrate retina cell fate. Birth Defects Res C Embryo Today 87:284–295.

Davis-Silberman N, Ashery-Padan R. 2008. Iris development in vertebrates; genetic and molecular considerations. Brain Res 1192:17–28.

Fuhrmann S. 2010. Eye morphogenesis and patterning of the optic vesicle. Curr Top Dev Biol 93:61–84.

Graw J. 2009. Mouse models of cataract. J Genet 88:469–486.

Sowden JC. 2007. Molecular and developmental mechanisms of anterior segment dysgenesis. Eye (London) 21:1310–1318.

Swaroop A, Kim D, Forrest D. 2010. Transcriptional regulation of photoreceptor development and homeostasis in the mammalian retina. Nat Rev Neurosci 11:563–576.

Wallace VA. 2011. Concise review: making a retina—from the building blocks to clinical applications. Stem Cells 29:412–417.

Chapter 20
Development of the Limbs

SUMMARY

The upper **limb buds** appear on day twenty-four as small bulges on the lateral body wall at about the level of C5 to T1. By the end of the fourth week, the upper limb buds have grown to form pronounced structures protruding from the body wall, and the lower limb buds first appear, forming at about the level of L1 to S1. Limb morphogenesis takes place from the fourth to the eighth weeks, with development of the lower limbs lagging slightly behind that of the upper limbs. Each limb bud consists of a **mesenchymal core** of mesoderm covered by an **epithelial cap** of ectoderm. Along the distal margin of the limb bud, the ectoderm thickens to form an **apical ectodermal ridge**. This structure maintains outgrowth of the limb bud along the **proximal-distal axis**.

By thirty-three days, the **hand plates** are visible at the distal end of the lengthening upper limb buds, and the lower limb buds have begun to elongate. By the end of the sixth week, the segments of the upper and lower limbs can be distinguished. **Digital rays** appear on the handplates and footplates during the sixth (upper limbs) and seventh (lower limbs) weeks. A process of **programmed cell death** occurs between the rays and accompanies freeing of the fingers and toes. By the end of the eighth week, all components of the upper and lower limbs are distinct.

The **skeletal elements** of the limbs develop by endochondral ossification in a proximodistal sequence from mesodermal condensations that first appear along the long axis of the limb bud during the fifth week. The cartilaginous precursors of the limb bones chondrify within this mesenchymal condensation, starting in the sixth week. Ossification of these cartilaginous precursors begins in the seventh to twelfth weeks.

The bones, tendons, and other connective tissues of the limbs arise from the lateral plate mesoderm, but the limb muscles and endothelial cells arise in the somitic mesoderm and migrate into the limb buds. In general, the muscles that form on the ventral side of the developing long bones become the flexors and pronators of the upper limbs and the flexors and adductors of the lower limbs. These muscles are innervated by ventral branches of the ventral primary rami of the spinal nerves. The muscles that form on the dorsal side of the long bones generally become the extensor and supinator muscles of the upper limbs and the extensor and abductor muscles of the lower limbs. These muscles are innervated by dorsal branches of the ventral primary rami. However, some muscles of the limbs shift their position dramatically during development, either by differential growth or by passive displacement during lateral rotation of the upper limb and medial rotation of the lower limb.

Clinical Taster

Freddie Musena M'tile (Musena means friend in Kenyan) was born in 2004 in Kenya with a condition called **tetra-amelia** (absence of all four limbs; Fig. 20-1). Children with birth defects are shunned in some cultures, and Freddie's biologic mother gave him up for adoption, fearing that her husband would kill him. A British charity worker and her Kenyan husband adopted him and brought him to the UK for treatment. The case received notoriety after Freddie was, for a time, denied a British visa. With donations obtained through Thalidomide UK, he was fitted with prosthetic devices to help him sit up, with future plans to fit him with artificial limbs. Unfortunately, Freddie died of a fungal infection after returning to Africa. By the time of his death, Freddie had become a national symbol in Kenya.

Although the cause of Freddie's birth defects is not certain, his biologic mother took medicine that was believed to have been **thalidomide**. Once banned after causing an estimated 12,000 cases of limb defects like Freddie's in the late 1950s and early 1960s, use of thalidomide is on the rise again. Originally prescribed in Europe and the UK to treat morning sickness during pregnancy, thalidomide is now used to treat leprosy, AIDS, and certain cancers (e.g., multiple myeloma). It is widely available in Third World countries, and Freddie's case helped raise awareness of the risks of thalidomide exposure during pregnancy, especially in countries where literacy rates are low.

The thalidomide epidemic that occurred now over fifty years ago led to concerns about methods used to validate the safety of new drugs. This resulted in new Food and Drug Administration (FDA) guidelines for drug testing—guidelines that remain in effect today.

Thalidomide is a potent **teratogen** that causes defects at single exposures as low as 100 mg. The exact mechanism by which thalidomide causes amelia (absent limbs) or phocomelia (hands or feet projecting directly from the shoulder or hip, respectively) is unknown. However, the drug's ability to inhibit angiogenesis (blood vessel formation) is a potentially strong mechanism. Disruption of blood supply has long been hypothesized to play a role in similar limb reduction defects.

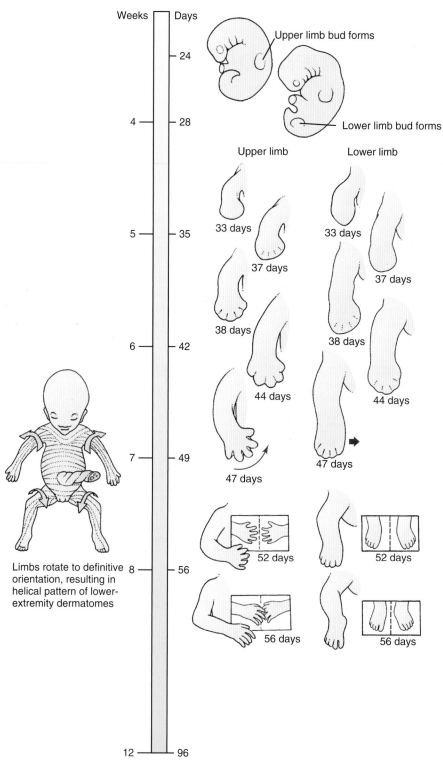

Weeks | Days

Upper limb bud forms

Lower limb bud forms

4 — 28

Upper limb   Lower limb

33 days   33 days

37 days   37 days

5 — 35

38 days   38 days

6 — 42

44 days   44 days

47 days   47 days

7 — 49

52 days   52 days

Limbs rotate to definitive orientation, resulting in helical pattern of lower-extremity dermatomes

8 — 56

56 days   56 days

12 — 96

Time line. Development of limbs.

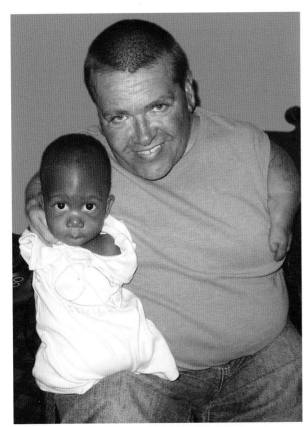

Figure 20-1. Freddie Musena M'tile meets Freddie Astbury, a thalidomide survivor of the original epidemic and President of Thalidomide UK. Freddie Musena M'tile was born in Kenya with tetra-amelia.

EPITHELIAL-MESENCHYMAL INTERACTIONS CONTROL LIMB OUTGROWTH

 Animation 20-1: Development of Limbs.
Animations are available online at StudentConsult.

Limb development takes place over a five-week period from the fourth to the eighth weeks. The upper limbs develop slightly in advance of the lower limbs, although by the end of the period of limb development, upper and lower limbs are nearly synchronized. Initiation of limb development starts with continued proliferation of the somatic lateral plate mesoderm in the limb regions of the lateral body wall (Fig. 20-2). The upper limb bud appears in the lower cervical region at twenty-four days, and the lower limb bud appears in the lower lumbar region at twenty-eight days. The origin of the limb buds is reflected in their final innervation (see later in this chapter and Chapter 10). Each limb bud consists of an outer ectodermal cap and an inner mesodermal core.

As each limb bud forms, the ectoderm along the distal tip of the bud is induced by the underlying somatic mesoderm to form a ridge-like thickening called the **apical ectodermal ridge** (AER) (see Fig. 20-2). This structure forms at the dorsal-ventral boundary of the limb bud and plays an essential role in the outgrowth of the limb.

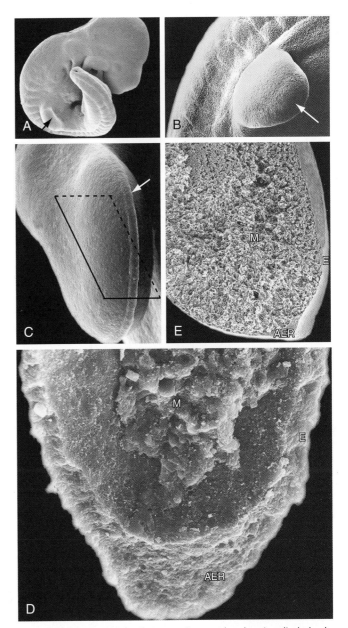

Figure 20-2. Scanning electron micrographs showing limb buds. The limb buds are formed from lateral plate mesoderm. *A,* Embryo with newly formed upper limb bud (arrow). *B,* By day twenty-nine, the upper limb bud (arrow) is flattened. *C,* Day thirty-two limb bud showing the apical ectodermal ridge (arrow) as a thickened crest of ectoderm at the distal edge of the growing upper limb bud. Rectangle indicates plane of sectioning shown in *E. D,* Limb bud ectoderm (*E*) removed from the bulk of the limb bud mesenchyme to show its internal face and attached mesenchymal core (*M*); note the thickened apical ectodermal ridge (AER). *E,* Limb bud sectioned at the level indicated by the rectangle in *C,* showing the inner mesenchymal core (*M*), the outer ectodermal cap (*E*), and the thickened apical ectodermal ridge (AER).

In the Research Lab

OVERVIEW OF PATTERNING OF LIMB BUD

Once the limb bud has formed, it differentiates with respect to three axes (Fig. 20-3). The **proximal-distal axis** runs from the shoulder or hip to the fingers or toes and consists of the **stylopod** (humerus or femur), **zeugopod** (radius and ulna or tibia and

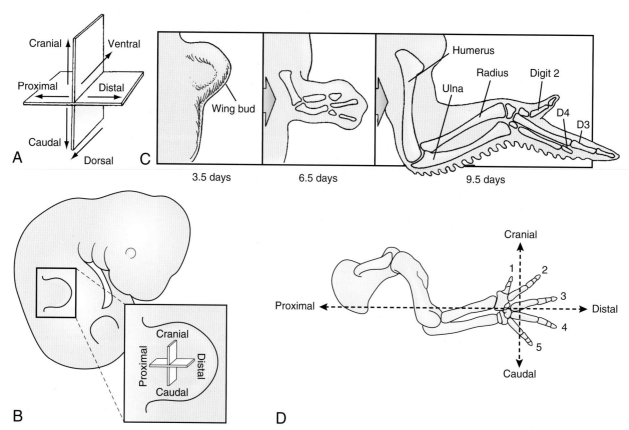

Figure 20-3. Axes and digits of the developing limb. *A,* The three axes of symmetry for limb development: cranial-caudal (anterior-posterior), dorsal-ventral, and proximal-distal. *B,* Drawing showing the mouse forelimb bud with two of the three axes labeled. *C,* Drawing showing development of the chick wing, which forms only three digits, numbered two (most cranial), three, and four (most caudal). Although this numbering scheme is widely used by embryologists for the digits of the chick wing and will be used in this text, recent evidence suggests that the three digits are actually evolutionarily equivalent to digits one, two, and three. *D,* Drawing of a skeleton of the mouse forelimb showing two of its axes and its five digits (number one through five, with one being most cranial); the autopod of the hindlimb also has five digits numbered correspondingly.

fibula), and **autopod** (the carpals and metacarpals or tarsal and metatarsals and the phalanges). Along the **cranial-caudal axis** (often called the anterior-posterior axis), the thumb (or big toe) is the most cranial digit, whereas the little finger (or little toe) is the most caudal digit. Along the **dorsal-ventral axis**, the knuckle side of the hand or the top of the foot is dorsal, whereas the palm of the hand or the sole of the foot is ventral. The limb bud develops from an apparently homogeneous cell population; thus, a cell in the limb bud must respond appropriately to its position relative to all three axes. Several questions arise: How does one part of the upper limb bud form the shoulder and another the forearm? How does one digital ray in the hand plate form an index finger and another the thumb? How do dorsal and ventral sides of the limb become differentiated from each other? Significant advances have been made toward answering these questions. We now know the key players that pattern the limb bud, and we can link these key players to mutations that cause human birth defects.

The cranial-caudal (anterior-posterior) axis is determined by signals from a small region of mesenchyme in the caudal part of the limb bud known as the **zone of polarizing activity** (ZPA), and this activity is mediated by Shh. Signals from the dorsal ectoderm (Wnt7a) determine the dorsal-ventral axis, whereas Fgfs and Wnts from the AER, together with retinoic acid in the lateral plate mesoderm, pattern the proximal-distal axis. These signals do not act in isolation to control patterning along the individual axes but are interdependent. For example,

Shh maintains expression of Fgfs in the AER and Wnt7a in the dorsal ectoderm. Conversely, Fgfs and Wnt7a maintain Shh expression in the ZPA, resulting in a positive feedback loop, promoting and coordinating patterning along each of the axes. During limb bud initiation, establishment of the dorsal-ventral axis is also necessary to correctly position the AER at the distal tip of the limb, whereas expression of Fgf8 in the AER acts together with other signals within the limb bud mesenchyme to initiate expression of Shh in the ZPA.

The position of the limb buds along the cranial-caudal axis of the body is specified by the expression of Hox genes in the lateral plate mesenchyme (see Chapter 8 for further coverage of Hox genes and craniocaudal patterning). The identity of the limb (arm vs. leg) is specified in the lateral plate mesoderm before limb bud initiation. The skeleton patterns the developing musculature, as in other regions of the body (e.g., the developing face; see Chapter 17).

The following paragraphs in this "In the Research Lab" detail development of the limb along the proximal-distal axis, including initiation of limb outgrowth. Development along the other two axes is covered in the next "In the Research Lab" in the sections entitled "Specification of Cranial-Caudal Axis" and "Specification of Dorsal-Ventral Axis."

GROWTH AND PATTERNING ALONG PROXIMAL-DISTAL AXIS

Classical embryologic experiments have shown that **proximal-distal outgrowth** is controlled by the apical ectodermal

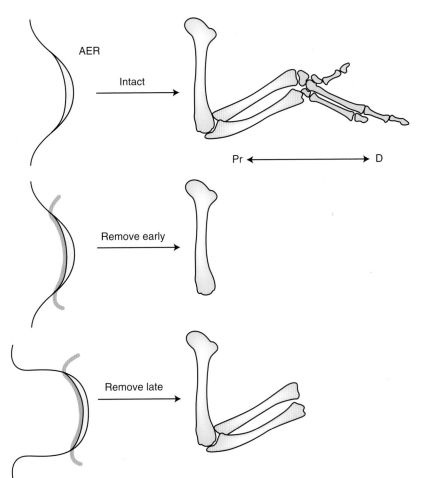

Figure 20-4. Skeletal development along the proximal (Pr)-distal (D) axis of a chick wing bud following removal of the apical ectodermal ridge (AER) at different stages of development.

ridge (AER). Removal of the AER results in the arrest of limb development, with the degree of development determined by the stage of development at which the AER was removed (Fig. 20-4). For example, in the chick, removal at stage 20 of development results in the formation of a limb truncated at the elbow joint, whereas removal slightly later at stage 24 leads to a limb lacking just the digits. Furthermore, in chick wingless and mouse limb deformity mutants, in which the AER develops initially but is not maintained, the limbs are truncated. Initiation of limb development without further maintenance occurs naturally in some species of snakes, whales, and dolphins. In these species, small hindlimb buds initially form. However, they do not develop, as the AER either does not form or is not maintained.

Several members of the Fgf family are expressed in the AER (Fgf4, 8, 9, and 17) (Fig. 20-5). These factors are key regulators of limb outgrowth. Beads soaked in Fgfs and transplanted to the tip of a limb bud following AER removal can proxy for the AER and maintain limb outgrowth. Moreover, there is redundancy in their function, such that several different Fgfs can proxy for the AER and for each other. For example, limbs lacking Fgf4, 9, or 17 are normal. Gene inactivation of Fgf8 in mice results in the formation of a slightly smaller limb bud, affecting growth of all limb segments. In these limbs, Fgf8 function is rescued by Fgf4, which is upregulated/sustained, but gene inactivation of both Fgf8 and Fgf4 results in increased apoptosis of the limb mesenchymal cells and reduces limb outgrowth.

Fgf signaling is essential for the *initiation* of limb development. Strikingly, application of an Fgf-soaked bead to the interlimb flank of an early chick embryo induces the formation of an extra limb (Fig. 20-6). At the forelimb level, Tbx5 induces Fgf10 expression in the presumptive forelimb mesenchyme. Fgf10 signaling in the mesoderm then induces Wnt3a (in the chick) in the overlying ectoderm. Wnt3a in turn induces Fgf8 in the presumptive AER, which maintains Fgf10 expression in the underlying mesenchyme and establishes a feedback loop between Fgf8 and Fgf10 to maintain limb outgrowth. The interplay between Wnt3a and Fgf8 continues throughout development of the limb, with misexpression of Wnt3a resulting in the induction of ectopic AER formation. Parallel processes occur in the mouse, where Wnt3/β-catenin signaling is required for both AER formation and maintenance.

How patterning is specified along the proximal-distal axis is still uncertain. One model that has been used for forty years to explain this patterning is called the **progress zone model**. The **progress zone** is defined as a narrow zone of mesenchyme about 300 μm in width underlying the AER, where cells are thought to acquire **positional information** that will inform them of their final **positional address** along the proximal-distal axis. Cells that exit the progress zone after a short residence are destined to form proximal structures such as the humerus or femur (i.e., elements of the stylopod). Cells with longest residence in the progress zone become the most distal structures, that is, the phalanges (i.e., elements of the autopod). How cells actually acquire positional information during residence in the progress zone is unknown. However, a timing mechanism in which a cell counts its number of mitotic divisions has been proposed.

Removal of the AER results in differences in the extent of cell death and cell proliferation in the limb bud mesenchyme

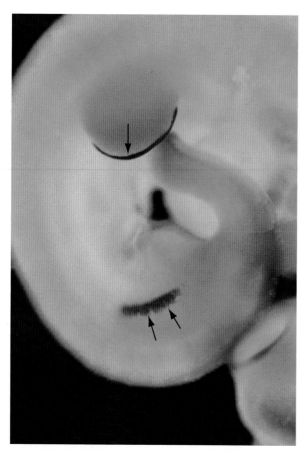

Figure 20-5. In situ hybridization showing that mRNA transcripts for Fgf8 are expressed in the ectoderm before limb bud outgrowth (two arrows mark expression in the hindlimb region near the bottom of the photograph) and then become discretely contained within the apical ectodermal ridge (single arrow) during later development. (The development of the forelimb bud is advanced with respect to that of the hindlimb bud.)

expression in the distal mesenchyme, which degrades retinoic acid. In Cyp26 mouse mutants, the distal markers are absent, whereas Meis1/2 expression is extended along the proximal-distal axis. As the limb bud grows, the cells in the middle will become out of range of both proximal and distal signals and will acquire a unique identity: the zeugopod.

Insight into the molecular mechanisms that regulate growth of each region of the limb bud has also been obtained. As described in Chapters 5, 8, and 17, four clusters of Hox genes are sequentially activated in vertebrates (including humans) following the 3′ to 5′ sequence along the DNA of the four respective chromosomes. Moreover, the most 5′ members of the Hoxd and Hoxa clusters (9 to 13) are initially coordinately expressed in nested cranial-caudal and proximal-distal domains within the growing limb bud (Fig. 20-8). This temporal and nested expression is known as **temporal and spatial colinearity** and is also seen during Hox expression and patterning of the developing somites (see Chapter 8). Ultimately, expression of each of the 5′ Hoxd genes (along with those of the Hoxa group) can be correlated with development of specific skeletal elements of upper and lower limb segments. For example, in the forelimb, Hoxd9 is expressed within the segment forming the scapula; Hoxd9 and Hoxd10 within the arm (containing the humerus); Hoxd9, Hoxd10, and Hoxd11 within the forearm and proximal wrist (containing ulna, radius, and proximal carpals); Hoxd9, Hoxd10, Hoxd11, and Hoxd12 within the distal wrist (containing distal carpals); and Hoxd9, Hoxd10, Hoxd11, Hoxd12, and Hoxd13 within the hand and fingers (containing metacarpals and phalanges; Fig. 20-9). These genes are required for growth of the different regions of the limb bud. The most 5′ Hox genes (8-11) are required for formation of the AER, whereas the Hox11-13 genes activate Shh expression in the ZPA.

The requirement for Hox genes in regional growth of the limb bud is directly shown by the knockouts of multiple paralogs of Hox genes in mice. For example, in forelimbs lacking Hoxa11 and Hoxd11 genes, the radius and ulna are severely affected (Fig. 20-10), whereas knockout of both Hoxa13 and Hoxd13 results in loss of the digits. Analysis of the Hoxa11/Hoxd11 mutants has shown reduced Fgf signaling, resulting in smaller skeletal condensations and delayed chondrocyte differentiation. Once these cartilaginous elements have formed, a growth plate defect significantly contributes to hypoplasia/aplasia of these elements at birth.

depending on the stage of removal. Removal early in development results in cell death encompassing the autopod and zeugopod (i.e., the radius and ulna or the tibia and fibula) progenitors, whereas later removal does not induce significant cell death but significantly decreases cell proliferation. Furthermore, reducing the levels of Fgf expression in the AER affects all skeletal elements. If the number of cell cycles determines cell fate, as suggested by the timing mechanism of positional information covered above, then the sequential reduction in Fgf signaling, which controls cell proliferation, should preferentially affect the autopod; it does not.

This conundrum is resolved with the **two-signal model** (Fig. 20-7). According to this model, limb bud cells are initially exposed to a proximal signal from the trunk (possibly retinoic acid produced by the enzyme Raldh2 in the flank mesenchyme) and a distal signal from the AER (Fgfs and Wnts). At an early stage of limb development, the entire limb bud is exposed to both signals; as a consequence, it expresses markers of the stylopod (the homeobox transcription factors Meis1 and Meis2) and autopod (e.g., the transcription factors, Ap1 and Msx1). As the limb grows out from the flank, only the proximal part of the limb continues to be exposed to retinoic acid and maintains Meis1/2 expression, whereas only the distal region is exposed to Fgf/Wnt signaling from the AER, which keeps the cells in an undifferentiated state. Fgfs also induce Cyp26

MORPHOGENESIS OF LIMB

Once the AER has been established, the limb continues to grow, with development occurring predominantly along the proximal-distal axis. Proliferation and growth are also slightly higher on the dorsal side of the limb bud, resulting in a ventral curvature of the developing limbs. Later development takes place as follows (Fig. 20-11).

Day thirty-three. In the upper limb, the **hand plate**, **forearm**, **arm**, and **shoulder** regions can be distinguished. In the lower limb, a somewhat rounded proximal part can be distinguished from a more tapering distal part that will form the foot.

Day thirty-seven. In the hand plate of the upper limb, a central **carpal region** is surrounded by a thinner crescentic rim, the **digital plate**, which will form the fingers. In the lower limb, the **thigh**, **leg**, and **foot** have become distinct.

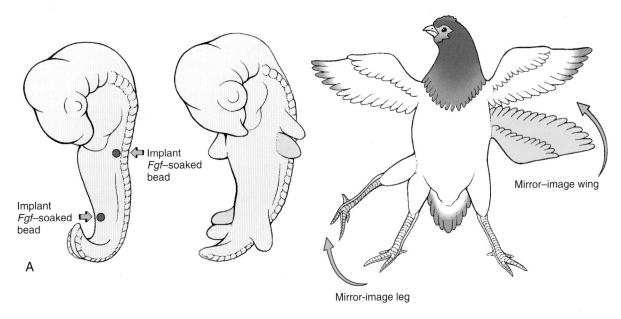

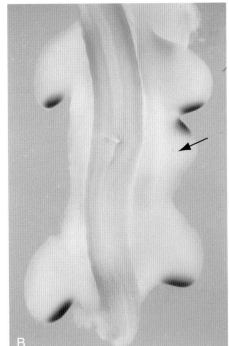

Figure 20-6. Fgf-soaked beads induce supernumerary limbs. *A,* Schematic drawing of the experimental procedure and the resulting induction of ectopic mirror-image legs/wings (shown in blue). *B,* Whole mount in situ hybridization shows Shh expression in the zone of polarizing activity in each limb bud (two wing buds, two leg buds, and a supernumerary bud) of a chick embryo two days after application of an Fgf bead. Arrow marks the induced supernumerary limb bud; note that Shh is expressed cranially rather than caudally (with respect to the embryo's cranial-caudal axis) within the supernumerary bud, resulting in the mirror-image orientation of the ectopic limb.

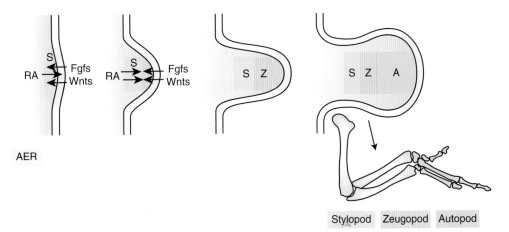

Figure 20-7. The two-signal model of patterning along the proximal-distal axis. RA, retinoic acid.

Day thirty-eight. Finger rays (more generally, digital rays) are visible as radial thickenings in the digital plate of the upper limb. The tips of the finger rays project slightly, producing a crenulated rim on the digital plate. A process of programmed apoptotic cell death between the digital rays will gradually sculpt the digital rays out of the digital plate by removing intervening tissue. This will free the fingers and toes. The lower limb bud has increased in length, and a clearly defined footplate has formed on the distal end of the limb.

Day forty-four. In the upper limb, the distal margin of the digital plate is deeply notched and the grooves between the finger rays are deeper. The bend where the elbow will form along the proximal-distal axis is becoming defined. **Toe rays** are visible in the digital plate of the foot, but the rim of the plate is not yet crenulated.

Day forty-seven. The entire upper limb has undergone **ventral flexion** (Fig. 20-12A; see also Fig. 20-11). The lower limb has also begun to flex toward the midline. The toe rays are more prominent, although the margin of the digital plate is still smooth (see Fig. 20-11).

Day fifty-two. The upper limbs are bent at the elbows, and the fingers have developed distal swellings called **tactile pads** (Fig. 20-12B; see also Fig. 20-11). The hands are slightly flexed at the wrists and meet at the midline in front of the cardiac eminence. The legs are longer, and the feet have begun to approach each other at the midline. The rim of the digital plate is notched.

Day fifty-six. All regions of the arms and legs are well defined, including the tactile pads on the toes (Fig. 20-12C). The fingers of the two hands overlap at the midline.

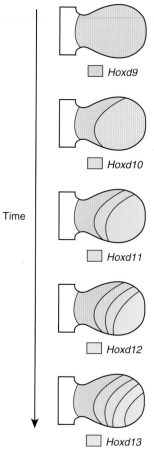

Time

Hoxd9

Hoxd10

Hoxd11

Hoxd12

Hoxd13

Figure 20-8. Progressive expression of Hoxd genes over time and space.

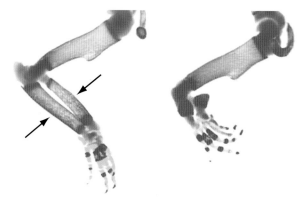

Figure 20-10. Aplasia of the radius and ulna (zeugopod) following gene inactivation of the Hox11 paralogs. Left, Wild-type mouse (arrows mark zeugopod); right, mutant mouse (i.e., forelimb lacks Hoxa11 and Hoxd11 expression).

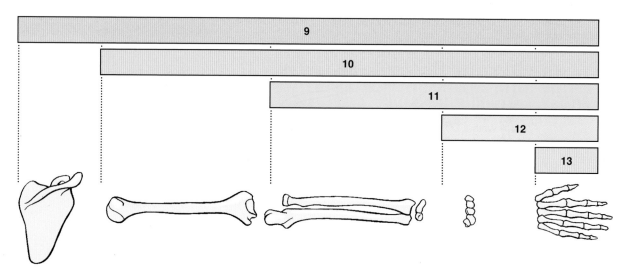

Figure 20-9. Hoxd gene expression patterns in relation to definitive segments of the upper limb.

In the Research Lab

SPECIFICATION OF CRANIAL-CAUDAL AXIS

The cranial-caudal (anterior-posterior) axis is determined by signals from a small region of mesenchyme in the caudal part of the limb bud known as the **zone of polarizing activity** (ZPA). Transplantation of the ZPA to the cranial portion of a chick limb bud induces mirror-image digit duplications (Fig. 20-13). Classic experiments originally showed that the number of ZPA cells transplanted or the length of exposure of the cranial limb bud cells to the ZPA signal determined the cranial-caudal identity of the digits that formed. If more ZPA cells were transplanted or cells were exposed for a longer time, the resulting ectopic digits would have a more caudal identity. This suggested that a **morphogen** is produced by the ZPA that diffuses across the limb's cranial-caudal axis. A high dose of the morphogen would induce the caudal digits, whereas progressively lower concentrations would induce the more cranial digits. In support of this, Sonic hedgehog (Shh) is expressed in the ZPA (Fig. 20-14A), and it diffuses across the limb. Moreover, ectopic expression of Shh at the cranial side of the limb bud induces digit duplications, and the identity of the digit correlates with the concentration of Shh applied.

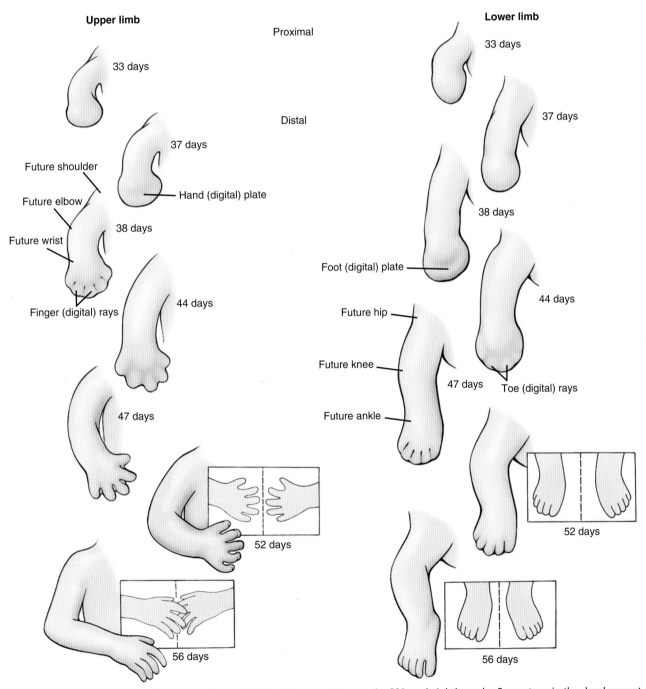

Figure 20-11. Development of the upper and lower limb buds occurs between the fifth and eighth weeks. Every stage in the development of the lower limb bud takes place later than in the upper limb bud.

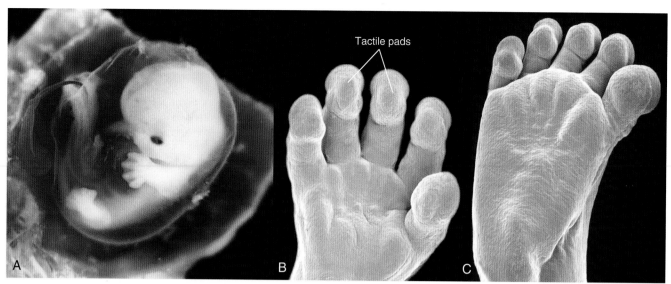

Figure 20-12. Human limbs during early development. *A,* By seven weeks, the digits are clearly visible in both upper and lower extremities. *B, C,* Scanning electron micrographs of a hand and foot, respectively, of a human embryo. Tactile pads are visible on the palmar side of the finger tips.

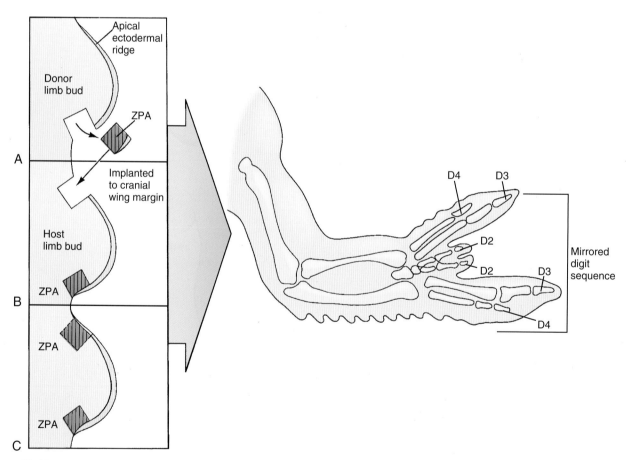

Figure 20-13. Transplantation of the zone of polarizing activity (ZPA) of a donor chick limb bud to the cranial edge of a host chick limb bud induces mirror-image polydactyly. *A, B, C,* Shows sequential steps in the transplantation process.

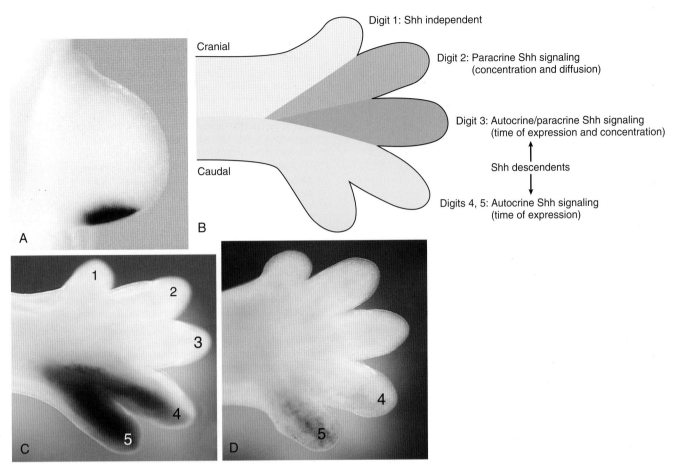

Figure 20-14. Cranial-caudal patterning of the limb bud. *A,* Expression of Shh (purple) in the zone of polarizing activity (ZPA) of the limb bud of a mouse embryo. *B,* The temporal-spatial model of Shh-mediated cranial-caudal patterning of the digits in the mouse limb. *C, D,* Fate maps of ZPA descendants when labeled at E10.5 and E11.5, respectively. Cells formerly in the ZPA express a reporter gene (brown), allowing them to be traced over time.

Additional experiments have challenged the idea that specification of the cranial-caudal axis of the limb bud involves only the simple diffusion of a morphogen. Instead, the **temporal-spatial gradient model** (Fig. 20-14*B*), based on these experiments (covered below), proposes that patterning of the digits is achieved by a combination of simple diffusion of a morphogen (namely, Shh) and differences encountered by target cells across the limb bud in the doses and durations of exposure to the morphogen. These events are analogous to those occurring in patterning of the dorsal-ventral axis of the neural tube, where both the dose and the length of exposure to Shh as it diffuses from the notochord and floor plate of the neural tube determine the eventual fate of the neuronal cell columns (see Chapters 4 and 9).

Specifically, the temporal-spatial model proposes that digit one of the mouse hand or foot develops independently of Shh signaling; digit two develops based on Shh concentration at the cranial limit of Shh diffusion (i.e., **paracrine** Shh signaling); digit three develops based on the length of exposure to Shh signaling and the dose of Shh signaling, and from being composed of both Shh descendants and non-descendants (i.e., both paracrine and **autocrine** Shh signaling); and digit four and five develop based on length of exposure to Shh signaling and from being composed entirely of Shh descendants (i.e., autocrine Shh signaling). Support for this model comes from two types of genetic fate mapping studies

In the first of these studies, the contributions of ZPA and non-ZPA regions of the limb bud to the digits were mapped. These

studies show that the ZPA descendants occupy the caudal one third of the limb bud and form digits three to five: *all* cells in digits four and five are derived from the ZPA, but cells in digit three arise from both ZPA and non–ZPA descendants (cells in digits one and two arise from non-ZPA descendants). Labeling the ZPA cells at different stages of development revealed that digit five arises from the ZPA after digit four; thus, because the ZPA is the source of Shh signaling, digit five is exposed to Shh signaling for the longest period of time (Fig. 20-14*C, D*).

In the second of these studies, the cells that receive an Shh signal (i.e., identified by their expression of Gli1, a transcriptional target of Shh) were mapped. These studies show that digits two to five respond to Shh signaling at some point during their development, and that digit one, the most cranial digit, develops independently of Shh signaling, which is consistent with the formation of one digit (digit one) in the Shh mutant hindlimb (Fig. 20-15*A, B*).

Combining the results of these two types of studies provides the basic tenets of the temporal-spatial model: (1) Shh diffuses from the ZPA as far cranially as digit two; thus, digit one develops independently of Shh signaling, but digit two depends on diffusion of Shh for its development, as it does not descend from the ZPA cells (which express Shh); (2) in contrast to digit two, digits three, four, and five arise in whole (digits four and five) or in part (digit three) from the Shh-expressing cells of the ZPA. As predicted from this model, altering the range that Shh can diffuse affects digit number.

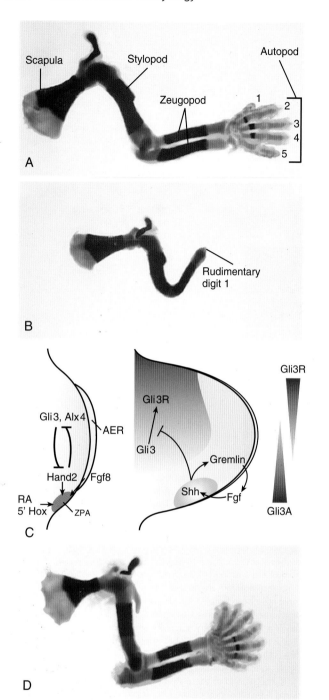

Figure 20-15. Roles for Shh signaling in the mouse forelimb. *A, B, D,* Skeletal structures in limbs of wild-type, Shh mutant, and Gli3 (Xt) mutant mice, respectively. *C,* Schemes showing signaling interactions during limb development that induce (left) and maintain (right) Shh expression. AER, apical ectodermal ridge; RA, retinoic acid; ZPA, zone of polarizing activity.

Removal of the cholesterol modification of Shh increases Shh diffusion and results in pre-axial polydactyly, whereas removal of the palmitic acid modification decreases Shh diffusion, which results in the loss of digit two (i.e., the digit that is solely dependent on Shh diffusion for its development).

Other experiments in which Shh expression was inactivated at different times of limb development have led to modification of the temporal-spatial model, called the **biphasic model**.

Inactivation of Shh at later phases of limb development reduces digit number but does not change digit identity in the digits that form. Therefore, it was argued that Shh has major and differing roles at two times in development: (1) patterning of the cranial-caudal axis of the limb bud during very early limb development by acting as a morphogen (phase I); and (2) control of expansion of the prespecified digit precursors via direct regulation of cyclins D1/E and cMyc, together with regulation of Fgf expression in the AER, which controls cell proliferation and cell survival of the underlying limb mesenchyme (phase II).

Because Shh has these two major roles, cranial-caudal patterning and outgrowth along the proximal-distal axis, Shh mutants are characterized by defective development of the caudal side of the limb (i.e., loss of caudal digits) and failure in limb outgrowth, resulting in a truncated limb (see Fig. 20-15*A, B*). In its later role, Shh maintains the expression of Fgfs in the AER via the expression of gremlin, a secreted Bmp antagonist that blocks the repressive actions of Bmps on AER function (Fig. 20-15*C*). In gremlin mouse mutants, Fgf4 and 8 expression is absent or reduced, respectively, again resulting in limb truncations. Fgfs in turn maintain Shh expression in the ZPA and Hox11-13 expression in the limb mesenchyme.

The limb bud is prepatterned across the cranial-caudal axis before expression of Shh. Gli3 and the aristaless-like 4 paired-type homeodomain protein, Alx4, function in the cranial mesenchyme to restrict expression of Hand2 to the caudal mesenchyme before Shh expression (see Fig. 20-15*C*). Shh expression is then activated in the caudal mesenchyme by the combined action of retinoic acid, the transcription factor Hand2, 5′ Hox genes, and Fgf8 signaling (see Fig. 20-15*C*). Strong's luxoid mutant, which is characterized by polydactyly, results from mutations in Alx4. In this mutant, the prepatterning that normally restricts Hand2 to the caudal limb bud does not occur. Consequently, an ectopic domain of Shh expression forms in the cranial mesenchyme (Fig. 20-16). Shh expression in the ZPA is regulated by the ZPA regulatory sequence (ZRS), a highly conserved 750-800 bp sequence in the Shh promoter, which is both necessary and sufficient to drive Shh expression. Some snakes and limbless amphibians lack the ZRS, explaining the absence of Shh expression and failure of limb outgrowth in these species. Hoxd11-13 and Hand2 bind directly to the ZRS. Shh expression is also directly suppressed in the anterior region of the limb bud by the Ets transcription factors Etv4 and Etv5, whereas the boundary of Shh expression is positioned by Ets1/Gabpα. Point mutations in the ZRS that alter the binding of the Ets transcription factors result in ectopic Shh expression in the cranial limb bud. These mutations cause polydactyly in mice, cats, chicks, and humans.

In the limb bud, Shh signaling is mediated by Gli3. In the absence of Shh, Gli3 is processed to its shorter form, which acts as a potent transcriptional repressor (Gli3R; R indicates the repressor form). In the presence of Shh signaling, this processing is prevented, and now the full-length Gli3 protein acts as a weak transcriptional activator (Gli3A; A indicates activator form). Gli3 is mutated in the Xt mouse mutant, which exhibits polydactyly with between six and nine morphologically indistinguishable digits (see Fig. 20-15*D*). As Gli3 function, which normally restricts Shh expression to the caudal mesenchyme, is absent, Shh is ectopically expressed in the cranial mesenchyme. However, unlike the polydactylous mutants discussed above, polydactyly is not the result of excess Shh signaling because compound Shh/Xt mutants have the same phenotype as Xt mutants. The double-compound mutant shows that failure of limb outgrowth in the Shh null mutant is due to ectopic Gli3R in the caudal mesenchyme. Therefore, in the absence of both functional Shh and Gli3,

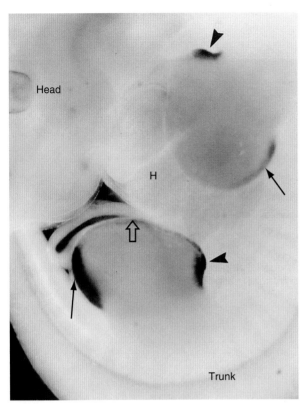

Figure 20-16. Gene expression in Strong's luxoid mouse mutant limb doubly labeled with probes for Shh and Fgf4. In situ hybridization showing Shh mRNA in its normal location in the zone of polarizing activity (solid arrows) in forelimb and hindlimb buds, and at an ectopic cranial location in each bud (arrowheads). Because of the ectopic expression of Shh, Fgf4, which is normally restricted to the caudal AER, is now extended throughout the craniocaudal extent of the AER (open arrow). H, heart.

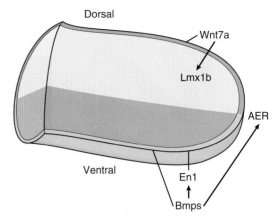

Figure 20-17. Schematic showing the signaling interactions that establish the dorsal-ventral pattern of the limb.

outgrowth can occur and the limb forms, but the digits are not patterned. Consequently, it can be concluded that number and patterning of the digits are actually determined by the levels of Gli3R.

SPECIFICATION OF DORSAL-VENTRAL AXIS

The third axis of the limb, the dorsal-ventral axis, is first regulated by signals from the mesenchyme and then from the ectoderm. If just the ectodermal covering of the limb bud is surgically rotated 180 degrees with respect to the mesenchyme, the dorsal-ventral polarity of the skeletal elements that are subsequently formed is reversed. Wnt7a, which is expressed in the dorsal ectoderm, is one regulator of dorsal-ventral patterning. In the Wnt7a knockout mouse, the paws are ventralized, with foot pads forming on the dorsal surface. Wnt7a activity is mediated by the Lmx1b homeobox gene, which is expressed in the dorsal mesenchyme. Lmx1b-mutant mouse limbs lack dorsal structures, whereas ectopic expression of Lmx1b in chick limb buds dorsalizes the limb. Mutation of LMX1B in humans leads to **nail-patella syndrome,** indicating that dorsal structures in the limb (i.e., nails and patellae) are mainly affected when this gene is not functional. Wnt7a also regulates Shh expression. Hence, in Wnt7a knockout mice, in addition to defects in dorsal-ventral patterning, abnormalities occur in limb outgrowth and development of the caudal digits. Likewise, mutations of WNT7A in humans result in hypoplastic/aplastic nails, ectopic dorsal palms, and

defects in caudal limb development (**Fuhrmann syndrome**). The homeobox transcription factor engrailed 1 is expressed in the ventral ectoderm and prevents the expression of Wnt7a in the ventral part of the limb, restricting positioning of the AER to the boundary of the dorsal-ventral axis. In the engrailed 1 null mouse, Wnt7a is ectopically expressed in the ventral ectoderm, the ventral limb bud is dorsalized, and ectopic or bifurcated AERs are formed. Bmp signaling in the ventral ectoderm induces engrailed 1 expression in the ventral ectoderm, gremlin expression in the mesenchyme, and initial expression of Fgf8 in the AER (Fig. 20-17). Thus, Bmp signaling initially establishes the dorsal-ventral axis together with the forward Shh-Fgf signaling loop that maintains outgrowth along the proximal-distal axis. This early role of Bmp in the induction of Fgf8 expression contrasts with its later role in limb development, which is to inhibit AER function (covered in next section of this "In the Research Lab").

CESSATION OF LIMB OUTGROWTH AND MORPHOGENESIS OF AUTOPOD

The AER is a transient embryonic structure that regresses when limb patterning has ceased. The AER initially regresses over the interdigital region but persists locally over the developing digits, which continue to elongate. Hence, once the digital rays have started to form, the number of phalanges and the length of the phalanges and digit identity are ultimately controlled by the duration of Fgf8 signaling. For example, maintaining Fgf expression by placing Shh beads into the interdigital mesenchyme or misexpressing a Bmp antagonist in the AER prolongs limb outgrowth and can increase the number of phalanges that form. In developing bat wings, a second phase of Shh expression prolongs digit outgrowth. Degeneration of the AER is the result of increased levels of Bmp signaling that inhibit Fg8 expression in the AER. The increase in Bmp signaling is due to loss of gremlin expression in the distal limb mesenchyme.

In the chick, the identity of each digit is modulated at this late stage of development by different levels of Bmp signaling from each region of adjacent caudal interdigital mesenchyme, which expresses Bmp2, 4, and 7. If this mesenchyme is removed, the immediately cranial digit will be cranialized. For example, removal of the interdigital mesenchyme between digits three and four will result in the morphologic transformation of digit three to a digit with the identity of digit two (i.e., a homeotic transformation). Furthermore, bisection of developing digit three with insertion of a piece of foil to prevent healing results in the formation of an

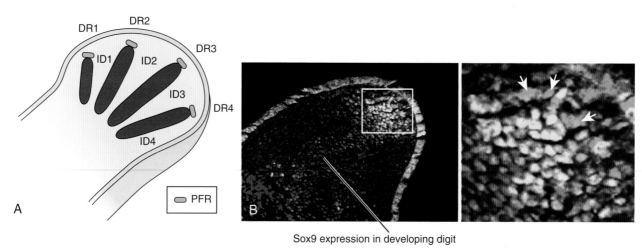

Figure 20-18. Bmp activity in the phalanx forming region (PFR; green region in *A* and green cells in *B*) determines digit identity. *A,* Drawing showing the autopod of the chick hindlimb. DR1-4, digital rays one-four; ID1-4, interdigital spaces one-four; the condensing digits are indicated in red. *B,* Section of the distal DR3 region in an E13.5 mouse embryo. Box is area enlarged in panel to the right. Green staining (arrows in enlargement) shows pSmad labeling (indicative of Bmp activity), and red staining shows Sox9 expression (marker of cartilage differentiation) in the forming digit 3. Sox9 expressing cells in the very distal region of the condensing digit also show pSmad activity (yellow).

ectopic digit: the caudal digit has the original identity (in this case, digit three), whereas the digit arising from the cranial part of the bisected digit has the characteristics of digit two. Bmp signaling maintains a subpopulation of cells in the distal mesenchyme (PFR, the phalanx forming region) that will give rise to the phalanges (Fig. 20-18). Each PFR is associated with a unique level of Bmp signaling. Reflecting the role of Bmp signaling during this late stage of development, many brachydactylies in humans are due to gene mutations that directly (e.g., GDF5/BMPR1B) or indirectly (e.g., IHH) affect the levels of Bmp signaling.

Removal of the interdigital mesenchyme involves **programmed cell death**, helping to free the digits and allowing the mobility required to carry out specialized tasks. This removal does not occur in the duck foot, which is specialized for swimming, and also does not occur in **soft tissue syndactyly**, which is a frequent clinical observation. Interdigital cell death requires Bmps, secreted metalloproteinases, Hoxd13, and retinoic acid signaling. Manipulation that increases Bmp activity leads to increased cell death in the interdigital necrotic zone (INZ), whereas decreasing Bmp activity in mouse mutants or expressing dominant negative Bmp receptors in the chick prevents INZ cell death and leads to digital webbing. Bmps, in part, mediate interdigital cell death by signaling to the AER to decrease the expression of cell survival factors, Fgf4 and 8. Therefore, excess Fgf signaling can result in syndactyly. This is seen in **Pfeiffer, Apert,** and **Jackson-Weiss syndromes,** which are due to constitutive activation of the FGF receptor, FGFR2. Hoxd13 regulates Raldh2 expression, which synthesizes retinoic acid in the interdigital mesenchyme. Decreased Raldh2 expression may contribute to the syndactyly observed in humans with HOXD13 mutations (see Fig. 20-23).

Other regions of programmed cell death are found within the AER, in the mesenchyme at the cranial limit of the AER, and in the mesenchyme between the radius and ulna or between the fibula and tibia. The developmental function of these regions of cell death is less clear, although the regions at the edges of the AER may determine the length of the AER and hence digit number.

In the Clinic

CONGENITAL ANOMALIES OF LIMBS

Humans exhibit a wide range of limb defects. In general, these fall into four categories. In **reduction defects**, part of the limb is missing, a condition called **meromelia** (Fig. 20-19*A*), or an entire limb is missing, a condition called **amelia** (Fig. 20-19*B*). In **duplication defects**, supernumerary limb elements are present. Examples include **polydactyly** (i.e., the presence of entire extra digits; Fig. 20-19*C*) and **triphalangeal thumb,** in which a third phalanx is present rather than just the normal two (Fig. 20-19*D*). In **dysplasias**, fusion of limb parts can occur, as in **syndactyly** (i.e., fusion of digits; Fig. 20-19*E*), or **disproportionate growth**, in which a part of the limb is abnormally larger, smaller, longer, or shorter, may be seen. In **deformations**, physical forces, for example, from **amniotic bands**, damage developing limbs (Fig. 20-19*F*). Table 20-1 lists a number of terms in common use to describe limb defects.

In addition to clinically significant defects of the limbs such as those just described, minor anomalies (variations of normal) are relatively common. Although a single **transverse palmar crease** (Fig. 20-20*A*) is often seen in infants with **trisomy 21 (Down syndrome)**, it is also found in 4% of normal newborns. Cutaneous syndactyly between toes two and three is considered a normal variant if the fusion extends less than one third the length of the toes (Fig. 20-20*B*).

Limb skeletal defects are very obvious during an ultrasound scan and may indicate a more widespread syndrome due to shared gene signaling networks. For example, 15% of polydactylies are associated with other defects and may indicate a defect in Shh signaling. A radial abnormality could indicate Holt-Oram syndrome, also characterized by cardiac abnormalities, TAR (thrombocytopenia-absent radius), or Fanconi's anemia. Sandal-gap deformity, where the big toe and second toe are wide apart, occurs in 45% of Down syndrome patients, although it is also a normal variant. Detection of limb abnormalities in the ultrasound scan may be the first step toward diagnosis of a syndrome at an early stage, which will aid parental counseling and in some instances may result in fetal therapies (see Chapter 6).

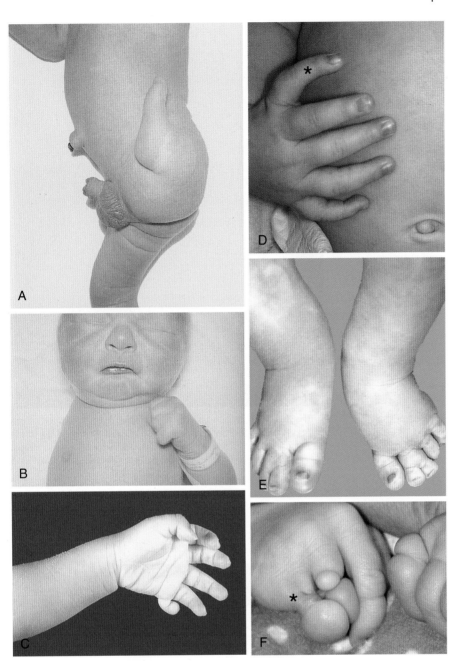

Figure 20-19. Limb defects in humans. *A,* Meromelia. In this example, the distal end of the infant's left lower limb has not completely formed. *B,* Amelia. In this example, the infant's entire right upper limb failed to form. *C,* Postaxial polydactyly (in this case, six digits). *D,* Right hand of an infant with a triphalangeal thumb (asterisk; three phalanges in digit one, rather than the normal two). *E,* Feet of an infant showing syndactyly; the bony elements of toes two and three are also fused. *F,* Hand of an infant with amniotic band–associated terminal limb defects. Note on the right hand, syndactyly (asterisk) proximal to the constriction and swelling distal to the constriction.

Genetic Causes of Limb Anomalies

Various gene mutations causing limb anomalies due to alterations in patterning, outgrowth, or cell differentiation have been characterized in humans. The generation of animal models has also highlighted the conservation of signaling pathways across species. For example, mutations in WNT3 (a member of the Drosophila Wingless family) have been linked to **tetra-amelia** in humans and other vertebrates, reflecting the requirement for Wnt signaling in limb bud initiation and outgrowth.

Shh is a central player in limb development, and it is not surprising that loss of SHH results in **acheiropodia**, a severe defect that includes absence of the hands and feet. This is due to a large (5-6 Kb) deletion in the LMBR1 gene, which is adjacent to the SHH gene and very likely disrupts the regulatory elements that control expression of SHH in the caudal limb bud. Shh expression in the ZPA is also regulated by a highly conserved ZPA regulatory sequence (ZRS), which promotes Shh expression in the ZPA while inhibiting ectopic Shh expression in the anterior mesenchyme. Point mutations in the ZRS that cause polydactyly, as a result of expansion of the ZPA or ectopic cranial limb bud expression, have been identified in humans as well as in other species. In humans these preaxial duplications range from the mildest phenotype of a **triphalangeal thumb** to more severe phenotypes of up to several additional digits (**polydactyly**) on the hands and/or feet (an example of such a severe duplication in humans, although of unknown genetic cause, is shown in Fig. 20-21).

Gli3, a component of Shh signaling, is essential for limb bud development. Gli3 heterozygous and homozygous mouse

TABLE 20-1 SOME COMMON TERMS FOR LIMB MALFORMATIONS

Term	Definition
Acheiropodia	Absence of the hands and feet
Adactyly	Absence of all digits on a limb
Amelia, ectromelia	Absence of one or more limbs
Arachnodactyly	Elongated digits
Brachydactyly	Shortened digits
Camptodactyly	Flexion contracture of a finger (often fourth or fifth), which cannot be fully extended
Clinodactyly	Curving of fifth finger toward the fourth
Ectrodactyly	Longitudinal divisions of the autopod into two parts, often with absence of central digits (also called split-hand or split-foot malformation)
Meromelia	Absence of part of a limb
Mesomelia	Shortened zeugopod
Oligodactyly	Absence of any number of fingers or toes
Phocomelia	Absence of proximal limb structures
Polydactyly	Presence of extra digits or parts of digits
Rhizomelia	Shortened stylopod
Syndactyly	Fusion of digits
Synostosis	Fusion of bones or intervening soft tissue
Triphalangeal thumb	A thumb with three rather than two phalanges

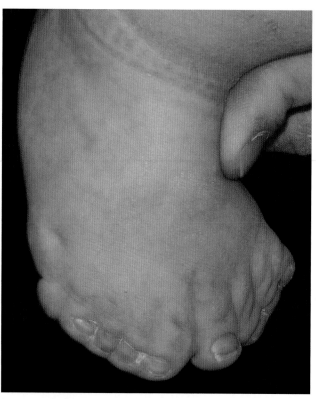

Figure 20-21. Foot of a child with mirror-imaged duplicated hands and feet (Laurin-Sandrow syndrome). Although the cause of the duplication is unknown in this syndrome, based on experiments in animal models, it is likely to involve ectopic SHH signaling in the cranial limb bud mesenchyme.

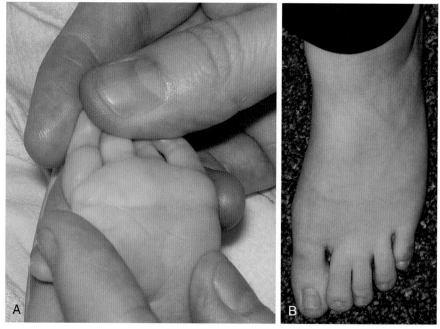

Figure 20-20. *A,* Single transverse palmar crease can occur in individuals with certain syndromes or can be a normal variant. *B,* Cutaneous syndactyly of toes two and three, without fusion of bony elements. This case would be considered a normal variant because cutaneous fusion extends less than one third the length of the toes. Compare this case to that shown in Figure 20-19*E.*

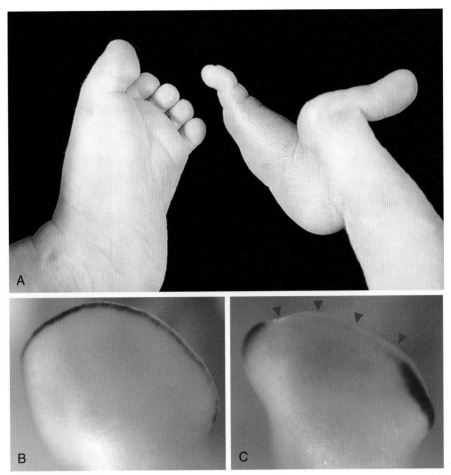

Figure 20-22. Split-foot anomaly. *A,* Photograph showing a child with a unilateral split-foot anomaly. *B, C,* Fgf8 expression in a wild-type mouse limb bud and in the Dlx5/6 double-mutant limb bud. Note the absence of Fgf8 expression in the central region of the apical ectodermal ridge (red arrowheads). Failure of this portion of the ridge to develop properly likely explains split-hand and split-foot anomalies, as shown in part *A.*

mutants have polydactylous limbs, showing that the level of expression of Gli3 controls digit number (see Fig. 20-15*D*). Mutations in GLI3 result in **Greig cephalopolysyndactyly**, **Pallister-Hall syndrome**, and **post-axial polydactyly type A**, all characterized by polydactyly. The Greig cephalopolysyndactyly syndrome is characterized by pre-axial and post-axial polydactyly of the feet and hands, respectively, and is due to loss of function of one copy of GLI3 (i.e., haploinsufficiency). In contrast, Pallister-Hall syndrome is characterized by central or insertional polydactyly, and mutant GLI3 proteins are thought to retain some GLI3 repressor activity.

Mesenchymal factors regulating Shh expression also result in limb defects. Mutation in TBX3 results in the autosomal dominant disorder **ulnar-mammary syndrome**. In this syndrome, the caudal side of the limb is affected, with reduction or complete loss of the ulna and posterior digits, as well as mammary gland defects. This phenotype is recapitulated in the Tbx3 mutant mouse, where analysis of the limb buds has shown that Shh is not expressed, explaining the loss of caudal limb structures. Two other T-Box transcription factors, Tbx4 and Tbx5, are restricted to the hindlimb and forelimb, respectively; this is reflected in the human syndromes resulting from mutations in these genes. Mutation in TBX4 causes **small patella syndrome**, whereas mutation in TBX5 results in **Holt-Oram syndrome**, which affects the forelimb (but not hindlimb) and heart. Mutation in PITX1, which regulates TBX4 expression, results in **congenital clubfoot** (see Fig. 20-25),

which can include patellar hypoplasia and tibial hemimelia.

Induction and maintenance of the AER are essential for limb outgrowth. Mutations in the transcription factor TP73L (also known as P63) result in **split-hand/split-foot type 4 syndrome** (Fig. 20-22*A*). These mutations can lead as well to **ectrodactyly-ectodermal dysplasia-clefting (EEC) syndrome**, which in part is also characterized by a split-hand and split-foot anomaly (a condition referred to as **ectrodactyly**). In p63 mouse mutants, the AER does not form appropriately and Fgf8 signaling is decreased, providing a potential mechanism, as the AER (or part of the AER) may degenerate prematurely. The transcription factors Dlx5 and Dlx6 are expressed in the AER, and a split-hand or split-foot anomaly is also seen in mouse Dlx5/6 double mutants. In these double mutants, analysis of AER markers clearly shows that the AER degenerates centrally, providing a mechanism for loss of the central digits (Fig. 20-22*B, C*). DLX5 mutations have also been identified in humans with split-hand and split-foot syndrome.

Reflecting their key roles in limb outgrowth and patterning, mutations in the Hox gene family have been identified in human syndromes. Mutation in HOXD13 results in **synpolydactyly and brachydactyly types D** and **E** (Fig. 20-23), whereas mutation in HOXA13 results in **hand-foot-genital syndrome**. HOXD11 mutations result in defects in more proximal limb structures in **radioulnar synostosis** (partial or full fusion of the radius and ulna with one another) with **amegakaryocytic thrombocytopenia syndrome**. The differential effects of

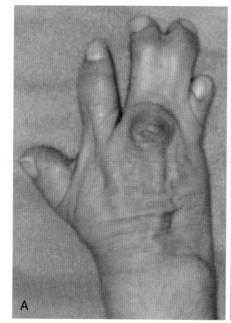

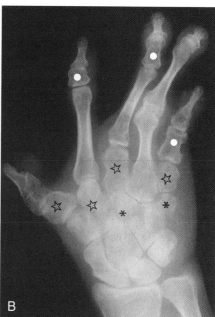

Figure 20-23. Hand (*A*) and radiograph (*B*) of a homozygous individual with a HOXD13 mutation. Note syndactyly of digits three-five, their single knuckle, transformation of metacarpals one, two, three, and five to short carpal-like bones (stars), two additional carpal bones (asterisks), and short second phalanges (white dots) in digits two, three, and five. The radius, ulna, and proximal carpal bones appear normal.

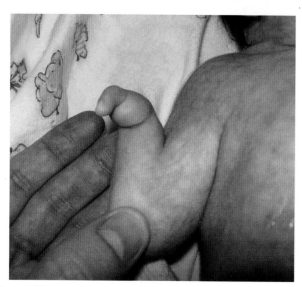

Figure 20-24. Severe upper limb defect in an infant with Cornelia de Lange syndrome. The autopod terminates in a single digit (monodactyly).

HOXD13 and HOXD11 mutations on the autopod and zeugopod reflect their differential requirements in patterning and growth of these regions of the limb (see Figs. 20-8, 20-9, 20-10).

A classical multiple malformation syndrome associated with limb anomalies is **Cornelia de Lange syndrome** (CdLS), first described in 1933. Most patients with this syndrome have upper limb anomalies ranging from small hands to severe limb reduction defects (Fig. 20-24). It was recently discovered that 50% of CdLS patients have mutations in the NIPBL gene (ortholog of the Drosophila nipped-B–like gene), which encodes a protein called DELANGIN. The function of this protein is unclear, but it seems to regulate the activity of other genes involved in development via its role in regulating chromatin organization.

Once specified, the skeletal elements must grow appropriately. Brachydactyly, shortening of the phalanges, is caused by a variety of mutations (GDF5, ROR2, IHH) that affect the generation and differentiation of chondrogenic precursors at the tip of the limb by decreasing Bmp signaling (see Fig. 20-18). Brachydactyly can also be caused by a defect in the growth plate that forms at the epiphyses of developing phalanges (e.g., gain of function FGFR3 mutations that decrease the number of proliferating chondrogenic precursors within the growth plate; see Chapter 8 for further coverage).

The mutations above illustrate the consequences of factors that change patterning and growth of the limb bud, but cell death must also occur within the interdigital mesenchyme to sculpt the limbs. Failure of cell death will result in syndactyly, which can be simple, just involving the soft tissues, or complex, involving bony fusions. All mutations in factors that control this cell death (FGFR2, HOXD13) are linked to syndactyly (see Fig. 20-23).

Non-Genetic Causes of Limb Defects

As with other regions of the body, genetic mutations and environmental causes can result in abnormalities. A variety of drugs and environmental **teratogens** have been shown to cause limb defects in experimental animals. Some of these agents are associated with limb defects in humans. Agents that influence general cell metabolism or cell proliferation are likely to cause limb defects if administered during the period of limb morphogenesis. Such agents include chemotherapeutic agents such as **5'-fluoro-2-deoxyuridine**, an inhibitor of thymidylate synthetase, and **acetazolamide**, a carbonic anhydrase inhibitor used in the treatment of glaucoma.

Other drugs that induce limb malformations in laboratory animals and humans are the anticonvulsants **valproic acid** and **phenytoin**, the anticoagulant **warfarin**, and (as discussed in the "Clinical Taster" for this chapter) the antileprosy, anticancer drug **thalidomide** (also used to treat HIV-related mouth and throat ulcers). Non-therapeutic drugs that can induce limb malformations include **alcohol** and **cocaine**. Children with **fetal alcohol syndrome** can have hypoplasia of the distal digits, joint contractures, and radial limb defects. Cocaine abuse in pregnancy is associated with limb reduction defects.

Fetal-maternal environmental factors associated with limb defects include **gestational diabetes, congenital varicella infection**, and **hyperthermia**. Limb defects can also result from physical factors. For example, a constricted uterine environment caused by **oligohydramnios** (insufficient amniotic fluid;

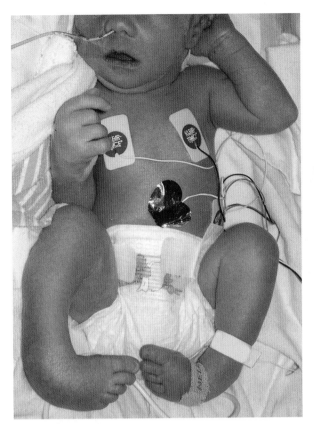

Figure 20-25. Newborn infant with bilateral talipes equinovarus deformity (clubfoot).

see Chapter 6) or reduced fetal movement can result in **clubfoot deformity (talipes equinovarus**; Fig. 20-25), and early **chorionic villus sampling** has been linked to an increased frequency of limb malformations. Vascular compromise in the fetus, due to vessel malformation or clots, has been proposed to be the cause of the unilateral limb anomalies seen in **Poland anomaly**.

TISSUE ORIGINS OF LIMB STRUCTURES

Quail-chick transplantation chimeras and genetically modified mice in which specific embryonic populations (e.g., neural crest) are permanently labeled with LacZ (covered in Chapter 5) have been used to study the cell populations that give rise to various tissues of the limbs. These studies have demonstrated that the lateral plate mesoderm gives rise to the **bones, ligaments, tendons,** and **dermis** of the limbs. In contrast, the limb **musculature** and **endothelial cells** migrate into the developing limb bud from the somites (covered in Chapter 8), and **melanocytes** and **Schwann cells** of the limb are derived from migrating neural crest cells (as occurs elsewhere in the body; covered in Chapter 4).

DIFFERENTIATION OF LIMB BONES

With the exception of the clavicle, which is in part a membrane bone, the limb skeletal elements form by endochondral ossification (covered in Chapter 8). The

mesenchyme of the limb buds first begins to condense in the fifth week. In general, the bones in the upper limb form slightly earlier than their counterparts in the lower limb. The proximal elements (i.e., the femur and humerus in the stylopod) differentiate first, and the distal elements (i.e., the digits in the autopod) differentiate last.

By the end of the fifth week, the mesenchymal condensation that will give rise to the proximal limb skeleton (scapula and humerus in the upper limb; pelvic bones and femur in the lower limb) is distinct. By the early sixth week, the mesenchymal rudiments of the distal limb skeleton are distinct in the upper and lower limbs, and chondrification commences in the humerus, ulna, and radius. By the end of the sixth week, carpal and metacarpal elements also begin to chondrify. In the lower limb, the femur, the tibia, and (to a lesser extent) the fibula begin to chondrify by the middle of the sixth week, and the tarsals and metatarsals begin to chondrify near the end of the sixth week. By the early seventh week, all skeletal elements of the upper limb except the distal phalanges of the second to fifth digits are undergoing chondrification. By the end of the seventh week, the distal phalanges of the hand have begun to chondrify, and chondrification is also under way in all elements of the lower limb except the distal row of phalanges. The distal phalanges of the toes do not chondrify until the eighth week.

The primary ossification centers of most of the limb long bones appear during weeks seven to twelve. By the early seventh week, ossification has commenced in the clavicle, followed by the humerus, radius, and ulna at the end of the seventh week. Ossification begins in the femur and tibia in the eighth week. During the ninth week, the scapula and ilium begin to ossify, followed in the next three weeks by the metacarpals, metatarsals, distal phalanges, proximal phalanges, and finally the middle phalanges. The ischium and pubis begin to ossify in the fifteenth and twentieth weeks, respectively, and ossification of the calcaneus finally begins at about sixteen weeks. Some of the smaller carpal and tarsal bones do not start ossification until early childhood.

Synovial joints (covered in Chapter 8) separate most of the skeletal elements. **Synchondroidal** or **fibrous joints**, such as those connecting the bones of the pelvis, also develop from interzones between forming bony elements, but the interzone mesenchyme simply differentiates into a single layer of fibrocartilage.

INNERVATION OF DEVELOPING LIMB

As described in Chapter 10, each spinal nerve splits into two main branches, the dorsal and ventral rami, shortly after it exits the spinal cord. The limb muscles are innervated by branches of the ventral rami of spinal nerves (Figs. 20-26, 20-27) C5 through T1/T2 (for the upper limb) and L4 through S3 (for the lower limb). Muscles originating in the dorsal muscle mass are served by dorsal branches of these ventral rami (arising from the LMCl neurons; covered in the following "In the Research Lab" entitled "Specification and Projection of Limb Motor Axons"), whereas muscles originating in the ventral muscle mass are served by ventral branches of the ventral rami (arising from the LMCm neurons; also covered in the following "In the Research Lab" entitled "Specification and Projection of Limb Motor Axons"). Thus, the innervation of a muscle shows whether it originated in the dorsal or the ventral muscle mass.

As illustrated in Figure 20-27, the motor axons that innervate the limbs perform an intricate feat of pathfinding to reach their target muscles. This is not dependent on muscles, as axons migrate almost normally in limbs lacking muscles. The ventral ramus axons destined for the limbs apparently travel to the base of the limb bud

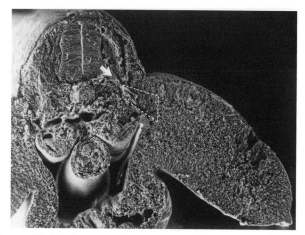

Figure 20-26. Scanning electron micrograph of a transversely sectioned embryo showing axons (arrow) entering the base of the limb bud (dotted area).

by growing along **permissive pathways**. The **growth cones** of these axons avoid or are unable to penetrate regions of dense mesenchyme or mesenchyme-containing glycosaminoglycans. The axons heading for the lower limb are thus deflected around the developing pelvic anlagen. In both the upper and lower limb buds, the axons from the nerves cranial to the limb bud grow toward the craniodorsal side of the limb bud, whereas the axons from the nerves caudal to the limb bud grow toward the ventrocaudal side of the limb bud (see Fig. 20-27).

Once the motor axons arrive at the base of the limb bud, they mix in a specific pattern to form the **brachial plexus** of the upper limb and the **lumbosacral plexus** of the lower limb. This zone thus constitutes a **decision-making region** for the axons (covered in the following "In the Research Lab" entitled "Specification and Projection of Limb Motor Axons").

Once the axons have sorted out in the plexus, the growth cones continue into the limb bud, presumably traveling along permissive pathways that lead in the general direction of the appropriate muscle compartment. Axons from the dorsal divisions of the plexuses tend to grow into the dorsal side of the limb bud and thus innervate mainly extensors, supinators, and abductor muscles; axons from the ventral divisions of the plexus grow into the ventral side of the limb bud and thus innervate mainly flexors, pronators, and adductor muscles. Over the very last part of an axon's path, axonal pathfinding is probably regulated by cues produced by the muscle itself. Similarly, local differences in cell

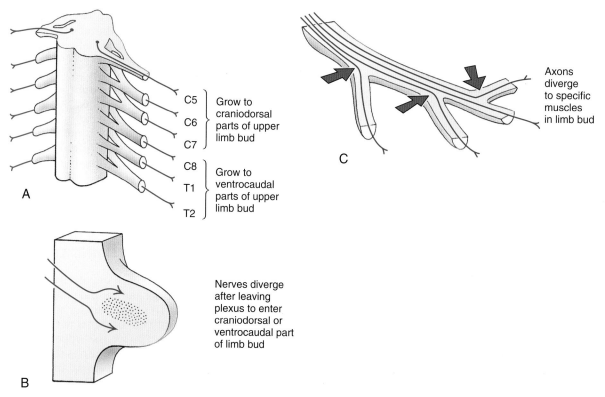

Figure 20-27. Growth of spinal nerve axons into the limb buds. *A, B,* Axons grow into the limb buds along permissive pathways. As the axons of the various spinal nerves mingle at the base of the limb buds to form the brachial and lumbosacral plexuses, each axon must "decide" whether to grow into the dorsal or ventral muscle mass. Factors that may play a role in directing axon growth include areas of dense mesenchyme or glycosaminoglycan-containing mesenchyme, which are avoided by outgrowing axons. *C,* Once the axons grow into the bud, decision points (arrows) under the control of "local factors" may regulate the invasion of specific muscle rudiments by specific axons.

surface molecules among muscle fibers most likely direct the final branching and distribution of axons within specific muscles.

As mentioned earlier in the chapter (see Fig. 20-11), the upper and lower limb buds rotate from their original orientation: basically, from a coronal orientation to a parasagittal orientation. Subsequently (between the sixth and eighth weeks), they also rotate around their long axis. The upper limb rotates laterally so that the elbow points caudally and the original ventral surface of the limb bud becomes the cranial surface of the limb. The lower limb rotates medially so that the knee points cranially and the original ventral surface of the limb bud becomes the caudal surface of the limb. As shown in Figure 20-28, this rotation causes the originally straight segmental pattern of lower limb innervation to twist into a spiral. The rotation of the upper limb is less extreme than that of the lower limb and is accomplished partly through caudal migration of the shoulder girdle. Moreover, some of the dermatomes in the upper limb bud exhibit overgrowth and come to dominate the limb surface.

In the Research Lab

SPECIFICATION AND PROJECTION OF LIMB MOTOR AXONS

A number of factors are thought to control axonal specification, migration, and projection, including the Lim and Hox homeobox proteins, Eph/ephrin signaling, Et-S transcription factors, and cell adhesion molecules such as type II cadherins and nCam. The motor neurons that innervate the limb bud form in the **lateral motor columns** (LMCs) within the neural tube in response to retinoic acid signaling from the paraxial mesoderm. The LMC has

two divisions consisting of LMCm (medial) and LMCl (lateral) neurons, which are distinguished by the differential expression of Lim homeobox proteins and project to the ventral and dorsal limb mesenchyme, respectively. LMCm neurons are Isl1 and Isl2 positive, whereas LMCl neurons express Lim1 and Isl2. Transplantation studies have shown that the axons have a remarkable ability to reach their appropriate targets. Thus, if the neural tube is shifted slightly along its cranial-caudal axis, the axons will still be able to project properly, being guided by a combination of local repulsive/attractive and chemoattractive cues.

LMCm and LMCl axons migrate along a common pathway to the plexus, where they pause and change their nearest neighbors: this resting period and the timing of subsequent ingrowth into the limb bud are determined by signals from the limb mesenchyme, such as ephrin and semaphorin 3A. At the junction of Lmxb1-expressing and non-expressing mesenchyme, a decision is made as to whether to enter the dorsal and ventral limb mesenchyme (Fig. 20-29A). LMCl neurons require Lim1 and its downstream target, EphA4, to project appropriately into the dorsal mesenchyme. EphA4 axons avoid the ventral mesenchyme, which expresses high levels of ephrin-A2 and ephrin-A5. In the absence of Lim1, the LMCl neurons project randomly (Fig. 20-29B). Likewise, in EphA4 mutant mice, the LMCl neurons project abnormally, but in this case, they all enter the ventral limb mesenchyme (Fig. 20-29C). In the converse situation, ectopic misexpression of EphA4 results in the LMCm neurons projecting dorsally. Similar repulsive interactions "force/guide" the LMCm neurons to enter the ventral mesenchyme: a subset of LMCm neurons express the secreted semaphorin co-receptor neuropilin 2 and avoid the semaphorin 3F-expressing dorsal mesenchyme. Loss of function of Lmx1b, which controls dorsal-ventral limb identity (covered in the preceding "In the Research Lab" in the section entitled "Specification of Dorsal-Ventral Axis,") results in the random projection of both LMCm and LMCl neurons (Fig. 20-29D).

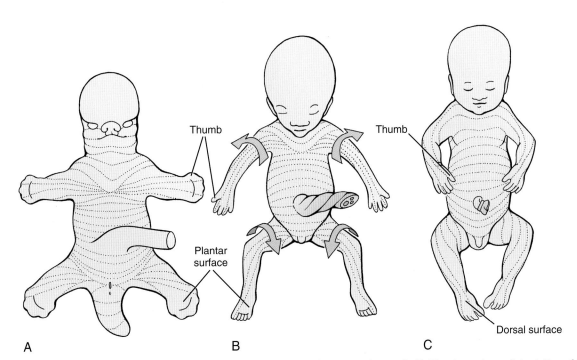

Figure 20-28. Rotation of the limbs. *A, B, C,* Indicate sequential stages in limb rotation (arrows in *B*). The dramatic medial rotation of the lower limbs during the sixth to eighth weeks causes the mature dermatomes to spiral down the limbs. The configuration of the upper limb dermatomes is partially modified by more limited lateral rotation of the upper limb during the same period.

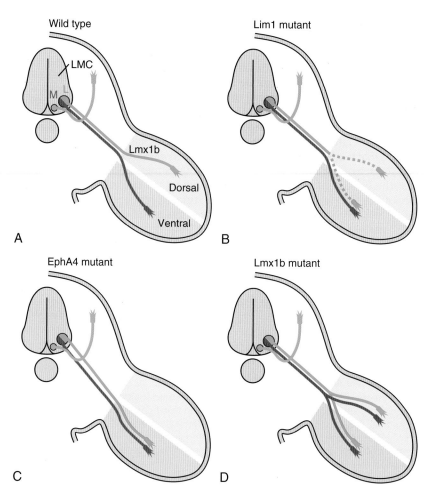

Figure 20-29. Motor columns and their axonal projections in wild-type and mutant mice as seen in drawings of transverse sections. The median motor column and its axonal projections are shown in green. They innervate muscles (not shown) adjacent to the vertebral column and derived from the corresponding segmental somitic myotome. The lateral motor column consists of two divisions: LMCm (purple) and LMCl (blue), with their axonal projections going to the dorsal and ventral regions of the developing limbs, respectively. *A,* Wild-type mouse. *B-D,* Lim1, EphA4, and Lmx1b mutant mice, respectively.

Embryology in Practice

WHEN THINGS DON'T FIT

A three-year-old boy is seen in the genetics clinic for limb and cardiac anomalies with the concern that he might have a congenital syndrome. The referring physician specifically requested evaluation of the boy for the "heart and hand" syndrome.

On examination, the boy is found to have symmetric upper limb anomalies (Fig. 20-30) consisting of absent thumbs, abnormal index fingers, short, curved fifth fingers, and lack of palmar creases. Both index fingers have circumferential nail formation (i.e., the nails encircled the tips of the digits). His forearms are short. He also has absent nipples and underdeveloped pectoralis muscles bilaterally. X-rays of his upper extremities show absence of bilateral radii and thumb bones and shortening of both ulnae. Echocardiography previously showed a moderately large atrial septal defect (ASD) and a small muscular ventricular septal defect (VSD). His lower extremities are normal.

In general, it is more common for limb defects to affect *either* the radial *or* ulnar elements, with both elements affected only in rare instances. Added to this is the unusual combination of heart defects and mammary abnormalities that do not fit together.

Radial ray anomalies with heart defects would suggest **Holt-Oram** (also known as "heart and hand") **syndrome**, caused by mutations in the TBX5 gene. However, absent nipples and ulnar ray anomalies are not seen in this syndrome and

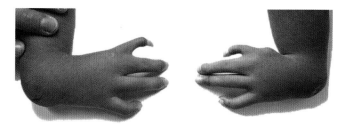

Figure 20-30. Upper limbs in a child with both Holt-Oram and ulnar-mammary syndromes.

would be more consistent with **ulnar-mammary syndrome**, caused by mutations in the TBX3 gene. Genetic testing for either or both of these genes could be considered equally.

While discussing the diagnostic approach to this seemingly disparate constellation of findings, an astute genetics fellow has a hypothesis. In looking up the genetic test information for the TBX3 and TBX5 genes, she notices that they map to the same chromosomal band. Querying the genome browser shows that these genes lie side by side on chromosome 12, spanning only 340 kilobases of DNA.

With this knowledge in hand, instead of single gene testing, she orders cytogenomic microarray analysis that uncovers a small deletion in this patient, confirming the diagnoses of *both* Holt-Oram and ulnar-mammary syndromes.

SUGGESTED READINGS

Anderson E, Peluso S, Lettice LA, Hill RE. 2012. Human limb abnormalities caused by disruption of hedgehog signaling. Trends Genet 28:364–373.

Bastida MF, Ros MA. 2008. How do we get a perfect complement of digits? Curr Opin Genet Dev 18:374–380.

Fernandez-Teran M, Ros MA. 2008. The apical ectodermal ridge: morphological aspects and signaling pathways. Int J Dev Biol 52: 857–871.

Hernandez-Martinez R, Covarrubias L. 2011. Interdigital cell death function and regulation: new insights on an old programmed cell death model. Dev Growth Differ 53:245–258.

Kao TJ, Law C, Kania A. 2012. Eph and ephrin signaling: lessons learned from spinal motor neurons. Semin Cell Dev Biol 23:83–91.

Polleux F, Ince-Dunn G, Ghosh A. 2007. Transcriptional regulation of vertebrate axon guidance and synapse formation. Nat Rev Neurosci 8:331–340.

Rabinowitz AH, Vokes SA. 2012. Integration of the transcriptional networks regulating limb morphogenesis. Dev Biol 368:165–180.

Stricker S, Mundlos S. 2011. Mechanisms of digit formation: human malformation syndromes tell the story. Dev Dyn 240:990–1004.

Suzuki T, Hasso SM, Fallon JF. 2008. Unique SMAD1/5/8 activity at the phalanx-forming region determines digit identity. Proc Natl Acad Sci USA 105:4185–4190.

Towers M, Tickle C. 2009. Growing models of vertebrate limb development. Development 136:179–190.

Zakany J, Duboule D. 2007. The role of Hox genes during vertebrate limb development. Curr Opin Genet Dev 17:359–366.

Zeller R, Lopez-Rios J, Zuniga A. 2009. Vertebrate limb bud development: moving towards integrative analysis of organogenesis. Nat Rev Genet 10:845–858.

Figure Credits

Cover photo. Courtesy of Dr. Robert E. Waterman and the University of New Mexico, Albuquerque.

Figure Intro-1. Adapted from Gasser RF. 1975. Atlas of Human Embryos. Harper and Row, New York.

Figure Intro-2. Courtesy of the Progeria Research Foundation and the child's parents.

Figure Intro-3. Courtesy of Drs. Kohei Shiota and Shigehito Yamada and Ms. Chigako Uwabe, Congenital Anomaly Research Center, Kyoto University Graduate School of Medicine.

Figure Intro-5. Adapted from Moore KL, Persaud TVN. 2003. The Developing Human. Clinically Oriented Embryology, Seventh Edition. Saunders, Philadelphia.

Table Intro-1. Adapted largely from O'Rahilly R, Müller F. 1987. Developmental Stages in Human Embryos. Carnegie Institute, Washington, DC, Publ. No. 637.

Figure 1-1. *B, C*, Adapted from Witschi E. 1948. Migration of the germ cells of human embryos from the yolk sac to the primitive gonadal folds. Contrib Embryol (No. 209) 32:67-80. Original source for scanning provided courtesy of Dr. John M. Optiz.

Figure 1-1. *D, E*, Courtesy of Drs. Peter Nichol and A. Shaaban.

Figure 1-4. Inset photo in *B* courtesy of Dr. Daniel S. Friend. *C*, Courtesy of Drs. Gary Schatten and Calvin Simerly.

Figure 1-7. *A*, From Phillips DM, Shalgi R. 1980. Surface architecture of the mouse and hamster zona pellucida and oocyte. J Ultrastruct Res 72:1-12. *B*, Courtesy of Dr. David M. Phillips.

Figure 1-8. *B*, Courtesy of Dr. Arthur Brothman.

Figures 1-9, 1-10. *A, B*, Courtesy of Dr. Sarah South.

Figure 1-10. *A*, Courtesy of Dr. Arthur Brothman. *B*, Courtesy of Dr. Sarah South.

Figure 1-11. Courtesy of Dr. Sarah South.

Figure 1-12. *B*, Courtesy of Drs. Gary Schatten and Calvin Simerly.

Figure 1-14. *B, C*, Courtesy of Dr. David M. Phillips.

Figure 1-15. Courtesy of Drs. Gary Schatten and Calvin Simerly.

Figure 1-16. From Boatman DE. 1987. In vitro growth of nonhuman primate pre- and peri-implantation embryos. In Bavister BD (ed): The Mammalian Preimplantation Embryo. Plenum, New York. Photos courtesy of Drs. Barry Bavister and D.E. Boatman.

Figure 1-17. From Nikas G, Asangla A, Winston RML, Handyside AH. 1996. Compaction and surface polarity in the human embryo in vitro. Biol Reprod 55:32-37. Photos courtesy of Dr. G. Nikas.

Figure 1-19. Courtesy of Dr. I. Santiago Alvarez.

Figure 1-20. Courtesy of Dr. Michael J. Tucker, Georgia Reproductive Specialists.

Figure 1-21. Courtesy of Dr. I. Santiago Alvarez.

Figure 2-7. From the Digitally Reproduced Embryonic Morphology (DREM) project, courtesy of Dr. Ray Gasser.

Figure 2-9. Courtesy of Dr. Tariq Siddiqi.

Figure 2-12. Adapted from Reik W, Walter J. 2001. Genomic imprinting: parental influence on the genome. Nat Rev Genet 2:21-32.

Figure 3-1. Adapted from Reuters.

Figure 3-5. From Sulik K, Dehart DB, Inagaki T, et al. 1994. Morphogenesis of the murine node and notochordal plate. Dev Dyn 201:260-278.

Figure 3-6. *A*, Adapted from Yost HJ. 2003. Left-right asymmetry: nodal cilia make and catch a wave. Curr Biol 13:R808-R809. *B*, Adapted from McGrath J, Somlo S, Makova S, et al. 2003. Two populations of node monocilia initiate left-right asymmetry in the mouse. Cell 114:61-73.

Figure 3-7. *C*, From Schoenwolf GC. 2001. Laboratory Studies of Vertebrate and Invertebrate Embryos. Guide and Atlas of Descriptive and Experimental Development. Eighth Edition. Prentice Hall, New Jersey.

Figure 3-9. From Tamarin A. 1983. Stage 9 macaque embryos studied by electron microscopy. J Anat 137:765-779.

Figure 3-14. From Schoenwolf GC. 2001. Laboratory Studies of Vertebrate and Invertebrate Embryos. Guide and Atlas of Descriptive and Experimental Development. Eighth Edition. Prentice Hall, New Jersey.

Figure 3-17. Courtesy of Dr. Olivier Pourquie. *A-F*, Adapted from McGrew MJ, Dale JK, Fraboulet S, Pourquie O. 1998. The lunatic fringe gene is a target of the molecular clock linked to somite segmentation in avian embryos. Curr Biol 8:979-982. *G-J*, Adapted from Dubrulle J, McGrew MJ, Pourquie O. 2001. FGF signaling controls somite boundary position and regulates segmentation clock control of spatiotemporal Hox gene activation. Cell 106:219-232.

Figure 3-18. Adapted from Pourquie O. 2004. The chick embryo: a leading model in somitogenesis studies. Mech Dev 121:1069-1079.

Figure 3-19. Adapted from Smith JL, Schoenwolf GC. 1998. Getting organized: new insights into the organizer of higher vertebrates. Curr Topics Dev Biol 40:79-110.

Figure 3-21. From Tamarin A. 1983. Stage 9 macaque embryos studied by electron microscopy. J Anat 137:765-779.

Figure 3-22. From the Digitally Reproduced Embryonic Morphology (DREM) project, courtesy of Dr. Ray Gasser.

Figure 3-23. *A,* Courtesy of Dr. Doug Melton. *B,* From Steinbeisser H, De Robertis EM, Ku M, et al. 1993. Xenopus axis formation: induction of goosecoid by injected X-wnt-8 and activin mRNAs. Development 118:499-507.

Figure 3-24. *A,* Courtesy of Dr. Mahua Mukhopadhyay. From Mukhopadhyay M, Shtrom S, Rodriguez-Esteban C, et al. 2001. Dickkopf1 is required for embryonic head induction and limb morphogenesis in the mouse. Dev Cell 1:423-434. *B,* Courtesy of William Shawlot. From Shawlot W, Behringer RR. 1995. Requirement for Lim1 in head-organizer function. Nature 374:425-430.

Figure 4-1. *A,* Courtesy of Dr. Janice L.B. Byrne. *B,* Courtesy of Dr. Earl Downey.

Figure 4-3. Courtesy of Dr. Arnold Tamarin.

Figure 4-4. *A,* Courtesy of Dr. Janice L.B. Byrne. *B-D,* Courtesy of Drs. Peter Nichol and A. Shaaban.

Figure 4-5. *B,* Courtesy of Dr. Kohei Shiota. From Yamada S, Uwabe C, Nakatsu-Komatsu T, et al. 2006. Graphics and movie illustrations of human prenatal development and their application to embryological education based on the human embryo specimens in the Kyoto collection. Dev Dyn 235:468-477. *C,* Adapted from Schoenwolf GC. 2001. Laboratory Studies of Vertebrate and Invertebrate Embryos. Guide and Atlas of Descriptive and Experimental Development. Eighth Edition. Prentice Hall, New Jersey. Courtesy of Dr. Robert E. Waterman.

Figure 4-6. Adapted from Schoenwolf GC. 2001. Laboratory Studies of Vertebrate and Invertebrate Embryos. Guide and Atlas of Descriptive and Experimental Development. Eighth Edition. Prentice Hall, New Jersey. From Colas JF, Schoenwolf GC. 2001. Towards a cellular and molecular understanding of neurulation. Dev Dyn 221:117-145.

Figure 4-8. Courtesy of Dr. Amel Gritli-Linde.

Figure 4-9. *A, C,* Courtesy of Dr. Takayuki Inagaki. *B,* Courtesy of Dr. John Carey.

Figures 4-11. *A, B;* **4-12.** *A, B;* **4-13.** *B,* Courtesy of Dr. John Kestle.

Figure 4-14. *A, B,* Courtesy of Dr. Takayuki Inagaki.

Figure 4-16. From Schoenwolf GC. 2001. Laboratory Studies of Vertebrate and Invertebrate Embryos. Guide and Atlas of Descriptive and Experimental Development. Eighth Edition. Prentice Hall, New Jersey. From Colas JF, Schoenwolf GC. 2001. Towards a cellular and molecular understanding of neurulation. Dev Dyn 221:117-145.

Figure 4-17. Photo courtesy of Drs. Antone Jacobson and Patrick Tam.

Figure 4-21. Redrawn from the data of D'Amico-Martel A, Noden DM. 1983. Contributions of placodal and neural crest cells to avian cranial peripheral ganglia. Am J Anat 166:445-468. Adapted from Baker C. 2005. Neural crest and cranial ectodermal placodes. In Rao MS, Jacobson M (eds): Developmental Neurobiology. Fourth Edition. Kluwer Academic/Plenum Publishers, New York.

Figure 4-23. Adapted from Farlie PG, McKeown SJ, Newgreen DF. 2004. The neural crest: basic biology and clinical relationships in the craniofacial and enteric nervous systems. Birth Defects Res C Embryo Today 72:173-189.

Figure 4-25. Adapted from Schoenwolf GC. 2001. Laboratory Studies of Vertebrate and Invertebrate Embryos. Guide and Atlas of Descriptive and Experimental Development. Eighth Edition. Prentice Hall, New Jersey.

Figure 4-26. Adapted from Brand-Saberi B, Christ B. 2000. Evolution and development of distinct cell lineages derived from somites. Curr Top Dev Biol 48: 1-42. Courtesy of Dr. Heinz Jacob.

Figure 5-1. *A,* Courtesy of Dr. Max Muenke. Adapted from El-Jaick KB, Powers SE, Bartholin L, et al. 2006. Functional analysis of mutations in TGIF associated with holoprosencephaly. Mol Genet Metab 90:97-111. *B,* Courtesy of Dr. Leslie Biesecker. Adapted from Biesecker LG. 2005. Mapping phenotypes to language: a proposal to organize and standardize the clinical descriptions of malformations. Clin Genet 68:320-326.

Figure 5-2. Courtesy of Dr. Susan Lewin and the child's family.

Figure 5-3. Courtesy of Dr. Roger A. Fleischman.

Figures 5-4, 5-5, 5-6, 5-7, 5-8, 5-9. Adapted from Wolpert L. 2002. Principles of Development. Oxford University Press, New York.

Figure 5-10. Adapted from Schoenwolf GC. 2001. Cutting, pasting and painting: experimental embryology and neural development. Nat Rev Neurosci 2:763-771.

Figure 5-11. *A-C,* Courtesy of Drs. Sophie Creuzet and Nichole Le Douarin. Adapted from Le Douarin NM. 2004. The avian embryo as a model to study the development of the neural crest: a long and still ongoing story. Mech Dev 121:1089-1102.

Figure 5-12. Adapted from Schoenwolf GC. 2001. Cutting, pasting and painting: experimental embryology and neural development. Nat Rev Neurosci 2:763-771.

Figures 5-13, 5-14. Adapted from Schoenwolf GC. 2001. Laboratory Studies of Vertebrate and Invertebrate Embryos. Guide and Atlas of Descriptive and Experimental Development. Eighth Edition. Prentice Hall, New Jersey.

Figure 5-15. Adapted from Schoenwolf GC. 2001. Cutting, pasting and painting: experimental embryology and neural development. Nat Rev Neurosci 2:763-771.

Figures 5-16, 5-17. Adapted from Nagy A, Gertsenstein M, Vintersten K, Behringer R. 2003. Manipulating the Mouse Embryo. A Laboratory Manual. Cold Spring Harbor, New York.

Figures 5-18, 5-19. Adapted from Wolpert L. 2002. Principles of Development. Oxford University Press, New York.

Figure 5-20. Adapted from Krumlauf R. 1993. Hox genes and pattern formation in the branchial region of the vertebrate head. Trends Genet 9:106-112.

Figure 5-21. Adapted from Kalthoff K. 2001. Analysis of Biological Development. McGraw-Hill Higher Education, New York. With permission from Prof. Klaus Kalthoff.

Figure 5-22. Adapted from Logan CY, Nusse R, 2004. The Wnt signaling pathway in development and disease. Annu Rev Cell Dev Biol 20:781-810.

Figure 5-23. Adapted from McMahon AP, Ingham PW, Tabin CJ. 2003. Developmental roles and clinical significance of hedgehog signaling. Curr Top Dev Biol 53:1-114.

Figure 5-24. Adapted from Massague J, Chen YG. 2000. Controlling TGF-beta signaling. Genes Dev 14:627-644.

Figure 5-25. Adapted from Wolpert L. 2002. Principles of Development. Oxford University Press, New York.

Figures 5-26, 5-27. Adapted from Gilbert SF. 2006. Developmental Biology. Eighth Edition. Sinauer Associates, Sunderland, Massachusetts.

Figure 5-28. Adapted from Maden M. 2002. Retinoid signalling in the development of the central nervous system. Nat Rev Neurosci 3:843-853.

Figure 6-1. Courtesy of Dr. Robert E. Waterman and the University of New Mexico School of Medicine, Albuquerque.

Figure 6-3. Adapted from Benirschke K. 1998. Remarkable placenta. Clin Anat 11:194-205.

Figure 6-4. From Castellucci M, Scheper M, Scheffen I, et al. 1990. The development of the human placental villous tree. Anat Embryol (Berl) 181:117-128.

Figure 6-7. *A, B,* Courtesy of Dr. Janice L. B. Byrne.

Figure 6-9. *A, B,* Courtesy of Drs. Peter Nichol and A. Shaaban.

Figure 6-10. Courtesy of the fetuses' parents.

Figure 6-11. Courtesy of Babies First Ultrasound, San Diego, California; www.bfiultrasound.com/default.html.

Figure 6-12. Courtesy of Dr. Gregorio Acacio, Hospital Israelita Albert Einstein, Sao Paulo, Brazil.

Figures 6-13, 6-14. Adapted from Jorde LB, Carey JC, Bamshad MJ, White RL. 2006. Medical Genetics. Third Edition, Updated Edition. Mosby, St Louis.

Figure 6-15. Adapted from Harrison MR, Adzick NS, Longaker MT, et al. 1990. Successful repair in utero of a fetal diaphragmatic hernia after removal of herniated viscera from the left thorax. N Engl J Med 322:1582-1584.

Figure 6-16. From Jones HW, Scott WW. 1958. Hermaphroditism, Genital Anomalies and Related Endocrine Disorders. Williams & Wilkins, Baltimore.

Table 6-1. Adapted from BabyCenter; http://www.babycenter.com/general/pregnancy/1290794.html.

Figure 7-1. Courtesy of Dr. Alan Rope.

Figure 7-2. Adapted from Holbrook KA, Dale BA, Smith LT, et al. 1987. Markers of adult skin expressed in the skin of the first trimester fetus. Curr Probl Dermatol 16:94-108.

Figure 7-3. Adapted from Foster CA, Bertram JF, Holbrook KA.1988. Morphometric and statistical analyses describing the in utero growth of human epidermis. Anat Rec 222:201-206.

Figure 7-4. Adapted from Wilson A, Radtke F. 2006. Multiple functions of Notch signaling in self-renewing organs and cancer. FEBS Lett 580:2860-2868.

Figure 7-5. Adapted from Fuchs E, Raghavan S. 2002. Getting under the skin of epidermal morphogenesis. Nat Rev Genet 3:199-209.

Figure 7-6. *A,* Courtesy of Drs. John Harper and Alan Irvine. Adapted from Irvine AD, Christiano AM. 2001. Hair on a gene string: recent advances in understanding the molecular genetics of hair loss. Clin Exp Dermatol 26:59-71. *B,* Adapted from Utto J, McGrath JA. 2007. Diseases of epidermal keratins and their linker proteins. Exp Cell Res 313:1995-2009.

Figure 7-8. *A,* Adapted from Holbrook KA. 1988. Structural abnormalities of the epidermally derived appendages in skin from patients with ectodermal dysplasia: insight into developmental errors. Birth Defects Orig Artic Ser 24:15-44. *B,* Adapted from Foster CA, Holbrook KA. 1989. Ontogeny of Langerhans cells in human embryonic and fetal skin: cell densities and phenotypic expression relative to epidermal growth. Am J Anat 184:157-164.

Figure 7-9. Adapted from Williams PL, Warwick R, Dyson M, Bannister LH. 1989. Gray's Anatomy. Churchill Livingstone, Edinburgh.

Figure 7-10. Adapted from Mikkola JL, Millar SE. 2006. The mammary bud as a skin appendage: unique and shared aspects of development. J. Mammary Gland Biol Neoplasia 11:187-203.

Figure 7-11. Adapted from Holbrook KA. 1988. Structural abnormalities of the epidermally derived appendages in skin from patients with ectodermal dysplasia: insight into developmental errors. Birth Defects Orig Artic Ser 24:15-44.

Figure 7-12. *A,* Courtesy of Dr. Irma Thesleff. Adapted from Pispa J, Thesleff I. 2003. Mechanisms of ectodermal organogenesis. Dev Biol 262:195-205. *B-D,* Courtesy of Drs. Elaine Fuchs and Ramanuj DasGupta. Adapted from DasGupta R, Fuchs E. 1999. Multiple roles for activated LEF/TCF transcription complexes during hair follicle development and differentiation. Development 126:4557-4568.

Figure 7-15. *A, B, C,* Adapted from Holbrook KA. 1988. Structural abnormalities of the epidermally derived appendages in skin from patients with ectodermal dysplasia: insight into developmental errors. Birth Defects Orig Artic Ser 24:15-44. *D, E, F,* Adapted from Seitz CS, Hamm H. 2005. Congenital brachydactyly and nail hypoplasia. Brit J Dermatol 152:339-1342. *G, H,* Courtesy of Dr. Alexandra L. Joyner. Adapted from Guo Q, Loomis C, Joyner AL. 2003. Fate map of mouse ventral limb ectoderm and the apical ectodermal ridge. Dev Biol 264:166-178.

Figure 7-16. Courtesy of Dr. Irma Thesleff. Adapted from Mikkola ML, Thesleff I. 2003. Ectodysplasin signaling in development. Cytokine Growth Factor Rev 14:211-224.

Figure 8-1. Courtesy of Dr. Lynn Jorde. From Jorde LB, Carey JC, Bamshad MJ, White RL, 2006. Medical Genetics. Third Edition, Updated Edition. Mosby, St Louis.

Figure 8-2. Courtesy of Dr. Michael Owen. Adapted from Otto F, Thornell AP, Crompton T, et al. 1997. Cbfa1, a candidate gene for cleidocranial dysplasia syndrome, is essential for osteoblast differentiation and bone development. Cell 89:765-771.

Figure 8-3. *A,* Adapted from Buckingham M, Bajard L, Chang T, et al. 2003. The formation of skeletal muscle: from somite to limb. J Anat 202:59-68. *B,* Adapted from Schoenwolf GC. 2001. Laboratory Studies of Vertebrate and Invertebrate Embryos. Guide and Atlas of Descriptive and Experimental Development. Eighth Edition. Prentice Hall, New Jersey. *C,* Adapted from Brand-Saberi B, Christ B. 2000. Evolution and development of distinct cell lineages derived from somites. Curr Top Dev Biol 48:1-42. Courtesy of Dr. Heinz Jacob.

Figure 8-5. Courtesy of Drs. Cathy Krull and Marianne Bronner-Fraser. Adapted from Krull CE, Lansford R, Gale NW, et al. 1997. Interactions of Eph-related receptors and ligands confer rostrocaudal pattern to trunk neural crest migration. Curr Biol 7:571-580.

Figure 8-10. Adapted from Hunt P, Krumlauf R. 1992. Hox codes and positional specification in vertebrate embryonic axes. Annu Rev Cell Biol 8:227-256.

Figure 8-11. A, Adapted from Wellik DM. 2007. *Hox* patterning of the vertebrate axial skeleton. Dev Dyn 236:2454-2463. B, Courtesy of Dr. Mario Capecchi. Adapted from Wellik DM, Capecchi MR. 2003. Hox10 and Hox11 genes are required to globally pattern the mammalian skeleton. Science 301:363-367. C, Courtesy of Dr. Moises Mallo. Adapted from Carapuco M, Novoa A, Bobola N, Mallo M. 2005. Hox genes specify vertebral types in the presomitic mesoderm. Genes Dev 19:2116-2121.

Figure 8-12. Adapted from Conlon RA. 1995. Retinoic acid and pattern formation in vertebrates. Trends Genet 11:314-319, p. 316, Fig. 2. Lohnes D. 2003. The Cdx1 homeodomain protein: an integrator of posterior signaling in the mouse. Bioessays 25:971-980.

Figure 8-13. A, Courtesy of Dr. Peter D. Turnpenny. Adapted from Whittock NV, Sparrow DB, Wouters MA, et al. 2004. Mutated MESP2 causes spondylocostal dysostosis in humans. Am. J Hum Genet 74:1249-1254. B, C, Courtesy of Drs. Ian Krantz and Kenro Kusumi. Adapted from Pourquie O, Kusumi K. 2001. When body segmentation goes wrong. Clin Genet 60:409-416.

Figure 8-15. Adapted from Buckingham M. 2006. Myogenic progenitor cells and skeletal myogenesis in vertebrates. Curr Opin Genet Dev 16:525-532.

Figure 8-16. A, B, Adapted from Kronenberg HM. 2003. Developmental regulation of the growth plate. Nature 423:332-336. B, Also adapted from Hartmann C, Tabin CJ. 2000. Dual roles of Wnt signaling during chondrogenesis in the chicken limb. Development 127:3141-3159.

Figure 8-18. Adapted from Francis-West PH, Abdelfattah A, Chen P, et al. 1999. Mechanisms of GDF-5 action during skeletal development. Development 126:1305-1315.

Figure 8-19. Courtesy of Drs. Frank Luyten and J. Terrig Thomas. Adapted from Thomas JT, Kilpatrick MW, Lin K, et al. 1997. Disruption of human limb morphogenesis by a dominant negative mutation in CDMP1. Nat Genet 17:58-64.

Figure 8-20. Courtesy of Dr. Bjorn Olsen. Adapted from Zelzer E, Olsen BR. 2003. The genetic basis for skeletal diseases. Nature 423:343-348.

Figure 8-22. Adapted from Chevallier A, Kieny M, Mauger A. 1977. Limb-somite relationship: origin of the limb musculature. J Embryol Exp Morphol 41:245-258.

Figure 8-23. A, Courtesy of Dr. C. Birchmeier. Adapted from Brohmann H, Jagla K, Birchmeier C. 2000. The role of Lbx1 in migration of muscle precursor cells. Development 127:437-445. B, Adapted from Buckingham M, Bajard L, Chang T, et al. 2003. The formation of skeletal muscle: from somite to limb. J Anat 202:59-68.

Figure 8-24. Adapted from Tzahor E. 2009. Heart and craniofacial muscle development: a new developmental theme of distinct myogenic fields. Dev Biol 327, 273-279.

Figure 8-25. Courtesy of Dr. Theodore Pysher.

Table 8-1. Data from Crafts RC. 1985. A Textbook of Human Anatomy. Third Edition. Churchill Livingstone, New York.

Figure 9-2. A, B, Adapted from Kiecker C, Lumsden A, 2005. Compartments and their boundaries in vertebrate brain development. Nat Rev Neurosci 6:553-564. C, Adapted from Rowitch DH. 2004. Glial specification in the vertebrate neural tube. Nat Rev Neurosci 5:409-419.

Figure 9-3. A, Adapted from Rakic P, 1982. Early developmental events: cell lineages, acquisition of neuronal positions, and areal and laminar development. Neurosci Res Prog Bull 20:439-451. B, Courtesy of Dr. Kathryn Tosney.

Figures 9-5, 9-10. Adapted from Williams PL, Warwick R, Dyson M, Bannister LH. 1989. Gray's Anatomy. Churchill Livingstone, Edinburgh.

Figure 9-12. Courtesy of Boston Children's Hospital, Dr. Benjamin Warf, and Ms. Meghan Weber.

Figure 9-16. Adapted from Roberts A, Taylor JSH. 1983. A study of the growth cones of developing embryonic sensory neurites. J Embryol Exp Morphol 75:31-47.

Figure 9-18. Adapted from Lambot MA, Depasse F, Noel JC, Vanderhaeghen P. 2005. Mapping labels in the human developing visual system and the evolution of binocular vision. J Neurosci 25:7232-7237.

Figure 9-19. From Colello RJ, Guillery RW. 1990. The early development of retinal ganglion cells with uncrossed axons in the mouse: retinal position and axomal course. Development 108:515-523.

Figure 9-20. Adapted from McLaughlin T, Hindges R, O'Leary DD. 2003. Regulation of axial patterning of the retina and its topographic mapping in the brain. Curr Opin Neurobiol 13:57-69.

Figure 9-21. G, Courtesy of Dr. Arnold Tamarin.

Figure 9-24. Courtesy of Dr. Andrew Lumsden.

Figure 9-27. Adapted from Bond J, Roberts E, Mochida GH, et al. 2002. ASPM is a major determinant of cerebral cortical size. Nat Genet 32:316-320.

Figure 10-1. A, B, From Bonkowsky JL, Johnson J, Carey JC, et al. 2003. An infant with primary tooth loss and palmar hyperkeratosis: a novel mutation in the NTRK1 gene causing congenital insensitivity to pain with anhidrosis. Pediatrics 112:e237-e241. Courtesy of Dr. Josh Bonkowsky.

Figure 10-2. Courtesy of Dr. Maya Sieber-Blum.

Figure 10-3. Courtesy of Dr. Carol Erickson.

Figure 10-5. B, Courtesy of Drs. James Weston and Michael Marusich.

Figure 10-6. Courtesy of Teri Belecky-Adams and Dr. Linda Parysek.

Figure 10-12. From Bridgman PC, Dailey ME. 1989. The organization of myosin and actin in rapid frozen nerve growth cones. J Cell Biol 108:95-109.

Figure 11-1. A, Courtesy of Drs. Kelsey Branchfield, Eric Domyan, and Xin Sun.

Figure 11-3. Courtesy of Dr. Kurt Albertine.

Figure 11-5. Courtesy of Dr. Ross Metzger.

Figure 11-6. Adapted from Peters K, Werner S, Liao X, et al. 1994. Targeted expression of a dominant negative FGF receptor blocks branching morphogenesis and epithelial differentiation of the mouse lung. EMBO J 13:3296-3301.

Figure 11-7. Courtesy of Dr. Mark Metzstein.

Figure 11-15. Courtesy of Children's Hospital Medical Center, Cincinnati, Ohio.

Figure 11-16. *A,* Courtesy of Dr. Janice L.B. Byrne. *B,* Courtesy of Dr. Lance Erickson.

Table 11-1. Adapted from Langston C, Kida K, Reed M, Thurlbeck WM. 1984. Human lung growth in late gestation in the neonate. Am Rev Respir Dis 129:607-613.

Figure 12-1. Adapted from Brand T. 2003. Heart development: molecular insights into cardiac specification and early morphogenesis. Dev Biol 258:1-19.

Figure 12-2. Adapted from Ladd AN, Yatskievych TA, Antin PB. 1998. Regulation of avian cardiac myogenesis by activin/TGFbeta and bone morphogenetic proteins. Dev Biol 204:407-419.

Figure 12-3. Adapted from Marvin MJ, DiRocco G, Gardiner A, et al. 2001. Inhibition of Wnt activity induces heart formation from posterior mesoderm. Genes Dev 15:316-327.

Figure 12-5. *A,* Adapted from Abu-Issa R, Kirby ML. 2007. Heart field: from mesoderm to heart tube. Ann Rev Cell Dev Biol 23:45-2368. *D,* Adapted from Hurle JM, Icardo JM, Ojeda JL. 1980. Compositional and structural heterogeneity of the cardiac jelly of the chick embryo tubular heart: a TEM, SEM and histochemical study. J Embryol Exp Morphol 56:211-223.

Figures 12-6, 12-8. Photos adapted from Kaufman MH. 1981. The role of embryology in teratological research, with particular reference to the development of the neural tube and the heart. J Reprod Fertil 62:607-623.

Figure 12-10. Adapted from Buckingham M, Meilhac S, Zaffran S. 2005. Building the mammalian heart from two sources of myocardial cells. Nat Rev Genet 6:826-835.

Figure 12-11. Adapted from van den Hoff M, Kruithof BPT, Moorman AFM. 2004. Making more heart muscle. BioEssays 26:248-261.

Figures 12-12, 12-13. From Manner J. 2000. Cardiac looping in the chick embryo: a morphological review with special reference to terminology and biomechanical aspects of the looping process. Anat Rec 259:248-262.

Figure 12-14. Courtesy of Children's Hospital Medical Center, Cincinnati, Ohio.

Figure 12-16. *A-C,* Drawn from data in Christoffels VM, Habets PE, Franco D. 2000. Chamber formation and morphogenesis in the developing mammalian heart. Dev Biol 223:266-278.

Figure 12-19. Adapted from Mjaatvedt CH, Markwald RR. 1989. Induction of an epithelial-mesenchymal transition by an in vivo adheron-like complex. Dev Biol 136:118-128.

Figure 12-20. Courtesy of Dr. Ray Runyan. From Person AD, Klewer SE, Runyan RB. 2005. Cell biology of cardiac cushion development. Int Rev Cytol 243:287-335.

Figure 12-21. *B, C,* Adapted from Icardo JM. 1988. Heart anatomy and developmental biology. Experientia 44:910-919.

Figure 12-22. *B,* Adapted from Hendrix MJC, Morse DE. 1977. Atrial septation. I. Scanning electron microscopy in the chick. Dev Biol 57:345-363.

Figure 12-25. Courtesy of Dr. Adriana Gittenberger-DeGroot.

Figure 12-26. Adapted from Mikawa T. 1999. Cardiac lineages. In Harvey RP, Rosenthal N (eds): Heart Development. Academic Press, New York.

Figure 12-29. From Anderson RH, Webb S, Brown NA. et al. 2006. Development of the heart: formation of the ventricular outflow tracts, arterial valves, and intrapericardial arterial trunks. Heart 89:1110-1118.

Figure 12-30. *A,* Adapted from Hurle JM, Colvee E, Blanco AM, 1980. Development of mouse semilunar valves. Anat Embryol 160:83-91.

Figure 12-31. Adapted from Kirby ML. 1988. Role of extracardiac factors in heart development. Experientia 44:944-951.

Figure 12-32. Adapted from Sizarov A, Ya J, de Boer BA, et al. Formation of the building plan of the human heart: morphogenesis, growth, and differentiation. Circulation 123:1125-1135.

Figure 12-33. *A, B,* Adapted from Manner J. 1992. The development of pericardial villi in the chick embryo. Anat Embryol 186:379-385.

Figures 12-34, 12-35. Courtesy of Dr. Adriana Gittenberger-DeGroot.

Figure 12-36. *B,* Courtesy of Dr. Margaret Kirby and the Medical College of Georgia, Augusta. *D,* Courtesy of Children's Hospital Medical Center, Cincinnati, Ohio.

Figure 12-37. *B,* Courtesy of Children's Hospital Medical Center, Cincinnati, Ohio.

Figure 13-1. *A, B,* Adapted from Eichmann A, Yuan L, Moyon D, et al. 2005. Vascular development: from precursor cells to branched arterial and venous networks. Int J Dev Biol 49:259-267.

Figures 13-2, 13-3. Adapted from Tavian M, Peault B. 2005. Embryonic development of the human hematopoietic system. Int J Dev Biol 49:243-250.

Figure 13-4. *A,* Adapted from Ody C, Vaigot P, Quéué P, et al. 1999. Glycoprotein IIb-IIIa is expressed on avian multilineage hematopoietic progenitor cells. Blood 93:2898-2906. *B,* Adapted from Corbel C, Salaün J. 2002. AlphaIIb integrin expression during development of the murine hematopoietic system. Dev Biol 243:301-311. *C,* Adapted from Emmel VE. 1916. The cell clusters in the dorsal aorta of mammalian embryos. Am J Anat 19:5141-5146. *D,* Adapted from Dieterlen-Lievre F, Le Douarin NM. 2004. From the hemangioblast to self-tolerance: a series of innovations gained from studies on the avian embryo. Mech Dev 121:1117-1128.

Figure 13-6. Adapted from Pardanaud L, Luton D, Prigent M, et al. 1996. Two distinct endothelial lineages in ontogeny, one of them related to hemopoiesis. Development 122:1363-1371.

Figure 13-8. Adapted from Dor Y, Porat R, Keshet E. 2001. Vascular endothelial growth factor and vascular adjustments to perturbations in oxygen homeostasis. Am J Physiol Cell Physiol 280:C1367-C1374.

Figure 13-9. Adapted from Rossant J, Howard L. 2002. Signaling pathways in vascular development. Annu Rev Cell Dev Biol 18:541-573.

Figure 13-10. *A, B,* Adapted from Bruckner AL, Frieden IJ. 2003. Hemangiomas of infancy. J Am Acad Dermatol 48:477-493.

Figure 13-14. Adapted from Bockman DE, Redmond ME, Kirby ML. 1989. Alteration of early vascular development after ablation of cranial neural crest. Anat Rec 225:209-217.

Figure 13-22. *A*, Adapted from Carlson BM. 1999. Human Embryology and Developmental Biology. Second Edition. Mosby St Louis. *B*, Adapted from Sadler TW (ed): Langman's Medical Embryology. Seventh Edition. Williams & Wilkins, Baltimore.

Figure 13-23. *D*, Courtesy of Children's Hospital Medical Center, Cincinnati, Ohio.

Figure 13-28. Adapted from Eichmann A, Yuan L, Moyon D, et al. 2005. Vascular development: from precursor cells to branched arterial and venous networks. Int J Dev Biol 49:259-267.

Figure 14-5. Adapted from Wells JM, Melton DA. 1999. Vertebrate endoderm development. Annu Rev Cell Dev Biol 15:393-410.

Figure 14-6. Adapted from Roberts DJ. 2000. Molecular mechanisms of development of the gastrointestinal tract. Dev Dyn 219:109-120.

Figure 14-10. Adapted from Jensen J. 2004. Gene regulatory factors in pancreatic development. Dev Dyn 229:176-200.

Figure 14-12. Adapted from Wilson ME, Scheel D, German MS. 2003. Gene expression cascades in pancreatic development. Mech Dev 120:65-80.

Figure 14-17. *B*, Courtesy of Dr. Natasza A. Kurpios.

Figure 14-22. Drawings adapted from those provided courtesy of Children's Hospital Medical Center, Cincinnati, Ohio.

Figure 14-24. Adapted from Radtke F, Clevers H. 2005. Self-renewal and cancer of the gut: two sides of a coin. Science 307:1904-1909.

Figure 14-25. Adapted from Logan CY, Nusse R. 2004. The Wnt signaling pathway in development and disease. Annu Rev Cell Dev Biol 20:781-810.

Figure 14-26. Adapted from Batlle E, Henderson JT, Beghtel H, et al. 2002. Beta-catenin and TCF mediate cell positioning in the intestinal epithelium by controlling the expression of EphB/ephrinB. Cell 111:251-263.

Figure 14-27. Adapted from Yang Q, Bermingham NA, Finegold MJ, Zoghbi HY, 2001. Requirement of Math1 for secretory cell lineage commitment in the mouse intestine. Science 294, 2155-2158.

Figure 14-28. Adapted from Sukegawa A, Narita T, Kameda T, et al. 2000. The concentric structure of the developing gut is regulated by Sonic hedgehog derived from endodermal epithelium. Development 127:1971-1980.

Figure 14-29. Adapted from Le Douarin NM. 2004. The avian embryo as a model to study the development of the neural crest: a long and still ongoing story. Mech Dev 121:1089-1102.

Figure 14-30. Courtesy of Children's Hospital Medical Center, Cincinnati, Ohio.

Figure 14-35. Courtesy of Dr. Janice L. B. Byrne.

Figure 15-3. Courtesy of Dr. Thomas J. Poole.

Figure 15-5. Courtesy of Drs. Odyssé Michos and Frank Constantini.

Figure 15-9. Adapted from Dressler G. 2002. Tubulogenesis in the developing mammalian kidney. Trends Cell Biol 12:390-395.

Figure 15-18. Adapted from Brauer PR. 2003. Human Embryology: The Ultimate USMLE Step 1 Review. Hanley & Belfus, Inc. (an imprint of Elsevier), Philadelphia.

Figure 16-2. From Evan AP, Gattone VC II, Blomgren PM. 1984. Application of scanning electron microscopy to kidney development and nephron maturation. Scan Electron Microsc 1:455-473.

Figure 16-3. Courtesy of Dr. Blanche Capel.

Figures 16-6, 16-9. Courtesy of Drs. Alex Combes and Peter Koopman.

Figure 16-10. From Miller A, Hong MK, Hutson JM. 2004. The broad ligament: a review of its anatomy and development in different species and hormonal environments. Clin Anat 17:244-251.

Figure 16-12. Adapted from Wilhelm D, Koopman P. 2006. The makings of maleness: towards an integrated view of male sexual development. Nat Rev Genet 7:620-631.

Figure 16-13. Courtesy of Dr. Alan Perantoni.

Figure 16-14. Adapted from Wilhelm D, Koopman P. 2006. The makings of maleness: towards an integrated view of male sexual development. Nat Rev Genet 7:620-631.

Figure 16-16. Courtesy of Dr. Blanche Capel. Adapted from Maatouk DM, DiNapoli L, Alvers, A, et al. 2008. Stabilization of β-catenin in XY gonads causes male-to-female sex-reversal. Human Mol Genet 17:2949-2955.

Figure 16-17. Adapted from Uhlenhaut NH, Jakob S, Anlag K, et al. 2009. Somatic sex reprogramming of adult ovaries to testes by FOXL2 ablation. Cell 139:1130-1142.

Figure 16-18. Adapted from Ludbrook LM, Harley VR. 2004. Sex determination: a 'window' of DAX1 activity. Trends Endocrinol Metab 15:116-121.

Figure 16-20. From Brauer PR. 2003. Human Embryology: The Ultimate USMLE Step 1 Review. Hanley & Belfus, Inc. (an imprint of Elsevier), Philadelphia.

Figure 16-21. *B-D*, Courtesy of Dr. Ashley Seifert. *B*, Adapted from Seifert AW, Bouldin CM, Choi K-S, et al. 2009. Multiphasic and tissue-specific roles of sonic hedgehog in cloacal septation and external genitalia development. Development 136:3949-3957. *C, D*, Adapted from Seifert AW, Harfe BD, Cohn MJ. 2008. Cell lineage analysis demonstrates and endodermal origin of the distal urethra and perineum. Dev Biol 318:143-152.

Figure 16-22. *B*, Adapted from Yamada G, Satoh Y, Baskin LS, Cunha GR. 2003. Cellular and molecular mechanisms of development of the external genitalia. Differentiation 71:445-460.

Figure 16-23. Courtesy of Dr. G. Yamada.

Figure 16-24. Adapted from Brauer PR. 2003. Human Embryology: The Ultimate USMLE Step 1 Review. Hanley & Belfus, Inc. (an imprint of Elsevier), Philadelphia.

Figure 16-26. *D*, Courtesy of Children's Hospital Medical Center, Cincinnati, Ohio.

Figure 16-28. *A, B, C*, Adapted from Brauer PR. 2003. Human Embryology: The Ultimate USMLE Step 1 Review. Hanley & Belfus, Inc. (an imprint of Elsevier), Philadelphia.

Figure 16-29. *D*, Courtesy of Children's Hospital Medical Center, Cincinnati, Ohio.

Figure 16-30. *A*, From Warkany J. 1971. Congenital Malformations. Notes and Comments. Year-Book Medical Publishers. Chicago. *B-D*, From Jones HW, Scott WW. 1958. Hermaphroditism, Genital Anomalies and Related Endocrine Disorders. Williams & Wilkins, Baltimore.

Figure 17-1. Courtesy of Dr. Alan Rope.

Figure 17-4. *A,* Adapted from McBratney-Owen B, Iseki S, Bamforth SD, et al. 2008. Development and tissue origins of the mammalian cranial base. Dev Biol 322:121-132. *B, C,* Courtesy of Dr. Sachiko Iseki.

Figure 17-6. *A,* Courtesy of Dr. David Billmire. *C,* Adapted from Morriss-Kay GM, Wilkie AO. 2005. Growth of the normal skull vault and its alteration in craniosynostosis: insights from human genetics and experimental studies. J Anat 207:637-653.

Figure 17-7. *A,* Courtesy of Dr. Andrew Wilkie. Adapted from Twigg SRF, Kan R, Babbs C, et al. 2004. Mutations of ephrin-B1 (*EFNB1*), a marker of tissue boundary formation, cause craniofrontonasal syndrome. Proc Natl Acad Sci U S A 101:8652-8657. *B,* Courtesy of Children's Hospital Medical Center, Cincinnati, Ohio.

Figure 17-8. *B,* Courtesy of Dr. Eiki Koyama. *C,* Courtesy of Dr. Jun Doshisha. Adapted from Aoto K, Shikata Y, Imai H, et al. 2009. Mouse Shh is required for prechordal plate maintenance during brain and craniofacial morphogenesis. Dev Biol 327:106-120.

Figure 17-9. *A-C,* Courtesy of Dr. Arnold Tamarin. *E,* Courtesy of Dr. Robert E. Waterman.

Figure 17-14. *A,* Adapted from Lumsden A, Keynes R, 1989. Segmental patterns of neuronal development in the chick hindbrain. Nature 337:424-428. *B,* Adapted from Kontges G, Lumsden A. 1996. Rhombencephalic neural crest segmentation is preserved throughout craniofacial ontogeny. Development 122:3229-3242.

Figure 17-15. *A,* Courtesy of Dr. Abigail Tucker. *B,* Courtesy of Dr. Moises Mallo. Adapted from Bobola N, Carapuco M, Ohnemus S, et al. 2003. Mesenchymal patterning by Hoxa2 requires blocking Fgf-dependent activation of Ptx1. Development 130:3403-3414.

Figure 17-16. *A,* Courtesy of Drs. Susan Reijntjes and Malcolm Maden. Adapted from Reijntjes S, Gale E, Maden M. 2004. Generating gradients of retinoic acid in the chick embryo: Cyp26C1 expression and a comparative analysis of the Cyp26 enzymes. Dev Dyn 230:509-517. *B,* Adapted from Mark M, Ghyselinck NB, Chambon P. 2004. Retinoic acid signalling in the development of branchial arches. Curr Opin Genet Dev 14:591-598.

Figure 17-17. *A, B,* Courtesy of Dr. Arnold Tamarin.

Figure 17-18. *A, C,* Courtesy of Dr. Arnold Tamarin.

Figure 17-19. *A, B,* Courtesy of Dr. Abigail Tucker. Adapted from Tucker AS, Lumsden A. 2004. Neural crest cells provide species-specific patterning information in the developing branchial skeleton. Evol Dev 6:32-40. *C,* Courtesy of Dr. Richard Schneider. Adapted from Eames BF, Schneider RA. 2005. Quail-duck chimeras reveal spatiotemporal plasticity in molecular and histogenic programs of cranial feather development. Development 132:1499-1509.

Figure 17-20. Courtesy of Dr. Michael Depew. Adapted from Depew MJ, Lufkin T, Rubenstein JL. 2002. Specification of jaw subdivisions by Dlx genes. Science 298:381-385.

Figure 17-21. *D,* Courtesy of Dr. Arnold Tamarin.

Figure 17-22. *B,* Courtesy of Dr. Arnold Tamarin.

Figure 17-23. Courtesy of Children's Hospital Medical Center, Cincinnati, Ohio.

Figure 17-28. *C,* Courtesy of Dr. Arnold Tamarin.

Figure 17-29. With permission from Dr. Robin Krimm. Adapted from Ma L, Lopez GF, Krimm RF. 2009. Epithelial-derived BDNF is required for gustatory neuron targeting during a critical developmental period. J Neurosci 29:3354-3364.

Figure 17-34. Adapted from Irving D, Willhite C, Burk D. 1986. Morphogenesis of isotretinoin-induced microcephaly and micrognathia studied by scanning electron microscopy. Teratology 34:141-153.

Figure 17-35. *E,* Courtesy of Dr. Abigail Tucker.

Figure 17-36. Courtesy of Drs. YiPing Chen and Yanding Zhang. Adapted from Zhang YD, Chen Z, Song YQ, et al. 2005. Making a tooth: growth factors, transcription factors, and stem cells. Cell Res 15:301-316.

Figure 17-37. Courtesy of Dr. Abigail Tucker.

Figure 17-38. *A-G,* Courtesy of Dr. Martyn Cobourne. *C, G,* Adapted from Cobourne MT, Sharpe PT. 2013. Disease of the tooth: the genetic and molecular basis of inherited anomalies affecting the dentition. WIREs Dev Biol 2:183-212.

Figure 17-39. *A, B,* Courtesy of Dr. Jodi L. Smith.

Figure 18-1. *A,* Courtesy of the family. *B,* Courtesy of Drs. Nancy Bonini and Derek Lessing.

Figure 18-2. *A,* Courtesy of Dr. Robert E. Waterman. *B, G,* Adapted from Kikuchi T, Tonosaki A, Takasaka T. 1988. Development of apical-surface structures of mouse otic placode. Acta Otolaryngol 106:200-207.

Figure 18-4. Courtesy of Dr. Doris K. Wu. Adapted from Morsli H, Choo D, Ryan A, et al. 1998. Development of the mouse inner ear and origin of its sensory organs. J Neurosci 18:3327-3335.

Figure 18-5. *A,* Courtesy of Dr. Suzanne L. Mansour and C. Albert Noyes. *B,* Adapted from Kelley MW. 2006. Regulation of cell fate in the sensory epithelia of the inner ear. Nat Rev Neurosci 7:837-849.

Figure 18-6. Adapted from Riccomagno MM, Takada S, Epstein DJ. 2005. Wnt-dependent regulation of inner ear morphogenesis is balanced by the opposing and supporting roles of Shh. Genes Dev 19:1612-1623.

Figure 18-8. *A, B,* Adapted from Barald KF, Kelley MW. 2004. From placode to polarization: new tunes in inner ear development. Development 131:4119-4130. *C,* Adapted from Frolenkov GI, Belyantseva IA, Friedman TB, Griffith AJ. 2004. Genetic insights into the morphogenesis of inner ear hair cells. Nat Rev Genet 5:489-498. *D,* Adapted from Kelley MW. 2006. Regulation of cell fate in the sensory epithelia of the inner ear. Nat Rev Neurosci 7:837-849.

Figure 18-10. Adapted from Kelley MW. 2006. Regulation of cell fate in the sensory epithelia of the inner ear. Nat Rev Neurosci 7:837-849.

Figure 18-11. *A,* Courtesy of Dr. Gregory Frolenkov. Adapted from Frolenkov GI, Belyantseva IA, Friedman TB, Griffith AJ. 2004. Genetic insights into the morphogenesis of inner ear hair cells. Nat Rev Genet 5:489-498. *B, C,* Courtesy of Dr. Jenny Murdoch. Adapted from Curtin JA, Quint E, Tsipouri V, et al. 2003. Mutation of Celsr1 disrupts planar polarity of inner ear hair cells and causes severe neural tube defects in the mouse. Curr Biol 13:1129-1133.

Figure 18-12. Adapted from Dahlen RT, Harnsberger HR, Gray SD, et al. 1997. Overlapping thin-section fast spin-echo MR of the large vestibular aqueduct syndrome. AJNR Am J Neuroradiol 18:67-75.

Figure 18-13. Adapted from Steel KP, Kros CJ. 2001. A genetic approach to understanding auditory function. Nat Genet 27:143-149.

Figure 18-14. *A*, Courtesy of Dr. Arnold Tamarin.

Figure 18-15. *A, B, C, D, F,* Courtesy of Dr. Roger E. Stevenson. Adapted from Carey JC. 2006. Ear. In Stevenson RE, Hall JG (eds): Human Malformations and Related Anomalies. Second Edition. Oxford University Press, London, pp. 327-371. *E,* Courtesy of Dr. John C. Carey and Meg Weist. Adapted from Kumar S, Marres HA, Cremers CW, Kimberling WJ. 1998. Autosomal-dominant branchio-otic (BO) syndrome is not allelic to the branchio-oto-renal (BOR) gene at 8q13. Am J Med Genet 76:395-401.

Figure 19-1. *A,* Courtesy of Dr. Robert E. Waterman. *C,* Adapted from Morriss-Kay GM. 1981. Growth and development of pattern in the cranial neural epithelium of rat embryos during neurulation. J Embryol Exp Morphol 65 Suppl:225-241. *E,* Adapted from Garcia-Porrero JA, Colvee E, Ojeda JL. 1987. Retinal cell death occurs in the absence of retinal disc invagination: experimental evidence in papaverine-treated chicken embryos. Anat Rec 217:395-401. *I,* Adapted from Morse DE, McCann PS. 1984. Neuroectoderm of the early embryonic rat eye. Scanning electron microscopy. Invest Ophthalmol Vis Sci 25:899-907.

Figure 19-3. *A, B,* Courtesy of Dr. Arnold Tamarin.

Figure 19-6. *A, B,* Courtesy of Dr. Sabine Fuhrmann. *C,* Adapted from Martinez-Morales JR, Rodrigo I, Bovolenta P. 2004. Eye development: a view from the retina pigmented epithelium. Bioessays 26:766-777. *D,* Adapted from Ashery-Padan R, Gruss P. 2001. Pax6 lights-up the way for eye development. Curr Opin Cell Biol 13:706-714.

Figure 19-7. *B,* Courtesy of Dr. Arnold Tamarin.

Figure 19-8. Adapted from Traboulsi EI. 2006. Eye. In Stevenson RE, Hall JG (eds): Human Malformations and Related Anomalies. Second Edition. Oxford University Press, London, pp. 297-325.

Figure 20-1. Courtesy of Freddie Astbury. Adapted from Thalidomide UK (www.thalidomideuk.com).

Figure 20-2. *A,* Courtesy of Dr. Robert E. Waterman. *B-D,* Adapted from Kelley RO. 1985. Early development of the vertebrate limb: an introduction to morphogenetic tissue interactions using scanning electron microscopy. Scan Electron Microsc (Pt 2):827-836.

Figure 20-3. *A, C,* Adapted from Alberts B, Johnson, A, Lewis J, et al. 2002. Molecular Biology of the Cell. Fourth Edition. Garland Science, New York.

Figure 20-4. Adapted from Mariani FV, Martin GR. 2003. Deciphering skeletal patterning: clues from the limb. Nature 423:319-325.

Figure 20-5. Courtesy of Drs. Sheila Bell and W. Scott.

Figure 20-6. *B,* Courtesy of Dr. Martin J. Cohn. Adapted from Cohn MJ, Izpisua-Belmonte JC, Abud H, et al. 995. Fibroblast growth factors induce additional limb development from the flank of chick embryos. Cell 80:739-746.

Figure 20-7. Adapted from Mariani FV, Martin GR. 2003. Deciphering skeletal patterning: clues from the limb. Nature 423:319-325.

Figure 20-8. Adapted from Izpisua-Belmonte JC, Duboule D. 1992. Homeobox genes and pattern formation in the vertebrate limb. Dev Biol 152:26-36.

Figure 20-9. Adapted from Davis AP, Witte DP, Hsieh-Li HM, et al. 1995. Absence of radius and ulna in mice lacking hoxa-11 and hoxd-11. Nature 375:791-795.

Figure 20-10. Courtesy of Dr. Mario Capecchi. Adapted from Wellik DM, Capecchi MR. 2003. Hox10 and Hox11 genes are required to globally pattern the mammalian skeleton. Science 301:363-367.

Figure 20-12. *A,* Courtesy of Dr. Arnold Tamarin. *B, C,* Courtesy of Dr. Robert E. Waterman.

Figure 20-13. Adapted from Alberts B, Johnson A, Lewis J, et al. 2002. Molecular Biology of the Cell. Fourth Edition. Garland Science, New York.

Figure 20-14. *A,* Courtesy of Dr. Rolf Zeller. Adapted from Panman L, Zeller R. 2003. Patterning the limb before and after SHH signalling. J Anat 202:3-12. *C, D,* Courtesy of Dr. Cliff Tabin. Adapted from Harfe BD, Scherz PJ, Nissim S, et al. 2004. Evidence for an expansion-based temporal Shh gradient in specifying vertebrate digit identities. Cell 118:517-528.

Figure 20-15. Courtesy of Dr. Rolf Zeller. Adapted from te Welscher P, Zuniga A, Kuijper S, et al. 2002. Progression of vertebrate limb development through SHH-mediated counteraction of GLI3. Science 298:827-830.

Figure 20-16. Adapted from Chan DC, Laufer E, Tabin C, Leder P. 1995. Polydactylous limbs in Strong's Luxoid mice result from ectopic polarizing activity. Development 121:1971-1978.

Figure 20-18. *B,* Courtesy of Dr. Sigmar Stricker. Adapted from Stricker S, Mundlos S. 2011. Mechanisms of digit formation: human malformation syndromes tell the story. Dev Dyn 240:990-1004.

Figure 20-19. *A, B, C, E,* Courtesy of Children's Hospital Medical Center, Cincinnati, Ohio. *D,* Courtesy of Dr. David Vischokil. *F,* Courtesy of Dr. John C. Carey.

Figures 20-20, 20-21. Courtesy of Dr. Irene Hung.

Figure 20-22. *A,* Courtesy of Children's Hospital Medical Center, Cincinnati, Ohio. *B, C,* Courtesy of Dr. Thomas Lufkin. Adapted from Kraus P, Lufkin T. 2006. Dlx homeobox gene control of mammalian limb and craniofacial development. Am J Med Genet A 140:1366-1374.

Figure 20-23. Courtesy of Muragaki Y, Mundlos S, Upton J, Olsen BR. 1996. Altered growth and branching patterns in synpolydactyly caused by mutations in HOXD13. Science 272:548-551.

Figures 20-24, 20-25. Courtesy of Dr. Irene Hung.

Figure 20-26. Adapted from Tosney KW, Landmesser LT. 1985. Development of the major pathways for neurite outgroth in the chick hindlimb. Dev Biol 109:193-214.

Figure 20-27. Adapted from Tosney KW, Landmesser LT. 1984. Pattern and specificity of axonal outgrowth following varying degrees of chick limb bud ablation. J Neurosci 4:2518-2527.

Figure 20-29. *A, B, D,* Adapted from Kania A, Johnson RL, Jessell TM. 2000. Coordinate roles for LIM homeobox genes in directing the dorsoventral trajectory of motor axons in the vertebrate limb. Cell 102:161-173. *C,* Adapted from Shirasaki R, Pfaff SL. 2002. Transcriptional codes and the control of neuronal identity. Annu Rev Neurosci 25:251-281.

Index

Page numbers followed by *f* indicate figures; *t*, tables; *b*, boxes.

Primary body, development of, 81
Primary bone collar, 188
Primary ciliary dyskinesia (PCD), 251b–252b
Primary ossification center, 187–188
Primitive groove, 59, 60f
Primitive node, 59, 60f
 neural plate formation and, 77
Primitive pit, 59, 60f
Primitive streak
 Brachyury expression in, 76b–77b, 77f
 formation of, 59–65, 60f–61f
Primordial germ cells (PGCs), 16–18,
 97b–99b. see also Gonocytes.
 apoptosis of, 16b–18b
 development of, molecular regulation of,
 16b–18b
 gonad formation stimulation by, 16–18
 migration into dorsal body wall, 16, 17f
 origin of, 16b–18b
 proliferation and survival of, 16b–18b
 in yolk sac, 16, 51
Processus vaginalis. see Vaginal process
Proctodeum, 372, 373f
Proepicardial organ, 267, 296–298
Progenitor cells, hematopoietic, 304, 306
Progeria, 5, 5f
Progesterone
 depot preparations of, 38b–41b
 in menstrual cycle, 33
Progesterone, placental, 143
Programmed cell death, 238b, 501,
 509b–514b
Progress zone, 503b–506b
Progress zone model, 503b–506b
Prokineticin2, Kallmann syndrome and,
 229b–230b
Proliferation, of retinal progenitor cells,
 494b–495b
Proliferative phase, of menstrual cycle, 33
Pronators, of upper limb, 192, 192t
Pronephroi, 375
Pronephros, 376–377, 378f
Proneural genes, 238b
Pronuclei, female and male, 34f–35f, 35
Prophase, 20–21, 20f, 21t
Prosencephalon, 95, 200, 201f
Prosomeres, 200–202
Prospective fate, of epiblast cells, 68–69
Prospective fate maps, 68–69, 70f
Prospective gut endoderm, 70f
Prospective potency, of epiblast cells, 68–69
Prostaglandin(s)
 ductus venosus and, 339
 placental, 143–144
Prostaglandin D2 (Pdg2), testes development
 and, 399b–401b
Prostate, 24
Prostate gland, 406, 406f, 407b–408b, 409f
Protanopes, 493–494
Proteinuria, 385b–386b
Proteoglycans, neural crest cell migration
 and, 97b–99b
Proto-oncogene, in neurofibromatosis type
 1, 238b
Prox1
 lens and, 495b
 lymphatic system and, 334b, 337f
 retinal progenitor cells and, 494b–495b
Proximal-distal axis, 501, 503b–506b
Proximal-distal outgrowth, 503b–506b
Prune belly syndrome, 86b, 195b
Pseudoglandular stage
 branching morphogenesis of lung during,
 258b–259b
 of lung development, 254t, 255

Pseudohermaphroditism
 female, 423b–427b
 male, 423b–427b, 425f–427f
Pseudopodia, 65
Psoriasis, 159b–160b
Pterygoid muscles, 444
Pthrp, chondrogenesis and, 189b–190b
Ptosis, 498b–499b
PTPN11, aortic coarctation and, 324b–327b
Puberty, 18–19
 failure to enter, 423b–427b
Pulmonary agenesis, 256b–258b
Pulmonary arterial-venous malformation,
 306b
Pulmonary artery, 267
Pulmonary hypertension, in hereditary
 hemorrhagic telangiectasia, 313b–314b
Pulmonary hypoplasia, 135b, 138, 256b–259b
 oligohydramnios and, 263b–265b
Pulmonary surfactant, 256b–258b
Pulmonary trunk stenosis, tetralogy of Fallot,
 298b–302b
Pulmonary veins, 267, 281f, 283
Pupil, 488
Pupillary membrane, formation of, 488,
 496–497
 persistence of, 498b–499b
Pupillary muscles, 497
Purkinje cell(s), 213
Purkinje cell layer, 213–214
Purkinje fibers, 296
Pycnodysostosis, 190b–191b
Pyloric atresia, 130
Pyloric stenosis, hypertrophic, infantile,
 369b–370b
Pyramidal cells, 227

Q

Quadratus lumborum muscle, 184b–185b

R

Rac1, in epithelial-to-mesenchymal
 transformation, 67b–68b
Radial arteries, 322, 325f
Radial axis, 364
Radial glia, 213–214, 213f–214f
Radioulnar synostosis, 514b–519b
Raldh-2 (retinaldehyde dehydrogenenase-2),
 of heart chamber, 279b–280b
Randomized laterality, 298b–302b
RAS-MAP kinase pathway, 12f
Rathke folds, 371–372
Rathke's pouch, 225, 226f
Rax, patterning of eye, 494b–495b
Receptors, for growth factors, 125
Reciprocal inductive signals, 380
Recombination, in meiosis, 20–21
Recreational drugs, teratogenic, 142
Rectocloacal canal, 388b–389b
Rectovesical fistula, 388b–389b
 development of, 392f
Rectus abdominis muscle, 185
Rectus muscles, 445
5α-reductase, 405
Reduction defects, 514b–519b
Reelin, Cajal-Retzius cells and, 227–228
Refsum disease, 242b
Reichert's cartilage, 441–442, 442f
Relaxin-like factor, testicular descent and,
 421b
Renal agenesis, 144
 bilateral, 375b, 381–382, 383b–385b
 and dysplasia, 385b–386b
 unilateral, 385b–386b

Renal arteries, 320, 322f
 accessory, 386–387
Renal-coloboma syndrome, 385b–386b
Renal columns, 382
Renal corpuscles, 377
Renal mesangial sclerosis, 385b–386b
Renal papilla, 382
Renal pelvis, 379–380, 381f
Renal plexus, 244
Renal pyramid, 382
Renal vesicle, development of, 382f
Reproductive efficiency, 38b–41b
Reproductive system
 development of, 394–428, 394b–396b
 embryonic male and female structures
 and, 398t
 male versus female development of,
 396–398, 399f
 timeline of, 395f
Resegmentation, of sclerotomes, 178–185,
 178f–180f, 178b–179b
Respiratory distress, 268b–269b
Respiratory distress syndrome, 256b–258b
Respiratory diverticulum, 251–254, 253f
Respiratory failure, surfactant deficiency and,
 256b–258b
Respiratory system, development of, 251–266
Respiratory tree
 development of, 252–260
 developmental abnormalities of,
 256b–258b, 257f
 induction of, 255b
 time line of development of, 252f
Ret
 Hirschsprung disease and, 370b–371b
 ureteric bud, 383b–385b
Rete testis, 394, 398, 400f
Reticular layer, 161
Retina
 axons of
 crossing of midline by, 220b–225b,
 222f–223f
 spatial targeting of, 220b–225b, 221f
 central artery of, 488, 496
 defects of, 498b–499b
 neural, 488
 cell pattern in, 220b–225b
 formation of, 492–496
Retinal dysplasia, 498b–499b
Retinal ganglion cells (RGCs), 220b–225b,
 495b
 axons of
 midline crossing of, 220b–225b,
 222f–223f
 spatial targeting of, 220b–225b, 221f
 mapping of visual space by, 220b–225b,
 222f
Retinal progenitor cells, proliferation
 and differentiation, regulation of,
 494b–495b
Retinaldehyde dehydrogenenase-2 (Raldh-2),
 of heart chamber, 279b–280b
Retinitis pigmentosa, 482b–484b
Retinoic acid, Hox gene regulation by,
 180b–183b
Retinoic acid receptors, cranialization of
 vertebral segments and, 180b–183b, 184f
Retinoic acid response elements (RAREs),
 hindbrain and, 447b–448b, 449f
Retinoid, neural plate and tube patterning
 and, 202b
Retinopathy of prematurity, 498b–499b
Retroperitoneal organs, 343–344, 346f
Reverse genetic approach, 114–115
Rh factors, erythroblastosis fetalis and,
 138–140